Merritt's Textbook of Neurology, ed 8
Edited by Lewis P. Rowland, MD
Philadelphia, Lea & Febiger, 1989
964 pp, illustrated, $67.50

The eighth edition of *Merritt's Textbook of Neurology*, like the seventh edition, is a multiauthored work. Many of the authors are among the leaders in their field and coverage of the subject matter is comprehensive for a single-volume work. The writing retains the direct, unadorned style and liberal use of tables that characterized the original work.

The book is organized into 3 sections, 22 chapters, and 162 subchapters. The first section is a 58-page review of signs and symptoms of neurological disorders. The second section concerns disorders of known etiology, and the third section deals with disorders of unknown etiology. Subchapters are individually authored and describe specific diseases or disorders. The figures are all in black and white but very clear. New in this eighth edition are photographs of magnetic resonance images, a section on neurovascular imaging, a section on the acquired immunodeficiency syndrome, material on Lyme disease, leptospirosis, Whipple's disease, hyperosmolar coma, respiratory failure, transient global amnesia, and the neurological complications of pregnancy. Other sections have been revised to reflect relevant scientific and clinical advances.

The index is extensive and well organized. A list of references is given at the end of each subchapter but they are not cited within the text. This design enhances readability and succinctness at the expense of utility as a reference source. The organization of the book, its size, and its writing style will make it useful as a reference for medical students, residents, and clinicians who need a convenient way to learn the fundamentals as well as the most important scientific details concerning clinical neurological entities. Overall, this book remains one of the best standard textbooks of neurology available in a single volume.

Michael E. Selzer, MD, PhD

Merritt's
TEXTBOOK OF NEUROLOGY

Merritt's
TEXTBOOK OF NEUROLOGY

edited by

LEWIS P. ROWLAND, M.D.

Columbia University College of Physicians and Surgeons
Neurological Institute of Presbyterian Hospital
Columbia-Presbyterian Medical Center
New York, New York

Eighth Edition

LEA & FEBIGER • Philadelphia • London
1989

Lea & Febiger
600 Washington Square
Philadelphia, PA   19106-4198
U.S.A.
(215) 922-1330

Lea & Febiger (UK) Ltd.
145a Croydon Road
Beckenham, Kent BR3 3RB
U.K.

First Edition, 1955; Reprinted 1955, 1957
Second Edition, 1959; Reprinted 1959, 1961
Third Edition, 1963; Reprinted 1964, 1966
Fourth Edition, 1967; Reprinted 1968, 1969, 1970
Fifth Edition, 1973; Reprinted 1974, 1975, 1977
Sixth Edition, 1979; Reprinted 1981
Seventh Edition, 1984; Reprinted 1985, 1987
Eighth Edition, 1989

LIBRARY OF CONGRESS
Library of Congress Cataloging-in-Publication Data

Merritt, H. Houston (Hiram Houston), 1902–1979.
   [Textbook of neurology]
   Merritt's textbook of neurology—8th ed. / edited by Lewis P. Rowland
      p.   cm.
   Includes bibliographies and index.
   ISBN 0-8121-1148-6
   1. Nervous system—Diseases. 2. Neurology. I. Rowland, Lewis P.
II. Title. III. Title: Textbook of neurology.
   [DNLM: Nervous System Diseases.   WL 100 M572t]
   RC346.M4 1989   616.8–dc19   DNLM/DLC
   for Library of Congress   88-9456
                                                 CIP

PRINTED IN THE UNITED STATES OF AMERICA

Print number: 5 4 3 2 1

Dedicated To
H. HOUSTON MERRITT
(1902–1979)

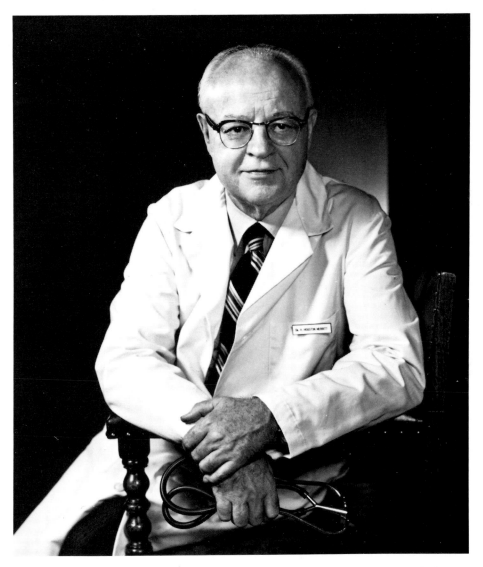

© Karsh, Ottawa.

*From the contributors to this book
and from all his students, everywhere*

Preface

The first edition of H. Houston Merritt's *Textbook of Neurology* appeared in 1955. He guided it through the sixth edition, and only in the last two revisions did he allow any of his colleagues to help. He did most of the work himself, even though he was disabled while the sixth edition was being prepared. Dr. Merritt died in 1979, just when the completed sixth edition was released for distribution.

The seventh edition was prepared by Dr. Merritt's students, including 30 who had become heads of departments and other distinguished professors throughout the United States. There were 70 contributors to a volume that had a twofold goal: to provide a historical document by Dr. Merritt's students, and to do that in a way that he would have approved of: making a textbook that would be useful. In preparing the seventh edition, we tried to retain as much of Dr. Merritt's writing as possible. In addition, the editor played an active role in trying to amalgamate the contributions of so many authors into a coherent volume.

The seventh edition was well received, and we were therefore encouraged to bring it up to date. Clinical neurology, like all other branches of medicine, is now advancing so rapidly that new editions will be needed at shorter intervals. Some of the changes in this, the eighth edition, are:

- Magnetic resonance imaging was just becoming available when the seventh edition appeared in 1984. No MRI photographs appeared in that volume, but this form of neuroimaging has become so important that the eighth edition is replete with new illustrations. We have also replaced old CT figures with examples made with technically improved scanners.
- Similarly, neurosonography was just beginning to have a major impact in 1984, and a new section on neurovascular imaging has been written for the current volume.
- In 1984, AIDS had just appeared on the scene; our chapter on that disease was added to the end of the book at the last moment. Now AIDS is an integral part of clinical neurology, and the section on AIDS has been moved to the chapter on infections of the nervous system. The neurologic aspects of AIDS are now recognized as a major consideration.
- New subjects for the current edition include Lyme disease, leptospirosis, Whipple disease, hyperosmolar coma, respiratory failure, transient global amnesia, and the neurologic complications of pregnancy. The impact of molecular genetics has been duly noted in the chapters on heritable diseases. We have tried to account for the emerging concepts of peroxisomal and mitochondrial diseases.
- Advances in clinical sciences or changing concepts have led to extensive revision of several sections, especially those on migraine, limb weakness, primary brain tumors, primitive neuroectodermal tumors, carcinomatous meningitis, lymphomas of the nervous system, paraneoplastic syndromes, head injury, adrenoleukodystrophy, chromosome abnormalities, thoracic outlet syndrome, peripheral neuropathies, and tropical myeloneuropathies, especially tropical spastic paraparesis.

However, those familar with the seventh edition should find themselves comfortable with the eighth edition. We have not tampered with the general organization of the book, and we have not tried to fix sections that were not broken. As time goes on, less and less of Dr. Merritt's taut writing will be in the book, but we have admired his nononsense approach and his desire to write directly, in plain words. It would still be difficult, we hope, for a literary sleuth to go through this book and decide where Dr. Merritt left off and the current authors began, or where the heavy hand of the neurologic editor left a mark.

Several contributors to the seventh edition were not able to provide revisions for this volume. We therefore thank the following authors for their earlier contributions, knowing that some of their words (and some of Dr. Merritt's) continue into the eighth edition: Howard Barrows, Patrick Bray, William Haas, T.R. Johns, Labe C. Scheinberg, and C.T. Vicale. Tragically, Elliot Weitzman died just as the seventh edition had gone to press; his remarkable chapter on sleep disorders has been maintained and updated by June Fry. We also regret to record the death of T.R. Johns, another leader of Neurology and dear friend.

We are indebted to many colleagues of the authors of different chapters for providing new illustrations. We are especially grateful for the help of Jacqueline Bello of the Radiology Division of the Neurological Institute of New York for updating and improving the quality of the radiologic images and adding more than 100 new images to the text. Sadek Hilal, Director of Neuroradiology at the same institution, was also generous in his support.

Shirley Susarchick and Sheila Crescenzo kept track of the chapters, retyped many, helped provide references, and generally guided the chapters through the editorial office to the publisher. As in the past, Edna Borea provided administrative guidance to everyone concerned.

At Lea & Febiger, Kenneth Bussy and David Amundson saw the manuscripts converted into this admirably produced volume.

This book is formally and properly dedicated to the memory of H. Houston Merritt. The editor also dedicates it to the memory of Mabel Carmichael Merritt and to the spouses and children of all the contributors, especially to Esther E. Rowland and our children, Andrew, Steven, and Judith.

New York, NY   Lewis P. Rowland, M.D.

Contributors

Editor for Radiology

Jacqueline A. Bello, M.D.
Assistant Professor of Radiology, Columbia University
College of Physicians and Surgeons
Assistant Attending Radiologist, Neurological Institute of
Presbyterian Hospital, Columbia-Presbyterian Medical
Center
New York, New York

Gary Abrams, M.D.
Associate Professor of Clinical Neurology, Columbia
University College of Physicians and Surgeons
Associate Attending Neurologist, Neurological Institute of
Presbyterian Hospital, Columbia-Presbyterian Medical
Center
New York, New York

Maxwell Abramson, M.D.
Chairman, Department of Otolaryngology, Columbia
University College of Physicians and Surgeons
Director, Otolaryngology Service, Presbyterian Hospital,
Columbia-Presbyterian Medical Center
New York, New York

Milton Alter, M.D., Ph.D.
Professor and Chairman, Department of Neurology, Temple
University School of Medicine
Chairman, Department of Neurology, Temple University
Hospital
Philadelphia, Pennsylvania

Alan M. Aron, M.D.
Professor of Clinical Neurology and Professor of Clinical
Pediatrics, Mt Sinai School of Medicine
Director of Child Neurology, Attending Neurologist, and
Attending Pediatrician,
Mt. Sinai Hospital
New York, New York

James Henry Austin, M.D.
Professor, Department of Neurology, University of Colorado
Health Sciences Center
Denver, Colorado

Mark L. Batshaw, M.D.
Chief, Division of Child Development and Rehabilitation,
University of Pennsylvania School of Medicine
Philadelphia, Pennsylvania

Myles M. Behrens, M.D.
Associate Professor of Clinical Ophthalmology, Columbia
University College of Physicians and Surgeons
Attending Ophthalmologist, Institute of Ophthalmology of
Presbyterian Hospital, Columbia-Presbyterian Medical
Center
New York, New York

Jacqueline A. Bello, M.D.
Assistant Professor of Radiology, Columbia University
College of Physicians and Surgeons
Assistant Attending Radiologist, Neurological Institute of
Presbyterian Hospital, Columbia-Presbyterian Medical
Center
New York, New York

Leonard Berg, M.D.
Professor of Clinical Neurology, Washington University
School of Medicine
St. Louis, Missouri

Carolyn B. Britton, M.D.
Assistant Professor of Neurology, Columbia University
College of Physicians and Surgeons
Assistant Attending Neurologist, Neurological Institute of
Presbyterian Hospital, Columbia-Presbyterian
Medical Center
New York, New York

John C.M. Brust, M.D.
Professor of Clinical Neurology, Columbia University College
of Physicians and Surgeons
Director, Department of Neurology, Harlem Hospital Center
New York, New York

Rosalie A. Burns, M.D.
Professor and Chairman, Department of Neurology, Medical
College of Pennsylvania
Director, Department of Neurology, Hospital of the Medical
College of Pennsylvania
Philadelphia, Pennsylvania

Sidney Carter, M.D.
Professor Emeritus of Neurology and Pediatrics, Columbia
University College of Physicians and Surgeons
Chief, Department of Neurology, Blythedale Children's
Hospital
Valhalla, New York

Abe M. Chutorian, M.D.
Professor of Clinical Neurology and Clinical Pediatrics,
Columbia University College of Physicians and Surgeons
Attending Neurologist, Neurological Institute and Babies
Hospital of Presbyterian Hospital, Columbia-Presbyterian
Medical Center
New York, New York

Lucien J. Cote, M.D.
Associate Professor of Neurology and Rehabilitation
Medicine, Columbia University College of Physicians and
Surgeons
Associate Attending Neurologist, Neurological Institute of
Presbyterian Hospital, Columbia-Presbyterian Medical
Center
New York, New York

Octavio de Marchena, M.D.
Assistant Professor of Clinical Neurology, Washington
University School of Medicine
St. Louis, Missouri

Darryl C. DeVivo, M.D.
Sidney Carter Professor of Neurology and Professor of
Pediatrics, Columbia University College of Physicians and
Surgeons
Director of Pediatric Neurology, Attending Neurologist, and
Attending Pediatrician, Neurological Institute and Babies
Hospital of Presbyterian Hospital, Columbia-Presbyterian
Medical Center
New York, New York

Salvatore DiMauro, M.D.
Professor of Neurology, Co-Director of the H. Houston
Merritt Clinical Research Center for Muscular Dystrophy
and Related Diseases, Columbia University College of
Physicians and Surgeons
New York, New York

Roger C. Duvoisin, M.D.
Professor and Chairman, Department of Neurology,
University of Medicine and Dentistry of New Jersey,
Robert Wood Johnson Medical School
New Brunswick, New Jersey

Stanley Fahn, M.D.
H. Houston Merritt Professor of Neurology, Columbia
University College of Physicians and Surgeons
Attending Neurologist, Neurological Institute of Presbyterian
Hospital, Columbia-Presbyterian Medical Center
New York, New York

Michael R. Fetell, M.D.
Associate Clinical Professor of Neurology, Columbia
University College of Physicians and Surgeons
Associate Attending Neurologist, Neurological Institute of
Presbyterian Hospital, Columbia-Presbyterian Medical
Center
New York, New York

Matthew E. Fink, M.D.
Assistant Professor of Clinical Neurology, Columbia
University College of Physicians and Surgeons
Associate Attending Neurologist, Neurological Institute of
Presbyterian Hospital, Columbia-Presbyterian Medical
Center
New York, New York

Robert A. Fishman, M.D.
Professor and Chairman, Department of Neurology,
University of California Medical School—San Francisco
San Francisco, California

John M. Freeman, M.D.
Professor of Neurology and Pediatrics, Johns Hopkins
Medical Institutions
Baltimore, Maryland

Arnold P. Friedman, M.D.
Adjunct Professor of Neurology, University of Arizona
College of Medicine
Tucson, Arizona

June M. Fry, M.D., Ph.D.
Assistant Professor of Neurology, Medical College of
Pennsylvania
Philadelphia, Pennsylvania

Sid Gilman, M.D.
Professor and Chairman, Department of Neurology,
University of Michigan
Ann Arbor, Michigan

Gilbert H. Glasser, M.D.
Professor, Department of Neurology, Yale University School
of Medicine
New Haven, Connecticut

Arnold P. Gold, M.D.
Professor of Clinical Neurology and Professor of Clinical
Pediatrics, Columbia University College of Physicians and
Surgeons
Attending Neurologist, Neurological Institute and Babies
Hospital of Presbyterian Hospital, Columbia-Presbyterian
Medical Center
New York, New York

Mark A. Goldberg, M.D., Ph.D.
Professor of Neurology, Professor of Pharmacology,
University of California Medical School–Los Angeles
Chairman, Department of Neurology, Harbor-UCLA Medical
Center
Torrance, California

David Goldblatt, M.D.
Professor of Neurology, University of Rochester School of
Medicine and Dentistry
Rochester, New York

Eli S. Goldensohn, M.D.
Professor of Neurology, Emeritus, Department of Neurology,
Columbia University College of Physicians and Surgeons
Professor of Neurology, Albert Einstein College of Medicine
Bronx, New York

Melvin Greer, M.D.
Professor and Chairman, Department of Neurology,
University of Florida College of Medicine
Gainesville, Florida

Sadek K. Hilal, M.D., Ph.D.
Professor of Radiology, Columbia University College of
*   Physicians and Surgeons*
Director of Neuroradiology, Neurological Institute of
*   Presbyterian Hospital, Columbia-Presbyterian Medical*
*   Center*
New York, New York

William G. Johnson, M.D.
Associate Professor of Clinical Neurology, Columbia
*   University College of Physicians and Surgeons*
Associate Attending Neurologist, Neurological Institute of
*   Presbyterian Hospital, Columbia-Presbyterian Medical*
*   Center*
New York, New York

Burk Jubelt, M.D.
Associate Professor of Neurology, Northwestern University
*   Medical School*
Associate Attending Neurologist, Northwestern Memorial
*   Hospital*
Chicago, Illinois

Robert Katzman, M.D.
Professor and Chair, Department of Neurosciences
University of California, San Diego
La Jolla, California

Charles Kennedy, M.D.
Professor of Pediatrics and Neurology, Georgetown
*   University School of Medicine*
Washington, DC

M. Richard Koenigsberger, M.D.
Director, Division of Pediatric Neurology, University of
*   Medicine and Dentistry of New Jersey*
Newark, New Jersey

Robert B. Layzer, M.D.
Professor of Neurology, University of California School of
*   Medicine—San Francisco*
San Francisco, California

Niels L. Low, M.D.
Pediatric Neurologist and Clinical Director, Blythedale
*   Children's Hospital*
Valhalla, New York

Elliott L. Mancall, M.D.
Professor and Chairman, Department of Neurology,
*   Hahnemann University*
Philadelphia, Pennsylvania

Joseph T. Marotta, M.D.
Attending Neurologist and Professor of Medicine, Wellesley
*   Hospital*
Toronto, Ontario

John H. Menkes, M.D.
Professor of Neurology and Pediatrics, University of
*   California School of Medicine—Los Angeles*
Los Angeles, California

James R. Miller, M.D.
Associate Professor of Clinical Neurology, Columbia
*   University College of Physicians and Surgeons*
Associate Attending Neurologist, Neurological Institute of
*   Presbyterian Hospital, Columbia-Presbyterian Medical*
*   Center*
New York, New York

Jay P. Mohr, M.D.
Sciarra Professor of Clinical Neurology, Columbia University
*   College of Physicians and Surgeons*
Attending Neurologist, Neurological Institute of Presbyterian
*   Hospital, Columbia-Presbyterian Medical Center*
New York, New York

Theodore L. Munsat, M.D.
Professor of Neurology, Tufts University School of Medicine
Boston, Massachusetts

Charles W. Olanow, M.D.
Professor of Neurology, University of South Florida College
*   of Medicine*
Tampa, Florida

Audrey S. Penn, M.D.
Professor of Neurology, Columbia University College of
*   Physicians and Surgeons*
Attending Neurologist, Neurological Institute of Presbyterian
*   Hospital, Columbia-Presbyterian Medical Center*
New York, New York

David E. Pleasure, M.D.
Professor of Neurology, Pediatrics, and Orthopedic Surgery,
*   University of Pennsylvania School of Medicine*
Philadelphia, Pennsylvania

Charles M. Poser, M.D.
Lecturer on Neurology, Harvard Medical School
Senior Neurologist, Beth Israel Hospital
Boston, Massachusetts

Leon D. Prockop, M.D.
Professor and Chairman, Department of Neurology,
*   University of South Florida College of Medicine*
Tampa, Florida

Isabelle Rapin, M.D.
Professor of Neurology and Pediatric Neurology, Albert
*   Einstein College of Medicine*
New York, New York

Neil H. Raskin, M.D.
Professor of Neurology, University of California School of
*   Medicine—San Francisco*
San Francisco, California

Ralph W. Richter, M.D.
Clinical Professor of Neurology, University of Oklahoma,
*   Tulsa Medical College*
Tulsa, Oklahoma

Roger N. Rosenberg, M.D.
Professor and Chairman, Department of Neurology,
*   University of Texas Health Sciences Center, Southwestern*
*   Medical School*
Dallas, Texas

Allen D. Roses, M.D.
Professor and Chief, Division of Neurology, Duke University
*   Medical Center*
Durham, North Carolina

Lewis P. Rowland, M.D.
*Henry and Lucy Moses Professor and Chairman, Department
of Neurology, Columbia University College of Physicians
and Surgeons*
*Director, Neurology Service, Neurological Institute of
Presbyterian Hospital, Columbia-Presbyterian Medical
Center*
New York, New York

Edward B. Schlesinger, M.D.
*Professor Emeritus of Neurological Surgery, Columbia
University College of Physicians and Surgeons*
*Consultant Emeritus, Neurological Institute of Presbyterian
Hospital, Columbia-Presbyterian Medical Center*
New York, New York

James F. Schwartz, M.D.
*Professor of Pediatrics and Neurology, Emory University
School of Medicine*
Atlanta, Georgia

Daniel Sciarra, M.D.
*Professor of Clinical Neurology, Columbia University College
of Physicians and Surgeons*
*Attending Neurologist, Neurological Institute of Presbyterian
Hospital, Columbia-Presbyterian Medical Center*
New York, New York

Chunilal P. Shah, M.D.
Chief of Neuroradiology, James A. Haley Veterans Hospital
*Assistant Professor, Departments of Neurology and
Radiology, University of South Florida College of Medicine*
Tampa, Florida

William A. Sibley, M.D.
*Professor, Department of Neurology, University of Arizona
College of Medicine*
Tucson, Arizona

Bertman E. Sprofkin, M.D.
*Clinicial Professor of Neurology and Associate Clinical
Professor of Neuropathology, Vanderbilt Medical School*
Nashville, Tennessee

Bennett M. Stein, M.D.
*Bryon Stookey Professor, Department of Neurosurgery,
Columbia University College of Physicians and Surgeons*
*Chairman, Neurosurgery Service Neurological Institute of
Presbyterian Hospital Columbia-Presbyterian Medical
Center*
New York, New York

Hartwell G. Thompson, M.D.
*Professor and Head, Department of Neurology, University of
Connecticut School of Medicine*
Farmington, Connecticut

James F. Toole, M.D.
*Walter Teagle Professor of Neurology and Director of Stroke
Center, Bowman Gray School of Medicine*
Winston-Salem, North Carolina

Leon A. Weisberg, M.D.
Professor of Neurology, Tulane Medical School
New Orleans, Louisiana

Elliot D. Weitzman, M.D.*
*Formerly Director, Institute of Chronobiology, New York
Hospital–Cornell Medical Center*
White Plains, New York

Harry H. White, M.D.
Attending Neurologist, Boone Hospital Center
Columbia, Missouri

Melvin D. Yahr, M.D.
*Henry P. and Georgette Goldschmidt Professor and
Chairman, Department of Neurology, Mount Sinai School
of Medicine*
New York, New York

Frank M. Yatsu, M.D.
*Professor and Chairman, Department of Neurology,
University of Texas Medical School in Houston*
Houston, Texas

Dewey K. Ziegler, M.D.
*Professor of Neurology, Department of Neurology,
University of Kansas College of Health Sciences and
Hospital School of Medicine*
Kansas City, Kansas

Earl A. Zimmerman, M.D.
*Professor and Chairman, Department of Neurology, Oregon
Health Sciences*
Portland, Oregon

---

*Deceased.

Contents

IV. Disorders of Cerebrospinal and Brain Fluids

V. Tumors

VI. Trauma

VII. Birth Injuries and Developmental Abnormalities

VIII.   Genetic Diseases of Recognized Biochemical Abnormality

NEUROLOGIC DISORDERS OF UNCERTAIN ETIOLOGY OR PATHOGENESIS

IX.   Cerebral Degenerations of Childhood

X.   Neurocutaneous Disorders

XI.   Cranial Nerve Disorders

XII.   Peripheral Neuropathies

XX. Intermittent or Paroxysmal Disorders

XXI. Systemic Diseases

XXII. Environmental Neurology

Signs and Symptoms of Neurologic Disease

Chapter I

Symptoms of Neurologic Disorders

1. DELIRIUM AND DEMENTIA
Robert Katzman

Delirium and dementia are two of the most common disorders of elderly patients, but both conditions may occur at any age. *Delirium* is the acute confusional state that may accompany infections, fever, metabolic disorders, and other medical or neurologic diseases. *Dementia,* in contrast, is usually chronic and progressive, and is usually caused by degenerative diseases of the brain or by multiple strokes. The most significant difference, however, is that delirium is manifested by a fluctuating mental state, whereas patients suffering from dementia are usually alert and aware until late in the course of the disease.

Delirium

The word *delirium* comes from the Latin word meaning "to leave the furrow (or track)." It is used to refer to a mental disturbance that is marked by clouding of consciousness, that is, reduced awareness of environment and inability to maintain attention; there is often restlessness and incoherence. Sometimes misinterpretations, illusions, and hallucinations occur. Characteristics that lead to the classification of a mental state as delirium include reduced and often fluctuating levels of alertness and awareness, and impairment of memory and intellectual function; the presence of a medical or neurologic condition to which the mental impairment is secondary; the disappearance of mental impairment if the primary medical or neurologic disorder is reversed; and the effect of the primary disorder on the brain, which is diffuse rather than focal.

Delirium is involved in a wide range of clinical states. In elderly patients with severe bronchopneumonia, delirium takes the form of lethargy and confusion; such patients lie quietly in bed despite the concomitant tachypnea. Delirium is a common secondary disorder in previously healthy patients who are suffering a severe febrile illness. *Delirium tremens* differs from other forms of delirium in that it occurs only in persons who are addicted to alcohol. It develops 24 to 48 hours after withdrawal from alcohol. The onset is marked by confusion, agitation, and hyperactivity. Memory is affected and hallucinations occur. Autonomic hyperactivity results in tachycardia and high fever. If untreated, delirium tremens can be fatal.

Delirium is treated as a medical emergency because the disease or drug intoxication to which it is secondary may be fatal if untreated. The following drugs have been known to cause delirium.

Atropine and related compounds
Barbiturates
Bromides
Chlordiazepoxide (Librium)
Chloral hydrate
Cimetidine
Clonidine
Cocaine
Diazepam (Valium)
Digitalis
Ethanol
Flurazepam (Dalmane)
Glutethimide (Doriden)
Haloperidol and other neuroleptics
Lithium
Meprobamate
Mephenytoin
Methyldopa
Phencyclidine hydrochloride (PCP)
Phenytoin
Prednisone
Propanolol
Tricyclic antidepressants

The fluctuating state of awareness in delirium

is accompanied by characteristic electroencephalographic (EEG) changes. The varying level of attention parallels slowing of the background EEG rhythms. Appropriate treatment of the underlying disease improves both the mental state and EEG of the patient. A patient with bronchopneumonia shows less confusion and a more normal EEG when given an oxygen mask. This finding has been incorporated into medicine so firmly that the steps needed to improve confusional states and altered levels of awareness in patients arriving in emergency rooms are among the first practical aspects of medicine learned.

Mental Status Examination. The mental status evaluation is an important part of every neurologic examination. It includes evaluation of awareness and consciousness, behavior, emotional state, content and stream of thought, and sensory and intellectual capabilities. Specific aspects of intellectual activity are most often impaired in organic disease of the brain. Evaluation of these aspects constitutes the mental status examination, which is important in the diagnosis of both delirium and dementia. Intellectual impairment is obvious in such florid conditions as delirium tremens or advanced dementia, but a cognitive deficit may not be evident in early cases of delirium or dementia unless the physician specifically tests mental status.

Traditionally, mental status examinations test *information* (e.g., where were you born? what is your mother's name? who is the President? when did World War II occur?), *orientation* (what place is this? what is the date? what time of day is this?), *concentration* (tested by using serial reversals, e.g. spell "world" backwards, name the months of the year backwards beginning with December), *calculation* (e.g., doing simple arithmetic, making change, counting backwards by 3's or 7's), *reasoning, judgment, and memory* (e.g., identify these three objects, please try to remember their names, I will state a name and address, please repeat after me and try to remember for a few minutes) (Table 1–1). The most important and sensitive items are probably orientation to time, serial reversals, and a memory phrase.

In addition to testing the mental status, it is necessary to test higher intellectual functions, including disorders of language (dysphasias), constructional apraxia (Fig. 1–1), right-left disorientation, inability to carry out complex commands, especially those requiring crossing the midline (e.g., touch your left ear with your right thumb), inability to carry out imagined acts (ideomotor apraxia, e.g., pretend that you have a book of matches and show me how you would light a match); unilateral neglect, or inattention on double stimulation. These abnormalities are often associated with more focal brain lesions, but may also be impaired in delirium or dementia. Examination of aphasia, apraxia, and agnosia is described in detail in Chapter 2.

Dementia

Dementia is characterized by progressive intellectual deterioration that is sufficiently severe to interfere with social or occupational functions. Memory, orientation, abstraction, ability to learn, visuospatial perception, and constructional praxis are all impaired in dementia. In contrast to patients with delirium, subjects with dementia are alert and aware until late in the course of the disease. Delirium is most often associated with intercurrent systemic diseases or drug intoxication, but dementia is usually due to a primary degenerative or structural disease of the brain. Alzheimer disease (see Section 111, The Dementias) accounts for over 50% of cases in both clinical and autopsy series (Table 1–2). Huntington disease (see Section 113, Huntington Disease and Other Forms of Chorea) is much less common, but is still an important cause in the presenium. Parkinsonism (see Section 118, Parkinsonism) is sometimes associated with dementia. Less common degenerative diseases include Pick disease (see Section 111), progressive supranuclear palsy (see Section 119, Progressive Supranuclear Palsy), and the hereditary ataxias (see Section 109, Hereditary Ataxias).

Twenty to 25% of cases of dementia are due to vascular disease. Contrary to earlier beliefs, dementia correlates less with the degree of cerebral arteriosclerosis than with the extent of destruction of cerebral hemisphere by multiple strokes; hence, the term *multi-infarct dementia* has come into use. Cognitive impairment becomes evident when 50 to 100 g of cerebral hemisphere is destroyed. The strokes may be due to thrombosis, emboli, or hemorrhages. Minute infarcts *(lacunae)* occur in the basal ganglia in the presence of hypertensive disease that involves brain arterioles; the resulting "lacunar state" sometimes gives rise to dementia. *Binswanger dementia* occurs when hypertensive vascular disease of brain arterioles results primarily in white-matter dis-

Table 1-1. Mental Status Examination

IMC*	MSQ†	MMS‡
1. What *year* is it now?	1. What is the name of this place?	ORIENTATION What is the (year) (season) (date) (day) (month)?
2. What *month* is it now?	2. Where is it located (address)?	Where are we: (state) (county) (town) (hospital) (floor)?
3. Memory phrase: Repeat phrase after me: John Brown, 42 Market Street, Chicago	3. What is today's date?	REGISTRATION Name three objects: take 1 second to say each. Then ask the patient to name all three after you have said them. Then repeat them until he learns all three.
4. About what *time* is it? (Within 1 hour)	4. What is the month now?	
5. *Count* backwards 20 to 1	5. What is the year?	
6. Say the months in reverse order	6. How old are you?	ATTENTION AND CALCULATION: Serial 7s. Stop after 5 answers. Alternatively spell "world" backwards.
7. Repeat the memory phrase	7. When were you born (month)?	RECALL Ask for the three objects repeated above.
	8. When were you born (year)?	LANGUAGE Name a pencil and a watch Repeat the following: "No ifs, ands, or buts" Follow a 3-stage command: "Take a paper in your right hand, fold it in half, and put it on the floor" Read and obey the following: "Close your eyes" "Write a sentence" "Copy design"
	9. Who is the President of the United States?	
	10. Who was the President before him?	

*Information Memory Concentration. (From Katzman R, Brown T, Fuld P, et al. Am J Psychiatry 1983; 140:734–739.) Normal 80-year-olds will make only one or two errors in the individual components of the memory phrase. The total number of errors on this test correlates highly with quantitive measures of pathology (number of plaques in cerebral cortex) in patients with Alzheimer's disease. Items 6 and 7 are the most sensitive to early changes in this disease.

†Mental Status Questionnaire. (From Kahn RL, Goldfarb AI, Pollack M, Peck A. Am J Psychiatry 1960; 117:326–328.) The MSQ has a long history of use primarily with nursing home patients. Subjects who make many errors on this test are usually moderately to severely demented.

‡Mini-Mental State. (From Folstein MF, Folstein S, McHugh P. J Psychiatr Res 1975; 12:189–198.) The MMS has come into widespread use because it closely mimics a clinical mental state examination and includes language items (naming, reading, and writing) and copying a design.

Please draw a clock. Put the hours on it and set the time at 3:30.

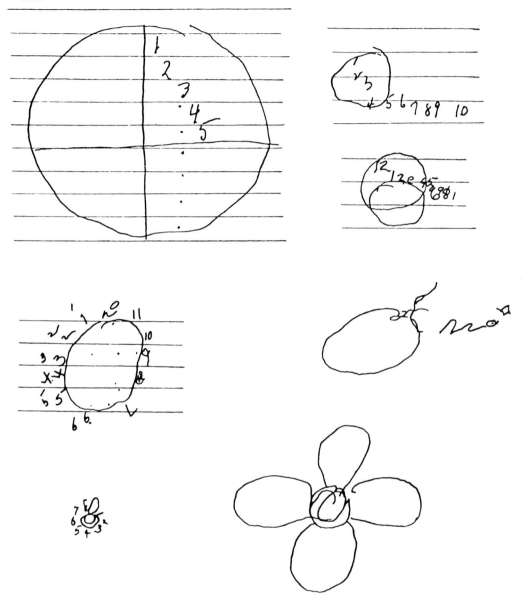

Fig. 1–1. A mental status examination question and examples of how several demented patients with Alzheimer disease responded.

ease including lacunae, cysts, and demyelination.

Intracranial mass lesions, including brain tumors and subdural hematomas, cause dementia without focal neurologic signs in as many as 5% of cases of dementia in some series. With the use of CT, these patients are rapidly identified and treated; future series of dementia cases will probably include fewer subjects with dementia caused by intracranial mass lesions.

The frequency of chronic communicating hydrocephalus (*normal pressure hydrocephalus*) as a cause of dementia in adults varies from 1 to 5% in different series. Diagnosis is usually straightforward when the hydrocephalus follows intracranial hemorrhage, head injury, or meningitis, but in idiopathic cases, it is often difficult to differentiate communicating hydrocephalus from ventricular enlargement due to brain atrophy.

At the turn of the century, the most common cause of dementia was neurosyphilis. Today, however, general paresis and other

Table 1–2. Diseases that Cause Dementia

	Clinical* Series		Autopsy† Series
Depressed/psychotic/no dementia	42		—
Patients with dementia	474		1000
Degenerative			
Alzheimer disease	267	56.3%	50.3%
Vascular/multi-infarct	40	8.4	22.3
Mixed	23	4.9	13.4
Other degenerative			
Huntington disease	26	5.5	—
Parkinson disease	7	1.5	1.0
Progressive supranuclear palsy	6	1.2	
Amyotrophic lateral sclerosis with dementia	3	0.6	
Progressive hemiatrophy	2	0.4	
Pick disease	1	0.2	2.1
Olivopontocerebellar atrophy			0.5
Epilepsy	1	0.2	
Metabolic/toxic/nutritional/alcoholism/ Wernicke/Korsakoff	17	3.6	1.1
Drug toxicity	8	1.7	
Metabolic (Thyroid/PA/hepatic/hypercalcemia)	8	1.7	
Infectious			
Creutzfeldt-Jakob disease	3	0.6	0.9
AIDS	24	5.1	
Other infections or inflammatory neuro-syphilis/multiple sclerosis/encephalitis	2	0.4	1.3
Vasculitis	3	0.6	
Hydrocephalus	8	3.8	1.1
Intracranial tumors	12	2.5	4.5
Post-traumatic/subdural	3	0.6	1.5

*Combined series (from Wells CE, ed. Dementia, 2nd ed. New York: Raven Press, 1977; Katzman R, personal series).
†Data from Jellinger K. Acta Neurol Belg 1976; 76:83–102.

forms of neurosyphilis are rare. The incidence of AIDS dementia is now rising rapidly in many metropolitan areas and may soon become the second or third most common cause of dementia in some localities. Creutzfeldt-Jakob disease is now the second most frequent cause of infectious dementia. Nonviral infections rarely present as chronic rather than acute encephalopathy. Fungal meningitis may occasionally present as dementia.

Nutritional, toxic, and metabolic causes of dementia are particularly important because they may be reversible. Korsakoff psychosis, usually found in alcoholics and attributed to thiamine deficiency, remains an important problem in our society. In contrast, the dementia of pellagra, a disorder produced by niacin and tryptophan deficiencies, has been almost entirely eliminated in the United States. Vitamin B_{12} deficiency occasionally causes dementia without anemia or spinal cord disease. Among the metabolic disorders that may present as dementia, hypothyroidism is the most important. Finally, prolonged administration of drugs may cause chronic intoxication (due to inability to metabolize the drug or to idiosyncratic reactions) that may be mistaken for dementia.

Differential Diagnosis. The first symptoms of patients with progressive dementia may include occasional forgetfulness, misplacing objects, and name-finding difficulties. Similar symptoms may occur in normal aging; however, these symptoms are minor and do not interfere with professional activities or the ability to live independently. In normal elderly patients, the symptoms are called "benign senescent forgetfulness." It is benign because follow-up has shown that the symptom complex does not lead to dementia. When dementia begins with similar symptoms, they are soon qualitatively different; the patient forgets not only details but important events. Moreover, mental status examinations (memory tests and serial reversals are most important here) are normal in the presence of benign senescent forgetfulness but abnormal in early dementia. More complete neuropsychologic examinations are occasionally needed to clarify this differential diagnosis.

Another difficult diagnostic problem is the differentiation of the patient with dementia and secondary depression from a patient with a primary depression and a secondary memory problem (*pseudodementia*) that will improve with treatment of the depression. The difficulty of this differentiation is dramatized by reports of 25 to 30% misdiagnosis in dementia series, in which the errors resulted chiefly from failure to recognize that older depressed individuals may show cognitive changes in mental status examination. In pseudodementia, the depression usually precedes the memory problem. The onset of the memory problem may be more abrupt than usually occurs in dementia and is often mild, tending to plateau. Neuropsychologic test results may be atypical for dementia. In pseudodementia, the EEG is usually normal. Whenever pseudodementia is suspected, vigorous treatment of the depression is indicated.

The differential diagnosis of dementia requires an accurate history and neurologic and physical examination. The history of a typical Alzheimer patient is one of an insidious onset and a slowly progressive, but relentless course in an otherwise healthy individual; the history of a patient with multi-infarct dementia may include an abrupt onset or stepwise development of the disease, a history of an obvious stroke, or the presence of hypertension or cardiac disease. A history of alcoholism should raise suspicion of Korsakoff psychosis.

Examination of the Alzheimer patient is usually normal except for primitive reflexes such as the snout reflex; the multi-infarct patient, on the other hand, often has evidence of hemiparesis or other focal neurologic signs; Huntington disease is readily recognized by the chorea and dysarthria. Parkinsonism patients are readily recognized by the typical gait, posture, bradykinesia, rigidity, and tremor; progressive supranuclear palsy is recognized by the limitation of vertical eye movements and extrapyramidal signs. Myoclonus occurs most often in Creutzfeldt-Jakob disease. Unsteadiness of gait is a hallmark of communicating hydrocephalus, but is even more severe in Creutzfeldt-Jakob disease, in the hereditary ataxias, and sometimes in Korsakoff psychosis.

The nature of the abnormality in higher function is important. All patients with dementia show abnormalities of recent memory. In Korsakoff psychosis, this loss of recent memory is the predominant finding and is often accompanied by confabulation. In the subcortical dementias (e.g., Huntington disease, progressive supranuclear palsy, and communicating hydrocephalus), memory impairment and psychomotor slowing are the most evident features. In contrast, patients with cortical dementias (e.g., Alzheimer or Pick disease, general paresis, Creutzfeldt-Jakob disease) and most patients with multi-infarct dementia show aphasia, agnosia, and apraxia in addition to memory loss and disorientation.

CT has become one of the most important diagnostic tools. Brain tumors, subdural hematomas, and hydrocephalus are readily diagnosed when it is used. Evidence of past strokes is sometimes visible. MRI is more sensitive than CT in demonstrating past strokes, but care must be used in interpreting changes in white matter intensity because intensity changes occur in normal aging and Alzheimer disease as well as in vascular dementia. The EEG is also helpful. In Alzheimer disease, there is usually a slowing of background rhythms. Periodic discharges are characteristic of Creutzfeldt-Jakob disease.

Blood tests are essential for diagnosis of dementia associated with endocrine disease and liver or kidney failure. It is also important to obtain thyroid function studies because hypothyroidism is a reversible cause of dementia. Vitamin B_{12} deficiency can be detected even in patients who are not anemic by determining serum vitamin B_{12} levels. Although neurosyphilis is rare today, it too is a reversible cause of dementia; a serologic test for syphilis is mandatory. Measurements of blood levels of drugs may detect intoxication.

Details of the differential diagnosis of diseases that cause dementia are provided in subsequent chapters. It is important to emphasize that an exhaustive evaluation of patients with dementia is warranted. Although we do not have effective treatment for the primary degenerative diseases, many other disorders that cause dementia are amenable to treatment that may arrest, if not reverse, the cognitive decline.

References

Cummings JL, Benson DB. Dementia: A Clinical Approach. London: Butterworths, 1983.

Diagnostic and Statistical Manual of Mental Disorders, 3rd ed. Washington DC, 1980; 104–112.

Folstein MF, Folstein S, McHugh P. "Mini-mental state": A practical method for grading the cognitive state of patients for the clinician. J Psychiatr Res 1975; 12:189–198.

Hachinski VC, Iliff LE, Ziljka E, et al. Cerebral blood flow in dementia. Arch Neurol 1975; 32:632–637.

Jellinger K. Neuropathological aspects of dementia resulting from abnormal blood and cerebrospinal fluid dynamics. Acta Neurol Belg 1976; 76:83–102.

Kahn RL, Goldfarb AI, Pollack M, Peck A, et al. Brief objective measures for the determination of mental status in the aged. Am J Psychiatry 1960; 117:326–328.

Katzman R, Brown T, Fuld P, et al. Validation of a short orientation-memory-concentration test of cognitive impairment. Am J Psychiatry 1983; 140:734–739.

Lipowski ZJ. Delirium (acute confusional state). JAMA 1987; 258:1789–1792.

Kral VA. Senescent forgetfulness: benign and malignant. Can Med Assoc J 1962; 86:257–260.

McHugh PR, Folstein MF. Psychopathology of dementia: implications for neuropathology. In: Katzman R, ed. Congenital and Acquired Disorders. New York: Raven Press, 1979; 17–30.

McKhann G, Drachman D, Folstein M, et al. Clinical diagnosis of Alzheimer's disease: Report of the NINCDS-ADRDA Work Groups under the auspices of Department of Health and Human Services Task Force on Alzheimer's Disease. Neurology 1984; 34:939–944.

NIA Task Force. Senility reconsidered. Treatment possibilities for mental impairment in the elderly. JAMA 1980; 244:259–263.

Romano J, Engel GL. Delirium. I. Electro-encephalographic data. Arch Neurol 1944; 51:356–377.

Wells CE, ed. Dementia, 2nd ed. New York: Raven Press, 1977.

Wolfson LW, Katzman R. Neurological Consultation at Age 80. In: Katzman R, Terry RD, eds. Neurology of Aging. Philadelphia: FA Davis, 1983.

2. APHASIA, APRAXIA, AND AGNOSIA

J.P. Mohr

Aphasia

Over 95% of right-handed people and most left-handed people are left-hemisphere dominant for speech and language. Right-hemisphere dominance for speech and language in a right-handed person is rare.

Disturbances in speech and language are usually caused by lesions in the region of the sylvian fissure of the dominant hemisphere. The farther from this zone that the lesion occurs, the less the disturbance in speech and language. The sylvian fissure comprises the opercular and insular regions, which are supplied by branches of the left sylvian artery.

The upper division of the sylvian artery supplies the insula and upper banks of the sylvian fissure; the lower division supplies the posterior temporal lobe and adjacent posterior parieto-occipital regions. Syndromes arising from arterial disease in the two divisions form the basis for most of our concepts of disturbed language, a group of disorders known as *aphasia.*

The most popular classification of aphasia is based on the classic view, in which the front half of the brain performs motor or executive functions, and the back half sensory or receptive functions, with the two regions connected by pathways in the white matter. Frontal lesions cause *motor aphasia,* those affecting the posterior regions cause *sensory aphasia,* and those interrupting the pathways between the frontal and posterior regions cause *conduction aphasia.* This formulation envisions a loop with its afferent portion from the eyes and ears through the visual and auditory system, an intrahemispheral portion through the white matter connecting the temporal with the frontal lobes (the arcuate fasciculus), and its efferent portion from the frontal lobes to the mouth and hand which, in its simplest function, permits words heard to be repeated aloud and words seen to be copied manually. The cortex grouped around the sylvian fissure is considered essential for these cross-modal transfers between the sensory and motor systems.

Meaning is thought to be conveyed to these shapes and sounds by access of the sylvian region to the rest of the brain through intrahemispheral and transcallosal pathways. Interruption of these pathways is postulated to produce *transcortical sensory aphasia,* in which words heard are repeated aloud or copied without comprehension, or *transcortical motor aphasia,* in which words can be repeated and words copied but no spontaneous communication by conversation or writing occurs. Other disconnections have also been proposed for pathways to or from the periphery, which would presumably be in the subcortical white matter. Disconnections of incoming pathways bearing visual lexical information would yield *pure alexia;* disconnections of those pathways conveying auditory material would cause *pure word deafness.* The combination of these two disconnections causes *subcortical sensory aphasia.* Disconnections of efferent pathways from the motor speech zones would produce *pure word mutism* or *subcortical motor aphasia.* Although these generalizations are broadly applicable as the major principles of cerebral organization, the uncritical acceptance of one theory forces the postulation of white-matter lesions and syndromes that occasionally prove misleading in efforts to diagnose the site and cause of a clinical disorder of speech and language. To avoid this problem, the discussion that follows emphasizes the clinical features that aid in local lesion diagnosis.

Motor Aphasias. A focal infarct involving any gyrus of the insula or the upper banks of the opercular cortex from the anterior inferior frontal region to the anterior parietal region disrupts the acquired skills involving the oropharyngeal, laryngeal, and respiratory systems that mediate speech, causing *acute mutism.* Writing may be preserved, although it is usually confined to a few simple words. Comprehension of words heard or seen is generally intact, because these functions are largely subserved by posterior regions. The smaller and more superficial the injury is, the briefer and less severe is the disruption in speech.

The speech that emerges within minutes or days of the onset of motor aphasia consists mostly of crude vowels *(dysphonia)* and poorly articulated consonants *(dysarthria).* Disturbed coordination *(dyspraxia)* of speaking and breathing alters the rhythm of speech *(dysprosody).* This faulty intonation, stress, and phrasing of words and sentences is known collectively as *speech dyspraxia.* The language conveyed through this speech is usually only slightly disturbed, but the grammatical forms used in speaking or writing are sometimes simplified.

The more anterior the lesion is along the operculum, the more speech dyspraxia predominates, especially with involvement of the inferior frontal region (Broca area), which is adjacent to the sensorimotor cortex. When the sensorimotor cortex itself is affected, dysarthria and dysphonia are more prominent than dysprosody and dyspraxia. These errors in pronunciation may make it impossible to understand the language conveyed by the patient's speech, but are not considered a sign of language disorder.

When infarcts occur more posteriorly along the sylvian operculum, the precise sensorimotor control over the positioning of the oropharynx is thought to be impaired, causing unusual mispronunciations as well as mild dysphasia. The disturbed pronunciation is not simple dysarthria; the faulty oropharyngeal positionings yield sounds that differ from those intended. The errors, analogous to the typing errors of a novice who is unfamiliar with the typewriter keyboard, are called *literal paraphasias.* The listener may mistake all utterances as language errors *(paraphasias),* or may be impressed with some of the genuine paraphasias and give it the name *conduction aphasia,* which blends with this disorder, but is usually due to a more posterior lesion. Until the speech errors are analyzed, the examiner may wonder how the patient's comprehension can be so intact when speech is so distorted.

The arrangement of the individual branches of the upper division of the sylvian artery favors the wide variety of focal embolic obstructions that produce this remarkable array of syndromes. The more specific the speech abnormality is, the more limited is the focal infarction. Because the sensorimotor cortex is part of the same arterial supply of the upper division of the middle cerebral artery, the larger infarcts usually cause contralateral hemiparesis and hemisensory syndromes, making the diagnosis of disease of the sylvian artery region fairly easy. Larger lesions (including those caused by occlusion of the trunk of the sylvian artery) spread over several gyri and cause a more severe clinical disorder.

Brain tumors are uncommon in the sylvian region and are usually large before motor aphasia appears, but the syndrome then approximates the later stages of major motor aphasia from infarction.

The larger the infarct is in breadth or depth, the longer is the delay before speech improves, and the more evident is dysphasia. In larger sylvian lesions, the dysphasia is most evident in the use of grammatical words, especially when the construction of sentences involves few nouns, or in tests that involve single letters, spelling, and subtleties of syntax. Problems with syntax occur not only in speaking and writing, but also in attempts to comprehend the meaning of words heard or seen. For example, the word "ear" is responded to more reliably than "are," "cat" more than "act," "eye" more than "I." The language content of spontaneously uttered sentences is condensed, missing many of the filler words, causing "telegraphic speech" or *agrammatism.* Agrammatism is an important sign of a major lesion of the operculum and insula.

In lesions involving many gyri, in most moderate and large hemorrhages, and in large neoplasms or abscesses big enough to produce unilateral weakness, the reduction of both speech and comprehension is profound and is called *total aphasia*. Within weeks or months in cases of infarction and hemorrhage, comprehension improves especially for nongrammatical forms, and speaking and writing seem to be affected more than listening and reading. This last syndrome, in which dysphasia is most evident in speaking and writing, is known as motor aphasia; the eponym *Broca's aphasia* is often used. This syndrome emerges from an initial syndrome of total aphasia as a late residual from a large lesion. It is not the usual acute syndrome of a circumscribed infarction, even when the lesion is confined to the pars opercularis of the inferior frontal gyrus (Broca's area).

Sensory Aphasias. A different set of acute symptoms follows occlusions in the region supplied by the lower division of the left sylvian artery, which irrigates the posterior half of the temporal lobe, and the posterior parietal and lateral occipital regions. Infarction is the usual cause for the discrete syndromes, while hemorrhage, epilepsy, and large infarcts may account for sudden major syndromes. Even large lesions in these areas, regardless of cause, are usually too remote from the operculum to affect the sensorimotor cortex; hemiparesis and speech disturbances (e.g., dysprosody, dysarthria, or mutism) are rarely found in conjunction.

In patients with large posterior lesions, the effects are almost the reverse of the insular-opercular syndromes: syntax is more preserved than semantics; the speech is filled with small grammatical words but the predicative words (i.e., words that contain the essence of the message) are omitted or distorted. The patient speaks easily, engages in simple conversational exchanges, and even appears to be making an effort to communicate; however, little meaning is conveyed in the partial phrases, disjointed clauses, and incomplete sentences. In the most severe form, speech is incomprehensible gibberish. When specific predicative words are called for, the patient hesitates. Words fail to occur to the patient *(omissions)*, are mispronounced as similar sounding words *(literal paraphasias)*, or are replaced by others that have a similar meaning *(verbal paraphasias)*. A similar disturbance affects attempts to understand the words heard or seen. These language disturbances may require prolonged conversation to be revealed in mild cases.

Because this disturbance in language contrasts with motor aphasia, it is often labeled as sensory aphasia, or *Wernicke aphasia*, but neither syndrome is purely motor or sensory.

The lower division of the sylvian artery gives off several closely grouped branches, making many of them susceptible to involvement by the same arterial occlusion that affects the sylvian artery, even if it is a relatively small embolus. This anatomic difference from the upper division of the sylvian artery accounts for the lower incidence of distinctive clinical variations. The posterior portions of the brain are also more compact than the anterior portions. As a result, large infarctions or mass lesions from hemorrhage, abscess, encephalitis, or brain tumors in the posterior brain tend to cause similar clinical disorders. Contralateral hemianopia usually implies a deep lesion; if there has been infarction, the lesion penetrates to the depths of the temporoparietal white matter. When hemianopia persists for more than about 1 week, the aphasia is likely to persist.

Focal lesions limited to the posterior temporal lobe usually produce part of the larger syndrome of sensory aphasia. Speech and language are only slightly disturbed, reading for comprehension may pass for normal, but auditory comprehension of language is grossly defective. Such cases were traditionally named *pure word deafness*, but spoken language usually contains verbal paraphasias and silent reading may also be disturbed. This syndrome might be better named the *auditory form of sensory aphasia*. It has a good prognosis and almost full clinical recovery occurs within weeks.

A similarly restricted dysphasia may affect reading and writing because of a more posteriorly placed focal lesion that damages the posterior parietal and lateral occipital regions. Reading comprehension and writing morphology are strikingly abnormal. This syndrome has been traditionally known as *alexia with agraphia*, but spoken language and auditory comprehension are also disturbed (although less than reading and writing). A better label might be the *visual form of sensory aphasia*. It also has a good prognosis.

The auditory and visual forms of Wernicke's aphasia are rarely produced by mass lesions from any cause and tend to blend in larger lesions. Whether the major syndrome of sensory aphasia is a unified disturbance or a synergistic result of several separate disorders has not been determined.

Amnestic Aphasia. Anomia, or *dysnomia*, is the term applied to errors in tests of naming. Analysis requires special consideration because the mere occurrence of naming errors is of less diagnostic importance than the type of error made. In all major aphasic syndromes, errors in language production cause dysnomia in the form of literal or verbal paraphasias. When the patient is asked to select among choices, the opportunities for error are limited to the choices available. However, in tests involving naming, there are no limits to possible responses. Errors often occur in naming tests, even in cases of mild dysphasia. For this reason, dysnomias accompanying literal or verbal paraphasias have little value as signs of focal brain disease.

Another pattern known as *amnestic dysnomia* has a greater localizing value. The patient acts as though the name has been forgotten, and may give functional descriptions instead. Invoking lame excuses, testimonials of prowess, claims of irrelevance, or impatience, the patient seems unaware that the amnestic dysnomia is a sign of disease. This pattern, known as *amnestic aphasia* when fully developed, is usually the result of disease of the deep temporal lobe gray and white matter. A frequent cause is Alzheimer disease, in which atrophy of the deep temporal lobe occurs early, and forgetfulness for names may be erroneously attributed to old age by the family. Identical symptoms may occur in the early stages of evolution of mass lesions from neoplasms or abscess, rarely as a sign of infarction in the deep temporal lobe. Amnestic aphasia is almost free of other disturbances in language, such as grammar, reading aloud, spelling and writing, unless the responsible lesion encroaches on the adjacent temporal parietal or sylvian regions. When due to a mass lesion, the syndrome often evolves into the full syndrome of Wernicke aphasia.

Thalamic Lesions and Aphasia. An acute deep lesion on the side of the dominant hemisphere may cause dysphasia if it involves the posterior thalamic nuclei that have reciprocal connections with the language zones. Large mass lesions or slowly evolving lesions from neoplasms that involve thalamic nuclei distort the whole hemisphere, making it difficult to recognize the components of the clinical picture. Small lesions are usually vascular, are most often hematomas, and are the usual cause of the sudden syndrome. As in delirium, consciousness fluctuates widely in this syndrome. As it fluctuates, language behavior varies from normal to spectacular usage. The syndrome may be mistaken for delirium due to metabolic causes (e.g., alcohol withdrawal). It is also important in the theory of language because the paraphasic errors are not due to a lesion that affects the cerebral surface, as was claimed traditionally. Prompt CT scanning usually demonstrates the thalamic lesion. The patient gradually improves, usually without any memory of the episode.

Apraxia

The term apraxia (properly known as *dyspraxia* because the disorder is rarely complete) refers to disturbances in the execution of learned movements other than those disturbances caused by any coexisting weakness. These disorders are broadly considered to be the body-movement equivalents of the dysphasias and, like them, have classically been categorized into motor, sensory, and conduction forms.

The motor form, known as *limb-kinetic* or *innervatory dyspraxia*, occurs as part of the syndrome of paresis caused by a cerebral lesion. The attempts to use the involved limbs reveal a disturbance in movement beyond that accounted for simply by weakness. Because attempted movements are disorganized, the patient appears clumsy or unfamiliar with the movements called for in tasks such as writing or using utensils. Although difficult to demonstrate, innervatory dyspraxia is a useful sign to elicit because it indicates that the lesion causing the hemiparesis involves the cerebrum, presumably including the premotor region and other association systems. Dyspraxias of this type are thought to be caused by a lesion involving the cerebral surface or the immediately adjacent white matter; apraxia is not seen in lesions that involve the internal capsule or lower parts of the neuraxis.

In *ideational dyspraxia*, movements of affected body parts appear to suffer a lack of basic plan, although individual familiar movements are carried out easily. This incompletely understood disorder is believed to be analogous to sensory aphasia (which features a breakdown of language organization despite continued utterance of individual words). The term is apparently derived from the simplistic notion that the lesion affects a brain region that contains the ideas for the chain of individual movements involved in complex behaviors such as feeding, dressing, or bathing. To the observer, the patient appears uncertain about what to do next and may be misdiagnosed as confused. The lesion causing ideational dyspraxia is usually in the posterior half of the dominant hemisphere. The coexisting sensory aphasia often directs diagnostic attention away from the dyspraxia which, like innervatory dyspraxia, is only rarely prominent enough to result in separate clinical recognition.

Ideomotor dyspraxia is the frequently encountered form of dyspraxia. The term is derived from the notion that the lesion disrupts the connections between the region of the brain containing the ideas and the region involved in the execution of the movements. The disturbance is analogous to so-called "conduction aphasia"; motor behavior is intact when executed spontaneously but faulty when attempted in response to verbal command. According to this formulation, disruption of the alleged pathways emanating from the posterior temporal region of the dominant hemisphere should cause ideomotor dyspraxia of the limbs of both sides of the body. For movements to be executed by the nondominant hemisphere in response to dictated commands that are processed by the dominant hemisphere, the lesion could involve the presumed white-matter pathways through the dominant hemisphere to its motor cortex, the motor cortex itself, or the white matter connecting to the motor cortex of the nondominant hemisphere through the corpus callosum. Because so many presumed pathways are involved, ideomotor dyspraxia is common. The syndrome is most frequently encountered in the limbs served by the nondominant hemisphere when the lesion involves the convexity of the dominant hemisphere. Concomitant right hemiparesis and dysphasias, usually of the motor type, often occupy the physician's attention so that the ideomotor dyspraxia of the nondominant limbs is unnoticed. The dysphasia may make it impossible to determine if ideomotor dyspraxia is present. When the dysphasia is mild, dyspraxia can be demonstrated by showing that the patient cannot make movements on command when he can mimic the behavior demonstrated by the examiner and execute it spontaneously at other times. The disturbances are most apparent for movements that involve the appendages (e.g., fingers, hands) or oropharynx, but axial and trunk movements are often spared.

Agnosia

Sometimes a patient with a brain lesion responds to common environmental stimuli as if they had never been encountered previously, even though the primary neural pathways of sensation function normally. This disorder is called an *agnosia* for the individual stimulus. Because the disturbance seen in response to a few stimuli is assumed to apply to others with similar properties, agnosias embrace specfic classes of stimuli (e.g., agnosia for colors) or more global disturbances for a form of sensation (e.g., visual or auditory agnosia). Such sweeping generalizations are usually unjustified in practice because careful examination often shows that the abnormality can be explained in some other way, including genuine unfamiliarity with the stimuli, faulty discrimination due to poor lighting, poor instructions by the examiner, or an overlooked end-organ failure (e.g., peripheral neuropathy, otosclerosis, cataracts). Faulty performance may also result from a dysphasia or dyspraxia. Errors arising from dysphasia are easily understood; dyspraxia may be more difficult to recognize. Sometimes it is not clear whether dyspraxia produces agnosia or vice versa. Posterior parietal lesions, arising from cardiac arrest, neoplasm, or infections, may impair the cerebral control of the precise eye movements involved in the practiced exploration of a picture or other complex visual stimulus; the resulting chaotic but conjugate eye movements prevent the victim from naming or interacting properly with the stimuli. This abnormality seems to be a form of cerebral blindness (which the patient may deny), and is an essential element of the *Balint syndrome,* which has had many other eponyms since the original description. Similar disturbances in skilled manual manipulation of objects may be documented in anterior parietal lesions that interfere with the ability to name or to use the object properly.

When all these variables have been taken into account, a small group of cases may remain in which the term agnosia may apply. Theories about the etiology of agnosia range over a considerable spectrum. At one end of the spectrum is the denial that such a state exists, the errors presumably resulting from a combination of dementia and impaired primary sensory processing; at the other end of the spectrum are postulates of anatomic disconnections due to lesions that lie between intact language areas and intact cerebral regions responsible for processing sensory input. Two claimed clinical subtypes of visual agnosia embrace these differing theories of agnosia: *apperceptive agnosia* refers to abnormality in the discrimination process and *associative agnosia* implies inability to link the fully discriminated stimulus to prior experience in order to name or to match the stimulus to others. Clinically, patients with apperceptive visual agnosia are said to fail tests of copying a stimulus or cross-matching a stimulus with others having the same properties (i.e., different views of a car), whereas patients with the associative form can copy and cross-match; neither type can name the stimulus as such. Disturbances of the ability to respond to stimuli have been described for colors (*color agnosia*) and for faces (*prosopagnosia*). Although the definition of agnosia requires that the victim treat the stimuli as unfamiliar, the errors often pass almost unnoticed (i.e., dark colors are misnamed for other dark colors, pictures of famous people are misnamed for each other). In the auditory system, a similar disturbance may occur with a normal audiogram in discrimination of sounds (*cortical deafness* or *auditory agnosia*), including words (*pure word deafness* or *auditory agnosia for speech*). An inability to recognize familiar objects by touch while still able to recognize them by sight is referred to as *tactile agnosia*.

In practical clinical terms, the clinical diagnosis of agnosia warrants consideration when the patient responds to familiar stimuli in an unusually unskillful manner, treats them as unfamiliar, or misnames them for other stimuli having similar hue, shape, or weight, yet does not show other signs of dysphasia or dyspraxia in other tests. The special testing is time-consuming, but often yields a diagnosis of a disorder arising from lesions of the corpus callosum, the deep white matter, or the cerebrum adjacent to the main sensory areas. The usual cause is atrophy or metastatic or primary tumor before more obvious defects occur in visual fields, motor function, and the like.

References

Balint R. Seelenlähmung des "Schauens," optische Ataxia, und räumliche Störung der Aufmerksamkeit. Monatschr Psychiatr Neurol 1909; 25:51–81.

Bogen JE, Bogen GM. Wernicke's region—where is it? Ann NY Acad Sci 1976; 280:834–843.

Brown JW. Aphasia, apraxia, and agnosia. Springfield: Charles C Thomas, 1972.

Damasio H, Damasio AR. The anatomic basis of conduction aphasia. Brain 1980; 103:337–350.

Geschwind N. Disconnection syndromes in animals and man. Brain 1965; 88:585–644.

Geschwind N. The apraxias: neural mechanisms of disorders of learned movement. Am Sci 1975; 63:188–195.

Geschwind N, Fusillo M. Color naming defects in association with alexia. Arch Neurol 1966; 15:137–146.

Graff-Radford NR, Damasio H, Yamada T, et al. Nonhemorrhagic thalamic infarction: clinical, neuropsychological and electrophysiological findings in four anatomical groups defined by computerized tomography. Brain 1985; 108:485–516.

Heilman KM, Valenstein E. Clinical Neuropsychology. New York: Oxford Press, 1979.

Leicester J, Sidman M, Stoddard LT, Mohr JP. The nature of aphasic responses. Neuropsychologia 1971; 9:141–155.

Ludlow CL, Rosenberg J, Fair C, et al. Brain lesions associated with nonfluent aphasia fifteen years following penetrating head injury. Brain 1986; 109:55–80.

Mazzochi F, Vignolo LA. Localisation of lesions in aphasia: clinical CT scan correlations in stroke patients. Cortex 1979; 15:627–653.

Mohr JP, Pessin MS, Finkelstein S, et al. Broca aphasia: pathologic and clinical aspects. Neurology 1978; 28:311–324.

Mohr JP. The vascular basis of Wernicke aphasia. Trans Am Neurol Assoc 1980; 105:133–137.

Naezer MA, Hayward RW. Lesion localization in aphasia with cranial computed tomography and Boston Diagnostic Aphasia Examination. Neurology 1978; 28:545–551.

Victor M, Angevine JB, Mancall EL, et al. Memory loss with lesions of the hippocampal formation. Arch Neurol 1961; 5:244–263.

Wyllie J. The Disorders of Speech. Edinburgh: Oliver & Boyd, 1894.

3. SYNCOPE AND SEIZURE
Dewey K. Ziegler

A common clinical problem is that of the patient who, in the absence of head trauma, has on one or more occasions repeatedly lost consciousness and promptly recovered. The term *syncope* has become somewhat ambiguous. Originally used to refer to loss of consciousness specifically due to cerebral ischemia, syncope now refers to episodes of diverse etiology and often difficult ascertainment. The latter meaning is used in this chapter.

Syncope is a common diagnostic problem in patients of all ages. Its prevalence has been reported to be as high as 47% in surveys of college students or young air force flying personnel, and equally high if not higher in the elderly. Prognosis varies from benign to ominous depending on etiology. Table 3–1 displays possible etiologies for brief episodes of loss of consciousness. The first principle in diagnosis of this common phenomenon is to

Table 3–1. Differential Diagnosis of Episodes of Transitory Loss of Consciousness of Rapid Onset

	Autonomic Dysfunction Before and During	Onset of Symptoms	Relation to Posture	Movement During Episode	EKG During Episode	Age of Patient	Recovery of Consciousness	Urinary Incontinence During Episode
"Reflex" vasodepressor syncope	Usually severe (pallor, sweating) preceding loss of consciousness	May be rapid or, not often, with premonitory sensation of "faintness"	Usually occurring with patient sitting or standing	Usually none; occasionally a few myoclonic jerks, tonic extension	Bradycardia, occasional dysrhythmia	Usually young	Rapid	Rare
Orthostatic hypotension	Frequent as in vasodepressor syncope except Shy-Drager syndrome	May be rapid or, not often, with premonitory sensation of "faintness"	Invariably erect posture	Usually none; occasionally a few myoclonic jerks, tonic extension	Tachycardia common	All ages	Rapid	Rare
Syncope of cardiac origin	Variable, not as severe as in vasodepressor syncope	May or may not be rapid	Inconstant	Usually none; occasionally a few myoclonic jerks, tonic extension	Dysrhythmia frequent; tachycardia block	All ages	Rapid	Rare
Seizure from cerebral dysfunction	Variable, rarely preceding loss of consciousness	Extremely rapid	None	Wide variety of involuntary movements	Usually normal or tachycardia	All ages	Often slow return to complete lucidity	Frequent
Hypoglycemia	Commonly pallor, bradycardia preceding and during syncope	Usually slow	None	Wide variety of involuntary movements or none	Usually bradycardia except in overt seizure; tachycardia	All ages	Variable; slow unless glucose administered	Frequent
Psychiatric episode	None	Slow or rapid	None	Wide variety of involuntary movements or none	Normal	Usually young	Slow or rapid	Rare

ascertain that the patient has experienced definite transient disturbance of consciousness. Many individuals refer to having "passed out" or having "had a spell" when, in actuality, consciousness was not lost or even impaired. Careful history-taking, with attention to the meaning patients attach to words, can usually differentiate other clinical states that may be confused with syncope.

Of these other states, possibly the most frequent is episodic vertigo. Patients often interpret the sudden violent sensation of movement of self or environment as loss of consciousness. The diagnostic problem is complicated because sudden vertigo is often accompanied by autonomic symptoms such as sweating, nausea, and occasionally the feeling of faintness. Conversely, in many types of vascular syncope, consciousness is impaired but not lost completely, a state for which the term "presyncope" has been coined. A prominent component of these symptoms may be a feeling of dizziness. It is often difficult to determine whether the patient is describing primary vestibular dysfunction or presyncope; the decision hinges on the prominence of the vertigo element in the symptoms.

Occasionally, transient attacks of loss of muscle tone in the legs can be mistaken in the history for syncope. Careful questioning, again, should dispel this possibility.

Transient disturbances of memory or normal consciousness can rarely be mistaken by patients for syncope. Episodes of hours of altered mental awareness occur in transient global amnesia. The prolonged duration of the episode and the, at least partially, normal speech and mental function during the episode differ from syncope.

Once the history of definite brief episodes of loss or impairment of consciousness has been established, there are four general classes of etiologic factors to be considered: vascular, epileptic, metabolic, and psychiatric. Diagnostic features helpful in distinguishing these causes of brief episodes of loss of consciousness are seen in Table 3–1.

Vascular Causes

For normal functioning, the brain requires that the heart deliver, at regular intervals, under adequate pressure, blood containing adequate quantities of oxygen and other nutrients. The heart, in turn, must receive the blood under adequate pressure from the peripheral vessels. Failure of any component of this mechanism may result in cerebral ischemia and syncope.

Vasovagal Syncope ("Fainting"). In this common phenomenon the loss of consciousness is brought about by precipitous fall in systemic blood pressure without compensatory rise in cardiac output. It is not known why the heart fails to respond by increasing output to the stimulus of fall in peripheral resistance. This failure has been ascribed to vagal inhibition (from which the term "vasovagal" derives), but the entire reaction can occur when vagal activity is blocked by atropine.

A characteristic sequence of events usually occurs. In the premonitory phase, the patient feels light-headed and apprehensive, with a strong but ill-defined sensation of malaise before consciousness is lost. Peripheral vasoconstriction imparts a pale or ashen appearance, and the pulse is rapid. Profuse sweating is often accompanied by hyperactivity of the gastrointestinal tract or urinary bladder, causing nausea or an urge to defecate or to urinate. Vision often becomes blurred and sometimes quite impaired, but there are no other specific abnormalities of special senses (i.e., there are no olfactory or auditory symptoms). Hyperventilation usually follows, resulting in hypocapnia, which may further lower cerebral blood flow. Attacks frequently occur when the individual is standing. A subject who is sitting or standing has a strong desire to lie down, or at least to lower the head below heart level; on occasion in mild attacks, this maneuver may reverse symptoms and abort a full attack.

If the attack proceeds, the patient loses tone in the muscles of the legs and trunk, falls, and loses consciousness. Pulse then slows, occasionally to the point of cardiac arrest. The period of unconsciousness characteristically lasts only a few minutes, during which time the patient continues to exhibit pallor and diaphoresis. In addition to hypotension and bradycardia, cardiac arrhythmias occasionally occur. The limbs usually remain completely flaccid. Occasionally, involuntary limb movements occur, usually consisting of a few brief myoclonic jerks. Rarely there is tonic extension of the trunk, especially when brain ischemia is prolonged; this phenomenon seems to be more common in children.

Pulse and blood pressure usually return rapidly to normal before symptoms completely disappear, and the return to consciousness is rapid and complete if the patient is allowed to remain recumbent. The patient may feel weak and briefly confused on recovery. No abnormal findings are present on physical examination in the interictal period. Urinary or bowel incontinence is rarely seen in syncope due to vasovagal attacks.

"Fainting" of this type is a syndrome of the young and tends to occur in individuals of some emotional lability. There are almost invariably, unlike all other kinds of syncope, precipitating stimuli or situations. These include severe pain, apprehension of pain or, as all who have seen melodrama know, confrontation with horrifying sights or sudden emotional shocks. Fainting after emotional stimuli seems more common in women, but syncope induced by pain is more common in men. A variety of background states may add to the likelihood of such syncope: fasting, overheated places, or prolonged standing, and marked fatigue.

Orthostatic Hypotension. Syncope may result from decrease in blood flow to the brain after rising from a supine or sitting to a standing position. A mild, orthostatic fall in blood pressure often occurs in normal individuals without causing symptoms. When, however, there is interference with the normal vascular reflexes that maintain blood flow to the brain with upright posture, syncope can result. The following are the common etiologies:

1. In American society, prescribed drugs may be the most common cause. These include phenothiazines, antihypertensive agents, diuretics, arterial vasodilators, levodopa, calcium channel blockers, tricyclic antidepressants, and lithium. Susceptibility varies markedly from one individual to another. The frail and elderly are particularly vulnerable to this effect. Use of phenothiazines to control agitation in an elderly patient often results in hypotension, syncope, a fall, and hip fracture.

2. Orthostatic hypotension may also follow prolonged standing, viral infection, or other illness requiring prolonged bed rest. Conditions that lead to debilitation or relatively low blood pressure also predispose to orthostatic hypotension: malnutrition, anemia, bleeding, or adrenal insufficiency.

3. In several diseases of the central and peripheral nervous system, orthostatic hypotension occurs because of failure of the vasomotor reflexes that are normally activated by standing. These include peripheral neuropathy, particularly diabetic neuropathy, diseases of the lateral columns of the spinal cord, e.g., syringomyelia and tabes dorsalis, and certain diseases characterized by progressive atrophy of neurons in multiple brain systems (the Shy-Drager syndrome). In one condition called "sympathotonic orthostatic hypotension," tachycardia accompanies the hypotension. It is thought that sympathetic nerves are intact, but that impaired alpha-receptor and excessive beta-receptor responses occur on standing.

Cardiac Disease. *Cardiac Arrhythmias.* The vasovagal attack is a common cause of vascular syncope only in the youthful, but temporary cardiac arrhythmias that impair cardiac output occur at all ages. There are a wide variety of such arrhythmias; they are particularly frequent in the elderly. Attacks can be produced by many types of cardiac disease.

When cardiac arrhythmia is suspected, the resting EKG is frequently normal. The most important next step in investigation is prolonged recording of the EKG, correlated with clinical symptoms. When this test demonstrates arrhythmias that are clearly accompanied by syncope, it is presumed that the cause of the symptom has been found. As in vasovagal syncope, episodes without total loss of consciousness (states mentioned previously as presyncope) may occur, but temporary cardiac arrhythmias are frequently asymptomatic. Concurrence of the symptoms with arrhythmia must exist to justify ascribing the episodes to a cardiac cause. Continuous recording for 48 or 72 hours, or even longer, is often necessary to capture the diagnostic period.

If temporary arrhythmia is established as the cause of syncope, invasive electrophysiologic cardiac studies are usually necessary to ascertain possible need for medication or a pacemaker. Occasionally the severity and frequency of arrhythmias on EKG are deemed sufficient to suggest the cause or the history of syncope in the absence of symptoms during EKG and to warrant proceeding with these further electrophysiologic cardiac studies—a difficult decision.

Other Cardiac Disease. Many types of cardiac disease, aside from those that cause arrhythmias, can produce syncope. These include myocardial infarction (in which syncope is rarely the presenting symptom) and a variety of lesions that in some way obstruct normal blood flow through the heart. These conditions include aortic and mitral stenosis, myxoma, congenital heart diseases, and pulmonary stenosis or emboli.

Certain clinical clues, positive and negative, suggest the existence of cardiac disease as the cause of syncope. This type of syncope, unlike the vasovagal syndrome or orthostatic hypotension, shows little relation to posture. Symptoms are usually of rapid onset. "Presyncopal" symptoms may occur alone, without complete loss of consciousness; patients often note abrupt onset of sensations of lightheadedness and confusion or apprehensiveness, but without any preceding or accompanying sweating or pallor. The patient is often aware of a chest sensation that is difficult to describe; pain may occur. In some patients, full syncope occurs without any premonitory symptoms. In cases of prolonged cardiac dysrhythmia, ill-defined symptoms may last much longer than they do in vasodepressor syncope.

Syncope after exertion is particularly characteristic of some types of cardiac disease, particularly those associated with obstruction of blood flow.

In patients with syncope of unknown cause, those with cardiac disease have a much higher subsequent mortality rate than those without. It is therefore important to identify patients who may be candidates for specific cardiac treatment.

Carotid Sinus Syncope. The carotid sinus can develop unusual sensitivity to normal pressure stimuli. This condition, the hyperactive carotid sinus, is found almost exclusively in the elderly and is probably related to atherosclerosis of the carotid sinus region. Because of this hyper-responsiveness to even slight pressure, syncope can be caused by tight collars or inadvertent pressure on the side of the neck. Two mechanisms of syncope may occur. The more common is bradycardia and, on occasion, cardiac arrest; less common is a fall in systemic blood pressure due to splanchnic vasodilation. These mechanisms may occur together. Whether there is a third "central" mechanism in which syncope occurs without bradycardia or fall in pressure is debatable.

As a diagnostic maneuver if hypersensitive carotid sinus is suspected, light massage to the neck area can be performed one side at a time. This maneuver should always be done with EKG monitoring and preferably with EEG as well.

Syncope from Other External Stimuli: Possible Vagal Mechanisms. Syncope has occurred in the course of a variety of events that provide stimuli to the central nervous system. In most cases when the cause has been investigated, bradycardia or cardiac arrhythmia has been discovered. Precipitating states include defecation, rectal examination, swallowing hot or cold liquids, venipuncture, or bronchoscopic examination. Other pathologic processes that have produced synope are mediastinal masses, pulmonary emboli, and gallbladder disease. It is thought that stimulation of the vagus by these varied phenomena results in reflex inhibition of normal heart rhythm, with resultant impaired cerebral perfusion.

Syncope can occur after emptying a distended urinary bladder. This syndrome is confined to men and may be the result of both vagal stimuli and orthostatic hypotension. It occurs especially after ingestion of excess fluid and alcohol.

Syncope after prolonged coughing (tussive syncope) may also result from a combination of factors. It is usually seen in stocky individuals with chronic lung disease. In children with asthma, it may mimic epilepsy. Increased intrathoracic pressure may decrease cardiac output, and vagal stimuli probably play a role. Sudden rise in intracranial pressure has also been reported. Syncope on weight lifting is probably due to similar mechanisms.

Hematologic Factors. Normal cerebral function demands not only adequate cardiac output and rhythm, but blood carrying adequate hemoglobin and oxygen. Severe deficiency in either can predispose to syncope.

Arterial Disease. A rare vascular cause of syncope is severe disease of the vertebral-basilar arterial system, usually of atherosclerotic origin. Episodic ischemia of the reticular formation of the brain stem is the presumptive cause of unconsciousness. These transient ischemic attacks (TIAs) usually occur in patients who at other times have one or more other manifestations of brain stem, cerebellar, or occipital lobe dysfunction (i.e., cranial nerve palsies, Babinski sign, ataxia, hemianopia, or cortical blindness). Whereas vasovagal syncope is a disease of the young, vertebral-basilar insufficiency is a disease of the elderly. There is usually little relationship to posture, and presyncopal symptoms are rare.

Migraine. Syncope may be preceded by severe headache. Rarely, such an attack is clearly convulsive in nature. In other cases, however, the patient is pale and flaccid, and the mechanism is presumably cerebral ischemia induced by vasoconstriction, or fall in blood pressure due to pain.

Epileptic Causes

GENERAL DIFFERENTIATION OF VASCULAR SYNCOPE FROM SEIZURE

The differentiation of vascular syncope from seizure is probably the most frequently encountered diagnostic problem in patients suffering spells of rapid loss of consciousness of brief duration.

Two kinds of seizures are most often confused with syncope: complex partial seizures and akinetic seizures. Seizures are discussed in detail elsewhere in this volume, but a few generalizations can be made about the differential diagnosis.

A few myoclonic jerks of the legs or arms may uncommonly be seen during a period of cerebral ischemia, particularly in adults. Even rarer is prolonged myoclonic jerking of arms and legs, or brief tonic extension of the body (convulsive syncope). The tonic-clonic attack associated with urinary incontinence is an extreme rarity unless cerebral ischemia is prolonged. The likelihood of the more severe manifestations (seizures, incontinence) increases if the patient's head is not immediately lowered at the onset of symptoms.

True seizures, unlike syncope due to cerebral ischemia, are never consistently related to head or body posture. Complex partial seizures (psychomotor seizures) commonly produce alterations in normal consciousness for which the patient has some memory. In these seizures, involuntary movements of some kind usually occur. They may affect the face, palate, trunk, or limbs. As in other seizures, urinary incontinence is common, and altered consciousness, unlike syncope, characteristically lasts several minutes. Confusion lasts at least several minutes after the attack.

Warning feelings described by patients as faintness or light-headedness are uncommon in seizures, and preictal diaphoresis is rare, in contrast to the sequence of events in syncope. Conversely, irritative special-sense phenomena (e.g., visual, olfactory, or auditory hallucinations), complex psychic sensations, and changes in emotional state are common in seizures, but not in syncope.

Simple loss of muscle tone with unconsciousness as a manifestation of a generalized seizure (akinetic seizure) is not common at any age and is particularly rare in adults. The period of unconsciousness is characteristically longer than in syncope. Postictal confusion is common.

Simultaneous recording of EEG and EKG is invaluable in these diagnostic problems. Finding a definite interictal spike abnormality in the temporal area on the EEG is strong evidence that spells of unconsciousness are complex partial seizures. Similarly, a generalized paroxysmal abnormality confirms the presence of generalized epilepsy. Long-term simultaneous recording may be needed. Demonstration of the characteristic EEG during an episode is proof that the cause was a seizure.

Table 3–2. Causes of Syncope (Yale Patients)*

Cause	Number of Patients
Vasovagal/psychogenic	80
Vasovagal episode	64
Gastrointestinal bleeding	6
Duodenal ulcer	3
Gastric ulcer	1
Gastritis	1
Diverticulosis	1
Postural hypotension	1
Diarrhea	5
Intravenous pyelographic dye reaction	1
Familial	1
Hyperventilation	2
Tussive syncope	2
Micturition syncope	1
Cardiac	15
Ventricular tachycardia	6
Complete heart block	3
Severe bradycardia	2
Myocardial infarction	2
Aortic stenosis	1
Rapid atrial fibrillation	1
Metabolic/drug	7
Hypoglycemia	3
Ethanol intoxication	3
Nitrate syncope	1
Central nervous system	5
Seizure	2
Vertebrobasilar insufficiency	3
Unknown	69
TOTAL	176

*From Eagle KA, Black HR, Cook E, Goldman L. Evaluation of prognostic classifications for patients with syncope. Am J Med 1985; 79:455–460.

Table 3–3. Causes of Syncope (Pittsburg Patients)*

Cause	Number of Patients
Cardiovascular	53
Ventricular tachycardia	20
Sick-sinus syndrome	10
Bradycardia	2
Supraventricular tachycardia	3
Complete heart block	3
Mobitz II atrioventricular block	2
Pacemaker malfunction	1
Carotid-sinus syncope	1
Aortic stenosis	5
Myocardial infarction	2
Dissecting aortic aneurysm	1
Pulmonary embolus	1
Pulmonary hypertension	2
Noncardiovascular	54
Vasodepressor syncope	9
Situational syncope (cough, micturition, defecation)	15
Drug-induced syncope	6
Orthostatic hypotension	14
Transient ischemic attacks	3
Subclavian steal syndrome	2
Seizure disorder	3
Vagal reaction with trigeminal neuralgia	1
Conversion reaction	1
Unknown	97
TOTAL	204

*From Kapoor WN, Karpf M, Wieand S, et al.: A prospective evaluation and follow-up of patients with syncope. N Engl J Med 1983; 309:197–203.

Metabolic Causes

Hypoglycemic States. Hypoglycemic states may present with feelings of faintness or dizziness, but rarely with rapid loss of consciousness and rapid recovery. Characteristic of hypoglycemia are states of impaired consciousness of varying degrees and altered behavior of insidious onset. Hypoglycemic states may last for less than an hour or several hours and are often associated with generalized seizures. Proof of the nature of the episodes is demonstrated by profound hypoglycemia at the time of the symptom and reversal of symptoms by glucose given intravenously. To explain severe symptoms such as syncope, blood sugar must be well into the abnormal range. It is usually incorrect to ascribe central nervous system dysfunction to borderline or mild degrees of hypoglycemia.

Table 3–4. Causes of Syncope*

Demonstrated at initial evaluation	
Vasovagal syncope	32
Situational syncope	32
Orthostatic hypotension	35
Drug-induced syncope	9
Transient ischemic attack	8
Psychiatric syncope	1
Seizure	1
Total	118
Suggested at initial evaluation	
Carotid sinus syncope	5
Aortic stenosis	8
Pulmonary embolus	2
Pulmonary hypertension	2
Subclavian steal	2
Dissecting aortic aneurysm	1
Total	20
Myocardial infarction	5
Overall total	143

*From Kapoor WN, Cha R, Peterson JR, et al.: Prolonged electrocardiographic monitoring in patients with syncope: importance of frequent or repetitive ventricular ectopy. Am J Med 1987; 82:20–28.

Psychiatric States

A variety of psychiatric states resemble syncope but show no evidence of physiologic dysfunction, i.e., no change in pulse or blood pressure, EKG, or EEG. The major diagnostic problem is differentiation from syncope, but the characteristic preictal diaphoresis and pallor of the latter are lacking. Unresponsiveness usually is more prolonged than in syncope. Hyperventilation also commonly occurs before or during anxiety episodes and often produces subjective states that the patient interprets as loss of consciousness. Unlike syncope patients, these individuals often respond to sensory stimuli while they are apparently unconscious. These states may be called manifestation of hysteria, Briquet syndrome, or malingering, depending on psychiatric judgment. The episodes usually occur in patients who show, at other times, other evidence of neurologic dysfunction that is characteristic of psychiatric conditions but that has no anatomic explanation (e.g., analgesia, bizarre motor dysfunction). Differentiation of these states from ictal or postictal components of complex partial seizures is frequently more difficult, often demanding observation under physiologic monitoring, and is discussed elsewhere in this volume.

Reports of the comparative frequency for the causes of syncope have varied; those of three large series are shown in Tables 3–2 through 3–4. One clear cause of variation is the source of the sample studied. Invariably, in large numbers of cases, the cause cannot be determined.

Treatment can be offered for many types of recurrent syncope, as described in the appropriate sections of this book and standard medical textbooks.

References

Bowder DB. Pallid syncope (reflex anoxic seizures). Arch Dis Child 1984; 59:1118–1119.

Eagle KA, Black HR, Cook FE, Goldman L. Evaluation of prognostic classifications for patients with syncope. Am J Med 1985; 79:455–460.

Haslam RHA, Freigang B. Cough syncope mimicking epilepsy in asthmatic children. Can J Neurol Sci 1985; 12:45–47.

Kapoor WN, Cha R, Peterson JR et al. Prolonged electrocardiographic monitoring in patients with syncope. Am J Med 1987; 82:20–28.

Kapoor WN, Karpf M, Wieand S, et al. A prospective evaluation and follow-up of patients with syncope. N Engl J Med 1983; 309:197–204.

Lin JT-Y, Ziegler DK, Lai C-W, Bayer W. Convulsive syncope in blood donors. Ann Neurol 1982; 11:525–528.

Lipsitz LA. Syncope in the elderly. Ann Intern Med 1983; 99:92–105.

Ormerod AD. Syncope. Br Med J 1984; 288:1219–1222.

Reiffel JA, Wang P, Bower R, et al. Electrophysiologic testing in patients with recurrent syncope: Are results predicted by prior ambulatory monitoring? Am Heart J 1985; 110:1146–1153.

Silverstein MD, et al. Patients with syncope admitted to medical intensive care units. JAMA 1982; 248:1185–1189.

4. COMA

John C.M. Brust

Consciousness, the awareness of self and environment, requires both arousal and mental content; the anatomic substrate includes both reticular activating system and cerebral cortex. *Coma* is a state of unconsciousness that differs from syncope in being sustained and from sleep in being less easily reversed. Cerebral oxygen uptake (cerebral metabolic rate of oxygen—$CMRO_2$) is normal in sleep or actually increases during the rapid eye movement (REM) stage, but $CMRO_2$ is abnormally reduced in coma.

Coma is clinically defined by the neurologic examination, especially responses to external stimuli. Terms such as *lethargy, obtundation, stupor,* and coma usually depend on the patient's response to normal verbal stimuli, shouting, shaking, or pain. These terms are not rigidly defined, and it is useful to record both the response and the stimulus that elicited it. It may occasionally be difficult or impossible to determine the true level of consciousness (e.g., when there is catatonia, severe depression, curarization, or akinesia plus aphasia).

Confusional state and *delirium* are terms that refer to a state of inattentiveness, altered mental content and, sometimes, hyperactivity rather than a decreased level of arousal; these conditions may presage or alternate with obtundation, stupor, or coma.

Examination and Major Diagnostic Procedures

In assessing a comatose patient, it is first necessary to detect and treat any immediately life-threatening condition: hemorrhage is stopped; the airway is protected, with intubation when necessary (including the prevention of apsiration in a patient who is vomiting); circulation is supported; and an EKG is performed to detect dangerous arrhythmia. If the diagnosis is unknown, blood is drawn for glucose determination, after which 50% dextrose is given intravenously, with parenteral thiamine. (Administering glucose alone to a thiamine deficient patient may precipitate Wernicke-Korsakoff syndrome.) When opiate overdose is a possibility, naloxone is given. If trauma is suspected, damage to internal organs and fracture of the neck should be taken into consideration until radiographs determine otherwise.

The next step is to ascertain the site and cause of the lesion. The history is obtained from whomever accompanies the patient, including ambulance drivers and police. Examination should include the following: the skin, nails, and mucous membranes (for pallor, cherry redness, cyanosis, jaundice, sweating, uremic frost, myxedema, hypo- or hyperpigmentation, petechiae, dehydration, decubiti, or signs of trauma); the breath (for acetone, alcohol, or fetor hepaticus); and the fundi (for papilledema, hypertensive or diabetic retinopathy, retinal ischemia, Roth spots, granulomas, or subhyaloid hemorrhages). Fever may imply infection or heat stroke; hypothermia may occur with cold exposure (especially in alcoholics), hypothyroidism, hypoglycemia, sepsis or, infrequently, a primary brain lesion. Asymmetry of pulses may suggest dissecting aneurysm. Urinary or fecal incontinence may signify an unwitnessed seizure, especially in patients who awaken spontaneously. The scalp should be inspected and palpated for signs of trauma (e.g., Battle sign), and the ears and nose are examined for blood or CSF. Resistance to passive neck flexion, but not to turning or tilting, suggests meningitis, subarachnoid hemorrhage, or foramen magnum herniation, but may be absent early in the course of the disorder and in patients who are deeply comatose. Resistance in all directions suggests bone or joint disease, including fracture.

In their classic monograph, Plum and Posner divided the causes of coma into supra- and infratentorial structural lesions and diffuse or metabolic diseases. By concentrating on motor responses to stimuli, respiratory patterns, pupils, and eye movements, the clinician can usually identify the category of coma.

The patient is observed in order to assess respiration, limb position, and spontaneous movements. Myoclonus or seizures may be subtle (e.g., twitching of one or two fingers or the corner of the mouth). More florid movements such as facial grimacing, jaw gyrations, tongue protrusion, or complex repetitive limb movements may defy ready interpretation. Asymmetric movements or postures may signify either focal seizures or hemiparesis.

Asymmetry of muscle tone suggests a structural lesion, but it is not always clear which side is abnormal. *Gegenhalten,* or paratonia, is resistance to passive movement that, in contrast to parkinsonian rigidity, increases with the velocity of the movement and, unlike clasp-knife spasticity, continues through the full range of the movement; it is attributed to diffuse forebrain dysfunction and is often accompanied by a grasp reflex.

Motor responses to stimuli may be appropriate, inappropriate, or absent. Even when patients are not fully awake, they may be roused to follow simple commands. Some patients who respond only to noxious stimuli (e.g., pressure on the sternum or supraorbital bone; pinching the neck or limbs; or squeezing muscle, tendon, or nailbeds) may make voluntary avoidance responses. The terms "decorticate" and "decerebrate" posturing are physiologic misnomers, but refer to hypertonic flexion or extension in response to noxious stimuli. In *decorticate rigidity,* the arms are flexed, adducted, and internally rotated and the legs are extended; in *decerebrate rigidity,* the arms and legs are all extended. These postures are most often associated with cerebral hemisphere disease, including metabolic encephalopathy, but may follow upper brain stem lesions or transtentorial herniation.

Flexor postures generally imply a more rostral lesion than does extensor posturing, and a better prognosis, but the pattern of response may vary with different stimuli or there may be flexion of one arm and extension of the other. When these postures seem to occur spontaneously, there may be an unrecognized stimulus (e.g., airway obstruction or bladder distention). With continuing rostrocaudal deterioration, there may be extension of the arms and flexion of the legs until, with lower brain stem destruction, there is flaccid unresponsiveness. Lack of motor response to any stimulus, however, should always raise the possibility of limb paralysis caused by cervical trauma, Guillain-Barré neuropathy, or the locked-in state.

Respiration. In *Cheyne-Stokes respiration* (CSR), periods of hyperventilation and apnea alternate in a crescendo-decrescendo fashion. The hyperpneic phase is usually longer than the apneic, so that arterial gases tend to show respiratory alkalosis; during periods of apnea, there may be decreased responsiveness, miosis, and reduced muscle tone. CSR occurs with bilateral cerebral disease, including impending transtentorial herniation, upper brain stem lesions, and metabolic encephalopathy. It usually signifies that the patient is not in imminent danger. On the other hand, short-cycle CSR *(cluster breathing),* with less smooth waxing and waning, is often an ominous sign of a posterior fossa lesion or dangerously elevated intracranial pressure.

Sustained hyperventilation is usually due to metabolic acidosis, pulmonary congestion, hepatic encephalopathy, or stimulation by analgesic drugs. Rarely it is the result of a lesion in the rostral brain stem. *Apneustic breathing,* consisting of inspiratory pauses, is seen with pontine lesions, especially infarction; it occurs infrequently with metabolic coma or transtentorial herniation.

Respiration that is variably irregular in rate and amplitude *(ataxic* or *Biot breathing)* indicates medullary damage, and may progress to apnea, which may also occur abruptly in acute posterior fossa lesions. Loss of automatic respiration with preserved voluntary breathing *(Ondine's curse)* occurs with medullary lesions; as the patient becomes less alert, apnea may be fatal. Other ominous respiratory signs are end expiratory pushing (like coughing) and "fish-mouthing" (i.e., lower-jaw depression with inspiration). Stertorous breathing (i.e., inspiratory noise) is a sign of airway obstruction.

Pupils. Pupillary abnormalities in coma may reflect an imbalance between inputs from the parasympathetic and sympathetic nervous systems or lesions of both. Although many people have slight pupillary inequality, anisocoria should be considered pathologic in a comatose patient. Retinal or optic-nerve damage does not cause anisocoria, even though there is an afferent pupillary defect. Parasympathetic lesions (e.g., oculomotor nerve compression in uncal herniation or after rupture of an internal carotid artery aneurysm) cause pupillary enlargement and, ultimately, full dilatation with loss of reactivity to light. Sympathetic lesions, either intraparenchymal (e.g., hypothalamic injury or lateral medullary infarction) or extraparenchymal (e.g., invasion of the superior cervical ganglion by lung cancer), cause the Horner syndrome with miosis. With involvement of both systems (e.g., midbrain destruction), one or both pupils are in midposition and are unreactive. It is uncertain whether the pin point but reactive pupils of pontine hemorrhage are caused by intra-axial sympathetic involvement or reticular formation lesions that dysinhibit the Edinger-Westphal nucleus.

With few exceptions, metabolic disease does not cause unequal or unreactive pupils. Fixed, dilated pupils after diffuse anoxia-ischemia carry a bad prognosis. Atropine-like drugs and glutethimide abolish pupillary reactivity; with anticholinergics the pupils are fully dilated and with glutethimide they are large or in midposition. Hypothermia and severe barbiturate intoxication can cause not only fixed pupils but a reversible picture that mimics brain death. Bilateral or unilateral pupillary dilation and unreactivity may accompany (or briefly follow) a seizure. In opiate overdose, miosis may be so severe that a very bright light and a magnifying glass are necessary to detect reactivity. Some pupillary abnormalities are local in origin (e.g., trauma or synechiae).

Eyelids and Eye Movements. Closed eyelids in a comatose patient mean that the lower pons is intact, and blinking means that reticular activity is taking place; however, blinking can occur with or without purposeful limb movements. Eyes that are conjugately deviated away from hemiparetic limbs indicate a destructive cerebral lesion on the side toward which the eyes are directed. Eyes turned toward paretic limbs may mean a pontine lesion, an adversive seizure or the wrong-way gaze paresis of thalamic hemorrhage. Eyes that are dysconjugate while at rest may mean paresis of individual muscles, internuclear ophthalmoplegia, or preexisting tropia or phoria.

When the brain stem is intact, the eyes may rove irregularly from side to side with a slow, smooth velocity; jerky movements suggest saccades and relative wakefulness. Repetitive smooth excursions of the eyes first to one side and then to the other, with 2- to 3-second pauses in each direction (*periodic alternating* or *ping pong gaze)* may follow bilateral cerebral infarction or cerebellar hemorrhage with an intact brain stem.

If cervical injury has been ruled out, oculocephalic testing (the *doll's eye maneuver)* is performed by passively turning the head from side to side; with an intact reflex arc (vestibular-brain stem-eye muscles), the eyes move conjugately in the opposite direction. A more vigorous stimulus is produced by irrigating each ear with 30 to 100 ml of ice water. A normal, awake person has nystagmus with the fast component in the direction opposite the ear stimulated, but a comatose patient with head elevated 30 degrees and with an intact reflex arc has deviation of the eyes toward the stimulus, usually for several minutes. Simultaneous bilateral irrigation causes vertical deviation, upward after warm water, and downward after cold water.

Oculocephalic or caloric testing may reveal intact eye movements, gaze palsy, individual muscle paresis, internuclear ophthalmoplegia, or no response. Cerebral gaze paresis can often be overcome by these maneuvers, but brain stem gaze palsies are usually fixed. Complete ophthalmoplegia may follow either extensive brain stem damage or metabolic coma but, except for barbiturate or phenytoin poisoning, eye movements are preserved early in metabolic encephalopathy. Unexplained dysconjugate eyes indicate a brain stem or cranial nerve lesion (including abducens palsy due to increased intracranial pressure).

Downward deviation of the eyes occurs with lesions in the thalamus or midbrain pretectum, and may be accompanied by pupils that do not react to light (*Parinaud syndrome)*. Downward eye deviation also occurs in metabolic coma, especially in barbiturate poisoning, and after a seizure. Skew deviation, or vertical divergence, follows lesions of the cerebellum or brain stem, especially the pontine tegmentum.

Retractatory and convergence nystagmus may be seen with midbrain lesions, but spontaneous nystagmus is rare in coma. *Ocular bobbing* (conjugate brisk downward movements from the primary position) usually follows destructive lesions of the pontine tegmentum (when lateral eye movements are lost), but may occur with cerebellar hemorrhage, metabolic encephalopathy, or transtentorial herniation. Unilateral bobbing (nystagmoid jerking) signifies pontine disease.

Tests

The EEG can distinguish coma from psychic unresponsiveness or locked-in state, although alpha-like activity in coma after brainstem infarction or cardiopulmonary arrest may make the distinction difficult. In metabolic coma, the EEG is always abnormal. Early in the course of metabolic encephalopathy, the EEG may be a more sensitive indicator of abnormality than the clinical state of the patient. The EEG may also reveal asymmetries or evidence of clinically unsuspected seizure activity. The definitive test, however, is CT, which should be performed before a spinal tap in patients with coma of unknown cause, particularly when an intracranial mass lesion is suspected. Preliminary studies suggest that magnetic resonance imaging is more sensitive than CT in detecting structural brain lesions in comatose patients, particularly those with head injury. Somatosensory and auditory evoked responses may reveal clinically unsuspected brain stem lesions and may have prognostic value after head injury.

Coma from Supratentorial Structural Lesions

Coma can result from bilateral cerebral damage or from sudden large unilateral lesions that functionally disrupt the contralateral hemisphere (diaschisis). CT studies indicate that with acute hemispheral masses, early depression of consciousness correlates more with lateral brain displacement than with transtentorial herniation. Eventually, however, downward brain displacement and rostrocaudal brain stem dysfunction can occur. Transtentorial herniation is divided into lateral (uncal) or central types. In *uncal herniation* (as in subdural hematoma), there is early compression of the oculomotor nerve by the inferiormedial temporal lobe, with ipsilateral pupillary enlargement. Alertness may

not be altered until the pupil is dilated, at which point there may be an acceleration of signs, with unilaterally and the bilaterally fixed pupils and oculomotor palsy, CSR followed by hyperventilation or ataxic breathing, flexor and then extensor posturing, and progressive unresponsiveness. Aqueductal obstruction and posterior cerebral artery compression may raise supratentorial pressure further. If the process is not halted, there ensues deep coma, apnea, bilaterally unreactive pupils, ophthalmoplegia, and eventually, circulating collapse and death. During the downward course of uncal herniaton, there may be hemiparesis ipsilateral to the cerebral lesion, attributed to compression of the contralateral midbrain peduncle against the tentorial edge (Kernohan's notch). The contralateral oculomotor nerve is occasionally compressed before the ipsilateral oculomotor nerve.

In *central transtentorial herniation* (as in thalamic hemorrhage), consciousness is rapidly impaired, pupils are of normal or small diameter and react to light and eye movements are normal. CSR, gegenhalten, and flexor or extensor postures are also seen. As the disorder progresses, the pupils become fixed in midposition, followed by the same sequence of unresponsiveness, ophthalmoplegia, and respiratory and postural abnormalities that are seen in uncal herniation.

The major lesions causing transtentorial herniation are traumatic (epidural, subdural, or intraparenchymal hemorrhage), vascular (ischemic or hemorrhagic), infectious (abscess or granuloma), and neoplastic (primary or metastatic). CT locates the lesion and often defines it. When the diagnosis is in doubt and CT is unavailable, cerebral arteriography is directed toward the side of the larger pupil.

Coma from Infratentorial Structural Lesions

Infratentorial structural lesions may compress or directly destroy the brain stem. Such lesions may also cause brain herniation, either transtentorially upward (with midbrain compression) or downward through the foramen magnum, with distortion of the medulla by the cerebellar tonsils. Abrupt tonsillar herniation causes apnea and circulatory collapse; coma is then secondary, for the medullary reticular formation probably has little direct role in arousal. In coma, *primary infratentorial structural lesions* are suggested by bilateral weakness, sensory loss, crossed cranial nerve with long tract signs, miosis, loss of lateral gaze with preserved vertical eye movements, dysconjugate gaze, ophthalmoplegia, short-cycle CSR, and apneustic or ataxic breathing. The clinical picture of pontine hemorrhage (i.e., sudden coma, pinpoint but reactive pupils, and no eye movement) is characteristic, but if the sequence of signs in a comatose patient is unknown, it may not be possible to tell whether the process began supratentorially or infratentorially. If the hemorrhage is in the posterior fossa, it may not be possible to find out where the lesion originated (e.g., cerebellar or pontine hemorrhage). Infrequent brain stem causes of coma include multiple sclerosis and central pontine myelinolysis.

Coma from Metabolic or Diffuse Brain Disease

In metabolic, diffuse, or multifocal encephalopathy, mental and respiratory abnormalities occur early; there is often tremor, asterixis, or multifocal myoclonus. Gegenhalten, frontal release signs (snout, suck, or grasp), and flexor or extensor posturing may occur. Except in glutethimide or atropine intoxication, the pupils remain reactive. The eyes may be deviated downward, but sustained lateral deviation or dysconjugate eyes argue against a metabolic disturbance. However, metabolic disease can cause both focal seizures and lateralizing neurologic signs, often shifting, but sometimes persisting (as in hypoglycemia and hyperglycemia).

Arterial gas determinations are useful in metabolic coma. Of the diseases listed in Table 4–1, psychogenic hyperventilation is more likely to cause delirium than stupor, but may coexist with hysterical coma. Mental change associated with metabolic alkalosis is usually mild.

Metabolic and diffuse brain diseases causing coma are numerous, but not unmanageably so. Most of the entities listed in Table 4–2 are described in other chapters.

Hysteria and Catatonia. Hysterical (conversion) unresponsiveness is rare and probably overdiagnosed. Indistinguishable clinically from malingering, it is usually associated with closed eyes, eupnea or tachypnea, and normal pupils. The eyelids may resist passive opening and, when released, close abruptly or jerkily rather than with smooth descent; lightly stroking the eyelashes causes lid-fluttering. The eyes do not slowly rove, but move with saccadic jerks, and ice-water caloric test-

Table 4–1. Causes of Abnormal Ventilation in Unresponsive Patients

Hyperventilation
  Metabolic acidosis
    Anion gap
      *Diabetic ketoacidosis
      *Diabetic hyperosmolar coma
      Lactic acidosis
      *Uremia
      Alcoholic ketoacidosis
      *Acidic poisons (ethylene glycol,
        methyl alcohol, paraldehyde)
    No anion gap
      Diarrhea
      Pancreatic drainage
      Carbonic anhydrase inhibitors
      NH_4Cl ingestion
      Renal tubular acidosis
      Ureteroenterostomy
  Respiratory alkalosis
    *Hepatic failure
    *Sepsis
    Pneumonia
    Anxiety (hyperventilation syndrome)
  Mixed acid-base disorders (metabolic acidosis and respiratory alkalosis)
    Salicylism
    *Sepsis
    *Hepatic failure

Hypoventilation
  Respiratory acidosis
    Acute (uncompensated)
      *Sedative drugs
      Brain stem injury
      Neuromuscular disorders
      Chest injury
      Acute pulmonary disease
    Chronic pulmonay disease
  Metabolic alkalosis
    Vomiting or gastric drainage
    Diuretic therapy
    Adrenal steroid excess (Cushing's syndrome)
    Primary aldosteronism
    Bartter's syndrome

*Common causes of stupor or coma.
(From Plum F, Posner JB. The Diagnosis of Stupor and Coma, 3rd ed. Philadelphia: FA Davis, 1980.)

ing causes nystagmus rather than sustained deviation. The limbs usually offer no resistance to passive movement, yet demonstrate normal tone. Unless organic disease or drug effect is also present, the EEG pattern is one of normal wakefulness.

In catatonia (which may occur with schizophrenia, depression, toxic psychosis, or other brain diseases), there may be akinetic mutism, grimacing, rigidity, posturing, cata-

Table 4–2. Diffuse Brain Diseases or Metabolic Disorders that Cause Coma

Deprivation of oxygen, substrate, or metabolic cofactor
  Hypoxia
  Diffuse ischemia (cardiac disease, decreased peripheral circulatory resistance, increased
    cerebrovascular resistance, widespread small-vessel occlusion)
  Hypoglycemia
  Thiamine deficiency (Wernicke-Korsakoff syndrome)
Disease of organs other than brain
  Liver (hepatic coma)
  Kidney (uremia)
  Lung (CO_2 narcosis)
  Pancreas (diabetes, hypoglycemia, exocrine pancreatic encephalopathy)
  Pituitary (apoplexy, sedative hypersensitivity)
  Thyroid (myxedema, thyrotoxicosis)
  Parathyroid (hypo- and hyperparathyroidism)
  Adrenal (Addison or Cushing disease, pheochromocytoma)
  Other systemic disease (cancer, porphyria, sepsis)
Exogenous poisons
  Sedative and narcotics
  Psychotropic drugs
  Acid poisons (e.g., methyl alcohol, ethylene glycol)
  Others (e.g., anticonvulsants, heavy metals, cyanide)
Abnormalities of ionic or acid-base environment of CNS
  Water and sodium (hypo- and hypernatremia)
  Acidosis
  Alkalosis
  Magnesium (hyper- and hypomagnesemia)
  Calcium (hyper- and hypocalcemia)
  Phosphorus (hypophosphatemia)
Disordered temperature regulation
  Hypothermia
  Heat stroke
CNS inflammation or infiltration
  Leptomeningitis
  Encephalitis
  Acute toxic encephalopathy (e.g., Reye syndrome)
  Parainfectious encephalomyelitis
  Cerebral vasculitis
  Subarachnoid hemorrhage
  Carcinomatous meningitis
Primary neuronal or glial disorders
  Creutzfeldt-Jakob disease
  Marchiafava-Bignami disease
  Adrenoleukodystrophy
  Gliomatosis cerebri
  Progressive multifocal leukoencephalopathy
Seizure and postictal states

(Modified from Plum F, Posner JB. The Diagnosis of Stupor and Coma, 3rd ed. Philadelphia: FA Davis, 1980.)

lepsy, or excitement. Respirations are normal or rapid, pupils are large but reactive, and eye movements are normal. The EEG is usually normal.

Locked-in Syndrome. Infarction or central pontine myelinolysis may destroy the basis pontis, producing total paralysis of the lower cranial nerve and limb muscles with preserved alertness and respiration. At first glance the patient appears unresponsive, but examination reveals voluntary vertical, and sometimes horizontal, eye movements, including blinking. (Even with facial paralysis, inhibition of the levator palpebrae can produce partial eye closure.) Communication is possible with blinking or eye movements to indicate "yes," "no," or letters.

Akinetic Mutism, Coma Vigil, and Vegetative State. The term *akinetic mutism* originally referred to a kind of stupor with a posterior

Table 4–3. Brain Death

Original criteria adopted by Harvard Ad Hoc Committee
  Unresponsive coma
  Apnea
  Absence of cephalic or spinal reflexes
  Isoelectric EEG
  Persistence of condition for at least 24 hours
  Absence of drug intoxication or hypothermia
Currently accepted criteria
  Unresponsive coma
  Apnea during 10 to 20 minutes of oxygenation
  Absence of cephalic reflexes with fixed pupils, but occasional presence of purely spinal
    reflexes
  Isoelectric EEG
  Conditions present for 30 minutes at least 6 hours after the onset of coma and apnea
  Diagnosis known: structural disease or irreversible metabolic disturbance; absence of drug
    intoxication or hypothermia

third ventricular tumor. With the term *coma vigil*, it has been used to describe a variety of states, including coma with preserved eye movements following midbrain lesions, psychomotor bradykinesia with frontal lobe disease, and isolated diencephalic and brain stem function after massive cerebral damage. For this last condition, the term *vegetative state* has been recommended, referring to patients who survive coma and assume sleep-wake cycles, normal respiratory and circulatory function, and primitive responses to stimuli, but without evidence of inner or outer awareness. Vegetative state may be either transient or persistent. The majority of comatose patients either die early or make varying degrees of recovery; those who enter the vegetative state may recover further. If there is no change after two weeks, however, improvement is unlikely.

Brain Death. Unlike vegetative state, in with the brain stem is intact, the term *brain death* means that neither the cerebrum nor the brain stem is functioning. The only spontaneous activity is cardiovascular, and the only reflexes are those mediated by the spinal cord. Criteria for brain death have been modified since the original report of the Ad Hoc Committee of the Harvard Medical School (Table 4–3). If the original criteria for brain death have been otherwise met, a patient can be declared brain dead despite the presence of spinally mediated reflexes such as tendon jerks, plantar responses, or simple withdrawal of a limb to painful stimuli. Apnea in the presence of adequate respiratory drive can be confirmed by disconnecting the patient from the respirator, with a catheter delivering oxygen at 6 L per minute to the trachea for 10 to 20 minutes, allowing Pa_{CO_2} to rise to between 50 and 60 mm Hg. In the United States, an EEG is required to demonstrate electrocerebral silence, but EEG is not considered necessary in the United Kingdom. Alternative confirmatory tests include four-vessel angiography or radioisotope cerebral angiography to document absence of cerebral blood flow.

Most workers believe that if criteria for brain death are present for six hours, the diagnosis is secure, which is an important consideration when organ transplantation is a possibility. (An exception is anoxic-ischemic brain damage, in which case at least 24 hours should elapse.) True brain death rarely lasts more than a few days and is always followed by circulatory collapse; however, the diagnosis must be certain. Drug intoxication must be excluded by the patient's history or by toxicologic studies. Hypothermia must not be present. Other possible explanations for unreactive pupils, absent oculovestibular reflexes, apnea, or absent motor activity must be ruled out.

In the United States, most states have passed statutes that equate brain death and legal death, but clinical criteria remain the responsibility of physicians.

References

Black PM. Brain death. N Engl J Med 1978; 299:338–384, 393–401.

Cant BR, Hume AL, Judson JA, Shaw NA. The assessment of severe head injury by short-latency somatosensory and brain-stem auditory evoked potentials. Electroencephalogr Clin Neurophysiol 1986; 65:185–195.

Drake B, Ashwal S, Schneider S: Determination of cerebral death in the pediatric intensive care unit. Pediatrics 1986; 78:107–112.

Fisher CM. Some neuro-ophthalmological observations. J Neurol Neurosurg Psychiatry 1967; 30:383–392.

Fisher CM. The neurological examination of the comatose patient. Acta Neurol Scand 1969; 45 (suppl 36):1–56.

Grindal AB, Suter C, Martinez AJ. Alpha-pattern coma: 24 cases with 9 survivors. Ann Neurol 1977; 1:371–377.

Guidelines for the determination of death: Report of the medical consultants on the diagnosis of death to the President's Commission for the Study of Ethical Problems in Medicine and Biomedical and Behavioral Research. Neurology 1982; 32:395–399.

Hansotia PL. Persistent vegetative state. Review and report of electrodiagnostic studies in eight cases. Arch Neurol 1985; 42:1048–1052.

Jenkins A, Teasdale G, Hadley MD, et al. Brain lesions detected by magnetic resonance imaging in mild and severe head injuries. Lancet 1986; 2:445–446.

Keane Jr. Ocular skew deviation. Arch Neurol 1975; 32:185–190.

Levy DE, Dates D, Coronna JJ, et al. Prognosis in nontraumatic coma. Ann Intern Med 1981; 94:293–301.

Malouf R, Brust JCM: Hypoglycemia: causes, neurological manifestations, and outcome. Ann Neurol 1985; 17:421–430.

Plum F, Posner JB. The Diagnosis of Stupor and Coma. 3rd ed. Philadelphia: FA Davis, 1980.

Ropper AH: Lateral displacement of the brain and level of consciousness in patients with an acute hemispheral mass. N Engl J Med 1986; 314:953–958.

Stewart JD, Kirkham TH, Mathieson G. Periodic alternating gaze. Neurology 1979; 29:222–224.

5. PAIN AND PARESTHESIAS

Hartwell G. Thompson
Lewis P. Rowland

All pain sensations are carried by nerves and therefore concern neurology; however, not all pain is relevant to neurologic diagnosis. The pain of any traumatic lesion is a separate concern. Pain in the thorax or abdomen almost always implies a visceral disorder rather than one of the spinal cord or nerve roots. Headache and other head pains, in contrast, are a major neurologic concern (see Section 8, Headache, and Section 144, Migraine). This section considers pain in the neck, low back, and limbs.

Pain syndromes often include another sensory aberration, *paresthesia,* which may arise from an abnormality anywhere along the sensory pathway from the peripheral nerves to the sensory cortex. Paresthesias are often described as a *pins-and-needles sensation* and are recognizable by anyone who has ever had an injection of local anesthetic for dental repairs. Central nervous system (CNS) disorders may cause particular kinds of paresthesias—focal sensory seizures with cortical lesions, spontaneous pain in the thalamic syndrome, or

bursts of paresthesias down the back or into the arms on flexing the neck *(Lhermitte symptoms)* in patients with multiple sclerosis or other disorders of the cervical spinal cord. Level lesions of the spinal cord may cause either a "band sensation" or "girdle sensation," a vague sense of awareness of altered sensation encircling the abdomen, or there may be a *sensory level* (i.e., altered sensation below the level of the spinal-cord lesion). Nerve root lesions or isolated peripheral nerve lesions may also cause paresthesias, but the most intense and annoying paresthesia encountered is multiple symmetric peripheral neuropathy (polyneuropathy). *Dysesthesia* is the term for the disagreeably abnormal sensations evoked when an area of abnormal sensation is touched; sometimes even the pressure of bedclothes cannot be tolerated by a patient with dysesthesia.

Beginning students are often confused by reports of paresthesias when the review of systems is recorded, or by nonanatomic patterns of abnormality in the sensory examination. Two general rules may help. First, if paresthesias do not persist, they are not likely to imply a neurologic lesion. (Pressure on a nerve commonly causes transient paresthesias in normal people who cross their legs, sit too long on a toilet seat, or drape an arm over the back of a chair, and many people have fleeting paresthesias of unknown cause and no significance.) Second, if paresthesias persist and no lesion is found, the patient should be reexamined.

Neck Pain. Most chronic neck pain is caused by bony abnormalities (cervical osteoarthritis or other forms of arthritis) or by local trauma. If pain remains local (i.e., not radiating into the arms) it is rarely of neurologic significance unless there are abnormal neurologic signs. It may be possible to demonstrate overactive tendon reflexes (clonus or Babinski signs) in a patient who has no symptoms other than neck pain. These signs could be evidence of compression of the cervical spinal cord and might be an indication for myelography to determine whether the offending lesion is some form of arthritis, tumor, or a congenital malformation of the cervical spine; however, it is rare to encounter neck pain as the only symptom of a compressive lesion.

Neck pain of neurologic significance is more commonly accompanied by other symptoms and signs, depending upon the location of the lesion: *radicular* distribution of pain is denoted by radiation down the medial (ulnar) or lateral (radial) aspect of the arm, sometimes down to the corresponding fingers. Cutaneous sensation is altered within the area innervated by the compromised root, or below the level of spinal end compression. The motor disorder may be evident by weakness and wasting of hand muscles innervated by the affected root, and the gait may be abnormal if there are corticospinal signs of cervical spinal cord compression. When autonomic fibers in the spinal cord are compromised, abnormal urinary frequency, urgency, or incontinence may occur, there may be bowel symptoms, and men may note sexual dysfunction. Reflex changes may be noted by the loss of tendon reflexes in the arms and overactive reflexes in the legs. Cervical pain of neurologic significance may be affected by movement of the head and neck and it may be exaggerated by natural Valsalva maneuvers in coughing, sneezing, or straining during bowel movements.

Cervical spondylosis is a more common cause of neck pain than spinal cord tumor, but it is probably not possible to make the diagnostic distinction without myelography because the pain may be similar in the two conditions. In young patients (i.e., younger than age 40), tumors, spinal arteriovenous malformations, and congenital anomalies of the cervico-occipital region are more common causes of neck pain than cervical spondylosis.

Low Back Pain. The most common cause of low back pain is herniated nucleus pulposus, but it is difficult to determine the exact frequency because acute attacks usually clear spontaneously and because chronic low back pain is colored by psychologic factors. The pain of an acute herniation of a lumbar disc is characteristically abrupt in onset, brought on by heavy lifting, twisting, or Valsalva maneuvers (sneezing, coughing, or straining during bowel movements). The patient may not be able to stand erect because paraspinal muscles contract so vigorously, yet the pain may be relieved as soon as the patient lies down, only to return again on any attempt to stand. The pain may be restricted to the low back or may radiate into one or both buttocks or down the posterior aspect of the leg to the thigh, knee, or foot. The distribution of pain sometimes gives a precise delineation of the nerve root involved, but this is probably true in a minority of cases. The pain of an acute lumbar disc is so stereotyped that the diagnosis can be made even if there are no reflex, motor, or sensory changes.

Chronic low back pain is a different matter. If neurologic abnormalities are present on examination, myelography is often indicated to determine whether the problem is caused by tumor, lumbar spondylosis with or without spinal stenosis, or arachnoiditis. If there are no neurologic abnormalities or if the patient has already had a laminectomy, chronic low back pain may pose a diagnostic and therapeutic dilemma. This is a major public health problem and it accounts for many of the patients who enroll in pain clinics.

Arm Pain. Pain in the arms takes on a different significance when there is no neck pain. Local pain arises from musculoskeletal diseases (e.g., bursitis or arthritis), which are now common because of widespread participation in sports by people who are not properly prepared.

Chronic pain may arise from invasion of the brachial plexus by tumors that extend directly from lung or breast tissue or that metastasize from more remote areas. The brachial plexus may also be affected by a transient illness (e.g., brachial plexus neuritis) that includes pain in the arm that is often poorly localized. The combination of pain, weakness, and wasting has given rise to the name *neuralgic amyotrophy.*

Thoracic outlet syndromes are another cause of pain in the arm that originates in the brachial plexus. Pain caused by thoracic outlet syndromes is often related to particular positions of the arm and is a cause of diagnostic vexation because there may be no abnormality on examination (see Section 60, Thoracic Outlet Syndrome); there are almost always vascular problems with secondary neurologic manifestations. P9 443

Single nerves may be involved in *entrapment neuropathies* that cause pain in the hands. The carpal tunnel syndrome of the median nerve is the best known entrapment neuropathy. The ulnar nerve is the most commonly affected at elbow, but may be subject to compression at the wrist. The paresthesias of entrapment neuropathies are restricted to the distribution of the affected nerve and differ from the paresthesias of areas innervated by nerve roots, although the distinction may be difficult to make if only a portion of the area supplied by a particular nerve root is affected.

Causalgia is the name given to a constant burning pain that is accompanied by trophic changes that include red glossy skin, sweating in the affected area, and abnormalities of hair and nails. The trophic changes are attributed to autonomic disorder. Causalgia was described in the nineteenth century in a monograph by Weir Mitchell, Morehouse, and Keen when they reviewed gunshot wounds and other nerve injuries of Civil War veterans. The basic mechanisms of causalgia are still poorly understood. The traumatic lesions of peripheral nerves are usually incomplete, and several nerves are often involved simultaneously. Causalgia usually follows high-velocity missile wound (bullets or shrapnel). It is less commonly caused by traction injury and is only rarely seen in inflammatory neuropathy or other types of peripheral nerve disease. The arms are more often involved than the legs, and the lesions are usually above the elbow or below the knee. Symptoms usually begin within the first few days following injury. Causalgic pain most often involves the hand. The shiny red skin, accompanied by fixed joints, is followed by osteoporosis. Both physical and emotional factors seem to play a role. Causalgia may be relieved by sympathectomy early in the course of treatment and may be due to *ephaptic transmission* through connections between efferent autonomic fibers at the site of partial nerve injury. This concept of "artificial synapses" after nerve injury has been widely accepted; however, there has been no convincing anatomic or physiologic corroboration.

Reflex sympathetic dystrophy refers to the local tissue swelling and bony changes that accompany causalgia. Similar changes may be encountered after minor trauma or arthritis of the wrist. In the shoulder-hand syndrome, inflammatory arthritis of the shoulder joint may be followed by painful swelling of the hand, with local vascular changes, disuse, and atrophy of muscle and bone. Sympathectomy has been recommended.

Leg Pain and Paresthesia. Leg pain due to occlusive vascular disease, especially with diabetes, varies markedly in different series but seems to be related to the duration of the diabetes and shows increasing incidence with age. Pain may be a major symptom of diabetic peripheral neuropathy of the multiple symmetric type. Diabetic mononeuritis multiplex, attributed to infarcts of the lumbosacral plexus or a peripheral nerve, is a cause of more restricted pain, usually of abrupt onset. Diabetic mononeuropathy may be disabling and alarming at the onset, but both pain and motor findings improve in a few months to 1 or 2 years. Nutritional neuropathy is an important cause of limb pain, especially in the

legs, in some parts of the world. This condition was striking in prisoner-of-war camps in World War II and has also been noted in patients on hemodialysis. Sudden fluid shifts may cause peripheral nerve disease symptoms for a time after dialysis.

Barring intraspinal disease, the most common neurologic cause of leg pain and paresthesias is probably multiple symmetric peripheral neuropathy. The paresthesias usually take on a glove-and-stocking distribution, presumably because the nerve fibers most remote from the perikaryon are most vulnerable. The feet are usually affected, sometimes alone or sometimes with the hands; the hands are rarely affected alone. Mixed sensorimotor neuropathies show motor abnormalities, with weakness and wasting as well as loss of tendon reflexes. Some neuropathies are purely sensory. Pain is characteristic of severe diabetic neuropathy, alcoholic neuropathy, amyloid neuropathy, and some carcinomatous neuropathies, but is uncommon in genetic neuropathy or Guillain-Barré syndrome. The pain of peripheral neuropathy, for unknown reasons, is likely to be more severe at night.

Entrapment neuropathy rarely affects the legs; however, diabetic mononeuropathy, especially femoral neuropathy, may cause pain of restricted distribution and abrupt onset, with later improvement of the condition that may take months.

Another major cause of leg pain is invasion of the lumbosacral plexus by tumor, but this is rarely an isolated event and other signs of the tumor are usually evident. The problem of distinguishing between spinal and vascular claudication is discussed in Section 58, Lumbar Spondylosis.

Limb pains and paresthesias are important in neurologic diagnosis not only because they persist for prolonged periods. They also become the object of symptomatic therapy by analgesics, tricyclic drugs, and monoamine oxidase (MAO) inhibitors (which may affect abnormal sensations by actions other than antidepressant effects), transcutaneous nerve stimulation, dorsal column stimulation, cordotomy, acupuncture, and other procedures. The long list of remedies attests to the limitations of each. Psychologic factors cannot be ignored in chronic pain problems.

References

Basbaum AI, Fields HL. Endogenous pain control mechanisms: review and hypothesis. Ann Neurol 1978; 4:451–462.

DeJong RN. The Neurologic Examination, 4th ed. New York: Harper & Row, 1979.

Fields HL. Pain. New York: McGraw-Hill Book Co, 1987.

Frymoyer JW. Back pain and sciatica. N Engl J Med 1988; 318:291–301.

Portenoy RK, Lipton RB, Foley KM. Back pain in the cancer patient: an algorithm for evaluation and management. Neurology 1987; 37:134–138.

Stimmel B. Pain, Analgesia, and Addiction: The Pharmacologic Treatment of Pain. New York: Raven Press, 1983.

Tahmoush AJ. Causalgia: redefinition as a clinical pain syndrome. Pain 1981; 10:187–197.

6. DIZZINESS AND HEARING LOSS

Maxwell Abramson

The peripheral auditory system comprises the outer ear, the middle ear (including the cochlea), and the eighth cranial nerve. Lesions of these structures cause three major symptoms: hearing loss, vertigo, and tinnitus. Vertigo usually implies a lesion of the inner ear or the vestibular portion of the eighth nerve. Tinnitus and hearing loss may arise from lesions anywhere in the peripheral or central auditory pathways.

Tinnitus

Tinnitus is an auditory sensation that arises within the head and is perceived in one or both ears, or inside the head. The sound may be continuous, intermittent, or pulsatile. Tinnitus should be divided into "objective" tinnitus (heard by the examiner as well as the patient) or "subjective" tinnitus, heard only by the patient. Objective tinnitus is uncommon, but it is associated with several serious conditions that mandate early diagnosis.

Objective Tinnitus. This condition results from intravascular turbulence, increased blood flow, or movement in the eustachian tube, soft palate, or temporomandibular joint. Bruits due to vascular turbulence may arise from aortic stenosis, carotid stenosis, arteriovenous malformations of the head and neck, vascular tumors (such as glomus jugulare), and aneurysms of the abdomen, chest, head, and neck. A continuous hum may result from asymmetrical enlargement of sigmoid sinus and jugular vein. Pulsatile objective tinnitus may result from high blood pressure, hyperthyroidism, or increased intracranial pressure. As part of the diagnostic evaluation of objective tinnitus, the stethoscope should be used for auscultation of the ear, head, and neck in all patients who note noises in the head or ear. Anyone with pulsatile tinnitus

should also have blood pressure and funduscopic evaluation.

Subjective Tinnitus. Unless of brief duration, subjective tinnitus results from damage or abnormality somewhere in the auditory system. The abnormality can be in the external ear, middle ear, inner ear, eighth nerve, or central auditory connections. Tinnitus may be an early warning signal, like pain arising from a lesion in or near a sensory peripheral nerve. For example, tinnitus after exposure to loud noise is due to cochlear injury, usually resulting in a temporary shift of the threshold in hearing sensitivity. Repeated exposure to noise may result in permanent cochlear damage and permanent hearing loss. Unilateral tinnitus is an early symptom of acoustic neuroma, often years before there is overt loss of hearing or unsteadiness of gait. Persistent tinnitus, therefore, requires otologic evaluation, including hearing tests. The basic hearing tests for evaluation of patients with tinnitus comprise pure tone and speech audiometry, as well as middle ear impedance measures, including tympanometry and measurement of the threshold and decay of the stapedial reflex. The tests help to differentiate the site of the lesion.

Hearing Loss

Hearing loss can be divided into two anatomic types based on the site of the lesion: *conductive* and *sensorineural.* Conductive hearing loss is due to middle ear disease. Sensorineural hearing loss is most often due to a lesion in the cochlea; less often, it is due to the cochlear nerve or, rarely, central connections.

Conductive Hearing Loss. This type of hearing loss results from anything in the external or middle ear that interferes with movement of the oval or round window. Patients with conductive hearing loss speak with a soft voice or with normal loudness because, to them, their own voices sound as load as background sounds in the environment. External ear or middle ear abnormalities are usually evident on physical examination except when there is ossicular fixation, for instance, with otosclerosis. In tuning fork tests, best carried out with a 256-Hz tuning fork, sound conveyed by bone conduction is as loud or louder than air conduction (*Rinne* test "negative"). In contrast, sound conveyed by air conduction is perceived as louder than bone conduction sound in patients with normal hearing or with sensorineural hearing loss. In conductive hearing loss, a tuning fork placed at midline of the head is heard louder in the ear on the side of the hearing loss (*Weber test* lateralizes to the abnormal side).

The diagnosis of conductive hearing loss can be confirmed by testing *middle ear impedance*, which measures the resistance of the middle ear to the passage of sound and can differentiate ossicular discontinuity from stiffness or mass effects that interfere with movement of the oval window. The severity of hearing loss and the conductive component should be assessed by audiometry, determining sound conduction by air and bone. Conductive hearing loss most commonly affects children and is usually due to otitis media with effusion. Conductive hearing loss should be treated vigorously in children because persistent hearing loss, even if slight, may interfere with speech and cognitive development. Chronic forms of conductive hearing loss can usually be restored to functional levels of hearing by reconstructive microsurgery. Hearing aids are also effective in rehabilitating patients with conductive hearing loss.

Sensorineural Hearing Loss. This condition is due to defects in the cochlea, cochlear nerve, or the brain stem and cortical connections. Patients with sensorineural hearing loss tend to speak with a loud voice because conduction of the voice through the head is reduced. Findings on physical examination are normal. Tuning fork tests show that air conduction exceeds bone conduction (positive Rinne test); in the Weber test, the tuning fork seems louder in the better ear. The patient's perception of the tuning fork, when it is placed against the mastoid, is less than the examiner's if the examiner has normal sensorineural hearing ("abnormal Schwabach test").

Patients with sensorineural hearing loss require a battery of audiometric tests to determine the site of abnormality. Patients with cochlear damage may show low-frequency hearing loss, a flat *audiometric configuration* or, more commonly, high-frequency hearing loss. The main causes are excessive exposure to noise, ototoxic drugs, age-related cochlear degeneration, congenital cochlear defects, and viral labyrinthitis. *Speech discrimination* remains relatively preserved compared to the extent of *pure-tone hearing loss*. The *stapedial reflex threshold*, as determined by *impedance measurements*, is present at reduced sensation levels; that pattern implies "recruitment," an

abnormal increase in loudness as the amplitude of the test sounds increases above the threshold. *Brain stem auditory-evoked responses* show a delay in the first brain stem wave, but a normal or shortened inter-peak latency.

Patients with damage to the cochlear nerve such as the *neural form of presbycusis* or compression of the nerve by an acoustic neuroma, usually show high-frequency hearing loss, as do patients with cochlear lesions. In nerve lesions, however, speech discrimination tends to be affected more severely than pure-tone hearing loss. The stapedial reflex either is absent or shows abnormal adaptation or decay. The test is carried out as part of impedance audiometry and is useful in determining the site of the lesion. Stapedial reflex threshold and decay, along with tympanometry, must be considered part of the diagnostic work-up for all patients with asymmetric sensorineural hearing loss. Brain stem auditory-evoked response testing in neural forms of hearing loss shows no waves at all, poorly formed waves, or increased inter-peak latency, either absolute or in comparison with the opposite ear.

Central lesions, such as recurrent small strokes or multiple sclerosis, often cause no detectable pure-tone hearing loss because the central auditory pathways are bilateral. Some patients, however, do note hearing loss. For them, hearing should be evaluated by *auditory brain stem response* testing, which may show bilateral conduction delay despite normal pure-tone hearing. Filtered speech or the voice discriminaton test may show abnormalities.

Most patients with sensorineural hearing loss can be helped by amplification; hearing aids are becoming smaller and more effective. The narrow range between signal and noise is being ameliorated by improved microcircuitry.

Dizziness

Dizziness is a term that encompasses three different sensations. *Vertigo* is a sense of movement usually due to an abnormality in the vestibular system. The subject feels that the person or the environment is moving (when it is not). Vertigo is aggravated by any movement of the head, and it persists in all positions: sitting, standing, or supine. *Dysequilibrium* is a feeling of unsteadiness or insecurity without rotation. Standing and walking are difficult. *Light-headedness* is a swimming, floating, giddy, or swaying sensation in the head or room. It is sometimes used to describe a state of impending faint or syncope. It usually occurs briefly before vasovagal syncope, but it may be persistent.

These varieties of dizziness must be separated from one another as well as psychomotor or complex partial seizures, and motor incoordination. These sensations are often described by the patient as dizziness. Each implies a different mechanism. *Syncope* is often the result of transient inadequacy of cerebral blood supply, oxygen, or glucose; before consciousness is lost, there is a feeling of faintness, weakness in the pit of the stomach, an urge to sit or lie down for relief, and darkening of vision. Either syncope or vertigo may be associated with the autonomic symptoms of perspiration, nausea, pallor, and tachycardia. The aura of *psychomotor or complex partial seizures* may include feelings of disorientation that are usually associated with feelings of unreality or brief lapses of memory. The report of an observer that the patient has been unresponsive or has shown automatisms is helpful in his distinction. *Motor incoordination,* which can be caused by cerebellar dysfunction, proprioceptive sensory loss, or ataxia of gait, may also lead to a feeling of insecurity about the environment; the resultant unsteady gait may be ascribed to dizziness. There may be overlap in these varieties of dizziness. Both seizures and transient loss of circulation to the brain may produce true vertigo, and vertigo may cause motor incoordination.

Several systems orient a person about body position and movement in the environment. These include: the visual system; the vestibular system with the semicircular canals that respond to changes in angular acceleration and the utricles and saccules that respond to linear acceleration and changes in relation to the pull of gravity; the auditory system, which senses position relative to direct or reflected sounds; the proprioceptive sensory system, which senses limb, body, and head posture through end-organs in muscle and tendon; and the exteroceptive sensory system, particularly touch, which provides cues about the body's relationship to gravity by the weight of clothes and the pressure of feet and buttocks against supporting surfaces. Dizziness results when a disorder in one of these systems causes insufficient, unbalanced, or abnormal sensory input so that there is a mismatch of information among the various sensory systems about the body's position or movement. Brain lesions can cause disordered integration of information from these systems, causing dizziness. The vestibular system is the one most frequently affected.

If vertigo is associated with nausea, veering gait, and a fear that moving the head or gazing in certain directions will aggravate symptoms, the physician should suspect a disorder of the semicircular canals or of the vestibular portion of the eighth nerve. On examination, symmetric nystagmus with a quick component in the same direction for all directions of gaze in which it is apparent, veering gait, and pastpointing also suggest a peripheral disorder of the vestibular system. By contrast, a central brain stem lesion is suggested by vertigo without associated symptoms or nystagmus. A cental brain stem lesion is also suggested by vertigo with asymmetric nystagmus, vertical nystagmus, or nystagmus in which the quick component changes with direction of gaze. The only exception is the bilateral cochlear disorder of drug toxicity in which the nystagmus may change with directions of gaze. The impression of a central CNS lesion is enhanced by symptoms or signs of lesions in other parts of the CNS.

COMMON CAUSES OF DIZZINESS OR HEARING LOSS

Benign Positional Vertigo. This condition is defined by vertigo that occurs only with a change in head position, usually after rolling over in bed, but it may be induced by rising from bed or chair, looking up, or turning the head. If vertigo occurs in bed or while the patient is sitting, it is not orthostatic hypotension. Postural vertigo occurs with the affected ear down, after a brief latent period, and it lasts less than 30 seconds. The vertigo fatigues rapidly and is extinguished if the change in position is repeated. Associated nystagmus is rotatory and upwards, reversing direction when the patient sits up. The syndrome may follow mild head injury, but is more often noted without apparent cause in middle-aged or elderly people.

Histologic evidence suggests that benign positional vertigo is due to "otoconia." The utricle or saccule becomes loose in the endolymphatic space, attaching to the posterior canal ampulla, making it sensitive to gravity, and giving rise to the term *cupulolithiasis.*

The symptoms are usually mild and transient. Recovery can be accelerated, if the symptoms are not too severe, by assuming the provocative position to enhance adaptation. More severe forms of benign positional vertigo may respond to drugs that suppress vestibular function such as meclizine or promethazine. Rarely, benign positional vertigo may be incapacitating; surgical section of the posterior ampillary nerve relieves the symptoms.

Because positional vertigo is not always vestibular in origin and not always benign, patients with positional vertigo should undergo tests, including electronystagmography, to insure that the nystagmus is transient, fatigable, and direction-constant. Types of nystagmus that do not meet these criteria include post-traumatic vertigo (originating from the labyrinth or central nervous system), alcohol-induced positional vertigo, and central lesions such as small strokes or tumors.

Vestibular Neuronitis. In this condition, vertigo occurs suddenly and severely with vomiting and nystagmus; it may last several days. There are no cochlear symptoms and audiologic tests are normal. Caloric tests show a reduced response on the affected side. The patient may feel unsteady for several weeks after an attack. Recurring attacks usually seem less severe than the first, and may continue for several months. The syndrome results from sudden loss of a function of one vestibular system; it is analogous to sudden loss of hearing. Vestibular neuronitis may follow an overt viral illness or may occur in an elderly patient to suggest small vessel obstruction. In most cases, however, the cause is unknown. The name *vestibular neuronitis* suggests a viral etiology and should be replaced by a descriptive term, such as *recurrent or acute vestibulopathy.* A brief course of vestibular suppressants followed by encouragement of physical activity may shorten the duration of disability by enhancing vestibular compensation.

Meniere Syndrome. This illness is characterized by recurrent attacks of tinnitus, hearing loss, and vertigo accompanied by a sense of pressure in the ear, distortion of sounds, and sensitivity to noises. The symptoms may not all occur at the same time in the same spell. Hearing loss or vertigo may even be absent for several years. The symptoms occur in clusters with variable periods of remission that may last for several years. Major attacks of vertigo last 5 to 30 minutes, with nausea and vomiting, and may force cessation of all usual activities. Minor spells are characterized by unsteadiness, giddiness, or light-headedness. Hearing loss begins as a low-frequency

cochlear type of hearing loss, improving between attacks. In severe cases, hearing loss becomes persistent and slowly progressive, usually flat in the configuration of audiometric tests. Symptoms are unilateral at first, but in 20 to 30% of the cases, depending on the length of follow-up, the other ear is ultimately affected. The pathogenesis is unknown.

A consistent histopathologic feature of Meniere's syndrome is an increase in endolymphatic volume with ballooning of the cochlear duct, utricle, and saccule. That configuration is called *endolymphatic hydrops.* As in other conditions characterized by increased extracellular fluid volume, symptoms are aggravated by salt-loading and may be helped by reducing dietary intake of salt or by giving diuretics. In the few patients who are incapacitated by major spells of vertigo, ablative surgery is used, either labyrinthectomy, when there is no useful hearing, or partial vestibular nerve section to spare the cochlear and facial nerves. Surgery to decompress the endolymphatic sac has been performed since 1927, but the technique is still controversial because no demonstrable beneficial effects have lasted longer than four or five years.

Meniere syndrome must be separated from congenital or tertiary syphilis, which also causes endolymphatic hydrops, vertigo, and hearing loss. In syphilis, hearing loss is progressive and usually bilateral. Cogan syndrome also resembles Meniere syndrome with endolymphatic hydrops, hearing loss, and vertigo. In Cogan syndrome, in addition, ocular inflammation occurs without evidence of syphilis. Cogan syndrome is thought to be an autoimmune condition, which may also be true of Meniere syndrome.

Perilymphatic Fistulas. Hearing loss, with or without vertigo, may follow sudden changes of pressure in the middle ear or CSF that may be due to weight-lifting, barotrauma of scuba diving, or even forcefully blowing the nose. Perilymph fistulas may arise spontaneously, especially in children with congenital defects of the inner ear. Stapedectomy also increases the risk of developing a perilymphatic fistula.

Cerebellopontine Angle Tumors. The most common tumor that grows in the cerebellopontine angle is the acoustic neuroma (schwannoma). By the time loss of corneal reflex, cerebellar signs, gross nystagmus, and facial weakness are seen, the tumor is large. Because the earliest symptoms are dizziness, tinnitus, and hearing loss, this tumor must always be considered in the evaluation of a patient with any of these symptoms. Early diagnosis is particularly important because improvement in microsurgical techniques has made it possible to remove the tumor completely without damaging the facial nerve and even to preserve useful hearing if the tumor is small. "Dizziness" is rarely true vertigo and does not occur in recurrent attacks; rather, there is a persistent sense of unsteadiness or light-headedness. All patients with tinnitus, hearing loss, or dizziness must have audiometric testing, including impedance testing with stapedial reflex evaluation. Impedance testing takes little time and provides the best guide for the use of more expensive tests. If the initial evaluation suggests a neural site of hearing loss, then electronystagmography with a caloric test and an auditory brain stem response test should be carried out. CT, combined with intravenous or intrathecal injections of contrast material, or MRI is then used to rule out or to establish the diagnosis of acoustic neuroma.

Drug Toxicity. Salicylates, aminoglycoside antibiotics, anticonvulsants, and alcohol can cause dizziness in the form of vertigo, dysequilibrium, and light-headedness. Tinnitus and hearing loss may also occur. These symptoms are bilateral and are often accompanied by ataxic gait as they variously affect the vestibular and cochlear apparatus. Sedatives (e.g., diazepam, phenobarbital), antihistamines, mood elevators, and antidepressants can also cause light-headedness and dysequilibrium. Recent intake of possibly toxic drugs should be reviewed with any dizzy patient. Cessation of use of the drug usually causes clearing of the symptoms in a few days, although vestibular damage due to aminoglycosides can result in permanent ataxia or hearing loss.

Craniocerebral Injuries. Loss of hearing, tinnitus, and vertigo (often postural) can be sequelae of head injury. Hearing loss may be due to a fracture in the middle ear or cochlea. Vertigo may be due to concussion or hemorrhage into the acoustic labyrinth. Postural vertigo may be a nonspecific reaction to concussion and part of the postconcussion syndrome.

Cardiac Arrhythmia. Cardiac arrhythmias sufficient to drop cardiac output can cause dizziness. The patient may not notice palpitations. If a cardiac arrhythmia is suspected, 24- to 48-hour continuous electrocardiographic (EKG) monitoring may help establish the relationship of arrhythmia to episodes of dizziness.

End-Organ Degeneration. With the increase in life expectancy, many patients now reach ages where degenerative losses cause dysequilibrium. Past a certain age (which is different for each patient), there is an almost linear decline in the number of hair cells in the acoustic labyrinth and the number of nerve fibers in the vestibular nerve; deterioration of other sensory systems (i.e., visual, proprioceptive, exteroceptive, and auditory) and the ability to integrate information from those sensory systems causes dysequilibrium in older patients. Older patients also lose cerebral adaptive functions and cannot compensate for the loss of sensory function.

Psychophysiologic Causes of Vertigo: Hyperventilation. Acute anxiety attacks or panic attacks can cause vertigo. It is not always easy to differentiate psychophysiologic cause and effect because vertigo can sometimes trigger acute anxiety or panic attacks. The history usually includes a period of external stress, fear of blacking out, fear of dying, shortness of breath, palpitations, tingling or weakess in the hands, mouth, or legs, and frequent or daily occurrence. Whirling vertigo is uncommon. These spells are often induced by hyperventilation. Asking the patient to hyperventilate for two minutes will evoke the typical symptoms. Patients with panic attacks may respond to antidepressant medication.

Other Causes of Dizziness. Dizziness may be a secondary effect of a variety of disorders, including the following:

Migraine (vertebral-basilar type)
Multiple sclerosis
Neurosyphilis
Cervical spondylosis
Sensory deprivation (e.g., polyneuropathy, visual impairment)
Vertebral-basilar insufficiency (e.g., TIA, infarction)
Cerebellar hemorrhage
Anemia
Orthostatic hypotension
Intralabyrinthine hemorrhage (e.g., leukemia, trauma)
Carotid-sinus syncope
Diabetes mellitus
Hypoglycemia

TAKING THE HISTORY

The first step in taking the patient's history is to determine whether the patient is suffering from vertigo, dysequilibrium, light-headedness, motor incoordination, seizure, syncope, or a combination of these. It is necessary to determine the time of onset, temporal pattern, associated symptoms, and factors that seem to precipitate, aggravate, or relieve symptoms. If there are episodes, the sequence of events needs to be known, including activities at onset, possible aura, quality, severity, sequence of symptoms, and the patient's response during the attack. Does the patient have to sit or lie down? Is consciousness lost? Can someone communicate with the patient during an attack? What other symptoms occur? After the attack, how does the patient feel? Can the patient remember the events that occurred during the attack? Can the patient function normally following an attack? These considerations suggest specific questions that must be asked in taking the history. The following list contains examples of the kinds of specific questions that should be put to the patient:

1. Is the dizziness precipitated by head movement? (Benign positional vertigo is characteristically precipitated by head movement, but orthostatic hypotension causes dizziness on rising from sitting or lying. Neck movements may precipitate dizziness in cervical osteoarthritis or muscle spasm. Head-turning may precipitate dizziness with carotid sinus syncope if the patient is wearing a tight collar.)
2. If there is vertigo, is it peripheral? Does the patient have a veering gait or an unsteady stance with nausea, perspiration, and tachycardia? In which direction does the vertigo occur?
3. Are cochlear and vestibular symptoms associated? (This pattern would suggest a peripheral lesion affecting both portions of the eighth nerve.)
4. Has there been recent head trauma?
5. Are there other neurologic symptoms such as visual changes, paralysis, sensory alterations, altered consciousness, or headaches? (These symptoms might suggest a more generalized neurologic disorder in which dizziness and hearing loss are only a part.)
6. Is there numbness in the hands and feet, visual impairment or history of diabetes or anemia? (Sensory loss in the elderly or chronically debilitated patient can lead to environmental disorientation that is interpreted as dizziness.)
7. Are there cardiac symptoms (e.g., tachycardia, palpitation, or anginal pain) that suggest cardiac disorder?
8. Are there psychiatric symptoms (e.g., thought disorders, delusions, hallucinations, bizarre behavior, or depression) that suggest dizziness of a psychic nature? Do symptoms of anxiety suggest possible hyperventilation?
9. After age 50, transient ischemic attacks (TIAs) may cause recurrent dizziness. Inquiry should include questions about other recurrent symptoms of vertebral-basilar ischemia, as well as risk factors (e.g., hypertension and cardiovascular disease).
10. Is there a familial history of dizziness or hearing loss?

Examination of the Ears

The external auditory meatus and the ear drum should be examined with an otoscope that is equipped with an enclosed or pneumatic head to which a rubber bulb is attached. Positive and negative pressure moves the tympanic membrane to evaluate possible presence of a small perforation, and the presence and character of middle ear fluid. The ossicles and medial structures of the middle ear can be seen as the tympanic membrane is pushed inward. The examiner must determine whether there is an obstruction of the external canal or whether there is blood, pus, or CSF in the canal. Scarring of the tympanic membrane can be seen, and the examiner can detect retraction pockets or retained keratin debris that may signify a cholesteatoma in the middle ear. Hearing should be evaluated with tuning forks (see hearing section) and with the examiner's voice. To test the hearing of one ear at a time, the opposite ear should be "masked" by a loud noise. One readily available masking noise is a suction catheter placed at the opposite ear. If the patient can hear a faint whisper, hearing is normal. Inability to hear a range of loudness from normal speech to a shout provides a rough guide to the severity of hearing loss.

Neurologic Examination. A complete physical and neurologic assessment is required for patients who complain of dizziness. The responsible system or anatomic location may be deduced by abnormalities found on examination. Nystagmus must be associated for direction, symmetry, and change with head position. A 30-diopter lens eliminates visual fixation and enhances nystagmus. The magnification produced makes it easier to observe the nystagmus. The cranial nerves around the eighth nerve must be assessed, including corneal reflex, abduction of the eye, and facial movement to evaluate possible cerebellopontine angle tumor.

Provocative Tests. The following provocative tests may precipitate dizziness and suggest the mechanism responsible:

Blood-pressure determination in a supine and then a standing position. A drop in system blood pressure exceeding 25 mm Hg suggests orthostatic hypotension as a possible cause for dizziness. The pulse response should be noted because tachycardia may not develop with central causes for orthostatic hypotension.

Valsalva maneuver to determine whether decreased cardiac output could be responsible for dizziness.

The *fistula test* is performed by alternately applying positive and negative pressure in the external ear canal, using a rubber bulb attached to an obturator or tight-fitting speculum of an otoscope. If there is vertigo with the fast component of nystagmus toward the tested ear, a perilymph fistula due to trauma or infection is probably present. The same pattern may be seen in patients with endolymphatic hydrops with ballooning of the saccular wall against the medial wall of the stapedial foot plate.

Positional testing used to evaluate the possibility of benign positional vertigo. The patient is seated on a table or on an armless bench and asked to keep is eyes wide open, staring at the examiner's nose. The head and upper body are rapidly brought backward, with the head extended 45° below the horizontal. After 30 seconds, the patient is rapidly brought to the upright position. This procedure is repeated with the head turned 90° to the right and then 90° to the left. Benign positional vertigo is characterized by a brief latency, rotatory nystagmus toward the downside ear, short duration, and rapid adaptation if the position is assumed repeatedly. Other forms of positional vertigo show persistence of nystagmus, lack of adaptation, and direction-changing nystagmus.

Caloric testing done in the office with 10 ml of cold tap water or 5 ml of ice water. If perforation and infection are not present, the head is extended backward, so the external meatus is in a vertical plane above the inner canthus of the eye and the cold water is instilled. Nystagmus is the normal result, and the duration of the fast component of nystagmus is compared in the two ears. The dizziness provoked by caloric testing can help differentiate vestibular and nonvestibular causes; if nystagmus and vertigo are milder on one side, there is "canal paresis," usually a sign of vestibular disease.

Sudden turning of the head to the left and right. The examiner should take care to separate the effects of neck-turning from the effects of head-turning by turning the head alone and then the body.

Hyperventilation for at least three minutes.

Carotid sinus massage. Care must be taken not to occlude the carotid artery or to massage both sides at the same time.

Electronystagmography (ENG). This test is particularly useful in comparing vestibular function of the two ears. The ENG can be combined with a bithermal caloric test and procedures that assess ocular pursuit, saccades, opticokinetic nystagmus, positional nystagmus, vestibulo-ocular reflexes (VOR) and visual-vestibular interactions. ENG is helpful in determining the site of dizziness. Examples of abnormalities that suggest CNS disease include: lack of suppression of caloric nystagmus by visual fixation, gross breakup of ocular-pursuit saccades, and abnormal opticokinetic nystagmus. Continuous EKG monitoring is used to rule out cardiac arrhythmias.

References

Baloh RW, Honrubia V. Clinical Neurophysiology of the Vestibular System. Contemporary Neurology Series. Philadelphia: F.A. Davis, 1979.

Barber HO. Current ideas on vestibular diagnosis. Otolaryngol Clin North Am Symp Adv Otolaryngol Diag 1978; 11/2:283–301.

Coles RRA, Hallan RS. Tinnitus and its management. Br Med Bull 1987; 43:983–998.

Dobie RA, Berlin CI. Influence of otits media on hearing and development. Ann Otol Rhinol Laryngol 1979; 88:48–56.

Drachman DA, Hart CW. A new approach to the dizzy patient. Neurology 1972; 22:323–334.

Gacek RR. Transection of the posterior ampullary nerve for the relief of benign paroxysmal positional vertigo. Ann Otol Rhinol Laryngol 1974; 83:596–605.

Grundfast KM, Bluestone CD. Sudden or fluctuating hearing loss and vertigo in children due to perilymph fistula. Ann Otol Rhinol Laryngol 1978; 87:761–779.

House JW, O'Connor AF (Eds). Handbook of Neurological Diagnosis. New York: Marcel Dekker, 1987.

Johnson EW. Auditory test results in 500 cases of acoustic neuroma. Arch Otolaryngol 1977; 103:152–158.

Schuknecht HF. Cupulolithiasis. Arch Otolaryngol 1969; 90:113–126.

Schuknecht HF. Pathology of the Ear. Cambridge: Harvard University Press, 1974.

7. IMPAIRED VISION
Myles M. Behrens

Impaired vision may be due to a lesion within the eyes, in the retrobulbar visual pathway (including the optic nerve and optic chiasm), or in the retrochiasmal pathway. The retrochiasmal pathway includes the optic tract, geniculate body (where synapse occurs), the visual radiation through the parietal and temporal lobes, and the occipital cortex. The pattern of visual loss may identify the site of the lesion. The course and accompanying symptoms and signs may clarify its nature.

Ocular Lesions. Impaired vision of ocular origin may be due to refractive error, to an opacity of the ocular media (which may be seen by external inspection or ophthalmoscopy), or to a retinal abnormality (e.g., retinal detachment, inflammation, hemorrhage, vascular occlusion). There may be associated local symptoms or signs such as pain or soft-tissue swelling.

Optic Nerve Lesions. A visual defect may originate in the optic nerve, particularly if the symptoms affect only one eye. The hallmarks of optic nerve dysfunction include blurred vision (indicated by decreased visual acuity), dimming or darkening of vsion (usually with decreased color perception), and decreased papillary reaction to light. This pupillary sign is not seen if the problem is media opacity, minor retinal edema, or nonorganic visual loss. It may be present to a mild degree in simple amblyopia.

The *relative afferent pupillary defect* indicative of an optic nerve lesion in one eye is best shown by the swinging-flashlight test. A bright flashlight is swung from one eye to the other just below the visual axis while the subject stares at a distant object in a dark room. When an eye with optic nerve dysfunction is illuminated, the pupil constricts in response to the light less quickly, less completely, and less persistently than the pupil of the normal fellow eye. If the expected constriction does not occur, or if the pupils actually dilate after the initial constriction to stimulation of one eye, the test is positive. Both pupils are equal in size at all times in purely afferent defects because there is hemidecussation of all afferent light input to the midbrain with equal efferent stimulation through both third nerves. Therefore, if one pupil is fixed to light because of an efferent defect, the other one can be observed throughout in performing this test.

The patient may be aware of, or the examiner may find, a *scotoma* (blind spot) in the visual field. This is often central or centrocecal (because the lesion affects the papillomacular bundle that contains the central fibers of the optic nerves), or altitudinal (because arcuate or nerve-fiber bundle abnormalities respect the nasal horizontal line, corresponding to the separation of upper and lower nerve-fiber bundles by the horizontal raphe in the temporal portion of the retina). These abnormalities are often evident on confrontation tests of the visual fields.

In a central scotoma of retinal origin (e.g., due to macular edema that affects photoreceptors), the patient may report that lines seem to be distorted *(metamorphopsia)* or objects may seem small *(micropsia).* Recovery of visual acuity may be delayed, e.g., in comparison to a normal fellow eye, after photostress, such as a flashlight stimulus for 10 seconds.

Bilateral optic nerve abnormalities, in particular those with centrocecal scotomas (Fig. 7–1), suggest a hereditary, toxic, nutritional, or demyelinating disorder; unilateral optic nerve disease is usually ischemic, inflammatory, or compressive. The course and associated symptoms and signs help to differentiate these possibilities.

Optic nerve infarction (anterior ischemic optic neuropathy) usually occurs in patients older than 50. The visual defect is usually primarily altitudinal, occasionally centrocecal, sudden in onset, and stable. There is pallid swelling of the optic disc with adjacent superficial hemorrhages. The swelling resolves in a month to six weeks, leaving optic atrophy and arteriolar narrowing on the disc (Fig. 7–2). The cause may be arteritis (giant cell or temporal arteritis, often with associated symptoms and signs) but is usually idiopathic, painless, and only rarely associated with carotid occlusive disease.

Optic neuritis usually occurs in young adults. It typically begins with a central or centrocecal scotoma and subacute progression of the defect that is followed by a gradual resolution; however, there may be residual optic atrophy. Initially, the disc may be normal (retrobulbar neuritis) or swollen (papillitis). Local tenderness or pain on movement of the eye is usually present and suggests such an intraorbital inflammatory disorder. The *Pulfrich phenomenon* is a stereo-illusion that may be caused by delayed conduction in one optic nerve, making it difficult to localize moving objects. This is not specific and may occur with retina or media defect. The *Ulthoff symptom* is exacerbation of a symptom after exercise or exposure to heat; it is not specific but occurs most often in demyelinating disorders. If, in a case suggesting optic neuritis, there is evidence of preexisting optic atrophy in either eye or optic neuropathy in the fellow eye, e.g., if the degree of relative afferent pupillary defect is less than anticipated, suggesting subclinical involvement of the other eye, demyelinating disease is also suggested.

In *compressive optic neuropathy*, there is usually steady progression of visual defect, although it may be stepwise or even remitting. The disc may remain relatively normal in appearance for months before primary optic atrophy is indicated fundoscopically by decrease in color of the disc, visible fine vessels on the disc, and peripapillary nerve fibers (best seen with a bright ophthalmoscope with red-free light). This form of optic atrophy must be distinguished from other specific types (e.g., glaucoma, in which the nerve head has an excavated or cupped appearance; post-papilledema (secondary) atrophy, with narrowing and sheathing of vessels and often indistinct margins; retinal pigmentary degeneration with narrowed vessels, which may also be seen after central retinal artery occlusion or optic nerve infarction; and congenital defects, such as coloboma or hypoplasia of the disc, with a small nerve head and a peripapillary halo that corresponds to the expected normal size of the disc).

Lesions of the Optic Chiasm. In a patient with optic neuropathy, recognition of an upper temporal hemianopic visual field defect (which may be asymptomatic) in the other eye is evidence of a chiasmal lesion that affects the anteriorly crossing lower fibers (see Fig. 7–1B). In contrast to optic nerve lesions, the majority of chiasmal lesions are compressive. The typical visual field defect is bitemporal hemianopia (see Fig. 7–1C). Because the macular fibers permeate the chiasm, any compressive lesion of the chiasm with a visual field defect is accompanied by temporal hemianopic dimming of red objects of any size in a pattern that respects the vertical line and permits secure confrontation testing.

Retrochiasmal Lesions. *Homonymous hemianopia* results from a retrochiasmal lesion. There may be varying awareness of the defect. It may be mistakenly attributed to the eye on the side of the defect, or the patient may be aware only of bumping into things on that side or of trouble reading (slowness and difficulty seeing the next word with right homonymous hemianopia, or difficulty finding the next line with a left hemianopia). The patient may ignore that side of the visual acuity test chart that corresponds to the hemianopia, but can see 20/20 unless there is another defect (see Fig. 7–1D).

With subtotal lesions, the congruity of the visual field defect in the two eyes helps in localization. Optic tract and geniculate lesions tend to have grossly incongruous visual field defects (see Fig. 7–1E). The further posterior the lesion is, the more congruous is the defect because the fibers from corresponding retinal loci in the two eyes converge on the same occipital locus.

With optic tract lesions anterior to the geniculate synapse, *optic atrophy* may develop. The eye with a temporal field defect develops a "bow-tie" pattern of atrophy, which may also occur with chiasmal lesions; the nasal portion of the disc is pale due to loss of the nasal fibers. The usual mild temporal pallor is more evident due to loss of the nasal half of the papillomacular bundle. (An imaginary vertical line through the macula corresponds to the vertical line that separates the nasal and temporal halves of the visual field.) There is a relatively pink appearance above and below where fibers from the temporal retina reach the disc.

With optic tract lesions, afferent pupillary input is impaired. When the lesion is grossly incongruous, a relative afferent pupillary defect may occur on the side with the greater deficit. It is found in the eye with the temporal hemianopia when homonymous hemianopia is total, because the temporal half-field is more extensive than the nasal half-field. The *Wernicke hemianopic pupillary phenomenon* may be difficult to elicit; pupillary constriction is more vigorous when the unaffected portion of retina is stimulated. When an optic tract lesion is close to and encroaches on the chiasm, visual acuity in the ipsilateral eye diminishes. There may be a relative afferent pupillary defect on that side as well.

Retrogeniculate lesions are not accompa-

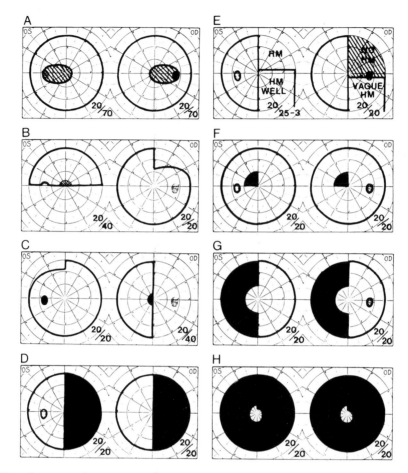

Fig. 7–1. *A.* Bilateral centrocecal scotoma. *B.* Inferior altitudinal defect with central scotoma O.S. and upper temporal hemianopic (junctional) defect O.D. *C.* Bitemporal hemianopia. *D.* Total right homonymous hemianopia. *E.* Incongruous right homonymous hemianopia. *F.* Congruous left homonymous hemianopic scotoma. *G.* Left homonymous hemianopia with macular sparing. *H.* Bilateral congruous homonymous hemianopia.

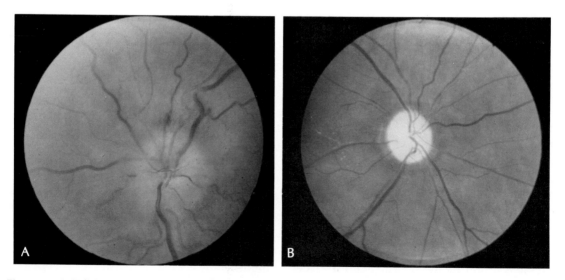

Fig. 7–2. *A.* Pallid swelling of the disc with superficial hemorrhages in a patient with acute anterior ischemic optic neuropathy. *B.* Optic atrophy with arteriolar narrowing after anterior ischemic optic neuropathy.

nied by clinical impairment of pupillary reactivity or optic atrophy. The homonymous hemianopic visual field defect tends to be superior when the temporal lobe radiations are affected, and the defect is denser below if the lesion is parietal. Occipital lesions result in precisely congruous defects, often scotomas with preserved peripheral vision (see Fig. 7–1E). If the scotoma is large enough, the area of preserved peripheral vision may be present only in the eye with the loss of temporal field (a preserved temporal crescent). This corresponds to the most anterior portion of the occipital cortex. The central portion of the visual field is represented in the posterior striate cortex, a marginal perfusion zone of both posterior and middle cerebral arteries. When the posterior cerebral artery is occluded, collateral supply from the middle cerebral artery may allow gross *macular sparing* (see Fig. 7–1G), preserving central vision. Homonymous hemianopia of occipital origin is often total. Isolated homonymous hemianopia is due to an infarct in 90% of the cases. *Cerebral blindness* (bilateral homonymous hemianopia—see Fig. 7–1H) may require distinction from hysterical blindness; opticokinetic nystagmus can be elicited in psychogenic disorders, but not after bilateral occipital lesions.

Irritative visual phenomena include formed visual hallucinations (usually of temporal lobe origin) and unformed hallucinations (usually of occipital origin) including the *scintillating homonymous scotoma* of migraine. *Amaurosis fugax* of one eye is occasionally due to vasospasm in migraine, but is usually due to ophthalmic-carotid hypoperfusion or embolization, or cardiogenic emboli. Formed or unformed hallucinations may be release phenomena when there is visual loss due to a lesion anywhere along the visual pathway. *Phosphenes* (light flashes) may occur in several kinds of optic nerve lesions, including demyelinating optic neuritis or they may occur with movement of the eye. Vitreal-retinal traction is a frequent and nonsinister cause of light flashes, especially with advancing age, although a retinal tear premonitory to retinal detachment may occur and must be ruled out.

Impairment of ocular motility is often a clue to diagnosis in many neurologic disorders. It may reflect a supra-, inter-, or infranuclear (fascicular or peripheral nerve) neurogenic lesion, neuromuscular transmission defect, myopathy, or mechanical restriction in the orbit. *Diplopia* (double vision) indicates malalignment of the visual axes if it is relieved by occlusion of either eye. Diplopia of monocular origin is psychogenic or due to a disturbance of the refractive media in the eye, e.g., astigmatism or opacity of the cornea or lens. Malalignment of the visual axes may occur in psychogenic convergence spasm (suggested by associated miosis due to the near response), in decompensation of strabismus (including convergence insufficiency, usually of no pathologic import), and less frequently, in divergence insufficiency (possibly due to bilateral sixth nerve paresis or, occasionally, increased intracranial pressure). The diplopia and malalignment of the visual axes in these cases are usually commitant, or equal in all directions of gaze. If strabismus begins in early childhood, there may be habitual suppression of the image of one eye, with impaired development of vision in that eye (termed *amblyopia*) rather than diplopia.

Incommitance, or inequality in the alignment of the visual axes in the direction of gaze, suggests limitation of action of one or more muscles. The deviation is generally greater if the paretic eye is fixing. The patient may lose one eye or adopt a head-turn or tilt to avoid diplopia (e.g., turning to the right when the right lateral rectus is limited, or tilting to the left if the right superior oblique is affected, to avoid the need for the intortional effect of that muscle). The patient may not be aware of either the diplopia or these adaptations.

To determine which muscle is impaired, the examiner obtains information from the history and examination (including use of a red glass). It is important to know whether the diplopia is vertical or horizontal, whether it is crossed (if the visual axes are divergent) or uncrossed (if convergent), whether greater near (if adducting muscles are involved) or at a distance (if abducting muscles are involved), and the direction of gaze in which the diplopia is maximal.

If the pattern of motility limitation conforms to muscles innervated by a single nerve, the lesion probably affects that nerve. With a third nerve palsy there is ptosis, limitation of action of the medial, inferior, and superior recti, and of the inferior oblique; that is, all the extraocular muscles are affected except the lateral rectus (sixth nerve) and superior oblique (fourth nerve). *Internal ophthalmoplega* (i.e., pupillary enlargement with defective constriction and defective accommodation) may be evident. When the ptotic lid is lifted, the eye is abducted (unless the sixth nerve is also affected) and on attempted downgaze the glove can be seen to intort (by observing nasal episcleral vessels) if the fourth nerve is intact. If more than one of these nerves is affected, the lesion is probably in the cavernous sinus, superior orbital fissure, or orbital apex. There may also be fifth nerve (ophthalmic division) and oculosympathetic defect *(Horner syndrome)*. The latter is indicated by relative miosis, mild ptosis, and incomplete and delayed dilation of the pupil. Such involvement is usually due to tumor, aneurysm, or inflammation, whereas isolated involvement of one of the ocular motor nerves may be ischemic.

Mechanical limitation of ocular motility may occur with orbital lesions, such as thyroid ophthalmopathy, orbital fracture, or tumor. It is indicated by limitation on forced duction, for example, an attempt to rotate the globe with forceps (traction test) or by elevation of intraocular pressure on the attempted movement with relatively intact velocity *saccades* (i.e., rapid eye movements). Other symptoms or signs of orbital lesions include proptosis (or enophthalmos in the case of fracture) beyond acceptable normal asymmetry of 2 mm, resistance to retropulsion, vascular congestion, tenderness, and eyelid abnormality other than ptosis (e.g., retraction, lid-lag, swelling).

Myasthenia gravis is suggested when affected muscles do not conform to the distribution of a single nerve and when symptoms vary, including diurnal fluctuation and fatigability. A demonstrable increase in the paresis or a slowing of saccades may occur after sustained gaze or repetitive movement (see Section 127, Myasthenia Gravis). Ptosis may similarly increase after sustained upward gaze, or a momentary lid-twitch may be seen on return of gaze from downward to straight ahead. There is no clinical abnormality of the pupils in myasthenia.

Analysis of saccadic function is of particular value in the analysis of supra- and internuclear ocular motility defects. The supranuclear control mechanisms of ocular movements include: the *saccadic system* of rapid conjugate eye movement of contralateral frontal lobe origin to achieve foveal fixation on a target (a combination of *pulse*, burst discharge in agonist with total inhibition of antagonist, and *step*, increased level of agonist and decreased level of antagonist discharge to maintain the new eccentric position); the *pursuit system* of slow conjugate movement of ipsilateral occipital lobe origin to maintain fo-

veal fixation on a slowly moving target; the *vestibular system* of slow conjugate movement to maintain stability of the retinal image if the head moves in relation to the environment; and the *vergence system* of dysconjugate slow movement to maintain alignment of the visual axes for binocular single vision. *Opticokinetic nystagmus* is the normal response to a sequence of objects moving slowly across the field of vision and can be considered a combination of pursuit and refixation saccades (to allow continuous pursuit, because vision is suppressed during the saccadic phase).

The polysynaptic saccadic pathway crosses at the level of the fourth-nerve nucleus to enter the *pontine paramedian reticular formation* (PPRF), where ipsilateral saccades and other horizontal movements are generated by stimulation of the sixth-nerve neurons and interneurons that travel up the opposite *medial longitudinal fasciculus* (MLF) to stimulate that third-nerve medial rectus subnucleus for conjugate gaze. Pathways for vertical movement seem to require bilateral stimuli. The immediate supranuclear apparatus for generating vertical gaze is in the midbrain.

General dysfunction of saccades (with limitation, slowing, or hypometria) is seen in several disorders including Huntington disease, hereditary cerebellar degeneration, progressive supranuclear palsy, and Wilson disease (see Chapter XIV, Movement Disorders). *Congenital ocular motor apraxia* is a benign abnormality of horizontal saccades that resolves with maturity. These infants are unable to perform horizontal saccades and substitute characteristic head thrusts past the object of regard, achieving fixation by the contraversive vestibular doll's head movement and then maintaining it while slowly rotating the head back. Focal dysfunction of saccades is manifested by lateral gaze paresis after contralateral frontal or ipsilateral pontine lesions; vestibular stimuli may overcome frontal gaze palsies but do not affect pontine lesions.

Internuclear ophthalmoplegia is the result of a lesion in the MLF that interrupts adduction in conjugate gaze (but convergence may be intact). Adduction nystagmus is seen in the contralateral eye. When the defect is partial, adducting saccades are slow, with resultant dissociation of nystagmus, again more marked in the abducting eye as when opticokinetic nystagmus (OKN) is elicited. When the lesion is unilateral, an ischemic lesion is likely; a bilateral syndrome implies multiple sclerosis. Vertical gaze-evoked nystagmus and *skew deviation* (one eye higher than the other) may be seen. The latter is a supranuclear vertical divergence of the eyes seen with brain stem or cerebellar lesions.

A unilateral pontine lesion that involves both the MLF and PPRF causes the combination of ipsilateral gaze palsy and internuclear ophthalmoplegia on contralateral gaze, a pattern called the *1½ syndrome*. The only remaining horizontal movement is abduction of the contralateral eye. The eyes are straight or exodeviated (if there is gaze preference away from the side of the gaze palsy). Superimposed esodeviation with related diplopia may occur if there is sixth nerve (fascicular) involvement as well.

Vertical gaze disorders are seen with midbrain lesions (the *sylvian aqueduct syndrome*). Characteristic dyssynergia on attempted upward saccades is best demonstrated by downward-moving OKN stimuli. Failure of inhibition leads to co-firing of oculomotor neurons with convergence-retraction nystagmus and related fleetingly blurred vision or diplopia. This may occur to a lesser extent with horizontal saccades as well, causing excessive adductor discharge and "pseudosixth nerve paresis." There is usually pupillary sluggishness in response to light (often with light-near dissociation) due to interruption of the periaqueductal afferent light input to the third nerve nuclei. Concomitant abnormalities include lid retraction (*Collier sign*), defective or excess accommodation or convergence, and skew deviation or monocular elevator palsy.

Oscillopsia is a sensation of illusory movement of the environment, unidirectional or oscillatory, and is seen with acquired nystagmus of various types. *Nystagmus* is an involuntary rhythmic oscillation of the eyes, generally conjugate and of equal amplitude, occasionally dysconjugate (as in the sylvian aqueduct syndrome) or dissociated in amplitude (as in internuclear ophthalmoplegia). The oscillations may be pendular or jerk in type, the latter more common in acquired pathologic nystagmus. In jerk nystagmus, the slow phase is operative and the fast phase is a recovery movement. The amplitude usually increases on gaze in the direction of the fast phase.

Horizontal and upward gaze-evoked nystagmus may be due to sedative or anticonvulsant drugs. Otherwise, *vertical nystagmus* indicates posterior fossa disease. Extreme end-gaze physiologic nystagmus, which may be of greater amplitude in the abducting eye, must be distinguished. It occurs only horizontally. *Jerk nystagmus* in the primary position, or rotary nystagmus, usually indicates a vestibular disorder that may be either central or peripheral. In a destructive peripheral lesion, the fast phase is away from the lesion; the same pattern is seen with a cold stimulus when the horizontal canals are oriented vertically (i.e., with the head elevated 30° in the supine position). *Downbeating nystagmus* in the primary position, often more marked on lateral gaze to either side, is often indicative of a lesion at the cervicomedullary junction. *Ocular bobbing* is usually associated with total horizontal pontine gaze palsy; it is not rhythmic, is coarser than nystagmus, may vary in amplitude, and is occasionally asymmetric; the initial movement is downward with a slower return. *Upbeating nystagmus* in the primary position may indicate a lesion of the cerebellar vermis or medulla, but most commonly the pons. *See-saw nystagmus* is vertically disconjugate with a rotary element, so that there is intortion of the elevating eye and simultaneous extortion of the falling eye. This pattern is often seen with parachiasm lesions, but is probably a form of alternating skew deviation due to involvement of vertical and tortional oculomotor control regions around the third ventricle. *Periodic alternating nystagmus* implies a nonsinister lesion of the lower brain stem; it is, in effect, a gaze-evoked nystagmus to either side of a null point that cycles back and forth horizontally. In the primary position there is nystagmus of periodically alternating direction. *Rebound nystagmus*, which may be confused with it, is a horizontal jerk nystagmus that is present in the primary position transiently after sustained gaze to the opposite side; it implies dysfunction of the cerebellar system.

Other ocular oscillations that follow cerebellar system lesions include *ocular dysmetria* (overshoot or terminal oscillation of saccades), *ocular flutter* (bursts of similar horizontal oscillation, actually "back-to-back" saccades without usual latency), *opsoclonus* (chaotic multidirectional conjugate saccades), and *fixation instability* (square-wave jerks), in which small saccades interrupt fixation, moving the eye away from the primary position and then returning after appropriate latency for a saccade. *Ocular myoclonus* is a rhythmic ocular oscillation that is often vertical and is often associated with synchronous palatal myoclonus.

When oscillopsia is monocular, there may be dissociated pathologic nystagmus of posterior fossa origin, including the jelly-like primarily vertical pendular nystagmus akin to myoclonus that is occasionally seen in multiple sclerosis. There may be benign myokymia of the superior oblique muscle, in which the patient is often aware of both a sensation of ocular movement and oscillopsia. Monocular nystagmus may also result from monocular visual loss in early childhood or from the insignificant and transient acquired entity of *spasmus nutans,* which is of uncertain etiology. It begins after four months of age and disappears within a few years. The nystagmus of spasmus nutans is asymmetric, rapid, and may be accompanied by head-nodding. It may be similar to congenital nystagmus. The latter begins at birth, persists, and is usually horizontal, either gaze-evoked or pendular, often with jerks to the sides, and there may be a null with head turn adopted for maximal visual acuity. It originates in a motor disorder, although it may be mimicked by the nystagmus of early binocular visual deprivation.

References

Behrens MM. Neuro-ophthalmic aspects of orbital disease. In: Duane TD, ed. Clinical Ophthalmology, vol 2. Hagerstown: Harper & Row, 1976.

Behrens MM. Neuro-ophthalmic motility disorders. Am Acad Ophthalmol Otolaryngol CETV videotape, 1975: Vol 1, No. 5.

Burde RM, Savino PJ, Trobe JD. Clinical Decisions in Neuro-Ophthalmology. St. Louis: C.V. Mosby, 1985.

Frisen L, Hoyt WF. Insidious atrophy of retinal nerve fibers in multiple sclerosis. Arch Ophthalmol 1974; 92:91–97.

Glaser JS. Neuro-Ophthalmology. Hagerstown: Harper & Row, 1978.

Leigh RJ, Zee DS. The Neurology of Eye Movement. Philadelphia: F.A. Davis, 1983.

Lessell S. Current concepts in ophthalmology: optic neuropathies. N Engl J Med 1978; 299:533–536.

Miller N, Walsh, Hoyt WF. Clinical Neuro-Ophthalmology, 4th ed. Baltimore: Williams & Wilkins, Vol. 1, 1982, Vol. 2, 1985.

Sharpe JA, Rosenberg MA, Hoyt WF, Daroff RB. Paralytic pontine exotrophia: a sign of acute unilateral pontine gaze palsy and internuclear ophthalmoplegia. Neurology 1974; 24:1076–1081.

Spector RH, Troost BT. The ocular motor system. Ann Neurol 1981: 9:517–525.

8. HEADACHE

Arnold P. Friedman

It has been estimated that headache is a complaint in more than half of the patients who visit physicians. Headache can result from intracranial or systemic diseases, personality or situational problems, or combinations of these factors. Most headaches are not due to catastrophic illness; however, meningitis, cerebral hemorrhage, and brain tumor do need immediate attention. Chronic headache probably arises most frequently from faulty adjustment to the environment; the nervous system is as sensitive to symbolic threats as it is to physical threats.

Headache always demands careful study. It may be indicative of an underlying disease that deserves treatment, or it may be the result of the disruptive effects of a psychologic disorder.

In general, the complaint of headache may be divided into two broad diagnostic categories. One group comprises the chronic recurring headaches: vascular headaches of the migraine type, muscular contraction (tension) headaches, or a combination of the two. When the sole complaint is headache, the diagnosis is made primarily by correct evaluation of the history.

The second category comprises headache due to intracranial lesions, systemic diseases, or local diseases of the eye and nasopharynx. In this group, diagnosis is made primarily by physical examination and laboratory findings.

The clinical approach must take into account the whole patient, including family, occupational, and social problems.

Pathophysiology

Headache may arise from stimulation of extracranial or intracranial structures. Extracranial pain-sensitive structures include the scalp, extracranial arteries, mucous membranes of nasal and paranasal spaces, external and middle ear, teeth, and muscles of the scalp, face, and neck. Pain due to disease of these structures is usually localized, but may spread to include a wide area of the head.

Intracranial pain-sensitive structures include the venous sinuses and tributaries, the parts of the dura at the base of the skull, the dural arteries (anterior and middle meningeal), the large arteries at the base of the brain leading to and coming from the circle of Willis, the upper cervical nerves and the fifth, ninth, and tenth cranial nerves. The brain parenchyma, the ependyma of the ventricles, the choroid plexus, the cranium, and much of the dura, arachnoid, and pia mater are insensitive to pain. The periosteum is locally sensitive to stretch.

Mechanisms. Possible basic mechanisms of headache in intracranial disease include: (1) traction due to direct or indirect displacement of pain-sensitive structures; (2) distention and dilatation of intracranial arteries; (3) inflammation in or about the pain-sensitive structures of the head; (4) distortion of pain-sensitive areas due to increased intraventricular pressure caused by lesions that obstruct CSF flow; and (5) direct pressure by an intracranial mass on certain cranial and cervical nerves. One or more of the mechanisms may be in operation in any given patient. Raised intracranial pressure itself does not cause headache; headaches were not induced in volunteers when their CSF pressure was raised by intrathecal injection of saline solution or when they inhaled carbon dioxide. Also postulated as mechanisms for headache have been distention of scalp arteries, sustained muscle contraction, and inflammation in or about these structures.

Pain Pathways. If the pain originates in structures above the tentorium, it is felt in the distribution of the fifth cranial nerve, in front of a line drawn vertically from the ears across the top of the head. Pain from structures in the posterior fossa is felt behind this line and is conveyed by the glossopharyngeal and vagus nerves by the upper cervical spinal roots. Pain arising from the posterior half of the sagittal sinus or the upper surface of the transverse sinus is transmitted over a branch of the first division (Arnold's nerve) of the trigeminal nerve and is referred to the frontal area; it is often retro-orbital. An accessory pathway for pain referred from supratentorial structures to the ear or frontotemporal areas may lie in the nervus intermedius of the facial nerve.

Although early reports indicated that dural stimulation elicits strictly unilateral referral of head pain, further investigations indicated that head pain of dural origin has limited clinical significance because there is no consistent referral pattern.

Pain fibers in the intraspinal portion of the descending trigeminal tract and nucleus descend into the upper two segments of the cervical cord where they are joined by similar fibers from the seventh, ninth, and tenth cranial nerves. Sensory fibers from the first three cervical dorsal roots ramify throughout this center and connect with trigeminal neurons in the nucleus of the spinal tract. After synapsing, the second-order neurons cross the midline and terminate in the opposite dorsal horn. This pattern explains why pain may be referred from a lesion in the upper neck to the head or vice versa.

Clinical Approach

Different possibilities are raised by the patient who presents with an acute onset of headache for the first time in his life. Severe headache of sudden onset, particularly if followed by impairment of consciousness or focal neurologic signs, suggests subarachnoid or intracerebral hemorrhage or meningitis. When headache appears for the first time after age 50, it is probably not migraine, tension, or a psychiatric disorder. If the headache recurs or is continuous, possible causes include cranial arteritis, intracranial mass, and meningeal inflammation.

The relationship of onset of headache to the time of day may indicate the underlying cause of the headache. For example, headache resulting entirely from hypertension (210 mm Hg systolic over 100 mm Hg diastolic) is usually present on awakening. Space-occupying lesions and migraine may cause headache early in the morning, whereas cluster headaches are frequently nocturnal, waking the patient after only a few hours of sleep. Headaches associated with frontal sinusitis may commence early in the morning; those due to maxillary sinusitis usually appear in the afternoon. Chronic sinusitis does not cause persistent headache. Onset of tension headache is generally not related to time of day; the patient may go to bed with the headache and wake up with it, or it may occur at any time of the day.

The site of the headache pain may be significant. Migraine tends to vary from side to side in different attacks and is commonly anterior. It is unilateral in two thirds of the patients and bilateral in the others. The possibility of an intracranial mass must be considered if recurring headache always affects the same side. The site of pain is usually not a reliable means of localizing cerebral tumors and may be misleading. As a generalization, intracranial lesions in the posterior fossa initially produce pain in the occipital nuchal region, whereas supratentorial lesions produce pain in the frontal, temporal, and parietal regions. In absence of papilledema, if the headache is one-sided, the site of the headache pain is the site of the lesion. Disease of the paranasal sinuses, teeth, eyes, or upper cervical vertebra induces pain that is referred in a regional, but not sharply localized, distribution that is fairly constant.

The quality of the pain may be important. A pulsatile, throbbing headache is of vascular origin whether due to the vasodilatation of migraine or to hypertension or fever. The pain of neuralgia occurs as transient, shock-like stabs of intense pain. Headaches associated with brain tumors usually have a steady aching quality and tend to be intermittent at first. The patient with tension headache usually complains of a constant, tight, pressing or band-like ache; throbbing is conspicuously absent. Intensity of the headache is not a reliable indication of the seriousness of the cause; pain may be moderate with an intracranial lesion and severe in a chronic anxiety state. Extremely severe headache of sudden onset always suggests subarachnoid hemorrhage. The symptoms accompanying the headache may also be an important guide to the underlying cause or type of headache.

Neurologic deficits usually accompany headache due to intracranial lesions. An infiltrating glioma, however, may extend throughout the hemisphere without causing headache because the large blood vessels are not disturbed until late in the course of the disease. Compression of the brain from a meningioma is more likely to cause seizures, focal cerebral symptoms, or progressive impairment of intellectual function before headache appears. Patients with subdural hematomas almost invariably present with headache because the increase in the size of the hematoma displaces the brain downward, stimulating pain-sensitive structures.

Headache associated with tumors metastatic to the brain can be deceptive. Headache is one of the most common manifestations of metastasis to the brain, but is not necessarily constant or severe. Headache is a common symptom with carcinomatosis of the meninges and may be present for several months before many other symptoms appear.

Patients with chronic meningitis (e.g., fungal, parasitic, or tuberculous) commonly have headache as an early complaint. Signs of meningeal involvement point toward the need for examination of the CSF.

Collagen-vascular disorders may present with headaches and bizarre focal or generalized neurologic signs. The patient should be carefully questioned about the relationship of the headache to daily patterns of living or to recent experiences. An intracranial vascular disturbance and accompanying headache, whether caused by hangover, fever, or intracranial tumor, are aggravated by jarring, sudden movements of the head, and Valsalva maneuvers (e.g., coughing, sneezing, or straining during defecation). Sexual intercourse may bring on a combined muscle-contraction and vascular headache and may precipitate subarachnoid hemorrhage.

Many headaches are brought on by psychologic stress factors. Before the clinician places the patient in this diagnostic category, it should be clear from the symptoms and motivations that psychologic factors are present. Lack of physical symptoms or signs and atypical features of the headache are not in themselves diagnostic of headache of this type. A direct relationship between the headache and emotional conflict or situational difficulties should be determined.

Examination of the head and neck, including inspection, palpation, percussion, and auscultation, must be performed on all headache patients. The neurologic examination must be complete. The cervical spine should be tested for tenderness and mobility.

Examination of the skull for local infections, hardened or tender arteries, bony swelling, and sensitive areas should be part of the routine examination. Palpation and auscultation of the major cranial arteries are important. There is some question about the diagnostic value of bruits, which are normally heard in children and sometimes heard in adults with no symptoms of cerebrovascular disease. Nevertheless, bruits may indicate carotid atherosclerosis or cerebrovascular malformation.

As part of the evaluation, ancillary studies are often advisable for headache patients when the diagnosis is obscure. Radiographic examinations of the skull and cervical spine are sometimes useful.

Principal Varieties of Headache

There are several ways of classifying headache. The most useful is based as far as possible on the mechanism of the pain. The pathophysiology of specific categories of headaches and clinical examples are briefly considered here.

Headaches from intracranial sources are most often produced by traction, displacement of intracranial arteries, or inflammation in or about pain-sensitive intracranial structures, chiefly the large arteries, veins, venous sinuses, and certain cranial nerves. This form of headache is evoked by an intracranial mass (tumor, abscess, aneurysm), nonspecific brain edema, meningitis, and other infections.

Headache may result from distention and dilatation of intracranial arteries associated with a number of systemic conditions, including fever, infection, hypoxia, nitrite and foreign protein administration, hypertension, electrolyte imbalance, and metabolic disorders.

Disease of the extracranial structures of the head that may give rise to headache and head pain includes glaucoma, errors of refraction, inflammatory processes in the eyes, nose, and ears, and cranial and neck structures that include involvement of the ligaments, muscles, and cervical nerve roots.

Some headaches are caused by contraction of the cervical or scalp muscles as a manifestation of emotional stress. This type of headache is called *tension, muscular contraction,* or *psychogenic.* The headache results from long-sustained contraction of the skeletal muscles of scalp, face, neck, and shoulders. Concurrent vascular and local chemical changes within the skeletal muscle are factors in producing the pain. The distinction between this type of headache and common migraine is often far from clear. In headache of this type, electromyograms frequently do not confirm the presence of excess muscle contraction.

Headache may occur as a manifestation of conversion mechanisms, hypochondriacal reaction, and delusional states.

Headache is a common sequel to minor or severe head injury. It may present intermittently for months or even years after a head trauma, but it usually disappears gradually. Headache localized to the site of the skull or scalp injury may be due to stimulation of traumatized nerve endings in the contused scalp. A variety of extracranial and intracranial mechanisms may be responsible, including sustained contraction of the muscles of the neck and scalp, vasodilatation, scar formation in the scalp or cranium, injury to structures of the neck, tissue distortion, contusion or bleeding in the meninges, and subdural hematoma. Psychologic mechanisms such as anxiety may play an important part in the pathogenesis of headache. (For a further discussion of headache, see Section 144, Migraine.)

Treatment and Management

In the treatment and management of a patient with headache, the physician is confronted with a broad spectrum of medical, surgical, and psychologic problems. Diagnosis is the first step in the management of headache. Treatment of headache as a symptom in the course of an already recognized disease is directed toward the fundamental pathophysiology. The choice of therapy depends on the specific problem and may entail operative therapy for remediable disturbances such as a brain tumor or removal of an allergic factor. Once the underlying cause has been determined and treatment started, the headache itself usually requires an appropriate analgesic.

The nonaddictive analgesics are effective for head pain of low intensity. For attacks of severe, persistent, muscle-contraction headache, the use of a non-narcotic, analgesic sedative with tranquilizer is effective. In combination, these drugs raise the pain threshold and reduce the anxiety and reaction to pain. Codeine sulfate (0.03 g) may be used alone or in combination with aspirin (0.3 to 0.6 g) if the pain is severe. Tranquilizers and sedatives in small doses are effective in treating the associated anxiety and tension. Antidepressants are most helpful in anxious and depressed patients. Because physical dependence on these agents may develop, these patients should be followed closely.

Surgical procedures for relief of chronic recurring headache (e.g., dorsal column stimulators, sensory rhizotomy) are usually not helpful.

"Autoregulatory" techniques have been advocated for treatment of chronic recurring headache, particularly migraine and muscle-contraction headache. One of the major autoregulatory techniques is biofeedback. Other relaxation techniques seem to provide temporary relief from their tension states; however, the underlying factors that produce tensions are not usually understood by the patient. Rather than getting at the cause of the tension, a reconditioning or covering technique substitutes for insight into the problem. The long-term results of these approaches to headache need proper evaluation.

References

Critchley M, et al. Headache: physiopathological and clinical concepts. Adv Neurol 1982; 33:1–405.

Dalessio D. Wolff's Headache and Other Head Pain, 4th ed. New York: Oxford University Press, 1980.

Ellertsen B, Kove H. MMPI patterns in chronic muscle pain, tension headache and migraine. Cephalalgia 1987; 7:65–71.

Friedman AP, Merritt HH. Headache: Diagnosis and Treatment. Philadelphia: FA Davis, 1959; 401.

Friedman AP, et al. Classification of headache. JAMA
    1962; 179:717–718.
Friedman AP, ed. Headache and related pain syndromes.
    Med Clin North Am 1978; 62:427–623.
Holmes DS, Burish TG. Effectiveness of biofeedback for
    treating migraine and tension headache in Review
    of the endera. J Psychosom Res 1983; 27:515–532.
Lance JW. Mechanism and Management of Headache,
    4th ed. London: Butterworths, 1982.
Rothner AD. Headaches in children: a review. Headache
    1978; 18:169–175.
Sjaastad O. 'Chronic daily headache' ('cefalea cronica
    quotidiana'). Cephalalgia 1985; 2(suppl):191–193.

9. INVOLUNTARY MOVEMENTS
Stanley Fahn

Although convulsions, fasciculations, and myokymia are involuntary movements, these disorders have special characteristics and are not classified with the types of abnormal involuntary movements to be described in this section. The disorders commonly called abnormal involuntary movements, or *dyskinesias*, are usually evident when the patient is at rest, are frequently increased by action, and disappear during sleep. There are exceptions to these generalizations. For example, palatal myoclonus may persist during sleep, and mild torsion dystonia may be present only during active voluntary movements (action dystonia), but not when the patient is at rest. The known dyskinesias are distinguished mainly by visual inspection of the patient. Electromyography (EMG) can occasionally be helpful by determining the rate, rhythmicity, and synchrony of the involuntary movements. Sometimes patients have dyskinesias that bridge the definitions of more than one disorder; this leads to compound terms such as choreoathetosis, which describes features of both chorea and athetosis.

Most abnormal involuntary movements are continuous or easily evoked, but some are intermittent or paroxysmal, such as tics and the *paroxysmal dyskinesias.* Gross movements of joints are visible, unlike the restricted muscle twitching of fasciculation or myokymia.

Tremors are rhythmic oscillatory movements. These result from alternating contractions of opposing muscle groups (e.g., parkinsonian tremor-at-rest) or from simultaneous contractions of agonist and antagonist muscles (e.g., essential tremor). A useful way clinically to divide tremor for aid in diagnosis is to determine whether the tremor is present under the following conditions: when the affected body part is at rest (as in parkinsonian disorders of the extrapyramidal system); with maintenance of posture (e.g., with arms outstretched in front of the body) as in essential tremor; with action (e.g., when writing or pouring water from a cup); or with intention (e.g., finger-to-nose maneuver) as in cerebellar disease (see Section 117, Benign Essential Tremor).

The term *myoclonus* refers to shock-like movements due to contractions or inhibitions (negative myoclonus) (see Section 114, Myoclonus). *Chorea* delineates brief, irregular contractions that, although rapid, are not as lightning-like as myoclonic jerks. In classic choreic disorders, such as Huntington disease and Sydenham chorea, the jerks affect individual muscles as random events that seem to flow from one muscle to another. They are not repetitive or rhythmical (see Section 113). *Ballism* is a form of chorea in which the choreic jerks are of very large amplitude, producing a flinging movement of the affected limbs. Chorea is presumably related to disorders of the caudate nucleus but sometimes involve other structures. Ballism is related to lesions of the subthalamic nucleus.

Dystonia is a syndrome of sustained muscle contraction frequently causing twisting and repetitive movements, or abnormal postures (see Section 116, Dystonia). Dystonia is represented by (1) sustained contractions of both agonist and antagonist muscles; (2) an increase of these involuntary contractions on attempting voluntary movement ("overflow"); (3) rhythmic interruptions (*dystonic tremor*) of these involuntary, sustained contractions when the patient attempts to oppose them; (4) inappropriate or opposing contractions during specific voluntary motor actions *(action dystonia);* and (5) *torsion spasms* that may be as rapid as chorea, but differ because the movements are continual and of a twisting nature, in contrast to the random and seemingly flowing movements of chorea. Torsion spasms may be misdiagnosed as chorea; the other characteristics frequently lead to the misdiagnosis of a conversion reaction.

Tics are patterned sequences of coordinated movements that appear suddenly and intermittently. The movements are occasionally simple and resemble a myoclonic jerk, but they are usually complex, ranging from head-shaking, eye-blinking, sniffing, and shoulder-shrugging to complex facial distortions, arm-waving, touching parts of the body, jumping movements, or making obscene gestures *(copropraxia).* Most often, tics are rapid

Table 9–1. Paroxysmal Kinesigenic Choreoathetosis and Paroxysmal Dystonia

Features	Kinesigenic Choreoathetosis	Dystonia
Genetics	Familial or sporadic	Familial or sporadic
Male:female ratio	4:1	2:1
Age at onset (years)	1–33, usually 5–15	1–22
Duration of attacks	<5 minutes	2 minutes to 4 hours
Maximum frequency	100/day	3/day
Precipitating factors	Sudden movements, startle	Fatigue, excitement, stress, alcohol, coffee
Response to anticonvulsants	Good	Poor

(Modified from Lance JW. Ann Neurol 1977; 2:285–293.)

and brief, but occasionally they can be sustained motor contractions (i.e., dystonic). In addition to motor tics, vocalizations can be a manifestation of tics. These range from sounds such as barking, throat-clearing, or squealing to verbalization, including the utterance of obscenities (*coprolalia*) and *echolalia* (repeating sounds or words). Motor and vocal tics are the essential features of the Gilles de la Tourette syndrome, which represents a severe form in the spectrum of tics.

One feature of tics is the compelling need felt by the patient to make the motor or phonic tic. Tics can be voluntarily controlled for brief intervals, but such a conscious effort is usually followed by more intense and frequent contractions. The milder the disorder, the more control the patient can exert. Tics can sometimes be suppressed in public. There is a wide spectrum of the severity and persistence of tics. Sometimes the tics are temporary and sometimes they are permanent.

Many people develop personalized mannerisms. These physiologic tics may persist after repeated performances of motor habits and have therefore been called "habit spasms." As a result, unfortunately, all tics have been considered by some physicians as habit spasms of psychic origin. Today, however, the trend is to consider pathologic tics a neurologic disorder.

Stereotypic movements are encountered in the syndrome of drug-induced *tardive dyskinesia* and refer to repetitive, rapid movements that have the speed of chorea (see Section 120, Tardive Dyskinesia). They most often affect the mouth; in *oro-lingual-buccal dyskinesia*, there are constant chewing movements of the jaw, writhing and protrusion movements of the tongue, and puckering movements of the mouth. Other parts of the body may also be involved.

Athetosis is a continual, slow, writhing movement of the limbs (distal and proximal),

trunk, head, face, or tongue. When these movements are brief, they merge with chorea (*choreoathetosis*). When the movements are sustained at the peak of the contractions, they merge with dystonia, and the term *athetotic dystonia* can be applied.

Akathitic movements are those of restlessness. They commonly accompany the subjective symptom of *akathisia*, an inner feeling of motor restlessness or the need to move. Today, akathisia is most commonly seen as a side effect of antipsychotic drug therapy, either as acute akathisia or tardive akathisia that often accompanies tardive dyskinesia. Akathitic movements (e.g., crossing and uncrossing the legs, caressing the scalp or face, pacing the floor, and squirming in a chair) can also be a reaction to stress, anxiety, boredom, or impatience; it can then be termed physiologic akathisia. Pathologic akathisia, in addition to that induced by antipsychotic drugs, can be seen in the encephalopathies of confusional states, and in some dementias. Picking at the bedclothes is a common manifestation of akathitic movements in the bedridden patients.

Two other neurologic conditions in which there are subjective feelings of the need to move are *tics* and the *restless legs syndrome*. The latter is characterized by formication in the legs, particularly in the evening when the patient is relaxing and sitting, or lying down and attempting to fall asleep. These sensations of ants crawling under the skin disappear when the patient walks around. This disorder is not understood but can respond to opioids.

Paroxysmal dyskinesias are syndromes in which the abnormal involuntary movements occur in a sudden burst. Three different paroxysmal dyskinetic disorders have been described; two of them are well characterized (Table 9–1). *Paroxysmal kinesigenic choreoathetosis* consists of brief (less than five minutes) bouts of choreoathetosis or dystonic postures induced by sudden movement. They can occur many times a day and respond to anticonvulsants. *Paroxysmal dystonia* is a sudden onset of sustained dystonic contractions lasting a few minutes to several hours. They occur less than four times a day, and are sometimes induced by fatigue, stress, excitement, and ingestion of alcohol and coffee. They do not respond well to phenytoin, carbamazepine, or barbiturates. A third type of paroxysmal disorder is the syndrome of *hyperekplexia* (excessive startle syndromes). These dramatic disorders have been given local names: Jumping Frenchmen of Maine, Myriachit, and Latah. Hyperekplexia can be hereditary or sporadic. There are excessive complex motor responses to a sudden tactile or verbal stimulus. Echolalia and echopraxia are sometimes seen.

References

Andermann F, Andermann E. Excessive startle syndromes: startle disease, jumping, and startle epilepsy. Adv Neurol 1986; 43:321–338.

Hening W, Walters A, Kavey N, Gidro-Frank S, Cote LJ, Fahn S, et al. Dyskinesias while awake and periodic movements in sleep in restless legs syndrome: Treatment with opioids. Neurology 1986; 36:1363–1366.

Lance JW. Familial paroxysmal dystonic choreoathetosis and its differentiation from related syndromes. Ann Neurol 1977; 2:285–293.

Marsden CD, Fahn S, eds. Movement Disorders. London: Butterworths, 1982.

Marsden CD, Fahn S, eds. Movement Disorders 2. Butterworth's International Medical Reviews. London: Butterworths, 1987.

10. WEAKNESS: THE SYNDROMES CAUSED BY WEAK MUSCLES

Lewis P. Rowland

Weakness implies that a muscle cannot exert normal force. Neurologists use the words *paralysis* or *plegia* to imply total loss of contractility; anything less than total is *paresis*. In practice, however, someone may mention a *partial hemiplegia*, which conveys the idea even if it is internally inconsistent.

Hemiplegia implies weakness of an arm and leg on the same side. *Crossed hemiplegia* is a confusing term, generally implying unilateral cranial nerve signs on one side and hemiplegia on the other side, a pattern seen with brain stem lesions above the decussation of the corticospinal tracts. *Monoplegia* is weakness of one limb; *paraplegia* means weakness of both legs.

In this section, I describe the syndromes that result from pathologically weak muscles so that a student new to neurology can find the sections of the book that describe specific diseases. There is more than one approach to this problem, because no single approach is completely satisfactory. Elaborate algorithms have been devised, but the flow chart may be too complicated to be useful unless it is run by a computer.

It may be simpler to determine first if there is pathologic weakness, then to find evidence of specific syndromes that depend on recognition of the following characteristics: distribution of weakness, associated neurologic abnormalities, tempo of disease, genetics, and age of the patient.

Recognition of Weakness or Pseudoweakness

Patients with weak muscles do not often use the word "weakness" to describe their symptoms. Rather they complain that they cannot climb stairs, rise from chairs, or run or they note footdrop (and may actually use that term). They may have difficulty turning keys or door knobs. If proximal arm muscles are affected, lifting packages, combing hair, or working overhead may be difficult. Weakness of cranial muscles causes ptosis of the eyelids, diplopia, dysarthria, dysphagia, or the cosmetic distortion of facial paralysis. These specific symptoms will be analyzed later.

Some people use the word "weakness" when there is no neurologic abnormality. For instance, aging athletes may find that they can no longer match the achievements of youth, but that is not pathologic weakness. Weakness in a professional athlete causes the same symptoms that are recognized by other people when the disorder interferes with the conventional activities of daily life. Losing a championship race, running the mile in more than four minutes, or jogging only five miles instead of a customary 10 are not symptoms of diseased muscles.

Others who lack the specific symptoms of weakness may describe "chronic fatigue." They cannot do housework; they have to lie down to rest after the briefest exertion. If they plan an activity in the evening, they may spend the entire day resting in advance. Employment may be in jeopardy. Myalgia is a common component of this syndrome, and there is usually evidence of depression.

Fading athletes and depressed, tired people with aching limbs have different emotional problems, but both groups lack the specific symptoms of muscle weakness, and they share two other characteristics: no abnormality appears on neurologic examination, and no true weakness is evident on manual muscle examination. That is, there is no weakness unless the examiner uses brute force. A vigorous young adult examiner may out-wrestle a frail octagenarian, but that does not imply pathologic weakness in the loser. Students and residents must use reasonable force in tests of strength against resistance.

Fatigue and similar symptoms may sometimes be manifestations of systemic illness due to anemia, malignant tumor, or acute infection. There is usually other evidence of the underlying disease, however, and that syndrome is almost never mistaken for a neurologic disorder.

Other patients have pseudoweakness. For instance, some patients attribute a gait disorder to weak legs, but it is immediately apparent, on examination or even before formal examination, that they have parkinsonism. Or a patient with peripheral neuropathy may have difficulty with fine movements of the fingers, not because of weakness but because of severe sensory loss. Or a patient may have difficulty raising one or both arms because of bursitis, not limb weakness. Or a patient with arthritis may be reluctant to move a painful joint. These circumstances are explained by findings on examination.

Examination may also resolve another problem in evaluating symptoms that might be due to weakness. Sometimes, when limb weakness is mild, it is difficult for the examiner to know how much resistance to apply, to know whether the apparent weakness is "real." Then, the presence or absence of wasting, fasciculation, or altered tendon reflexes may give the crucial clues. Symptomatic weakness is usually accompanied by some abnormality on examination. Even in myasthenia gravis, symptoms may fluctuate in intensity, but there are always objective signs of abnormality on examination if the patient is currently having symptoms. There is a maxim: "A normal neurologic examination is incompatible with the diagnosis of symptomatic myasthenia gravis."

Finally, examination may uncover the patient with deliberate pseudoweakness that may be due to deceit, deliberate or otherwise. Hysterical patients, Münchausen patients, or other malingerers who feign weakness all lack specific symptoms. Or they may betray inconsistencies in the history because they can participate in some activities but not in others that involve the same muscles. On examination, their dress, cosmetic facial makeup, and behavior may be histrionic. In walking they may stagger dramatically, but do not fall or injure themselves by bumping into furniture. In manual muscle tests, they abruptly give way or they shudder in tremor rather than apply constant pressure. "Misdirection of effort" is one way to describe that behavior. Some simply refuse to participate in the test. The extent of disorder may be surprising, however. We and others have seen psychogenic impairment of breathing that led to use of a mechanical ventilator.

Patterns of Weakness

In analyzing syndromes of weakness, the examiner uses several sources of information for the differential diagnosis. The pattern of weakness and associated neurologic signs delimit some of the anatomic possibilities, to answer the question *Where* is the lesion? The age of the patient and the tempo of evolution aid in deciding *what* is the lesion.

The differential diagnosis of weakness encompasses much of clinical neurology, so the reader will be referred to other sections for some of the discussion. For instance, the first task in the analysis of a weak limb is to determine whether the lesion is due to a lesion of the upper or lower motor neuron, a distinction that is made on the basis of clinical findings. Overactive tendon reflexes with clonus, Hoffmann signs, and Babinski signs denote an upper motor neuron disorder. Lower motor neuron signs include muscle weakness, wasting, and fasciculation, with loss of tendon reflexes. These distinctions may seem crude, but they have been passed as reliable from generation to generation of neurologists.

If the clinical signs imply a lower motor neuron disorder, the condition could be due to problems anywhere in the motor unit (motor neuron or axon, neuromuscular junction, or muscle). This determination is guided by principles stated in Section 129. Diseases of the motor unit are also discussed in that section, so the following discussion will be concerned primarily (but not entirely) with central lesions.

Hemiparesis. If there is weakness of the arm and leg on the same side, and signs imply a central lesion, the lesion could be in the cervical spinal cord or in the brain. Pain in the neck or in the distribution of a cervical dermatome might be clues to the site of the lesion. Facial weakness may occur with the hemiparesis, placing the lesion in the brain and above the nucleus of the seventh cranial nerve, a change in mentation or speech may indicate that the lesion is cerebral, not cervical. Sometimes, however, there are no definite clinical clues to the site of the lesion, and the examiner must rely on CT, EEG, CSF findings, or myelography to determine the site and nature of the lesion together.

The course of hemiparesis gives clues to the nature of the disorder. The most common cause in adults is cerebral infarction or hemorrhage. Abrupt onset, prior transient attacks, and progression to maximal severity within 24 hours in a person with hypertension or advanced age are indications that a stroke has occurred. If no cerebral symptoms are present, there could conceivably be transverse myelitis of the cervical spinal cord, but that condition would be somewhat slower in evolution (days rather than hours) and more likely to involve all four limbs. Similarly, multiple sclerosis is more likely to be manifest by bilateral corticospinal signs than a pure hemiplegia.

If hemiparesis of cerebral origin progresses for days or weeks, it is reasonable to suspect a cerebral mass lesion, whether the patient is an adult or a child. If the patient has had focal seizures, that possibility is the more likely. In addition to brain tumors, other possibilities include arteriovenous malformation, brain abscess, or other infections. AIDS is a constant consideration. Metabolic brain disease usually causes bilateral signs with mental obtundation and would be an unusual cause of hemiparesis, even in a child.

Hemiparesis of subacute evolution could arise in the cervical spinal cord if there were, for instance, a neurofibroma of a cervical root. That condition would be signified by local pain in most cases and, because there is so little room in the cervical spinal canal, bilateral corticospinal signs would probably be present.

In general, hemiparesis usually signifies a cerebral lesion rather than one in the neck, and the cause is likely to be denoted by the clinical course, and by CT or other brain-imaging.

Paraparesis. *Paresis* means weakness, and *paraparesis* is used to describe weakness of both legs. However, the term has also been extended to include gait disorders caused by

lesions of the upper motor neuron, even when there is no weakness on manual muscle examination. The disorder is then attributed to *spasticity,* or the clumsiness induced by malfunction of the corticospinal tracts. In adults, the most common cause of that syndrome, "spastic paraparesis of middle life," is multiple sclerosis. The differential diagnosis includes tumors in the region of the foramen magnum, Chiari malformation, cervical spondylosis, arteriovenous malformation, and primary lateral sclerosis. The diagnosis cannot be made on clinical grounds alone and requires information from CSF examination (protein, cells, gamma globulin, oligoclonal bands), evoked potentials, CT, MRI, and myelography.

When there are cerebellar or other signs, in addition to bilateral corticospinal signs, the disorder may be multiple sclerosis or an inherited disorder such as olivopontocerebellar degeneration. The combination of lower motor neuron signs in the arms and upper motor neuron signs in the legs is characteristic of amyotrophic lateral sclerosis; the same syndrome has been attributed without proof to cervical spondylosis. That pattern may also be seen in syringomyelia, but it is exceptional to find syringomyelia without typical patterns of sensory loss.

Other clues to the nature of spastic paraparesis include cervical or radicular pain in neurofibromas or other extra-axial mass lesions in the cervical spinal canal. Or there may be concomitant cerebellar signs or other indication of multiple sclerosis.

It is said that brain tumors in the parasagittal area may cause isolated spastic paraparesis by compressing the leg areas of the motor cortex in both hemispheres. However, this possibility seems more theoretical than real, because no well-documented cases have been reported.

Chronic paraparesis may also be due to lower motor neuron disorders. Instead of upper motor neuron signs, there is flaccid paraparesis, with loss of tendon reflexes in the legs. This differential diagnosis includes motor neuron diseases, peripheral neuropathy, and myopathy as described in Section 129.

Paraparesis of acute onset (days, rather than hours or weeks) presents a different problem in diagnosis. If there is back pain and tendon reflexes are preserved or there are frank upper motor neuron signs, a compressive lesion may be present. As the population ages, metastatic tumors become an increasingly more common cause. In children or young adults, the syndrome may be less ominous, even with pain, because the disorder is often due to acute transverse myelitis. This may be seen in children or adults and, in addition to the motor signs, a sensory level usually designates the site of the lesion. Myelography is needed to make this differentiation. In the elderly, a rare cause of acute paraplegia is infarction of the spinal cord. That syndrome is also seen in surgical procedures that require clamping of the aorta.

If the tendon reflexes are lost and there is no transverse sensory level in a patient with an acute paraparesis, the most common cause is Guillain-Barré syndrome, at any age from infancy to the senium. Sensory loss may facilitate that diagnosis, but sometimes little or no sensory impairment occurs. Then, the diagnosis depends upon examination of the CSF and EMG. The Guillain-Barré syndrome, however, may also originate from diverse causes. In developing countries, acute paralytic poliomyelitis is still an important cause of acute paraplegia. Rarely, an acute motor myelitis may be due to some other virus.

The "reverse" of paraplegia would be weakness of the arms with good function in the legs, or *bibrachial paresis.* Lower motor neuron syndromes of this nature are seen in some cases of amyotrophic lateral sclerosis (with or without upper motor neuron signs in the legs). The arms hang limply at the side while the patient walks with normal movements of the legs. Similar patterns may be seen in some patients with myopathy of unusual distribution. It is difficult to understand how a cerebral lesion could cause weakness of the arms without equally severe weakness of the legs, but that is the "man-in-the-barrel syndrome," seen in comatose patients who survive a bout of severe hypotension. The lesion is not known but could be bilateral and prerolandic.

Monomelic Paresis. If one leg or one arm is weak, the presence of pain in the low back or the neck may point to a compressive lesion. Whether acute or chronic, herniated nucleus pulposus is high on the list of possibilities if radicular pain is present. Acute brachial plexus neuritis (neuralgic amyotrophy) is another cause of weakness in one limb, with pain; a corresponding syndrome of the lumbosacral plexus is much less common. Peripheral nerve entrapment syndromes may also cause monomelic weakness and pain, but the pain is local, not radicular. Mononeuritis

multiplex may also cause local pain, paresthesia, and paresis.

In painless syndromes of isolated limb weakness in adults, motor neuron disease is an important consideration if there is no sensory loss. Sometimes, in evaluating a limb with weak, wasted, and fasciculating muscle, the examiner is surprised because tendon reflexes are preserved or even overactive, instead of being lost. That apparent paradox implies lesions of both upper and lower motor neurons, almost pathognomonic of amyotrophic lateral sclerosis. That disease may be asymmetric in the early stages.

It is theoretically possible for strokes or other cerebral lesions to cause monomelic weakness with upper motor neuron signs. However, that is almost never seen. Weakness due to a cerebral lesion may be more profound in the arm, but abnormal signs are almost always present in the leg, too, that is, the syndrome is really a hemiparesis.

Neck Weakness. Difficulty holding up the head is seen in some patients with diseases of the motor unit, probably never in patients with upper motor neuron disorders. Usually, patients with neck weakness also have symptoms of disorder of the lower cranial nerves (dysarthria and dysphagia) and often also of adjacent cervical segments, as manifest by difficulty raising the arms. Amyotrophic lateral sclerosis and myasthenia gravis are probably the two most common causes.

Rarely, there is isolated weakness of neck muscles, with difficulty holding the head up but no oropharyngeal or arm symptoms. "Floppy head syndrome," however, is a disabling disorder and is usually due to one of three conditions: motor neuron disease, myastheia gravis, or polymyositis. We have seen one with a Chiari malformation. Some cases, however, are idiopathic.

Weakness of Cranial Muscles. The syndromes due to weakness of cranial muscles are discussed in Sections 7 (Impaired Vision) and 59 (Injury to Cranial and Peripheral Nerves). The major problems in differential diagnosis involve the site of local lesions that affect individual nerves of ocular movement, facial paralysis, or the vocal cords. Pseudobulbar palsy due to upper motor neuron lesions must be distinguished from bulbar palsy due to lower motor neuron disease and then almost always a form of amyotrophic lateral sclerosis. This distinction depends upon associated signs of upper or lower motor neuron lesion. Myasthenia gravis can affect the eyes, face, or oropharynx (but only exceptionally the vocal cords); in fact, the diagnosis of myasthenia gravis is doubtful if there are no cranial symptoms. Brain stem syndromes in the aging population may be due to stroke, meningeal carcinomatosis, or brain stem encephalitis.

References

Asher R. Munchausen syndrome. Br Med J 1954; 1.

Ashizawa T Rolak LA, Hines M. Spastic pure motor monoparesis. Ann Neurol 1986; 20:638–641.

Hopkins A, Clarke C. Pretended paralysis requiring artificial ventilation. Br Med J 1987; 294:961–962.

Kennedy HG. Fatigue and fatigability. Lancet 1987; 1:1145.

Knopman DS, Rubens AB. The value of CT findings for the localization of cerebral functions. The relationship between CT and hemiparesis. Arch Neurol 1986; 43:328–332.

Lange DJ, Fetell MR, Lovelace RE, Rowland LP. The floppy-head syndrome. Ann Neurol 1986; 20:133A.

Marsden CD. Hysteria—a neurologist's view. Psychol Med 1986; 16:277–288.

Maurice-Williams RS, Marsh H. Simulated paraplegia; an occasional problem for the neurosurgeon. J Neurol Neurosurg Psychiatry 1985; 48:826–831.

McHardy KC. Clinical algorithms; weakness. Br Med J 1984; 1:1591–1594.

Sage JI, Van Uitert RL. Man-in-the-barrel syndrome. Neurology 1986; 36:1102–1103.

Seyal M, Pedley TA. Sensory evoked potentials in adult-onset progressive spastic paraparesis. NY State J Med 1984; 84:68–71.

11. GAIT DISORDERS
Sid Gilman

The stance and gait of a patient may immediately suggest specific disorders of motor or sensory function, or even specific diseases. Particular types of gait disorder are so characteristic of some diseases that the diagnosis may be obvious (e.g., Parkinson disease).

In normal locomotion, one leg and then the other alternately supports the erect moving body. Each leg undergoes periods of acceleration and deceleration as body weight is transferred from one foot to the other. When the moving body passes over the supporting leg, the other leg swings forward in preparation for its next support phase. One foot or the other constantly contacts the ground and, when support of the body is transferred from the trailing leg to the leading leg, both feet are on the ground momentarily.

Any form of bipedal walking includes two basic requirements: continuous ground reaction forces that support the body's center of gravity, and periodic movement of each foot from one position of support to the next in the direction of progression. As a consequence of these basic requirements, certain displacements of the body segments occur regularly in walking. To start walking, a person raises one foot and accelerates the leg forward; this is the *swing phase* of walking. Muscle action in the supporting leg causes the center of gravity of the body to move forward, creating a horizontal reaction force at the foot. The greater this reaction force, the greater the acceleration of the body because the amount of force is equal to the body mass multiplied by the amount of acceleration. The swing phase ends when the leg that has swung forward is placed on the ground, which is when the *stance phase* of walking begins. During the stance phase, weight is transferred to the opposite leg and another swing phase can begin. The major groups of muscles of the leg are active at the beginning and end of the stance and swing phases. As the body passes over the weight-bearing leg, it tends to be displaced toward the weight-bearing side, causing a slight side-to-side movement. In addition, the body rises and falls with each step. The body rises to a maximum level during the swing phase and descends to a minimum level during the stance phase. As the body accelerates upward, there is an increase in the vertical floor reaction to a value that exceeds body weight. The vertical floor reaction falls to a minimum during downward acceleration, reducing the total vertical reaction to a value less than body weight.

Examining Stance and Gait

When examining a patient's stance and gait, the physician should observe the walking patient from the front, back, and sides. The patient should rise quickly from a chair, walk normally at a slow pace and then at a fast pace, and then turn around. The patient should walk on his or her toes or heels, and in tandem (i.e., placing the heel of one foot immediately in front of the toes of the opposite foot, attempting to move in a straight line). The patient should stand with the feet together and the head erect, first with open eyes and then with closed eyes, to determine whether balance can be maintained.

When a person walks normally, the body should be held erect with the head straight and the arms hanging loosely at the sides, each moving rhythmically forward with the opposite leg. The shoulders and hips should be approximately level. The arms should swing equally. The steps should be straight and about equal in length. The head should not be tilted and there should be no appreciable scoliosis or lordosis. With each step, the hip and knee should flex smoothly and the angle should dorsiflex with a barely perceptible elevation of the hips as the foot clears the ground. The heel should strike the ground first and the weight of the body should be transferred successively onto the sole of the foot and then to the toes. The head and then the body should rotate slightly with each step, without lurching or falling.

Each person walks in a characteristic fashion. There are gross similarities among people, but a person's gait reflects physical characteristics and personality traits. Among the variables are speed, stride length, characteristics of the walking surface, and the type of footwear worn. Perhaps more important are the person's aspirations, motivations, and attitudes. For some situations, speed is the most important factor. In other situations, safe arrival or the minimal expenditure of energy may be more important. Some people learn to walk gracefully or in the least obtrusive manner and as a consequence may expend extra energy. Others learn to walk ungracefully but as effectively as possible for the amount of energy expended. The manner of walking may provide clues to personality traits (e.g., aggressiveness, timidity, self-confidence, aloofness).

The Gait in Hemiparesis. Hemiparetic patients usually stand and walk with the affected arm fixed and the leg extended. In walking, patients have difficulty flexing the hip and knee and dorsiflexing the ankle; the paretic leg swings outward at the hip to avoid scraping the foot on the floor. The leg is held stiffly and rotates in a semicircle, first away from and then toward the trunk, with a circumduction movement. Despite the circumduction, the foot may scrape the floor so that the toe and outer side of the sole of the shoe become worn first. The upper body often rocks slightly to the opposite side during the circumduction movement. The arm on the hemiparetic side usually moves little during walking, remaining adducted at the shoulder, flexed at the elbow, and partially flexed at the wrist and fingers; loss of the swinging motion of the arm may be the first sign of insidious hemiparesis.

The Gait in Paraparesis. The gait of patients with spastic paraparesis is characterized by slow, stiff movements at the knees and hips,

with evidence of considerable effort. The legs are usually maintained extended or slightly flexed at the hips and knees and are often adducted at the hips. In some patients, the legs may cross with each step, causing a *scissors gait*. The steps are short and the patient may move the trunk from side to side in attempts to compensate for the slow and stiff movements of the legs. The legs circumduct at the hips and the feet scrape the floor so that the soles of the shoes become worn at the toes.

The Gait in Parkinsonism. Parkinson disease patients stand in a posture of general flexion with the spine bent forward, the head bent downward, the arms moderately flexed at the elbows, and the legs slightly flexed. Patients stand immobile and rigid, with a paucity of automatic movements of the limbs and a mask-like fixed facial expression with infrequent blinking. Although the arms are held immobile, there is a tremor that involves the fingers and wrists at 4 to 5 cycles per second. When these patients walk, the trunk bends even further forward; the arms remain immobile at the sides of the body or become further flexed and carried somewhat ahead of the body. The arms do not swing. As the patients walk forward, the legs remain bent at the knees, hips, and ankles. The steps are short so that the feet barely clear the ground and the soles of the feet shuffle and scrape the floor. The gait, with characteristically small steps, is termed *marche à petits pas*. Forward locomotion may lead to successively more rapid steps and the patient may fall unless assisted; this increasingly rapid walking is called *festination*. If the patients are pushed forward or backward they may not be able to compensate with flexion or extension movements of the trunk. The result is a propulsive or retropulsive series of steps. Parkinsonian patients can sometimes walk with surprising rapidity for brief intervals.

Patients often have difficulty when they start to walk after standing still or sitting in a chair. They may take several very small steps that cover little distance before taking longer strides. The walking movements may stop involuntarily and the patient may freeze on attempts to pass through a doorway or into an elevator.

Cerebellar Disease. Patients with disease of the cerebellum stand with the legs farther apart than is normal, and may develop *titubation*, a coarse fore-and-aft tremor of the trunk. Often they cannot stand with the legs so close that the feet are touching; they sway or fall in attempts to do so, whether the eyes are open or closed. They walk cautiously, taking steps of varying length, some shorter and others longer than usual. They may lurch from one side to another. Because of this unsteady or *ataxic gait,* which is attributed to poor balance, they fear walking without support and want to hold onto objects in the room, such as a bed or a chair, moving cautiously between these objects. When gait ataxia is mild, it may be exaggerated when patients attempt tandem-walking in a straight line, successively placing the heel of one foot directly in front of the toes of the opposite foot. The patients commonly lose balance and must quickly place one foot to the side to avoid falling.

When disease is restricted to the vermal portions of the cerebellum, disorders of stance and gait may appear without other signs of cerebellar dysfunction such as limb ataxia or nystagmus. This pattern is seen in alcoholic cerebellar degeneration. Diseases of the cerebellar hemispheres, unilateral or bilateral, may also affect gait. With a unilateral cerebellar-hemisphere lesion, ipsilateral disorders of posture and movement accompany the gait disorder. Patients usually stand with the shoulder on the side of the lesion lower than the other; there is accompanying scoliosis. The limbs on the side of the cerebellar lesion show decreased resistance to passive manipulation *(hypotonia).* On walking, these patients stagger and progressively deviate to the affected side. This can be demonstrated by asking them to walk around a chair. As the patients rotate toward the affected side, they tend to fall into the chair; rotating toward the normal side, they move away from the chair in a spiral. The affected leg shows marked ataxia in walking or other tests of coordinated movement. Patients with bilateral cerebellar-hemisphere disease show a disturbance of gait similar to that seen in disease of the vermis, but signs of cerebellar dysfunction also appear in coordinated limb movements.

The Gait in Sensory Ataxia. Another characteristic gait disorder results from loss of proprioception in the legs due to lesions of the afferent fibers in peripheral nerves, dorsal roots, dorsal columns of the spinal cord, or medial lemnisci. These patients are unaware of the position of the limbs and, consequently, have difficulty standing or walking. They usually stand with the legs spread widely apart. If asked to stand with feet together and eyes open, they remain stable, but when the eyes are closed, they sway and often fall *(Romberg sign).* They walk with the legs spread widely apart, watching the ground carefully. In stepping, they lift the legs higher than necessary at the hips and fling them abruptly forward and outward. The steps vary in length and may cause a characteristic sound as the foot slaps the floor. They usually hold the body somewhat flexed, often using a cane for support. If vision is impaired and these patients attempt to walk in the dark, the gait disturbance worsens.

Hysterical Gait Disorders. Hysterical disorders of gait may appear in association with hysterical paralysis of one or both legs. The gait is usually bizarre, easily recognized, and unlike any disorder of gait evoked by organic disease. In some patients, however, hysterical gait disorders may be difficult to identify. In hysterical hemiplegia, patients drag the affected leg along the ground behind the body and do not circumduct the leg or use it to support weight, as in hemiplegia due to an organic lesion. At times, the hemiplegic leg may be pushed ahead of the patient and used mainly for support. The arm on the affected side does not develop the flexed posture commonly seen with hemiplegia from organic causes, and the hyperactive tendon reflexes and Babinski sign on the hemiplegic side are missing.

Hysterical paraplegic patients usually walk with one or two crutches or lie helplessly in bed with the legs maintained in rigid postures or, at times, completely limp. The term *astasia-abasia* refers to patients who cannot stand or walk but who can carry out natural movements of the limbs when lying in bed. At times, patients with hysterical gait disorders walk only with seemingly great difficulty, but they show normal power and coordination when lying in bed. On walking, patients cling to the bed or the furnishings of the room. If asked to walk without support, patients may lurch dramatically while managing feats of extraordinary balance to avoid falling. They may fall, but only when a nearby physician or family member can catch them or when soft objects are available to cushion the fall. The gait disturbance is often dramatic, with the patient lurching wildly in many directions and finally falling, but only when other people are watching the performance. They demonstrate remarkable agility in their rapid postural adjustments when they attempt to walk.

The Gait in Cerebral Palsy. The term cerebral palsy includes several different motor abnormalities that usually result from perinatal injury. The severity of the gait disturbance varies depending upon the nature of the lesion. Mild limited lesions may result in exaggerated tendon reflexes and extensor plantar responses with a slight degree of talipes equinovarus but no clear gait disorder. More severe and extensive lesions often result in bilateral hemiparesis; patients stand with the legs adducted and internally rotated at the hips, extended or slightly flexed at the knees, with plantar flexion at the ankles. The arms are held adducted at the shoulders and flexed at the elbows and wrists. Patients walk slowly and stiffly with plantar flexion on the feet, causing them to walk on the toes. Bilateral adduction of the hips causes the knees to rub together or to cross, causing the scissors gait.

The gait in patients with cerebral palsy can be altered by movement disorders. Athetosis is common and consists of slow, serpentine movements of the arms and legs between the extreme postures of flexion-with-supination and extension-with-pronation. On walking, patients with athetotic cerebral palsy show involuntary limb movements that are accompanied by rotary movements of the neck and constant grimacing. The limbs usually show the double hemiparetic posture described previously; however, superimposed upon this posture may be partially fixed asymmetric limb postures with, for example, flexion with supination of one arm and extension with pronation of the other. Asymmetric limb postures commonly occur in association with rotated postures of the head, generally with extension of the arm on the side to which the chin rotates and flexion of the opposite arm.

The Gait in Chorea. *Chorea* literally means the dance, and refers to the gait disorder seen most often in children with Sydenham chorea, or adults with Huntington disease. Both conditions are characterized by continuous and rapid movements of the face, trunk, and limbs. Flexion, extension, and rotatory movements of the neck occur with grimacing movements of the face, twisting movements of the trunk and limbs, and rapid piano-playing movements of the digits. Walking generally accentuates these movements. In addition, sudden forward or sideward thrusting movements of the pelvis and rapid twisting movements of the trunk and limbs result in a gait that resembles a series of dancing steps.

The Gait in Dystonia Musculorum Deformans. The first symptom of this disorder often consists of an abnormal gait, resulting from inversion of one foot at the ankle. Patients walk on the lateral side of the foot initially; as the disease progresses, this problem worsens and patients develop other postural abnormalities that include elevation of one shoulder, elevation of a hip, and twisted postures of the trunk. Intermittent spasms of the trunk and limbs then interfere with walking. Eventually, there is torticollis, tortipelvis, lordosis, or scoliosis. Finally, patients may become unable to walk.

The Gait in Muscular Dystrophy. In muscular dystrophy, weakness of the muscles of the trunk and the proximal leg muscles produces a characteristic stance and gait. In attempting to rise from the seated position, patients flex the trunk at the hips, put their hands on their knees, and push the trunk upward by working the hands up the thighs. This sequence is termed *Gowers sign.* Patients stand with exaggerated lumbar lordosis and a protruberant abdomen because of weakness of the abdominal and paravertebral muscles. Patients walk with the legs spread widely apart and have a characteristic waddling motion of the pelvis that results from weakness of the gluteal muscles. The shoulders often slope forward and winging of the scapulae may be seen as the patients walk.

The Gait in Frontal Lobe Disease. Patients with bilateral frontal lobe disease have a characteristic gait disorder. Patients stand with the feet spread widely apart and take a first step only after a long delay. Several small shuffling steps may cover a short distance, followed by a few steps of moderate amplitude, after which patients stop walking again. This cycle is then repeated. The gait disorder commonly occurs in association with dementia and grasp, suck, and snout reflexes. Usually the patients do not have muscular weakness, tendon reflex anormalities, sensory changes, or extensor plantar responses. Patients can perform the individual limb movements required for walking if asked to mimic walking movements while lying supine. The disorder is considered a form of apraxia, a disturbance in the coordinated performance of a motor function in the absence of weakness of the muscles required for the function.

The Gait in Lower Motor-Neuron Disorders. Diseases of the motor neurons or peripheral nerves characteristically cause distal weakness, and foot drop is a common manifestation. In motor neuron disease itself or in heritable neuropathies (e.g., Charcot-

Marie-Tooth disease), the disorder is likely to be bilateral. If there is a compressive lesion of one peroneal nerve, the process may be unilateral. In either case, patients cannot dorsiflex the foot in walking as is normal each time the swinging leg begins to move. As a result, the toes are scuffed along the ground. To avoid this awkwardness, the patient raises the knee higher than usual, resulting in a "steppage" gait. If proximal muscles are affected (in addition to or instead of distal muscles), the gait also has a waddling quality.

References

Gilman S, Bloedel J, Lechtenberg R. Disorders of the Cerebellum. Philadelphia: FA Davis, 1981.

Grillner S. Neurobiological bases of rhythmic motor acts in vertebrates. Science 1985; 228:143.

Herman RM, Grillner S, Stein PSG, Stuart DG, eds. Neural Control of Locomotion. New York: Plenum Press, 1976.

Stein RB, Pearson KG, Smith RS, Redford, JB, eds. Control of Posture and Locomotion. New York: Plenum Press, 1973.

12. SIGNS AND SYMPTOMS IN NEUROLOGIC DIAGNOSIS
Lewis P. Rowland

An anonymous sage once said that 90% of the neurologic diagnosis depends on the patient's medical history and that the remainder comes from the neurologic examination and laboratory tests. Sometimes, of course, findings in blood tests or CT are pathognomonic, but students have to learn which tests are appropriate and when to order them. It is therefore necessary to know which diagnostic possibilities are reasonable considerations for a particular patient. In considering these different diagnostic possibilities, specific symptoms are not the only ingredient in analyzing the patient's history, as I shall discuss briefly in this section.

It is commonly taught that neurologic diagnosis depends on answers to two questions that are considered separately and in sequence. First, *where is the lesion?* Is it in the cerebrum, basal ganglia, brain stem, cerebellum, spinal cord, peripheral nerves, neuromuscular junction, or muscle? Second, *what is the nature of the disease?* If the site of the lesion can be determined, the number of diagnostic possibilities is reduced to a manageable number. However, an experienced clinician is likely to deal with both questions simultaneously; site and disease are identified

at the same time. Sometimes the process is reversed. To take an obvious example, if a patient suddenly becomes speechless or awakens with a hemiplegia, the diagnosis of stroke is presumed. The location is then deduced from findings on examination, and both site and process are ascertained by CT. If there are no surprises in the CT (e.g., demonstration of a tumor or vascular malformation), further laboratory tests might be considered to determine the cause of an ischemic infarct.

The specific natures of different symptoms and findings on examination are discussed in the preceding sections of this chapter and in teaching manuals on the neurologic examination. Other considerations that influence diagnosis are briefly discussed here.

Age of Patient. The symptoms and signs of a stroke may be virtually identical in a 10-year old, a 25-year-old, and a 70-year-old; however, the diagnostic implications are vastly different for each patient. Some brain tumors are more common in children and others are more common in adults. Progressive paraparesis is more likely to be due to spinal cord tumor in a child, whereas in an adult, it is more likely to be due to multiple sclerosis. Focal seizures are less likely to be fixed in pattern and are less likely to indicate a specific structural brain lesion in a child than in an adult. Myopathic weakness of the legs in childhood is more likely to be caused by muscular dystrophy than polymyositis; the reverse is true in patients older than 25. Muscular dystrophy rarely begins after age 35. Multiple sclerosis rarely starts after age 55. Hysteria is not a likely diagnosis when neurologic symptoms start after age 50. (These ages are arbitrary, but the point is that age is a consideration in some diagnoses.)

Sex. Only a few diseases are gender-specific. X-linked diseases (e.g., Duchenne musclar dystrophy) occur only in boys or, rarely, in girls with chromosome disorders. Among young adults, autoimmune diseases are more likely to affect women, especially systemic lupus erythematosus and myasthenia gravis, although young men are also affected in some cases.

Women are exposed to the neurologic complications of pregnancy and may be at increased risk of stroke because of oral contraceptives. Men are more often exposed to head injury.

Ethnicity. Stating the race of the patient in every case history is an anachronism of modern medical education. In neurology, race is important only when sickle cell disease is considered. Malignant hypertension and sarcoidosis may be more prevalent in blacks, but whites are also susceptible. However, other ethnic groups are more susceptible to particular diseases: Tay-Sachs disease, familial dysautonomia, and Gaucher disease in Ashkenazi Jews; thyrotoxic periodic paralysis in Japanese and perhaps in other Asians; nasopharyngeal carcinoma in Chinese; Marchiafava-Bignami disease in Italian wine drinkers (a myth?); and hemophilia in descendants of the Romanoffs. Ethnicity is rarely important in diagnosis.

Socioeconomic Considerations. Ghetto dwellers, whatever their race, are prone to the ravages of alcoholism, drug addiction, and trauma. Impoverishment is also accompanied by malnutrition, infections, and the consequences of medical neglect. Within the ghetto and in other social strata, the AIDS epidemic has generated concern about the risk factors of male homosexuals, intravenous drug users, prostitutes, and recipients of blood transfusions. For most other neurologic disorders, however, race, ethnicity, sex, sexual orientation, and socioeconomic status do not affect the incidence.

Tempo of Disease. Seizures, strokes, and syncope are all abrupt in onset, but differ in manifestations and duration. Syncope is the briefest. There are usually sensations that warn of the impending loss of consciousness. After fainting, the patient begins to recover consciousness in a minute or so. A seizure may or may not be preceded by warning symptoms. It can be brief or protracted, and is manifested by alteration of consciousness or by repetitive movements, stereotyped behavior, or abnormal sensations. A stroke due to cerebral ischemia or hemorrhage "strikes out of the blue" and is manifested by hemiparesis or other focal brain signs. The neurologic disorder that follows brain infarction may be permanent or the patient may recover partially or completely in days or weeks. If the signs last less than 24 hours, the episode is called a transient ischemic attack (TIA). Sometimes it is difficult to differentiate a TIA from the postictal hemiparesis of a focal motor seizure, especially if the seizure was not witnessed. Another syndrome of abrupt onset is subarachnoid hemorrhage, in which the patient often complains of "the worst headache of my life"; this is sometimes followed by loss of consciousness.

Symptoms of less than apoplectic onset may progress for hours (intoxication, infection, or subdural hematoma), days (Guillain-Barré syndrome), or longer (most tumors of the brain or spinal cord). The acute symptoms of increased intracranial pressure or brain herniation are sometimes superimposed on the slower progression of a brain tumor. Progressive symptoms of brain tumor may be punctuated by seizures. Heritable or degenerative diseases tend to progress very slowly, becoming most severe only after years of increasing disability (e.g., Parkinson disease or Alzheimer disease).

Remissions and exacerbations are characteristic of myasthenia gravis, multiple sclerosis, and some forms of peripheral neuropathy. Bouts of myasthenia tend to last for weeks at a time; episodes in multiple sclerosis may last only days in the first attacks, then tend to increase in duration, and to leave more permanent neurologic disability. These diseases sometimes become progressively worse, without remissions.

The symptoms of myasthenia gravis vary in a way that differs from any other disease. The severity of myasthenic symptoms may vary from minute to minute. More often, however, there are differences in the course of a day (usually worse in the evening than in the morning, but sometimes vice versa), or from day to day.

Some disorders characteristically occur in bouts that usually last minutes or hours, rarely longer. Periodic paralysis, migraine headache, cluster headaches, and narcolepsy are examples of such disorders.

To recognize the significance of these differences in tempo, it is necessary to have some notion of the different disorders.

Duration of Symptoms. It may be of diagnostic importance to know how long the patient has had symptoms before consulting a physician. Long-standing headache is more apt to be a tension or vascular headache, but headache of recent onset is likely to imply intracranial structural disease and should never be underestimated. Similarly, seizures or drastic personality change of recent onset implies need for CT and other studies to evaluate possible brain tumor or encephalopathy.

Medical History. It is always important to know whether there is any systemic disease in the patient's background. Common disorders, such as hypertensive vascular disease or diabetes mellitus, may be discovered for the first time when the patient is examined because of neurologic symptoms. Because they are common, these two disorders may be merely coincidental, but depending on the neurologic syndrome, either diabetes or hypertension may actually be involved in the pathogenesis of the neural signs. If the patient is known to have a carcinoma, metastatic disease is assumed to be the basis of neurologic symptoms until proven otherwise. If the patient is taking medication for any reason, the possibility of intoxication must be considered. Cutaneous signs may point to neurologic complications of von Recklinghausen disease or other phakomatoses, or may suggest lupus erythematosus or some other systemic disease.

Identifying Site of Disorder. Aspects of the history may suggest the nature of the disorder; specific symptoms and signs suggest the site of the disorder. *Cerebral disease* is implied by seizures or by focal signs that can be attributed to a particular area of the brain; hemiplegia, aphasia, or hemianopia are examples. Generalized manifestations of cerebral disease are seizures, delirium, and dementia. *Brain stem disease* is suggested by cranial nerve palsies, cerebellar signs of ataxia of gait or limbs, tremor, or dysarthria. Dysarthria may be due to incoordination in disorders of the cerebellum itself or its brain stem connections. Cranial nerve palsies or the neuromuscular disorder of myasthenia gravis may also impair speech. Ocular signs have special localizing value. Involuntary movements suggest *basal ganglia disease.*

Spinal cord disease is suggested by spastic gait disorder and bilateral corticospinal signs, with or without bladder symptoms. If there is neck or back pain, a compressive lesion should be suspected; if there is no pain, multiple sclerosis is likely. The level of a spinal compressive lesion is more likely to be indicated by cutaneous sensory loss than by motor signs. The lesion that causes spastic paraparesis may be anywhere above the lumbar segments.

Peripheral nerve disease usually causes both motor and sensory symptoms (e.g., weakness and loss of sensation). The weakness is likely to be more severe distally, and the sensory loss may affect only position or vibration sense. A more specific indication of peripheral neuropathy is loss of cutaneous sensation in a "glove-and-stocking" distribution.

Neuromuscular disorders and diseases of muscle cause limb or cranial muscle weakness without sensory symptoms. If limb weakness and loss of tendon jerks are the only signs (with no sensory loss), electromyography and muscle biopsy are needed to determine whether the disorder is one of motor neurons, peripheral nerve, or muscle.

The following sections consider the diseases that cause these symptoms and signs.

References

Dejong RN: Neurological Examination, 4th ed. New York: Harper & Row, 1979.

Fried R. The hyperventilation syndrome: research and clinical treatment. Baltimore, Johns Hopkins University Press, 1987.

Mayo Clinic and Foundation. Clinical Examinations in Neurology, 5th ed. Philadelphia: WB Saunders Co., 1981.

Neurologic Disorders of Known Etiology

Chapter II

Infections of the Nervous System

13. BACTERIAL INFECTIONS
James R. Miller
Burk Jubelt

The parenchyma, coverings, and blood vessels of the nervous system may be invaded by virtually any pathogenic microorganism. It is customary, for convenience of description, to divide the syndromes produced according to the chief site of the lesion. This division is an arbitrary one because the inflammatory process frequently involves more than one of these structures.

Involvement of the meninges by pathogenic microorganisms is known as *leptomeningitis*, because the infection and inflammatory response are generally confined to the subarachnoid space and the arachnoid and pial tissues. Cases are subdivided into two groups, acute and subacute meningitis, according to the severity of the inflammatory reactions, which in part is related to the nature of the infecting organism.

Acute Purulent Meningitis

Bacteria may gain access to the ventriculo-subarachnoid space by way of the blood in the course of septicemia or as a metastasis from infection of the heart, lung, or other viscera. The meninges may also be invaded by direct extension from a septic focus in the skull, spine, or parenchyma of the nervous system (e.g., sinusitis, otitis, osteomyelitis, brain abscess). Organisms may gain entrance to the subarachnoid space through compound fractures of the skull and fractures through the nasal sinuses or mastoid or following neurosurgical procedures. They rarely may be introduced when lumbar puncture is performed to remove fluid or to inject contrast media, anesthetics, antibiotics, or drugs. The pathology, symptoms, and clinical course of patients with acute purulent meningitis are similar regardless of the causative organisms. The diagnosis and program of therapy depend on the isolation and identification of the organisms and the determination of the source of the infection.

Acute purulent meningitis may be the result of infection with almost any pathogenic bacteria. Isolated examples of infection by the uncommon forms are recorded in the literature, but Hemophilus influenzae, Neisseria meningitidis, and Streptococcus pneumoniae account for most cases. In recent years, there has been an increase in the incidence of cases in which no organism can be isolated. These patients now comprise the fourth major category of purulent meningitis. This may be due to the administration of therapy prior to admission to the hospital and the performance of lumbar puncture. In the neonatal period, Escherichia coli and group B streptococci are the most common causative agents. Approximately 60% of the postneonatal bacterial meningitis of children is due to H. influenzae. The overall fatality rate from bacterial meningitis is now 10% or less. Many deaths occur during the first 48 hours of hospitalization.

For convenience, special features of the common forms of acute purulent meningitis are described separately. Neonatal infections are discussed in Section 64.

MENINGOCOCCAL MENINGITIS

Meningococcal meningitis or acute cerebrospinal fever was described by Vieusseux in 1805, and the causative organism was identified by Weichselbaum in 1887. It occurs almost constantly in sporadic form and at irregular intervals in epidemics. Epidemics are especially likely to occur when there are large shifts in population as in time of war.

Pathogenesis. The meningococci (Neisseria meningitidis) may gain access to the meninges directly from the nasopharynx through the cribriform plate or by way of the blood. The fact that organisms can be cultured from the blood or from cutaneous lesions before the appearance of meningitis is strong evidence that the infection takes place through the blood by way of the choroid plexus in many, if not all, cases. In addition, the ventricular fluid may be teeming with organisms before infection of the meninges is evident.

Pathology. In acute fulminating cases, death may occur before there are any significant pathologic changes in the nervous system. In the usual case, in which death does not occur for several days after the onset of the disease, an intense inflammatory reaction occurs in the meninges. The inflammatory reaction is especially severe in the subarachnoid spaces over the convexity of the brain around the cisterns at the base of the brain; it may extend a short distance along the perivascular spaces into the substance of the brain and spinal cord. The inflammatory reaction rarely breaks into the parenchyma. Meningococci, both intra- and extracellular, are found in the meninges and CSF. With progress of the infection, the pia-arachnoid becomes thickened and adhesions may form. Adhesions at the base may interfere with the flow of CSF from the fourth ventricle and may produce hydrocephalus. Inflammatory reaction and fibrosis of the meninges along the roots of the cranial nerves are thought to be the cause of the cranial nerve palsies that are seen occasionally. Damage to the auditory nerve often occurs suddenly, and the auditory defect is usually permanent. This condition may result from extension of the infection to the inner ear or thrombosis of the nutrient artery. In addition, facial paralysis frequently occurs after the meningeal reaction has subsided. Signs and symptoms of parenchymatous damage (e.g., hemiplegia, aphasia, cerebellar signs) are infrequent and are probably due to infarcts as the result of thrombosis of inflamed arteries or veins.

With effective treatment, and in some cases without treatment, the inflammatory reaction in the meninges subsides and no evidence of the infection may be found at autopsy in patients who die months or years later.

Incidence. Meningococcus is the causative organism in about 20% of all cases of bacterial meningitis in the United States. Serogroup B is now the most commonly reported type (50%) causing meningitis. Although both the sporadic and epidemic forms of the disease may attack individuals of all ages, children and young adults are predominantly affected. The normal habitat of the meningococcus is the nasopharynx, and the disease is spread by carriers or by individuals with the disease. A polysaccharide vaccine for groups A, C, Y, and W-B5 meningococci has reduced the incidence of meningococcal infection among military recruits.

Symptoms. The onset of meningococcal meningitis, similar to that of other forms of meningitis, is accompanied by chills and fever, headache, nausea and vomiting, pain in the back, stiffness of the neck, and prostration. The occurrence of herpes labialis, conjunctivitis, and a petechial or hemorrhagic skin rash is common with meningococcal infections. At the onset, the patient is irritable. In children, there is frequently a characteristic sharp shrill cry (meningeal cry). With progress of the disease, the sensorium becomes clouded and stupor or coma may develop. Occasionally, the onset may be fulminant and accompanied by deep coma. Convulsive seizures are often an early symptom, especially in children, but focal neurologic signs are uncommon. Acute fulminating cases with severe circulatory collapse are relatively rare.

Signs. The patient appears acutely ill, and may be confused, stuporous, or semicomatose. The temperature is elevated at 101° or 103° F, but it may occasionally be normal at the onset. The pulse is usually rapid and the respiratory rate is increased. Blood pressure is normal except in acute fulminating cases when there may be profound hypotension. A petechial rash may be found in the skin, mucous membranes, or conjunctiva, but never in the nail beds. It usually fades in three or four days. There is rigidity of the neck with positive Kernig and Brudzinski signs. However, these signs may be absent in newborns, elderly, or comatose patients. Increased intracranial pressure causes bulging of an unclosed anterior fontanelle and periodic respiration. The reflexes are often decreased but may occasionally be increased. Cranial nerve palsies and focal neurologic signs are uncommon, and usually do not develop until several days after the onset of the infection. The optic discs are normal, but papilledema may develop if the meningitis persists for more than a week.

Laboratory Data. The white blood cells in peripheral blood are increased with counts usually in the range of 10,000 to 30,000 per mm³, but they occasionally may be normal or higher than 40,000 per mm³. The urine may contain albumin, casts, and red blood cells. Meningococci can be cultured from the nasopharynx in most cases, from the blood in over 50% of the cases in the early stages, and from the skin lesions when these are present.

The CSF is under increased pressure, usually between 200 and 500 mm H_2O. The CSF is cloudy or purulent and contains a large number of cells, predominantly polymorphonuclear leukocytes. The cell count in the fluid is usually between 2,000 and 10,000 per mm³. Occasionally, it may be less than 100 and infrequently more than 20,000 per mm³. The protein content is increased. The sugar content is decreased, usually to levels below 20 mg/dl. Gram-negative diplococci can be seen intra- and extracellularly in stained smears of the fluid, and meningococci can be cultured on the appropriate media in over 90% of untreated cases. Particle agglutination procedures are more sensitive than the older counterimmunoelectrophoresis for detection of bacterial antigens and may indicate the etiologic agent sooner when the CSF is tested. However, they cannot be relied upon for definite diagnosis because of relatively low specificity and sensitivity. For meningococcus, the capsular polysaccharide is the antigen detected. In unusual instances, the CSF may demonstrate minimal or no increase in cell count and no bacteria on the Gram stain, but N. meningitidis may be isolated. Clear CSF in a patient with suspected bacterial meningitis should be carefully cultured.

Complications and Sequelae. The complications and sequelae include those commonly associated with an inflammatory process in the meninges and its blood vessels (i.e., convulsions, cranial nerve palsies, focal cerebral lesions, damage to the spinal cord or nerve roots, hydrocephalus), and those that are due to involvement of other portions of the body by meningococci (e.g., panophthalmitis and other types of ocular infection, arthritis, purpura, pericarditis, endocarditis, myocarditis, pleurisy, orchitis, epididymitis, albuminuria or hematuria, adrenal hemorrhage). Disseminated intravascular coagulation may complicate the meningitis. Complications may also arise from intercurrent infection of the upper respiratory tract, middle ear, and lungs. Any of the aforementioned complications may leave permanent residua, but the most common sequelae are due to injury of the nervous system. These include deafness, ocular palsies, blindness, changes in mentality, convulsions, and hydrocephalus. With the methods of treatment available at present, complications and sequelae of the meningeal infection are rare, and the complications due to the involvement of other parts of the body by the meningococci or other intercurrent infections are more readily controlled.

Diagnosis. Meningococcal meningitis can be diagnosed with certainty only by the isolation of the organism from the CSF. However, the diagnosis can be made with relative certainty before the organisms are isolated in a patient with headache, vomiting, chills and fever, neck stiffness, and a petechial cutaneous rash, especially if there is an epidemic of meningococcal meningitis or if there has been exposure to a known case of meningococcal meningitis.

To establish the diagnosis of meningococcal meningitis, cultures should be made of the skin lesions, nasopharyngeal secretions, blood, and CSF. Because meningococci are particularly sensitive to chilling and freezing, it is important that inoculation of the appropriate media be made promptly, preferably directly from the lumbar puncture needle. In addition, a tube containing 5 to 10 ml of CSF can be incubated for subculture after a few hours. The diagnosis can be established in most cases by examination of smears of the sediment of the CSF after application of the Gram stain.

Prognosis. The mortality rate of untreated meningococcal meningitis varied widely in different epidemics, but was usually between 50% and 90%. With present-day therapy, however, the overall mortality rate is about 10% and the incidence of complications and sequelae is low.

Features of the disease that influence the mortality rate are the age of the patient, bacteremia, day of treatment, complications, and general condition of the individual. The lowest fatality rates are seen in patients between the ages of 5 and 10, and in patients without bacteremia who are treated early in the course of the disease. The highest mortality rates occur in infants, in elderly debilitated individuals, in those who are treated late in the course of the disease, and in those with extensive hemorrhages into the adrenal gland.

Treatment. Aqueous penicillin G or ampicillin administered intravenously is the treatment of choice. If the patient is allergic to penicillin, chloramphenicol is the preferred alternative drug. The duration of treatment should be 5 to 7 days after the patient becomes afebrile. The CSF should be examined 24 to

48 hours after the initiation of treatment to assess the effectiveness of the medication. Post-treatment examination of the CSF is not a meaningful criterion of recovery, and the CSF need not be re-examined if the patient is clinically well.

Fluid balance and hydration should be monitored by the measurement of central venous pressure. Dehydration is common and fluids should be replaced by intravenous administration. Hyponatremia may be due to excessive fluid intake or inappropriate secretion of antidiuretic hormone.

If hypovolemic shock occurs, volume expansion with isotonic electrolyte solution is indicated. Vasopressors may be required. Heparinization should be considered if intravascular clotting occurs.

Phenytoin, diazepam, or phenobarbital can be used to control recurrent convulsive seizures. Cerebral edema may require the use of osmotic diuretics or the administration of corticosteroids, but only if there is evidence of early or impending cerebral herniation.

Persons who have had intimate contact with meningococcal meningitis patients may be given rifampin as a prophylactic measure.

HEMOPHILUS INFLUENZA MENINGITIS

Infections of the meninges by H. influenzae were reported as early as 1899. At present, it is the most common (around 50%) type of acute bacterial meningitis. It is predominantly a disease of infancy and early childhood; over 50% of the cases occur within the first two years of life and 90% before the age of 5. H. influenzae is the cause of about 30% of the cases of bacterial meningitis in the 5- to 10-year age-group. It is about equal in frequency to meningococcus and S. pneumoniae. After that it is decidedly rarer than the other two agents (Table 13–1). In infants and children, H. influenzae meningitis is usually primary.

In adults it is more commonly secondary to acute sinusitis, otitis media, or fracture of the skull. It is associated with CSF rhinorrhea, immunologic deficiency, diabetes mellitus, and alcoholism. Currently, cases tend to occur in the autumn and spring, with fewest occurring in the summer months.

The pathology of H. influenzae meningitis does not differ from that of other forms of acute purulent meningitis. In patients with a protracted course localized pockets of infection in the meninges or cortex, internal hydrocephalus, degeneration of cranial nerves, and focal loss of cerebral substance secondary to thrombosis of vessels may be found.

The symptoms and physical signs of H. influenzae meningitis are similar to those of other forms of acute bacterial meningitis. The disease usually lasts 10 to 20 days. It may occasionally be fulminating, and frequently it is protracted and extends over several weeks or months.

The CSF changes are similar to those described for the other acute meningitides. The organisms can be cultured from the CSF. Blood cultures are often positive early in the disease.

Complications and sequelae are common in untreated cases owing to the protracted course of the disease. These include paralysis of extraocular muscles, deafness, blindness, hemiplegia, recurrent convulsions, and mental deficiency.

The mortality rate in untreated cases in H. influenzae meningitis in infants is over 90%. The prognosis is not so grave in adults, in whom spontaneous recovery is more frequent. Adequate treatment has reduced the mortality rate to about 10%, but sequelae are not uncommon.

The diagnosis of H. influenzae meningitis is based on the isolation of the organisms

Table 13–1. Total Number of Bacterial Meningitis Cases and Fatality Rates From 27 Participating States

Organism	Cases Reported	% of Total	Case Fatality Rate
Hemophilus influenzae	6,756	48.3	6.0
Neisseria meningitidis	2,742	19.6	10.3
Streptococcus pneumoniae	1,865	13.3	26.3
Group B streptococcus	476	3.4	22.5
Listeria monocytogenes	265	1.9	28.5
Other	1,043	7.5	33.7
Unknown	827	5.9	16.4
Total	13,974	99.9	....

(From Sclech WF, et al. JAMA 1985; 253:1749–1754.)

from the CSF and blood. The type of organism can be determined by means of capsular swelling with specific rabbit antiserum. H. influenzae antigen may be demonstrated in CSF by particle agglutination. Although there are six known types, most of the infections in infants are due to type b.

The continuing emergence of organisms resistant to antibiotics and the rapid introduction of new antibiotics to combat these changes render textbook recommendations of specific antibiotics of doubtful utility. Ampicillin-resistant strains of H. influenzae have spread so widely that ampicillin alone is no longer a reliable therapy. A combination of ampicillin and chloramphenicol has been used, but third-generation cephalosporins (such as ceftriaxone) seem to provide a useful alternative with fewer side effects.

Subdural effusion, which may occur in infants with any form of meningitis, is most commonly seen in connection with H. influenzae meningitis. Persistent vomiting, bulging fontanelles, convulsion, focal neurologic signs, and persistent fever should lead to consideration of this complication. Prompt relief of the symptoms usually follows evacuation of the effusion by tapping the subdural space through the fontanelles. Persistent or secondary fever without worsening of meningeal signs may be due to an extracranial focus of infection, such as a contaminated urinary or venous catheter, or to drug administration.

PNEUMOCOCCAL MENINGITIS

The pneumococcus (Streptococcus pneumoniae) is about equal in frequency to meningococcus as a cause of meningitis, except that it is more frequent in the elderly. Meningeal infection is usually a complication of otitis media, mastoiditis, sinusitis, fractures of the skull, upper respiratory infections, and infections of the lung. Alcoholism, asplenism, and sickle cell disease predispose patients to developing pneumococcal meningitis. The infection may occur at any age, but more than 50% of the patients are less than 1 or over 50 years of age.

The clinical symptoms, physical signs, and laboratory findings in pneumococcal meningitis are the same as those of other forms of acute purulent meningitis. The diagnosis is usually made without difficulty because the CSF contains large numbers of the organisms. When gram-positive diplococci are seen in smears of the CSF or its sediment, a positive quellung reaction serves to identify both the pneumococcus and its type. Particle agglutination of CSF and serum may be helpful in demonstrating pneumococcal antigen.

Before the introduction of sulfonamides, the mortality rate in pneumococcal meningitis was almost 100%. It is now approximately 20 to 30%. The prognosis for recovery is best in cases that follow fractures of the skull and those with no known source of infection. The mortality rate is especially high when the meningitis follows pneumonia, empyema, or lung abscess, or when a persisting bacteremia indicates the presence of an endocarditis. The triad of pneumococcal meningitis, pneumonia, and endocarditis (Austrian syndrome) has a particularly high fatality rate.

Aqueous penicillin given intravenously is the drug of choice in the treatment of pneumococcal meningitis. The treatment should be continued for 12 to 15 days. Chloramphenicol is an alternative drug for adults. The primary focus of infection should be eradicated by surgery if necessary. Persistent CSF fistulas following fractures of the skull must be closed by craniotomy and suturing of the dura. Otherwise the meningitis will almost certainly recur.

STAPHYLOCOCCAL MENINGITIS

Staphylococci (S. aureus and S. epidermidis) are a relatively infrequent cause of meningitis. Meningitis may develop as a result of spread from furuncles on the face or from staphylococcal infections elsewhere in the body. It is sometimes a complication of cavernous sinus thrombosis, epidural or subdural abscess, and neurosurgical procedures involving shunting to relieve hydrocephalus. Endocarditis may be found in association with staphylococcal meningitis. Intravenous treatment with a penicillinase-resistant penicillin (nafcillin or oxacillin) is the preferred treatment. Therapy must be continued for two to four weeks. In nosocomial infections or other situations in which resistance to oxacillin is likely, treatment with vancomycin is appropriate. Complications such as ventriculitis, arachnoiditis, and hydrocephalus may occur. The original focus of infection should be eradicated. Laminectomy should be performed immediately when a spinal epidural abscess is present, and cranial subdural abscess should be drained through craniotomy openings.

STREPTOCOCCAL MENINGITIS

Infection with the streptococcus accounts for 1 to 2% of all cases of meningitis. Streptococcal meningitis is usually caused by group A organisms. The symptoms are not distinguished from other forms of meningitis. Members of other groups may occasionally be isolated from CSF. It is always secondary to some septic focus, most commonly in the mastoid or nasal sinuses. Treatment is the same as outlined for the treatment of pneumococcal meningitis together with surgical eradication of the primary focus.

MENINGITIS DUE TO OTHER BACTERIA

Meningitis in the newborn infant is most often caused by coliform gram-negative bacilli, especially Escherichia coli and group B hemolytic streptococci. It often accompanies septicemia and may show none of the typical signs of meningitis in children and adults. Instead, the infant shows irritability, lethargy, anorexia, and bulging fontanelles. Meningitis due to gram-negative enteric bacteria also occurs frequently in immunosuppressed or chronically ill, hospitalized adult patients and in persons with penetrating head injuries, neurosurgical procedures, congenital defects, or diabetes mellitus. In these circumstances, meningitis may be difficult to recognize because of altered consciousness related to the underlying illness.

A third-generation cephalosporin and an aminoglycoside are currently used for treatment of gram-negative meningitides. If Pseudomonas aeruginosa is present or suspected, ceftazidime is preferred. If initial response is poor, intraventricular administration of the aminoglycoside can be considered. Care must also be taken to insure that the organism is sensitive to the agents chosen; if not, some other antibiotic should be selected. Gram-negative bacillary meningitis has a high mortality (40 to 70%) and a high morbidity.

Meningitis due to Listeria monocytogenes may occur in adults with chronic diseases (e.g., renal disease with dialysis or transplantation, cancer, connective tissue disorders, chronic alcoholism) as well as in infants. A laboratory report of "diphtheroids" seen on Gram stain or isolated in culture should suggest the possible presence of Listeria monocytogenes. Listeria septicemia occurs in about 65% of patients. The treatment of choice for Listeria monocytogenes meningitis is ampicillin or aqueous penicillin. The illness has a mortality rate of 30 to 60% with the highest fatality rate among the elderly with malignancies.

ACUTE PURULENT MENINGITIS OF UNKNOWN CAUSE

Patients may have clinical symptoms indicative of an acute purulent meningitis but with atypical CSF findings. These patients have usually manifested nonspecific symptoms and have often been treated for several days with some form of antimicrobial therapy in dosages sufficient to modify the CSF abnormalities, but not sufficient to eradicate the infection. Their symptoms are of longer duration, they have less marked alterations of mental status, and they die later in their hospitalization than patients with proven bacterial meningitis. In these cases, the CSF pleocytosis is usually only moderate (500 to 1,000 cells/mm^3 with predominance of polymorphonuclear leukocytes), and the sugar content is normal or only slightly decreased. Organisms are not seen on stained smears and are cultured with difficulty. Repeated lumbar puncture may be helpful in arriving at the correct diagnosis. Antibiotics should be selected on the basis of epidemiologic or clinical factors. The age of the patient and the setting in which the infection occurred are the primary considerations. In patients with partially treated meningitis and in those with meningitis of unknown etiology, the drugs of choice, in general, are ampicillin (in adults); ampicillin and chloramphenicol (in children); and ampicillin and gentamicin (in neonates or when gram-negative organisms are suspected). Some third-generation cephalosporins are currently being studied as alternatives in these situations, particularly when resistance to the older antibiotics is suspected on epidemiologic grounds. Therapy should be modified if an organism different from that originally suspected is isolated or if the clinical response is less than optimal. The mortality and frequency of neurologic complications of these patients are similar to those of patients in whom the responsible bacteria have been identified.

RECURRENT BACTERIAL MENINGITIS

Repeated episodes of bacterial meningitis signal a host defect, either in local anatomy or in antibacterial and immunologic defenses. They usually follow trauma; several years may pass between the trauma and the first bout of meningitis. Streptococcus pneumoniae is the usual pathogen. Bacteria may enter the subarachnoid space through the cribriform plate, a basilar skull fracture, erosive bony changes in the mastoid, congenital dermal defects along the craniospinal axis, penetrating head injuries, or neurosurgical procedures. CSF rhinorrhea or otorrhea is often present, but may be transient. It may be detected by testing for a significant concentration of glucose in nasal or aural secretions. Treatment of recurrent meningitis is similar to that for first bouts. Cryptic CSF leaks can be demonstrated by polytomography of the frontal and mastoid regions by monitoring the course of radioiodine-labeled albumin instilled intrathecally or by CT after intrathecal injection of metrizamide. Patients with recurrent pneumococcal meningitis should be vaccinated with pneumococcal vaccine. Long-term prophylactic treatment with penicillin should be considered. Surgical closure of CSF fistulas is indicated to prevent further episodes of meningitis.

Subacute Meningitis

Subacute meningitis is usually due to infection with tubercle bacilli or mycotic organisms. The clinical syndrome differs from that of acute purulent meningitis in that the onset of symptoms is usually less acute, the degree of inflammatory reaction less severe, and the course more prolonged.

TUBERCULOUS MENINGITIS

Tuberculous meningitis differs from that caused by most of the other common bacteria in that the course is more prolonged, the mortality rate is higher, the CSF changes are less severe, and treatment is less effective in preventing sequelae.

Pathogenesis. Tuberculous meningitis is always secondary to tuberculosis elsewhere in the body. The primary focus of infection is usually in the lungs, but it may be in the lymph glands, bones, nasal sinuses, gastrointestinal tract, or any organ in the body. The onset of meningeal symptoms may coincide with signs of acute miliary dissemination or there may be clinical evidence of activity in the primary focus; however, meningitis is sometimes the only manifestation of the disease.

It has been claimed that the meningitis is almost always secondary to rupture of a cerebral tubercle into the ventriculosubarachnoid spaces. Tubercles in the nervous system of any appreciable size are rare in the United States. This fact does not mean, however, that the meningitis may not result from dissemination of the bacteria from minute or microscopic tubercles near the meningeal surfaces. In some cases, meningitis may be a manifestation of an acute miliary dissemination from other viscera, suggesting that the meningitis is due to lodgement of bacteria directly in the meninges or choroid plexus.

Pathology. The meninges on the surface of the brain and the spinal cord are cloudy and thickened, but the process is usually most intense at the base of the brain. A thick collar of fibrosis may form around the optic nerves, cerebral peduncles, and basilar surface of the pons and midbrain. The ventricles are moderately dilated and the ependymal lining is covered with exudate or appears roughened (granular ependymitis). Minute tubercles may be visible in the meninges, choroid plexus, or cerebral substances.

On microscopic examination, the exudate in the thickened meninges is composed chiefly of mononuclear cells, lymphocytes, plasma cells, macrophages, and fibroblasts with an occasional giant cell. The inflammatory process may extend for a short distance into the cerebral substance where minute granulomas may also be found. Proliferative changes are frequently seen in the inflamed vessels of the meninges, producing a panarteritis. These arteritic changes may lead to thrombosis of the vessel and formation of infarcts in the cerebral substances.

Incidence. Although tuberculous meningitis may occur at any age, it is most common in childhood and early adult life. In areas with a high incidence of tuberculosis, tuberculous meningitis is seen most commonly in infants and young children. In areas of low incidence, such as the United States, tuberculous meningitis is more common in adults. Approximately 20% of the cases develop before the age of 5 and over 80% occur before the age of 40. It is rare in patients younger than 6 months.

Symptoms. The onset is usually subacute, with headache, vomiting, fever, bursts of irritability, and nocturnal wakefulness as the most prominent symptoms. Anorexia, loss of weight, and abdominal pain may be present. The prodromal stage lasts for two weeks to three months in most cases. In young children, a history of close contact with a person known to have tuberculosis is a diagnostic help. Stiffness of the neck and vomiting become evident within a few days. Convulsive seizures are not uncommon in children during the first days of the disease. The headache becomes progressively more severe; there is bulging of the fontanelles in infants. The pain often causes the infant to emit a peculiarly shrill cry (meningeal cry). With progress of the disease, patients become stuporous or comatose. Blindness and signs of damage to other cranial nerves may appear, or there may be convulsive seizures or focal neurologic signs.

Physical Findings. The physical findings in the early stages are those associated with meningeal infection (i.e., fever, irritability, stiffness of the neck, and Kernig and Brudzinski signs). Tendon reflexes may be exaggerated or depressed. Signs of increased intracranial pressure and focal brain damage are rarely present at the onset. The initial irritability is gradually replaced by apathy, confusion, lethargy, and stupor. Papilledema, cranial nerve palsies, and focal neurologic signs are common in the late stages of the disease. There may be external ophthalmoplegia, usually incomplete, unilateral, and involving chiefly the oculomotor nerve. Ophthalmoscopy may demonstrate choroid tubercles. Clinical evidence of tuberculosis elsewhere in the body is usually present.

Convulsions, coma, and hemiplegia occur as the disease advances. The temperature, which is only moderately elevated (100° to 102° F) in the early stages, rises to high levels before death. The respiratory and pulse rates are increased. In the terminal stages, respirations become irregular and of the Cheyne-Stokes type.

Diagnosis. The diagnosis of tuberculous meningitis can be established by recovery of the organisms from the CSF. The CSF findings are, however, quite characteristic and a presumptive diagnosis can be made when the typical abnormalities are present. These include: increased pressure; slightly cloudy or ground-glass appearance of the CSF with formation of a clot on standing; moderate pleocytosis of 25 to 500 cells/mm³, with lymphocytes as the predominating cell type; increased protein content; decreased sugar content with values in the range of 20 to 40 mg/dl; a negative serologic test for syphilis; and absence of growth when the CSF is inoculated on routine culture media. Although none of the above abnormalities is diagnostic, their occurrence in combination is usually pathognomonic, and is sufficient evidence to warrant intensive therapy until the diagnosis can be confirmed by stained smears of the sediment or pellicle or by culture of the CSF. Smears of the CSF sediment demonstrate

acid-fast bacilli in 20 to 30% of patients on single examination; with repeated examinations, the yield of positive smears is increased to 75%.

Other diagnostic aids include a thorough search for a primary focus, including radiographs of the chest and tuberculin skin tests. Patients with tuberculous meningitis may have hyponatremia due to inappropriate secretion of antidiuretic hormone. CT of the brain in tuberculous meningitis may disclose enhancing exudates in the subarachnoid cisterns, hydrocephalus, areas of infarction, and associated tuberculomas.

Tuberculous meningitis must be differentiated from other forms of acute and subacute meningitis, viral infections, and meningeal reactions to septic foci in the skull or spine.

Acute purulent meningitis is characterized by a high cell count and the presence of the causative organisms in the CSF. Preliminary antibiotic therapy of purulent meningitis may cause the CSF findings to mimic those of tuberculous meningitis.

The CSF in syphilitic meningitis may show changes similar to those of tuberculous meningitis. The normal or relatively normal sugar content and the positive serologic reactions make the diagnosis of syphilitic meningitis relatively easy.

The clinical picture and CSF findings in cryptococcus meningitis may be identical with those of tuberculous meningitis. The differential diagnosis can be made by finding the budding yeast organisms in the counting chamber or in stained smears, by detecting cryptococcal antigen in CSF by the latex agglutination test, and by obtaining a culture of the fungus. Much less frequently, other mycotic infections may involve the meninges.

Meningeal involvement in the course of viral infections such as mumps, lymphocytic choriomeningitis, or other forms of viral encephalitis may give a clinical picture similar to that of tuberculous meningitis. In these cases, the CSF sugar content is usually normal.

Diffuse involvement of the meninges by metastatic tumors (carcinoma or sarcoma) or by gliogenous tumors may produce meningeal signs. The CSF may contain a number of lymphocytes and polymorphonuclear leukocytes and a reduced sugar content. The triad of mental clarity, lack of fever, and hyporeflexia suggests neoplastic meningitis. A protracted course or the finding of neoplastic cells in the CSF excludes the diagnosis of tuberculous meningitis.

CNS sarcoidosis may also cause meningitis with CSF changes similar to those of tuberculous meningitis. Failure to detect microbes by smear or culture and a protracted course are clues to the diagnosis of sarcoidosis. Leptomeningeal biopsy may be needed to establish the diagnosis, but, most patients show systemic signs of sarcoidosis in lymph nodes, liver, lung, or muscle (see Section 18, Sarcoidosis).

Prognosis and Course. The natural course of the disease is death in six to eight weeks. With early diagnosis and appropriate treatment, the recovery rate approaches 90%. Delay in diagnosis is associated with rapid progression of neurologic deficits and a poorer prognosis. Prognosis is worst at the extremes of life, particularly in the elderly. The presence of cranial nerve abnormalities on admission, confusion, lethargy, and elevated CSF protein concentration are associated with a poor prognosis. The presence of active tuberculosis in other organs or of miliary tuberculosis does not significantly affect the prognosis if antitubercular therapy is given. Relapses occasionally occur after months or even years in apparently cured patients.

Sequelae. Minor or major sequelae occur in about 25% of the patients who recover. These vary from minimal degree of facial weakness to severe intellectual and physical disorganization. Physical defects include deafness, convulsive seizures, blindness, hemiplegia, paraplegia, and quadriplegia. Intracranial calcifications may appear two to three years after the onset of the disease.

Treatment. Treatment should be started immediately without waiting for bacteriologic confirmation of the diagnosis in a patient with the characteristic clinical symptoms and CSF findings. It is generally agreed that the prognosis for recovery and freedom from sequelae are directly related to the promptness of the initiation of therapy. As initial form of therapy, isoniazid supplemented with rifampin and ethambutol is used and continued for 18 to 24 months. Intramuscular injections of streptomycin may be used. Corticosteroids may prove beneficial in the early phases of the disease when there is evidence of subarachnoid block or impending cerebral herniation. Peripheral neuropathy secondary to isoniazid treatment can be prevented by giving pyridoxine. Intrathecal therapy is not indicated.

Subdural and Epidural Infections

CEREBRAL SUBDURAL EMPYEMA

A collection of pus between the inner surface of the dura and the outer surface of the arachnoid of the brain is known as *subdural empyema.*

Etiology. Subdural empyema may result from the direct extension of injection from the middle ear, the nasal sinuses, or the meninges. It may develop as a complication of compound fractures of the skull, or in the course of septicemia. An acute attack of sinusitis just before the development of subdural empyema is common. The mechanism of the formation of subdural empyema following compound fractures of the skull is easily understood, but the factors that lead to subdural infection rather than leptomeningitis or cerebral abscess in patients with infections of the nasal sinuses or mastoids are less clear. Chronic infection of the mastoid or paranasal sinuses with thrombophlebitis of the venous sinuses or osteomyelitis and necrosis of the cranial vault commonly precedes the development of the subdural infection.

The infection is most often due to streptococcus. Other bacteria frequently recovered from subdural pus are staphylococci and gram-negative enteric organisms.

Pathology. The pathologic findings depend on the mode of entry of the infection into the subdural space. In traumatic cases, there may be osteomyelitis of the overlying skull, with or without accompanying foreign bodies. When the abscess is secondary to infection of the nasal sinuses or middle ear, thrombophlebitis of the venous sinuses or osteomyelitis of the frontal or temporal bone is a common finding. Dorsolateral and interhemispheric collections of pus are common; collections beneath the cerebral hemispheres are uncommon. After paranasal infections, subdural pus forms at the frontal poles and extends posteriorly over the convexity of the frontal lobe. After ear infection, the subdural pus passes posteriorly and medially over the falx to the tentorium and occipital poles. The brain beneath the pus is molded in a manner similar to that seen in cases of subdural hematoma. Thrombosis or thrombophlebitis of the superficial cortical veins, especially in the frontal region, is common and produces a hemorrhagic softening of the gray and white matter drained by the thrombosed vessels. The subarachnoid spaces beneath the subdural empyema are filled with a purulent exudate, but there is no generalized leptomeningitis in the initial stage.

Incidence. Subdural empyema is a relatively rare form of intracranial infection, occurring less than half as frequently as brain abscess. It may develop at any age, but is most common in children and young adults. Males are more frequently affected than females.

Symptoms and Signs. Symptoms include those associated with the focus or origin of the infection and those due to the intracranial extension. Local pain and tenderness are present in the region of the infected nasal sinus or ear. Orbital swelling is usually present when the injection is secondary to frontal sinus disease. Chills, fever, and severe headache are common initial symptoms of the intracranial involvement. Neck stiffness and Kernig sign are present. With progress of the infection, the patient lapses into a confused, somnolent, or comatose state. Thrombophlebitis of the cortical veins is manifested by jacksonian or generalized convulsions and by the appearance of focal neurologic signs (e.g., hemiplegia, aphasia, paralysis of conjugate deviation of the eyes, cortical sensory loss). In the late stages, the intracranial pressure is increased and papilledema may occur. The entire clinical picture may evolve in as little as a few hours or as long as 10 days.

Laboratory Data. A marked peripheral leukocytosis is usually present. Radiographs of the skull may show evidence of infection of the mastoid or nasal sinuses or of osteomyelitis of the skull. The CSF is under increased pressure. It is usually clear and colorless, and there is a moderate pleocytosis, varying from 25 to 500 cells/mm^3 with 10 to 80% polymorphonuclear leukocytes. In some patients, the CSF cellular response may be composed chiefly of lymphocytes or mononuclear cells; other patients may not show any cells in the CSF. The protein content is increased, with values commonly in the range of 75 to 150 mg/dl. The sugar content is normal and the CSF is sterile unless the subdural infection is secondary to a purulent leptomeningitis. Spinal puncture should be done with caution because instances of transtentorial herniation within eight hours after lumbar puncture have been described in this condition. Lumbar puncture should be avoided if the diagnosis can be established in other ways.

CT of the head characteristically demonstrates a crescent-shaped area of hypodensity at the periphery of the brain and mass displacement of the cerebral ventricles and midline structures. There usually is contrast enhancement between the empyema and cerebral cortex. CT may fail, however, to define the pus collection in some patients with typical clinical presentations. The combination of CT and cerebral angiography is considered the radiographic procedure of choice.

EEG is unreliable in the diagnosis of subdural empyema. The value of radionuclide scanning is limited.

Diagnosis. The diagnosis of subdural empyema should be considered whenever meningeal symptoms or focal neurologic signs develop in patients presenting evidence of a suppurative process in nasal sinuses, mastoid process, or other cranial structures.

Subdural empyema must be differentiated from other intracranial complications of infections in the ear or nasal sinus. These include extradural abscess, sinus thrombosis, and brain abscess. The presence of focal neurologic signs and neck stiffness is against the diagnosis of extradural abscess. In addition, patients are not as acutely ill with an infection limited to the extradural space.

The differential diagnosis between subdural empyema and septic thrombosis of the superior longitudinal sinus is difficult because focal neurologic signs and convulsive seizures are common to both conditions. In fact, thrombosis of sinus or its tributaries is a frequent complication of subdural empyema. Factors in favor of the diagnosis of sinus thrombosis are a septic temperature and the absence of signs of meningeal irritation. Subdural empyema can also be confused with viral encephalitis or various types of meningitis. The diagnosis may be obscured by early antibiotic therapy.

Brain abscess can be distinguished by the relatively insidious onset and the protracted course.

Clinical Course. The mortality rate is high (25 to 40%) because of failure to make an early diagnosis. If the disorder is untreated, death commonly follows the onset of focal neurologic signs within 6 days. Uncontrollable cerebral edema contributes to a lethal outcome. The causes of death are dural venous sinus thrombosis, fulminant meningitis, and multiple intracerebral abscesses. With prompt evacuation of the pus and chemotherapy, recovery is possible even after focal neurologic signs have appeared. Gradual improvement of the focal neurologic signs is to be expected after recovery from the infection. However, seizures, hemiparesis and other focal deficits may be long-term sequelae.

Treatment. The treatment of subdural empyema is prompt surgical evacuation of the pus through trephine operation, carefully avoiding passage through the infected nasal sinuses. Systemic therapy with penicillin and chloramphenicol or other antimicrobials is begun before surgery and continued until the infection is brought under control. Antibiotics are commonly instilled into the subdural space at the time of operation. Treatment of cerebral edema is also a necessity.

INTRACRANIAL EPIDURAL ABSCESS

Abscesses confined to the epidural space are frequent and are almost always associated with overlying infection in the cranial bones. Penetration from chronic sinusitis or mastoiditis is most common, but infection following head trauma or neurosurgery may also cause this problem. Frequently intracranial epidural abscess is associated with deeper penetration of the infection and subdural empyema, meningitis, or intraparenchymal abscess. Severe headache, fever, malaise, and findings referable to the initial site of infection are the features of isolated intracranial epidural abscess. Focal neurologic findings are rarely present. Diagnosis is made most easily by CT scanning which usually demonstrates a characteristic extradural defect (Fig. 13–1), but sometimes a small abscess is difficult to detect. Repeat scanning is necessary if headache persists despite antibiotic treatment of an infected sinus or other focus. Evaluation of cerebrospinal fluid is not of great help. The protein may be modestly elevated and a mild pleocytosis may be present, but organisms are not seen on gram stain and cultures are routinely negative. Lumbar puncture is certainly to be discouraged until after it has been established by scanning that significant mass effect is not present. The role of MRI scanning is yet to be determined. As with most abscesses, surgical drainage is usually necessary to ensure cure. However, if it appears from the scan and lack of neurologic findings that the infection is confined to the epidural space, trephination may suffice and a craniotomy can be avoided. Appropriate antibiotic treatment is mandatory and is the same as that for subdural empyema, because the sources of infection are similar. It is not clear whether irrigation of the epidural space with antibiotic is useful.

SPINAL EPIDURAL ABSCESS

Spinal epidural abscess is a collection of purulent material located outside the dura mater within the spinal canal. Infections of the spinal epidural space are accompanied by fever, headache, pain in the back, weakness of the lower extremities and, finally, complete paraplegia.

Etiology. Infections may reach the fatty tissue in the spinal epidural space by one of three routes: (1) direct extension from inflammatory processes in adjacent tissues, such as decubitus ulcers, carbuncles, or perinephric abscesses; (2) metastasis through the blood from infections elsewhere in the body; and (3) perforating wounds, spinal surgery, or lumbar puncture. The first route of infection accounts for most cases. The primary site of infection is often a furuncle on the skin, but septic foci in the tonsils, teeth, lungs, uterus, or other organ may metastasize to the epidural fat. Chronic debilitating diseases, diabetes mellitus, immunosuppressive therapy, and heroin abuse are contributing factors.

Staphylococcus aureus accounts for 50 to 60% of epidural abscesses. Other bacteria responsible include E. coli, other gram-negative organisms, and hemolytic and anaerobic streptococci.

Pathology. No region of the spine is immune to infection, but the midthoracic vertebrae are most frequently affected. The character of the osteomyelitis in the vertebra is similar to that encountered in other bones of the body. The laminae are most commonly involved, but any part of the vertebra, including the body, may be the seat of the infection. The infection in the epidural space may be acute or chronic.

In acute cases, which are by far the most common, a purulent necrosis of the epidural fat extends over several segments of the entire length of the cord. The pus is usually posterior to the spinal cord, but may be on the anterior surface. When the infecting organism is of low virulence, the infection may localize and assume a granulomatous nature.

The lesions in the spinal cord depend on the extent to which the infection has progressed before treatment is begun. Necrosis in the periphery of the cord may result from pressure of the abscess, or myelomalacia of one or several segments may occur when the veins or arteries are thrombosed. There is ascending degeneration above and descending degeneration below the level of the necrotic

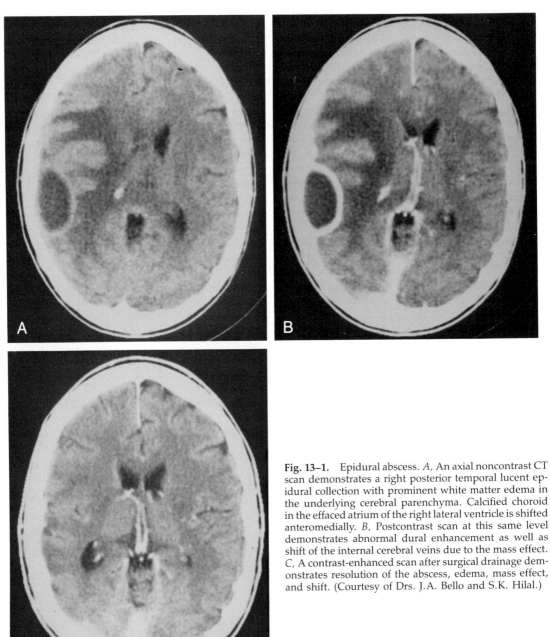

Fig. 13–1. Epidural abscess. *A,* An axial noncontrast CT scan demonstrates a right posterior temporal lucent epidural collection with prominent white matter edema in the underlying cerebral parenchyma. Calcified choroid in the effaced atrium of the right lateral ventricle is shifted anteromedially. *B,* Postcontrast scan at this same level demonstrates abnormal dural enhancement as well as shift of the internal cerebral veins due to the mass effect. *C,* A contrast-enhanced scan after surgical drainage demonstrates resolution of the abscess, edema, mass effect, and shift. (Courtesy of Drs. J.A. Bello and S.K. Hilal.)

lesion. The substance of the spinal cord may occasionally be infected by extension through the meninges, with the formation of a spinal cord abscess.

Incidence. Spinal epidural abscesses account for approximately 1 of every 20,000 admissions to United States hospitals. They can occur at all ages; 60% affect adults between 20 and 50 years of age.

Symptoms and Signs. The symptoms of acute spinal epidural abscess develop suddenly, several days or weeks following an infection of the skin or other parts of the body. The preceding infection may occasionally be so slight that it is overlooked. Severe back pain is usually the presenting symptom. Malaise, fever, neck stiffness, and headache may be present or follow in a few days. Usually within hours, but sometimes not for several weeks, initial symptoms are followed by radicular pain. If the abscess is untreated, muscular weakness and paralysis of the legs may develop suddenly.

Fever and malaise are usually present in the early phase; lethargy or irritability develops as the disease progresses. There is neck stiffness and a Kernig sign. Local percussion tenderness over the spine is an important diagnostic sign. Tendon reflexes may be increased or decreased, and the plantar responses may be extensor. With thrombosis of the spinal vessels, a flaccid paraplegia occurs with complete loss of sensation below the level of the lesion and paralysis of the bladder or rectum. Immediately after the onset of paraplegia, tendon reflexes are absent in the paralyzed extremities. There is often erythema and swelling in the area of back pain.

In chronic cases in which the infection is localized and there is granuloma formation, the neurologic signs are similar to those seen with other types of extradural tumors. Fever is rare; weakness and paralysis may not develop for weeks or months.

Laboratory Data. In acute cases, leukocytosis is present in the blood. The erythrocyte sedimentation rate is usually elevated. Radiographs of the spine are usually normal, but may show osteomyelitis or a contiguous abscess (Fig. 13–2).

Myelography is almost invariably abnormal. Complete extradural block is found in 80% of patients; the others demonstrate partial block. It is critically important to consider the possibility of epidural abscess in any case of acute or subacute myelopathy, because lumbar puncture may penetrate the pus and

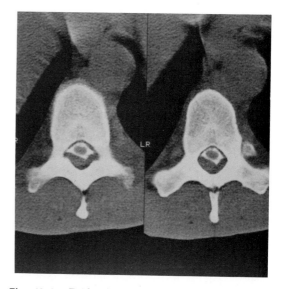

Fig. 13–2. Epidural abscess. Axial CT myelography demonstrates abnormal epidural soft tissue density posterior to and deforming the thecal sac, with anterior displacement of the cord at this lower thoracic level. (Courtesy of Dr. S.K. Hilal.)

carry infection into the subarachnoid space. When complete block or a lower thoracic-lumbar abscess is suspected, myelography should be performed by cervical puncture. The needle should be advanced slowly and suction applied with a syringe as the epidural space is approached. If the abscess has extended to the level of the puncture, pus may be withdrawn for culture and the procedure terminated.

Epidural abscesses can be demonstrated by spinal CT, with or without use of intravenous contrast material. Until the reliability of this procedure is fully established, myelography should still be performed if CT does not demonstrate an abscess that is clinically suspected. The value of MRI for this diagnosis has yet to be determined.

CSF pressure is normal or increased and there is complete or almost complete subarachnoid block. The CSF is xanthochromic or cloudy in appearance. There is usually a slight or moderate pleocytosis in the CSF, varying from a few to several hundred cells/mm^3. Rarely, no cells may be present. The protein content is increased with values commonly between 100 and 1,500 mg/dl. The CSF sugar content is normal and CSF cultures are sterile unless meningitis has developed.

Diagnosis. A presumptive diagnosis can be made when subarachnoid block is found in a patient with back and leg pain of acute onset with back tenderness and signs of meningeal irritation. This is true when there is a history of recent pyogenic infection. The diagnosis should be made before signs of transection of the cord develop.

Acute spinal epidural abscess must be differentiated from acute or subacute meningitis, acute poliomyelitis, infectious polyneuritis, acute transverse myelitis, multiple sclerosis and epidural hematoma. The clinical, CSF and myelography findings are sufficient to differentiate these conditions.

Chronic epidural abscess may be confused with chronic adhesive arachnoiditis or tumors in the epidural space.

The diagnosis of granulomatous infection is rarely made before operation. The signs are those of chronic cord compression. Operation is indicated by the presence of these signs and evidence of spinal subarachnoid block.

Course and Prognosis. If treatment is delayed in acute spinal epidural abscess, complete or incomplete transection syndrome almost invariably develops. Flaccid paraplegia, sphincter paralysis, and sensory loss below the level of the lesion persist throughout the life of the individual.

The mortality rate is approximately 30% in the acute cases and 10% in the chronic cases. Death may occur in acute cases as a direct result of the infection or secondary to complications. Total recovery may occur in patients who do not have total paralysis or who have weakness lasting less than 36 hours. Fifty percent of patients paralyzed for 48 hours or more progress to permanent paralysis and death.

Treatment. The treatment of spinal epidural abscess is prompt surgical drainage by laminectomy. Antibiotics should be administered before and after the operation. Aerobic and anaerobic cultures should be obtained at operation. The area of suppuration should be irrigated with an antibiotic solution. Delay in draining the abscess may result in permanent paralysis. Little improvement can be expected in acute cases with signs of transection if the operation is performed after they occur because these signs are caused by softening of the spinal cord secondary to thrombosis of the spinal vessels. In chronic cases where compression of the cord plays a role in the production of the signs, considerable improvement in the neurologic symptoms and signs may be expected after the operation.

When there is back pain with minimal or no neurologic abnormality, surgery may not be needed, but epidural aspiration for culture is used to guide antibiotic therapy, followed by CT monitoring of the course. This is potentially perilous because progression of neurologic dysfunction can be rapid and irreversible. Close observation and immediate surgical drainage are necessary if neurologic deterioration occurs.

Leprosy

Leprosy (Hansen disease) is a chronic disease due to infection by Mycobacterium leprae, which has a predilection for the skin and the peripheral nerves. The bacillus has this predilection for mucous membranes and skin, including superficial nerves, because these are the cooler areas of the body where the temperature is ideal for multiplication. Two major clinical types are recognized: lepromatous and tuberculoid.

Etiology. Mycobacterium leprae is an acid-fast, rod-shaped organism morphologically similar to the tubercle bacillus. The organism can be demonstrated in the cutaneous lesion and is sometimes present in the blood of lepromatous patients. The disease is transmitted by direct contact, which must be intimate and prolonged because the contagiousness is low. The portal of entry is probably through abrasions in the skin or mucous membranes of the upper respiratory tract. The incubation period is long, averaging three to four years in children and longer in adults. Transmission from patients with tuberculoid leprosy is rare.

Pathology. The affected nerve trunks are diffusely thickened or are studded with nodular swellings. There is an overgrowth of connective tissue with degeneration of the axon and myelin sheath. Bacilli are present in the perineurium and endoneural septa. They have also been found in dorsal root ganglia, spinal cord, and brain, but they do not produce any significant lesions within the CNS. Degenerative changes in the posterior funiculi of the cord, which are found in some cases, can be attributed to the peripheral neuritis.

Incidence. Leprosy is most common in tropical and subtropical climates, and it is estimated that 10 to 20 million people are infected. The disease is prevalent in South and Central America, China, India, and Africa. It is uncommon in Europe or North America. In the United States, the disease is mostly confined to Louisiana, Texas, Florida, Southern California, Hawaii, and New York. The number of new cases in the United States has increased in recent years because of immigration from endemic areas.

Children are especially susceptible to the disease, but it may occur in adults. In childhood, the disease is evenly distributed between the two sexes, but among adults, men are more frequently affected than women.

Symptoms and Signs. In most cases, a mixture of cutaneous and peripheral nerve lesions occurs. Neurologic involvement is more frequent and occurs early in the tuberculoid form. The earliest manifestation of neural leprosy is an erythematous macule, the lepride. This lesion grows by peripheral extension to form an annular macule. The macule has an atrophic, depigmented center that is partially or completely anesthetic. These lesions may attain an enormous size and cover the major portion of one extremity or the torso. Infection of the nerve may result in the formation of nodules or fusiform swelling along its course. Although any of the peripheral nerves may be affected, the disease has a predilection for the ulnar, great auricular, posterior tibial, common peroneal, and the fifth and seventh cranial nerves. These nerves are involved at locations where their course is superficial. Repeated attacks of neuralgic pains often precede the onset of weakness or sensory loss.

Cranial Nerves. Involvement of the fifth nerve is manifested by the appearance of patches of anesthesia on the face. Involvement of the entire sensory distribution of the nerve or its motor division is rare. Keratitis, ulceration, and blindness may ensue as results of injury to the anesthetic cornea. Complete paralysis of the facial nerve is rare, but weakness of a portion of one or several muscles is common. The muscles of the upper half of the face are most severely affected. Partial paralysis of the orbicularis and other facial muscles may result in lagophthalmos, ectropion, and facial asymmetry. Involvement of the oculomotor or other cranial nerves is rare.

Motor System. Weakness and atrophy develop in the muscles innervated by the affected nerves. There is wasting of the small muscles of the hands and feet, with later extension to the forearm and leg, but the proximal muscles are usually spared. Clawing of the hands or feet is common, but wrist-drop and foot-drop are late manifestations. Fasciculations may occur and contractures may develop.

Sensory System. Cutaneous sensation is impaired or lost in the distribution of the affected nerves in a somewhat irregular or patchy fashion. Various types of dissociated sensory impairment are seen. The sensory impairment may be of a nerve or root distribution, but more commonly it is of a glove-and-stocking type. Deep sensation, pressure pain, the appreciation of vibration, and position sense are usually spared or are less severely affected than superficial cutaneous sensation.

Reflexes. Tendon reflexes are usually preserved until late advanced stages of nerve damage when they are reduced or lost. The abdominal skin reflexes and plantar responses are normal.

Other Signs. Vasomotor and trophic disturbances are usually present. Anhydrosis and cyanosis of the hands and feet are common. Trophic ulcers develop on the knuckles and on the plantar surface of the feet. There may be various arthropathies as well as resorption of the bones of the fingers, starting in the terminal phalanges and progressing upward. The skin shrinks as digits become shorter and finally the nail may be attached to a small stump.

Laboratory Data. There are no diagnostic changes in the blood, although mild anemia and an increased erythrocyte sedimentation rate may be seen. As many as 33% of lepromatous patients have false-positive serologic tests for syphilis. The only CSF abnormality is a slight increase in the protein content.

Diagnosis. The diagnosis of leprosy is made without difficulty from the characteristic skin and neuritis lesions. The clinical picture may occasionally have a superficial similarity to that of syringomyelia, hypertrophic interstitial neuritis, or von Recklinghausen disease. The correct diagnosis is usually not difficult if the possibility of leprosy is kept in mind and scrapings from cutaneous lesions and nerve biopsy specimens are examined for acid-fast bacilli.

Course and Prognosis. The prognosis in the neural form (primarily tuberculoid) of the disease is less grave than in the cutaneous form (primarily lepromatous), in which death within 10 to 20 years is the rule. Neural leprosy is not necessarily fatal. The progress of the neuritis is slow and the disease may come to a spontaneous arrest or be controlled by therapy. Incapacitation may result from the paralyses and disfigurement.

Treatment. Dapsone (4,4-diamino-diphenylsulphone, DDS), a folate antagonist, is the primary drug for treatment. Therapy must be continued for years, if not for life, especially for lepromatous leprosy. In lepromatous disease, because of the development of drug resistance, multiple-drug therapy is now recommended. Rifampin or clofazimine is combined with dapsone. Patients with sulfone-resistant bacilli are best treated with rifampin and clofazimine.

Rickettsial Infections

Rickettsiae are obligate intracellular parasites about the size of bacteria. They are visible in microscopic preparations as pleomorphic coccobacilli. Each of the rickettsiae pathogenic for humans is capable of multiplying in arthropods as well as in animals and humans. They have a gram-negative-like cell wall and an internal structure similar to bacteria (i.e., with a prokaryotic DNA arrangement and ribosomes). Diseases due to rickettsiae are divided into five groups on the basis of their biologic properties and epidemiologic features: (1) typhus, (2) spotted fever, (3) scrub typhus, (4) Q fever, and (5) trench fever. Invasion of the nervous system is common only in infections with organisms of the first three groups.

TYPHUS FEVER

Three types of infection with rickettsiae of the typhus group are recognized: (1) primary louse-borne epidemic typhus; (2) its recrudescent form, Brill-Zinsser disease; and (3) flea-borne endemic murine typhus.

Pathology. The pathologic changes are most severe in the skin, but the heart, lungs, and CNS are also involved. The brain is edematous and minute petechial hemorrhages are present. The characteristic microscopic lesions are small round nodules composed of elongated microglia, lymphocytes, and endothelial cells. These are scattered diffusely throughout the nervous system in close relation to the smaller vessels. Vessels in the center of the lesions show severe degenerative changes. The endothelial cells are swollen and the lumen may be occluded. In addition to the microglial nodules, there is a mild degree of perivascular infiltration in the meninges and parenchyma.

Incidence. Since its recognition as a disease entity in the sixteenth century, typhus has been known as one of the great epidemic diseases of the world. It is especially prevalent in war times or whenever there is a massing of people in camps, prisons, or ships.

Epidemic typhus (caused by R. prowazekii) is spread among humans by the human body louse (Pediculus humanus corporis). Outbreaks of epidemic typhus last occurred in the United States in the nineteenth century. The freedom of the population from lice explains the absence of epidemics in the United States. Sporadic cases in the U.S. have been associated with flying squirrel contact. The location of the disease is now limited to the Balkans and Middle East, North Africa, Asia, Mexico, and the Andes. In the epidemic form, all age groups are affected.

Rickettsiae may remain viable for as long as 20 years in the tissues of recovered patients without manifest symptoms. Brill-Zinsser disease is a recrudescence of epidemic typhus that occurs years after the initial attack and may cause a new epidemic.

Murine typhus (R. typhi) is worldwide in distribution and is distributed to humans by fleas. The disease is most prevalent in Southeastern and Gulf-Coast states and among individuals whose occupations bring them into rat-infested areas. The disease is most common in the late summer and fall months. Control of rats and their fleas has resulted in a marked reduction of murine typhus in the U.S.

Symptoms and Signs. The incubation period lasts about 15 days. The onset of symptoms is abrupt, with fever, prostration, and muscular aches and pains. The skin eruption appears on the third to seventh day as pink, erythematous macules, profusely scattered over the trunk and limbs. Symptoms of involvement of the nervous system are present in practically all cases. Intractable and persistent headache, neck stiffness, and delirium are early manifestations. Later there may be various degrees of coma, convulsive seizures, and signs of focal damage to the cerebrum, spinal cord, or cranial and peripheral nerves. Coarse tremors may appear. Urinary and fecal incontinence are seen in moderately or severely ill patients.

Laboratory Data. The white cell count in the blood is usually normal. Proteinuria, hematuria, and oliguria commonly occur. Agglutinating antibodies for Proteus OX19 (Weil-Felix reaction) appear in the serum after the fifth day except in Brill-Zinsser disease. CSF pressure is usually normal but may be slightly increased. The CSF is clear but contains a small or moderate number of white cells (25 to 200/mm^3), usually lymphocytes. The CSF protein content is slightly increased, but the sugar is normal.

Diagnosis. A presumptive diagnosis of typhus fever can be made on the basis of the characteristic skin rash and signs of involvement of the nervous system. The diagnosis is established by the Weil-Felix reaction, which becomes positive in the fifth to eighth day of the disease. The titer rises in the first few weeks of the convalescence and then falls. Antibodies to specific rickettsiae can be demonstrated by complement fixation, microagglutination, or immunofluorescence reactions.

Course and Prognosis. The course of typhus fever usually extends over two to three weeks. Death from epidemic typhus usually occurs between the ninth and eighteenth day of illness. In patients who recover, the temperature begins to fall after 14 to 18 days and reaches normal levels in two to four days. Complications include bronchitis and bronchopneumonia, myocardial degeneration, gangrene of the skin or limbs, and thrombosis of large abdominal, pulmonary, or cerebral vessels.

The prognosis of epidemic typhus depends on the patient's age and immunization status. The disease is usually mild in children younger than 10. After the third decade, mortality increases steadily with each decade. Death is usually due to the development of pneumonia, circulatory collapse, and renal failure. The mortality rate in murine typhus in the United States is low (less than 1%). There are no neurologic residua in patients who recover.

Treatment. Chloramphenicol, tetracycline, and doxycycline are effective agents in the treatment of rickettsial infections. Supportive measures include parenteral fluids, sedation, analgesics for headache, oxygen, and skin care. The vector must be removed from the patient's body and surroundings by appropriate measures.

ROCKY MOUNTAIN SPOTTED FEVER

Rocky Mountain spotted fever is an acute endemic febrile disease produced by infection with the Rickettsia rickettsii. It is transmitted to humans by various ticks, the most common of which are the Dermacentor andersoni (wood tick) in the Rocky Mountain and Pacific Coast states and Dermacentor variabilis (dog tick) in the East and South. Rabbits, squirrels, and other small rodents serve as hosts for the ticks and are responsible for maintaining the infection in nature. Diseases of the Rocky Mountain spotted fever group are present throughout the world.

Pathology. The lesions of spotted fever are similar to those of typhus. In addition to the glial nodules and perivascular infiltration, minute areas of focal necrosis in the nervous system are common as the result of thrombosis of small arterioles.

Incidence. The disease has been reported from almost all states, as well as from Canada, Mexico and South America. Approximately 1000 cases are reported annually in the United States, mostly from rural areas. Most cases are seen during the period of maximal tick activity—the late spring and early summer months.

Symptoms and Signs. A history of tick bite is elicited in 80% of affected patients. The incubation period varies from 3 to 12 days. The onset is usually abrupt, with severe headache, fever, chills, myalgias, arthralgias, restlessness, prostration and, at times, delirium and coma. A rose-red, maculopapular rash appears between the second and sixth day (usually on the fourth febrile day) on the wrists, ankles, palms, soles, and forearms. The rash rapidly spreads to the legs, arms, and chest. The rash becomes petechial and fails to fade on pressure by about the fourth day.

Neurologic symptoms occur early and are frequently a prominent feature. Headache, restlessness, insomnia, and back stiffness are common. Delirium of coma alternating with restlessness is present during the height of the fever. Tremors, athetoid movements, convulsions, opisthotonos, and muscular rigidity may occur. Retinal venous engorgement, retinal edema, papilledema, retinal exudates, and choroiditis may occur. Deafness, visual disturbances, slurred speech, and mental confusion may be present and may persist for a few weeks following recovery.

Laboratory Data. The laboratory findings are similar to those of typhus fever, except that leukocytosis in the blood is more common. Proteinuria and hematuria are commonly found. The CSF is usually normal. A few patients have a mild to moderate CSF pleocytosis. Eosinophilic meningitis has been reported.

Diagnosis. The diagnosis is made on the basis of the development of the characteristic rash and other symptoms of the disease following exposure to ticks. Clinical distinction from typhus fever may be impossible. The onset of the rash in distal parts of the limbs favors a diagnosis of Rocky Mountain spotted fever. In rare instances, however, neurologic signs may present before the rash appears. A rise in antibody titer during the second week of illness can be detected by specific complement fixation, immunofluorescence and microagglutination tests, or by the Weil-Felix reaction with Proteus OX19 and OX2.

Course and Prognosis. In patients who recover, the fever falls at about the end of the third week, although mild cases may become afebrile before the end of the second week. Convalescence may be slow, and residuals of damage to the nervous system may persist for several months.

In untreated cases, the overall case fatality is about 20%. Prognosis depends on the severity of the infection, host factors (e.g., age, the presence of other illness), and the promptness with which antimicrobial treatment is started.

Treatment. Control measures include personal care and vaccination. Tick-infested areas should be avoided. If exposure is necessary, high boots, leggings, or socks should be worn outside the trouser legs. Body and clothing should be inspected after exposure, and attached ticks should be removed with tweezers. The hands should be carefully washed after handling the ticks. Workers whose occupations require constant exposure to tick-infested regions should be vaccinated yearly, just before the advent of the tick season.

The treatment of Rocky Mountain spotted fever is the prompt administration of a tetracycline antibiotic or chloramphenicol. Any patient seriously considered to have Rocky Mountain spotted fever should be treated promptly while diagnostic tests proceed.

SCRUB TYPHUS

Scrub typhus is an infectious disease caused by R. tsutsugamushi (R. orientalis), which is transmitted to humans by the bite of larval trombiculid mites (chiggers). It resembles the other rickettsial diseases and is characterized by sudden onset of fever, cutaneous eruption, and the presence of an ulcerative lesion (eschar) at the site of attachment of the chigger.

Epidemiology. The disease is limited to eastern and southeastern Asia, India, and northern Australia and adjacent islands.

Pathology. In the brain, there is a vasculitis and perivasculitis similar to those found in other organs. In addition, there is lymphocytic infiltration of the meninges, perivascular cuffing in the parenchyma, and the formation of glial nodules similar to those of epidemic or murine typhus.

Symptoms and Signs. The disease begins abruptly, following an incubation period of 10 to 12 days, with fever, chills and headache. The headache increases in intensity and may become severe. Conjunctival congestion, moderate generalized lymphadenopathy, deafness, apathy, and anorexia are common symptoms. Delirium, coma, restlessness, and muscular twitchings are present in severe cases. A primary lesion (the eschar) is seen in nearly all cases and represents the former site of attachment of the infected mite. There may be multiple eschars. The cutaneous rash appears between the fifth and eighth day of the disease. The eruption is macular or maculopapular and nonhemorrhagic. The trunk is involved first with later extension to the limbs.

Laboratory Data. The white blood cell count may be normal or low in the early stages, but a slight leukocytosis is not uncommon in the second week. Occasional clotting disturbances, including disseminated intravascular coagulation, have been reported. There is a moderate pleocytosis and an increase in CSF protein content.

Diagnosis. The diagnosis is made on the basis of the development of typical symptoms, the presence of the characteristic eschar, and a rising titer to Proteus OXK in the Weil-Felix test during the second week of illness. Immunofluorescence testing with specific antigens may be diagnostic.

Course and Prognosis. In fatal cases, death usually occurs in the second or third week as a result of pneumonia, cardiac failure, or cerebral involvement. In the preantibiotic era mortality could reach 60% depending on geographic locale and virulence of the strain. Deaths are rare with appropriate antibiotic treatment.

In patients who recover, the temperature begins to fall at the end of the second or third week. Permanent residua are not common, but the period of convalescence may extend over several months.

Treatment. The treatment of scrub typhus is the same as that described for typhus fever.

Other Bacterial Infections

BRUCELLOSIS

Brucellosis (undulant fever) is a disease with protean manifestation due to infection with short, slender, rod-shaped, gram-negative microorganisms of the genus Brucella. The infection is transmitted to man from animals, usually cattle or swine. The illness is prone to occur in slaughterhouse workers, livestock producers, veterinarians, and persons who ingest unpasteurized milk or milk products. An acute febrile illness is characteristic of the early stages of the disease. The common symptoms include chilly sensations, sweats, fever, weakness, and generalized malaise; 70% of patients experience body aches and nearly 50% complain of headache. However, physical signs of lymphadenopathy, splenomegaly, hepatomegaly, and tenderness of the spine are infrequent, occurring in less than a fourth of cases. This is followed by the subacute and chronic stages in about 15 to 20% of patients with localized infection of the bones, joints, lungs, kidneys, liver, lymph nodes, and other organs.

Involvement of the nervous system is rare. A few cases have been reported with symptoms and signs of optic neuritis, meningo-encephalitis, meningomyelitis, or peripheral neuritis.

The CSF in reported cases is under increased pressure, with a pleocytosis varying from a few to several hundred cells. The protein content is moderately to greatly increased, and the sugar content is decreased. The CSF has increased gamma globulin levels and often contains Brucella-agglutinating antibodies.

In a few patients with CNS involvement that came to autopsy, there was a subacute meningitis with perivascular infiltrations, thickening of the vessels in the brain and spinal cord, and degenerative changes in the white and gray matter. Organisms have been cultured from the CSF of a few cases.

The diagnosis is made from a history of previous symptoms of the disease, culture of the organisms from the blood or CSF, and serologic testing.

Treatment is with tetracycline for six weeks and streptomycin for two weeks. The prolonged treatment produces a lower relapse rate.

BEHÇET SYNDROME

An inflammatory disorder of unknown cause, characterized by the occurrence of relapsing uveitis and recurrent genital and oral ulcers, was described by Behçet in 1937. The disease may involve the nervous system, skin, joints, peripheral blood vessels, and other organs. Evidence of CNS involvement is present in 25 to 30% of patients. Neurologic symptoms antedate the more diagnostic criteria of aphthous stomatitis, genital ulcerations, and uveitis in only 5% of cases. Pathologic confirmation of cerebral involvement has been obtained in a few cases. The disease appears to have a predilection for young adult men.

Etiology and Pathology. The cause of Behçet syndrome is unknown. No infectious agent has been consistently isolated, although there have been several reports of a virus having been recovered from patients with the disease. Lymphocytes from Behçet syndrome patients inhibit the growth of herpes simplex virus, and RNA complementary to herpes simplex virus has been detected in patients' mononuclear cells. Circulating immune complexes of the IgA and IgG variety may be detected in patients' serums. The disease is associated with HLA-B5 tissue type in Japan and the Mediterranean nations.

In patients studied at necropsy, there was a mild inflammatory reaction in the meninges and in the perivascular spaces of the cerebrum, basal ganglia, brain stem, and cerebellum, and degenerative changes in the ganglion cells. Inflammatory changes were also found in the iris, choroid, retina, and optic nerve.

Incidence. The disease is common in northern Japan, Turkey, and Israel; the incidence in Japan is 1 per 10,000. The syndrome is less commonly seen in the United States. An annual incidence of 1 per 300,000 was determined for Olmstead County, Minnesota. The age of onset is in the third and fourth decades of life; men are more frequently affected than women. The exact incidence of neurologic symptoms is not known, but it approximates 10% of affected individuals.

Symptoms and Signs. The ocular signs include keratoconjunctivitis, iritis, hypopyon, uveitis, and hemorrhage into the vitreous. Ocular symptoms occur in 90% of patients. These may progress to total blindness in one or both eyes. The cutaneous lesions are in the nature of painful recurrent and indolent ulcers, which are most commonly found on the genitalia or the buccal mucosa. Virtually all patients have recurrent oral aphthous ulcers. Arthritis occurs in about 50% of patients. Furunculosis, erythema nodosum, thrombophlebitis, and nonspecific skin sensitivity are also common. Patients with Behçet syndrome often develop a pustule surrounded by erythema at the site of a needle puncture; when present, the finding is considered virtually pathognomonic.

Any portion of the nervous system may be affected. Cranial nerve palsies are common. Other symptoms and signs include papilledema, convulsions, mental confusion, coma, aphasia, hemiparesis, quadriparesis, pseudobulbar palsy, and evidence of involvement of the basal ganglia, cerebellum, or spinal cord.

Laboratory Data. A low-grade fever is common during the acute exacerbations of the disease. This may be accompanied by an elevation of the sedimentation rate, anemia, and a slight leukocytosis in the blood. A polyclonal increase in serum gamma globulin may be present. Coagulation profile may disclose elevated levels of fibrinogen and factor VIII.

The CSF pressure may be slightly increased. There is a pleocytosis of a mild or moderate degree, and a moderate increase in the protein content. CSF sugar, when reported, has been normal. The serologic tests for syphilis are negative in the blood and CSF. Elevation of the CSF gamma globulin content has been reported. CSF cultures have been negative. Mild diffuse abnormalities may be found on the EEG. CT may demonstrate lesions of decreased density that may be contrast enhancing.

Diagnosis. The diagnosis is based on the occurrence of signs of a meningoencephalitis in combination with the characteristic cutaneous and ocular lesions. The disease may simulate multiple sclerosis with multifocal involvement of the nervous system including the brain stem, cerebellum, and corticospinal tract. Syphilis is excluded by the negative serologic tests. Sarcoidosis is excluded by the absence of other signs of this disease, lack of characteristic histologic changes in biopsied lymph node, liver, or other tissues, a negative Kveim-Siltzbach skin test, and the presence of serum angiotensin-converting enzyme.

Course. The course of the disease is characterized by a series of remissions and exacerbations extending over a number of years. During the period of remission, all the symptoms may improve greatly. Unilateral amblyopia or complete blindness may result from the ocular lesions. Residuals of the neurologic lesions are not uncommon.

Neurologic and posterior uveal tract lesions indicate a poor prognosis. Death has occurred from the disease, chiefly when the CNS became involved. Permanent remission of symptoms has not been reported.

Treatment. Various antibiotics, chemotherapy, and corticosteroids have been used in the treatment, but there is no evidence that any of these forms of therapy have any effect on the course of the disease. When the neurologic components of the disease are life-threatening, immunosuppressive therapy may be considered. Therapy is difficult to assess because of the variable natural course.

VOGT-KOYANAGI-HARADA SYNDROME

A relatively rare disease characterized by uveitis, retinal hemorrhages and detachment, depigmentation of the skin and hair, and signs of involvement of the nervous system was reported by Vogt, Koyanagi, and Harada in the 1920s. The dermatologic signs include poliosis and canities (patchy whitening of eyelashes, eyebrows, and scalp hair), alopecia (patchy loss of hair), and vitiligo (patchy depigmentation of skin).

The nervous system is affected in practically all cases. The neurologic symptoms are caused by an inflammatory adhesive arachnoiditis. The most common patient complaint is headache, sometimes accompanied by dizziness, fatigue, and somnolence. Neurosensory deafness, hemiplegia, ocular palsies, psychotic manifestations, and meningeal signs may occur. The CSF is under increased pressure. There is a moderate degree of lymphocytic pleocytosis. The CSF protein content is normal or slightly elevated; an elevated gamma globulin has been reported. The CSF glucose level is normal.

The period of activity of the process lasts for 6 to 12 months and is followed by a recrudescence of the ophthalmic and neurologic signs.

The cause of the disease is unknown. It has been suggested that it is caused by a viral infection, but proof for this is lacking. The eye lesions are similar to those of sympathetic ophthalmia.

There is no specific therapy, but some reports suggest that administration of corticosteroids may be of value.

MOLLARET MENINGITIS

Patients with recurrent episodes of benign aseptic meningitis were first described by Mollaret in 1944. The disease is characterized by repeated short-lived, spontaneous remitting attacks of headache, and nuchal rigidity. Between attacks, the patient enjoys good health. The meningitis episodes usually last two or three days. Most are characterized by a mild meningitis without associated neurologic abnormalities. Transient neurologic disturbances (coma, seizures, syncope, diplopia, dysarthria, disequilibrium, facial paralysis, anisocoria, and extensor plantar responses) have been reported. The patient's body temperature is moderately elevated with a maximum of 104° F (40° C). Neck stiffness and the signs of meningeal irritation are present. The first attack may appear at any age between childhood and late adult years. Both sexes are equally affected. The episodes usually last for three to five years.

During the attacks, there is a CSF pleocytosis and a slight elevation of the protein content. The CSF sugar content is normal. The cell counts range from 200 to several thousand/mm³; most of the cells are mononuclear. Large fragile endothelial cells are found in the CSF in the early phases of the disease; their presence is variable and is not considered essential for the diagnosis.

Proposed etiologic agents in individual cases have included Herpes simplex type I, epidermoid cyst, and Histoplasmosis, but none have been found with consistency. It is therefore not possible to determine whether Mollaret meningitis is a syndrome of multiple etiologies of a disease that excludes known causes.

The differential diagnosis of the condition includes recurrent bacterial meningitis, recurrent viral meningitis, sarcoidosis, hydatid cyst, fungal meningitis, intracranial tumors, Behçet syndrome, and the Vogt-Koyanagi-Harada syndrome. The latter two conditions may be differentiated by eye and skin lesions and associated findings.

Patients with Mollaret meningitis always recover rapidly and spontaneously without specific therapy. There is no effective therapy for shortening the attack or preventing fresh attacks.

ASEPTIC MENINGEAL REACTION

Aseptic meningeal reaction (sympathetic meningitis, meningitis serosa) is a term used to describe those cases with evidence of a meningeal reaction in the CSF in the absence of any infecting organism. Three general classes of cases fall into this category: (1) those in which the meningeal reaction is due to a septic or necrotic focus within the skull or spinal canal (parameningeal infection); (2) those in which the meningeal reaction is due to the introduction of foreign substances (e.g., air, dyes, drugs, blood) into the subarachnoid space; and (3) those in association with connective tissue disorders.

The symptoms that are present in the patients in the first group are those associated with the infection or morbid process in the skull or spinal cavity. Only occasionally are there any symptoms and signs of meningeal irritation.

In the second group of patients, where the meningeal reaction is due to the introduction of foreign substances into the subarachnoid space, fever, headache, and stiffness of the neck may occur. The appearance of these symptoms leads to the suspicion that an actual infection of the meninges has been produced by the inadvertent introduction of pathogenic organisms. The normal sugar content of the CSF and the absence of organisms on culture establish the nature of the meningeal reaction.

An aseptic meningeal reaction may complicate the course of systemic lupus erythematosus and periarteritis nodosa. In certain instances, the meningeal reaction in systemic lupus erythematosus patients may be induced by nonsteroidal anti-inflammatory drugs or azathioprine. An aseptic meningeal reaction may also occur in the Sjögren syndrome.

The findings in the CSF that are characteristic of an aseptic meningeal reaction are an increase in pressure, a varying degree of pleocytosis (10 to 4,000 cell/mm³), a slight or moderate increase in the protein content, a normal sugar content, and the absence of organisms on culture. (Exceptionally, and without explanation, the aseptic meningeal reaction of systemic lupus erythematosus may be accompanied by low CSF sugar values.) With a severe degree of meningeal reaction, the CSF may be purulent in appearance and may contain several thousand cells/mm³ with a predominance of polymorphonuclear leukocytes. With a lesser degree of meningeal reaction, the CSF may be normal in appearance or only slightly cloudy and may contain a moderate number of cells (10 to several hundred/mm³), with lymphocytes being the predominating cell type in the CSF with less than 100 cells/mm³.

The pathogenesis of the changes in the CSF is not clearly understood. The septic foci in the head that are more commonly associated with an aseptic meningeal reaction are septic thrombosis of the intracranial venous sinuses, osteomyelitis of the spine or skull, extradural, subdural, or intracerebral abscesses or septic cerebral emboli. Nonseptic foci of necrosis are only rarely accompanied by an aseptic meningeal reaction. Occasionally patients with an intracerebral tumor or cerebral hemorrhage that is near to the ventricular walls may show the similar changes in the CSF.

The diagnosis of an aseptic meningeal reaction in patients with a septic or necrotic focus in the skull or spinal cord is important in that it directs attention to the presence of this focus and the necessity for appropriate surgical and medical therapy before the meninges are actually invaded by the infectious process or before other cerebral or spinal complications develop.

MENINGISM

Coincidental with the onset of any of the acute infectious diseases in childhood or young adult life, there may be headache, stiffness of the neck, Kernig sign and, rarely, delirium, convulsions, or coma. The appearance of these symptoms may lead to the tentative diagnosis of an acute meningitis or encephalitis.

Meningism refers to the syndrome of headache and signs of meningeal irritation in patients with an acute febrile illness, usually of a viral nature, in whom the CSF is commonly under increased pressure but normal in other respects. The condition may prove diagnostically confusing.

There is no completely satisfactory explanation for the syndrome. Acute hypotonicity of the patient's serum, inappropriate secretion of antidiuretic hormone, and an increased formation of CSF have been considered as possible causes. The characteristic findings on lumbar puncture are a slight or moderate increase in pressure, a clear, colorless CSF that contains no cells, and a moderate reduction in the protein content of the CSF.

The condition is brief in duration. Spinal puncture, which is usually performed as a diagnostic measure in these cases, is the only therapy necessary for the relief of the symptoms. The reduction of pressure by the removal of CSF results in the disappearance of symptoms. Rarely is more than one puncture necessary.

MYCOPLASMA PNEUMONIAE INFECTION

Mycoplasmas, originally called pleuro-pneumonia-like organisms (PPLO), lack a cell wall. Individual mycoplasmas are bounded by a unit membrane that encloses the cyto-plasm, DNA, RNA, and other cellular components. They are the smallest of free-living organisms and are resistant to penicillin and other cell-wall active antimicrobials.

Of mycoplasmas that infect humans, mycoplasma pneumoniae is the only species that has been clearly shown to be a significant cause of disease. It is a major cause of acute respiratory disease, including pneumonia. A variety of neurologic conditions have been described in association with M. pneumoniae infection. These include meningitis, encephalitis, postinfectious leukoencephalitis, acute cerebellar ataxia, transverse myelitis, ascending polyneuritis, radiculopathy, cranial neuropathy, and acute psychosis. The most common neurologic condition appears to be meningitis or meningoencephalitis with alterations in mental status. The CSF usually contains polymorphonuclear leukocytes and mononuclear cells in varying proportions. The CSF has a normal or mildly elevated protein content and a normal glucose level. Bacterial, viral, and mycoplasma cultures of the CSF are usually sterile.

The neurologic features associated with M. pneumoniae infection are so diverse that the correct diagnosis cannot be made on clinical grounds alone. Cold isohemagglutinins for human Type-O erythrocytes can be detected in about 50% of patients during the second week of illness; they are the first antibodies to disappear. Specific antibodies can also be demonstrated.

Tetracycline and erythromycin are the drugs of choice for M. pneumoniae infections of a severe nature. It is not known if neurologic complications benefit from antimicrobial treatment.

LEGIONELLA PNEUMOPHILIA INFECTION

Legionella pneumophilia is a poorly staining gram-negative bacterium that either does not grow or grows very slowly on most artificial media. The organism was first isolated from fatal cases of pneumonia among persons attending an American Legion Convention in Philadelphia in 1976 (Legionnaires' disease). The bacterium is acquired by inhalation of contaminated aerosols or dust from air-conditioning systems, water, or soil.

Symptoms and Signs. Pneumonia is the most typical systemic manifestation of infection. Upper respiratory infection, a severe influenza-like syndrome (Pontiac fever), and gastrointestinal disease may also occur.

A number of neurologic conditions have

been described in association with L. pneumophilia infection (Legionnaires' disease, legionellosis). They include acute encephalomyelitis, pronounced cerebellar deficit, chorea, and peripheral neuropathy. Confusion, delirium, and hallucinations are common symptoms. The pathophysiology of these syndromes is unclear because bacteria have rarely been demonstrated in the CNS. Myoglobinuria and elevated serum creatine kinase levels have also been reported.

Laboratory Data. L. pneumophilia is rarely recovered from pleural fluid, sputum, or blood; it can frequently be isolated from respiratory secretions by transtracheal aspiration or bronchoalveolar lavage and lung biopsy tissue. A retrospective diagnosis can be made by a significant rise in specific serum antibodies detected by immunofluorescence.

Treatment. The treatment of choice is administration of erythromycin. Relapses are uncommon if treatment is continued for 14 days. When relapses occur, they usually respond to a second course of the antibiotic. Fluid volume should be maintained with intravenous fluids; hypoxic patients should be given oxygen.

The true incidence of neurologic involvement in Legionnaires' disease is still unknown. The neurologic deficit is known to be reversible, but little exact information about recovery is available.

Whipple Disease

Whipple disease was originally described as a gastrointestinal disorder associated with arthralgia. It is caused by a bacilliform bacterium, and infection is evident in several organs. The organism has not been successfully cultured, and the disease has not been reproduced in animals. Therefore, little is known about the organism or pathophysiology of the illness. The role of T-cell-mediated immune defects is uncertain. Whipple disease has been described in connection with AIDS and other conditions of immune depression. There have been cases of CNS disease without evidence of infection elsewhere.

The bacillus has morphologic features of both gram-positive and gram-negative organisms, but it is usually gram-positive. It appears both intracellularly and extracellularly; infected macrophages are characteristically present. In most tissues, however, infection is not restricted to macrophages alone. Infected cells stain strongly with periodic acid-Schiff (PAS). Examination by electron microscopy demonstrates that the areas of intense PAS-staining are packed with bacilli, some degenerated. These areas usually have a distinctive sickle shape. Cells containing them are referred to as SPCs (sickle particle cells).

The epidemiology of Whipple disease is not understood. There seems to be a predominance in elderly men of the systemic disorder, but this is less obvious in the cases reported with primarily CNS manifestations. The symptoms of the systemic disease are weight loss, abdominal pain, diarrhea (often with steatorrhea), and arthralgia. Arthralgia often antedates the gastrointestinal symptoms. Malabsorption may be prominent. Low-grade fever, lymph adenopathy, and increased skin pigmentation also occur.

General laboratory studies usually reveal steatorrhea, impaired xylose absorption, anemia, and hypoalbuminemia. However, diagnosis is usually made by jejunal biopsy to demonstrate the PAS-staining macrophages. Because PAS-positive macrophages may be found in other diseases and in other tissues of apparently normal individuals, confirmation of the diagnosis is facilitated by detection of the actual bacillus with appropriate strains or electron microscopy.

The neurologic disorder is usually a progressive encephalopathy, characterized by memory loss, personality change, and cognitive dysfunction. Seizures have been described. Focal findings may suggest discrete lesions and include ophthalmoplegia, motor and sensory signs, ataxia, and evidence of hypothalamic dysfunction, including hypersomnolence and hormone deficiencies. Peripheral neuropathy has also been described.

Cases without arthralgia or gastrointestinal symptoms are particularly difficult to diagnose. CSF examination has been reported as normal or has showed moderate pleocytosis (about 200 cells, mostly mononuclear) or protein levels up to 100 to 200 mg/dl. IgG elevation has been reported, but it is not known if oligoclonal bands are present. CT usually demonstrates focal lesions, particularly in cases diagnosed antemortem without obvious systemic findings. Biopsy of these lesions has provided the diagnosis in several cases. The role of MRI has not been defined.

Diagnosis is confirmed by findng PAS-containing macrophages in the brain and by demonstrating the bacillus in these cells. Infection of neural cells has not been demonstrated. If the organism has been detected in a small bowel biopsy, then cerebral biopsy is not necessary. Therapeutic trials without definite diagnosis have been attempted, but carry the usual pitfalls of misdiagnosis and mistreatment. This is particularly important because response to treatment of CNS manifestations has varied in documented cases. Treatment of CNS Whipple disease has included different antibiotics such as penicillin and tetracycline. Trimethoprim-sulfamethoxazole is now considered the antibiotic of choice. The variability in results is probably due to irreversibly destroyed tissue. Treatment must be prolonged because recurrence has followed months of treatment and apparent resolution of disease.

References

Acute Bacterial Meningitis

Benson CA, Harris AA. Acute neurologic infections. Med Clin North Am 1986; 70:987–1011.

Cherubin CE, Marr JS, Sierra MF, Becker S. Listeria and gram-negative bacillary meningitis in New York City, 1972–1979. Frequent causes of meningitis in adults. Am J Med 1981; 71:199–209.

Davey PG, Cruikshank JK, McManus IC, Mahood B, Snow MH, Geddes AM. Bacterial meningitis—ten years' experience. J Hyg (Lond.) 1982; 88:383–401.

Dodge PR, Swartz MN. Bacterial meningitis—a review of selected aspects. II. Special neurologic problems, postmeningitic complications and clinicopathological corrections. N Engl J Med 1965; 272:954–960, 1003–1010.

Durack DT, Spanos A. End-of-treatment spinal tap in bacterial meningitis. JAMA 1982; 248:75–78.

Geiseler PJ, Nelson KE, Levin S, Reddi KT, Moses VK. Community-acquired purulent meningitis: A review of 1,316 cases during the antibiotic era, 1954–1976. Rev Infect Dis 1980; 2:725–745.

Mancebo J, Domingo P, Blanch L, Coll P, Net A, Nolla J. Post-neurosurgical and spontaneous gram-negative bacillary meningitis in adults. Scand J Infect Dis 1986; 18:533–538.

Marton KI, Gean AD. The spinal tap: a new look at an old test. Ann Intern Med 1986; 104:840–848.

Murphy DJ. Group A streptococcal meningitis. Pediatrics 1983; 71:1–5.

Overall JC Jr. Neonatal bacterial meningitis. J. Pediatr 1970; 76:499–511.

Overturf GD. Pyogenic bacterial infections of the CNS. Neurol Clin 1986; 4:69–90.

Sanford JP. Guide to Antimicrobial Therapy. West Bethesda: Antimicrobial Therapy, 1987.

Sangster G, Murdoch J McC, Gray JA. Bacterial meningitis 1949–79. J Infect Dis 1982; 5:245–255.

Schlech WF, Ward JI, Band JD, Hightower A, Fraser DW, Broome CV. Bacterial meningitis in the United States, 1978 through 1981; The National Bacterial Meningitis Surveillance Study. JAMA 1985; 253:1749–1754.

Swartz MN, Dodge PR. Bacterial meningitis—a review of selected aspects. I. General clinical features, special problems and unusual meningeal reactions mimicking bacterial meningitis. N Engl J Med 1965; 272:725–731, 779–787, 898–902.

Whitby M, Finch R. Bacterial meningitis; rational selection and use of antibacterial drugs. Drugs 1986; 31:266–278.

Subacute Meningitis
Tuberculous Meningitis

Alvarez S, McCabe WR. Extrapulmonary tuberculosis revisited: a review of experience at Boston City and other hospitals. Medicine 1984; 63:25–55.

Blargava S, Gupta AK, Tandon PN. Tuberculous meningitis—a CT study. Br J Radiol 1982; 55:189–196.

Kennedy DH, Fallon RJ. Tuberculous meningitis. JAMA 1979; 241:264–268.

Kingsley DP, Hendrickse WA, Kendall BE, Swash M, Singh V. Tuberculous meningitis: role of CT in management and prognosis. J Neurol Neurosurg Psychiat 1987; 50:30–36.

Kocen RS, Parsons M. Neurological complications of tuberculosis: some unusual manifestations. Q J Med 1970; 39:17–30.

Sheller JR, Des Prez RM. CNS tuberculosis. Neurol Clin 1986; 4:143–158.

Stockstill MT, Kauffman CA. Comparison of cryptococcal and tuberculous meningitis. Arch Neurol 1983; 40:81–85.

Sumaya CV, Simek M, Smith MHD, Seidemann MF, Ferriss GS, Rubin W. Tuberculous meningitis in children during the isoniazid era. J Pediatr 1975; 87:43–49.

Traub M, Colchester ACF, Kingsley DPE, Swash M. Tuberculosis of the central nervous system. Q J Med 1984; 53:83–100.

Subdural and Epidural Infections
Cerebral Subdural Empyema

Dunker RO, Khakoo RA. Failure of computed tomograph scanning to demonstrate subdural empyema. JAMA 1981; 246:1116–1118.

Kaufman DM, Miller MH, Steigbigel NH. Subdural empyema: analysis of 17 recent cases and review of the literature. Medicine (Baltimore) 1975; 54:485–498.

Kaufman DM, Litman N, Miller MH. Sinusitis: induced subdural empyema. Neurology 1983; 33:123–132.

Luken MG III, Whelan MA. Recent diagnostic experience with subdural empyema. J Neurosurg 1980; 52:764–771.

Renaudin JW, Frazee J. Subdural empyema—importance of early diagnosis. Neurosurgery 1980; 7:477–479.

Sadhu VK, Handel SF, Pinto RS, Glass TF. Neuroradiologic diagnosis of subdural empyema and CT limitations. AJNR 1980; 1:39–44.

Intracranial Epidural Abscess

Lott T, el Gammal T, Dasilva R, Hanks D, Reynolds J. Evaluation of brain and epidural abscesses by computed tomography. Radiology 1977; 122:371–376.

Silverberg AL, DiNubile MJ. Subdural empyema and cranial epidural abscess. Med Clin NA 1985; 62:361–374.

Smith HP, Hendrick EB. Subdural empyema and epidural abscess in children. J Neurosurg 1983; 58:392–397.

Spinal Epidural Abscess

Baker AS, Ojemann RG, Swartz MN, Richardson EP Jr. Spinal epidural abscess. N Engl J Med 1975; 293:463–468.

Danner RL, Hartman BJ. Update of spinal epidural abscess: 35 cases and review of the literature. Rev Infect Dis 1987; 9:265–274.

Enberg RN, Kaplan RJ. Spinal epidural abscess in children. Early diagnosis and immediate surgical drainage is essential to forestall paralysis. Clin Pediatr 1974; 13:247–253.

Kaufman DM, Kaplan JG, Litman N. Infectious agents in spinal epidural abscesses. Neurology 1980; 30:844–850.

Ravicovitch MA, Spallone A. Spinal epidural abscesses. Surgical and parasurgical management. Eur Neurol 1982; 21:347–357.

Verner EF, Musher DM. Spinal epidural abscess. Med Clin NA 1985; 69:375–384.

Leprosy

Brandsma W. Basic nerve function assessment in leprosy patients. Lepr Rev 1981; 52:111–119.

Browne SG. Leprosy—clinical aspects of nerve involvement. In: Hornabrook RW, ed. Topics on Tropical Neurology. Philadelphia: FA Davis, 1975:1–6.

Canizares O. Diagnosis and treatment of leprosy in the United States. Med Clin North Am 1965; 49:801–816.

Charosky CB, Gatti JC, Cardama JE. Neuropathies in Hansen's disease. Int J Lepr Other Mycobact Dis 1983; 51:576–586.

Cochrane RG, Davey TF. Leprosy in theory and practice, 2nd ed. Baltimore: Williams & Wilkins, 1964.

Dastur DK. Leprosy (an infectious and immunological disorder of the nervous system). In: Vinken PJ, Bruyn GW, Klawans HL, eds. Handbook of Clinical Neurology (vol 33). New York: Elsevier-North Holland, 1978:421–468.

Gelber RH, Zacharia AG. Bilateral ulnar nerve abscess in lepromatous leprosy; a first encounter. Int J Lepr Other Mycobact Dis 1986; 54:480–482.

Pedley JC, Harman DJ, Waudby H, McDougall AC. Leprosy in peripheral nerves: histopathological findings in 119 untreated patients in Nepal. J Neurol Neurosurg Psychiatry 1980; 43:198–204.

Reichart PA, Šrisuwan S, Metah D. Lesions of the facial and trigeminal nerve in leprosy; an evaluation of 43 cases. Int J Oral Surg 1982; 11:14–20.

Rickettsial Infections

Harrell GT. Rickettsial involvement of the nervous system. Med Clin North Am 1953; 37:395–422.

Woodward TE. Rickettsial diseases in the United States. Med Clin North Am 1959; 43:1507–1535.

Typhus Fever

Herman E. Neurological syndromes in typhus fever. J Nerv Ment Dis 1949; 109:25–36.

Miller ES, Beeson PB. Murine typhus fever. Medicine 1946; 25:1–15.

Rocky Mountain Spotted Fever

Bell WE, Lascari AD. Rocky Mountain spotted fever. Neurological symptoms in the acute phase. Neurology 1970; 20:841–847.

Crennan JM, Van Scoy RE. Eosinophilic meningitis caused by Rocky Mountain spotted fever. Am J Med 1986; 80:288–289.

D'Angelo LJ, Winkler WG, Bregman DJ. Rocky Mountain spotted fever in the United States, 1975–1977. J Infect Dis 1978; 138:273–276.

Helmick CG, Bernard KW, D'Angelo LJ. Rocky Mountain spotted fever: clinical, laboratory, and epidemiological features of 262 cases. J Infect Dis 1984; 150:480–488.

Katz DA, Dworzack DL, Horowitz EA, Bogard PJ. Encephalitis associated with Rocky Mountain spotted fever. Arch Pathol Lab Med 1985; 109:771–773.

Massey EW, Thames T, Coffey CE, Gallis HA. Neurologic complications of Rocky Mountain spotted fever. South Med J 1985; 78:1288–1290, 1303.

Miller JQ, Price TR. The nervous system in Rocky Mountain spotted fever. Neurology 1972; 22:561–566.

Scrub Typhus

Ripley MS. Neuropsychiatric observations on tsutsugamushi (scrub typhus). Arch Neurol Psychiatry 1946; 56:42–54.

Other Bacterial Infections

Brucellosis

Araj GF, Lulu AR, Saadah MA, Mousa AM, Strannegard L-L, Shakir RA. Rapid diagnosis of central nervous system brucellosis by ELISA. J Neuroimmunol 1986; 12:173–182.

Fincham RW, Sahs AL, Joynt RJ. Protean manifestations of nervous system brucellosis. Case histories of a wide variety of clinical forms. JAMA 1963; 184:269–275.

Labrisseau A, Maravi E, Aguilera F, Martinez-Lage JM. The neurological complications of brucellosis. Can J Neurol Sci 1978; 5:369–376.

Young EJ. Human brucellosis. Rev Infect Dis 1983; 5:821–842.

Behçet's Syndrome

Alema G. Behçet's disease. In: Vinken PJ, Bruyn GW, Klawans HL, eds. Handbook of Clinical Neurology, vol 34. New York: Elsevier-North Holland, 1978:475–512.

Behçet H. Über rezidivierende Aphthose durch ein Virusverursachte Geschwur am Mund, am Auge und an den Genitalien. Dermatol Monatsschr 1937, 105:1152–1157.

Chajek T. Fainaru M. Behçet's disease. Report of 41 cases and a review of the literature. Medicine (Baltimore) 1975; 54:179–196.

Dobkin BH. Computerized tomography findings in neuro-Behçet's disease. Arch Neurol 1980; 37:58–59.

Iragui VJ, Maravi E. Behçet syndrome presenting as cerebrovascular disease. J Neurol Neurosurg Psychiatry 1986; 49:838–840.

Motomura S, Tabira T, Kuroiwa Y. A clinical comparative study of multiple sclerosis and neuro-Behçet's syndrome. J Neurol Neurosurg Psychiatry 1980; 43:210–213.

O'Duffy JD, Goldstein NP. Neurologic involvement in seven patients with Behçet's disease. Am J Med 1976; 61:170–178.

Wolf SM, Schotland DL, Phillips LL. Involvement of nervous system in Behçet's syndrome. Arch Neurol 1965; 12:315–325.

Yazici H, Tuzun Y, Pazarli H, Yurdakul S, Ozyazgan Y, Ozdogan H, Serdaroglu S, et al. Influence of age on onset and patient's sex on the prevalence and severity of manifestations of Behçet's syndrome. Ann Rheum Dis 1984; 43:783–789.

Vogt-Koyanagi-Harada Syndrome

Pattison EM. Uveomeningoencephalitic syndrome (Vogt-Koyanagi-Harada). Arch Neurol 1965; 12:197–205.

Reed H. Uveo-Encephalitis. World Neurol 1960; 1:173–178.

Riehl J-L, Andrews JM. Uveomeningoencephalitic syndrome. Neurology 1966; 16:603–609.

Mollaret Meningitis

Galdi AP. Benign recurrent aseptic meningitis (Mollaret's meningitis). Case report and clinical review. Arch Neurol 1979; 36:657–658.

Hermans, PE, Goldstein NP, Wellman WE. Mollaret's meningitis and differential diagnosis of recurrent meningitis. Am J Med 1972; 52:128–140.

Mollaret, P. La méningite endothélio-leucocytaire multirecurrente bénigne. Syndrome nouveau ou maladie nouvelle? Rev Neurol (Paris) 1944; 76:57–76.

Steel JG, Dix RD, Baringer JR. Isolation of herpes simplex virus type I in recurrent Mollaret meningitis. Ann Neurol 1982; 11:17–21.

Tyler KL, Adler D. Twenty-eight years of benign recurring Mollaret meningitis. Arch Neurol 1983; 40:42–43.

Aseptic Meningeal Reaction

Alexander EL, Alexander GE. Aseptic meningoencephalitis in primary Sjögren's syndrome. Neurology 1983; 33:593–598.

Canoso JJ, Cohen AS. Aseptic meningitis in systemic lupus erythematosus. Arthritis Rheum 1975; 18:369–374.

Meningism

Fishman RA. Cerebrospinal Fluid in Diseases of the Nervous System. Philadelphia: WB Saunders Co, 1980.

Mycoplasma Pneumoniae Infection

Decaux G, Szyper M. Ectors M, Cornil A, Franken L. Central nervous complications of mycoplasma pneumoniae. J Neurol Neurosurg Psychiatry 1980; 43:883–887.

Fisher RS, Clark AW, Wolinsky JS, Parhad IM, Moses H, Mardiney MR. Postinfectious leukoencephalitis complicating *Mycoplasma pneumoniae* infection. Arch Neurol 1983; 40:109–113.

Pönka A. Central nervous system manifestations associated with serologically verified *Mycoplasma pneumonia* infection. Scand J Infect Dis 1980; 12:175–184.

Legionella Pneumophilia Infection

Harris LF. Legionnaires' disease associated with acute encephalomyelitis. Arch Neurol 1981; 38:462–463.

Heath PD, Booth L, Leigh PN, Turner AM. Legionella brain stem encephalopathy and peripheral neuropathy without preceding pneumonia (letter). J Neurol Neurosurg Psychiatry 1986; 49:216–218.

Johnson JD, Raff MJ, Van Arsdall JA. Neurologic manifestations of Legionaires disease. Medicine 1984; 63:303–310.

Pendelbury WW, Perl DP, Winn WC Jr, McQuillen JB. Neuropathologic evaluation of 40 confirmed cases of "Legionella" pneumonia. Neurology 1983; 33:1340–1344.

Shetty KR, Cilyo CL, Starr BD, Harter DH. Legionnaires' disease with profound cerebellar involvement. Arch Neurol 1980, 37:379–380.

Weir AI, Bone I, Kennedy DH. Neurological involvement in legionellosis. J Neurol Neurosurg Psychiatry 1982; 45:604–608.

Whipple Disease

Adams M, Rhyner PA, Day J, DeArmond S, Smuckler EA. Whipple's disease confined to the central nervous system. Ann Neurol 1987; 21:104–108.

Ambler MW, Homans AC, O'Shea PA. An unusual central nervous system infection in a young immuno-compromised host. Arch Pathol Lab Med 1986; 110:497–501.

Feurle GE, Volk B, Waldherr R. Cerebral Whipple's disease with negative jejunal histology. N Engl J Med 1979; 300:907–908.

Halperin JJ, Landis DMD, Kleinman GM. Whipple disease of the nervous system. Neurology 1982; 32:612–617.

Jankovic J. Whipple's disease of the central nervous system in AIDS. N Engl J Med 1986; 315:1029–1030.

Johnson L, Diamond I. Cerebral Whipple's disease. Diagnosis by brain biopsy. Am J Clin Pathol 1980; 74:486–490.

Ludwig B, Bohl J, Haferkamp G. Central Nervous System Involvement in Whipple's Disease. Neuroradiology 1981; 21:289–293.

Pollock S, Lewis PD, Kendall B. Whipple's disease confined to the nervous system. J Neurol Neurosurg Psychiatry 1981; 44:1104–1109.

Rhyser RJ, Locksley RM, Eng SC, Dobbins WO, Schoenknecht FD, Rubin CE. Reversal of dementia associated with Whipple's disease by trimethoprim-sulfamethaxazole, drugs that penetrate the blood-brain barrier. Gastroenterology 1984; 86:745–752.

Schmitt BP, Richardson H, Smith E, Kaplan R. Encephalopathy complicating Whipple's disease. Failure to respond to antibiotics. Ann Intern Med 1981; 94:51–52.

Swash M, Schwartz MS, Vandenburg MJ, Pollock DJ. Myopathy in Whipple's disease. Gut 1977; 18:800–804.

14. FOCAL INFECTIONS

Leonard Berg
Octavio de Marchena

Osteomyelitis and Malignant External Otitis

Involvement of the bones at the base of the skull by infectious processes may be accompanied by osteomyelitis with or without abscess formation. Infections of the mastoid process or temporal bone may cause cranial nerve palsies, particularly of the facial and acoustic nerves. Paralysis of the lower cranial nerves develops when the occipital bone is affected.

In recent years, a number of patients have been reported with infection of the external auditory canal by Pseudomonas aeruginosa with spread to the local subcutaneous tissues, the parotid gland, the temporomandibular joint, the masseter muscle, and the temporal bone. A necrotizing osteomyelitis of the base of the skull develops and causes the neurologic manifestations. The high mortality rate (40%) has led to the use of the term "malignant" for this form of otitis.

The patients are usually elderly and diabetic, but severely ill children may be affected. Symptoms and signs include pain in the ear, with or without a purulent discharge, swelling of the parotid gland, trismus and paralysis of the sixth, seventh, eighth, tenth, eleventh, and twelfth nerves. Death is usually related to the development of meningitis.

CT and MRI can demonstrate bony involvement. In addition, MRI can show inflammatory changes in the soft tissues. Radionuclide gallium and technetium scans offer useful information for management along with the other imaging procedures.

Prolonged intravenous administration of gentamicin and carbenicillin has resulted in arrest or cure of the disease. Surgical debridement is sometimes necessary.

Brain Abscess and Subdural Empyema

BRAIN ABSCESS

Encapsulated or free pus in the substance of the brain following an acute purulent infection is known as brain abscess. Abscesses may vary in size from a microscopic collection of inflammatory cells to an area of purulent necrosis involving the major part of one hemisphere. Abscess of the brain has been known for over 200 years, but surgical treatment started with Macewen in 1880.

Etiology. Brain abscesses arise either as direct extension from infections within the cranial cavity (e.g., mastoid, nasal sinuses, osteomyelitis of the skull), from infections secondary to fracture of the skull or neurosurgical procedures, or as metastases from infection elsewhere in the body. Brain abscess is rarely a complication of bacterial meningitis, except in infants. Infections in the middle ear or mastoid process may spread to the cerebellum or temporal lobe through involvement of the bone and meninges or through the blood vessels or nerves, with or without extradural or subdural infection or thrombosis of the lateral sinus. Infection from the mastoid process may metastasize through the blood to other portions of the brain, thus explaining the occurrence of an abscess in one hemisphere secondary to disease in the contralateral mastoid process. Infection in the frontal ethmoid or, rarely, the maxillary sinuses spreads to the frontal lobes through erosion of the skull. Subdural or extradural infection or thrombosis of the venous sinuses may be present in addition.

Metastatic abscesses of the brain are commonly secondary to suppurative processes in the lungs (e.g., bronchiectasis, lung abscess). Less frequently, they may follow bacterial endocarditis. Other sources of infection include the tonsils and upper respiratory tract, from which the infection may reach the brain along the carotid sheath. Infections elsewhere than in the heart or lungs occasionally metastasize to the brain. The route of infection in such cases is not clear. Congenital heart disease and pulmonary arteriovenous fistulas (as in hereditary hemorrhagic telangiectasia) both predispose to brain abscess. In each of these two disorders, infected venous blood bypasses the pulmonary filter and gains access to the cerebral arterial system.

Abscesses of the brain secondary to cranial trauma are due to the introduction of infected missiles or tissues into the brain substance through compound fractures of the skull. These are far less common than in former years. In children, penetration of a lead pencil tip through the thin squamous portion of the temporal bone has resulted in formation of brain abscess around the foreign material.

The infecting organism may be any of the common pyogenic bacteria, but Staphylococcus aureus, Streptococcus viridans, hemolytic streptococcus, Enterobacteriaceae, and anaerobes such as Bacteroides are most commonly found. In young infants, gram-negative organisms are the most frequent offenders. Pneumococci, meningococci, and Hemophilus influenzae, which are the major causes of bacterial meningitis, are rarely recovered from brain abscesses. The abscess is often sterile by the time the operation is performed, but the failure to culture an organism often results from inadequate techniques for demonstrating anaerobes. Brain abscess is an infrequent complication of infection with fungi (e.g., Nocardia) or parasites (e.g., Entamoeba histolytica). In immunocompromised hosts, abscesses are caused by a wide variety of organisms that are otherwise rarely pathogenic. Abscesses caused by Toxoplasma gondii, Aspergillus, Candida, and other unusual organisms are being seen more frequently.

Pathology. The pathologic changes in brain abscess are similar regardless of whether the infection extends to the brain directly from epidural or subdural infection, by retrograde thrombosis of veins, or by metastasis through the arterial system (Fig. 14–1). In the first stage, there is suppurative inflammation of brain tissue *(purulent cerebritis)*. The inflammation then proceeds to necrosis. When host defenses control the spread of the infection, the macroglia and fibroblasts proliferate in an attempt to surround the infected and necrotic tissue. Granulation tissue and fibrous encapsulation develop. Edema of the adjacent portion of the cerebrum or of the entire hemisphere is a common finding (Figs. 14–1 and 14–2).

Incidence. Brain abscesses were quite common in the first half of this century, but the introduction of effective therapy for purulent infection of the mastoid process and nasal sinuses has greatly reduced the incidence of all intracranial complications of these infections including brain abscess. Brain abscesses are rare and constitute less than 2% of all intracranial surgery. Brain abscess may occur at any age, but it is more common in the first to third decades of life, as a result of the high incidence of mastoid and nasal sinus disease in those years.

Symptoms and Signs. The symptoms of brain abscess are those of any expanding lesion in the brain, but headache is particularly prominent. Symptoms of infection are lacking unless the focus that gave rise to the abscess is still active. Chills and fever are distinctly rare except when there is an embolic lesion in the brain secondary to acute endocarditis.

Edema of neighboring brain tissue rapidly increases intracranial pressure. Headache, nausea, and vomiting are early symptoms. Convulsions, focal or generalized, are common.

The body temperature is normal or subnormal except when fever results from other complications or activity of the septic source of the abscess. The pulse and respiratory rate are normal unless intracranial pressure is greatly increased. Many patients develop papilledema. Inequality in the degree of papilledema in the two eyes has no lateralizing value. Signs of injury to the third or sixth cranial nerve as a result of increased intracranial pressure are occasionally seen. Focal signs include: hemiparesis or hemiplegia when the abscess is in the cerebral hemispheres; torpidity and mental confusion, especially with abscesses in the frontal lobe; hemianopic and aphasic disturbances, particularly anomia, when the temporal or parietooccipital lobes are involved; and ataxia, intention tremor, nystagmus, and other symptoms of cerebellar and vestibular dysfunction when the abscess is in the cerebellum. Not infrequently, however, the signs of an abscess in the cerebrum or cerebellum are limited to those resulting from increased intracranial pressure.

Abscesses in the brain stem are rare, and the diagnosis is usually established at necropsy. Fever, headache, cranial nerve palsies, hemiparesis, dysphagia, and vomiting were the common manifestations in the 38 patients collected from the literature by Weickhardt.

Laboratory Data. Examination of the blood

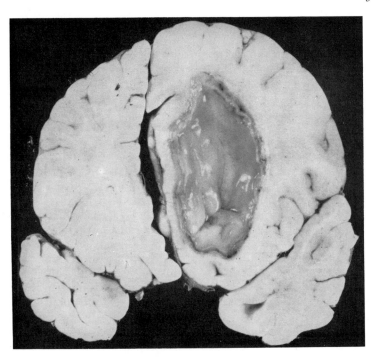

Fig. 14–1. Brain abscess. Fresh abscess in frontal lobe secondary to pulmonary infection. (Courtesy of Dr. Abner Wolf.)

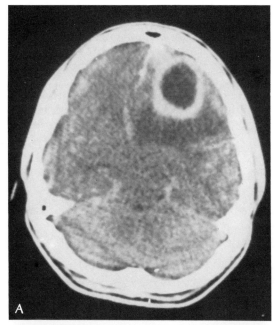

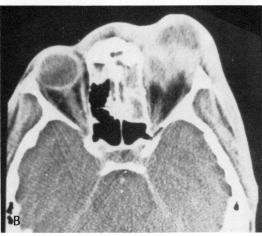

Fig. 14–2. Brain abscess. *A*, A frontal lobe abscess is delineated on CT by ring enhancement and surrounding edema. *B*, The lesion originated in ethmoid sinusitis, and orbital cellulitis occurred on the same side. (Courtesy of Drs. S.K. Hilal and S.R. Ganti.)

and urine is normal unless there is activity in the septic focus or unless complications are present.

Although the following older data on the results of CSF examination provided valuable information in earlier years, the availability of CT and the hazards of lumbar puncture in the presence of brain abscess contradict its use for diagnostic purposes, unless acute meningitis is suspected. The changes in the CSF are related to the size, location, and stage of development of the abscess, and to the pres-

ence or absence of acute meningitis. When acute meningitis is present, the CSF findings are those commonly seen in acute purulent meningitis. The discussion here is confined to those patients in whom bacterial infection of the meninges is present. The CSF changes are essentially those of an expanding intracranial lesion (increased pressure) plus those that accompany an aseptic meningeal reaction. The pressure is elevated in almost all patients. In the series reported by Merritt and Fremont-Smith, it was over 200 mm/H$_2$O in 70% and greater than 300 mm/H$_2$O in 60%. The CSF is usually clear and colorless, but it may be cloudy or turbid in the early stages. A fine clot may form in CSF with a high cell count. The cell count is directly related to the stage of encapsulation of the abscess and its nearness to the meningeal or ventricular surfaces. The cell count varies from normal to a thousand or more cells per mm^3. In early unencapsulated abscesses near the ventricular or subarachnoid spaces, the cell count is high, with a high percentage of polymorphonuclear leukocytes. The cell count is normal or only slightly increased when the abscess is firmly encapsulated. The cell count in 34 patients examined at various stages of the disease varies between 4 and 800 cells with an average of 135 cells/mm^3. Extension of the abscess to the meninges or ventricles is accompanied by an increase in the cell count and other findings of acute meningitis. Rupture of an abscess into the ventricles is signaled by a sudden rise of pressure and the presence of free pus in the CSF with a cell count of 20,000 to 50,000/mm^3. The protein content is moderately increased (between 45 and 200 mg/dl) in about 75% of the patients with unruptured abscesses. The CSF sugar content is normal. A decrease in sugar content below 40 mg/dl indicates that the meninges have been invaded by bacteria.

The EEG changes are similar to those found in cases with other space-occupying lesions. Radionuclide scan is usually positive, but false-negative results have been reported.

Radiographs of the skull may show separation of sutures in infants or children and an increase in the convolution markings. In adults, there may be displacement of the pineal calcification and, when increased intracranial pressure is chronic, enlargement of the sella turcica and thinning of the clinoid processes ("secondary sella"). CT permits accurate localization of cerebritis or abscess and serial assessment of the size of the lesion, its demarcation, the extent of surrounding edema, and total mass effect. In early cerebritis, there is an ill-defined lesion of low density on the CT scan, often with patchy contrast enhancement in the periphery. A ring of enhancement with a lucent center soon forms. The ring becomes increasingly well-defined with surrounding edema (Fig. 14–3).

Diagnosis. Brain abscess can be diagnosed without difficulty when convulsions, focal neurologic signs, or increased intracranial pressure develop in a patient with congenital heart disease or with acute or chronic infection in the middle ear, mastoid process, nasal sinuses, heart, or lungs. In the absence of any obvious focus of infection, the diagnosis may be difficult and may require CT or cerebral angiography. The characteristic progression

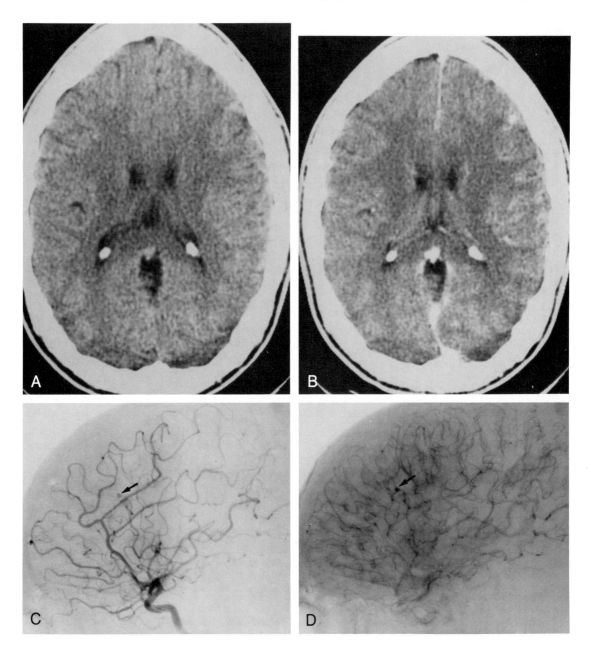

Fig. 14–3.   Mycotic aneurysm, secondary to aortic valve endocarditis. *A,* Axial noncontrast and *(B),* contrast-enhanced CT scans demonstrate punctate left frontal enhancement consistent with a mycotic aneurysm. *C,* Early and *(D),* later arterial phase subtraction films from a selective left internal carotid angiogram confirm the diagnosis, demonstrating an abnormal punctate collection of contrast that *persists.* (Courtesy of Drs. J.A. Bello and S.K. Hilal.)

of CT changes over a few days is helpful, but angiography can contribute by demonstrating that the mass is avascular in its central bulk (Fig. 14–4).

The common differential diagnoses that must be considered are brain tumor, extra-dural or subdural abscess, sinus thrombosis, meningitis, mycotic aneurysm, and encephalitis, especially that due to Herpes simplex. Most of these conditions can be differentiated

by the history of the development of symptoms and the results of EEG and CT.

The diagnosis of meningitis is readily established by examination of the CSF. The differential between brain tumor and abscess cannot be made before operation in many cases. The presence of an active focus of infection in the mastoid process or nasal sinuses and a pleocytosis in the CSF are strong evidence for the diagnosis of an abscess. Sub-

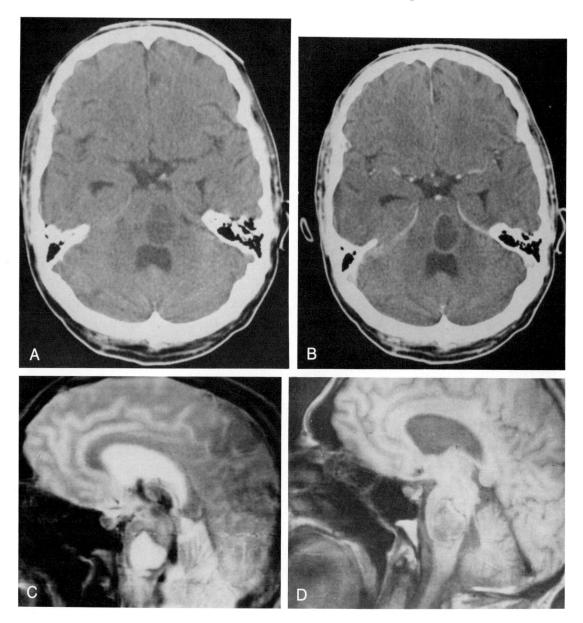

Fig. 14–4. Brainstem abscess. *A,* Axial noncontrast CT scan demonstrates a round low-density left pontine lesion with mass effect on the fourth ventricle. *B,* Ring enhancement of the lesion after contrast is typical of an abscess. *C,* Sagittal T_2 weighted and *(D),* sagittal T_1 weighted MRI scans demonstrate the lesion to be cystic-isointense to CSF signal (compare to signal within the lateral ventricle). Note definition of the abscess rim in *D.* The sagittal MRI scans are useful in planning a surgical approach through the fourth ventricle. (Courtesy of Drs. J.A. Bello and S.K. Hilal.)

dural or, rarely, epidural infections in the frontal regions may give signs and symptoms exactly the same as those of an abscess in the frontal lobe and, in many cases, the differential diagnosis cannot be made. The presence of fever with focal seizures favors the diagnosis of subdural rather than intraparenchymal abscess.

Thrombosis of the lateral sinus often follows middle ear or mastoid process infection and may be accompanied by convulsions and signs of increased intracranial pressure, making the differentiation between this condition and abscess of the temporal lobe or cerebellum difficult. The presence of focal neurologic signs (e.g., hemiplegia, hemianopia, aphasia) favors the diagnosis of an abscess. Similarly, chronic increased intracranial pressure may follow thrombosis or ligation of the lateral sinus. This condition is often described under the terms "otitic hydrocephalus" or "hypertensive meningeal hydrops." The increased intracranial pressure with papilledema results from interference with the drainage of blood from the brain.

Mycotic aneurysm may cause a syndrome of aseptic meningitis in the setting of bacterial endocarditis. CT excludes an abscess, but angiography is necessary to identify the aneurysm before rupture. Herpes simplex encephalitis presents with headache, fever, an acute temporal lobe or frontal lobe syndrome, and CSF changes indicative of aseptic meningeal reaction (sometimes with xanthochromia and red cells). On CT, the temporal lobe is swollen, with irregular lucency and patchy contrast enhancement.

Treatment. The introduction of CT has revolutionized the management of brain abscess. Not only has CT made it possible to diagnose and localize cerebritis or abscess in the proper clinical setting, it also permits choice of treatment and provides appropriate monitoring of the patient's response. Prior to CT, the treatment of brain abscess was surgery in various forms, including incision and drainage through a trephine opening, marsupialization, packing the cavity, and complete extirpation. Surgery with both pre- and postoperative antibiotics is still the best treatment for many patients, especially those with abscesses that are large and readily accessible or abscesses close to the ventricles into which the lesion may rupture. Stupor is an indication for surgery.

Through the use of CT, it has been shown that single or multiple lucent lesions with contrast enhancing rings have diminished in size and eventually disappeared with courses of appropriate antibiotics, usually given for four to six weeks. If the bacterial cause and its sensitivity to antibiotics are not known (from the site of primary infection elsewhere), the usual recommendation is to use one of the penicillins plus chloramphenicol. An alternative regimen is the combination of metronidazole and cefotaxime. Both have good CNS penetration, and the combination covers anaerobic bacteria, staphylococci, streptococci, Hemophilus spp., and Enterobacteriaceae. The benefits and risks of concurrent corticosteroid therapy are still debated.

The clinical and CT responses are closely monitored to assess the effectiveness of medical therapy or the need for surgical intervention. Even lesions that have thick, well-developed ring enhancement on CT may disappear with medical management (see Fig. 14–2). Because the ring disappears, it is unlikely that this radiologic sign represents a fibrous capsule. These totally reversible lesions may be forms of suppurative cerebritis, which in former years would have been attacked surgically after allowing time on antibiotics "for the capsule to develop."

CT has also improved surgical management by permitting accurate localization, assessment of risk of rupture into ventricle, proper selection of type of surgical procedure and its timing, opportunity to choose a more limited operation with lower morbidity, and accurate monitoring of response to treatment.

Prognosis. The outcome of untreated brain abscess is, with rare exceptions, death. The mortality in surgically treated cases varies depending on various factors: location and degree of encapsulation of the abscess, site of the original infection, presence of complications, and presence of single or multiple abscesses. The mortality rate in the 99 patients reported by Loeser and Scheinberg was approximately 45%. Mortality in other pre-CT series varied from 35 to 55%. The highest mortality rate occurred in patients whose primary infection was in the lungs. In recent small series managed with CT, the mortality has been less than 10%.

Sequelae of brain abscess include recurrence of the abscesss, development of new abscess if the primary focus still exists, residual focal neurologic defects, and the development of continuation of recurrent convulsive seizures. Prophylactic treatment with phenobarbital or phenytoin should be given for at least a year to all patients who have been treated for an abscess in the cerebral hemisphere.

SUBDURAL EMPYEMA

Subdural empyema is a collection of pus in the subdural space that can present with symptoms similar to those of brain abscess. Subdural infection usually results from contiguous spread of infection, with sinusitis the most common source. Otitic infection, head trauma, and cranial surgery also contribute to this condition. Polymicrobial infection is common with pathogens similar to those of brain abscess, including microaerophilic streptococci and anaerobic organisms. Once the infection develops, it may spread over the convexities and along the falx, although loculation is common. Associated complications include cortical vein thrombosis, brain or epidural abscess, and meningitis. Patients present with headache, fever and, in 80 to 90% of instances, focal neurologic signs. The combination of fever and focal seizures is particularly suggestive of this disorder.

Lumbar puncture is considered risky because of the mass effect produced by the empyema. When performed, it is rarely diagnostic unless an associated bacterial meningitis is present. The CT scan reveals a crescent-shaped area of hypodensity along the dura or adjoining the falx. There is usually mass effect and contrast enhancement of the margin of the hypodensity. Angiography can be helpful by demonstrating inward displacement of vessels from the inner surface of the skull.

In contrast to brain abscess, subdural infection requires drainage by burr hole and/or craniotomy. Intravenous antibiotics are given depending on the organism identified or, if unknown, with the same antibiotics used in brain abscess. Anticonvulsants are frequently required. The use of steroids to reduce brain edema is common but remains controversial.

References

Osteomyelitis and Malignant External Otitis

Case Records of the Massachusetts General Hospital. Malignant external otitis. N Engl J Med 1983; 308:443–451.

Chandler JR. Malignant external otitis: further considerations. Ann Otol Rhinol Laryngol 1977; 86:417–428.

Curtin HD, Wolf P, May M. Malignant external otitis: CT evaluation. Radiology 1982; 145:383–388.

Damiani JM, Damiani KK, Kinney SE. Malignant external otitis with multiple cranial nerve involvement. Am J Otol 1979; 1:115–120.

Dinapoli RP, Thomas JE. Neurologic aspects of malignant external otitis: report of three cases. Mayo Clin Proc 1971; 46:339–344.

Gherini SG, Brackmann DE, Bradley WG. Magnetic resonance imaging and computerized tomography in malignant external otitis. Laryngoscope 1986; 96:542–548.

Lucente FE, Parisier SC, Som PM. Complications of the treatment of malignant external otitis. Laryngoscope 1983; 93:279–281.

Meyers BR, Mendelson MH, Parisier SC, Hirschman SZ. Malignant external otitis. Comparison of monotherapy vs combination therapy. Arch Otolaryngol Head Neck Surg 1987; 113:974–978.

Parisier SC, Lucente FE, Som PM, Hirschman SZ, Arnold LM, Roffman JD. Nuclear scanning in necrotizing progressive "malignant" external otitis. Laryngoscope 1982; 92:1016–1020.

Reiter D, Bilaniuk LT, Zimmerman RA. Diagnostic imaging in malignant otitis externa. Otolaryngol Head Neck Surg 1982; 90:606–609.

Schwarz GA, Blumenkrantz MJ, Sundmaker WLH. Neurologic complications of malignant external otitis. Neurology 1971; 21:1077–1084.

Brain Abscess and Subdural Empyema

Alderson D, Strong AJ, Ingham HR, Selkon JB. Fifteen-year review of the mortality of brain abscess. Neurosurgery 1981; 8:1–6.

Armstrong D, Wong B. Central nervous system infections in immunocompromised hosts. Am Rev Med 1982; 33:293–308.

Atkinson EM. Abscess of the Brain: Its Pathology, Diagnosis and Treatment. London: Medical Publications, 1934.

Bell WE. Treatment of bacterial infections of the central nervous system. Ann Neurol 1981; 9:313–327.

Brewer NS, MacCarty CS, Wellman WE. Brain abscess: a review of recent experience. Ann Intern Med 1975; 82:571–576.

Britt RH, Enzmann DR, Yeager AS. Neuropathological and computerized tomographic findings in experimental brain abscess. J Neurosurg 1981; 55:590–603.

Clark DB. Brain abscess and congenital heart disease. Clin Neurosurg 1966; 14:274–287.

Courville CB, Nielsen JM. Fatal complications of otitis media: with particular reference to intracranial lesions in a series of 10,000 autopsies. Arch Otolaryngol 1934; 19:451–501.

Curless RG. Neonatal intracranial abscess: two cases caused by Citrobacter and a literature review. Ann Neurol 1980; 8:269–272.

Harvey FH, Carlow TJ. Brainstem abscess and the syndrome of acute tegmental encephalitis. Ann Neurol 1980; 7:371–376.

Idriss ZH, Gutman LT, Kronfol NM. Brain abscesses in infants and children. Clin Pediatr 1978; 17:738–746.

Kagawa M, Takeshita M, Yatō S, Kitamura K. Brain abscess in congenital cyanotic heart disease. J Neurosurg 1983; 58:913–917.

Kaplan K. Brain abscess. Med Clin North Am 1985; 69:345–359.

Kaufman DM, Litman N, Miller MH. Sinusitis-induced subdural empyema. Neurology 1983; 33:123–132.

Loeser E Jr, Scheinberg L. Brain abscesses: a review of ninety-nine cases. Neurology 1957; 7:601–609.

Macewen W. Pyogenic Infective Diseases of the Brain and Spinal Cord: Meningitis, Abscess of Brain, Infective Sinus Thrombosis. Glasgow: James Maclehose & Son, 1893

Maurice-Williams RS. Open evacuation of pus: a satisfactory surgical approach to the problem of brain abscess? J Neurol Neurosurg Psychiatry 1983; 46:697–703.

Merritt HH, Fremont-Smith F. The Cerebrospinal Fluid. Philadelphia: WB Saunders, 1938: 150–152.

Neu HC. Brain abscess. In Goldensohn ES, Appel SH, eds: Scientific Approaches to Clinical Neurology. Philadelphia: Lea & Febiger, 1977: 452–460.

Rosenblum ML, Hoff JT, Norman D, Weinstein PR, Pitts L. Decreased mortality from brain abscesses since the advent of computerized tomography. J Neurosurg 1978; 49:658–668.

Shaw MDM, Russell JA. Cerebellar abscess: a review of 47 cases. J Neurol Neurosurg Psychiatry 1975; 38:429–435.

Silverberg AL, DiNubile MJ. Subdural empyema and cranial epidural abscess. Med Clin North Am 1985; 69:361–374.

Smith HP, Hendricks EB. Subdural empyema and epidural abscess in children. J Neurosurg 1983; 58:392–397.

Turner AL, Reynolds FE. Intracranial Pyogenic Disease: A Pathological and Clinical Study of the Pathways of Infection from the Face, Nasal and Paranasal Air-Cavities. London: Oliver, 1931.

Weickhardt GD, Davis RL: Solitary abscess of the brainstem. Neurology 1964; 14:918–925.

Weisberg LA. Cerebral computerized tomography in intracranial inflammatory disorders. Arch Neurol 1980; 37:137–142.

Weisberg LA. Nonsurgical management of focal intracranial infection. Neurology 1981; 31:575–580.

Whelan MA, Hilal SK. Computed tomography as a guide in the diagnosis and follow-up of brain abscesses. Radiology 1980; 135:663–671.

15. VIRAL INFECTIONS

Burk Jubelt
James R. Miller

Although rabies has been known since ancient times and acute anterior poliomyelitis was recognized as a clinical entity in 1840, our knowledge of the role of viruses in the production of neurologic disease is of recent origin. In 1804, Zinke showed that rabies could be produced in a normal dog by inoculation of saliva from a rabid animal, but the filterable nature of rabies virus was not demonstrated until 1903. In 1908, Landsteiner and Popper produced a flaccid paralysis in monkeys by the injection of an emulsion of spinal cord from a fatal case of poliomyelitis. In the 1930s, filterable viruses were recovered from patients with epidemic encephalitis (arboviruses) and aseptic meningitis (lymphocytic choriomeningitis virus). With the use of electron microscopic tissue culture and immunologic techniques, many additional viruses that infect the nervous system have been recovered and characterized.

Although the list of viruses that cause human disease in epidemic or sporadic forms is extensive, viral infections are not a common cause of neurologic disease. Most viral infections of the central nervous system are uncommon complications of systemic illnesses caused by common human pathogens. After viral multiplication in extraneural tissues, dissemination to the CNS occurs by the hematogenous route or by spread along nerve fibers.

Viruses are *classified* according to their nucleic acid content, size, sensitivity to lipid solvents (enveloped versus nonenveloped), morphology, and mode of development in cells. The principal division is made according to whether the virus contains RNA or DNA. Members of almost every major animal virus group have been implicated in the production of neurologic illness in animals or humans (Table 15–1). The nature of the lesions produced varies with the virus and the conditions of infection. They may include neoplastic transformation, system degeneration, or congenital defects, such as cerebellar agenesis and aqueductal stenosis, as well as the inflammatory and destructive changes often considered typical of viral infection. In addition, the concept that a viral infection causes only an acute illness that quickly follows infection of the host has been challenged by demonstration that, in slow viral infections, illness may not appear until many years after exposure to the agent. It is useful to distinguish between CNS viral infections of an acute or chronic (slow) nature.

Acute Viral Infections

CNS VIRAL SYNDROMES

Acute viral infection of the nervous system can be manifest clinically in three forms: viral (aseptic) meningitis, encephalitis, or myelitis (Table 15–2). Viral meningitis is usually a self-limited illness characterized by signs of meningeal irritation such as headache, photophobia, and neck stiffness. Encephalitis entails involvement of parenchymal brain tissue as indicated by convulsive seizures, alterations in the state of consciousness, and focal neurologic abnormalities. When both meningeal and encephalitic findings are present, the term *meningoencephalitis* may be used. Viral infections may also localize to the parenchyma of the spinal cord resulting in myelitis. Myelitis may occur from infection of spinal motor neurons (paralytic disease, poliomye-

Table 15–1. Viral Infections of the Nervous System

RNA-Containing Viruses:	*Representative Viruses Responsible for Neurologic Disease*
Picornavirus (enterovirus)	Poliovirus
	Coxsackievirus
	Echovirus
	Enterovirus 70 and 71
	Enterovirus 72 (hepatitis A)
Togavirus (arbovirus)	Equine encephalomyelitis (Eastern, Western, Venezuela)
	St. Louis encephalitis
	Japanese encephalitis
	Tick-borne encephalitis
	Rubella
Bunyavirus (arbovirus)	California encephalitis
Orbivirus (arbovirus)	Colorado tick fever
Orthomyxovirus	Influenza
Paramyxovirus	Measles (subacute sclerosing panencephalitis)
	Mumps
Arenavirus	Lymphocytic choriomeningitis
Rhabdovirus	Rabies
Retrovirus	Human immunodeficiency virus (acquired immunodeficiency syndrome)
DNA-Containing Viruses:	
Herpesviruses	Herpes simplex
	Varicella-zoster
	Cytomegalovirus
	Epstein-Barr (infectious mononucleosis)
Papovavirus	Progressive multifocal leukoencephalopathy
Poxvirus	Vaccinia
Adenovirus	Adenovirus serotypes

litis), sensory neurons, autonomic neurons (bladder paralysis), or demyelination of white matter (transverse myelitis). When both encephalitis and myelitis occur, the term *encephalomyelitis* is used. The CSF findings in these three acute viral syndromes are usually similar, consisting of an increase in pressure, pleocytosis of varying degree, a moderate protein content elevation, and a normal sugar content.

Common biologic properties of members of a specific virus group may dictate how they attack the CNS and the type of disease they produce. For example, individual picornaviruses, such as poliovirus and echovirus, can cause similar clinical syndromes. Members of specific virus groups also show different predilections for cell types or regions of the nervous system. Thus, members of the myxovirus group attack ependymal cells, and herpes simplex virus shows preference for frontal and temporal lobes.

Table 15–2. Specific Etiology of Acute CNS Syndromes of Viral Etiology (Walter Reed Army Institute of Research 1958–1963)

	Aseptic Meningitis	*Encephalitis*	*Paralytic Disease*	*Total*
Mumps	28	11	1	40
LCM*	7	0	0	7
Herpes simplex	2	7	0	9
Poliovirus	18	5	66	89
Coxsackievirus A	18	1	0	19
Coxsackievirus B	71	4	0	75
Echovirus	55	3	1	59
Arbovirus	3	5	0	8

*Lymphocytic choriomeningitis.
(From Buescher, et al. Res Publ Assoc Re Nerv Ment Dis 1968; 44:147.)

The tendency for a disease to appear in an epidemic or sporadic form may also be related to the biologic properties of the virus. Most epidemic forms of meningitis, encephalitis, or myelitis are due to infection with picornaviruses or togaviruses. The picornaviruses (enteroviruses) are relatively acid- and heat-resistant, which results in fecal-hand-oral transmission during the hotter months of the year. Many togaviruses require a multiplication phase in mosquitoes or ticks before they can infect people; human epidemics occur when climatic and other conditions favor a large population of infected insect vectors. Neurologic diseases due to members of other virus groups usually occur sporadically or as isolated instances that complicate viral infections of other organs or systems.

Diagnosis. Knowledge of whether the illness is occurring in an epidemic setting and of the seasonal occurrence of the different forms of acute viral infections may indicate the methods to be used in detecting the infective agent. Infection with the picornaviruses or arboviruses tends to occur in the summer and early fall; other viruses, such as mumps, occur in late winter or spring.

The diagnosis can be made by a combination of virus isolation (inoculation of blood, nasopharyngeal washings, feces, CSF, or tissue suspensions into susceptible animals or tissue culture systems) and serologic tests. Infectious virus particles in human fluids and tissues are usually few in number, and many viruses are easily disrupted and inactivated even at room temperature; tissues and fluids to be used for virus isolation studies should therefore be frozen unless they can be immediately transferred to the laboratory in appropriate transport media.

The ability to recover virus from the CSF varies according to the nature of the agent. Some viruses, such as mumps virus, can frequently be isolated from the CSF, whereas other viruses, such as poliovirus and herpes simplex type 1, are rarely recovered.

Serologic tests are applicable to all known acute viral diseases of the nervous system. Serum should be frozen and kept at a low temperature until the tests are made. The diagnosis of an acute viral infection and the establishment of the type of virus rest upon the development of antibodies to the infection, traditionally a fourfold antibody rise. It is therefore necessary to show that antibodies are not present or are present only in low titer in the early stage of the illness and that they are present in high titer at a proper interval after the onset of symptoms. Several to many days are usually required for the development of antibodies; serum removed in the first few days of the illness can therefore serve as the control. Serum withdrawn in the convalescent stage, three to five weeks after the onset of the illness, may be used to determine whether antibodies have developed. If the antibodies are present in equal titer in both specimens, it can be stated that the acute illness was not due to the virus tested. When there is no change in titer, positive tests merely indicate that the individual has at some time in the past had an infection with this type of virus.

If brain tissue from the patient is available in fatal cases or by brain biopsy, further studies can define the responsible virus. Brain sections can be analyzed by immunostaining techniques (fluorescence antibody, peroxidase antiperoxidase) to determine if specific viral antigens are present. Electron microscopy may indicate the presence of virus particles or components of specific morphology. Suspensions of brain and spinal cord can be injected into susceptible animals and tissue culture cell lines. In special instances, tissue cultures can be initiated from brain tissue itself. Such brain cell cultures can then be examined for the presence of viral antigens or infective virus. If an agent is recovered, final identification can be made by neutralization with known specific antiserum.

Treatment. There is as yet no fully adequate therapy for viral infections of the nervous system. The single possible exception is the use of DNA inhibitors in the treatment of herpesvirus infections.

Immunization procedures with either live attenuated vaccines or inactivated virus are available for rabies, poliomyelitis, mumps, influenza, rubella, and measles. Immunization against the arboviruses has not been given adequate human trial and has been used mainly to protect laboratory workers.

Although we can anticipate that effective antiviral chemotherapeutic agents will become available in the future, vector control and mass immunization now seem to be the most practical means for effective control.

PICORNAVIRUS (ENTEROVIRUS) INFECTIONS

Picornaviruses are small, nonenveloped RNA viruses that multiply in the cytoplasm of cells. They are the smallest RNA viruses, hence the name "pico (small) RNA virus."

Human picornaviruses can be divided into two subgroups: the enteroviruses, which are found primarily in the gastrointestinal tract, and the rhinoviruses, which are found in the nasopharynx. The enteroviruses comprise the *polioviruses, coxsackieviruses,* and *echoviruses,* all of which are capable of producing inflammation in the CNS. More recently identified enteroviruses have been named *unclassified enteroviruses 68 to 72.* Enterovirus 72 is the official name of hepatitis A virus. CNS disease has occurred with enteroviruses 70 to 72.

The picornaviruses cannot be inactivated by most agents. The enteroviruses are resistant to the acid and bile of intestinal contents and may survive for long periods in sewage or water. Picornaviruses grow only in primate cells and are highly cytocidal. Virus particles may form crystalline arrays in the cytoplasm of cells that are recognized as acidophilic inclusions in histologic preparations.

Poliomyelitis

Acute anterior poliomyelitis (infantile paralysis, Heine-Medin disease) is an acute generalized disease caused by poliovirus infection characterized by destruction of the motor cells in the spinal cord and brain stem, and the appearance of a flaccid paralysis of the muscles innervated by the affected neurons.

Although the disease has probably occurred for many centuries, the first clear description was given by Jacob Heine in 1840, and the foundation of our knowledge of the epidemiology of the disease was laid by Medin in 1890. The studies of Landsteiner, Popper, Flexner, Lewis, and others in the first decade of this century proved that the disease was caused by a virus.

Invasion of the nervous system occurs as a relatively late and infrequent manifestation. Orally ingested virus multiplies in the pharynx and ileum, probably in lymphoid tissue of the tonsils and Peyer's patches. The virus then spreads to cervical and mesenteric lymph nodes and can be detected in the blood shortly thereafter. Viremia is accompanied by no symptoms or by a brief minor illness. It is still not definitely known how the virus gains access to the nervous system in paralytic cases. The most likely possibility is via direct spread from the blood at defective areas of the blood-brain barrier. Less likely is neural spread from the intestine or from neuromuscular junctions.

The virus has a predilection for the large motor cells, causing chromatolysis with acidophilic inclusions and necrosis of the cells. The necrotic cells are phagocytized by leukocytes. Degeneration of the neurons is accompanied by an inflammatory reaction in the adjacent meninges and in the perivascular spaces and by secondary proliferation of the microglia. Recovery may occur in partially damaged cells, but the severely damaged cells are phagocytized and removed. The degenerative changes are most intense in the ventral horn cells, and the motor cells in the medulla; however, the neurons in the posterior horn, the posterior root ganglion, and elsewhere in the CNS may be involved to a lesser degree. The inflammatory reaction may also be present in the white matter (Fig. 15–1). Although the pathologic changes are most intense in the spinal cord and medulla, any portion of the nervous system may be affected, including the midbrain, cerebellum, basal ganglia, and cerebral cortex. The selective affinity of the virus for the large motor cells is manifest by the predominance of the involvement of the motor area of the cerebral cortex. Degeneration of the peripheral nerves follows destruction of the motor cells. With subsidence of the destructive process, the inflammatory reaction disappears. Fibrous astrocytes proliferate in an attempt to fill the defect caused by the loss of nerve cells. This is often incomplete and there may be shrinkage of the spinal cord or cyst formation in the ventral horns.

Epidemiology. Acute anterior poliomyelitis is worldwide in distribution, but is more prevalent in temperate climates. It may occur in sporadic, endemic, or epidemic form at any time of the year, but is most common in late summer and early fall.

Acute anterior poliomyelitis was formerly the most common form of viral infection of the nervous system. Prior to 1956, between 25,000 and 50,000 cases occurred annually in the United States.

Since the advent of an effective vaccine, the incidence of the disease has decreased dramatically in the United States as well as in other developed countries. In fact, paralytic poliomyelitis is becoming a clinical rarity except for isolated cases and small epidemics in areas where the population has not been vaccinated. Figure 15–2, taken from the United States Public Health Service poliomyelitis surveillance reports, shows the magnitude of the decrease of incidence of reported cases of poliomyelitis in the United States in the years between 1935 and 1964. The incidence has

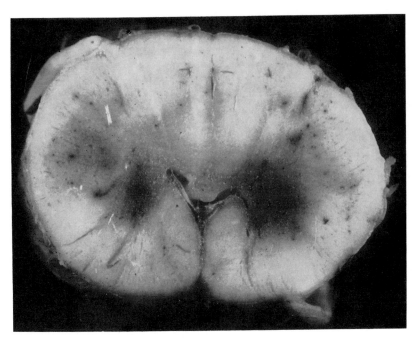

Fig. 15–1. Acute anterior poliomyelitis. Congestion and inflammation in gray and white matter of cervical cord. (Courtesy of Dr. Abner Wolf.)

remained low to date. A similar decrease has been reported in other countries in which vaccination has been practiced on a large scale. However, paralytic poliomyelitis is still a significant health problem in developing areas of the world. Worldwide in 1984 there were 24,275 cases of paralytic poliomyelitis reported to the World Health Organization. During the 12-year period from 1973 to 1984, there were 138 cases of paralytic poliomyelitis

in the United States; 105 were vaccine-associated and 33 were due to wild-type virus. Fourteen of the vaccine-associated cases occurred in immunodeficient children often as chronic rather than as acute CNS disease.

Three antigenically distinct types of poliovirus have been defined. All three types can cause paralytic poliomyelitis or viral meningitis, but type I appears to be most often associated with paralytic disease.

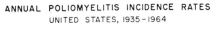

ANNUAL POLIOMYELITIS INCIDENCE RATES
UNITED STATES, 1935–1964

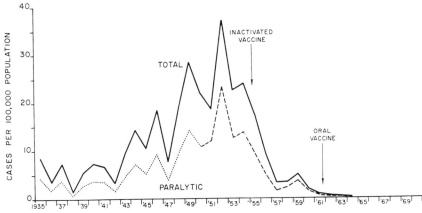

Fig. 15–2. Annual poliomyelitis incidence rates in the United States, 1935–1964. Paralytic cases prior to 1951 assumed to be 50% of total. After 1951, cases reported as unspecified were prorated among paralytic and nonparalytic cases. (From National Morbidity Reports.)

The disease may occur at any age. It is rare before the age of 6 months. In the late nineteenth and early twentieth centuries, poliomyelitis changed from an endemic to an epidemic disease. In the early epidemics, 90% of paralytic cases occurred in people less than 5 years old. As epidemics recurred, there was a shift of paralytic cases in older individuals, so that the majority of cases occurred in children more than 5 years old and in teenagers. Paralysis was also seen more frequently in young adults.

The virus is present in the oropharynx during the first week of the disease. It can be demonstrated in the feces for a longer period and has been isolated from them as long as 19 days before the onset of paralytic symptoms, as well as in healthy contacts during an epidemic. In fatal human cases, the virus has usually been recovered from the brain and spinal cord. It can be detected in the pharyngeal wall, but more readily in the intestinal wall and its contents.

Prophylaxis. Oral vaccination with live attenuated virus (Sabin) is effective in the prevention of paralytic infections. Antibody response is dependent on multiplication of attenuated virus in the gastrointestinal tract. Significant antibody levels develop more rapidly and persist longer than those that follow immunization with formalized polioviruses (Salk). Live attenuated vaccine is also capable of spreading and thus immunizing contacts of vaccinated individuals. The recommended procedure is to give three immunizing doses of trivalent oral vaccine within the first year of life beginning at 6 to 12 weeks of age. A fourth dose may be given before the child enters school.

Symptoms. The symptoms at the onset of poliomyelitis are similar to those of any acute infection. In about 25% of the cases, these initial symptoms subside in 36 to 48 hours and the patient is apparently well for 2 to 3 days until there is a secondary rise in temperature (dromedary type) accompanied by symptoms of meningeal irritation. In most cases, this second phase of the illness directly follows the first without any intervening period of freedom from symptoms. The headache increases in severity and muscle soreness appears, most commonly in the neck and back. Drowsiness or stupor occasionally develops, but the patient is irritable and apprehensive when aroused. Convulsions are occasionally seen at this stage in infants.

Paralysis, when it occurs, usually develops between the second and fifth day after the onset of signs of involvement of the nervous system, but it may be the initial symptom or, in rare instances, may be delayed for as long as 2 to 3 weeks. After the onset of paralysis, there may be extension of the motor loss for 3 to 5 days. Further progress of signs and symptoms rarely occurs after this time. The fever lasts for 4 to 7 days and subsides gradually. The temperature may return to normal before the development of paralysis or while the paralysis is advancing. Limb muscles are usually involved but, in severe cases, respiratory and cardiac muscles may be affected.

Acute cerebellar ataxia, isolated facial nerve palsies, and transverse myelitis have been observed in poliovirus-infected individuals.

Laboratory Data. There is a leukocytosis in the blood. CSF pressure may be increased. A CSF pleocytosis develops in the period before the onset of the paralysis. Initially, polymorphonuclear cells predominate, but a shift to lymphocytes occurs within several days. The CSF protein content is slightly elevated except in the cases with a severe degree of paralysis, when it may be elevated to 100 to 300 mg/dl and may persist for several weeks.

Diagnosis. Acute anterior poliomyelitis can be diagnosed without difficulty in most cases by the acute development of an asymmetric flaccid paralysis accompanied by the characteristic changes in the CSF. A presumptive diagnosis can be made in the preparalytic stage and in nonparalytic cases during an epidemic. The diagnosis can be suspected in patients who have not been vaccinated or have defects in their immune response. The diagnosis of poliovirus infection can be established with certainty by recovery of the virus from stool, throat washings, CSF, or blood. Recovery of virus from the throat or feces requires the additional demonstration of a fourfold rise in the patient's antibody level in complement fixation or neutralization tests before a specific viral diagnosis can be made. Poliovirus is recovered only rarely from the CSF.

Prognosis. Fewer than 10% of patients die from the acute disease. Death is usually due to respiratory failure or pulmonary complications. The mortality rate is highest in the bulbar form of the disease, where it is often greater than 50%. The prognosis is poor when the paralysis is extensive or when there is a slow progress of paralysis with exacerbations and involvement of new muscles over a period of days. The prognosis with regard to return of function depends on the extent of paralysis, as muscle groups only partially paralyzed are more likely to recover.

About 25% of patients have developed new symptoms 30 to 40 years after the acute poliomyelitis. These new symptoms have been collectively referred to as the *post-polio syndrome*. Some of these patients develop a slowly progressive weakness with atrophy and fasciculations, called *post-poliomyelitis progressive muscular atrophy* (PPMA).

Treatment. Treatment in the preparalytic stage is essentially supportive. Muscle paralysis that results in stretching or malposition may require the application of removable splints. Fluid, vitamin, and electrolyte intake should be maintained intravenously if indicated. When the muscle tenderness has subsided, gentle massage, together with active and passive movements, is given to relax muscles and prevent contractures. These procedures should be discontinued if they produce pain or fatigue the patient. Attention should be given to the bladder and bowel. Catheterization may be necessary for a few days and enemas are advisable if the abdominal muscles are weakened.

Treatment of patients with paralysis of respiratory muscles or bulbar involvement requires great care. The patient should be watched carefully for signs of respiratory embarrassment, and as soon as these become apparent, mechanical respiratory assistance should be given immediately. The development of anxiety in a previously calm patient is a serious warning of cerebral anoxia and may precede labored breathing or cyanosis. When patients are reassured and given artificial respiratory assistance, the chances of recovery are greatly increased. The use of the respirator should be continued in bulbar cases until the respiratory centers have recovered. If the respiratory difficulty is due to paralysis of intercostal muscles and the diaphragm, the patient may need the aid of a respirator every day for varying periods over several months.

Treatment in the convalescent stage and thereafter consists of physiotherapy, muscle re-education, application of appropriate corrective appliances, and orthopedic surgery. Rehabilitation of the severely paralyzed patient requires facilities available only in special institutes for rehabilitation, as well as the ingenuity of the physician and the patient's courage and persistence.

Coxsackieviruses

In 1948, Dalldorf and Sickles inoculated specimens obtained from patients with suspected poliomyelitis into the brains of newborn mice and discovered the coxsackieviruses. Two subgroups, A and B, can be distinguished by their effects on suckling mice. In mice, group A viruses cause myositis leading to flaccid paralysis and death. Group B viruses cause encephalitis, myocarditis, pancreatitis and necrosis of brown fat; animals develop tremors, spasms, and paralysis before death. Twenty-three group A and six group B serotypes are currently recognized.

When they involve the human nervous system, both group A and group B coxsackieviruses most frequently cause aseptic meningitis. Occasionally, coxsackievirus infection causes encephalitis, and rarely paralytic disease or acute cerebellar ataxia are seen. Group A coxsackieviruses can cause herpangina and hand-foot-and-mouth disease. Group B coxsackieviruses cause pericarditis, myocarditis, and epidemic myalgia (pleurodynia, Bornholm disease).

The symptoms and signs of meningeal involvement are similar to those that follow infection with other viruses that cause aseptic meningitis. The onset may be acute or subacute with fever, headache, malaise, nausea, and abdominal pain. Stiffness of the neck and vomiting usually begin 24 to 48 hours after the initial symptoms. There is a mild or moderate fever. Muscular paralysis, sensory disturbances, and reflex changes are rare. Paralysis, when present, is mild and transient. Meningeal symptoms occasionally occur in combination with myalgia, pleurodynia, or herpangina.

The CSF pressure is normal or slightly increased. There is a mild or moderate pleocytosis in the CSF, ranging from 25 to 250/mm³ with 10 to 50% polymorphonuclear cells. The protein content is normal or slightly increased and the sugar content is normal.

Diagnosis of infection with coxsackievirus can be established only by recovering the virus from the feces, throat washings, or CSF and by demonstrating an increase in viral antibodies in the serum. Meningitis due to one of the coxsackieviruses cannot be distinguished from the other viral agents that cause aseptic meningitis except by laboratory studies. It is differentiated from meningitis due to pyogenic bacteria and yeast by the relatively low cell count and the normal sugar content in the CSF.

Echoviruses

This group of picornaviruses was originally isolated in cell culture from the feces of apparently normal persons. They were considered "orphans" because they lacked a parent disease. The designation *ECHO* was derived from the first letter of the term *Enteric Cytopathogenic Human Orphans*. Thirty-two serotypes are now recognized. Many strains cause hemagglutination of human type O erythrocytes.

The echoviruses cause gastroenteritis, macular exanthema, and upper respiratory infections. Echovirus 9 infections may cause a petechial rash that may be confused with meningococcemia. When the nervous system is infected, the syndrome of aseptic meningitis usually results.

The clinical picture of infection with the echoviruses is similar to that of nonparalytic poliomyelitis. Children are more frequently affected than adults. The main features are fever, coryza, sore throat, vomiting, and diarrhea. A rubelliform rash is often present. Headache, neck stiffness, lethargy, irritability, and slight muscular weakness indicate involvement of the nervous system and suggest the possibility of acute anterior poliomyelitis. The disease usually runs a benign course that subsides in 1 or 2 weeks.

Cerebellar ataxia has been reported in children as the result of echovirus infection. The onset of ataxa is acute; the course is benign with remission of the symptoms within a few weeks. Oculomotor nerve paralysis with pupillomotor fiber sparing and other cranial nerve palsies have rarely been observed in conjunction with echovirus infection. Echoviruses can cause a persistent CNS infection in children with agammaglobulinemia; this is an echovirus-induced meningoencephalitis that is often associated with a dermatomyositis-like syndrome. It can be treated with immune globulin.

The CSF pleocytosis may vary from several hundred to a thousand or more cells/mm³, but is usually less than 500/mm³. Early in the infection, there may be as many as 90% polymorphonuclear leukocytes; within 48 hours, however, the response becomes completely mononuclear. The CSF protein content is normal or slightly elevated. The sugar content remains normal.

The echoviruses are commonly recovered from feces, throat swabs, and CSF. Human or simian kidney cells are used in virus isolation. Virus typing is carried out by neutralization of hemagglutination-inhibition tests. Neutralizing antibodies are present in the serum one week after the onset of illness and persist for months or years.

Enteroviruses 70, 71 and 72

Newly recognized enteroviruses are now named as unclassified enteroviruses. Several of these new enteroviruses have caused CNS infections. Enterovirus 70 causes epidemics of acute hemorrhagic conjunctivitis (AHC), which initially occurred in Africa and Asia. More recently, outbreaks of AHC have occurred in Latin America and the southeastern United States. Neurologic abnormality occurs in about 1 in 10,000 or 15,000 cases of AHC, primarily in adults. The most common neurologic picture is a polio-like syndrome of flaccid, asymmetric, and proximal paralysis of the legs accompanied by severe radicular pains. Paralysis is permanent in over half the cases. Isolated cranial nerve palsies (primary facial nerve), pyramidal tract signs, bladder paralysis, vertigo, and sensory loss have been reported. Because neurologic involvement usually occurs about two weeks after the onset of AHC, it may be difficult to isolate the virus at the time neurologic signs are seen. Thus, diagnosis often depends on serologic studies. The neurologic disorder has rarely been seen without the preceding conjunctivitis.

Enterovirus 71 has been recognized as causing outbreaks of hand-foot-and-mouth disease. Upper respiratory infections and gastroenteritis also occur. Neurologic involvement may occur in up to 25% of cases with children and teenagers primarily affected. Neurologic manifestations include aseptic meningitis, cerebellar ataxia, and various forms of poliomyelitis (flaccid monoparesis, bulbar polio). Most of these cases have occurred in Europe and Asia. Two cases of transient paralysis were seen in a recent outbreak in New York. Diagnosis can be made by virus isolation from throat, feces, or vesicles and by neutralization antibody studies.

Enterovirus 72 (hepatitis A virus) apparently has caused primarily encephalitis as a distinct entity, although hepatic encephalitis is obviously more common. EV 72 has also been associated with transverse myelitis.

TOGA- AND ARBOVIRUSES

The arboviruses (*arthropod-borne*) are small, spherical, ether-sensitive viruses that contain RNA. Over 400 serologically distinct arboviruses are currently recognized. Most but not all arboviruses are now officially classified as togaviruses. Although the term *ar-*

bovirus is no longer an official taxonomic term, it is still useful for viruses that are transmitted by vectors. These viruses develop within the cytoplasm of infected cells, often within vacuoles. The virus particle contains an electron-dense core surrounded by a lipoprotein envelope that has projections. Many togaviruses agglutinate erythrocytes of newborn chicks or adult geese within restricted pH ranges. Togaviruses can be divided into groups on the basis of their cross-reactivity in hemagglutination-inhibition or complement-fixation tests.

Most togaviruses multiply in a blood-sucking arthropod vector. In their natural environment, these viruses alternate between an invertebrate vector and a mammal. Mosquitoes and ticks are the most common vectors. Birds seem to be the principal natural hosts, but wild snakes and some rodents are probably a secondary reservoir. People and horses are incidental hosts and human or horse infection terminates the chain of infection.

Approximately 80 arboviruses are known to cause human disease. The spectrum of disease produced is broad, ranging from hemorrhagic fevers (yellow fever) to arthralgias, rashes, and encephalitis.

Arboviruses are difficult to isolate in the laboratory. The virus may be recovered from blood during the early phases (2 to 4 days) of the illness. In nonfatal cases, the diagnosis usually depends on the demonstration of a fourfold rise in antibodies during the course of the illness. The virus may be isolated from the tissues at necropsy by the intracerebral inoculation of infant mice and susceptible tissue culture cells.

Arbovirus infection of the nervous system may result in viral meningitis or more frequently in moderate or severe encephalitis. Diseases due to arboviruses typically occur in late summer and early fall.

Equine Encephalomyelitis

Etiology. Three distinct types of equine encephalomyelitis are now recognized to occur in the United States. They are due to three serologically distinct alphaviruses (formerly group A arboviruses): eastern equine encephalitis (EEE), western equine encephalitis (WEE), and Venezuelan equine encephalitis (VEE). Infection with these viruses was thought to be limited to horses until 1932 when Meyer reported an unusual type of encephalitis in three men who were working in close contact with affected animals. The first cases in which EEE virus was recovered from

human brain tissue were reported from Massachusetts in 1938 by Fothergill and co-workers. Many arboviruses take their name from the location in which they were first isolated. They are not confined, however, by specific geographic boundaries. WEE virus infection is now known to occur in all parts of the United States, although most frequently in the western two thirds of the country. EEE is usually localized to the Atlantic and Gulf coasts and the Great Lakes areas. Cases of EEE have been reported in regions west of the Mississippi River, as well as in Central and South America and the Philippines.

Pathology. In EEE, the brain is markedly congested and there are widespread degenerative changes in the nerve cells. The meninges and perivascular spaces of the brain are intensely infiltrated with polymorphonuclear leukocytes and round cells. In some areas, the accumulation of these cells is so great that they give the appearance of small abscesses. Focal vasculitic lesions often with thrombus formation may occur. Destruction of myelin is prominent only near the necrotic foci. The lesions are found in both the white and gray matter and are most intensive in the cerebrum and brain stem; however, they may also be present in the cerebellum and spinal cord.

In contrast to EEE, the pathology of WEE is characterized by a lesser degree of inflammatory reaction, which is primarily mononuclear, a paucity of changes in the nerve cells, more extensive areas of demyelination, and greater frequency of petechial hemorrhage.

Incidence. Equine encephalomyelitis is a rare human infection, tending to occur as isolated cases or in small epidemics. Epizootics in horses may precede the human cases by several weeks. Equine encephalomyelitis mainly affects infants, children, and adults over 50 years of age. Inapparent infection is common in all age groups.

Symptoms. Infection with the EEE virus is characterized by the sudden onset of drowsiness, stupor, or coma with convulsive seizures, headache, vomiting, neck stiffness, and high fever. Cranial nerve palsies, hemiplegia, and other focal neurologic signs are common.

The symptoms of infection with WEE and VEE are less severe. The onset is acute, with general malaise and headache occasionally followed by convulsions, nausea, and vomiting. There is moderate fever and neck stiffness. The headaches increase in severity and there is drowsiness, lethargy, or coma. Paresis and cranial nerve palsies may occur.

Laboratory Data. Leukocytosis may occur in the blood, especially in infections with EEE; white blood cell counts as high as 35,000 have been reported.

The CSF changes are greatest in EEE where the pressure is always moderately or greatly increased. The CSF is cloudy or purulent, containing 500 to 3000 cells/mm³ with a predominance of polymorphonuclear leukocytes. The protein content is increased but the sugar content is normal. With abatement of the acute stage, the cell count drops and lymphocytes become the predominating cell type, although polymorphonuclear cells persist as a significant fraction.

The CSF changes in the WEE and VEE are less severe. The pressure is usually normal and the cellular increase is moderate, with counts varying from normal to 500 cells/mm³, with mononuclear cells as the predominating cell type.

Diagnosis. Isolation of equine encephalomyelitis viruses from blood and CSF of patients during life has been accomplished infrequently in the early phases of the disease. It cannot be considered a practical diagnostic method. The hemagglutination-inhibition, complement-fixation, and neutralization tests are the serologic methods of choice for patients who recover. In fatal cases the diagnosis can be established by isolation of the virus from brain. Togavirus particles have been recognized in brain specimens examined by means of electron microscopy.

Equine encephalomyelitis must be differentiated from the other acute infectious diseases of the nervous system, including acute and subacute meningitides, encephalomyelitis following the acute exanthemata, aseptic meningeal reaction associated with infections in the skull, brain abscess, and other virus infections of the nervous system.

The acute and subacute meningitides are excluded by the normal sugar content and the absence of bacteria in the CSF. Encephalomyelitis following acute exanthemata, aseptic meningeal reaction accompanying infections in the skull, and brain abscess are excluded by the absence of the usual associated findings in these conditions. Differentiation from other virus encephalomyelitides can only be made by isolation of the virus or by serologic tests.

Course and Prognosis. The mortality rate in EEE is over 50%. The duration of the disease varies from less than one day in fulminating cases to over four weeks in less severe cases. In patients who recover, sequelae such as mental deficiency, cranial nerve palsies, hemiplegia, aphasia and convulsions are common. Children under 10 years of age are more likely to survive the acute infection, but also have the greatest chance of being left with severe neurologic disability.

The fatality rate in WEE is 10% or less. Sequelae among young infants are frequent and severe, but are uncommon in adults who recover from the illness. The mortality rate in VEE is less than 0.5%; nearly all deaths have occurred in young children.

Treatment. Treatment in the acute stage of the disease is entirely supportive. Vaccines against the equine encephalomyelitis viruses have been produced; their use should be confined to laboratory workers and others who are subject to unusual exposure to the virus. Vaccination on a large-scale community program is not indicated because of the low incidence of the disease.

St. Louis Encephalitis

The first outbreak of acute encephalitis in which a virus was definitely established as the causative agent was the epidemic that occurred in St. Louis in 1933. This type of encephalitis had probably existed in this area prior to 1933; sporadic cases of encephalitis had occurred in St. Louis in July and August during the previous 14 years, and a small epidemic (38 cases) of encephalitis occurred in Paris, Illinois in 1932. Neutralization tests on the serum of recovered patients of this epidemic proved it to be due to a virus identical to that of the St. Louis epidemic of 1933. Since 1933 repeated outbreaks have occurred in the United States with increasing frequency and widening geographic distribution. St. Louis encephalitis is the most common form of arbovirus encephalitis in the United States.

The virus responsible for St. Louis encephalitis is a mosquito-transmitted flavivirus (formerly group B arbovirus). Epidemics follow two epidemiologic patterns: rural and urban. Rural epidemics tend to occur in the western United States. The rural cycle involves birds as the intermediate host, similar to WEE. Urban epidemics occur primarily in the Midwest, Mississippi River Valley, and eastern United States. The urban outbreaks can be abrupt and extensive because humans are the intermediate hosts. St. Louis encephalitis primarily affects the elderly. As with other arboviruses, disease in humans usually appears in midsummer to early fall.

Pathology. Grossly, there is a mild degree of vascular congestion and occasional petechial hemorrhages. The characteristic microscopic changes are a slight infiltration of the meninges and blood vessels of the brain and spinal cord with mononuclear cells, focal accumulation of inflammatory and glial cells in the substance of the brain, and degenerative changes in the neurons. Both gray and white matter are affected, but the nuclear masses of the thalamus and midbrain are more affected than the cortex.

Symptoms and Signs. Infection with St. Louis encephalitis virus usually results in inapparent infection. Symptoms in these abortive cases are so mild that they are diagnosed only by the development of viral antibodies.

About 75% of patients with clinical manifestations have encephalitis; the others have aseptic meningitis or nonspecific illness. Almost all patients over 40 years of age with symptoms develop encephalitic signs.

The onset of neurologic symptoms may be abrupt or may be preceded by a prodromal illness of three or four days' duration, characterized by headache, myalgia, fever, sore throat, or gastrointestinal symptoms. The headache increases in severity, and neck stiffness develops. Other common signs include increase or diminution of tendon reflexes, moderately coarse intention tremor of the fingers, lips, and tongue, ataxia, and absence of abdominal skin reflexes. In the more severe cases, there may be delirium, coma or stupor, disturbance of vesical and rectal sphincters, focal neurologic signs and, rarely, cranial nerve palsies.

The temperature is elevated (100° to 104° F) from the onset and falls in 10 days to 2 weeks. The pulse is increased in proportion to the fever. Bradycardia is rare.

Laboratory Data. A mild to moderate leukocytosis occurs in the blood. The CSF is usually abnormal. There is a mild pleocytosis in most cases, averaging approximately 100 cells/mm^3. Cell counts as high as 500 or more have been reported. Lymphocytes are the predominating cell type, although a few polymorphonuclear cells may be found early in the disease. The sugar content is normal. Hyponatremia due to inappropriate secretion of antidiuretic hormone occurs in a fourth to a third of cases.

Diagnosis. Encephalitis due to infection with the St. Louis virus can be diagnosed only by isolation of the virus from blood, CSF, or brain tissue, or by the development of antibodies. It must be differentiated from the subacute meningitides and other forms of viral encephalitis. The differential diagnosis from tuberculous and other meningitides can be made from the examination of the CSF. Differentiation from other forms of viral encephalitis depends on the results of serologic tests.

Course and Prognosis. The disease runs an acute course in most cases and results in death or recovery within two to three weeks. Occasionally, the symptoms may be of longer duration. The mortality rate in the 1933 epidemic in St. Louis was 20%. Mortality has varied from 2 to 12% in subsequent epidemics. Cranial nerve palsies, hemiplegia, and other focal neurologic signs are more common in cases with prolonged coma or confusion.

The most common sequela of St. Louis encephalitis are headaches, insomnia, easy fatigability, and nervousness occurring three to five months after the illness appears. Residuals and cranial nerve palsies, hemiplegia, and aphasia are found in some cases. Epileptiform attacks or behavior changes in children are rare.

Treatment. There is no specific treatment for the encephalitis due to St. Louis virus.

Japanese Encephalitis

Japanese encephalitis was first identified as a distinct disease after a large epidemic in 1924, although a form of encephalitis had appeared in Japan almost every summer and had been recognized as early as 1871. The causative agent is a mosquito-transmitted flavivirus (formerly group B arbovirus). The disease has a characteristic seasonal occurrence, with the worst outbreaks in hot, dry weather. It is most common in Japan, but is also found in neighboring regions and India. The changes in the nervous system include degeneration of the ganglion cells in the cerebellum, cerebral cortex, basal ganglia, and substantia nigra and, to a lesser extent, in the medulla and spinal cord. The leptomeninges are infiltrated with lymphocytes and the vessels in the substance of the nervous system are surrounded by monocytes and macrophages. Focal necrosis and glial nodules are not uncommon.

The clinical picture and laboratory findings are similar to those of St. Louis encephalitis. The disease is most common in children, and the mortality rate in some epidemics has been as high as 60%. This figure is undoubtedly too high because most mild cases are not admitted to a hospital.

Severe neurologic residuals and mental defects are common, especially in the young. The diagnosis may be established by isolation of the virus from the blood, CSF, or cerebral tissue, and by appropriate antibody tests, including the new CSF ELISA test. There is no specific treatment. An inactivated vaccine has been used in Japan, China and Korea and has recently become available in the United States.

California Encephalitis

Human neurologic disease associated with California encephalitis virus was first recognized in the early 1960s. Subsequently, La-Crosse virus, also a member of the California virus serogroup, has been shown to cause most of these infections. Infection occurs most frequently in midwestern states, but it also occurs along the eastern seaboard. These viruses are now known to be one of the more important causes of encephalitis in the United States. The California virus serogroup is now classified among the bunyaviruses, a group of enveloped viruses with segmented, helical, circular ribonucleoproteins.

The virus is transmitted by woodland mosquitoes. The virus cycle involves small woodland animals but not birds. Consequently, rural endemic rather than epidemic disease usually occurs. The disease occurs in the late summer and early fall and nearly all patients are children. Infants under one year of age and adults are rarely affected. Headache, nausea and vomiting, changes in sensorium, meningeal irritation, and upper motor neuron signs have been commonly reported. The peripheral blood count is usually elevated. The CSF contains an increased number of lymphocytes and shows the other findings typical of viral meningitis or encephalitis.

The case fatality is low (less than 1%). Recovery usually occurs within 7 to 10 days. Emotional lability, learning difficulties, and recurrent seizures have been reported as sequelae.

The diagnosis can be established by serologic studies. Neutralizing and hemagglutination-inhibition antibodies appear shortly after the onset of the disease; complement-fixing antibodies can be detected 10 to 12 days after initial symptoms.

Other Arbovirus Encephalitides

Colorado tick fever (CTF) is caused by an orbivirus, and transmitted by wood ticks with small animals as the intermediate host. It is confined to the geographic area of the tick in the Rocky Mountains. Infection often involves hikers, foresters, or vacationers in the spring and summer. Three to six days after a tick bite, a febrile illness with headache and myalgias develops. About 50% of the patients have a biphasic fever pattern. A peripheral leukocytosis is usually seen. Aseptic meningitis occurs in about 20% of the cases. This is a benign disease; encephalitis and permanent sequela are almost never seen. Diagnosis can be readily made by virus isolation from the blood or by serology.

Tick-borne encephalitis (TBE) viruses are togaviruses (flavivirus group) that are closely related and are transmitted by wood ticks. Disease is seen primarily in the northern latitude woodlands of Siberia and Europe. The Siberian strains cause a severe encephalitis (Russian spring-summer encephalitis virus). The European and Scandinavian strains (Central European encephalitis) tend to cause a milder encephalitis that can present as a biphasic illness with recrudescence several weeks after the initial influenza-like illness. A case of TBE has been seen in Ohio after foreign tick exposure. Powassan virus, a member of the TBE complex, has been isolated from a few patients with encephalitis in the United States and Canada. Clinical infections are severe but very rare because the ticks that transmit the virus only rarely attack humans. A related virus, louping ill, causes a sporadic, mild encephalitis in the British Isles.

Other arboviruses that have caused occasional epidemics of encephalitis include West Nile and Rift Valley fever in the Middle East and Murray Valley encephalitis in Australia.

Rubella

Rubella (German measles) is the cause of an exanthematous disease that can produce marked neurologic damage in the unborn child of a mother infected during pregnancy (congenital rubella syndrome). Gregg, an Australian ophthalmologist, was the first to correlate the occurrence of congenital cataracts among newborn babies with maternal rubella infection during the first trimester of pregnancy. Congenital rubella is now known to produce a variety of defects including deafness, mental retardation, and cardiac abnormalities. The frequency of congenital defects is highest in the first trimester of pregnancy and fall as gestation advances.

Rubella virus was originally isolated by demonstrating that monkey-kidney cells infected with the virus became resistant to superinfection with picornaviruses. Subsequently the virus was shown to grow and produce cytopathogenic changes in a number of continuous cell lines, making it possible to characterize the properties of the virus and to develop a vaccine. Rubella virus is now classified as a togavirus, although it is not an arbovirus. It is an enveloped virus that contains RNA and agglutinates erythrocytes from pigeons, geese, and day-old chicks.

Rubella virus induces a chronic persistent infection in the fetus. For a long time after birth, infants may shed virus from the nasopharynx, eye, or CSF. Virus production continues despite the development of neutralizing and hemagglutinating antibodies by the infected child.

The lesions in the nervous system are those of a chronic leptomeningitis with infiltration of mononuclear cells, lymphocytes, and plasma cells. Small areas of necrosis and glial cell proliferation are seen in the basal ganglia, midbrain, pons, and spinal cord. Microscopic vasculitis and perivascular calcification can also occur.

The infant with rubella encephalitis is usually lethargic, hypotonic, or inactive at birth or within the first few days or weeks after birth. Within the next several months, the child may develop restlessness, head retraction, opisthotonic posturing, and rigidity. Seizures and a meningitis-like illness may occur. The anterior fontanelle is usually large; microcephaly occurs infrequently. The child may have other associated defects such as deafness, cardiovascular anomalies and congestive heart failure, cataracts, thrombocytopenia, and areas of hyperpigmentation about the navel, forehead, and cheeks. Improvement of varying degrees may be noted after the first 6 to 12 months of life.

The CSF contains an increased number of cells as well as a moderately increased protein content. Rubella virus can be recovered from the CSF of approximately 25% of the patients and may persist in the CSF for more than a year after birth.

Specific diagnosis can be made by recovery of the virus from throat swab, urine, CSF, leukocytes, bone marrow, and lens. Evidence of infection can be made by serologic tests. A rubella-specific IgM serologic test can be used for diagnosis in the newborn.

The primary method of treatment is prevention of fetal infection. Live rubella vaccine should be given to all children between one year of age and puberty. Adolescent girls and nonpregnant women should be given vaccine if they are shown to be susceptible to rubella by serologic testing.

Rubella virus can also cause several uncommon neurologic syndromes. Postinfectious encephalomyelitis occurs with acquired rubella; a chronic or slow viral infection termed "progressive rubella panencephalitis" occurs rarely.

MYXOVIRUS INFECTIONS

Mumps Meningitis and Encephalomyelitis

Mumps is a disease caused by a paramyxovirus that has predilection for the salivary glands, mature gonads, pancreas, breast, and the nervous system. The virus causes hemagglutination of erythrocytes of fowl, humans, and other species. It produces hemolysis and contains complement-fixing components. There is only one serotype. Like other paramyxoviruses, mumps virus develops from the cell surface by a budding process.

Clinical evidence of involvement of the nervous system occurs in the form of a mild meningitis or encephalitis in a small percentage of the cases. Other neurologic complications of mumps include an encephalomyelitis with cranial and peripheral nerve palsies, myelitis, and peripheral neuritis. It is not clear whether these neurologic complications of mumps are caused by direct action of the virus or whether they are due to allergic or other factors, as is thought to be the case with similar complications following vaccination and various infectious diseases (postinfectious encephalomyelitis).

Pathology. The pathology of mumps meningitis and encephalitis has not been clearly elucidated because of the low mortality rate. The pathologic changes are limited to an infiltration of the meninges and cerebral blood vessels with lymphocytes and mononuclear cells. The morbid changes in cases of encephalomyelitis following mumps are exactly the same as those found following other infectious diseases, namely, perivenous demyelinization with infiltration of the vessels of the brain and spinal cord by lymphocytes and phagocytic microglia.

Incidence. The incidence of neurologic complications of mumps varies greatly in different epidemics, ranging from a low of less than 1% to a high of about 10%. A slight pleocytosis may be found in the CSF with little or no clinical evidence of meningitis, and a few cases have been reported in which meningeal symptoms were the only indication of infection ("mumps sine parotide"). Holden and his associates performed a lumbar puncture on the fourth day in 100 consecutive cases of mumps. Mumps meningitis was diagnosed in 33 of the 100 patients on the basis of the presence of headache, drowsiness, and neck stiffness. A pleocytosis greater than 10 cells/mm³ was present in all but five of their 33 cases. In four additional cases, there was a pleocytosis in the CSF without any neurologic symptoms.

Although the two sexes are equally susceptible to mumps, neurologic complications are three times more frequent in boys. Children are commonly affected, but epidemics may occur in young adults living under community conditions best exemplified by army camps. Most cases of mumps encephalitis in the United States appear to occur in the late winter and early spring.

Symptoms. In most cases, the symptoms of involvement of the nervous system are those of meningitis (i.e., headache, drowsiness, and neck stiffness). These symptoms commonly appear 2 to 10 days after the onset of the parotitis. They may occasionally precede the onset of swelling of the salivary glands. Only about 50% of the patients with mumps meningitis and encephalitis have parotitis. The symptoms are benign and disappear within a few days.

Complications. Deafness is the most common sequel of mumps. The loss of hearing, which is unilateral in more than 65% of the cases, may develop gradually or it may have an abrupt onset accompanied by vertigo and tinnitus. The deafness that follows mumps seems to be due to damage to the membranous labyrinth. Orchitis, oophoritis, pancreatitis, and thyroiditis also may occur.

Myelitis, polyneuritis, encephalitis, optic neuritis, and other cranial nerve palsies may develop 7 to 15 days after the onset of the parotitis. These complications are similar to those that develop after other infectious diseases and are considered to be an example of so-called postinfectious encephalomyelitis.

A few cases of hydrocephalus have been reported in children who have had mumps virus infections. The hydrocephalus seems to be due to aqueductal stenosis induced by mumps virus.

Laboratory Data. In mumps meningitis, the blood usually shows a relative lymphocytosis and a slight leukopenia. The CSF is under slightly increased pressure. The CSF is clear and colorless except when a high cell count is present, at which time it may be slightly opalescent. The cell count is increased, usually in the range of 25 to 500 cells/mm³, but occasionally the counts may be as high as 3,000 cells/mm³. Lymphocytes usually constitute 90 to 96% of the total, even in CSF with a high cell count, but polymorphonuclear leukocytes may occasionally predominate in the early stages. The degree of pleocytosis is not related to the severity of symptoms, and it may persist for 30 to 60 days. Inclusions of viral nucleocapsid-like material have been recognized by electron microscopic observation of CSF cells from patients with mumps meningitis. The protein content is normal or moderately increased and mumps-specific oligoclonal IgG may be present. The sugar content is usually normal, but may show a moderate reduction in 5 to 10% of cases. Mumps virus can be recovered from the CSF in a significant number of patients.

Diagnosis. Mumps meningitis is diagnosed on the basis of meningeal symptoms and a pleocytosis in the CSF in a patient with mumps. In patients who develop neurologic symptoms during an epidemic of mumps and who show no evidence of involvement of the salivary glands, the diagnosis cannot be made with certainty unless the virus can be recovered from the CSF or there is a significant increase in the complement fixation antibodies in the serum. Virus can usually be recovered from the saliva, throat, urine, and CSF.

Mumps meningitis must be differentiated from other forms of meningitis, especially tuberculous and fungal, if the CSF glucose is low. A normal sugar content and the absence of organisms in the CSF are important in excluding acute purulent, tuberculous, or fungal meningitis.

Since licensure of the live attenuated mumps vaccine in 1967, the incidence of mumps has decreased to less than 5% of the prevaccine level. CNS complications from the vaccine, if they occur at all, are rare.

Subacute Measles Encephalitis

Measles virus causes a wide spectrum of neurologic disease ranging from subclinical involvement and postinfectious encephalomyelitis (acute measles encephalitis) within days after the onset of a measles exanthem to chronic subacute sclerosing panencephalitis (SSPE) (see Chronic Viral Infections). Toxic encephalopathy and acute infantile hemiplegia have rarely occurred with measles infections, but these seem to be complications of severe febrile illnesses of childhood and are not specific syndromes caused by measles. Subacute measles encephalitis (measles inclusion body encephalitis, immunosuppressive measles encephalitis) occurs as an opportunistic infection in immunosuppressed or immunodeficient patients. Most of these cases have occurred in children, but a few have occurred in adults. Several cases have been reported in patients with no obvious immune defects. A history of measles exposure 1 to 6 months before the onset of neurologic disease can usually be obtained. The disease is characterized by generalized and focal seizures including epilepsia partialis continua, occasional focal deficits, and a progressive deterioration of mental function leading to coma and death in several weeks to four or five months. Routine CSF tests are normal. Pathology reveals numerous inclusions in neurons and glia with microglial activation but minimal perivascular inflammation.

RHABDOVIRUS INFECTION

Rabies

Rabies (hydrophobia, lyssa, rage) is an acute viral disease of the CNS that is transmitted to humans by the bite of an infected (rabid) animal. It is characterized by a variable incubation period, restlessness, hyperesthesia, convulsions, laryngeal spasms, widespread paralysis, and almost invariably death.

Etiology. Rabies virus is an enveloped bullet-shaped virus that contains single-stranded RNA. Because of its characteristic morphology, rabies has been classified among the rhabdo (rod-shaped) viruses. The virus appears capable of infecting every warm-blooded animal. Rodents are used for laboratory investigations, and the virus replicates in a number of tissue culture cell lines. The virus of rabies is present in the saliva of infected animals and is transmitted to humans by bites or abrasions of the skin. After inoculation, the virus replicates in muscle cells and then travels to the CNS by way of both sensory and motor nerves by axonal transport. After CNS invasion, dissemination of virus is rapid, with early selective involvement of limbic system neurons. The disease is usually caused by the bite of a rabid dog, but it may be transmitted by cats, wolves, foxes, raccoons, skunks, and other domestic or wild animals. Cases have been reported in which the infection was transmitted by both vampire and insectivorous bats.

Several cases of airborne transmission of rabies have occurred in spelunkers of bat-infested caves and in laboratory workers. Unusual human-to-human transmission has occurred in two patients who were recipients of corneal transplants.

The incubation period usually varies between 1 and 3 months with the extremes of 10 days and more than a year. In general, the incubation period is directly related to the severity of the bite or bites and their location. The period is shortest when the wound is on the face and longest when the leg is bitten.

Pathology. The pathology of rabies is that of a generalized encephalitis and myelitis. There is perivascular infiltration of the entire CNS with lymphocytes and, to a lesser extent, polymorphonuclear leukocytes and plasma cells. The perivascular infiltration is usually mild, and may be focal or diffuse. Diffuse degenerative changes occur in the neurons. Pathognomonic of the disease is the presence of cytoplasmic eosinophilic inclusions, with central basophilic granules that are found in neurons (Negri bodies—Fig. 15–3). These are usually found in pyramidal cells of the hippocampus and cerebellar Purkinje cells, but they may be seen in neurons of the cortex and other portions of the CNS, as well as in the spinal ganglia. These inclusions contain rabies virus antigen as demonstrated by immunofluorescence. Rabies virus nucleocapsids have been found in electron microscopic studies of the inclusions. These inclusion bodies are occasionally absent. There are proliferative changes in the microglia with the formation of rod cells, which may be collected into small nodules (Babès nodules). The degenerative changes in the neurons may be quite severe with little or no inflammatory reaction. This is especially apt to occur in cases with a long incubation period.

Incidence. The incidence of rabies is inversely proportional to the diligence of public health authorities in the control of rabid animals. The disease is almost nonexistent in Great Britain, where strict regulations are enforced. It is becoming a clinical rarity in the

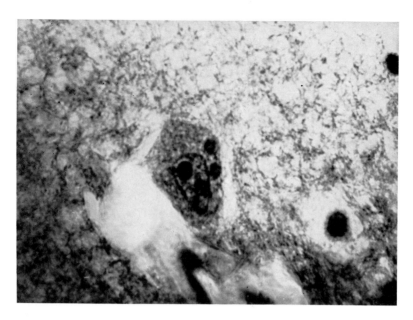

Fig. 15–3. Rabies: Inclusion bodies (Negri bodies) in cytoplasm of ganglion cell of cerebral cortex.

United States and most of the countries of Central Europe, but it is still common in southeastern Europe and Asia. There have been 21 cases of human rabies in the United States from 1974 to 1984.

The incidence of the disease in individuals who have been bitten by rabid dogs is low (15%), but it is high (40%) when the bite is inflicted by a rabid wolf. The incidence is highest when the wounds are severe and near the head. It is low when the bite is inflicted through clothing, which cleans some or most of the infecting saliva from the teeth.

Symptoms. The onset is denoted by pain or numbness in the region of the bite, in about half of cases. Other initial symptoms include fever, apathy, drowsiness, headache, and anorexia. This period of lethargy passes rapidly into a state of excitability in which all external stimuli are apt to cause localized twitchings or generalized convulsions. There may be delirium with hallucinations and bizarre behavior (thrashing, biting, severe anxiety). A profuse flow of saliva occurs; spasmodic contractions of the pharynx and larynx are precipitated by any attempt to consume liquid or solid food. As a result, the patient violently refuses to accept any liquids; hence, the name hydrophobia. The body temperature is usually elevated and may reach 105° to 107° F in the terminal stages. The stage of hyperirritability gradually passes over into a state of generalized paralysis and coma. Death results from paralysis of respiration.

The disease may occasionally begin with paralysis (paralytic form or dumb rabies), without convulsive phenomena or laryngeal spasm. The paralysis is a flaccid type and may start in one limb and spread rapidly to involve the others. The paralysis is more often symmetric than asymmetric. Symptoms and signs of a transverse myelitis may develop.

Laboratory Data. There is a leukocytosis in the blood, and albumin may be present in the urine. The CSF is under normal pressure and a lymphocytic pleocytosis is present, varying from 5 to several hundred/mm³ in only about 50% of the cases. The protein content is usually increased.

Diagnosis. Rabies is often diagnosed from the appearance of the characteristic symptoms after the bite of a rabid animal. The diagnosis can occasionally be made by fluorescent antibody staining of corneal smears or skin biopsies from the back of the neck, although both false-negative and false-positive results occur. Serum and CSF should also be tested for rabies antibodies. Negative results for these tests do not rule out the possibility of rabies. Virus isolation from the saliva, throat, and CSF should also be attempted, although this is rarely successful. The only sure way of making the diagnosis while the patient is alive is by brain biopsy. The differential diagnosis includes all forms of encephalitis and those viruses causing lower motor neuron paralysis for the paralytic form of rabies.

Course and Prognosis. The disease is almost always fatal and usually runs its course in 2 to 10 days. Death within 24 hours of the onset of symptoms has been reported. A few cases with recovery have been reported.

Treatment. There is no specific antiviral therapy. Treatment is therefore entirely prophylactic, and includes both passive antibody and vaccine. Passive immunization is by use of human immune rabies globulin. Immune globulin is infiltrated into the wound and given intramuscularly. If human gamma globulin is not available, equine rabies antiserum can be used after appropriate tests for horse serum sensitivity. The administration of globulin of serum should be followed by a full course of active immunization, preferably with human diploid cell vaccine.

Serum sickness is common after the injection of the horse serum and should be treated with antihistamines. Neurologic complications are rare with the human diploid cell vaccine. Encephalomyelitis and polyneuritis are common with the older nervous tissue vaccines.

ARENAVIRUS INFECTIONS

Lymphocytic Choriomeningitis

Lymphocytic choriomeningitis (LCM) is a relatively benign viral infection of the meninges and CNS. The clinical features of the disease were described by Wallgren in 1925 (under the term *aseptic meningitis*). The disease is of historic importance because it was the first in which a virus was proved to be the cause of a benign meningitis with a predominance of lymphocytes in the CSF.

Etiology and Incidence. In 1934, Armstrong and Lillie recovered a hitherto undescribed virus from the brain of a patient who had died of encephalitis during the St. Louis epidemic in 1933. This virus produced an infiltration of round cells in the meninges and choroid plexus of experimental animals. Armstrong and Lillie designated it as the virus of experimental lymphocytic choriomeningitis. In 1935, Traub found that this same virus was carried by apparently healthy mice. The role of the virus in human disease was established by Rivers and Scott in 1935, when they isolated it from the CSF of two patients with the clinical syndrome described by Wallgren. LCM virus is an RNA virus. It is the cause of only about 1 to 5% of cases of viral meningitis. The vast majority of such cases are due to infection of the meninges by enteroviruses and mumps virus.

The portal of entry is probably the respiratory tract. Virus multiplication first occurs in the respiratory epithelium. Some patients develop symptoms of an upper respiratory illness or of an influenza-like illness. Mice are the major reservoir of the virus and are implicated as the intermediate host. Both pet and laboratory hamsters may be a source of infection.

The virus attacks all age groups, but most frequently affects older children and young adults. The two sexes are equally affected. The disease is most common in the winter when mice move indoors.

Pathology. The pathology of the disease has not been adequately studied because of the low mortality rate. In addition, most reports lack confirmatory viral studies. Changes in fatal cases include infiltration of the meninges and choroid plexus with lymphocytes, perivascular infiltration in the brain substance, and degenerative changes in the ganglion cells. Proliferation of the arachnoid with the formation of an adhesive arachnoiditis (Barker and Ford) and focal lesions in the brain and spinal cord (Howard) have been reported.

Symptoms and Signs. Invasion of the blood by the virus of lymphocytic choriomeningitis may produce symptoms of a systemic influenza-like illness with or without evidence of involvement of the CNS. Onset of the infection is characterized by fever, headache, malaise, myalgias, and symptoms of upper respiratory infection or pneumonia. The meningeal symptoms usually develop within a week after the onset. Occasionally there is a remission in the prodromal symptoms, and the patient is apparently in good health when meningeal symptoms develop.

Severe headache, nausea, and vomiting mark the beginning neurologic involvement, most often aseptic meningitis. The temperature is moderately elevated (99° to 104° F). The usual signs of meningitis (stiff neck, Kernig and Brudzinski signs) are present. The parenchyma may occasionally be involved (encephalitic or meningoencephalitic forms) with drowsiness, stupor, and confusion. Papilledema, oculomotor and facial palsies, and signs of focal lesions in the brain or a transverse lesion of the spinal cord have been reported. In the encephalitic form, convalescence is prolonged, but good restoration of function usually occurs in the damaged tissue. Death may occur, but is rare.

Laboratory Data. In the early influenza-like stages, leukopenia and thrombocytopenia may be seen. Later, the leukocyte count may be elevated with a predominance of polymorphonuclear leukocytes. The CSF is under increased pressure and is clear and colorless. The CSF contains an excess of cells, varying from less than a hundred to several thousand/mm³. Lymphocytes constitute almost 100% of the cells. Eosinophilia has been reported. The protein content is increased. The sugar content is usually normal, but may be reduced.

Diagnosis. A presumptive diagnosis of lymphocytic choriomeningitis can be made on the basis of the characteristic history (prodromal symptoms followed by meningitis) and the CSF findings. A definitive viral diagnosis may be made by recovery of the virus from blood or CSF, but in most cases, the diagnosis is made by seroconversion. Complement-fixing antibodies are usually detectable 1 to 2 weeks after the onset of disease; neutralizing antibodies appear after 6 to 8 weeks.

Differential Diagnosis. Lymphocytic choriomeningitis must be differentiated from other diseases that are associated with lymphocytic pleocytosis in the CSF, including tuberculous meningitis, fungal meningitis, syphilitic meningitis, leptospirosis, lyme disease, listeria monocytogenes, mycoplasma, rickettsia, toxoplasmosis, meningitis caused by other viruses, and parameningeal infections. The differential diagnosis can be made in most of these conditions by the characteristic clinical and CSF findings and by the results of serologic tests.

Course and Prognosis. The duration of the meningeal symptoms varies from 1 to 4 weeks with an average of 3 weeks. The mortality rate is low, and complete recovery is the rule except in the rare patients with encephalitis in whom residuals of focal lesions in the brain or spinal cord may be present.

Treatment. There is no specific treatment.

Other Arenaviruses

Junin (Argentinian hemorrhagic fever) and Machupo (Bolivian hemorrhagic fever) viruses and Lassa fever virus of Africa cause severe hemorrhagic fevers. Although hemorrhage and shock are the usual causes of death from these severe systemic infections, it is not unusual to see neurologic involvement.

ADENOVIRUSES

Adenoviruses are nonenveloped (ether-resistant), icosahedral DNA-containing viruses of which there are more than 30 serotypes. These viruses were not discovered until 1953 when they were isolated from tissue culture of surgically removed tonsils and adenoids, thus the name. Adenoviruses can be spread by both respiratory and gastrointestinal routes and cause a variety of clinical syndromes. Respiratory infection is most often seen, manifested by coryza, pharyngitis and, at times, pneumonia. Pharyngoconjunctival fever, epidemic keratoconjunctivitis, pertussis-like syndrome, and hemorrhagic cystitis are other manifestations. Most infections occur in children; about 50% of these infections are asymptomatic. Epidemics of respiratory diseases have also been common among military personnel.

Neurologic involvement has occurred mostly in children as an encephalitis or meningoencephalitis and is quite rare. Only a few pathologic studies have been performed, and the encephalitis appears to be of the primary type with virus invasion of the brain. Histologic changes include perivascular cuffing and mononuclear cell parenchyma infiltrates, but in some cases, little or no inflammation is seen. Virus has been isolated from the brain and CSF in several cases. The encephalitis is usually of moderate to severe intensity with meningism, lethargy, confusion, coma, and convulsions. Ataxia has also been reported. Death occurs in up to 30% of the cases. CSF pleocytosis often, but not always, occurs and can be polymorphonuclear or mononuclear. The protein content may be normal or elevated. Diagnosis can be made by serology or by isolation of virus from the CSF, throat, respiratory secretions, and feces. There is no specific treatment.

An unusual case of adenovirus encephalitis occurring as a subacute infection in an adult with lymphoma has been reported. Perivascular inflammation, activation of microglia, and neuronal intranuclear inclusions occurred. On electron microscopy, adenovirus-like particles were seen in the inclusions and virus was isolated from the brain.

HERPESVIRUS INFECTIONS

The herpesvirus group is composed of DNA-containing viruses that contain a lipid envelope and multiply in the nucleus of the cell. Members of this group share the common feature of establishing latent infections. Herpesviruses may remain quiescent for long periods of time, being demonstrable only sporadically or not at all until a stimulus triggers reactivated infection. Within cells, accumulations of virus particles can often be recognized in the nucleus in the form of acidophilic inclusion bodies. Members of the herpesvirus group that are associated with neurologic disease include herpes simplex, varicella-zoster, cytomegalovirus, and the Epstein-Barr (EB) virus.

Herpes Simplex Encephalitis

Encephalitis caused by herpes simplex virus (HSV) is the single most important cause of fatal sporadic encephalitis in the United States. Early diagnosis is crucial because there is effective antiviral treatment for this encephalitis.

Etiology. Two antigenic types of herpes simplex virus (herpesvirus hominis) are distinguished by serologic testing. The type 1 strains (HSV-1) are responsible for almost all cases of herpes simplex encephalitis in adults and cause oral herpes. Type 2 strains (HSV-2) cause genital disease. In the neonatal period, HSV-2 encephalitis occurs as part of a disseminated infection or as localized disease and is acquired during delivery. In adults, HSV-2 is spread by venereal transmission and causes aseptic meningitis.

Incidence and Pathogenesis. HSV-1 is transmitted by respiratory or salivary contact. Primary infection usually occurs in childhood or adolescence. It is usually subclinical or may present as stomatitis, pharyngitis, or respiratory disease. About 50% of the population has antibody to HSV-1 by age 15, whereas 50 to 90% of adults have antibody depending on socioeconomic status. HSV-1 encephalitis can occur at any age, but more than half of the cases occur in patients more than 20 years of age. This finding suggests that encephalitis most often occurs from endogenous reactivation of virus rather than from primary infection. Neurologic involvement is a rare complication of reactivation. During the primary infection, virus becomes latent in the trigeminal ganglia. Years later, nonspecific stimuli cause reactivation, which is usually manifested as herpes labialis (cold sores). Presumably, virus can reach the brain through branches of the trigeminal nerve to the basal meninges, resulting in localization of the encephalitis to the temporal and orbital frontal lobes. Alternatively, serologic studies suggest

that about 25% of cases of HSV-1 encephalitis occur as part of a primary infection. Experimental studies indicate that this could occur by spread of virus across the olfactory bulbs to the orbital frontal lobes and subsequently the temporal lobes. The encephalitis is sporadic without seasonal variations. HSV-1 encephalitis occurs rarely as an opportunistic infection in the immunocompromised host.

Except when infantile infection occurs at delivery, HSV-2 is spread by sexual contact. Thus, primary infection usually occurs during the late teenage or early adult years. As noted previously, HSV-2 causes aseptic meningitis in adults, which probably occurs as part of the primary infection. Similar to HSV-1, opportunistic infections may also occur in immunocompromised patients.

Pathology. In fatal cases, intense meningitis and widespread destructive changes occur in the brain parenchyma. Necrotic, inflammatory, or hemorrhagic lesions may be found. These lesions are maximal, most often in the frontal and temporal lobes. There is often an unusual degree of cerebral edema accompanying the necrotic lesions. Eosinophilic intranuclear inclusion bodies (Cowdry type A inclusions) are present in neurons. These inclusions containing viral antigen and herpesvirus particles have been recognized on electron microscopic examination.

Symptoms and Signs. The most common early symptoms and signs in herpes simplex encephalitis are fever and headache. The onset is most often abrupt and may be ushered in by major motor or focal seizures. However, the encephalitis may evolve more slowly with expressive aphasia, paresthesias, or mental changes preceding more severe neurologic signs. Most patients have a temperature between 101° and 104° F at the time of admission. Nuchal rigidity or other signs of meningeal irritation are often found. Mental deficits include confusion and personality changes varying from withdrawal to agitation with hallucinations. A progressive course ensues within hours to several days, with an increasing impairment of consciousness and the development of focal neurologic signs. Rarely, the course may be subacute or chronic, lasting several months. Focal signs such as hemiplegia, hemisensory loss, and aphasia are considered distinguishing features of herpes encephalitis, but are seen in only about 50% of affected patients on initial examination. Herpetic skin lesions are seen in only a few cases, but are also seen with other diseases. A history of cold sores is not helpful because the incidence is similar to that of the general population.

Laboratory Data. There is a moderate leukocytosis in the blood. The CSF pressure may be moderately or greatly increased. The pleocytosis in the fluid varies from less than 10 to 1,000 cells/mm^3; lymphocytes or occasionally polymorphonuclear leukocytes may predominate. Red blood cells are frequently seen, but their presence or absence is not diagnostic. The CSF sugar content is usually normal, but may be low. Virus is rarely recovered from the CSF. In 5 to 10% of cases, the initial CSF examination is normal.

The EEG is usually abnormal with diffuse slowing or focal changes over temporal areas; periodic complexes against a slow-wave background may be seen. The EEG is the most likely test to show early focal abnormalities. Both radioisotope brain scan and angiography may reveal focal lesions of the temporal lobe. CT may demonstrate low-density abnormality, mass effect, or liner contrast enhancement in over 90% of the patients, but it may be entirely normal during the first week of disease. Thus, CT cannot be relied upon alone for early diagnosis. An MRI scan may reveal focality during the first week of disease when the CT scan is normal.

Diagnosis. Early definitive diagnosis can be established only by recovery of virus or demonstration of viral antigen in brain. Because patients may show a rise in antibody titer with recurrent herpes simplex cutaneous lesions or with inapparent infection, a fourfold rise in the serum antibody titer to herpesvirus may occur in patients with encephalitis from other causes. Fluctuations in antibody level may also occur with reactivated infection, and there may be uncertainty about the significance of a positive serologic response.

The diagnosis can be made, in a substantial proportion of patients, by examining tissue obtained by brain biopsy. Craniotomy and open biopsy are the procedures of choice as they allow better visualization of the biopsy area and therapeutic decompression. Characteristic intranuclear inclusions, positive immunohistochemical staining, or the finding of typical herpes virions on electron microscopic examination indicate herpesvirus infection. Inoculation of brain biopsy suspensions into susceptible rodents and tissue cultures may result in recovery of the virus. The appearance of herpes antibodies in the CSF is a useful retrospective diagnostic test, but these an-

tibodies occur too late in the disease to aid therapy. Because herpes simplex encephalitis has a high mortality rate, and because the outcome of therapy is affected by the patient's level of consciousness, diagnostic measures leading to the demonstration of the virus should be initiated as soon as possible when the disease is suspected.

The differential diagnosis of HSV-1 encephalitis includes: other viral and postinfectious encephalitides; bacterial, fungal, and parasitic infections; and tumors. Brain abscess is often the most difficult diagnosis to exclude. About 25% of biopsy-negative patients have another treatable disease. Thus, empirical treatment without biopsy is usually not indicated.

Prognosis and Treatment. The disease appears fatal in approximately 70% of the cases. Recovery may be complete in mild cases, but patients who survive the acute disease are usually left with severe neurologic residuals. Measures to decrease life-threatening brain edema, including the administration of adrenal corticosteroids, appear indicated. Several presumably therapeutic agents (e.g., iododeoxyuridine, cytosine arabinoside) are not efficacious and have marked toxicity. Vidarabine, a DNA polymerase inhibitor, has been demonstrated to decrease mortality to 28%, as compared to 70% for patients receiving placebo. Recently, acyclovir has been demonstrated to be more efficacious than vidarabine in two controlled trials. It selectively inhibits virus-specific polymerase and has less toxicity than vidarabine. Acyclovir is now the drug of choice for HSV encephalitis. As with vidarabine, outcome depends on the patient's age and level of consciousness.

Herpes Zoster

Herpes zoster (shingles) is a viral disease that produces inflammatory lesions in the posterior root ganglia and is characterized clinically by the appearance of pain and a skin eruption in the distribution of the affected ganglia. Signs and symptoms of involvement of the motor roots or the CNS are also present in a small percentage of the patients.

Etiology. The virus of herpes zoster is identical to varicella virus, the causative agent of chickenpox. The varicella-zoster virus is a large enveloped DNA-containing virus that has the same structure as other herpesviruses. The agent can be cultured in human tissue culture cells, where it tends to remain bound to cells. Varicella virus recovered from chickenpox patients is identical to herpes zoster virus recovered from patients with shingles by all serologic tests. Children can catch chickenpox from exposure to adults with shingles, but adults are subject to zoster only if they have had chickenpox earlier in life. Epidemiologic considerations led Hope-Simpson to speculate that zoster infection is a reactivation of latent varicella-zoster virus originally acquired in a childhood attack of chickenpox. Although varicella-zoster virus can remain latent within tissues in the same manner as herpes simplex virus, there is no antigenic similarity between the two viruses.

Herpes zoster frequently occurs in connection with systemic infections, immunosuppressive therapy, and localized lesions of the spine or nerve roots (e.g., acute meningitides, tuberculosis, Hodgkin disease, metastatic carcinoma, trauma to the spine). In some cases the cutaneous eruption is at the same segment as the localized lesion of the spine, but in others it is at an entirely different level. It is most probable that systemic disease or local lesions of the spine or nerve roots merely serve to activate the infection.

Pathology. Although the symptoms are usually confined to the distribution of one or two sensory roots, the pathologic changes are usually more widespread. The affected ganglia of the spinal or cranial nerve roots are swollen and inflamed. The inflammatory reaction is chiefly of a lymphocytic nature, but a few polymorphonuclear leukocytes or plasma cells may also be present. Some of the cells of the ganglion are swollen and others are degenerated. The inflammatory process commonly extends to the meninges and into the root entry zone (posterior poliomyelitis). Not infrequently, some inflammatory reaction occurs in the ventral horn and in the perivascular space of the white matter of the spinal cord. The pathologic changes in the ganglia of the cranial nerves and in the brain stem are similar to those in the spinal root and spinal cord.

Incidence. Herpes zoster is a relatively common disease with an incidence that varies from 1 to 5 cases/1,000 people each year. Rates are higher in patients with malignancies and in those receiving immunosuppressive therapy. Symptoms of involvement of the nervous system, with the exception of pain, are rare, only occurring in about 10% of patients. The disease may occur at any time of life, but is more common in middle or later life.

Symptoms and Signs. The disease may begin with headaches, malaise, and fever, but more commonly the initial symptom is a neuralgic pain or dysesthesia in the distribution of the affected root. The pain is followed in 3 to 4 days by reddening of the skin and appearance of clusters of vesicles in part of the area supplied by the affected roots. These vesicles, which contain clear fluid, may be discrete or may coalesce. Within 10 days to 2 weeks, the vesicles are covered with a scab, which after desquamation leaves a pigmented scar. These scars are usually replaced by normally colored skin in the ensuing months. Permanent scarring may occur if there is ulceration or secondary infection of the vesicles. Coincidental to the eruption, there is swelling of the lymph nodes that drain the affected area. This adenopathy is usually painless and subsides with the skin rash.

Herpes zoster is primarily an infection of the spinal ganglion, but the cranial ganglia are affected in about 20% of the cases. The thoracic, lumbar, cervical, and sacral segments are involved in descending order of frequency. The involvement is almost always unilateral, but both sides may be involved in one or more segments.

Among the less common symptoms are impairment of cutaneous sensation and muscular weakness in the distribution of the affected root, headache, neck stiffness, and confusion. The latter symptoms indicate involvement of the meninges. Weakness of intercostal muscles may be present and not be noted. Involvement of the cervical or lumbar segments may be accompanied by weakness and occasionally subsequent atrophy of isolated muscle groups in the arm or leg (zoster paresis). The rare involvement of sacral segments may result in bladder paralysis with urinary retention or incontinence. Oculomotor palsies may also occur.

Ophthalmic Zoster. Involvement of the trigeminal ganglion occurs in about 20% of the cases. Any division of the ganglion may be involved, but the first division (ophthalmic) is by far the most commonly affected. The seriousness of the involvement of this ganglion is due to the changes that develop in the eyes secondary to panophthalmitis or scarring of the cornea. There may be a temporary or permanent paresis of the muscles supplied by the oculomotor nerves as a complication of ophthalmic zoster.

Geniculate Herpes. Otic zoster with involvement of the geniculate ganglion (Ramsay Hunt syndrome), although rare, assumes prominence because of paralysis of the facial muscles. The rash is usually confined to the tympanic membrane and the external auditory canal. It may spread to involve the outer surface of the lobe of the ear and, when combined with cervical involvement, vesicles are found on portions of the neck. The facial paralysis is identical to that of Bell palsy. Loss of taste over the anterior two thirds of the tongue occurs in more than one half of cases. Partial or complete recovery is the rule. Involvement of the ganglia of Corti and Scarpa is accompanied by tinnitus, vertigo, nausea, and loss of hearing.

Complications. Although there is a lymphocytic pleocytosis in the CSF, meningeal symptoms are uncommon. Signs of involvement of the tracts of the spinal cord in the form of a Brown-Séquard syndrome or a transverse or ascending myelitis have occurred. Mental confusion, ataxia, and focal cerebral symptoms have been attributed to involvement of the brain by the varicella-zoster virus (herpes zoster encephalitis). Polyneuritis of the so-called infectious or Guillain-Barré type has been reported as a sequel of herpes zoster. A more recently recognized complication of ophthalmic zoster is the acute contralateral hemiplegia and at times other ipsilateral hemispheric deficits such as aphasia that occur several weeks to several months later. Arteritis, apparently with viral invasion, develops in the carotid and other vessels ipsilateral to the zoster ophthalmicus, resulting in hemispheric infarction.

Other complications of herpes zoster include injury to the eyes, scarring of the skin, facial or other palsies, and *postherpetic neuralgia*. The latter is most common in elderly debilitated patients and affects chiefly the ophthalmc or intercostal nerves. The pains are persistent and are sharp and shooting in nature. The skin is sensitive to touch. These pains may persist for months or years and are often refractory to all forms of treatment.

Laboratory Data. The abnormalities in the laboratory findings are confined to the CSF. Even in uncomplicated herpes zoster, there is an inconstant lymphocytic pleocytosis, which may be found before the onset of the rash. The CSF may be normal in many of the cases, with symptoms of involvement of only one thoracic segment, but it is usually abnormal when the cranial ganglia are involved or when paralysis of other neurologic signs are present. The cell count varies from 10 to several hundred/mm^3 with lymphocytes as the predominating cell type. The protein content is normal or moderately increased. The sugar content is normal.

Diagnosis. Herpes zoster is diagnosed without difficulty when the characteristic rash is present. In the pre-eruptive stage, the pain may lead to the erroneous diagnosis of disease of the abdominal or thoracic viscera. The possibility of herpes zoster should be considered in all patients with root pains of sudden onset that have existed for less than four days. Difficulties in diagnosis may also be encountered when the vesicles are widespread or when they are scant or entirely absent (zoster sine herpete). It is possible that herpes zoster may cause intercostal neuralgia or facial palsy without any cutaneous eruption, but a careful search usually reveals a few vesicles.

If necessary, varicella-zoster virus may be isolated from vesicle fluid by inoculation into susceptible human or monkey cells and identified by serologic means. Virus may also be detected by electron microscopic examination of vesicular fluid and immunohistochemical staining of cells from vesicular scrapings.

Treatment. There is still no effective means of preventing herpes zoster. The treatment of uncomplicated zoster includes only the use of analgesics and nonspecific topical medications for the rash. The use of topical antiviral agents is of questionable benefit. Although antibiotics have no effect on the virus, they may be indicated to control secondary infection. In double-blind trials, several of the new antiviral agents (e.g., vidarabine, acyclovir), when used systemically, have been demonstrated to decrease pain, virus shedding, and healing time of acute herpes zoster. These agents do not seem to prevent postherpetic neuralgia, but do decrease viral dissemination and its complications. For this reason, these agents are indicated for the systemic complications, especially in immunosuppressed patients, and for zoster encephalomyelitis and arteritis. Because the arteritis may be due to an allergic response, it has been treated with a combination of corticosteroids and an antiviral agent. Zoster immune globulin is useful in prophylaxis of varicella in immunosuppressed children, but is not helpful for zoster.

Postherpetic neuralgia is difficult to treat. It is refractory to the usual analgesics. Sectioning the affected posterior roots is usually not successful in relieving pain. Corticosteroids have been shown to decrease the incidence of postherpetic neuralgia, but had no effect on the resolution of acute zoster. Their use would seem risky because of immuno-suppression and possible virus dissemination. Amitriptyline, carbamazepine, and phenytoin are the mainstays of therapy.

Cytomegalovirus Infection

Cytomegalic inclusion body disease is an infection that occurs in utero by transplacental transmission. The responsible agent is cytomegalovirus (CMV), a member of the herpesvirus group that is among the common parasites of humans. The virus can only be grown in cultured human cells. Multiplication is slow and much of the newly formed virus remains cell-associated. CMV infection results in the appearance of large, swollen cells that often contain large eosinophilic intranuclear and cytoplasmic inclusions.

Intrauterine infection of the nervous system may result in stillbirth or prematurity. The cerebrum is affected by a granulomatous encephalitis with extensive subependymal calcification. Hydrocephalus, hydranencephaly, microcephaly, cerebellar hypoplasia, or other types of developmental defects of the brain may be found. Convulsive seizures, focal neurologic signs, and mental retardation are common in infants that survive. Jaundice with hepatosplenomegaly, purpuric lesions, and hemolytic anemia may be present. Periventricular calcification is often seen in radiographs of the skull. Affected infants often succumb in the neonatal period, but prolonged periods of survival are possible. Subclinical or "silent" congenital infections may result in deafness and developmental abnormalities. There can also be progressive nervous system damage and, presumably, a persistent infection for months after birth.

CMV infections may also occur in adults, producing a mononucleosis-like syndrome, but involvement of the nervous system is uncommon in the adult form of the disease. Infection with CMV in 12 of 34 patients who died following renal transplantation and immunosuppression was reported by Schneck. Often, this CNS involvement in immunosuppressed patients is asymptomatic, although fatal encephalitis has occurred. The encephalitis has a subacute or chronic course. CMV infection has been implicated as a cause of infectious polyneuritis.

CMV can be recovered from urine, saliva, or liver biopsy specimens. Complement-fixation and neutralization tests are available. A presumptive diagnosis can be made by looking for typical cytomegalic cells in stained preparations of urinary sediment or saliva.

Vidarabine and acyclovir are not efficacious for treating neonates with congenital infections. These drugs have been reported to be beneficial in a few adult infections, but this is not usual.

Epstein-Barr Virus Infection

Infectious mononucleosis (glandular fever) is a systemic disease of viral origin with involvement of the lymph nodes, spleen, liver, skin and, occasionally, the CNS. It occurs sporadically and in small epidemics. It is most common in children and young adults. The usual symptoms and signs are headache, malaise, sore throat, fever, enlargement of the lymph nodes in the cervical region, occasionally enlargement of the spleen, and changes in the blood. Unusual manifestations include a cutaneous rash, jaundice, and symptoms of involvement of the nervous system.

Epstein-Barr (EB) virus is a herpesvirus that was originally isolated from African children with Burkitt lymphoma. Patients with heterophil-positive infectious mononucleosis develop antibodies to EB virus during the course of their illness, demonstrating that EB virus is the cause of infectious mononucleosis.

Although neurologic complications rank first as a cause of death, there have been few autopsy studies of the brain in fatal cases of infectious mononucleosis. Acute cortical inflammation similar to that seen in other viral infections has been observed. Atypical cells, probably lymphocytes, have been found in the inflammatory exudate.

The exact incidence of involvement of the nervous system is unknown, but it is probably less than 1%. A lymphocytic pleocytosis in the CSF may be found in the absence of any neurologic symptoms or signs. Severe headache and neck stiffness may be the initial or only symptoms of cerebral involvement (aseptic meningitis). Signs of encephalitis (delirium, convulsions, coma, and focal deficits) are rare manifestations. Optic neuritis, paralysis of the facial and other cranial nerves, acute autonomic neuropathy, infectious polyneuritis (Guillain-Barré syndrome), and transverse myelitis have been reported in a few cases. Acute cerebellar ataxia has also been associated with infectious mononucleosis.

The CNS manifestations may appear early in the course of the disease in the absence of any other findings, or their onset may be delayed until the convalescent stage. The prognosis is excellent with complete remission of symptoms in all cases except those with respiratory paralysis in severe polyneuritis.

In the laboratory examination, the important findings are a leukocytosis in the blood with an increase in the lymphocytes and the appearance of abnormal mononuclear cells (atypical lymphocytes). Liver function tests are often abnormal and heterophil antibody is present in 90% of patients. With involvement of the meninges, a lymphocytic pleocytosis is in the CSF (10 to 600 cells/mm³) with or without a slight increase in protein content. The sugar content is normal and the CSF serologic tests for syphilis are negative. False-positive tests for syphilis are occasionally obtained on the serum.

The diagnosis is established by the appearance of neurologic symptoms in patients with other manifestations of the disease. The differential diagnosis includes mumps and other viral diseases that cause a lymphocytic meningeal reaction. The differential diagnosis can be made by a study of the blood and the heterophil antibody reaction, and by measurement of the antibody response to EB virus antigens. Oropharyngeal excretion of EB virus can also be determined. These tests should be performed on all cases of lymphocytic meningitis in which the diagnosis is obscure.

There is no specific therapy. Treatment with steroids may be indicated in certain patients with severe pharyngotonsillitis or other complications.

ACUTE DISSEMINATED ENCEPHALOMYELITIS

Acute disseminated encephalomyelitis (ADE) may occur in the course of various infections, particularly the acute exanthematous diseases of childhood, and following vaccination against smallpox and rabies, thus the terms post- or parainfectious and postvaccinal encephalomyelitis. The clinical symptoms and the pathologic changes are similar in all of these cases, regardless of the nature of the acute infection.

Etiology and Pathogenesis. The list of diseases that may be accompanied or followed by signs and symptoms of an encephalomyelitis is probably not yet complete, but it includes: measles, rubella, varicella-zoster, smallpox, mumps, influenza, parainfluenza, infectious mononucleosis, typhoid, mycoplasma infections, upper respiratory and other obscure febrile disease, as well as vaccination against smallpox, measles, or rabies. Reactions in the nervous system may also follow inoculations with typhoid vaccine and with sera, particularly that against tetanus. In these latter conditions, the clinical picture is more likely to be that of a mononeuritis or generalized polyneuritis.

The pathogenesis of ADE is not known. Because the condition occurs in the course of diseases that are known to be of viral origin or follows vaccination against viral diseases, it was natural to assume that the changes in the nervous system were due to direct involvement by either the virus of the disease itself or by some other virus activated by the infection. However, virus usually has not been isolated from the nervous system of these cases.

Other theories include damage by a toxin elaborated by the virus or, more likely, an allergic or autoimmune reaction. Various mechanisms have been proposed by which a virus might trigger an immune-mediated reaction against CNS myelin to cause a disease similar to experimental allergic encephalomyelitis. This could possibly involve the systemic interaction of a virus with the immune system without viral invasion of the nervous system.

Pathology. Little or no change occurs in the external appearance of the brain or spinal cord. On sectioning, many small yellowish-red lesions are present in the white matter of the cerebrum, cerebellum, brain stem, and spinal cord. The characteristic feature of these lesions is a loss of myelin, with relative sparing of the axis cylinders. The lesions in the brain are oval or round and usually surround a distended vein. In cross sections of the spinal cord, they tend to extend in a radial manner from the gray matter to the periphery of the cord (Fig. 15–4). The lesions are usually found in large numbers in almost all parts of the CNS, but in some cases they may be concentrated in the white matter of the cerebrum; in others the cerebellum, brain stem, or spinal cord may be most severely affected. On microscopic examination, there is perivenular lymphocytic and mononuclear cell infiltration and demyelination. On myelin stained specimens, there is destruction of myelin sheaths within the lesions, with a fairly sharp margin between the affected and normal areas. Axis cylinders are affected to a much lesser extent than the myelin sheaths. Phagocytic microglial cells may also be found within the lesion and in the perivascular space of adjacent ves-

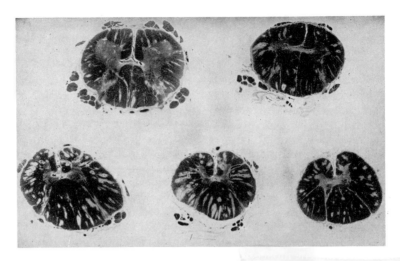

Fig. 15–4. Acute postinfectious encephalomyelitis. Radial streaks of demyelination in spinal cord (myelin sheath stain).

sels. Although the lesions are concentrated in the white matter, a few patches may be found in the gray matter. Nerve cells in these areas may occasionally be destroyed or may show various degenerative changes. ADE is a monophasic disease as lesions have a similar age of onset.

Acute hemorrhagic leukoencephalitis appears to be a fulminant form of ADE. Pathologic lesions are similar to those of ADE with the addition of microscopic hemorrhages and perivascular polymorphonuclear cell infiltrates.

Incidence. Previously, smallpox vaccination (vaccinia virus) was one of the more frequent causes of postinfectious or postvaccinal encephalomyelitis. The exact frequency has not been accurately established because of the wide range reported, varying from more than 1 case/100 to less than 1 case/100,000 vaccinees. Because smallpox has apparently been eradicated as a natural disease, vaccination is no longer recommended. Thus, vaccinia virus is no longer a common cause of postinfectious encephalomyelitis. The smallpox virus (variola virus) also probably caused this syndrome in the past.

The incidence of encephalomyelitis following vaccination against rabies with the old nerve-tissue-prepared vaccines ranged as high as 1/600 persons with a mortality rate of 10 to 25%. With the duck-embryo vaccine, this complication has decreased to approximately 1/33,000 recipients. This complication has not been reported with the new human diploid cell vaccine, although several cases of Guillain-Barré syndrome have occurred.

Damage to the nervous system with the acute exanthemata occurs most commonly following measles, where the incidence is approximately 1/1,000 cases. However, in countries using measles vaccination, measles is no longer a common cause of postinfectious encephalomyelitis. The incidence following measles vaccine is only about 1 per million recipients. Postinfectious encephalomyelitis following rubella or mumps was much less frequent than that seen with natural measles, but even this occurrence has been decreased with vaccination. Varicella infections are now one of the more common causes of postinfectious encephalomyelitis, although the exact incidence is not known. Nonspecific upper respiratory infections are probably the most common cause now.

Symptoms and Signs. The symptoms and signs of ADE are related to the portion of the nervous system that is most severely damaged. Because any portion of the nervous system may be affected, it is not surprising that variable clinical syndromes may occur. In some cases, there are signs and symptoms of generalized involvement (ADE), but one or more portions of the neuraxis may suffer the brunt of the damage, resulting in various clear-cut clinical syndromes: meningeal, encephalitic, brain-stem, cerebellar, spinal cord, and neuritic.

Symptoms of involvement of the meninges (i.e., headaches, stiffness of the neck) are common early in the course of all types. In some cases, no further symptoms are present. In others, these initial symptoms and signs may be followed by evidence of damage to the cerebrum. In the encephalitic form, there may be convulsions, stupor, coma, hemiplegia, aphasia, or other signs of focal cerebral involvement. Cranial nerve palsies, especially *optic neuritis,* or signs and symptoms of cerebellar dysfunction predominate in a few cases. More common than brain stem or cerebellar involvement, however, are signs and symptoms of injury of the spinal cord. This may be disseminated in the cord or more commonly may take the form of an acute transverse myelitis.

Acute transverse myelitis or acute transverse myelopathy (ATM) is a syndrome of multiple causes. It may be acute, developing over hours to several days, or subacute, developing over one to two weeks. The most common picture is a transverse myelitis, interrupting both motor and sensory tracts at one level, usually thoracic. It usually begins with localized back or radicular pain followed by the abrupt onset of bilateral paresthesias of the legs, an ascending sensory level, and a paraparesis that often progresses to paraplegia. Urinary bladder and bowel involvement occurs early and is prominent. In general, patients with rapid progression and flaccidity below the level of the lesion have the worst prognosis. The syndrome may also take the form of an ascending myelitis, a diffuse or patchy myelitis, or a partial myelitis (Brown-Séquard syndrome, anterior spinal artery distribution lesion, posterior column myelopathy). Only about one fourth to one third of the cases of ATM are caused by viral infections or vaccinations via a demyelinating process. Less frequently, a complete transverse myelitis has been caused by direct virus invasion of the cord, e.g., poliovirus or herpes zoster. Other less frequent causes of ATM include systemic lupus erythematosus, other vasculitides, other causes of spinal cord infarction, multiple sclerosis, and trauma. Idiopathic ATM is most frequent. Obviously, it is important to exclude cord compression by epidural abscess or tumor, intrinsic cord bacterial or fungal infections, or tumors and treatable vascular diseases.

Acute cerebellar ataxia constitutes about half the cases of postinfectious encephalomyelitis following varicella, whereas cerebral and spinal involvement is more common with measles and vaccinia.

Other parainfectious syndromes may also be seen. Acute toxic encephalopathy and Reye syndrome are seen more frequently after varicella, influenza, and rubella. Peripheral nerve involvement with an acute ascending paralysis of the Guillain-Barré type is more frequent with rabies vaccine, especially with the older preparations, and after influenza and upper respiratory infections. Brachial neuritis is the usual neurologic complication of antitetanus vaccine.

Laboratory Data. The CSF pressure is usually normal, but it may be slightly elevated. There is a mild to moderate increase in the white cells: 15 to 250 cells/mm^3 with lymphocytes as the predominating cell type. The protein content is normal or slightly elevated (35 to 150 mg/dl). The sugar content is within normal limits. The CSF myelin basic protein level is usually increased. The EEG is abnormal in practically all cases. There is an increase in the amount of slow frequency waves, usually of 4 to 6 Hz with high voltage. The abnormalities are usually generalized and symmetric on both sides of the head, but focal or unilateral changes may be found. The abnormalities persist for several weeks after apparent clinical recovery. Persisting abnormalities correlate well with permanent neurologic damage or convulsive disorders. After several days, the CT scan may show diffuse or scattered low-density lesions in the white matter, some of which may enhance with contrast. MRI scanning may reveal an increased signal intensity.

Diagnosis. Because there is no specific diagnostic test, the diagnosis of postinfectious or postvaccinal encephalomyelitis should be considered when neurologic signs develop 4 to 21 days following vaccination, the onset of one of the acute exanthemata, or an upper respiratory tract infection. The differential diagnosis includes practically all of the acute infectious diseases of the nervous system, particularly the acute or subacute encephalitis, and acute diffuse multiple sclerosis.

Prognosis and Course. The mortality rate is high (10 to 30%) in the patients with severe involvement of the cerebrum in measles, rubella, vaccinia, or after rabies vaccination. It is low in the cases of acute cerebellar ataxia or with involvement only of the peripheral nerves. Death may occur as a result of cerebral damage in the acute stage or following intercurrent infections, bedsores, or urinary sepsis in late stages. In patients who survive, the neurologic signs usually improve considerably, with about 90% having complete recovery. Postencephalitic sequelae, such as parkinsonism, do not occur; as a rule, there are no new symptoms after recovery from an acute attack. Behavior disorders, mental deterioration, or convulsive seizures may occur as sequelae in children. Sequelae are most frequently seen with measles.

Treatment. A number of reports suggest that the administration of adrenocorticotropic hormone or corticosteroids reduces the severity of the neurologic defects.

Chronic Viral Infections

Chronic or slow viral infections that result in chronic neurologic disease can be caused by conventional viruses or the unconventional transmissible spongiform encephalopathy agents. The conventional agents cause chronic inflammatory or demyelinating disease; in humans, these include subacute sclerosing panencephalitis (SSPE), progressive rubella panencephalitis, and progressive multifocal leukoencephalopathy (PML). In SSPE, a chronic inflammatory disease is caused by a defect in the production of measles virus, which results in a cell-associated infection. With progressive rubella panencephalitis, both inflammation and demyelination may be seen. The pathogenic mechanisms have not yet been defined, but the virus does not appear to be defective. PML is a noninflammatory demyelinating disease that occurs in immunocompromised hosts; it is caused by an opportunistic papovavirus infection. Animal models of inflammatory and demyelinating diseases caused by conventional agents include "old dog encephalitis" induced by canine distemper virus (a myxovirus-like measles), visna virus (retrovirus) leukoencephalitis of sheep, and Theiler virus (picornavirus) demyelinating disease of mice.

The unconventional transmissible spongiform encephalopathy agents cause noninflammatory degenerative diseases. Three human diseases, kuru, Creutzfeldt-Jakob disease (CJD), and Gerstmann-Sträussler-Scheinker (GSS) disease, are caused by these agents. Kuru is a disease that occurs only in New Guinea. It was the first human chronic neurologic disease that was transmitted to experimental animals. Creutzfeldt-Jakob disease is a neurologic degenerative disease that presents with dementia and occurs throughout the world. GSS disease is a familial illness characterized by ataxia and later dementia. Animal models for these agents include scrapie of sheep and transmissible mink encephalopathy. These transmissible spongiform agents are unusual. They do not cause cytopathic changes in cell culture, and no virus-like particles have been observed by electron microscopy. It is difficult to purify the agents from diseased tissue. They are markedly resistant to ionizing radiation, ultraviolet exposure, and chemical treatments that inactivate conventional viruses. These agents may not contain nucleic acids, but may be composed only of proteins, and thus may not truly be viruses. A sialoglycoprotein of 27,000 by 30,000 Daltons (27–30) has been associated with scrapie transmissibility and recently has been identified in the brains of CJD and GSS disease patients. This protein has been referred to as the *prion* protein (PrP) 27–30. Prion is the term coined to indicate that these agents may be "proteinaceous infectious particles." In scrapie, a single gene codes for this protein, and the gene is found in normal as well as infected brains. Thus, this protein may actually be an abnormal host protein. In addition, purified scrapie and CJD prions aggregate into amyloid-like bifringent rods. Filamentous scrapie-associated fibrils (SAF) have been found by electron microscopic examination of scrapie-infected animal brains and CJD brain samples. It is unclear whether PrP 27–30 or SAF are forms of the infectious agent or just pathologic reaction products. Another peculiarity of these agents is their inability to provoke an immune response in the host after either natural or laboratory infection.

SUBACUTE SCLEROSING PANENCEPHALITIS

Subacute sclerosing panencephalitis (SSPE, Dawson disease, subacute inclusion body encephalitis) is a disease caused by a defective measles virus characterized by progressive dementia, incoordination, ataxia, myoclonic jerks, and other focal neurologic signs. The disease was first described by Dawson in 1933 and 1934 as "subacute inclusion encephalitis" and thought to be of viral origin because of the presence of type A intranuclear inclusions. Numerous cases have been reported since that date, but recovery of a viral agent was not possible until the advent of specialized techniques of viral isolation. The cases reported by Pette and Doring in 1939 as "nodular panencephalitis" and by Van Bogaert in 1945 as "subacute sclerosing leukoencephalitis" appear to be the same disease. The abbreviation *SSPE* was coined by a combination of the three terms.

Pathology. In severe long-standing cases, the brain may feel unduly hard. A perivascular infiltration occurs in the cortex and white matter with plasma and other mononuclear cells. Patchy areas of demyelinization and gliosis occur in the white matter and deeper layers of the cortex. The neurons of the cortex, basal ganglia, pons, and inferior olives show degenerative changes. Intranuclear and intracytoplasmic eosinophilic inclusion bodies are found in neurons and glial cells. When examined with the electron microscope, these inclusions are seen to be composed of hollow tubules similar to nucleocapsids of paramyxoviruses. When these inclusions are stained by the fluorescent antibody method, positive staining reaction for measles virus is obtained.

Incidence. Children younger than 12 years of age are predominantly affected, although a few cases in adults in their 20s have been reported. Boys are more often affected than girls, and more cases have occurred in rural than in urban settings. The incidence of SSPE has decreased about tenfold since the introduction of the live attenuated measles vaccine. After natural measles infection, the incidence of SSPE is 5 to 10 cases per million clinical measles infections. After vaccine, the rate is less than one case per million vaccine recipients.

Symptoms. The disease has a gradual onset without fever. Forgetfulness, inability to keep up with school work, and restlessness are common early symptoms. These are followed in the course of weeks or months by incoordination, ataxia, myoclonic jerks of the muscles of the trunk and limbs, apraxia, and loss of speech; seizures and dystonic posturing may occur. Vision and hearing are preserved until the terminal stage, in which there is a rigid quadriplegia simulating complete decortication. Cranial nerve palsies may appear, and patches of chorioretinitis have been reported in occasional cases.

Laboratory Data and Diagnosis. Elevated levels of measles antibody can be found in serum and CSF. The CSF is under normal pressure and the cell count is normal or rarely only slightly increased. The protein content is normal, but a striking increase in the CSF immunoglobulin content is found even in an otherwise normal fluid. Oligoclonal IgG bands representing measles virus-specific antibodies can be demonstrated by agarose electrophoresis of CSF. The EEG often shows a widespread abnormality of the cortical activity with a "burst suppression" pattern of high-amplitude slow wave (or spike and slow wave) complexes occurring at a rate of one every 4 to 20 seconds synchronous with or independent of the myoclonic jerks (Fig. 15–5). CT may show cortical atrophy and focal or multifocal low-density lesions of the white matter.

Virus isolation was accomplished by establishing tissue culture cell lines from brain biopsies obtained from affected patients. These cultures contained measles virus antigen as demonstrated by fluorescent antibody staining and could be made to shed an infectious virus that was serologically indistinguishable from measles virus by cocultivation with other established tissue culture cell lines.

Pathogenesis. A defect in measles virus production seems to occur because the viral M (membrane) protein cannot be found in the brain tissue of affected patients. The M protein is necessary for alignment of nucleocapsids under viral proteins in the cell membrane so that budding of virus can take place. Thus, in SSPE there is no budding and no release of extracellular virus. There is accumulation of measles virus nucleocapsids within cells (cell-associated infection), and virus spread occurs by cell fusion. Why and how the M protein deficiency occurs are unclear. As has been demonstrated in tissue culture, brain cells may be incapable of synthesizing the M protein. Another possibility is that selective antibody pressure might somehow cause a restricted cell-associated infection because over half of the patients with SSPE have had an acute measles infection before reaching two years of age, when maternal antibody may still have been present. Antibody pressure resulting in cell-associated infection has been demonstrated in tissue culture and experimental animals.

Course, Prognosis, and Treatment. The course of the disease is prolonged, usually lasting several years. Both rapidly progressive disease, leading to death in several months, and protracted disease, lasting over 10 years, have occurred. Spontaneous long-term improvement or stabilization occurs in about 10% of the cases. The variable course makes it difficult to evaluate therapeutic modalities. There is no definite specific therapy. Empirical treatment with isoprinosine may slow disease progression. Intrathecal interferon may induce remissions. No controlled studies have been performed.

PROGRESSIVE RUBELLA PANENCEPHALITIS

Rubella virus, like measles virus, has been recognized to cause a slowly progressive pan-

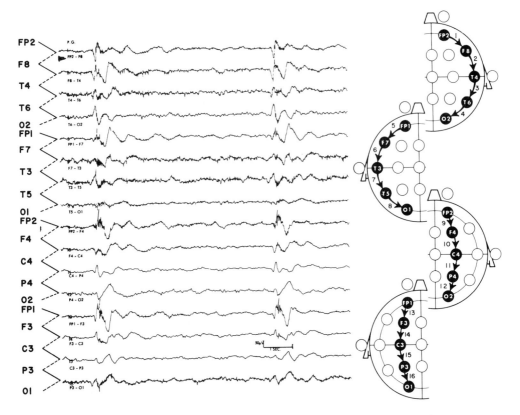

Fig. 15–5. Subacute sclerosing panencephalitis. Multiphasic long duration sharp wave discharges repeat every 7 seconds in a 14-year-old boy. In this condition, periodic discharges recur regularly at 4 to 20 second intervals.

encephalitis. This is a rare disease of children and young adults. Fewer than a dozen cases have been reported. Most cases have occurred in patients with the congenital rubella syndrome, but several cases have appeared following postnatally acquired rubella. No cases have been ascribed to rubella vaccine. The pathogenic mechanisms of the disease have not been well defined. There does not appear to be a defect in rubella virus production as occurs in SSPE. Unlike measles virus, rubella virus does not have an M protein. Because of the recognition that immune complexes are in the serum and CSF, it is possible that immune complex deposition in vascular endothelium may be the primary pathogenic mechanism.

The pathologic condition is characterized by inflammation and demyelination. The inflammation consists of lymphocytic and plasma cell infiltration of the meninges and perivascular spaces of the gray and white matter. Extensive demyelination with atrophy and gliosis of the white matter is usually seen. Any part of the brain may be affected, but changes are often most prominent in the cer-

ebellum. Inclusion bodies and virus particles have not been identified. Vasculitis involving arterioles with fibrinoid degeneration and mineral deposition is seen. Arterioles may be thrombosed. There are adjacent microinfarcts. IgG deposits have been demonstrated in histologically normal vessels.

The disease usually presents in the second decade of life. Until that time, infected children continue to develop regardless of whether they have congenital defects. The disease usually begins with dementia manifested by deterioration of school performance and behavior problems similar to those of early SSPE. Progressive cerebellar ataxia is the other most prominent neurologic sign. Gait ataxia is initially seen, but the arms subsequently become involved. Later, pyramidal tract involvement (with spasticity, dysarthria, dysphagia, hyperactive reflexes, and Babinski signs) is seen. Optic atrophy and retinopathy, similar to that seen in congenital rubella, occur. Seizures and myoclonus have been reported, but are not prominent features. Symptoms and signs suggestive of infection (headache, fever, and nuchal rigidity) are not seen.

Routine blood counts and chemical profiles are normal. The EEG demonstrates diffuse slowing. A burst-suppression pattern similar to that of SSPE is rarely seen. CT may demonstrate ventricular enlargement, which is most prominent in the fourth ventricle because of cerebellar atrophy. For this reason, the cisterna magna may also be quite prominent. The CSF is under normal pressure. There is usually a moderate lymphocytic pleocytosis with up to 40 cells/mm^3, but the fluid may occasionally be acellular. The protein is increased in the range of 60 to 150 mg/dl with the IgG fraction being up to 50% of this. Most of the IgG is composed of oligoclonal bands directed against rubella virus. Conventional serologic techniques demonstrate elevated serum and CSF antibody titers against rubella virus. The virus is difficult to recover. It has been isolated in only two cases, one from brain biopsy material and another from peripheral blood leukocytes. Both were obtained by cocultivation.

The diagnosis can easily be made in a patient with the congenital rubella syndrome. In postnatally acquired cases, SSPE is the other major diagnostic consideration. Other dementing illnesses of childhood should be considered; however, the combined data of the clinical picture (especially when ataxia ensues), the CSF findings, and serology should be diagnostic. The course is protracted over many years with periods of stabilization and even partial remission. No treatment for the disease is known. Isoprinosine has not altered disease progression.

PROGRESSIVE MULTIFOCAL LEUKOENCEPHALOPATHY

Progressive multifocal leukoencephalopathy (PML) is a rare subacute demyelinating disease caused by an opportunistic papovavirus. The disease usually occurs in patients with defective cell-mediated immunity. Cases have primarily occurred in patients with reticuloendothelial diseases, such as Hodgkin disease, other lymphomas, and leukemia. Cases have also occurred in patients with carcinoma, sarcoidosis, and in those immunosuppressed therapeutically. In most of these disorders, PML is a rare complication; it is probably most common in AIDS patients. A few cases occurring in the apparent absence of an underlying disease have been described.

The pathologic condition is characterized by the presence of multiple, in part confluent, areas of demyelination in various parts of the nervous system, accompanied at times by a mild degree of perivascular infiltration. These multifocal areas of demyelination are most prominent in the subcortical white matter, whereas involvement of cerebellar, brain stem, or spinal cord white matter is less common. As the disease progresses, the demyelinated areas coalesce to form large lesions. Hyperplasia of astrocytes into bizarre giant forms that may resemble neoplastic cells is found. There is a loss of oligodendroglia with relative sparing of axons in the lesions. Eosinophilic intranuclear inclusions are seen in oligodendroglial cells at the periphery of the lesions. Electron microscopic studies have shown that these inclusions are composed of papovavirus particles (Fig. 15–6). It is presumed that the demyelination is due to destruction of oligodendroglia by the virus. Most cases have been caused by the JC strain and several by the SV-40 strain. Isolation of these agents required special techniques of cocultivating brain cultures from patients with permissive cell lines; human fetal brain tissue could also be used to induce virus replication.

The clinical manifestations are diverse and are related to the location and number of the lesions. Onset is subacute to chronic with hemiplegia, sensory abnormalities, and other focal signs of lesions in the cerebral hemispheres. Cranial nerve palsies, ataxia, and spinal cord involvement are less common. Dementia usually ensues. A definite diagnosis can be made only by pathologic investigation. Virus isolation techniques are difficult and time-consuming. More rapid identification can be made by immunofluorescence or by immune electron microscopy. The CSF is usually normal. The EEG often demonstrates nonspecific diffuse or focal slowing. CT may reveal multiple lucencies in the white matter. MRI may also demonstrate white matter abnormalities, but they are less characteristic than the CT lucencies. Serology is not helpful because most people have been exposed to the JC strain in the first two decades of their lives.

The symptoms and signs are progressive and death usually ensues in a few months. A prolonged course over several years has occurred rarely.

There have been reports of treatment with DNA inhibitors, such as cytarabine and vidarabine, but the results are not encouraging.

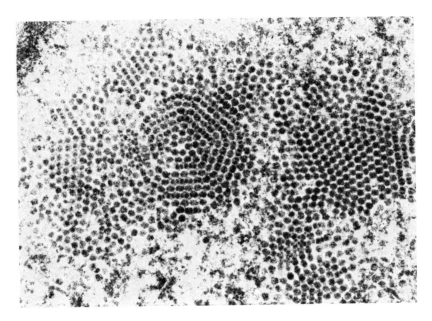

Fig. 15–6. Papovavirus-like particles present in glial nucleus in progressive multifocal leukoencephalopathic brain. (×65,000) (Courtesy of Dr. G. M. Zu Rhein.)

For patients receiving immunosuppressive drugs, it might be reasonable to stop this therapy to restore immune competence.

KURU

This progressive and fatal neurologic disorder occurs exclusively among natives of the New Guinea Highlands. It is manifested by incoordination of gait, severe truncal and limb ataxia, abnormal involuntary movements resembling myoclonus or chorea, convergent strabismus and, later in the disease, dementia. The illness terminates fatally in 4 to 24 months. Eighty percent of adults afflicted are women. Cannibalism appears to have been the principal mode of transmission. The incidence of kuru has markedly declined with the suppression of cannibalism. Neuropathologic changes include widespread neuronal loss, neuronal and astrocytic vacuolization, and astrocytic proliferation. These changes are most prominent in the cerebellum, where gross atrophy may be seen. The cerebrum and brain stem are involved to a lesser degree.

The similarity between the clinical and neuropathologic changes of kuru with those seen in scrapie-afflicted sheep led Gajdusek and Gibbs to attempt to infect higher primates with brain suspensions. Inoculation of chimpanzees was followed by the appearance of a kuru-like disease 14 months to several years later; subpassage to other chimpanzees produced a similar neurologic disease. Thus,

kuru is important from a historical perspective because it was the first human slow virus infection to be recognized.

CREUTZFELDT-JAKOB DISEASE

In 1920 and 1921, Creutzfeldt and Jakob described a progressive disease of the cortex, basal ganglia, and spinal cord that developed in middle-aged and elderly adults. Creutzfeldt-Jakob disease (spastic pseudosclerosis, cortico-striato-spinal degeneration) is caused by a transmissible spongiform encephalopathy agent. The disease is relatively rare, with an incidence of about one case per million people annually. This incidence is the same throughout the world except for the high incidence reported among Libyan Jews. Approximately 10 to 15% of cases occur in a familial pattern.

Pathology. The pathologic condition is essentially degenerative with cerebral atrophy evident grossly. Microscopic findings are similar to other spongiform encephalopathies with neuronal loss, astrocytosis, and the development of cytoplasmic vacuoles in neurons and astrocytes (status spongiosis—Fig. 15–7). There is no inflammation. The cortex and basal ganglia are most affected, but all parts of the neuraxis may be involved (Table 15–3).

Symptoms and Signs. The clinical features include the gradual onset of dementia in middle or late life, but occasionally in early adult-

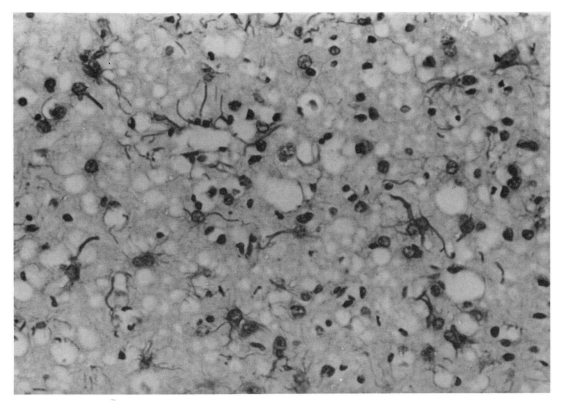

Fig. 15–7. Creutzfeldt-Jakob Disease. Section from cortex showing status spongiosis of the neuropil, loss of neurons and prominent astrocytosis. (PTAH stain ×120) (Courtesy of Dr. Mauro C. Dal Canto.)

hood. Vague prodromal symptoms of anxiety, fatigue, dizziness, headache, impaired judgement, and unusual behavior may occur. Once memory loss is recognized, it usually progresses rapidly and other characteristic signs appear, sometimes abruptly. The most frequent signs, aside from dementia, are those of pyramidal tract disease (weakness and stiffness of the limbs with accompanying reflex changes), extrapyramidal signs (tremors, rigidity, dysarthria, and slowness of movements), and myoclonus, which is often stimulus-sensitive. Other signs include

amyotrophy, cortical blindness, seizures, and those of cerebellar dysfunction (Table 15–4). None of the usual signs of an infection is seen.

Table 15–4. Manifestations of Creutzfeldt-Jakob Disease in 124 Patients

	%	
Mental deterioration	100	
Dementia		94
Abnormal behavior		45
Aphasia, apraxia, agnosia		39
Movement disorder	90	
Myoclonus		84
Other (chorea, tremor)		32
Abnormal EEG	77	
"Periodic" (l/sec)		40
Extrapyramidal signs	60	
Cerebellar signs	56	
Pyramidal signs	44	
Visual loss	40	
Lower motor neuron signs	12	
Seizures	9	
Sensory loss	7	
Cranial nerve signs	2	

Table 15–3. Distribution of Lesions in 72 Autopsy-Proven Cases of Creutzfeldt-Jakob Disease

Location	No. of Cases	%
Cortex	72	100
Basal ganglia	65	90
Corticospinal tracts	24	33
Motor neurons	27	38
Thalamus	48	67
Cerebellum	38	53

(Modified from Siedler H, Malamud N. J Neuropathol Exp Neurol 1963; 22:381–402.)

(From Brown P, Cathala F, Sadowsky D, Gajdusek DC. Ann Neurol 1979; 6:430–437.)

Laboratory Data. Routine blood counts and chemistries are normal. The CSF is usually normal, although the protein content may rarely be elevated. Recently, abnormal proteins have been identified in the CSF of CJD patients by two-dimensional electrophoresis. Periodic complexes of spike or slow wave activity with intervals of 0.5 to 2.0 seconds are characteristic of the EEG in the middle and late stages of the disease (Fig. 15–8). CT may reveal cerebral atrophy with enlarged ventricles and widened sulci; this is usually late in the course of the disease.

Course and Prognosis. The disease runs a rapid course with death usually occurring within a few months to a year. The course may rarely be prolonged over a number of years. There is no specific treatment.

Transmissibility and Biohazard Potential. As with kuru, neurologic illness can be produced in chimpanzees by the inoculation of brain suspensions prepared from the brains of Creutzfeldt-Jakob patients. The neuropathologic changes found in these chimpanzees resemble those observed in patients with Creutzfeldt-Jakob disease. The illness has also been transmitted experimentally to a variety of simian species as well as to cats, hamsters, goats, guinea pigs, rats, and mice.

The mode of transmission of Creutzfeldt-Jakob disease is unknown. The agent has been detected in most internal organs (lung, liver, kidney, spleen, and lymph nodes), cornea, and blood, but it has not been detected in saliva or feces. Only a low level of infectivity has been detected in the urine. These findings suggest a lack of significant spread by respiratory, enteric, or sexual contact. Failure to find an increased incidence in physicians, laboratory workers, and spouses also suggests that these usual modes of transmission are not of major importance. Isolation of Creutzfeldt-Jakob patients does not seem necessary except for secretions and body fluids as done with cases of hepatitis. Inadvertent human-to-human transmission has been reported following corneal transplantation, the use of inadequately sterilized stereotactic brain electrodes, use of natural human growth hormone preparations, and the use of a human dura mater graft. Thus, caution must be exercised in operating rooms and pa-

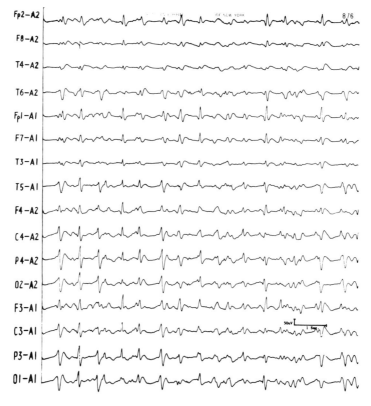

Fig. 15–8. Creutzfeldt-Jakob disease. Record of a 65-year-old man shows spikes of sharp waves at intervals of 0.7 second throughout the recording. Such periodicity with 0.5- to 2.0-second intervals occurs in the middle and late stages and may be absent in the early stages of the disease.

thology laboratories, and in the preparation of brain-derived biologicals. Medical personnel should avoid contact of open sores or conjunctiva with these tissues. Caution should be taken to avoid accidental percutaneous exposure to CSF, blood, or tissue. Special sterilization of surgical instruments and all types of needles are required. Because the transmissible spongiform encephalopathy agents are highly resistant to ordinary physical or chemical treatment (routine autoclaving or formalin), special autoclaving procedures or special inactivating agents, including sodium hypochlorite (household bleach), are required.

GERSTMANN-STRÄUSSLER-SCHEINKER (GSS) DISEASE

GSS disease has been proposed as the third human disease caused by the transmissible spongiform encephalopathy agents. It has also been referred to as the Gerstmann-Sträussler syndrome. Several aspects appear to separate GSS disease from CJD, although some cases of GSS disease are probably variants of CJD. GSS disease is a familial illness, although it is not clear if it is inherited (passed vertically) or due to genetic susceptibility to the agent. GSS disease has a lengthy course with a range of 2 to 10 years being common. Clinically it begins with ataxia; dementia eventually supervenes. Because of brain stem involvement, patients often appear to have an olivopontocerebellar degeneration. Pathologically there is usually spongiform change and amyloid plaque deposition in the cerebellum, cerebrum, and brain stem. There is also degeneration of the spinocerebellar and corticospinal tracts. As with CJD, there is no treatment.

ENCEPHALITIS LETHARGICA

Encephalitis lethargica (sleeping sickness, von Economo disease) is a disease of unknown cause that occurred in epidemic form in the years 1917 to 1928. Clinically, the disease was characterized by signs and symptoms of diffuse involvement of the brain and by the development of various sequelae in a large percentage of the recovered patients. Although the disease spread rapidly over the entire world, it is apparently extinct at present, at least in epidemic form. The disease is important because patients who are suffering from its sequelae are still living and there is always the possibility that it may occur in epidemic form again.

Encephalitis lethargica affected patients of all ages and affected both sexes evenly, including people of all races and occupations. Familial incidence was uncommon; it was not possible to trace the spread of the disease by contact with an affected individual.

The etiology of encephalitis lethargica is unknown. It is presumed that the disease was due to a virus, but proof is lacking. Because of the concurrence of encephalitis lethargica and the pandemic of influenza beginning in 1918, there has been speculation about a common etiology; this has not been resolved but is probably unlikely.

The pathologic lesions in the subacute stages were similar to other encephalitides with inflammation in the meninges, around blood vessels, and in the parenchyma (both gray and white matter) of the brain and spinal cord. Acute degenerative changes of neurons also occurred.

Symptoms and Signs. The symptoms were usually of acute or subacute onset. Fever was usually present at the onset, but sometimes did not develop until later. It was usually mild and lasted only a few days. In fatal cases, a rise to 107° or more often occurred in the terminal stages.

Headache was present in a large percentage of cases. Lethargy was one of the most common early symptoms. It lasted only a few days in some cases, but in others persisted for weeks or months. The lethargy occasionally alternated with insomnia and delirium, or there was a reversal in the sleep rhythm.

Disorders of eye movements, the most frequent sign of localized damage to the nervous system, were present in about 75% of the patients. They varied from transient diplopia to complete paralysis of one or more ocular muscles. Psychic disturbances characteristic of an acute oganic psychosis were not uncommon.

Although hemiplegia or monoplegia was occasionally seen, the most frequent motor symptoms were those associated with disease of the basal ganglia. Choreic, athetoid, dystonic, myoclonic, and tic-like movements were often present in the acute stages. Rigidity and alternating tremors, sometimes present at this stage, were more commonly a sequel of the disease. Intention tremor and other cerebellar symptoms were present in a few cases.

Laboratory Data. A lymphocytic pleocytosis in the CSF was generally present during the first few weeks, but it usually disappeared within two months. The protein content was abnormal in about 50% of the patients, usually being less than 100 mg/dl.

Diagnosis. The diagnosis of encephalitis lethargica is, for all practical purposes, not justified at present. In the light of present knowledge, the diagnosis may be justified in any patient with signs and symptoms of encephalitis with special features of disturbed sleep rhythm and diplopia in the acute stage, and the development of signs of injury of the basal ganglia at that time or in subsequent years.

Course and Prognosis. In the average case, the duration of the acute stage was about four weeks. The acute stage was sometimes much longer and merged gradually into the so-called postencephalitic phase of the disease. The mortality rate was about 25% and was highest among infants and the elderly. The frequency of sequelae is unknown.

Sequelae. In some instances, symptoms were merely a continuation of those present in the acute stage. In others, the symptoms developed after an interval of several months or many years during which the patient was apparently well.

The parkinsonian syndrome that develops after encephalitis lethargica is similar to that of the idiopathic type (paralysis agitans); in many cases a differential diagnosis is not possible. Some features, however, point to postencephalitic origin. These include the development of parkinsonism in childhood or early adult life and the presence of symptoms that are uncommon in other forms of parkinsonism, such as grimaces, torticollis, torsion spasms, myoclonus, oculogyric crises, facial and respiratory tics, and bizarre postures and gaits.

Behavior disorders and emotional instability without evidence of intellectual impairment were common sequelae in children. They occurred in about 30% of the patients, most of whom had no evidence of parkinsonism, and tended to remit with the passage of years.

References

General

Bell WE, McCormick WF. Neurologic Infections in Children, 2nd ed. Philadelphia: WB Saunders, 1981.

Evans AS, ed. Viral Infections of Humans, 2nd ed. New York: Plenum Press, 1982.

Fields BN, ed. Virology. New York: Raven Press, 1985.

Gadjusek DC. Slow virus infections of the nervous system. N Engl J Med 1967; 276:392–400.

Hanshaw JB, Dudgeon JA. Viral Diseases of the Fetus and Newborn, 2nd ed. Philadelphia: WB Saunders, 1985.

Jackson A, Johnson RT. Viral meningitis and encephalitis. In: Vinken PJ, Bruyn GW, Klawans HL, McKendall RR, eds. Handbook of Clinical Neurology (Vol. 52). New York: Elsevier-North Holland, 1988.

Johnson KP, ed. Symposium on neurovirology. Neurol Clin 1984; 2:177–413.

Johnson RT. Viral Infections of the Nervous System. New York: Raven Press, 1982.

Johnson RT, Mims CA. Pathogenesis of virus infections of the nervous system. N Engl J Med 1968; 278:23–30, 84–92.

Kennard C, Swash M. Acute viral encephalitis: its diagnosis and outcome. Brain 1981; 104:129–148.

Landsteiner K, Popper E. Uebertragung der Poliomyelitis acuta auf Affen. Z Immunitatsf Exp Therap 1909; 2:377–390.

Lennette EH, Magoffin RL, Knouf EG. Viral central nervous system disease. An etiologic study conducted at the Los Angeles County General Hospital. JAMA 1962; 179:687–695.

Lennette EH, Schmidt NJ, eds. Diagnostic Procedures for Viral, Rickettsial and Chlamydial Infections, 5th ed. Washington, DC: American Public Health Association, 1979.

Lepow ML, Coyne N, Thompson LB, Carver DH, Robbins FC. A clinical, epidemiologic and laboratory investigation of aseptic meningitis during the four-year period 1955–1958. II. The clinical disease and its sequelae. N Engl J Med 1962; 266:1188–1193.

Meyer HM Jr, Johnson RT, Crawford IP, Dascomb HE, Rogers NG. Central nervous system syndromes of "viral" etiology. A study of 713 cases. Am J Med 1960; 29:334–347.

Nicolosi A, Hauser WA, Beghi E, Kurland LT. Epidemiology of central nervous system infections in Olmsted County, Minnesota, 1950–1981. J Infect Dis 1986; 154:399–408.

Vinken PJ, Bruyn CW, Klawans HL, McKendall RR, eds. Viral disease. Handbook of Clinical Neurology (Vol. 52). New York. Elsevier-North Holland, 1988.

Picornavirus (Enterovirus) Infections

Center for Disease Control. Enterovirus surveillance, summary 1970–1979. November, 1981.

Chonmaitree T, Menegus MA, Powell KR. The clinical relevance of 'CSF viral culture': a two-year experience with aseptic meningitis in Rochester, NY. JAMA 1982; 247:1843–1847.

Grist NR, Bell EJ, Assuad F. Enteroviruses in human disease. Prog Med Virol 1978; 24:114–157.

Jubelt B, Lipton HL. Enterovirus infections of the nervous system. In: Vinken PJ, Bruyn GW, Klawans HL, McKendall RR, eds. Handbook of Clinical Neurology (Vol. 52). New York: Elsevier-North-Holland, 1988.

Sells CJ, Carpenter RL, Ray G. Sequelae of central-nervous-system enterovirus infections. N Engl J Med 1975; 293:1–4.

Singer JI, Maur PR, Riley JP, Smith PB. Management of central nervous system infections during an epidemic of enteroviral aseptic meningitis. J Pediatr 1980; 96:559–563.

Wilfert CM, Thompson RJ, Sundner TR, O'Quinn A, Zeller J, Blacharsh J. Longitudinal assessment of children with enteroviral meningitis during the first three months of life. Pediatrics 1981; 67:811–815.

Poliomyelitis

Anonymous. Late sequela of poliomyelitis. Lancet 1986; 2:1195–1196.

Bodian D. Emerging concept of poliomyelitis infection. Science 1955; 122:105–108.

Centers for Disease Control. Poliomyelitis surveillance, summary, 1980–1981. December, 1982.

Centers for Disease Control. Imported paralytic poliomyelitis—United States, 1986. MMWR 1986; 35:671–674.

Davis LE, Bodian D, Price D, Butler IJ, Vicker JH. Chronic progressive poliomyelitis secondary to vaccination of an immunodeficient child. N Engl J Med 1977; 297:241–245.

Horstmann DM, Quinn TC, Robbins FC, eds. International symposium on poliomyelitis control. Rev Infect Dis 1984; 6 (Suppl 2):S301–S600.

Hovi T, Cantell K, Huovilainen A, et al. Outbreak of paralytic poliomyelitis in Finland: widespread circulation of antigenetically altered poliovirus type 3 in a vaccinated population. Lancet 1986; 1:1427–1432.

Jubelt B, Cashman NR. Neurological manifestations of the post-polio syndrome. Crit Rev Neurobiol 1987; 3:199–220.

Nathanson N, Martin JR. The epidemiology of poliomyelitis: enigmas surrounding its appearance, epidemicity and disappearance. Am J Epidemiol 1979; 110:672–692.

Nkowane BM, Wassilak SGF, Orenstein WA, et al. Vaccine-associated paralytic poliomyelitis: United States 1973–1984. JAMA 1987; 257:1335–1340.

Paul JR. History of Poliomyelitis. New Haven: Yale University Press, 1971.

Price RW, Plum F. Poliomyelitis. In: Vinken PJ, Bruyn GW, Klawans HL, eds. Handbook of Clinical Neurology (vol 34). New York: Elsevier-North Holland, 1978; 93–132.

Sabin AB. Pathogenesis of poliomyelitis. Reappraisal in the light of new data. Science 1956; 123:1151–1156.

Wyatt HV. Poliomyelitis in hypogammaglobulinemics. J Infect Dis 1972; 128:802–806.

Coxsackieviruses

Chalhub EG, DeVivo DC, Siegel BA, Gado MH, Feigin RD. Coxsackie A9 focal encephalitis associated with acute infantile hemiplegia and porencephaly. Neurology 1977; 27:574–579.

Dalldorf G, Sickles GM. An unidentified filterable agent isolated from the feces of children with paralysis. Science 1948; 108:61–62.

Farmer K, MacArthur BA, Clay MM. A follow up study of 15 cases of neonatal meningoencephalitis due to coxsackie virus B5. J Pediatr 1975; 87:568–571.

Feldman W, Larke RPB. Acute cerebellar ataxia associated with isolation of coxsackie virus type A9. Can Med Assoc J 1972; 106:1104–1107.

Heathfield KWG, Pilsworth R, Wall BJ, Corsellis JA. Coxsackie B5 infections in Essex, 1965, with particular reference to the nervous system. Q J Med 1967; 36:579–595.

Kaplan MH, Klein SW, McPhee J, Harper RG. Group B coxsackievirus infections in infants younger than three months of age: a serious illness. Rev Infect Dis 1983; 5:1019–1032.

McLeod DL, Beale AJ, McNaughton GA, Rhodes AJ. Clinical features of aseptic meningitis caused by coxsackie B virus. Lancet 1956; 2:701–703.

Echoviruses

Erlendsson K, Swartz T, Dwyer JM. Successful reversal of echovirus encephalitis in X-linked hypogammaglobulinemia by intraventricular administration in immunoglobulin. N Engl J Med 1985; 312:351–353.

Hayes RE, Cramblett HG, Kronfol HJ. ECHO virus and meningoencephalitis in infants and children. JAMA 1969; 208:1657–1660.

Herternstein JR, Sarnat HB, O'Connor DM. Acute unilateral oculomotor paralysis associated with ECHO 9 viral infections. J Pediatr 1976; 89:79–81.

Jarvis WR, Tucker G. Echovirus type 7 meningitis in young children. Am J Dis Child 1981; 135:1009–1012.

Karzon DT, Hayner NS, Winkelstein W, Barron AL. An epidemic of aseptic meningitis syndrome due to ECHO virus type 6. II. A clinical study of ECHO 6 infection. Pediatrics 1962; 29:418–431.

McAllister RM, Hummeler K, Coriell LL. Acute cerebellar ataxia. Report of a case with isolation of type 9 ECHO virus from the cerebrospinal fluid. N Engl J Med 1959; 261:1159–1162.

McKinney RE, Katz SL, Wilfert CM. Chronic enteroviral meningoencephalitis in agammaglobulinemic patients. Rev Infect Dis 1987; 9:334–356.

Wenner HA, Abel D, Olson LC, Burry VF. A mixed epidemic associated with echovirus types 6 and 11; virologic, clinical and epidemiologic studies. Am J Epidemiol 1981; 114:369–378.

Enteroviruses 70 and 71

Anonymous. Neurovirulence of enterovirus 70. Lancet 1982; 1:373–374.

Centers for Disease Control. Case of paralytic illness associated with enterovirus 71 infection. MMWR 1988; 37:107–114.

Chonmaitree T, Menegus MA, Schheruish-Swierkosz EM, Schwalenstocker E. Enterovirus 71 infection: report of an outbreak with two cases of paralysis and a review of the literature. Pediatrics 1981; 67:489–493.

Chumakov M, Voroshilova M, Shindarovl, et al. Enterovirus 71 isolated from cases of epidemic poliomyelitis-like disease in Bulgaria. Arch Virol 1979; 60:329–340.

Ishimarv Y, Nakano S, Yamaoka K, Takami S. Outbreaks of hand, foot, and mouth disease by enterovirus 71: high incidence of complication disorders of central nervous system. Arch Dis Child 1980; 55:583–588.

Vejjajiva A. Acute hemorrhagic conjunctivitis with neurologic complications. In: Vinken PJ, Bruyn GW, Klawans HL, McKendall RR, eds. Handbook of Clinical Neurology (Vol. 52). New York: Elsevier-North Holland.

Wadia NH, Wadia PN, Katrak SM, Misra VP. A study of the neurological disorder associated with acute haemorrhagic conjunctivitis due to enterovirus 70. J Neurol Neurosurg Psychiatry, 1983; 46:599–610.

Toga- and Arboviruses

Aguilar MJ, Calanchini PR, Finley KH. Perinatal arbovirus encephalitis and its sequelae. Res Publ Assoc Nerv Ment Dis 1968; 44:216–235.

Centers for Disease Control. Arboviral infections of the central nervous system—United States, 1987. MMWR 1988; 37:506–515.

Grimstad PR. Mosquitoes and the incidence of encephalitis. Adv Virus Res 1983; 28:357–438.

Rennels MB, Arthropod-borne virus infections of the central nervous system. Neurol Clin 1984; 2:241–254.

Equine Encephalomyelitis

Ayres JC, Feemster RF. The sequelae of Eastern equine encephalomyelitis. N Engl J Med 1949; 240:960–962.

Bastian FO, Wende RD, Singer DB, Zeller RS. Eastern equine encephalomyelitis: histopathologic and ultrastructural changes with isolation of the virus in a human case. Am J Clin Pathol 1975; 64:10–13.

Earnest MP, Goolishian HA, Calverley JR, Hays RD, Hill HR. Neurologic, intellectual, and psychologic sequelae following western encephalitis. Neurology 1971; 21:969–974.

Ehrenkranz NJ, Sinclair MC, Buff E, Lyman DO. The natural occurrence of Venezuelan equine encephalitis in the United States. N Engl J Med 1970; 282:298–302.

Ehrenkranz NJ, Ventura AK. Venezuelan equine encephalitis virus infection in man. Annu Rev Med 1974; 25:9–14.

Finely KH, Fitzgerald LH, Richter TW, Riggs N, Shelton JT. Western encephalitis and cerebral ontogenesis. Arch Neurol 1967; 16:140–164.

Goldfield M, Sussman O. The 1959 outbreak of eastern encephalitis in New Jersey. I. Introduction and description of outbreak. Am J Epidemiol 1968; 87:1–10.

Rozdilsky B, Robertson HE, Charney J. Western encephalitis: report of eight fatal cases, Saskatchewan epidemic, 1965. Can Med Assoc J 1968; 98:79–86.

St. Louis Encephalitis

Brinker KR, Paulson G, Monath TP, Wise G, Fass RJ. St. Louis encephalitis in Ohio, September 1975: clinical and EEG studies in 16 cases. Arch Intern Med 1979; 139:561–566.

Monath TP, ed. St. Louis Encephalitis. Washington, DC: American Public Health Association, 1980.

Nelson DB, Kappus KD, Janowski HT, Buff E, Wellings, FM, Schneider NJ. St. Louis encephalitis—Florida 1977. Am J Trop Med Hyg 1983; 32:412–416.

Powell KE, Kappus KD. Epidemiology of St. Louis encephalitis and other acute encephalitides. Adv Neurol 1978; 19:197–215.

Reyes MG, Gardner JJ, Poland JD, Monath TP. St. Louis encephalitis: quantitative histologic and immunofluorescent studies. Arch Neurol 1981; 38:329–334.

Southern PM, Smith JW, Luby JP, Barnett JA, Sanford JP. Clinical and laboratory features of epidemic St. Louis encephalitis. Ann Intern Med 1969; 71:681–689.

Japanese Encephalitis

Burke, DS, Lorsomrudee W, Leake CJ, et al. Fatal outcome in Japanese encephalitis. Am J Trop Med Hyg 1985; 34:1203–1210.

Dickerson RB, Newton JR, Hansen JE. Diagnosis and immediate prognosis of Japanese B encephalitis. Am J Med 1952; 12:277–288.

Johnson RT, Intralawan P, Puapanwatton S. Japanese encephalitis: identification of inflammatory cells in cerebrospinal fluid. Ann Neurol 1986; 20:601–695.

Lewis L, Taylor HG, Sorem MB, Norcross JW, Kindsvatter VH. Japanese B encephalitis. Arch Neurol Psychiatry 1947; 57:430–463.

Monath TP. Japanese encephalitis—a plague of the Orient. N Engl J Med 1988; 319:641–643.

Richter RW, Shimpjyo S. Neurologic sequelae of Japanese B encephalitis. Neurology 1961; 11:553–559.

California Virus Encephalitis

Balfour HH, Siem RA, Bauer H, Quie PG. California arbovirus (LaCrosse) infections. Pediatrics 1973; 52:680–691.

Calisher CH, Thompson WH, eds. California serogroup viruses. New York: Alan R Liss, Inc., 1983.

Centers for Disease Control. LaCrosse encephalitis in West Virginia. MMWR 1988; 37:79–82.

Chun RWM, Thompson WH, Grabow JD, Mathews CG. California arbovirus encephalitis in children. Neurology 1968; 18:369–375.

Clark GG, Pretula HL, Langkop CW, Martin RJ, Calisher CH. Occurrence of LaCrosse (California serogroup) encephalitis viral infections in Illinois. Am J Trop Med Hyg 1983; 32:838–843.

Hilty MD, Haynes RE, Azimi PH, Cramblett MG. California encephalitis in children. Am J Dis Child 1972; 124:530–533.

Hurwitz ES, Schell W, Nelson D, Washburn J, LaVenture M. Surveillance for California encephalitis group virus illness in Wisconsin and Minnesota, 1978. Am J Trop Med Hyg 1983; 32:595–601.

Young DJ. California encephalitis virus: a report of three cases and a review of the literature. Ann Intern Med 1966; 65:419–428.

Other Arbovirus Encephalitides

Bennett NM. Murray Valley encephalitis, 1974: clinical features. Med J Aust 1976; 2:446–450.

Cruse RP, Rothner AD, Erenberg G, Calisher CH. Central European tick-borne encephalitis: an Ohio case with a history of foreign travel. Am J Dis Child 1979; 133:1070–1071.

Embil JA, Camfield P, Artsob H, Chase DP. Powassan virus encephalitis resembling herpes simplex encephalitis. Arch Intern Med 1983; 143:341–343.

Gadoth N, Weitzman S, Lehmann EE. Acute anterior myelitis complicating West Nile fever. Arch Neurol 1979; 36:172–173.

Goodpasture HC, Poland JD, Francy DB, Bowen GS, Horn KA. Colorado tick fever: clinical, epidemiologic, and laboratory aspects of 228 cases in Colorado in 1973–1974. Ann Intern Med 1978; 88:303–310.

Meegen JM, Niklasson B, Bengtsson E. Spread of Rift Valley fever virus from continental Africa. Lancet 1979; 2:1184–1185.

Smorodintsev AA. Tick-borne spring-summer encephalitis. Prog Med Virol 1958; 1:210–247.

Rubella

Burke JR, Hinman R, Krugman S. International symposium on prevention of congenital rubella infection. Rev Infect Dis 1985; 7(Suppl 1):S1–S215.

Centers for Disease Control. Rubella and congenital rubella syndrome—New York City. MMWR 1986; 35:770–779.

Desmond MM, Wilson GS, Melnick JL, et al. Congenital rubella encephalitis. J Pediatr 1967; 71:311–331.

Ishikawa A, Murayama T, Sakuma N, et al. Computed cranial tomography in congenital rubella syndrome. Arch Neurol 1982; 39:420–421.

Miller E, Cradock-Watson JE, Pollock TM. Consequence of confirmed maternal rubella at successive stages of pregnancy. Lancet 1982; 2:781–784.

Rorke LB, Spiro AJ. Cerebral lesions in congenital rubella syndrome. J Pediatr 1967; 70:243–255.

Waxham NR, Wolinsky JS. Rubella virus and its effects on the central nervous system. Neurol Clin 1984; 2:367–385.

Myxovirus Infections

Mumps Meningitis and Encephalomyelitis

Johnstone JA, Ross CAC, Dunn M. Meningitis and encephalitis associated with mumps infection: a 10 year study. Arch Dis Child 1972; 47:647–651.

Jubelt B. Enterovirus and mumps virus infections of the nervous system. Neurol Clin 1984; 2:187–213.

Koskiniemi M, Donner M, Pettay O. Clinical appearance and outcome in mumps encephalitis in children. Acta Paediatr Scand 1983; 72:603–609.

Levitt LP, Rich RA, Kinde SW, Lewis AL, Gates EH, Bond JO. Central nervous system mumps: a review of 64 cases. Neurology 1970; 20:829–834.

McLean DDM, Bach RD, Larke PR, McNaughton GA. Mumps meningoencephalitis, Toronto 1963. Can Med Assoc J 1964; 90:458–462.

Schwartz GA, Yang DC, Noone EL: Meningoencephalomyelitis with epidemic parotitis. Arch Neurol 1964; 11:453–462.

Taylor FB Jr, Toreson WE. Primary mumps meningoencephalitis. Arch Intern Med 1963; 112:216–221.

Thompson JA. Mumps: a cause of acquired aqueductal stenosis. J Pediatr 1979; 94:923–924.

Wilfert CM. Mumps meningoencephalitis with low cerebrospinal fluid glucose, prolonged pleocytosis, and elevation of protein. N Engl J Med 1969; 280:855–859.

Subacute Measles Encephalitis

Agamanolis DP, Tan JS, Parker DL. Immunosuppressive measles encephalitis in a patient with a renal transplant. Arch Neurol 1979; 36:686–690.

Chadwick DW, Martin S, Buxton PH, Tomlinson AH. Measles virus and subacute neurological disease: an unusual presentation of measles inclusion body encephalitis. J Neurol Neurosurg Psychiatry 1982; 45:680–684.

Rhabdovirus Infection

Rabies

Anderson LJ, Nicholson KG, Tauxe RV, Winkler WG. Human rabies in the United States, 1960 to 1979: epidemiology, diagnosis and prevention. Ann Intern Med 1984; 100:728–735.

Baer GM, Fishbein DB. Rabies post-exposure prophylaxis. N Engl J Med 1987; 316:1270–1272.

Baer GM, Shaddock JH, Houff SA, Harrison AK, Gardner JJ. Human rabies transmitted by corneal transplant. Arch Neurol 1982; 39:103–107.

Bernard KW, Smith PW, Kader FJ, Moran MJ. Neuroparalytic illness and human diploid cell rabies vaccine. JAMA 1982; 248:3136–3138.

Centers for Disease Control. Rabies surveillance 1986. MMWR 1987; 36, suppl. 35.

Chopra JS, Banerjee AK, Murthy JMK, Pal SR. Paralytic rabies: a clinico-pathological study. Brain 1980; 103:789–802.

Dupont JR, Earle KM. Human rabies encephalitis, a study of forty-nine fatal cases with a review of the literature. Neurology 1965; 15:1023–1034.

Hemachudha T. Rabies. In: Vinken PJ, Bruyn GW, Klawans HL, McKendall RR, eds. Handbook of Clinical Neurology (Vol. 52). New York: Elsevier-North Holland, 1988.

Hemachudha T, Phanaphak P, Johnson RT, Griffin DE, Ratanavongsiri J, Siriprasomsup W. Neurologic complication of Semple-type rabies vaccine: clinical and immunologic studies. Neurology 1987; 37:550–556.

Miller A, Nathanson N. Rabies: recent advances in pathogenesis and control. Ann Neurol 1977; 2:511–519.

Porras C, Barboza JJ, Fuenzalida E, Adaros HL, Oviedo AM, Furst J. Recovery from rabies in man. Ann Intern Med 1976; 85:44–48.

Sung JH, Hayano M, Mastri AR, Okagaki T. A case of human rabies and ultrastructure of the negri body. J Neuropathol Exp Neurol 1976; 35:541–559.

Warrell DA, Davidson NM, Pope MN, et al. Pathophysiology studies in human rabies. Am J Med 1976; 60:180–190.

Arenavirus Infections

Lymphocytic Choriomeningitis

Armstrong C, Lille RD. Experimental lymphocytic choriomeningitis of monkeys and mice produced by a virus encountered in studies of the 1933 St. Louis encephalitis epidemic. Public Health Rep 1934; 49:1019–1027.

Biggar RJ, Woodall JP, Walter PD, Haughie GE. Lymphocytic choriomeningitis outbreak associated with pet hamsters: fifty-seven cases from New York State. JAMA 1975; 232:494–500.

Chesney PJ, Katcher ML, Nelson DB, Horowitz SD. CSF eosinophilia and chronic lymphocytic choriomeningitis virus meningitis. J Pediatr 1979; 94:750–752.

Colmore JP. Severe infections with the virus of lymphocytic choriomeningitis. JAMA 1952, 148:1199–1201.

Farmer TW, Janeway CA. Infections with virus of lymphocytic choriomeningitis. Medicine 1942; 21:1–53.

Lehmann-Grube F. Lymphocytic choriomeningitis virus and other arenavirus infections of the nervous system. In: Vinken PJ, Bruyn GW, Klawans HL, McKendall RR, eds. Handbook of Clinical Neurology (Vol. 52). New York: Elsevier-North Holland, 1988.

Rivers TM, Scott TFM. Meningitis in man caused by a filtrable virus. Science 1935; 81:439–440.

Thacker WL, Lewis VF. Prevalence of lymphocytic choriomeningitis virus antibodies in patients with acute central nervous system disease. J Infect 1982; 5:309–310.

Vanzee BE, Douglass RG, Betts RF, Bauman AW, Fraser DW, Hinman AR. Lymphocytic meningitis in university hospital personnel: clinical features. Am J Med 1975; 58:803–809.

Warkel RL, Rinaldi CF, Bancroft WH, et al. Fatal acute meningoencephalitis due to lymphocytic choriomeningitis virus. Neurology 1973; 23:198–203.

Adenoviruses

Chou SM, Roos R, Burrell R, Gutmann L, Harley JB. Subacute focal adenovirus encephalitis. J Neuropathol Exp Neurol 1973; 32:34–49.

Davis D, Henslee J, Markesbery WR. Fatal adenovirus meningoencephalitis in a bone marrow transplant patient. Ann Neurol 1988; 23:385–389.

Kelsey SD. Adenovirus meningoencephalitis. Pediatrics 1978; 61:291–293.

Kim KS, Gohd RS. Acute encephalopathy in twins due to adenovirus type 7 infection. Arch Neurol 1983; 40:58–59.

Roos R. Adenovirus infections of the nervous system. In: Vinken PJ, Bruyn GW, Klawans HL, McKendall RR, eds. Handbook of Clinical Neurology (Vol. 52). New York: Elsevier-North Holland, 1988.

Simila S, Jouppila R, Salmi A, Pohjonen K. Encephalomeningitis in children associated with an adenovirus type 7 epidemic. Acta Paediatr Scand 1970; 59: 310–316.

West TE, Papasian CJ, Park BH, Parker SW. Adenovirus type 2 encephalitis and concurrent Epstein-Barr virus infection in an adult man. Arch Neurol 1985; 42:815–817.

Herpesvirus Infections

Herpes Simplex Encephalitis

Britton CB, Mesa-Tejada R, Fenoglio CM, Hays AP, Garvey GG, Miller JR. A new complication of AIDS: thoracic myelitis caused by herpes simplex virus. Neurology 1985; 35:1071–1074.

Davis LE, Johnson RT. An explanation for the localization of herpes simplex encephalitis? Ann Neurol 1979; 5:2–5.

Dix RD, Waitzman DM, Follansbee S, et al. Herpes simplex virus type 2 encephalitis in two homosexual men with persistent lymphadenopathy. Ann Neurol 1985; 17:203–206.

Dutt MK, Johnston IDA. Computerized tomography and EEG in herpes simplex encephalitis: their value in diagnosis and prognosis. Arch Neurol 1982; 39:99–102.

Klapper PE, Laing I, Lonson M. Rapid non-invasive diagnosis of herpes encephalitis. Lancet 1981; 2:607–609.

Koskiniemi M, Vaheri A, Taskinen E. Cerebrospinal fluid alterations in herpes simplex encephalitis. Rev Infect Dis 1984; 6:608–618.

McKendall RR. Herpes simplex virus infections. In: Vinken PJ, Bruyn GW, Klawans HL, McKendall RR, eds. Handbook of Clinical Neurology (Vol. 52). New York: Elsevier-North Holland, 1988.

Morawetz RB, Whitley RJ, Murphy DM. Brain biopsy for suspected herpes encephalitis: 40 cases. Neurosurgery 1983; 12:654–657.

Sage, JI, Weinstein MP, Miller DC. Chronic encephalitis possibly due to herpes simplex virus: two cases. Neurology 1985; 35:1470–1472.

Schlageter N, Jubelt B, Vick NA. Herpes simplex encephalitis without CSF leukocytosis. Arch Neurol 1984; 41:1007–1008.

Schroth G, Gawehn J, Thron A, Vallbracht A, Voigt K. Early diagnosis of herpes simplex encephalitis by MRI. Neurology 1987; 37:179–183.

Skoldenberg B, Forsgren M, Alestig K, et al. Acyclovir versus vidarabine in herpes simplex encephalitis. Randomized multicentered study in consecutive Swedish patients. Lancet 1984; 2:707–711.

Whitley RJ, Alford CA, Hirsch MS, et al. Vidarabine versus acyclovir therapy in herpes simplex encephalitis. N Engl J Med 1986; 314:144–149.

Whitley RJ, Soong S-J, Hirsch MS, et al. Herpes simplex encephalitis: vidarabine therapy and diagnostic problems. N Engl J Med 1981; 304:313–318.

Whitley RJ, Soong S-J, Linneman C Jr, et al. Herpes simplex encephalitis: clinical assessment. JAMA 1982; 247:317–320.

Herpes Zoster

Aleksic SN, Budzilovich GN, Lieberman AN. Herpes zoster oticus and facial palsy (Ramsay Hunt Syndrome): clinico-pathologic study and review of literature. J Neurol Sci 1973; 20:149–159.

Applebaum E, Krebs, SI, Sunshine A. Herpes zoster encephalitis. Am J Med 1962; 32:25–31.

Balfour HH Jr, Bean B, Laskin DL, et al. Acyclovir halts progression of herpes zoster in immunocompromised patients. N Engl J Med 1983; 308:1448–1453.

Bean B, Braun C, Balfour HH Jr. Acyclovir therapy for acute herpes zoster. Lancet 1982; 2:118–121.

Eaglstein WH, Katz R, Brown JA. The effect of early corticosteroid therapy on the skin eruption and pain of herpes zoster. JAMA 1970; 211:1682–1683.

Eidelberg D, Sotrel A, Horoupian S, et al. Thrombotic cerebral vasculopathy associated with herpes zoster. Ann Neurol 1986; 19:7–14.

Gilden DH. Varicella-zoster virus infections. In: Vinken PJ, Bruyn GW, Klawans HL, McKendall RR, eds. Handbook of Clinical Neurology (Vol. 52). New York: Elsevier-North Holland, 1988.

Hope-Simpson RE: The nature of herpes zoster: a long term study and a new hypothesis. Proc R Soc Med 1965; 58:9–20.

Jemsek J, Greenberg SB, Tabor L, et al. Herpes zoster-associated encephalitis: clinicopathologic report of 12 cases and review of the literature. Medicine 1983; 62:81–97.

Mulder RR, Lumish RM, Corsello GR. Myelopathy after herpes zoster. Arch Neurol 1983; 40:445–446.

Portenoy RK, Duma C, Foley KM. Acute herpetic and postherpetic neuralgia: clinical review and current management. Ann Neurol 1986; 20:651–664.

Ragozzino MW, Melton LJ III, Kurland LT, Chu CP, Perry HO. Population-based study of herpes zoster and its sequelae. Medicine 1982; 61:310–316.

Ryder JW, Croen K, Kleinschmidt-DeMasters BK, et al. Progressive encephalitis three months after resolution of cutaneous zoster in a patient with AIDS. Ann Neurol 1986; 19:182–188.

Thomas JE, Howard FM Jr. Segmental zoster paresis—a disease profile. Neurology 1972; 22:459–466.

Watson CP, Evans RJ, Reed K, Merskey H, Goldsmith L, Warsh J. Amitriptyline versus placebo in postherpetic neuralgia. Neurology 1982; 32:671–673.

Cytomegalovirus

Bale JF Jr. Human cytomegalovirus infection and disorders of the nervous system. Arch Neurol 1984; 41:310–320.

Bale JF Jr, Jordon C. Cytomegalovirus infections. In: Vinken PJ, Bruyn GW, Klawans HL, McKendall RR, eds. Handbook of Clinical Neurology (Vol. 52). New York: Elsevier-North Holland 1988.

Bray PE, Bale JF, Anderson RE, Kern ER. Progressive neurological disease associated with chronic cytomegalovirus infection. Ann Neurol 1981; 9:499–502.

Dorfman LJ. Cytomegalovirus encephalitis in adults. Neurology 1973; 23:136–144.

Duchowny M, Caplan L, Siber G. Cytomegalovirus infection of the adult nervous system. Ann Neurol 1979; 5:458–461.

MacDonald H, Tobin JO. Congenital cytomegalovirus infection: a collaborative study on epidemiological, clinical, and laboratory findings. Dev Med Child Neurol 1978; 20:471–472.

Masdeu JC, Small CB, Weiss L, Elkin CM, Llena J, Mesa-Tejada R. Multifocal cytomegalovirus encephalitis in AIDS. Ann Neurol 1988; 23:97–99.

Schmitz M, Enders G. Cytomegalovirus as a frequent cause of Guillain-Barré syndrome. J Med Virol 1977; 1:21–27.

Schneck SA. Neuropathological features of human organ transplantation. Probably cytomegalovirus infection. J Neuropathol Exp Neurol 1965; 24:415–429.

Stagno S, Pass RF, Dworsky ME, et al. Congenital cytomegalovirus infection: the relative importance of primary and recurrent maternal infection. N Engl J Med 1982, 306:945–949.

Epstein-Barr Virus

Davie JC, Ceballos R, Little SC. Infectious mononucleosis with fatal neuronitis. Arch Neurol 1963; 9:265–272.

DeSimone PA, Snyder D. Hypoglossal nerve palsy in

infectious mononucleosis. Neurology 1978; 28:844–847.

Erzurum S, Kalavsky SM, Watanakanakorn C. Acute cerebellar ataxa and hearing loss as initial symptoms of infectious mononucleosis. Arch Neurol 1983; 40:760–762.

Gautier-Smith PC. Neurological complications of glandular fever (infectious mononucleosis). Brain 1965; 88:323–334.

Gottlieb-Stematsky T, Arlazoroff A. Epstein-Barr virus infection. In: Vinken PJ, Bruyn GW, Klawans HL, McKendall RR, eds. Handbook of Clinical Neurology (Vol. 52). New York: Elsevier-North Holland, 1988.

Grose C, Henle W, Henle G, Feorino PM. Primary Epstein-Barr virus infections in acute neurologic disease. N Engl J Med 1975; 292:392–395.

Russell J, Fisher M, Zivin JA, Sullivan J, Drachman DA. Status epilepticus and Epstein-Barr virus encephalopathy. Arch Neurol 1985; 42:789–792.

Schnell RG, Dyck PJ, Walter EJ, Bowie BM, Klass DW, Taswell HF. Infectious mononucleosis: neurologic and EEG findings. Medicine 1966; 45:51–63.

Silverstein A, Steinberg G, Nathanson M. Nervous system involvement in infectious mononucleosis: the heralding and/or major manifestation. Arch Neurol 1972; 26:353–358.

Sworn MJ, Urich H. Acute encephalitis in infectious mononucleosis. J Pathol 1970; 100:201–205.

Acute Disseminated Encephalomyelitis

Arnason BGW. Neuroimmunology. N Engl J Med 1987; 316:406–408.

Berman M, Feldman S, Ater M, Zilber N, Kahana E. Acute transverse myelitis: incidence and etiologic considerations. Neurology 1981; 31:966–971.

Decaux G, Szyper M, Ectors M, Cornil A, Franken L. Central nervous system complications of mycoplasma pneumoniae. J Neurol Neurosurg Psychiatry 1980; 43:883–887.

Fenichel GM. Neurological complications of immunization. Ann Neurol 1982; 12:119–128.

Hirtz DG, Nelson KB, Ellenberg JH. Seizures following childhood immunizations. J Pediatr 1983; 102:14–18.

Holliday PL, Baver RB. Polyradiculoneuritis secondary to immunization with tetanus and diphtheria toxoids. Arch Neurol 1983; 40:56–57.

Johnson KP, Wolinsky JS, Ginsberg AH. Immune mediated syndromes of the nervous system related to virus infections. In: Vinken PJ, Bruyn GW, Klawans HL., eds. Handbook of Clinical Neurology (Vol. 34). New York: Elsevier-North Holland, 1978: 391–434.

Johnson RT, Griffin DE, Hirsch RL, et al. Measles encephalitis—clinical and immunological studies. N Engl J Med 1984; 310:137–141.

Miller HG, Stanton JB, Gibbons JL. Para-infectious encephalomyelitis and related syndromes. Q J Med 1956; 25:427–505.

Peters ACB, Versteeg J, Lindeman J, Bots GTAM. Varicella and acute cerebellar ataxia. Arch Neurol 1978; 35:769–771.

Spillane JD, Wells CEC. The neurology of Jennerian vaccination. A clinical account of neurological complications which occurred during the smallpox epidemic in South Wales in 1962. Brain 1964; 87:1–44.

Sulkava R, Rissanen A, Pyhala R. Post-influenzal encephalitis during the influenza A outbreak of 1979/1980. J Neurol Neurosurg Psychiatry 1981; 44:161–163.

Tyler HR. Neurological complications of rubeola (measles). Medicine 1957; 36:147–167.

Ziegler DK. Acute disseminated encephalitis: some therapeutic and diagnostic considerations. Arch Neurol 1966; 14:476–488.

Chronic Viral Infections

Subacute Sclerosing Panencephalitis

Begeer JH, Haaxma R, Snoek JW, Boonstra S, Le Coultre R. Signs of focal posterior cerebral abnormality in early subacute sclerosing panencephalitis. Ann Neurol 1986; 19:200-202.

Cape CA, Martinez AJ, Robertson JT, Hamilton R, Jabour JT. Adult onset of subacute sclerosing panencephalitis. Arch Neurol 1973; 28:124–127.

Case Records of the Massachusetts General Hospital (Case 25-1986). N Engl J Med 1986; 314:1689–1700.

Dawson JR. Cellular inclusions in cerebral lesions of epidemic encephalitis. Arch Neurol Psychiatry 1934; 31:685–700.

Freeman JM. The clinical spectrum and early diagnosis of Dawson's encephalitis. J Pediatr 1969; 75:590–603.

Griffith JF. Subacute sclerosing panencephalitis and lymphocytes. N Engl J Med 1985; 313:952–954.

Hall WW, Choppin PW. Measles-virus proteins in the brain tissue of patients with subacute sclerosing panencephalitis; absence of the M protein. N Engl J Med 1981; 304:1152–1155.

Horta-Barbosa L, Fuccillo DA, Sever JL, Zeman W. Subacute sclerosing panencephalitis: isolation of measles virus from a brain biopsy. Nature 1969; 221:974.

Panitch HS, Gomez-Plascencia J, Norris FH, Cantell K, Smith RA. Subacute sclerosing panencephalitis treatment with intraventricular interferon. Neurology 1986; 36:562–566.

Payne FE, Baublis JV, Itabashi HH. Isolation of measles virus from cell cultures of brain from a patient with subacute sclerosing panencephalitis. N Engl J Med 1969; 281:585–589.

Risk WS, Haddad FS. The variable natural history of subacute sclerosing panencephalitis: a study of 118 cases from the Middle East. Arch Neurol 1979; 36:610–614.

Swoveland P, Johnson KP, Rammohan KW. Subacute sclerosing panencephalitis and other paramyxovirus infections. In: Vinken PJ, Bruyn GW, Klawans HL, McKendall RR, eds. Handbook of Clinical Neurology (Vol. 52). New York: Elsevier-North Holland, 1988.

Tellez-Nagel J, Harter DH. Subacute sclerosing leukoencephalitis: ultrastructure of intranuclear and intracytoplasmic inclusions. Science 1966; 154:899–901.

Zilber N, Rannon L, Alter M, Kahana E. Measles, measles vaccination, and the risk of subacute sclerosing panencephalitis (SSPE). Neurology 1983; 33:1558–1564.

Progressive Rubella Panencephalitis

Coyle PK, Wolinsky JS. Characterization of immune complexes in progressive rubella panencephalitis. Ann Neurol 1981; 9:557–562.

Townsend JJ, Brainger JR, Wolinsky JS, et al. Progressive rubella panencephalitis: late onset after congenital rubella. N Engl J Med 1975; 292:990–993.

Townsend JJ, Stroop WG, Baringer JR, Wolinsky JS, McKerrow JH, Berg BO. Neuropathology of progressive rubella panencephalitis after childhood rubella. Neurology 1982; 32:185–190.

Weil ML, Itabashi HH, Cremer NE, Oshiro LS, Lennette EH, Carnay L. Chronic progressive panencephalitis due to rubella virus simulating subacute sclerosing panencephalitis. N Engl J Med 1975; 292:994–998.

Wolinsky JS. Progressive rubella panencephalitis. In: Vinken PJ, Bruyn GW, Klawans HL, McKendall RR, eds. Handbook of Clinical Neurology (Vol 52). New York: Elsevier-North Holland, 1988.

Wolinsky JS, Dau PC, Buimovici-Klein E, et al. Progressive rubella panencephalitis: immunovirological studies and results of isoprinosine therapy. Clin Exp Immunol 1979; 35:397–404.

Progressive Multifocal Leukoencephalopathy

Astrom KE, Mancall EL, Richardson EP. Progressive multifocal leukoencephalopathy: a hitherto unrecognized complication of chronic lymphatic leukemia and Hodgkin's disease. Brain 1958; 81:93–111.

Brooks BR, Walker DL. Progressive multifocal leukoencephalopathy. Neurol Clin 1984; 2:299–313.

Krupp LB, Lipton RB, Swerdlow ML, Leeds NE, Llena J. Progressive multifocal leukoencephalopathy: clinical and radiologic features. Ann Neurol 1985; 17:344–349.

Miller JR, Barrett RE, Britton CB, et al. Progressive multifocal leukoencephalopathy in a male homosexual with T-cell immune deficiency. N Engl J Med 1982; 307:1436–1438.

Padgett BL, Walker DL, ZuRhein GM, Eckroade RJ. Cultivation of papova-like virus from human brain with progressive multifocal leuconcephalopathy. Lancet 1971; 1:1257–1260.

Richardson EP Jr. Progressive multifocal leucoencephalopathy. N Engl J Med 1961; 265:815–823.

Richardson EP Jr. Progressive multifocal leucoencephalopathy 30 years later. N Engl J Med 1988; 318:315–317.

Smith CR, Sima AAF, Salit IE, Gentili F. Progressive multifocal leukoencephalopathy: failure of cytarabine therapy. Neurology 1982; 32:200–203.

ZuRhein GM, Chou SM. Particles resembling papovaviruses in human cerebral demyelinating disease. Science 1965; 148:1477–1479.

Kuru

Gajdusek DC. Unconventional viruses and the origin and disappearance of kuru. Science 1977; 197:943–960.

Gajdusek DC, Gibbs CJ, Alpers M. Experimental transmission of a kuru-like syndrome to chimpanzees. Nature 1966; 209:794–796.

Gajdusek DC, Zigas V. Degenerative disease of the central nervous system in New Guinea: the endemic occurrence of "kuru" in the native population. N Engl J Med 1957; 257:974–978.

Gajdusek DC, Zigas V. Kuru. Clinical, pathological, and epidemiological study of an acute progressive degenerative disease of the central nervous system among natives of the Eastern Highlands of New Guinea. Am J Med 1959; 26:442–469.

Hadlow WJ. Scrapie and kuru. Lancet 1959; 2:289–290.

Hornabrook RW. Kuru—a subacute cerebellar degeneration: the natural history and clinical features. Brain 1968; 91:53–74.

Prusiner SB, Gajdusek DC, Alpers MP. Kuru with incubation periods exceeding two decades. Ann Neurol 1982; 12:1–9.

Creutzfeldt-Jakob Disease

Brown P, Cathala F, Raubertas RF, Gajdusek DC, Castaigne P. The epidemiology of Creutzfeldt-Jakob disease: conclusion of a 15-year investigation in France

and review of the world literature. Neurology 1987; 37:895–904.

Brown P, Rodgers-Johnson P, Cathala F, Gibbs CJ Jr, Gajdusek DC. Creutzfeldt-Jakob disease of long duration: clinicopathological characteristics, transmissibility, and differential diagnosis. Ann Neurol 1984; 16:295–304.

Committee on health care issues, American Neurological Association. Precautions in handling tissues, fluids, and other contaminated materials from patients with documented or suspected Creutzfeldt-Jakob disease. Ann Neurol 1986; 19:75–77.

Davanipour Z, Alter M, Sobel E, Asher D, Gajdusek DC. Creutzfeldt-Jakob disease: possible medical risk factors. Neurology 1985; 35:1483–1486.

DeArmond SJ, Mobley WC, DeMott DL, Barry RA, Beekstead JH, Prusiner SB. Changes in the localization of brain prion proteins during scrapie infection. Neurology 1987; 37:1271–1280.

Duffy P, Wolf J, Collins G, De Voe AG, Streenten B, Cowen D. Possible person-to-person transmission of Creutzfeldt-Jakob disease. N Engl J Med 1974; 290:692–693.

Fields BN. Powerful prions? N Engl J Med 1987; 317:1597–1598.

Gibbs CJ, Gajdusek DC, Asher DM, et al. Creutzfeldt-Jakob disease (spongiform encephalopathy) transmission to the chimpanzee. Science 1968; 161:388–389.

Harrington MG, Merril CR, Asher DM, Gajdusek DC. Abnormal proteins in the cerebrospinal fluid of patients with Creutzfeldt-Jakob disease. N Engl J Med 1986; 315:279–283.

Masters CL, Harris JO, Gajdusek DC, Gibbs CJ Jr, Bernouilli C, Asher DM. Creutzfeldt-Jakob disease: patterns of worldwide occurrence and the significance of familial and sporadic clustering. Ann Neurol 1979; 5:177–188.

Prusiner SB. Slow virus infections of the nervous system. In: Vinken PJ, Bruyn GW, Klawans HL, McKendall RR, eds. Handbook of Clinical Neurology (Vol. 52). New York: Elsevier-North Holland, 1988.

Siedler H, Malamud N. Creutzfeldt-Jakob's disease. Clinicopathologic report of 15 cases and review of the literature. J Neuropathol Exp Neurol 1963; 22:381–402.

Tinter R, Brown P, Hedley-Whyte T, Rappaport B, Piccardo CP, Gajdusek DC. Neuropathologic verification of Creutzfeldt-Jakob disease in the exhumed American recipient of human pituitary growth hormone: epidemiologic and pathogenetic implications. Neurology 1986; 36:932–936.

Gerstmann-Sträussler-Scheinker (GSS) Disease

Masters CL, Gajdusek DC, Gibbs CJ Jr. Creutzfeldt-Jakob disease virus isolations from the Gerstmann-Sträussler syndrome with an analysis of the various forms of amyloid plaque deposition in the virus-induced spongiform encephalopathies. Brain 1981; 104:559–588.

Vinters HV, Hudson AJ, Kaufmann JCE. Gerstmann-Sträussler-Scheinker disease: autopsy study of a familial case. Ann Neurol 1986; 20:540–543.

Encephalitis Lethargica

Anonymous. Encephalitis lethargica. Lancet 1981; 2:1396–1397.

Association for Research in Nervous and Mental Disease. Acute epidemic encephalitis (lethargic encephalitis). New York: Paul B Hoeber, 1921.

Howard RS, Lees AJ. Encephalitis lethargica: a report of four recent cases. Brain 1987; 110:19–33.

Ravenholt RT, Foege WH. 1918 influenza, encephalitis lethargica, parkinsonism. Lancet 1982; 2:860–864.

Riley HA. Epidemic encephalitis. Arch Neurol Psychiatry 1930; 24:574–604.

Von Economo C. Encephalitis lethargica. Wein Klin Wochenschr 1917; 30:581–585.

Yahr MD. Encephalitis lethargica (Von Economo's disease, epidemic encephalitis). In: Vinken PJ, Bruyn GW, Klawans HL, eds. Handbook of Clinical Neurology (Vol. 35). New York: Elsevier-North Holland, 1978: 451–457.

16. ACQUIRED IMMUNODEFICIENCY SYNDROME

Carolyn B. Britton

James R. Miller

Burk Jubelt

The acquired immunodeficiency syndrome (AIDS), an invariably fatal illness, is characterized by a severe deficiency of cell-mediated immunity that predisposes affected individuals to opportunistic infections and unusual malignant tumors. The underlying immune deficiency is caused by infection of T-helper (T_4) lymphocytes and possibly other cells of the immune system by a retrovirus known as the human immunodeficiency virus (HIV).

Before the discovery of HIV, the diagnosis of illness depended on evidence of secondary opportunistic infection or unusual neoplasia to fulfill the criteria for AIDS established by the US Centers for Disease Control (CDC). It is now recognized that AIDS patients are only a minor proportion of those infected by HIV. Serologic studies have demonstrated that asymptomatic carriers of the virus constitute a far larger proportion of those infected. An acute self-limited illness sometimes occurs at the onset of infection. Some HIV carriers have chronic lymphadenopathy, but are otherwise well. In others, designated as having AIDS-related complex (ARC), lymphadenopathy is associated with weight loss and minor infections related to immune deficiency. Some syndromes, such as progressive encephalopathy, may be a direct effect of HIV infection rather than immunosuppression and the secondary illnesses characteristic of AIDS. The CDC has proposed a classification for HIV infection (Table 16–1) that accounts for all the recognized illnesses associated with this infection.

Incidence. The first cases of AIDS were reported in 1981. However, the disease had been seen in the United States several years earlier, and retrospective serologic studies have indicated that HIV was introduced before 1975. The number of cases has increased every year. As of December 1987, slightly over 48,000 AIDS cases had been reported to the CDC. At first, the doubling time of reported cases was about six months, but had fallen to 13 months by late 1986.

Ninety-seven percent of all AIDS patients have been in specific populations who have a defined risk behavior. Sixty-six percent have been homosexual or bisexual men. Seventeen percent have been heterosexual intravenous (IV) drug users. Homosexual or bisexual men who also used IV drugs have comprised 8%. Four percent have been heterosexual sex partners of people with AIDS (or at risk for AIDS). Another 1% have been individuals who received blood transfusions or specific clotting factors for coagulation disorders such as hemophilia. Other recipients of transfused blood have accounted for 2%. AIDS has been reported in every state in the United States, but most cases occur in large urban populations.

The illness is known worldwide and is prevalent in Central Africa, where heterosexual spread is the predominant mode of transmission. Serologic evidence suggests high infection rates among certain populations of major cities (prostitutes; persons with other sexually transmitted diseases and/or frequent sexual contacts) and low or nondetectable infection rates in most rural African populations studied. Although disease-reporting is incomplete, the evidence of an African origin for HIV is less certain than previously thought.

AIDS in Children. By the end of 1987, there were 737 patients with AIDS who were children under the age of 13. Seventy-seven percent of them came from families in which one or both parents had AIDS or a defined risk behavior for exposure to HIV. Six percent had coagulation disorders and 13% had received blood transfusions.

Etiology. Serologic evidence as well as characteristics of the virus indicates that the cause of AIDS is infection with HIV. The nomenclature of this organism is still not firmly decided. The World Health Organization has suggested the name human immune deficiency virus. However, some earlier names are still in use: human T-cell lymphotropic virus-III (HTLV-III) or lymphadenopathy-associated virus (LAV). Neither name is satisfactory. "HTLV-III" suggests a taxonomic relationship with other HTLV viruses that is not

Table 16–1.   Classification of HIV Infections

GROUP   I: Acute infection (transient symptoms with seroconversion)
GROUP   II: Asymptomatic infection (seropositive only)
GROUP III: Persistent generalized lymphadenopathy
GROUP IV: Other disease
  Subgroup A. Chronic constitutional disease
  Subgroup B. Neurologic disease
  Subgroup C. Specified secondary infections
    Category C–1. Diseases listed in the CDC definition for AIDS
    Category C–2. Other specified secondary infections
  Subgroup D. Specified secondary cancers (includes cancers fulfilling CDC definition of AIDS)
  Subgroup E. Other conditions

(From Centers for Disease Control, Morbidity and Mortality Weekly Report. 1986; 35:334–339)

consistent with viral structure or genome homology. "LAV" obscures the relationship to many manifestations of the infection. The discovery of other viruses similar to HIV that also appear to cause immunodeficiency in humans has led to the designation of HIV as HIV-I.

HIV is closely related to the lentiviruses. Visna virus, which causes a slowly progressive demyelinating syndrome in ovines, was previously the best known virus of that group.

Pathogenesis. The primary abnormality in AIDS is a severe cellular immunodeficiency attributed to infection of T_4 helper cells by HIV. In cultured T_4 cells, HIV infection results in syncytia formation, cytopathic effect, and cell death. However, in infected humans HIV can be detected only in about 10% of T_4 cells at any time. It is therefore not clear how the infection leads to the profound reduction in T-helper cell number and function. The effect on T_4 cells results in reversal of the T-helper to T-suppressor cell ratio, cell-mediated immune anergy, depressed lymphoproliferative response to mitogens, and reduced natural killer cell activity.

Both macrophages and B cells may also be infected by HIV. Infection in these cells may contribute to other immunologic abnormalities that are not primarily related to T_4 cell dysfunction: hypergammaglobulinemia, impaired antibody responses to new antigens (especially encapsulated bacteria), and increased blood levels of immune complexes. Antilymphocyte antibodies correlate with seropositivity for HIV.

The HIV genome is integrated into the cellular genome, but is also found free within infected cells. The infection is probably permanent. Most seropositive individuals in epidemiologic studies have been asymptomatic. Some have the constitutional symptoms and minor illnesses of ARC. It is unknown whether all infected patients eventually develop overt AIDS, but epidemiologic evidence indicates that an asymptomatic carrier state may last for several years before typical clinical syndromes appear. Asymptomatic individuals are at least as infectious as patients with overt disease.

Normal antigenic activation of infected lymphocytes is the postulated trigger for expression of viral genes and viral reproduction. The activation presumably leads to the cytopathic effects on lymphocytes and then the illness. Groups at greatest risk for AIDS are all frequently exposed to foreign antigens as well as to the virus.

The loss of cellular immune functions increases susceptibility to opportunistic infections and rare neoplasia. Pneumocystis carinii pneumonia (PCP) is the most common opportunistic infection, occurring in about 60% of cases. Multiple infections are common, especially in patients without PCP (21% of cases). Opportunistic systemic infections include mycobacteriosis (both tuberculosis and diseases caused by atypical species, particularly of the avium-intracellular group), fungal infections (candidiasis, cryptococcosis, aspergillosis, histoplasmosis), other viral infections (cytomegalovirus—CMV, disseminated herpes simplex virus—HSV), and parasitic infections (toxoplasmosis, cryptosporidiosis, strongyloidiasis, isosporiasis). CNS infections have been caused by mycobacteria, Cryptococcus, Candida, aspergilli, CMV, papovavirus (progressive multifocal leukoencephalopathy), Toxoplasma, and Strongyloides.

Kaposi sarcoma is the most common tumor, but systemic and central nervous system lymphomas also occur.

CNS Pathogenesis. In addition to neurologic illness caused by opportunistic infections and lymphoma, HIV itself is probably an important cause of neurologic disease. The evidence includes production of specific antibodies to HIV within the neuraxis and recovery of infectious virus from brain or CSF.

In situ hybridization studies have detected viral nucleic acid in the brain only in macrophages and not in neurons or astroglia. Macrophages may be important in bringing HIV through the blood-brain barrier, but HIV can also infect vascular endothelium. Immunofluorescence studies for viral-specific proteins indicate that HIV may be present in basal ganglia cells and suggest a somewhat broader distribution of virus than the genome detection studies suggest. Some glial lines have also been injected experimentally in cell culture.

However, the current evidence of limited presence of HIV in the brain does not satisfactorily explain the progressive encephalopathy that is an important feature of HIV infection. Indirect effects of the virus on nerve cells have been postulated, including blockade of cell surface receptors by viral or viral-induced protein. Alternatively, neuronal or glial cell functions may be affected by a restricted infection with the presence of a low level of virus that is difficult to detect.

Clinical Syndrome. Symptoms and signs of AIDS depend upon the particular opportunistic infection or neoplasm that occurs. However, the entire spectrum of illness caused by HIV infection has been broadened by recognition that infected patients may be ill, but may not have clinical features by which AIDS was originally defined.

Acute infection with HIV may be asymptomatic or may be manifest by a transient nonspecific mononucleosis-like illness with fever, malaise, gastrointestinal symptoms, myalgia, sore throat, diarrhea, and generalized adenopathy. This syndrome occurs days or weeks after exposure and is accompanied by the appearance of antibodies to HIV. CNS infection may be the first evidence of HIV infection because aseptic meningitis associated with seroconversion has occurred.

After the initial infection, an asymptomatic state or persistent generalized adenopathy may be present. ARC may develop with recurrent fever, fatigue, weight loss, oral candidiasis, and diarrhea in addition to lymphadenopathy. ARC progresses to typical AIDS without exception. Immune-mediated syndromes, especially autoimmune thrombocytopenic purpura, are also seen in HIV-infected individuals.

Neurologic complications are common and occur eventually in at least 60% of HIV-infected patients with clinical illness. Neurologic symptoms are the first manifestations of disease in 10 to 20% of patients. Clinical involvement has occurred at all levels of the neuraxis. Meningitis, subacute encephalopathy (progressive dementia), focal brain lesions, retinopathy, cranial or peripheral neuropathy, movement disorders, myelopathy, and polymyositis have all been noted. Pathologically detected cerebral lesions are more common than clinically observed manifestations, probably because the CNS disease is obscured by overwhelming systemic illness. Neurologic involvement may be related to direct effects of HIV, secondary infections, or neoplasms. It is often difficult to ascribe a particular problem to a specific agent because multiple pathogens may be present, each alone capable of causing the clinical syndrome.

Meningitis in AIDS may be caused by viruses, fungi, mycobacteria, or tumor cells. Cryptococcal meningitis is most common. HIV infection may cause aseptic meningitis, sometimes recurrent, and sometimes with cranial neuropathy. The virus has been isolated from CSF. Meningovascular syphilis may occur. Metastatic leptomeningeal lymphoma causes a chronic meningitis that may also cause cranial neuropathy.

The most common cerebral syndrome of viral etiology is subacute encephalopathy or encephalitis, also known as "AIDS dementia." The syndrome is characterized by the insidious onset of cognitive, behavioral, and motor impairment. Early symptoms include impaired memory, diminished concentration, mental slowness, confusion, apathy, social withdrawal, loss of libido, poor balance, and leg weakness. In some cases, psychiatric disorders or behavioral changes are dominant and include organic psychosis that mimics schizophrenia or depression. Acute mania has also been described. Commonly, a severe ill-defined anxiety state is present. Some patients reach a plateau of fixed mental impairment, but most progress in weeks or months to a state of severe dementia, mutism, incontinence, paraplegia and, occasionally, myoclonus.

The cerebral syndrome may be either the initial or only clinical manifestation of HIV infection. It is attributed to direct viral infection of the nervous system, and the virus has been isolated from brain, spinal cord, and CSF of affected patients. However, as mentioned previously, direct infection of neural tissues has not yet been established.

CSF is normal or shows a mild pleocytosis and protein elevation. Oligoclonal bands are often present. CSF gamma globulin content may be increased, presumably because there is intrathecal synthesis of antibody against HIV. CT shows cortical atrophy, attenuation of white matter, and enlarged ventricles. MRI often shows widespread white matter disease with increased signal on T_2-weighted scans. Postmortem examination of brain and spinal cord reveals cortical atrophy, microglial nodules, and multinucleated giant cells of mononuclear cells. Focal demyelination and vacuolation of white matter are also found. There is little correlation between the severity of clinical manifestations and the degree of pathologic change.

Subacute encephalopathy has also been attributed to several secondary pathogens, including cytomegalovirus (CMV), atypical mycobacterium (MAI), and Toxoplasma, and also to primary lymphoma. These pathogens may coexist with HIV encephalomyelitis.

Focal or multifocal neurologic syndromes may be caused by infections, neoplasms, or vascular complications. Common infections are toxoplasmosis, progressive multifocal leukoencephalopathy (PML), fungal and mycobacterial granulomas, and herpes simplex virus (HSV) encephalitis. Rarely, bacterial abscesses are present. Neoplasms that cause focal signs include primary lymphoma, metastatic systemic lymphoma, and metastatic Kaposi sarcoma. Vascular complications may be due to hemorrhage or infarction. Hemorrhage may be a complication of thrombocytopenia or tumor, and infarction may be due to nonbacterial thrombotic endocarditis or herpes zoster arteritis.

Cranial neuropathies have been associated with recurrent HIV meningitis or other viral infections such as herpes zoster or CMV, cryptococcosis, mycobacteriosis, and leptomeningeal lymphoma. Isolated Bell's palsy may be due to acute HIV infection. Infectious retinopathy is caused by CMV, Toxoplasma, or Candida. A noninfectious retinopathy with cotton-wool spots is due to microvascular damage from circulating immune complexes.

A progressive myelopathy may occur that appears to be due to HIV. It is most common in AIDS patients with opportunistic infections. The clinical findings are progressive spastic paraparesis with hyperreflexia and Babinski signs, ataxia, and incontinence. Co-existent peripheral neuropathy may result in burning paresthesias, areflexia, and loss of extensor plantar responses. Pathologic changes resemble B_{12} deficiency with vacuolar change and demyelination of the anterior, lateral, and posterior columns, most severe in the thoracic cord. Microglial nodules are also observed. HIV has been cultured from spinal cord and is the putative cause, although it is uncertain whether there is direct infection, immune injury, or metabolic pertubation.

Myelitis may also be caused by direct viral infection with HSV, CMV, or varicella zoster (VZV). Anterior horn cell (AHC) lesions have also been noted. In the best documented case, AHC involvement was associated with severe CMV radiculopathy. B cell neoplasms, such as lymphoma or plasmacytoma, cause myelopathy by cord compression.

Peripheral nerve disorders in AIDS include distal symmetric sensorimotor neuropathy, inflammatory neuropathy with either mononeuropathy multiplex or a distal symmetric disorder, acute Guillain-Barré syndrome, or polyradiculopathy. Cranial neuropathy may coexist. Clinical manifestations include burning paresthesias, distal weakness and atrophy, paraparesis, sensory changes, and areflexia. Sphincter function may be affected. Demyelinating, axonal, and mixed lesions are described pathologically. Associated possible etiologic pathogens are HIV, CMV, and VZV. HIV may also be directly related because it has been cultured from sural nerve. CSF may show a mild to moderate mixed pleocytosis, mild protein elevation, oligoclonal bands, and elevated gamma globulin. Some patients improve spontaneously. It is not clear whether specific clinical syndromes of peripheral neuropathy can be attributed to direct virus infection or to immune reactions.

Movement disorders reported in AIDS include myoclonus, parkinsonian tremor and rigidity, supranuclear ophthalmoparesis, dystonia, chorea, ballismus, and segmental myoclonus. One patient with supranuclear ophthalmoparesis, myoclonus, and parkinsonism had CNS Whipple disease with a negative jejunal biopsy. The diagnosis was made only at autopsy. Myopathy and necrotizing myositis of uncertain cause have also been reported.

Laboratory Tests. Virtually all patients with clinically apparent AIDS have serum antibodies to HIV virus. An ELISA assay is the usual screening test. This test requires confirmation, however, to ensure specificity by radioimmunoprecipitation of the serum with labeled viral proteins or by immunostaining of viral proteins that have been separated into a characteristic pattern by electrophoresis with the serum (western blots). The serology test is not required to make the diagnosis when the clinical disorder is typical.

In the early stages of the viral infection, HIV serology may be negative. Therefore, for acute viral syndromes (such as aseptic meningitis) in patients with known risk factors, lack of antibodies does not preclude the diagnosis. A convalescent titer should be obtained at least six weeks later. HIV serology may also be useful when there are neurologic findings without obvious stigmata of AIDS. Care must be taken in interpreting the result because, at this early stage in understanding the neurology of HIV infection, neurologic abnormalities may not necessarily be related to an asymptomatic HIV infection.

Other laboratory studies useful in evaluating patients with HIV infection include T cell quantitation and the T_4/T_8 cell ratio. Serologic studies and isolation attempts for other infectious agents associated with the AIDS syndrome are also useful. Elevated IgM titers to these pathogens are seldom found, either because the immune suppression is present or because the infection is a reactivation of a previously contained or latent infection. IgG titers are often low and may even be absent despite active infection.

Diagnostic Evaluation. In addition to HIV serology and T cell laboratory studies, cutaneous anergy and lymphopenia are consistently found in patients with AIDS. Serum gamma globulins are usually elevated and circulating immune complexes may be detected. Pulmonary lesions may be detected by chest radiograph. Gallium scan is also useful in identifying inflammatory pulmonary lesions such as PCP that are not apparent on roentgenographic examination. Biopsy of lymph nodes or skin lesions with appropriate cultures may be diagnostic of lymphoma, Kaposi sarcoma, or mycobacterial or fungal infections. Cerebral aspergillosis is associated with pulmonary infection. Candida and bacterial brain abscesses are often associated with systemic infection and may be diagnosed by blood culture.

Neurologic Evaluation. EEG may show focal or diffuse slowing. It may suggest a metabolic cause of encephalopathy rather than cerebral infection or neoplasm if triphasic waves are present.

CSF analysis and culture may be diagnostic in fungal, mycobacterial, or lymphomatous meningitis. Viruses (including HIV) are infrequently cultured from CSF, but may sometimes be detected by immune stains of sedimented CSF cells.

The CSF formula has been variable. It may be normal or mildly deranged and unrepresentative of the intensity of infection. Detection of oligoclonal bands is a sensitive, but not infallible, indication of CNS infection, but it is not known if the bands are specific for HIV and other infecting organisms. Antibodies specific for HIV in the CSF have, however, been demonstrated by radioimmune assay, and production of HIV antibodies in the neuraxis is suggested by comparison to titers in serum.

CT is helpful in distinguishing focal from diffuse brain lesions. Enhancing lesions with mass effect are seen with toxoplasmosis, lymphoma, and abscesses. Nonenhancing white matter lesions are seen in PML and, sometimes, in Aspergillus infection. MRI may detect lesions that are not apparent on CT. MRI is especially useful in HIV encephalopathy, by showing extensive white matter abnormalities when the CT may be normal or may only demonstrate a variable degree of atrophy.

Brain biopsy is required for definite diagnosis of cerebral lesions. Selection of the biopsy site should be guided by the results of CT or MRI. A presumptive diagnosis of toxoplasmosis may be based on CT evidence of multiple abscesses or a deep abscess that involves the basal ganglia (where biopsy would not be feasible) and response to appropriate treatment (Fig. 16–1). Myelography should be considered for spinal cord syndromes, particularly if the CSF protein is over 100 mg/dl. CSF examination, viral titers, and viral cultures of blood and urine for HIV, CMV, EMG, and biopsy may be helpful in evaluating peripheral neuropathies and myopathies.

Treatment, Course, and Prognosis. AIDS is a progressive, eventually fatal disease. Life may be prolonged by appropriate treatment of secondary infections and neoplasms, but without correction of the underlying HIV infection and immunodeficiency, response to treatment is impaired. Relapse, new infections, or malignant tumors are inevitable. Often there is a continual accrual of complicating illnesses.

Unsuccessful attempts have been made to treat HIV infection by antiviral agents, to im-

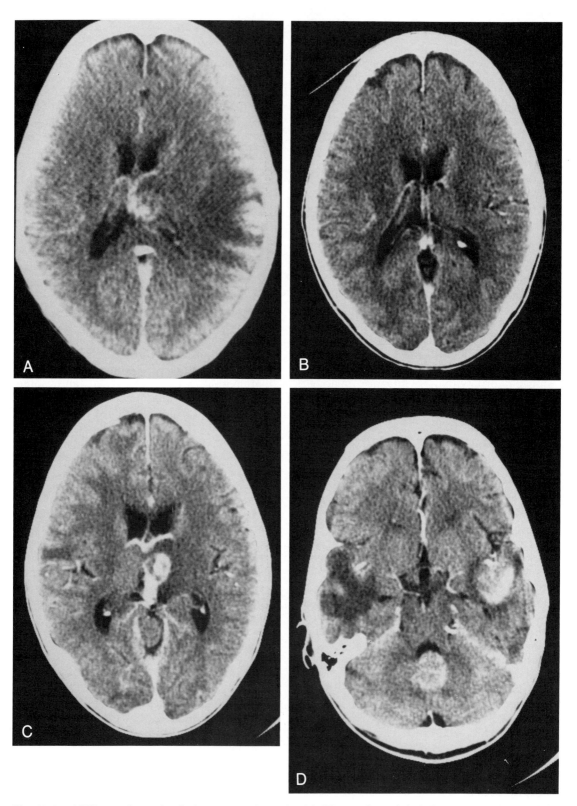

Fig. 16–1. AIDS, toxoplasmosis. *A,* A contrast-enhanced axial CT scan shows left thalamic parietal and nodular enhancing lesions with adjacent edema and mass effect consistent with toxoplasmosis. *B,* A follow-up contrast-enhanced scan six weeks later demonstrates resolution of the lesions and mass effect with therapy. Contrast-enhanced axial CT scans obtained at the same *(C),* and lower *(D)* levels 11 weeks later demonstrate recurrent nodular and ring enhancement in the left thalamus with adjacent edema and mass effect. The edema in the right frontal and temporal regions, in *C* and *D,* is related to another lesion. Additional enhancing lesions are present in the left temporal region and vermis *(D).* (Courtesy of Drs. J.A. Bello and S.K. Hilal.)

prove the immune status of AIDS patients, or to prevent development of immune deficiency in asymptomatic HIV infection. However, one drug that disrupts the life cycle of the AIDS virus has shown promise in early clinical trials and has been released for treatment in specific circumstances. The drug, 3'-azido-3-deoxythymidine (AZT, Zidovudine), apparently blocks viral replication by incorporation into the DNA copy of the viral RNA genome and termination of DNA synthesis. Short-term results indicate that the drug suppresses viral replication, improves immune function, and may induce spontaneous remission of some secondary infections or may allow more successful treatment of the infection. The major adverse side effect is bone marrow depression with anemia and leukopenia that often require repeated transfusion or drug holidays. Relapse of secondary problems may occur when treatment must be discontinued. The medication has not cured HIV infection, but some patients have had prolonged remissions of secondary complications and substantial clinical improvement.

AZT penetrates the blood-brain barrier and may be effective against HIV in the CNS. An effect on HIV encephalopathy is not yet certain, but preliminary studies have been encouraging. Penetration of the blood-brain barrier may also be an important consideration, because the presence of HIV in the CNS may provide a protected reservoir of infection. That aspect has implications for the development of future anti-HIV drugs.

Development of a vaccine promises to be the best method to limit the current pandemic. The genetic variability of the viral surface proteins is a formidable obstacle. In the meantime, careful monitoring of blood products for infection, restricted sexual contacts and, perhaps, the use of condoms are important means of limiting the spread of HIV infection.

Secondary infections and malignant tumors may be appropriately treated but are rarely cured. Sulfadiazine and pyrimethamine are effective treatment for toxoplasmosis, but chronic treatment may be needed to prevent relapse. Acyclovir is the preferred treatment for herpes simplex or varicella zoster. Radiation therapy is of temporary benefit in primary brain lymphoma or leptomeningeal lymphoma. Cryptococcus infection responds to antifungal therapy, but relapse is common with cessation of treatment. There is no effective treatment for CMV, PML, or MAI infections, but combined chemotherapy may temporarily control MAI.

Precautions for Clinical and Laboratory Services. Strict observation of contamination procedures is mandatory for clinical and laboratory services. The precautions are similar to those for hepatitis B infection, which has similar venereal and parenteral transmission characteristics. The hospital patient with known or suspected HIV infection should be isolated, and precautions should be observed in the handling of all wastes, body fluids, and surgical specimens. Gloves should be worn to prevent direct mucous-membrane contact with blood, excretions, secretions, and tissues of infected patients. Goggles or glasses should be used when heavy aerosol contamination with blood or other secretions is anticipated (e.g., in the operating room).

The CDC is prospectively following 735 health care workers who have had needlestick injuries or extensive mucous membrane exposure. Five persons with needle injuries are seropositive for HIV; in two of them, seroconversion was documented after the injury. Three additional individuals with skin or mucous membrane exposure converted to seropositivity after the apparent exposure. To date, none of these workers is ill. The risk to health care workers is obviously small, considering the large number of similar contacts that go unreported. Nonetheless, it is clear that strict precautions must be observed, in the handling of needles, instruments, and infected body fluids.

Unlike some other organisms that infect the CNS, such as the agent of Creutzfeldt-Jakob disease, HIV is readily inactivated by heat and standard sterilization solutions including 70% alcohol. Special sterilization procedures are unnecessary for this conventional enveloped virus.

References

Barton NW, Safai B, Nielsen SL, Posner JB. Neurological complications of Kaposi's sarcoma. An analysis of 5 cases and a review of the literature. J Neurooncol 1983; 1:333–346.

Behar R, Wiley C, McCutchan JA. Cytomegalovirus polyradiculoneuropathy in acquired immune deficiency syndrome. Neurology 1987; 37:557–561.

Bishburg E, Sunderam G, Reichman LB, Kapila R. Central nervous system tuberculosis with the acquired immunodeficiency syndrome and its related complex. Ann Intern Med 1986; 105:210–213.

Britton CB, Mesa-Tejada R, Fenoglio CM, Hays AP, Garvey GG, Miller JR. A new complication of AIDS: thoracic myelitis caused by herpes simplex virus. Neurology 1985; 35:1071–1074.

Carne CA, Tedder RS, Smith A, Sutherland S, Elkington

SG, Daly HM, Preston FE, Craske J. Acute encephalopathy coincident with seroconversion for anti-HTLV-III. Lancet 1985; 2:1206–1208.

Clavel F, Guétard D, Brun-Vézinet F, Chamaret S, Rey M, Santos-Ferreira MO, Laurent AG, Dauguet C, Katlama C, Rouzioux C, Klatzmann D, Champalimaud JL, Montagnier L. Isolation of a new human retrovirus from West African patients with AIDS. Science 1986; 233:343–346.

Cornblath DR, McArthur JC, Kennedy PG, Witte AS, Griffin JW. Inflammatory demyelinating peripheral neuropathies associated with human T-cell lymphotrophic virus type III infection. Ann Neurol 1987; 21:32–40.

Curran JW, Hardy AM, Jaffee HW, Darrow WW, Dowdle WR. The epidemiology of AIDS: current status and future prospects. Science 1985; 229:1352–1357.

Curran JW, Jaffe HW, Hardy AM, Meade Morgan W, Selik RM, Dondero TS. Epidemiology of HIV Infection and AIDS in the United States. Science 1988; 239:610–616.

de la Monte SM, Ho DD, Schooley RT, Hirsch MS, Richardson EP. Subacute encephalomyelitis of AIDS and its relation to HTLV-III infection. Neurology 1987; 37:562–569.

Eidelberg D, Sotrel A, Vogel H, Walker P, Kleafield J, Crumpacker CS. Progressive polyradiculopathy in acquired immunodeficiency syndrome. Neurology 1986; 36:912–916.

Epstein LG, Sharer LR, Joshi VV, Fojas MM, Konigsberger MR, Oleske JM. Progressive encephalopathy in children with acquired immunodeficiency syndrome. Ann Neurol 1985; 17:488–496.

Epstein LG, Sharer LR, Oleske JM, Connor EM, Goudsmit J, Bagdon L, Robert-Guroff M, Koenigsberger MR. Neurologic manifestations of human immunodeficiency virus infection in children. Pediatrics 1986; 78:678–687.

Gabuzda DH, Hirsch MS. Neurologic manifestations of infection with human immunodeficiency virus. Clinical features and pathogenesis. Ann Intern Med 1987; 107:383–391.

Gabuzda DH, Ho D, de la Monte SM, Hirsch MS, Rota TR, Sobel RA. Immunohistochemical identification of HTLV-III antigen in brains of patients with AIDS. Ann Neurol 1986; 20:289–295.

Gallo RC, Salahuddin SZ, Popovic M, Shearer GM, Kaplan M, Haynes BF, Palker TJ, Redfield R. Frequent detection and isolation of cytopathic retroviruses (HTLV-III) from patients with AIDS and at risk for AIDS. Science 1984; 224:500–503.

Gartner S, Markovits P, Markovitz DM, Betts RF, Popovic M. Virus isolation from and identification of HTLV-III/LAV-producing cells in brain tissue from a patient with AIDS. JAMA 1986; 256:2365–2371.

Gyorkey F, Melnick JL, Gyorky P. Human immunodeficiency virus in brain biopsies of patients with AIDS and progressive encephalopathy. J Infect Dis 1987; 155:870–876.

Ho DD, Rota TR, Schooley RT, Kaplan JC, Allan JD, Groopman JE, Resnick L, Felsenstein D. Isolation of HTLV-III from cerebrospinal fluid and neural tissues of patients with neurologic syndromes related to the acquired immunodeficiency syndrome. N Engl J Med 1985; 313:1493–1497.

Hollander J, Levy JA. Neurologic abnormalities and recovery of human immunodeficiency virus from cerebrospinal fluid. Ann Intern Med 1987; 106:692–695.

Koenig S, Gendelman HE, Orenstein JM, Dal-Canto MC,

Pezeshkpour GH, Yungbluth M, Janotta F, Aksamit A. Detection of AIDS virus in macrophages in brain tissue from AIDS patients with encephalopathy. Science 1986; 233:1089–1093.

Levy RM, Bredesen DE, Rosenblum ML. Neurological manifestations of the acquired immunodeficiency syndrome (AIDS): experience at UCSF and review of the literature. J Neurosurg 1985; 62:475–495.

Luft BJ, Brooks RG, Conley FK, McCabe RE, Remington JS. Toxoplasmic encephalitis in patients with acquired immune deficiency syndrome. JAMA 1984; 252:913.

McArthur JC. Neurologic manifestations of AIDS. Medicine 1987; 66:407–437.

Miller JR, Barrett RE, Britton CB, Tapper ML, Bahr GS, Bruno PJ, Marquardt MD, Hays AP. Progressive multifocal leukoencephalopathy in a male homosexual with T-cell immune deficiency. N Engl J Med 1982; 307:1436–1438.

Nath A, Jankovic J, Pettigrew LC. Movement disorders and AIDS. Neurology 1987; 37:37–41.

Navia BA, Cho ES, Petito CK, Price RW. The AIDS dementia complex: II. Neuropathology. Ann Neurol 1986; 19:525–535.

Navia BA, Jordan BD, Price RW. The AIDS dementia complex: I. Clinical features. Ann Neurol 1986; 9:517–526.

Navia BA, Price RW. The acquired immunodeficiency syndrome dementia complex as the presenting or sole manifestation of human immunodeficiency virus infection. Arch Neurol 1987; 44:65–69.

Petito CK, Cho ES, Lemann W, Navia BA, Price RW. Neuropathology of acquired immundeficiency syndrome (AIDS): an autopsy review. J Neuropathol Exp Neurol 1986; 45:635–646.

Petito CK, Navia BA, Cho ES, George DC, Price RW. Vacuolar myelopathy pathologically resembling subacute combined degeneration in patients with the acquired immunodeficiency syndrome. N Engl J Med 1985; 312:874–879.

Piette AM, Tusseau F, Vignon D, Chapman A, Parrot G, Leibowitch J, Montagnier L. Acute neuropathy coincident with seroconversion for anti-LAV/HTLV-III (Letter). Lancet 1986; 1:852.

Piot P, Plummer FA, Mhalu FS, Lamboray J-L, Chin J, Mann JM. AIDS: An International Perspective. Science 1988; 239:573–579.

Post MJ, Sheldon JJ, Hensley GT, Soila K, Tobias JA, Chan JC, Quencer RM, Moskowitz LB. Central nervous system disease in acquired immunodeficiency syndrome: Prospective correlation using CT, MR imaging, and pathologic studies. Radiology 1986; 158:141–148.

Price RW, Brew B, Sidtis J, Rosenblum M, Scheck AC, Cleary P. The brain in AIDS: central nervous system HIV-1 infection and AIDS dementia complex. Science 1988; 239:597–604.

Resnick L, diMarzo-Veronese F, Schupbach J, Tourtellotte WW, Ho DD, Muller F, Shapshak P, Vogt M. Intra-blood-brain-barrier synthesis of HTLV-III-specific IgG in patients with neurologic symptoms associated with AIDS or AIDS-related complex. N Engl J Med 1985; 313:1498–1504.

Shaw GM, Harper ME, Hahn BH, Epstein LG, Gajdusek DC, Price RW, Navia BA, Petito CK. HTLV-III infection in brains of children and adults with AIDS encephalopathy. Science 1985; 227:177–182.

Snider WD, Simpson DM, Nielsen S, Gold JW, Metroka CE, Posner JB. Neurological complications of acquired immune deficiency syndrome: analysis of 50 patients. Ann Neurol 1983; 14:403–418.

So YT, Beckstead JH, Davis RL. Primary central nervous system lymphoma in acquired immune deficiency syndrome: a clinical and pathological study. Ann Neurol 1986; 20:566–572.

Update: Acquired immunodeficiency syndrome. United States. MMWR 1986; 35:757–766.

Wiley CA, Schrier RD, Nelson JA, Lampert PW, Oldstone M. Cellular localization of human immunodeficiency virus infection within the brains of acquired immune deficiency syndrome patients. Proc Natl Acad Sci USA 1986; 83:7089–7093.

Yankner BA, Sklonik PR, Shoukimas GM, Gabuzda DH, Sobel RA, Ho DD. Cerebral granulomatous angiitis associated with isolation of human T-lymphotropic virus type III from the central nervous system. Ann Neurol 1986; 20:362–364.

Yarchoan R, Berg G, Brouwers P, Fischl MA, Spitzer AR, Wichman A, Grafman J. Response of human immunodeficiency virus associated neurological disease to 3'-azido-3'deoxythymidine. Lancet 1987; 1:132–135.

Ziegler JL, Beckstead JA, Volberding PA, Abrams DI, Levine AM, Lukeis RJ, Gill PS, Burkes RL. Non-Hodgkin's lymphadenopathy and the acquired immunodeficiency syndrome. N Engl J Med 1984; 311:565–570.

17. FUNGAL INFECTION

Leon D. Prockop

Fungal infection, or mycosis, of the CNS results in one or more tissue reactions: meningitis, meningoencephalitis, abscess or granuloma formation, and arterial thrombosis. Subacute or chronic meningitis or meningoencephalitis are most common, but granulomatous lesions and abscesses typify the response to some fungi; thrombotic occlusions occur with other fungal infections. The lungs, skin, and hair are usually the primary site of involvement by fungi.

Fungi exist in two forms: molds and yeasts. Molds are composed of tubular filaments that are sometimes branched and are called hyphae. Yeasts are unicellular organisms that have a thick cell wall that is surrounded by a well-defined capsule. Infecting fungi comprise two groups: pathogenic and opportunistic.

The pathogenic fungi are those few species that can infect a normal host after inhalation or implantation of the spores. Naturally, chronically ill or other immunologically compromised individuals are more susceptible to infection than normal persons; acquired immunodeficiency syndrome (AIDS) has become a major cause of fungal infection. In nature, fungi grow as saprophytic soil-inhabiting mycelial units that bear spores. During infection, they adapt to higher temperatures and lower oxidation-reduction potentials of tissues. They also overcome host defenses by increased growth rate and by relative insensitivity to host defense mechanisms (e.g., phagocytosis).

The pathogenic fungi cause histoplasmosis, blastomycosis, coccidioidomycosis, and paracoccidioidomycosis. The first three are endemic to some areas of North America, and the last to areas of Central and South America. Neurologic disorders are rare in patients with systemic North American blastomycosis or histoplasmosis. Coccidioidomycosis is a more common disease, especially in Arizona and California, and meningitis is a dreaded, often fatal, complication.

The second group of systemically infecting fungi, the opportunistic organisms, is not thought to incite infection in the normal host. These diseases include: aspergillosis, candidiasis, cryptcoccosis, mucormycosis (phycomycosis), and nocardiosis, and even rarer fungal diseases. With some of these fungi, minor changes in host defenses may cause disease (e.g., candidal overgrowth in mucous membranes). With most opportunistic fungi, the CNS is infected only after there have been major changes in the host, such as extensive use of antimicrobial agents that destroy normal nonpathogenic bacterial flora; administration of immunosuppressive agents or corticosteroids that lower the host's resistance; and systemic illness such as Hodgkin disease, leukemia, diabetes mellitus, AIDS, or other diseases that interfere with the host's immune reactions. Prolonged therapeutic use of deep venous lines also seems to be a contributing factor.

Except in some regions of Asia, CNS manifestations of aspergillosis are uncommon. CNS nocardiosis is rare. Athough clinically apparent meningeal infection with candida is rare, candidiasis has become an increasingly common postmortem brain finding that is often not appreciated clinically. In autopsy studies, candidiasis occurs in compromised patients and produces intracerebral microabscesses and noncaseating granulomas without diffuse leptomeningitis. In contrast to most mycoses, in which neurologic disease is secondary to systemic involvement, cryptococcal meningitis may be a primary infection. Although this fungus is considered opportunistic, the factors that predispose to cryptococcal infection in some apparently normal individuals are unknown.

In mucormycosis, primary infection of the nasal sinuses and eye often extends to the brain or cranial nerves in the compromised patient. Rare fungal causes of neurologic disorders include: allescheriosis, alternariasis, cephalosporiosis, cladosporiosis, diplorhinotrichosis, drechsleriasis, fonsecaeasis, madurellosis, paecilomycosis, penicilliosis, sporotrichosis, streptomycosis, torulopsiasis, trichophytosis, and ustilagomycosis.

Diagnosis of fungal infections is often difficult and depends on the alertness of the physician. The characteristic findings in the radiographs of the lungs and other organs, skin tests, antibody tests of serum and CSF, and isolation of organisms from lesions and CSF are important diagnostic aids. Brain CT and MRI scans may document mass lesions caused by granulomas or abscess. Likewise, in meningitis, CT or MRI may demonstrate obliteration of subarachnoid spaces or hydrocephalus, which are findings that are useful in management and prognosis.

Treatment of human fungal infections is at best unsatisfactory. The administration of penicillin and other commonly used antimicrobial agents is useless and may lead to spread of the infection, with the exception of infection by actinomycosis and nocardiosis. Actinomycosis is curable by either tetracycline antibiotics or penicillin and nocardiosis by sulfonamides. Hydroxystilbamidine is effective in the treatment of blastomycosis. Amphotericin B is the most effective therapeutic preparation for most neurologic fungal disease, although important roles for 5-fluorocytosine, micronazole, and ketoconazole are being recognized.

Cryptococcosis

Cryptococcosis is the most common mycotic infection that directly involves the CNS. The disease may simulate tuberculous meningitis, brain tumor, encephalitis, or psychosis.

Pathogenesis. Cryptococcus neoformans (Torula histolytica or Torulopsis neoformans) is a fungus found throughout the world. Infections by the small yeast-like spherule have been described under various terms such as torulosis, yeast meningitis, and European blastomycosis. Although the skin and mucous membranes may be the primary site of infection, the respiratory tract is usually the portal of entry. The organism has been recovered in fruit, milk, soil, wasps' nests, some grasses and plants, human skin and mucous membranes, and the manure of pigeons and other birds. The last serves as a reservoir from which human infection may occur.

In 30 to 50% of reported cases, cryptococcosis is associated with debilitating diseases such a lymphosarcoma, reticulum-cell sarcoma, leukemia, Hodgkin disease, multiple myeloma, sarcoidosis, tuberculosis, diabetes mellitus, renal disease, and lupus erythematosus. CNS infection may occur independently of, or in association with, evidence of systemic disease. However, by the time the diagnosis of systemic cryptococcosis is firmly established, 70% of patients have neurologic abnormalities.

Pathology. The changes in the nervous system include infiltration of the meninges with mononuclear cells and the cryptococcus organisms. The organisms may be scattered diffusely throughout the parenchyma of the brain with little or no local inflammatory reaction. An abscess in the brain or small granulomas are occasionally formed in the meninges of the brain or spinal cord.

Symptoms and Signs. Symptomatic onset of nervous-system involvement is subacute. Meningeal symptoms usually predominate, but occasionally focal neurologic signs or mental symptoms are in the foreground. The usual clinical picture is that of subacute meningitis or encephalitis. The diagnosis of tuberculous meningitis is often entertained until attention is directed to the correct diagnosis by the peculiar appearance of some of the "cells" in the CSF. The diagnosis of yeast meningitis has been established by culture of the organism on Sabouraud medium.

Large granulomas in the cerebrum, cerebellum, or brain stem cause the same clinical syndromes as other expanding lesions in these sites. Prior to the availability of CT, the diagnosis of a granuloma was rarely made before operation. Nonetheless, definitive diagnosis can be made only when the meningeal involvement is also present and the organisms are recovered from the CSF.

Laboratory Data. The CSF findings in infections with cryptococci are similar to those of tuberculous meningitis. The CSF is usually under increased pressure. There is a slight or moderate pleocytosis from 10 to 500 cells/mm^3. The protein content is increased. The sugar content is decreased, with values commonly between 15 mg and 35 mg. The diagnosis is made by finding the organisms in the counting-chamber centrifuge sediment of the fluid (Fig. 17–1), by growth on Sabouraud

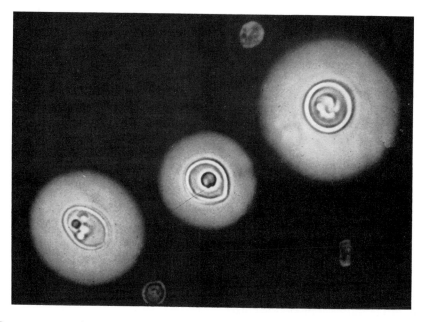

Fig. 17–1. Cryptococcus neoformans meningitis. Fresh preparation of sediment from CSF stained with India ink. The capsule is three times the diameter of the cell. (Courtesy of Dr. Margarita Silva.)

medium, or by the results of animal inoculation. The organisms may also be cultured from the urine, blood, stool, sputum, and bone marrow. The organisms are usually visible on smear or growth in cultures. Diagnosis can be established by the detection of cryptococcal antigen in serum and CSF.

Course. The disease in untreated cases is usually fatal within a few months, but may occasionally last for several years (Fig. 17–2) with recurrent remissions and exacerbations. Occasionally, yeast organisms in the CSF have been noted for three years or longer. Spontaneous cure has been reported in a few cases. Treatment with amphotericin B has a definite beneficial effect. Butler and his associates reported improvement in 31 of 36 treated cases. Seventeen of the 31 patients who showed improvement remained well, three died of unrelated causes, and 11 had one or more relapses of meningitis.

Treatment. The commonly used antimicrobial agents have no appreciable effect on the course of the infection. Some success has been reported with the administration of amphotericin B and 5-fluorocytosine. Combined treatment must be used to prevent failure due to emergence of flucytosine resistance. Amphotericin B administration by cisternal injection or into the lateral ventricle through an Ommaya reservoir has been used. Sterility of the CSF is probably the best end-point of suc-

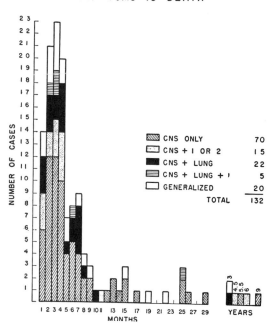

Fig. 17–2. Duration of life in 132 cases of untreated cryptococcal meningitis. The stippled area referred to as 1 and 2 in the figure indicates cases in which skin or bones were also involved. (Courtesy of Dr. Charles Carton.)

cessful treatment. The course of treatment should be repeated if there is a relapse.

Side effects of the administration of amphotericin B include thrombophlebitis, nausea and vomiting, fever, anemia, hypokalemia, and elevation of the blood urea level. Aspirin and antihistamines, blood transfusions, and temporary reduction in the drug dosage are of value in control of side effects.

Mucormycosis

Cerebral mucormycosis (phycomycosis) is an acute, rarely curable disease that is caused by fungi of the class Phycomycetae, especially of the genera Rhizopus. It is a common contaminant of laboratory cultures that is not ordinarily pathogenic. Cases have been reported in all parts of the United States, Canada, and England. The disease is probably worldwide. It usually occurs as a complication of diabetes mellitus or blood dyscrasia, particularly leukemia. The use of antibiotics and adrenocortical steroids may also predispose to mucormycosis.

The fungi enter the nose and, in susceptible persons, cause sinusitis and orbital cellulitis. Subsequently, they may penetrate arteries to produce thrombosis of the ophthalmic and internal carotid arteries and later invade veins and lymphatics. There are ocular, cerebral, pulmonary, intestinal, and disseminated forms of the disease.

Proptosis, ocular palsies, and hemiplegia are common neurologic signs that are associated with the involvement of the orbital and internal carotid arteries. The organisms may invade the meninges to cause meningitis or may extend into the brain and produce a mycotic encephalitis.

Diagnosis is made by examination of the sputum, CSF, or exudate of tissue from the nasal sinuses. Culture of rhizopus is corroborative but not diagnostic because it is a common contaminant.

A dramatic improvement in prognosis has been noted in recent years, with 73% survival of cases diagnosed since 1970 compared to 6% before then. Treatment consists of the administration of amphotericin B and control of predisposing factors (e.g., diabetes). Local drainage and early surgery of the necrotic tissue to prevent disease from spreading should be performed.

References

General

Bauman JM, Osenbach R, Hartshorne MF, Youngblood L, Crooks L, Landry AJ, Cawthon, MA. Positive indium-111 leukocyte scan in nocardia brain abscess. J Nucl Med 1986; 27:60–62.

Chaparas SD. The immunology of mycobacterial infections. CRC Crit Rev Microbiol 1982: 9:139–197.

Duma RJ. Therapy of fungal and amebic infections of the central nervous system. In: Sande MA, Smith AL, Root RK, eds. Bacterial Meningitis. New York: Churchill Livingston, 1985; 219–252.

Goodpasture HC, Hershberger RE, Barnett AM, Peterie JD. Treatment of central nervous system fungal infection with ketoconazole. Arch Intern Med 1985; 145:879–880.

Hawkins C, Armstrong D. Fungal infections in the immunocompromised host. Clin Haematol 1984; 13:599–630.

Malik R, Malhotra V, Gondal R, Bechar PC, Malik TK, Kumar S. Mycopathology of cerebral mycosis. Acta Neurochir 1985; 78:161–163.

Rippon JW. Mycosis. In: Vinken PJ, Bruyn GW, eds. Handbook of Clinical Neurology, vol 35. Amsterdam: Elsevier-North Holland, 1978: 371–381.

Salaki JS, Louria DB, Chmel H. Fungal and yeast infections of the central nervous system. Medicine 1984; 63:108–132.

Salfelder K. Atlas of Deep Mycoses. Philadelphia: W.B. Saunders Co., 1980.

Walsh TJ, Hier DB, Caplan LR. Fungal infections of the central nervous system: comparative analysis of risk factors and clinical signs in 57 patients. Neurology 1985; 35:1654–1657.

Actinomycosis

Causey WA. Actinomycosis. In: Vinken PJ, Bruyn GW, eds. Handbook of Clinical Neurology, vol 35. Amsterdam: Elsevier-North Holland, 1978: 383–394.

Millan JM, Escudero L, Roger RL, de la Fuente M, Diez I. Actinomycotic brain abscess: CT findings, J Comput Assist Tomogr 1985; 9:976–978.

Aspergillosis

Centeno RS, Bentson JR, Mancuso AA. CT scanning in rhinocerebral mucormycosis and apergillosis. Radiology 1981; 140:383–389.

Mikhael MA, Rushovich AM, Ciric I. Magnetic resonance imaging of cerebral aspergillosis. Comput Radiol 1985; 9:85–89.

Rhine WD, Arvin AM, Stevenson DK. Neonatal aspergillosis. Clin Pediatr 1986; 25:400–403.

Saravia-Gomez J. Aspergillosis of the central nervous system. In: Vinken PJ, Bruyn GW, eds. Handbook of Clinical Neurology, vol 35. Amsterdam: Elsevier-North Holland, 1978: 395–400.

Walsh TJ, Hier DB, Caplan LR. Aspergillosis of the central nervous system: clinicopathological analysis of 17 patients. Ann Neurol 1985; 18:574–582.

Blastomycosis

Benzel EC, King JW, Mirfakhraee M, West BC, Misra RD, Hadden TA. Blastomycotic meningitis. Surg Neurol 1986; 26:192–196.

Leers WD. North American blastomycosis. In: Vinken PJ, Bruyn GW, eds. Handbook of Clinical Neurology, vol 35. Amsterdam: Elsevier-North Holland, 1978: 401–411.

Candida (Moniliasis)

Parker JC, McCloskey JJ, Lee RS. Human cerebral candidosis: a postmortem evaluation of 19 patients. Hum Pathol 1981; 12:23–28.

Smego RA, Perfect JR, Durack DT. Combined therapy with amphotericin B and 5-fluorocytosine for candida meningitis. Rev Infect Dis 1984; 6:791–801.

Tveten L. Candidosis. In: Vinken PJ, Bruyn GW, eds. Handbook of Clinical Neurology, vol 35. Amsterdam: Elsevier-North Holland, 1978: 413–442.

Coccidioidomycosis

Bouza E, Dreyer JS, Hewitt WL, Meyer RD. Coccidioidal meningitis; an analysis of thirty-one cases and review of the literature. Medicine 1981; 60:139–172.

DeFelice R, Galgiani JN, Campbell SC, Palpant SD, Friedman BA, Dodge RR, Weinberg MG, et al. Ketoconazole treatment of nonprimary coccidioidomycosis. Am J Med 1982; 72:681–687.

Goldstein E, Lawrence RM. Coccidioidomycosis of the central nervous system. In: Vinken PJ, Bruyn GW, eds. Handbook of Clinical Neurology, vol 35. Amsterdam: Elsevier-North Holland, 1978: 443–457.

Young RF, Gade G, Grinnell V. Surgical treatment for fungal infections in the central nervous system. J Neurosurg 1985; 63:371–381.

Histoplasmosis

Lawrence RM, Goldstein E. Histoplasmosis. In: Vinken PJ, Bruyn GW, eds. Handbook of Clinical Neurology, vol 35. Amsterdam: Elsevier-North Holland, 1978: 503–515.

Wheat J, French M, Batteiger B, Kohler R. Cerebrospinal fluid histoplasma antibodies in central nervous system histoplamosis. Arch Intern Med 1985; 145:1237–1240.

Nocardiosis

Causey WA, Lee R. Nocardiosis. In: Vinken PJ, Bruyn GW, eds. Handbook of Clinical Neurology, vol 35. Amsterdam: Elsevier-North Holland, 1978: 517–530.

Felice GA, Simpson GL. Management of nocardia infections. In: Remington JS, Swartz MR, eds. Current Clinical Topics in Infectious Diseases, vol 5. New York: McGraw-Hill, 1984: 49–64.

Paracoccidioidomycosis

Saravia-Gomez J. Paracoccidioidomycosis of the central nervous system. In: Vinken PJ, Bruyn GW, eds. Handbook of Clinical Neurology, vol 35. Amsterdam: Elsevier-North Holland, 1978: 531–539.

Uncommon Fungal Diseases

Fetter BF, Klintworth GK. Uncommon fungal diseases of the nervous system. In: Vinken PJ, Bruyn GW, eds. Handbook of Clinical Neurology, vol 35. Amsterdam: Elsevier-North Holland, 1978: 557–575.

Cryptococcosis

Brown RW, Clarke RJ, Gonzales MF. Cytologic detection of cryptococcus neoformans in cerebrospinal fluid. Acta Cytol 1985; 29:151–153.

Daunt N, Jayasinghe LS. Cerebral torulosis: clinical features and correlation with computed tomography. Clin Radiol 1985; 36:485–490.

De Wytt CN, Dickson PL, Holt GW. Cryptococcal meningitis. A review of 32 years experience. J Neurol Sci 1982; 53:283–292.

Diamond RD, Bennett JE. Prognostic factors in cryptococcal meningitis: a study in 111 cases. Ann Intern Med 1974; 80:176–181.

Fujita NK, Reynard M, Sapico FL, Guze LB, Edwards JE Jr. Cryptococcal intracerebral mass lesions: the role of computed tomography and nonsurgical management. Ann Intern Med 1981; 94:382–388.

Garcia CA, Weisberg LA, Lacorte WSJ. Cryptococcal intracerebral mass lesions: CT-pathologic considerations. Neurology 1985; 35:731–734.

Polsky B, Depman MR, Gold JW, Galicich JH, Armstrong D. Intraventricular therapy of cryptococcal meningitis via a subcutaneous reservoir. Am J Med 1986; 81:24–28.

Sabetta JR, Andriole VT. Cryptococcal infection of the central nervous system. Med Clin North Am 1985; 69:333–344.

Stockstill MT, Kauffman CA. Comparison of cryptococcal and tuberculous meningitis. Arch Neurol 1983; 40:81–85.

Weenink HR, Bruyn GW. Cryptococcosis of the nervous system. In: Vinken PJ, Bruyn GW, eds. Handbook of Clinical Neurology, vol 35. Amsterdam: Elsevier-North Holland, 1978: 459–502.

Mucormycosis

Dhermy P. Phycomycosis (mucormycosis). In: Vinken PJ, Bruyn GW, eds. Handbook of Clinical Neurology, vol 35. Amsterdam: Elsevier-North Holland, 1978: 541–555.

Gamba JL, Woodruff WW, Djang WT, Yeates AE. Craniofacial mucormycosis: assessment with CT. Radiology 1986; 160:207–212.

Morduchowicz G, Shmueli D, Shapira Z, Cohen SL, Yussim A, Block CS, Rosenfeld JB, Pitlik SD. Rhinocerebral mucormycosis in renal transplant recipients. Rev Infect Dis 1986; 8:441–446.

Parfrey NA. Improved diagnosis and prognosis of mucormycosis. Medicine 1986; 65:113–123.

Rangel-Guerra R, Martinez HR, Saenz C. Mucormycosis. Report of 11 cases. Arch Neurol 1985; 42:578–581.

---

18. SARCOIDOSIS
Leon D. Prockop

Sarcoidosis (Besnier-Boeck-Schaumann disease) is a generalized disease of unknown cause, perhaps infectious, that is characterized by the development of small nodules (follicles or tubercles). Numerous clinical syndromes result, depending on the organ involved by the granulomatous process. The lungs, skin, lymph nodes, bones, eyes, and parotid glands are most commonly affected. Neurosarcoidosis primarily affects the leptomeninges, but any portion of the brain or spinal cord may be involved. Cranial and peripheral nerve lesions or myopathy may occur, and multiple sites are affected in some patients.

Pathology. The characteristic lesions are small nodules composed of lymphocytes, endothelial cells, and giant cells (Fig. 18–1). Although some believe that sarcoidosis is an atypical form of tuberculosis, tubercle bacilli are found only when active tuberculosis is also evident. In these cases, tubercle bacilli

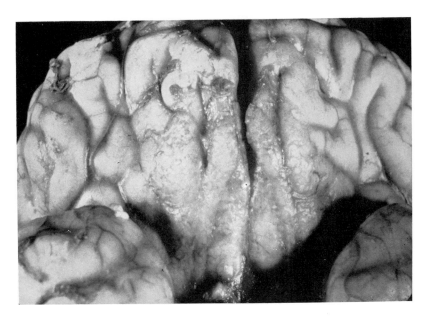

Fig. 18–1.   Sarcoidosis. Lesions in the meninges at the base of the frontal lobe. (Courtesy of Dr. Abner Wolf.)

may be found in the pre-existing sarcoid lesion. Several nonspecific immunologic abnormalities have been noted. Cutaneous anergy, a manifestation of depressed cellular immunity, is common.

Incidence. Sarcoidosis is found throughout the world. The prevalence in the industrialized nations varies by sex, geographic location, and race, but averages 3 to 50 cases/ 100,000 population. Although the exact incidence of neurosarcoidosis is also unknown, reported frequencies vary from 1 to 27% of all cases of sarcoidosis; the average is 5%. Median age of onset of neurologic symptoms was 44 in 50 patients (range 10 to 69) in one series. Autopsy studies indicate that many cases are not detected clinically. Clinical concepts are based mainly on single reports or small series of advanced cases that may give incomplete information of a disease with a fluctuating course.

Symptoms and Signs. The first symptoms of generalized sarcoidosis may be neurologic, with headache, vertigo, facial weakness, hemiparesis, ataxic gait, paresthesias, impaired memory, seizures, psychic alteration, or impaired vision (Table 18–1).

Symptoms and signs relate to site of involvement. The cranial nerves are commonly affected in the following order of frequency: VII, VIII, II, III, IV or VI, and I. Facial paralysis usually occurs in association with uveitis and parotitis (uveoparotid fever). Syndromes include aseptic meningitis, hydrocephalus, hy-

pothalamic dysfunction, and diffuse encephalopathy with vasculopathy. Seizures, which imply poor prognosis, occur in up to 22% of patients with neurosarcoidosis. Any of the peripheral nerves may be affected alone or in combination with other peripheral or cranial nerves, with resulting weakness, atrophy, and loss of sensory and tendon reflexes. The syndrome may be that of mononeuritis multiplex or symmetrical polyneuropathy.

Chronic adhesive arachnoiditis or nodule formation may develop in the dura or arachnoid, especially in the posterior fossa.

After meningeal involvement, single or multiple parenchymal lesions may occur in the cerebral hemisphere, basal ganglia, brain stem, cerebellum, or spinal cord. The appropriate focal neurologic symptoms and signs are seen in these patients. Dementia may be the first manifestation.

Sarcoid lesions in muscles may be found on biopsy with no clinical symptoms; however, myopathic limb weakness may be seen.

Laboratory Data. Moderate fever is an inconstant feature. A mild leukocytosis and eosinophilia are sometimes present. Anemia may occur. The serum globulin content is elevated in about 50% of cases; the serum calcium in about 30%. The skin-tuberculin reaction is negative. Circulating immune complexes, especially glycol precipitable immunoglobulins, have been associated with neurosarcoidosis. Serum angiotensin-converting enzyme (ACE) levels are abnormally

Table 18–1. Comparative Frequencies of Clinical Manifestations in Neurosarcoidosis

Clinical Manifestations	Oksanen 1969–1983		Stern et al 1975–1980		Delaney 1970–1975	
			Number (%) of Patients			
Cranial neuropathy	21	(42)	24	(73)	11	(48)
Intramedullary disease Mass or focal lesion						
Hypothalamus	5	(10)	5	(15)	6	(26)
Other intracranial	17	(34)	0	(0)	8	(35)
Intraspinal	5	(10)	2	(6)	2	(9)
Encephalopathy, vasculopathy	15	(30)	0	(0)	11	(48)
Seizures	9	(18)	0	(0)	5	(22)
Aseptic meningitis	4	(8)	6	(18)	6	(26)
Hydrocephalus	3	(6)	3	(9)	4	(17)
Peripheral neuropathy	9	(18)	2	(6)	1	(4)
Myopathy	5	(10)	4	(12)	2	(9)

increased in many patients with active untreated sarcoidosis. There may be a disproportionate frequency of HLA-B8 antigen in patients with sarcoidosis. Contrast-enhanced CT and MRI of brain or spinal cord may be of diagnostic value. Signs of meningitis or meningoencephalitis are accompanied by CSF abnormalities commonly seen in any subacute meningitis: the pressure is increased, there is a mild pleocytosis (10 to 200 cells, mainly lymphocytes), and protein content is increased up to 2,000 mg/dl. The CSF sugar content may be decreased (15 to 40 mg/dl), but no organisms are recovered. A slight pleocytosis and increased total protein and gamma globulin fraction content in the CSF may be found without clinical evidence of meningeal involvement. CSF ACE, variably elevated in systemic disease, is abnormal in about half of those with neurosarcoidosis. Fluctuations in CSF levels of ACE seem to correlate with the clinical course.

Diagnosis. The diagnosis of sarcoidosis as the cause of neurologic signs and symptoms is usually made without difficulty when there are cutaneous or lymph node manifestations. Biopsy of nodules confirms the diagnosis. Granulomas may also be found by biopsy of muscle or liver. In addition, the ocular manifestations and the radiographic appearance of lung and bone lesions are sufficiently characteristic to be of diagnostic value. However, unless the disease is present in other organs, it is difficult to diagnose neurologic sarcoidosis. Helpful clues include a history of uveitis, Bell palsy, or other manifestations of the disease. The cutaneous Kveim test has been of diagnostic value, but the requisite sarcoid antigen (from affected lymph nodes) is not generally available.

The differential diagnosis includes epidemic parotitis, Hodgkin disease, leprosy, syphilis, cryptococcosis, tuberculosis, multiple sclerosis, and a variety of cerebral mass lesions. These conditions can usually be excluded by the clinical picture, biopsy of the nodules, radiographic findings, and other laboratory tests.

Course and Prognosis. Sarcoidosis is generally a benign disease, tending to involve one or more organ systems for many years. Acute monophasic and chronic progressive or relapsing neurosarcoidosis occurs. Acute episodes tend to subside spontaneously. As a rule, recovery of peripheral or cranial nerve palsies is slow. Remission from meningeal or parenchymatous involvement may be complete. Increased intracranial pressure may be fatal.

Treatment. No specific therapy is known. Antibiotics have no proven effect. Radiotherapy has been advocated. ACTH and the adrenal steroids seem to have a beneficial effect on neurologic lesions as well as on those in other organs.

References

Delaney P. Neurological manifestations in sarcoidosis: review of the literature, with a report of 23 cases. Ann Intern Med 1977; 87:336–345.

Jabs DA, Johns CJ. Ocular involvement in chronic sarcoidosis. Am J Ophthalmol 1986; 102:297–301.

James DG, Neville E, Siltzbac LE, Teiriaf J, Battesti JP, Sharma OP, Hosoda Y, et al. A worldwide review of sarcoidosis. NY Acad Sci 1976; 278:321–400.

Johns CJ, Schonfeld SA, Scott PP, et al. Longitudinal study of chronic sarcoidosis with low dose maintenance corticosteroid therapy. Outcome and complications. Ann NY Acad Sci 1986; 465:702–712.

Leeds NE, Zimmerman RD, Elkin CM, Nussbaum M, LeVan AM. Neurosarcoidosis of the brain and meninges. Semin Roentgenol 1985; 20:387–392.

Oksanen V. Neurosarcoidosis: clinical presentations and course in 50 patients. Acta Neurol Scand 1986; 73:283–290.

Oksanen V, Fyhrquist F, Somer H, Gronhagen-Riska C. Angiotensin converting enzyme in cerebrospinal fluid: a new assay. Neurology 1985; 35:1220–1223.

Oksanen V, Gronhagen-Riska C, Fyhrquist F, Somer H. Systemic manifestations and enzyme studies in sarcoidosis with neurologic involvement. Acta Med Scand 1985; 218:123–127.

Pentland B, Mitchell JD, Cull RE, Ford MJ. Central nervous system sarcoidosis. Q J Med 1985; 56:457–465.

Saint-Remy JR, Mitchell DN, Cole PJ. Variation in immunoglobulin levels and circulating immune complexes in sarcoidosis. Correlation with extent of disease and duration of symptoms. Am Rev Respir Dis 1983; 127:23–27.

Stern BJ, Krumholz A, Johns C, Scott P, Nissim J. Sarcoidosis and its neurological manifestations. Arch Neurol 1985; 42:909–917.

Uddenfeldt P, Bjelle A, Olsson T, Stjernberg N, Thunell M. Musculo-skeletal symptoms in early sarcoidosis. Twenty-four newly diagnosed patients and a two-year follow-up. Acta Med Scand 1983; 214:279–284.

19. SPIROCHETE INFECTIONS: NEUROSYPHILIS

Lewis P. Rowland

Definition. Neurosyphilis comprises the several different syndromes that are due to infection of the brain or spinal cord by the spirochete Treponema pallidum (Table 19–1). It is not known how much of the damage is caused by direct effects of the pathogenic organism, and how much by immune responses or other mechanisms.

History. Neurosyphilis has been recognized for about 100 years. During that time, the disease has played an important role in the evolution of modern neurology. "Dementia paralytica," or paretic neurosyphilis, was described in 1882 by Bayle. It was the first psychiatric disease or "mental disorder" for which specific cerebral pathology and specific cause were found. In 1892 Wilhelm Erb described the spinal cord disorder tabes dorsalis. At about the same time, Quincke introduced the lumbar puncture procedure and examination of the CSF became an important way to detect syphilitic infection of the nervous system, even before symptoms or signs were evident. The organism was histologically identified in brain by Noguchi and Moore in 1913. There was no effective treatment until 1918, when Wagner van Jauregg introduced malarial fever therapy for dementia paralytica. He was awarded the Nobel

Prize for that work. The introduction of arsenical drug therapy for treatment of syphilis was also historically of great importance, because it was the first planned use of a drug to attack an invading organism without significantly interfering with the well-being of the host (Ehrlich's "magic bullet" concept). Arsphenamine was useful in early syphilis, but it was not very effective once neurosyphilis had been established. Fever therapy did arrest the disease at that stage, but it was crude, unpleasant, and generated complications. Safer and more effective therapy came with the introduction of penicillin in 1945.

Epidemiology. A generation ago, this venereal disease accounted for a large proportion of patients admitted to neurologic services and also to psychiatric hospitals. With the introduction of penicillin after World War II, there were major changes. Early infection was cured before infection of the nervous system was established; neurosyphilis was prevented. An unknown number of cases were also prevented by the widespread use of penicillin to treat symptomatic gonorrhea, as well as many other concurrent infections of people with unrecognized syphilis. There was another factor: the development of more sensitive tests to detect early infection. Neurosyphilis plummeted as a cause of first admissions to mental hospitals from 5.9/100,000 population in 1942 to 0.1/100,000 in 1965. New cases became so rare that many hospitals discarded routine testing to detect syphilis.

In addition to the decline in incidence of neurosyphilis, other changes have occurred. The incidence of tabes has declined. Whether the incidence of meningitis has also declined is uncertain because figures conflict in two recent series. An apparent increase in taboparesis may be due to more sophisticated and more widespread use of neuropsychologic tests. Some clinicians have stated that the routine use of penicillin has led to increased prevalence of atypical forms of neurosyphilis that are more difficult to recognize. However, it now seems likely that clinical expression is similar to traditional teaching, but there may have been a shift in the relative proportions of different forms (Table 19–2).

Another important consideration is the relationship of syphilis to AIDS. The concomitant occurrence of the diseases probably reflects the importance of venereal transmission in the spread of both. The possibility that immunosuppression induced by the human im-

Table 19–1.   Classification of Neurosyphilis

Type	Clinical Symptoms	Pathology
I. Asymptomatic	No symptoms. CSF abnormal	Various. Chiefly leptomeningitis; arteritis or encephalitis may be present
II. Meningeal and vascular		
Cerebral meningeal		
Diffuse	Increased intracranial pressure; cranial nerve palsies	Leptomeningitis with hydrocephalus; degeneration of cranial nerves; arteritis
Focal	Increased intracranial pressure; focal cerebral symptoms and signs of slow onset	Granuloma formation (gumma)
Cerebrovascular	Focal cerebral symptoms and signs of sudden onset	Endarteritis with infarcts
Spinal meningeal and vascular	Paresthesias, weakness, atrophy, and sensory loss in limbs and trunk	Admixture of endarteritis and meningeal infiltration and thickening with degeneration of nerve roots and substance of the cord—myelomalacia
III. Parenchymatous		
Tabetic	Pains, paresthesias, crises, ataxia, impairment of pupillary reflexes, loss of tendon reflexes, impaired proprioceptive sensation, and trophic changes	Leptomeningitis and degenerative changes in posterior roots, dorsal funiculi, and brain stem
Paretic	Personality changes, convulsions, and mental deterioration. Physical deterioration in late stages	Meningoencephalitis
Optic atrophy*	Loss of vision, pallor of optic discs	Leptomeningitis and atrophy of optic nerves

*Rarely occurs alone. Usually found in tabetic or paretic neurosyphilis.
(From Merritt HH, Adams RD, Solomon HC. Neurosyphilis. New York: Oxford University Press, 1946.)

Table 19–2.   Frequency of Different Forms of Symptomatic Neurosyphilis

	Preantibiotic Era			Antibiotic Era	
	1	2	3	4	5
Tabetic	45	48	45	15	11
Paretic	17	18	8	12	4
Taboparetic	4	7	9	23	23
Vascular	15	19	9	19	61
Meningeal	8	8	19	23	0
Eighth nerve	2	—	—	—	—
Optic neuritis	4	—	—	—	—
Spinal cord	4	—	10	8	—
Miscellaneous	1	—	—	—	—

(1) Merritt, Adams, Solomon, 1946 (457 patients).
(2) Kierland et al, 1942 (2,019 patients).
(3) Wolters, 1987 (518 patients, 1930–1940).
(4) Wolters, 1987 (121 patients, 1970–1984).
(5) Burke, Schaberg, 1985 (26 patients).

munodeficiency virus (HIV) has augmented the occurrence or modified the clinical appearance of syphilis during co-infection is currently under study.

The decline in incidence of neurosyphilis in the antibiotic era led some to speculate that syphilis would vanish. However, after stabilizing at relatively low levels the incidence began to rise, especially in the population of homosexual men. The incidence of all forms of syphilis fell from 72/100,000 population in 1943 to 4/100,000 in 1956. It has now increased to about 12/100,000. A decade ago, in California, the incidence of neurosyphilis was about the same as that for Huntington disease and about half that of multiple sclerosis. The incidence of neurosyphilis has again risen, however, while the incidence of the others has remained the same. Neurosyphilis is still a disease of concern.

Pathology. In early neurosyphilis, lymphocytes and other mononuclear cells infiltrate the meninges. These inflammatory reactions also involve the cranial nerves and provoke axonal degeneration. When the inflammation involves small meningeal vessels with endothelial proliferation, occlusion may cause ischemic necrosis of brain and spinal cord tissue. This process may cause demyelination, myelomalacia of the periphery of the cord, or transverse myelitis.

The pathology of dementia paralytica develops slowly. After an inflammatory meningeal reaction, lymphocytes and plasma cells infiltrate small cortical vessels and sometimes extend into the cortex itself. The cortical inflammatory response provokes loss of cortical neurons and glial proliferation. Spirochetes can be demonstrated in the cortex in dementia paralytica, but only rarely in other forms of neurosyphilis.

In tabes dorsalis the mononuclear inflammation of meninges and blood vessels is followed by insidious degeneration of the posterior roots and posterior fiber columns of the spinal cord (Fig. 19–1) and, at times, the cranial nerves.

Asymptomatic Neurosyphilis. In asymptomatic neurosyphilis, primary infection has been evident or serologic evidence of syphilis is present in the serum, and the CSF is also abnormal. The incidence of asymptomatic neurosyphilis was about 30% of all cases of syphilis in the preantibiotic era, and it probably has not changed much since then. However, it is uncertain whether the CSF should be examined in all cases of syphilis; CSF is no

longer examined routinely in many centers because the treatment dosage regularly given is that recommended for asymptomatic neurosyphilis. Nevertheless, asymptomatic neurosyphilis is defined by findings in the CSF, so the incidence of this form of syphilis will not be known if the CSF is not examined in all cases.

The pathology of asymptomatic neurosyphilis is not known. When CSF examination was routine, the prevalence of asymptomatic cases depended partly on the duration of infection, increasing rapidly in the first two years, then decreasing because two outcomes were possible. Either a symptomatic form of neurosyphilis appeared, or the infection was overcome and the CSF returned to normal.

Cerebral Meningeal Neurosyphilis. When the cerebral meninges are affected, the clinical picture is that of acute or subacute meningitis, often with cranial nerve palsies. A few patients also have focal neurologic signs because of simultaneous syphilitic arteritis. The interval between primary infection and meningeal symptoms and signs may be a few months or several years, usually within one year of the primary infection and coincident with the secondary rash in about 10%.

Symptoms are caused by three pathologic mechanisms: (1) increased intracranial pressure and hydrocephalus from blockade of CSF pathways; (2) cranial nerve palsies from nerve damage by infection; and (3) focal cerebral signs from thrombosis of small cerebral vessels adjacent to the inflamed meninges. The meningeal signs usually disappear even without treatment, but cranial nerve palsies persist. Treatment at this point is essential to prevent paresis or tabes dorsalis.

Cerebrovascular Syphilis. Syphilitic endarteritis may cause small infarcts in the brain or spinal cord. In the preantibiotic era, many of the middle-aged patients with syphilis who also had a stroke could have had atherosclerotic vascular disease. In one of the two postantibiotic series (see Table 19–2), the relative incidence of vascular syphilis rose dramatically, but younger patients were affected, making it more likely that syphilis was responsible.

The clinical syndromes also differ from atherosclerotic cerebrovascular disease, because evidence of focal lesions may be preceded by weeks or months of personality changes that may pose a problem in psychiatric diagnosis. Persistent headache may be noted. Addition-

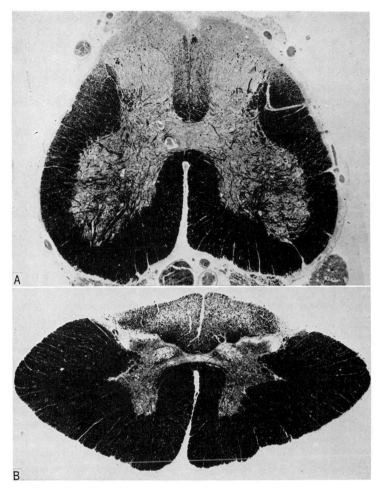

Fig. 19–1. Tabes dorsalis. Degeneration of the posterior column in the sacral and thoracic cord (myelin sheath stain). (From Merritt HH, Adams RD, Solomon HC. Neurosyphilis. New York: Oxford University Press, 1946.)

ally, the onset of focal signs may not be apoplectic, progressing instead for several days. The clinical impression may be one of "encephalopathy" rather than "stroke."

Men are affected more often than women. The symptoms usually appear 5 to 30 years after the primary luetic infection, but the interval seems to be much shorter in young men who have both AIDS and vascular neurosyphilis. In one young man, signs of meningovascular syphilis appeared within four months of the primary infection.

The diagnosis of meningeal or vascular syphilis of the spinal cord depends on symptoms and signs of myelopathy in combination with CSF changes of syphilis. It is usually a progressive syndrome without a clear level of spinal cord disease, but it may sometimes cause transverse myelitis. Meningeal or vascular syphilis of the spinal cord must be distinguished from other disorders of the spinal cord, as well as from tabes dorsalis. Syphilis has not been implicated as a cause of motor neuron disease, and it may be doubted that syphilis ever causes the syndrome of pure spastic paraplegia (spastic paraplegia of Erb). Usually, sensory and sphincter abnormalities are present as well as motor disorder, without a clear upper level of pathology.

Antisyphilitic treatment reverses the symptoms and signs of meningomyelitis unless there has been spinal cord infarction, which leaves permanent disability. Gummas of the spinal cord have not been seen recently, but they did not respond to drug therapy or excision in the past.

Gumma. A gumma is a syphilitic granuloma, usually avascular, and often forming a mass lesion that is separable from the surrounding brain. It may be attached to the dura and has been classified as a localized form of meningeal neurosyphilis. Early, there are inflammatory components and, later, the lesion becomes fibrotic. The symptoms and findings are usually those of a brain tumor. The widespread use of CT may indicate that this kind of lesion is not rare.

Paretic Neurosyphilis. This form of neurosyphilis has also been called *dementia paralytica, general paresis of the insane,* or *syphilitic meningoencephalitis.*

Spirochetes cause the chronic meningoencephalitis. The leptomeninges are opalescent to opaque, thickened, and adherent to the cortex (Table 19–3). The cortical gyri are atrophic (Fig. 19–2). The sulci are widened and filled with CSF. When the brain is sectioned, the ventricles are enlarged. The walls are covered with sand-like granulations termed *granular ependymitis* (Figs. 19–3, 19–4).

Clinical symptoms of paretic neurosyphilis are protean (Table 19–4) and may mimic functional or organic mental disorders as well as minor and major psychoses. The most common presenting symptom is uncomplicated dementia, with progressive loss of memory, impaired judgment, and emotional lability. Mental faculties decline severely in all cases. In the final stages there is limb weakness, hence the term general paresis of the insane, and convulsive seizures may occur (Table 19–5).

If untreated, paretic neurosyphilis is fatal in three to five years. Penicillin is an effective treatment for neurosyphilis, but the ultimate clinical results depend on the nature and extent of neuropathology when treatment is started. If inflammatory reaction is the only cause of the cerebral dysfunction, cure is likely. If spirochetal infection has already destroyed enough cerebral neurons, the infec-tion may be arrested but cerebral functions will not be restored.

Tabes Dorsalis. Tabes dorsalis, also called progressive *locomotor ataxia,* is clinically manifested by lancinating or lightning-like pains, progressive ataxia, loss of tendon reflexes, variable loss of proprioception, and dysfunction of bowel, bladder, and genital organs.

At first, lymphocytes and plasma cells infiltrate the spinal leptomeninges and intraspinal portion of the dorsal roots. Then the lumbar and sacral dorsal roots and dorsal funiculi of the spinal cord shrink. The column of Goll degenerates, with infrequent changes in cervical dorsal roots (see Fig. 19–1). The optic and other cranial nerves may be infiltrated and shrink in some cases.

The chief signs of tabes dorsalis are loss of tendon reflexes at the knees and ankles, impaired vibratory and position sense in the legs, and abnormal pupils (Table 19–6).

In 94% of patients with tabes dorsalis, the pupils are irregular, unequal, or show impaired responses to light. In 48%, Argyll Robertson pupils are present, with loss of the light reaction, but with preservation of pupillary constriction in accommodation. Other findings may include impaired superficial and deep sensation, weakness, wasting and hypotonia of muscles, optic atrophy with visual loss, other cranial nerve palsies, and trophic changes, including Charcot joints or "mal perforant." Dysfunction of bowel, bladder, or genitals is also frequent.

Tabes dorsalis is seldom fatal. Ataxia or blindness may be incapacitating. Atonic bladder may lead to urinary tract infection and death.

Tabes dorsalis may arrest spontaneously or may be arrested by treatment, but the lancinating pains and ataxia often continue.

Congenital Neurosyphilis. Congenital syphilis has been recognized since the sixteenth century. Clauston described congenital dementia paralytica in 1877 and Hemak described congenital tabes in 1885. The spirochete from the mother infects the fetus between the fourth and seventh months of pregnancy. The mother who has had syphilis for a longer time is less likely to give birth to an infected infant. The incidence of congenital neurosyphilis in North America has continued to decline with the improved detection and treatment of syphilis in adults and it is now rare. The clinical types are similar to those in adults except that tabes dorsalis is uncommon. Additional features of congenital

---

Table 19–3. Pathology of Paretic Neurosyphilis*

Macroscopic
   Thickening of opacity of the meninges
   Widening of cerebral sulci
   Dilatation of the cerebral ventricles
   Granular ependymitis

Microscopic
   Inflammatory reaction—perivascular and meningeal
   Degenerative changes in parenchyma
   Degenerative and reactive changes (rod cells) in glia
   Deposition of iron pigment
   Presence of spirochetes

*Changes localized to or most severe in the front and temporal poles.

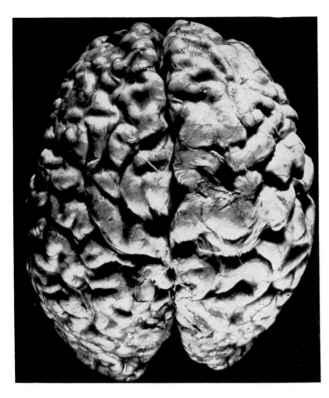

Fig. 19–2. Paretic neurosyphilis. Thickening of the meninges and atrophy of the cerebral convolutions. (From Merritt HH, Adams RD, Solomon HC. Neurosyphilis. New York: Oxford University Press, 1946.)

neurosyphilis are hydrocephalus and the Hutchinson triad (interstitial keratitis, deformed teeth, and hearing loss), but the triad is seldom complete. Use of penicillin is similar to that in the treatment of adults. Although the infection may be arrested, the pre-existing damage and neurologic signs may persist.

Diagnosis of Neurosyphilis. The diagnosis of active neurosyphilis, symptomatic or asymptomatic, depends on the documentation of one or both of two kinds of abnormalities in the CSF: those that are found in "routine" analysis of CSF cells or protein and those that relate to serologic tests for syphilis.

In active infections, there is a CSF *pleocytosis* of 200 to 300 cells, mostly lymphocytes but

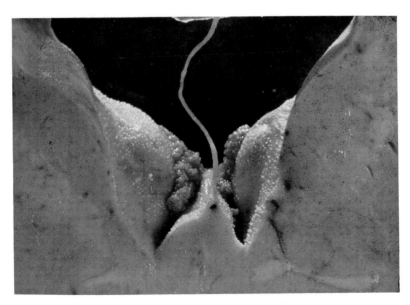

Fig. 19–3. Paretic neurosyphilis. Granular ependymitis of the floor of lateral ventricles. (From Merritt HH, Adams RD, Solomon HC. Neurosyphilis. New York: Oxford University Press, 1946.)

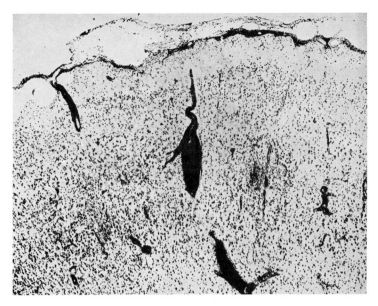

Fig. 19–4. Paretic neurosyphilis. Inflammatory reaction in the meninges and in the perivascular spaces of the cortical vessels (Nissl stain). (From Merritt HH, Adams RD, Solomon HC. Neurosyphilis. New York: Oxford University Press, 1946.)

Table 19–4.   Symptoms of Paretic Neurosyphilis

Early Stage	Late Stage
Irritability	Impaired memory
Fatigability	Defective judgment
Conduct slump	Depression or elation
Personality changes	Lack of insight
Headaches	Confusion and disorientation
Forgetfulness	
Tremors	Poorly systematized delusions
	Seizures
	Transient paralysis or aphasia

Table 19–5.   Neurologic Signs of Paretic Neurosyphilis

Common
  Relaxed, expressionless facies
  Tremors of facial and lingual muscles
  Dysarthria
  Impairment of handwriting
  Hyperactive tendon reflexes

Rare
  Focal signs, e.g., hemiplegia, hemianopia
  Optic atrophy
  Eye muscle palsies
  Absent reflexes
  Babinski toe sign

with some plasma cells. The CSF *total protein* content and the amount of *gamma globulin* increase; the CSF glucose content is normal. Oligoclonal bands and an elevated percentage of IgG may be found in CSF and reflect the immunologic response previously detected by the colloidal gold test, which was less reliable and nonspecific. Without further testing the presence of oligoclonal bands is also nonspecific, but immunologic procedures can demonstrate that the bands represent antibodies reactive with treponemal antigens and might be useful in cases where the diagnosis is particularly troubling (Vartdal et al., 1982).

There are two types of serologic tests for syphilis. First, the nonspecific tests detect antibodies against lipid antigens called *reagin.* The antigen is a mixture of cardiolipin, lecithin, and cholesterol. The first of these was the Wassermann test, followed by the Kolmer test. Now, the most widely used test of this class is the *Venereal Disease Research Laboratory (VDRL) test*, a flocculation test that is done on a slide. Compared to other tests, it is relatively simple to perform and reproducible. The rapid plasma reagin (RPR) card test is another version.

The other category of test is specific in that it depends on the demonstration of antibody against Treponema pallidum itself, or components of the organism. The standard test in the United States is the fluorescent treponemal antibody absorption (FTA-ABS) test.

Table 19–6. Symptoms and Signs in Tabetic Neurosyphilis. Analysis of 150 Cases

Symptoms	%	Signs	%
Lancinating pains	75	Abnormal pupils	94
Ataxia	42	Argyll Robertson	48
Bladder disturbance	33	Other abnormalities	64
Paresthesias	24	Reflex abnormalities	
Gastric or visceral crises	18	Absent ankle jerks	94
Visual loss	16	Absent knee jerks	81
Rectal incontinence	14	Absent reflexes	11
Deafness	7	Romberg's sign	55
Impotence	4	Impaired sensation	
		Impaired vibratory sense	52
		Impaired vision	43
		Impaired touch and pain	13
		Optic atrophy	20
		Ocular palsy	10
		Charcot joints	7

(From Merritt HH, Adams RD, Solomon HC. Neurosyphilis. New York: Oxford University Press, 1946.)

Another test, used in some centers, is the *microhemagglutination test for T. pallidum (MHA-TP)*. In these hemagglutination tests, sensitized sheep erythrocytes are coated with lysed T. pallidum to provide the antigen.

The FTA-ABS test is an important one for serum. This specific test is used to show that a reactive VDRL test is actually due to syphilis. In late latent syphilis, the blood VDRL may even be negative when the FTA-ABS is positive, but false positive reactions may occur under those circumstances. Nevertheless, there is no currently acceptable form of the FTA-ABS test for use on CSF. The following discussion of CSF tests is therefore restricted to the VDRL.

In general, the diagnosis of active CNS syphilis depends on finding both a positive CSF-VDRL test and CSF pleocytosis. There are few false positive CSF-VDRL tests; it is a highly specific indicator of neurosyphilis. However, it may be insensitive and is said to be negative in many cases of neurosyphilis. The problem, in a patient with a negative VDRL test in CSF, is to prove that the condition is truly neurosyphilis, and that would depend on the individual circumstances. If the clinical syndrome were typical of a standard form of neurosyphilis, it might be appropriate to make the diagnosis despite a negative CSF-VDRL test. If the syndrome were atypical, however, skepticism might be in order.

Because the CSF-VDRL titer may persist despite adequate treatment for neurosyphilis, evaluation of therapy depends more on changes in cell count and protein. The cell count should return to normal within 6 to 12 weeks. The protein content declines more slowly.

Whether CSF should be examined in all asymptomatic patients with positive blood serology is being debated. As indicated in Table 19–7, it seems reasonable to have this baseline data before commencing on a course of treatment.

Treatment of Neurosyphilis. The treatment of neurosyphilis begins with the treatment of early syphilis. The standard treatment has been a single intramuscular injection of 2.4 million units of penicillin G benzathine. In early studies, the failure rates ranged from 0 to 7%, but there have been no recent studies to document the present rate of efficacy.

Moreover, there is no prompt and reliable way to determine the adequacy of treatment. Instead, the patient must return for repeated testing at 3, 6, and 12 months, or until the patient becomes seronegative.

Criteria for treatment failure include the following: (1) Clinical signs of syphilis persist. (2) There is a fourfold rise in VDRL titer. (3) The VDRL is positive after one year in patients treated for primary syphilis or two years after treatment for secondary syphilis.

The occasional failure of this regimen was documented when symptoms of neurosyphilis appeared five months after a patient with secondary syphilis received the standard dose of penicillin G benzathine. To avoid that problem, a fourth criterion for retreatment is being considered: There should be a fourfold drop in VDRL titer at three months, and an eightfold drop at six months.

Penicillin G benzathine does not provide therapeutic levels of the drug in CSF. For es-

Table 19–7. Recommendations for Use of Diagnostic Tests for Syphilis

Immediate Diagnostic or Therapeutic Action	Further Investigation or Action
Primary syphilis	
Dark-field or direct fluorescent test	VDRL titer for follow-up
Secondary syphilis	
VDRL titer	VDRL titer for follow-up
*Selected asymptomatic persons**	
VDRL titer	MHA-TP or FTA-ABS if VDRL positive
Adequacy of treatment for early or late syphilis	
VDRL titer 3, 6, 12 mos. after treatment	Retreat if high titer does not fall by 12 mos. or if titer increases after initial fall
Seropositive persons†	
CSF-VDRL, CSF cell count	Treat for neurosyphilis if CSF-VDRL positive or pleocytosis
Follow-up after treatment for asymptomatic neurosyphilis	
CSF cell count 6 wks., 3 mos., and 6 mos. after treatment	CSF cell count at 12 mos., 24 mos. if normal at 6 mos.
Suspected syphilis‡	
Treat as for early syphilis	VDRL titer 1, 3, and 6 mos. after treatment

*Includes all pregnant women; proven contacts of people with infectious syphilis; and people in high-risk groups.

†Includes people with neurologic abnormalities; before treatment with nonpenicillin regimens; before retreatment after treatment failure.

‡Includes women with newly discovered syphilis seropositivity late in pregnancy; infants of mothers with inadequately treated syphilis; proven contacts of those with infectious syphilis.

(From Hart G. Syphilis tests in diagnostic and therapeutic decision making. Ann Intern Med 1986; 104:368–376.)

tablished neurosyphilis, therefore, the recommended therapy is intravenous administration of aqueous penicillin G, 24 million units daily for three weeks or aqueous penicillin G, 2 million units daily with 2 g of probenecid given orally each day. The probenecid enhances serum levels of penicillin by reducing renal excretion.

Penicillin may provoke allergic reactions of rash or anaphylaxis. The Jarisch-Herxheimer fever reaction may occur with any form of antisyphilitic treatment but seems to be less common in neurosyphilis. For patients who are allergic to penicillin, there are two effective alternatives. Doxycycline, 300 mg orally, can be given in divided doses daily for 30 days. Alternatively, tetracycline can be used in a dosage of 500 mg four times daily for 14 days.

Gummas have responded to treatment with penicillin alone, penicillin plus steroids, and even steroids alone. If the clinical circumstances make that diagnosis likely, and if the clinical condition of the patient permits, a trial of conservative treatment is warranted. If the diagnosis is doubtful, or if the circumstances dictate more immediate attention, biopsy and excision may be appropriate.

Under any circumstances, patients with both AIDS and any form of syphilis should be treated with a regimen recommended for neurosyphilis.

After a course of therapy, quantitative blood serology is determined at three-month intervals and usually shows a decline in titer if it was previously elevated. Clinical neurologic examination should be performed regularly. The CSF is examined at 6 and 12 months. If not normal, CSF is reexamined in two years. After three years, if the patient has improved and is clinically stable, and the CSF and serologic tests are normal, neurologic and CSF examinations are discontinued.

Retreatment is recommended with high doses of intravenous penicillin G in the following situations: if the clinical neurologic findings progress without finding another cause, especially if CSF pleocytosis persists; if the CSF cell count is not normal at six months; if the VDRL test in serum or CSF fails to decline or shows a fourfold increase; or if the first course of treatment was suboptimal.

References

Adie WJ. Argyll-Robertson pupils, true and false. Br Med J 1931; 2:136–138.

Argyll-Robertson D. Four cases of spinal miosis with remarks on the action of light on the pupil. Edinburgh Med J 1869; 15:487–493.

Berry CD, Hooton TM, Collier AC, Lukehart SA. Neurologic relapse after benzathine penicillin therapy for secondary syphilis in a patient with HIV infection. N Engl J Med 1987; 316:1587–1589.

Bowsher D, Rennie I, Lahueria J, Nelson A. Tabes dorsalis with tonic pupils and lightning pains relieved by sodium valproate. J Neurol Neurosurg Psychiatry 1987; 50:239–241.

Brown ST. Update on recommendations for the treatment of syphilis. Rev Infect Dis 1982; 4(Suppl): S837–S841.

Burke JM, Schaberg DR. Neurosyphilis in the antibiotic era. Neurology 1985; 35:1368–1371.

Crimenez-Roldan S, Benito C, Martin M. Dementia paralytica: deterioration from communicating hydrocephalus. J Neurol Neurosurg Psychiatry 1979; 42:501.

Dacas J, Robson HB. CSF penicillin levels during therapy for latent syphilis. JAMA 1981; 246:2583–2584.

Dans PE, Cafferty L, Otter SE, Johnson RJ. Inappropriate use of the CSF VDRL test to exclude neurosyphilis. Ann Intern Med 1986; 104:86–89.

Erb WH. Über syphilitische Spinalparalyse. Neurol Centralbl 1892; 11:161–168.

Fichter RR, Aral SO, Blount JH, Zaidi AA, Reynolds GH, Darrow WW. Syphilis in the United States, 1967–1979. Sex Transm Dis 1983; 10:77–80.

Fleet WS, Watson RT, Ballinger WE. Resolution of a gumma with steroid therapy. Neurology 1986; 36:1104–1107.

Guinam ME. Treatment of primary and secondary syphilis: defining failure at 3- and 6-month follow-up. JAMA 1987; 257:359–360.

Hahn RD, Cutler JC, Curtis AC, et al. Penicillin treatment of asymptomatic central nervous system syphilis. I. Probability of progression to symptomatic neurosyphilis. Arch Dermatol 1956; 74:355–366.

Harrigan EP, MacLaughlin TJ, Feldman RG. Transverse myelitis due to meningovascular syphilis. Arch Neurol 1984; 41:337–338.

Hart G. Syphilis tests in diagnostic and therapeutic decision making. Ann Intern Med 1986; 104:368–376.

Hillbom M, Kinnunen E. New cases of neurosyphilis in Finland. Acta Med (Scand) 1982; 211:55–58.

Holmes MD, Brant-Zawadzki MM, Simon RP. Clinical features of meningovascular syphilis. Neurology 1984; 34:553–556.

Hotson JR. Modern neurosyphilis: a partially treated chronic meningitis. West J Med 1981; 135:191–200.

Jaffe HW, Kabins SA. Examination of CSF in patients with syphilis. Rev Infect Dis 1982; 4(suppl):S842–S847.

Johns DR, Tierney M, Felsenstein D. Alteration in the natural history of neurosyphilis by concurrent infection with HIV. N Engl J Med 1987; 316:1569–1572.

Kierland RR, O'Leary PA, Van Doren E. Symptomatic neurosyphilis. Ven Dis Inform 1942; 22:360–377.

Merritt HH, Adams RD, Solomon HC. Neurosyphilis. New York: Oxford University Press, 1946.

Noguchi H, Moore JW. A demonstration of treponema pallidium in the brain of general paresis. J Exp Med 1913; 17:232–238.

Nordenbo AM, Sorensen PS. The incidence and clinical presentations of neurosyphilis in Greater Copenhagen, 1974–1978. Acta Neurol (Scand) 1981; 63:237–246.

Simon RP. Neurosyphilis: an update. West J Med 1981; 134:87–91.

Spielmeyer W. Zur Pathogenese der Tabes. Z Gesamte Neurol Psychiatr 1923; 84:257–265. 1924; 91:627–632. 1925; 97:287–328.

Vartdal F, Vandvik B, Michaelsen T, et al. Neurosyphilis: Intrathecal synthesis of oligoclonal antibodies to Treponema pallidum. Ann Neurol 1982; 11:35–40.

Wagner-Jauregg J. Über die Einwirkung der Malaria auf die Progressive Paralyse. Psychiatr Neurol Wochenschr 1918–1919; 20:132–151.

Wilner E, Brody JA. Prognosis of general paresis after treatment. Lancet 1968; 2:1370–1371.

Wolters EC. Neurosyphilis: a changing diagnostic problem? Eur Neurol 1987; 26:23–28.

20. SPIROCHETE INFECTIONS: LEPTOSPIROSIS
James R. Miller

Leptospirosis is caused by a group of closely related spirochetes belonging to the genus Leptospira. The organisms that cause human disease are now thought to belong to a single species, L. interrogans, with subtypes such as canicola, Pomona, and icterohaemorrhagiae recognized serologically. Over 170 serovariants are arranged in 18 serogroups.

Previously, specific serovariants were linked with particular clinical syndromes. However, different serovariants have been associated with the same or different clinical presentations. Humans are incidental hosts for these spirochetes, which are enzootic in both wild and domestic animals including cats, dogs, and cattle. Animals can become clinically sick, and asymptomatic carriers can excrete the spirochete in urine for months or years. Human infection comes from contact with infested animal tissue or urine or by exposure to contaminated ground water, soil, or vegetation. Leptospira can survive for prolonged periods outside of hosts in appropriate environmental conditions. The spirochete is thought to enter humans through mucocutaneous abrasions; it is not known if the organism can penetrate intact skin. Infection is not limited to specific human populations, but the incidence is probably higher in those who work with animal tissue such as slaughterhouse employees, farmers, biological laboratory workers, and persons preparing foods.

Symptoms usually appear abruptly one to two weeks after exposure, with chills, fever, myalgia, headache, and meningismus. Gastrointestinal symptoms include nausea, emesis, anorexia, and diarrhea. There can be cough and chest pain. Cardiac manifestations, including bradycardia and hypotension, can be severe. Conjunctival suffusion is typical, but not constant. There can be pharyngeal injection, cutaneous hemorrhages, or maculopapular rash. Hepatosplenomegaly and lymphadenopathy can occur. In the acute first stage there is septicemia and the organism can be isolated from CSF.

A second wave of symptoms can appear after the acute illness has apparently resolved. Original symptoms recur, sometimes with meningeal signs. Rarely, encephalitis, myelitis, optic neuritis, or peripheral neuritis can develop. During the second phase of illness IgM antibody to the Leptospira microorganisms and immune complexes can be found. Because the spirochete can no longer be isolated at this time, it is thought that the clinical illness of this phase is immune-mediated.

Leptospiral infection can be manifest clinically as aseptic meningitis. Although the agent can be recovered early in the syndrome, pleocytosis is not found until the second phase. Usually cell counts are in the range of 10 to several hundred, but they can be higher. Neutrophils might be present early, but mononuclear cells predominate from the outset. Unlike most forms of viral meningitis, CSF protein can exceed 100 mg/dL in leptospirosis. Probably all pathogenic serovariants can cause aseptic meningitis; the most common are canicola, icterohemorrhagiae, and Pomona.

Other specific syndromes associated with leptospiral infection are pretibial (Fort Bragg) fever, myocarditis, and Weil syndrome. Pretibial fever, first described at an American military base during World War II, is characterized by an erythematous macular rash over the tibias. Splenomegaly is also a feature. The rash occurs in the early phase of an otherwise typical leptospiral infection.

Weil syndrome is characterized by hepatomegaly and unusually severe jaundice, often with azotemia and proteinuria. Disseminated visceral and cutaneous hemorrhage can also occur. Bleeding is attributed primarily to vasculitis, but thrombocytopenia and hypoprothrombinemia can contribute. Mental changes are frequent and could be the result of cerebral infection, metabolic derangement, or intracerebral petechial hemorrhages. Weil syndrome was originally related to icterohaemorrhagiae, but other serotypes also have been found to cause it.

Leptospiral infection, particularly when it appears as an aseptic meningitis, can be diagnosed only with a high index of suspicion.

Culture of the organism is possible if special facilities are available. Dark-field examination of blood, urine, or CSF is unreliable. Serologic studies usually confirm the clinical diagnosis, but the antibody is not detected until the second phase of the illness.

A variety of antibiotics have been used effectively to treat leptospiral infection. They must be administered early in the illness. High-dose penicillin is most generally used; tetracycline is the alternative for those who are allergic to penicillin. Spontaneous recovery is the rule for younger patients without other illnesses. Mortality is over 50% after age 50, however, and is usually associated with severe liver disease and jaundice.

References

Andrew AD, Marrocco GR. Leptospirosis in New England 1977; JAMA 238:2027–2028.

Arean VM. The Pathologic Anatomy and Pathogenesis of Fatal Human Leptospirosis (Weil's Disease). 1962; Am J Pathol 40:393–423.

Edwards GA, Domm BM. Human Leptospirosis. 1960; Medicine 39:117–156.

Feigin RD, Anderson DC. Human Leptospirosis. 1975; CRC Crit Rev Clin Lab Sci 5:413–467.

Heath CW, Alexander AD, Galton MD. Leptospirosis in the United States. 1965; N Engl J Med 273:857–864.

21. SPIROCHETE INFECTIONS: LYME DISEASE
James R. Miller

In 1975 a cluster of arthritis cases in children was recognized in Old Lyme, Connecticut. Many patients had a history of a migratory rash called erythema chronicum migrans (ECM), and some had neurologic or myocardial dysfunction. Affected adults were seen as well. The syndrome has been attributed to a previously unrecognized spirochete that is transmitted to humans by ixodid ticks. The spirochete has some characteristics of treponemes, but it is classified among the borreliae (Borrelia burgdorferi). In the northeastern United States the vector, Ixodes damminis, regularly infests deer and mice. However, other animals are also hosts for the tick.

The disease occurs throughout the United States in regions where ixodid ticks are found. The extent of human disease is unknown, but in the Lyme area, antibodies are found in 4% of the population. In Europe, a closely related or identical spirochete is associated with a similar clinical disorder called *Bannwarth syndrome* or *tick-borne meningopolyneuritis* (Garin-Bujadoux, Bannwarth). Although the manifestations of the disease were described in Europe earlier in the century and were associated with ixodid ticks, the nature of the infection was determined only after the spirochete was identified in North America. The disease has also been found in Australia.

The spirochete is most frequently transmitted to humans by the nymph stage of the tick, which is active in early summer, but transmission earlier or later can occur from contact with the adult arthropod. B. burgdorferi can also be isolated from the tick larva, but it is difficult to recover from infected humans.

The course of human infection has been divided into three stages, but overlaps in symptoms and in timing are common. Usually a migrating erythematous ring (ECM) develops 3 to 32 days after exposure; the center of the rash is at the site of the tick bite. Smaller secondary rings often appear later, and their centers are less indurated than that of the primary lesion. At this stage, headache, myalgia, stiff neck, and even cranial nerve palsies (almost invariably the seventh nerve) can occur, but CSF is usually normal. ECM usually resolves in three to four weeks, although transitory erythematous blotches and rings that do not migrate can occur later.

More prominent neurologic and cardiac manifestations are seen in the second stage, several weeks after the onset of ECM. Heart problems are usually confined to conduction defects, but there may be myopericarditis with left ventricular dysfunction. Meningeal symptoms and signs constitute the major features of the neurologic illness, with headache and stiff neck. Fever is not a regular feature. Radiculitis, multiple or isolated, is common and can cause severe root pain or focal weakness. Cranial nerves, usually the seventh, are frequently involved. Both sides of the face can become paralyzed, simultaneously or sequentially. Polyneuritis or mononeuritis multiplex can also occur. Identifying the cause requires a sensitive index of suspicion in areas where the disease is endemic. Neurologic disease can also occur without a previous ECM or recognized tick bite.

In original descriptions, ataxia, altered consciousness, and myelitis were noted. Later, however, CNS manifestations have been less prominent, with decreased concentration, irritability, emotional lability, and memory and sleep disorders most usually noted. Because the disease is not fatal, the lesions that cause the neurologic syndromes have not been defined. Immune complex vasculitis might play a role.

The third stage of Lyme disease is characterized by chronic arthritis in patients with HLA-DR2 antigen. It usually appears several months after the original infection, but it can be present at the time of the subacute neurologic disease. The spirochete has not been isolated from joint fluid, and the arthritis could be an autoimmune disorder, although successful treatment of the arthritis with an antibiotic has been reported.

Although neurologic disorder has been mostly associated with the subacute second stage of the disease, there might be a chronic encephalomyelopathy with CT and MRI evidence of white matter disease. The syndrome is one of progressive long-tract dysfunction that might include optic nerve and sphincters. Response to antibiotic treatment has not been impressive. A syndrome of acral dysasthesias has recently been described in the late stage of Lyme disease. There is electrophysiologic evidence of a neuropathic process, and the sensory symptoms respond to appropriate antibiotic therapy for the spirochete.

Diagnosis. The combination of meningitis, radiculitis, and neuritis without fever occurs in virtually no other circumstance. If the appropriate history of tick exposure and ECM is obtained, the diagnosis is assured. However, partial syndromes and absence of appropriate early findings might require differentiation from a wide variety of illnesses, from herniated disc to other causes of acute aseptic or subacute meningitis. CT is normal, and EEGs are usually normal or nonspecific. CSF pressure is normal. Abnormalities in the CSF formula are usually, but not always, present (Table 21–1). Oligoclonal bands, however, have been detected uniformly. Borrelia burgdorferi has been isolated from the CSF, a rare technical feat that cannot be relied on for routine diagnosis. Demonstration of elevated levels of spirochete-specific IgM or IgG in the serum by immunofluorescent techniques constitutes the basis of diagnosis.

Treatment. Oral tetracycline has been successful in the early stage characterized by ECM. This regimen usually prevents the appearance of later stages. Neurologic involvement was first treated successfully with high-dose penicillin given intravenously for 10 days. Without penicillin, neurologic symptoms lasted for a mean of 30 weeks. With the antibiotic, symptoms resolve as it is being administered. Motor disorders last a mean of

Table 21–1.   CSF Analysis in Lyme Disease Encephalomyelitis

Test	CSF
Opening pressure*	Normal
Total white cells/mm³	166 (15–700)†
Percent lymphocytes	93 (40–100)
Glucose (mg/dL)‡	49 (33–61)
Protein (mg/dL)	79 (8–400)
IgG/albumin ratio (N = 20)	0.18 (0.9–0.44)
Oligoclonal bands (N = 4)	Present
Myelin basic protein (N = 5)	Absent
VDRL (N = 20)	Negative

*N = 38 except where noted
†Median (range)
‡Serum glucose = 95 (87–113)
(From Pachner AR, Steere AC. Neurology 1985; 35:47–53.)

seven to eight weeks irrespective of antibiotic treatment. Sporadic reports indicate that high-dose tetracycline or ceftriaxone treatment might be effective and should be used if the patient is allergic to penicillin. More thorough studies are needed. It is recommended that isolated nerve palsies associated with elevated spirochete antibody be treated with doses appropriate for ECM therapy.

References

Ackermann R, Horstrup P, Schmidt R. Tick-borne meningopolyneuritis (Garin-Bujadoux, Bannwarth). Yale J Biol Med 1984; 57:485–490.

Bendig JW, Ogilvie D. Severe encephalopathy associated with Lyme disease. Lancet 1987; 1:681–682.

Broderick JP, Sandok BA, Mertz LE. Focal encephalitis in a young woman 6 years after the onset of Lyme disease: tertiary Lyme disease? Mayo Clin Proc 1987; 62:313–316.

Halperin JJ, Little BW, Coyle PK and Dattwyler RJ. Lyme disease: cause of a treatable peripheral neuropathy. Neurology 1987; 37:1700–1706.

Pachner AR, Steere AC. The triad of neurologic manifestations of Lyme disease: meningitis, cranial neuritis and radiculoneuritis. Neurology 1985; 35:47–53.

Reik L, Burgdorfer W, Donaldson JO. Neurologic abnormalities in Lyme disease without erythema chronicum migrans. Am J Med 1986; 81:73–78.

Shrestha M, Grodzicki RL, Steere AC. Diagnosing early Lyme disease. Am J Med 1985; 78:235–240.

Steere AC, Grodzicki RL, Kornblatt AN, Craft JE, Barbour AG, Burgdorfer W, Schmid GP, et al. The spirochetal etiology of Lyme disease. N Engl J Med 1983; 308:733–740.

Steere AC, Hutchinson GJ, Rahn DW, Sigal LH, Craft JE, DeSanna ET, Malawista SE. Treatment of the early manifestations of Lyme disease. Ann Intern Med 1983; 99:22–26.

Steere AC, Malawista SE, Snydman DR, et al. Lyme arthritis: an epidemic of oligoarticular arthritis in children and adults in three Connecticut communities. Arthritis Rheum 1977; 20:7–17.

Steere AC, Pachner AR, Malawista SE. Neurological abnormalities of Lyme disease: successful treatment with high-dose intravenous penicillin. Ann Intern Med 1983; 99:767–772.

Weder B, Wiedersheim P, Matter L, Steck A, Otto F. Chronic progressive neurological involvement in Borrelia burgdorferi infection. J Neurol 1987; 234:40–43.

---

22. PARASITIC INFECTIONS

Burk Jubelt
James R. Miller

Disease caused by parasites is uncommon in the United States and other developed countries. However, in tropical and less developed areas, parasitic infections exact a heavy toll on society. Because systemic infections are common in tropical areas, CNS infections are often seen. Poverty and poor living conditions play a significant role in the pathogenesis of these infections, but an appropriate climate for vectors to facilitate transmission is also necessary. The combination of increased international travel to and immigration from endemic areas has increased the likelihood of encountering tropical parasitic infections in the United States. Indigenous parasites have recently been encountered more frequently because of long-term survival of immunosuppressed patients who have increased susceptibility to infection.

Parasitic infections can be divided into two categories: those caused by worms (helminths) and those caused by protozoa. Helminths are large, complex organisms that frequently elicit allergic responses (eosinophilia) and more often cause focal, rather than diffuse, involvement of the nervous system. Helminths are divided into roundworms (nematodes), flukes (trematodes), and tapeworms (cestodes). Protozoa are small (microbial size) single-cell organisms that more frequently cause diffuse encephalitic, as opposed to focal, involvement of the nervous system. Protozoa do not elicit allergic reactions or cause eosinophilia.

Helminthic Infection

TRICHINOSIS (TRICHINELLOSIS)

Trichinosis is an acute infection caused by the roundworm *Trichinella spiralis*. Infection is acquired by eating larvae in raw or undercooked pork. Bear and walrus meat have also been incriminated. Involvement of the CNS in patients with trichinosis, which is estimated to occur in 10 to 17% of the cases, may be manifested by confusion, delirium, and focal neurologic signs.

Pathology. The pathologic changes in the nervous system include the presence of filiform larvae in the cerebral capillaries and in the parenchyma, perivascular inflammation, petechial hemorrhages, and granulomatous nodules.

Symptoms and Signs. Trichinosis manifests as a systemic infection due to larval migration with fever, headache, muscle pain and tenderness, periorbital edema, and subconjunctival hemorrhages. Gastrointestinal symptoms are less frequent, occurring in only about 25% of cases. Neurologic symptoms may develop any time within the first few weeks of the infection. There may be a severe encephalitis with confusion, coma, seizures, and evidence of focal damage to the cerebrum or cerebellum, with monoplegia, hemiplegia, quadriplegia, cerebellar ataxia, or bulbar palsy. Edema of the optic nerve, meningeal signs, spinal cord involvement, and neuropathies may also occur. Loss of tendon reflexes, which may occur in the absence of other neurologic symptoms, is often due to the muscular involvement.

Laboratory Data. The most significant laboratory finding is a leukocytosis and eosinophilia in the blood. Muscle enzymes may also be elevated. The CSF may be normal or there may be a slight lymphocyte pleocytosis, but a few eosinophils may occasionally be present. Red blood cells and xanthochromia may be seen. The protein and pressure are often elevated. The parasites are found in the CSF of approximately 30% of patients.

Diagnosis. The diagnosis is usually not difficult when neurologic symptoms appear in one or more of a group of individuals who have eaten infected pork and show the other manifestations of the disease (gastrointestinal symptoms, tenderness of the muscles, and edema of the eyelids). Difficulty is encountered in the isolated cases in which the infection results from the ingestion of meat preparations that supposedly contain no pork, or where the other manifestations of the infection are lacking. Trichinosis should be considered an etiologic factor in all patients with encephalitis of obscure nature. Repeated examination of the blood for eosinophilia and elevated muscle enzymes, biopsy of the muscles, and the specific skin and serologic tests should establish the diagnosis.

Prognosis. Recovery within a few days or weeks is the rule except when there is profound coma or evidence of severe damage to the cerebrum. The disease has been reported to have a 10% mortality. Recovery is usually accompanied by complete or almost complete remission of the neurologic signs. Recurrent convulsive seizures have been reported as a late sequel of the cerebral infection.

Treatment. The treatment is symptomatic. The administration of corticosteroids and thiabendazole has been recommended. Mebendazole and flubendazole have also been used.

SCHISTOSOMIASIS (BILHARZIASIS)

Involvement of the nervous system by the ova of trematodes is rare. In most reported cases, the lesions were associated with infection with Schistosoma japonicum, but isolated cases of S. haematobium and S. mansoni have also been recorded. The mechanism by which the ova are deposited in the nervous system is not understood. S. japonicum has a predilection for the cerebral hemispheres; S. haematobium and S. mansoni more frequently affect the spinal cord. These predilections appear to relate to the location of the adult worms from where ova are released. S. japonicum resides in mesenteric venules, but the occurrence of ectopic worms in cerebral venules may explain the high incidence of cerebral involvement. S. mansoni primarily resides in the inferior mesenteric venules whereas S. haematobium is found in the vesical plexus.

Pathology. The presence of the ova in the nervous system causes an inflammatory exudate containing eosinophils and giant cells, necrosis of the parenchyma, and deposition of calcium. The juxtaposition of numerous small lesions may result in formation of a large granulomatous tumor.

Incidence. S. japonicum occurs mainly in Asia and in the tropics. World War II gave occasion to observe it in United States troops. S. mansoni is prevalent in Puerto Rico and other Caribbean areas. S. haematobium occurs in Africa. The onset of symptoms may occur within a few months of exposure or it may be delayed for one to two years. Relapses may occur several or many years after the original infection. The CNS is involved in 3 to 5% of the cases.

Symptoms. Cerebral schistosomiasis may be acute or chronic. Acute cases usually present as a diffuse fulminating meningoencephalitis with fever, headache, confusion, memory loss, lethargy, and coma. Focal or generalized seizures, hemiplegia, and other focal neurologic signs are common. The chronic cerebral form usually simulates the clinical picture of a tumor with localizing signs and increased intracranial pressure with papilledema. Granulomatous masses in the spinal cord almost always present acutely with signs and symptoms of an incomplete transverse lesion, with or without spinal subarachnoid block, depending on the size of the lesion. Granulomatous root involvement may also occur.

Laboratory Data. There is leukocytosis with an increase in eosinophils in the blood, although this may not be the case with the chronic cerebral form. The CSF pressure may be increased with large intracerebral lesions, and partial or incomplete subarachnoid block may occur with spinal lesions. A slight or moderate pleocytosis in the CSF (sometimes with eosinophils) and an increased protein content may occur. Spinal cord lesions may be demonstrated by myelography, CT, or MRI.

Diagnosis. The diagnosis is established from the history of gastrointestinal upset, eosinophilia in the blood, and the presence of ova in the stool or urine. Skin tests, serologic tests, and biopsy of the rectal mucosa are also of value in the establishment of the diagnosis.

Treatment. The broad spectrum drug praziquantel is now available in the United States and is the drug of choice. It is effective against all three human schistosomes. Newer species-specific alternative drugs are metrifonate, which is effective against S. haematobium, and oxamniquine, which is effective against S. mansoni. Oral steroids may also be of benefit to decrease swelling. Anticonvulsive drugs should be given to control the seizures. Surgical excision of the large granulomatous lesions may be required. Decompressive laminectomy may be beneficial when there is a subarachnoid block.

ECHINOCOCCUS (HYDATID CYSTS)

Echinococcus is a tissue infection of humans caused by the larvae of Echinococcus granulosus, a tapeworm parasite of the dog family. There is an intermediate phase of development with hydatid cyst formation in other mammals. Sheep and cattle are usually the intermediate hosts, but humans may be infected, especially by ova shed in dog feces. The disease is most common in countries where herd dogs assist with sheep and cattle raising. It is rare in the United States.

The cysts are most commonly found in the liver and the lungs. If the embryos pass the pulmonary barrier, cyst formation may occur in any organ. The brain is involved in about 2% of the cases and neurologic symptoms may develop in patients with cysts in the skull or spine.

Cerebral cysts are usually single. They are most common in the cerebral hemispheres, but may develop in the ventricles or cerebellum. The infestation may occur at any age, but is most common in children from rural areas.

The signs and symptoms that develop with cysts in the brain are similar to those of tumor in the affected region. Seizures and increased intracranial pressure may also occur. Involvement of the spine may result in spinal cord compression. The diagnosis of hydatid cyst as the cause of cerebral symptoms is rarely made before operation. CT and angiography, rather than ventriculography, should be used to localize the lesions, because of the danger of puncturing the cyst. Needle biopsy is also precluded. Rupture of a cyst results in allergic manifestations, including anaphylaxis. Eosinophilia is uncommon except after cyst rupture. Liver enzymes are usually normal. Serologic tests are positive in about 50% of infected individuals.

Treatment is complete surgical removal without puncturing the cyst. Drug treatment with albendazole or possibly praziquantel or mebendazole may decrease the size of cysts and prevent allergic reactions and secondary hydatidosis at the time of operation.

Several other Echinococcus species have rarely infected the human CNS. A variant of E. granulosus has a sylvatic cycle with wild animals as the main hosts and occurs in Canada and Alaska. E. multilocularis primarily involves the lungs (alveolar hydatid disease) with rodents as the intermediate hosts and wolves, foxes, coyotes, dogs, and cats as the definitive hosts. It occurs in the northern hemispheres of the world. Unlike E. granulosus, which produces large single cystic lesions, E. multilocularis produces masses of small cystic lesions. Treatment is similar to that for E. granulosus.

CYSTICERCOSIS

Cysticercosis is the result of encystment of the larvae of Taenia solium, the pork tapeworm, in the tissues. The infestation is acquired by ingestion of the ova through autoinfection by anal-oral transfer, fecal contamination of food, or autoinfection by reverse peristalsis of proglottids into the stomach. The larvae are not acquired by eating infected pork, and cysticercosis regularly occurs in vegetarians in edemic areas. Ingestion of infected pork results in the adult tapeworm infection.

Incidence. CNS involvement occurs in 50 to 70% of all cases. Virtually all symptomatic patients have CNS involvement. Cerebral cysticercosis is common in Mexico, Central and South America, Southeast Asia, China and India. The disease has recently become relatively common in the Southwestern United States because of immigration from Mexico. The disease may occur in other areas where a reservoir of infected pigs exists. In Mexico, cerebral cysticercosis is found in 2 to 4% of the population in unselected autopsy studies. It may be the single most common cause of neurologic disease.

Pathology. Typical cysts measure 5 to 10 mm and may be discrete and encapsulated or delicate, thin-walled, and multicystic. The miliary form with hundreds of cysticerci is most common in children. Meningeal cysts cause a chronic CSF pleocytosis. Live encysted larvae in the parenchyma cause little inflammation. Inflammation occurs when the larvae die, usually years after ingestion, and often correlates with the onset of symptoms.

Symptoms and Signs. Clinical manifestations can be divided into three basic types depending on anatomic site: parenchymal, meningitic, and intraventricular. The most common presenting manifestations are seizures, increased intracranial pressure, and meningitis.

In the parenchymal form, symptoms are related to the site of encystment. Cortical cysts frequently give rise to focal or generalized seizures. Other focal deficits may appear suddenly or may be more chronic. Signs include hemiparesis, sensory loss, hemianopsia, aphasia, or ataxia from cerebellar cysts. Stroke, which occurs secondary to vessel involvement, and dementia are occasionally seen.

The meningitic form may be the result of the rupture or death of an arachnoidal cyst or its transformation into the racemose form of the organism, which can enlarge within the basal cisterns and cause obstructive hydrocephalus. Symptoms of meningeal involvement vary from mild headache to a syndrome of chronic meningitis with meningism and communicating hydrocephalus. Spinal involvement may occur and may evolve into arachnoiditis and complete spinal subarachnoid block.

Cysts in the third or fourth ventricle obstruct the flow of CSF and can result in obstructive hydrocephalus. The cyst may move within the ventricular cavity and produce a "ball-valve" effect, resulting in intermittent symptoms. Sudden death may occur in these patients, occasionally without prior symptoms.

Laboratory Data and Diagnosis. The diagnosis of cysticercosis should be considered in all patients who have ever resided in endemic areas and who have epilepsy, meningitis, or increased intracranial pressure. CT is useful in evaluating such patients. Hydrocephalus may be observed and the exact site of obstruction determined. Intravenous contrast material may demonstrate intraventricular cysts, but MRI or ventriculography may be required. Parenchymal cysts may calcify, revealing single or multiple punctate calcifications on CT. Viable cysts appear as small, lucent areas that may be enhanced either diffusely or in a ring pattern after the infusion of intravenous contrast material (Fig. 22–1).

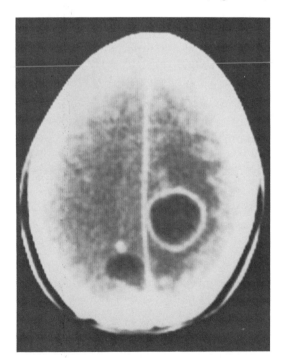

Fig. 22–1. Cerebral cysticercosis. CT scan. Patient with partial seizures and normal examination. A large lucent lesion with rim enhancement is seen on the left. A nonenhancing lucency with small calcification appears in the right parietal region. Other smaller lesions are seen bilaterally. (Courtesy of Drs. Verity Grinnell and Mark A. Goldberg.)

CSF examination may be normal or may reveal a moderate pleocytosis and elevated pressure. In more severe meningitis, the CSF may contain several hundred to several thousand white blood cells (usually mononuclear), elevated protein content, and low glucose, presenting a clinical picture similar to that for fungal or tuberculous meningitis. Eosinophilic meningitis is occasionally seen, but is uncommon. The presence of eosinophilia in the blood suggests another parasitic infestation and does not occur in pure neurocysticercosis. Measurement of complement-fixing antibody in CSF or serum is sometimes helpful, but false-negative results are common. Newer, more specific serologic tests include indirect hemagglutination and ELISA tests. The presence of calcified nodules in skeletal muscle is common among Indians, but is unusual in cases originating in Latin America.

Treatment. Ventricular shunting is usually adequate for treatment of hydrocephalic forms of this disorder. Usually, seizures can be controlled with standard anticonvulsants. Intractable seizures may develop, and surgical removal of cysts may be beneficial. Corticosteroids have been used to relieve the meningitic symptoms, but their value has not been established. Niclosamide can be used if there is a persistent intestinal infestation, but does not affect the encysted larvae. Praziquantel appears to be the first effective drug against the cysts. It is effective in stopping the progression of the parenchymal form of cysticercosis. It is less effective for the chronic meningitic form with arachnoiditis. Concomitant use of corticosteroids may be required to prevent severe inflammatory reactions and edema in response to the dying cysticerci.

EOSINOPHILIC MENINGITIS

The human nervous system may be invaded by the nematode rat lungworm, Angiostrongylus cantonensis, which uses a molluscan intermediate host and invades the domestic rat and other rodents in the course of its life cycle. Infection in humans is usually due to the ingestion of raw snails, shrimp, crabs, and fish, which serve as transport hosts. Cases have been reported from Hawaii, the Philippines, Southeast Asia and, recently, Cuba.

Involvement of the human nervous system is characterized by an acute meningeal reaction and there may be encephalitis, encephalomyelitis, or radiculomyeloencephalitis. Involvement of cranial nerves (especially six

and seven) and spinal roots is common. Severe dysesthetic pains, probably from posterior root inflammation, occur in about 50% of the patients. The infection is most common in children. The lesions in the nervous system are due to destruction of tissue by the parasite and to necrosis and aneurysmal dilatation of cerebral vessels, resulting in small or large hemorrhages. The disease commonly takes the form of an acute meningitis with a CSF pleocytosis of 100 to 200 cells/mm³ with many eosinophils. A peripheral blood eosinophilia is almost always seen. Serologic and skin tests are available. Usually the disease is self-limited. In the severe cases, death may be the result of small or large hemorrhagic lesions in the brain. There is no specific therapy.

Not all cases of eosinophilic meningitis are due to A. cantonensis infestation; other parasitic infections, coccidioidomycosis, foreign bodies, drug allergies, and neoplasms may also cause this syndrome. Rarely, another nematode of the Far East, Gnathostoma spinigerum, has caused eosinophilic meningitis. It has also caused the clinical syndromes of radiculomyeloencephalitis and meningoradiculomyelitis.

PARAGONIMIASIS

Paragonimiasis is the disease caused by the lung flukes Paragonimus westermani and P. mexicanus. Other Paragonimus species may occasionally infect humans. These trematodes commonly infect humans in Africa, Southeast Asia, South Pacific areas, and Central and South America. Infection occurs by eating uncooked or poorly cooked crustaceans. Immature flukes exist in the intestines and spread through the body, occasionally reaching the brain and spinal cord. Pulmonary and intestinal symptoms are the most common. Pulmonary involvement includes chronic cough, hemoptysis, and cavitary lesions on chest radiographs, thus simulating tuberculosis.

CNS involvement occurs in 10 to 15% of affected patients. Symptoms and signs of cerebral involvement include fever, headache, meningoencephalitis, focal and generalized seizures, dementia, hemiparesis, visual disturbances, and other focal manifestations. Acute purulent (meningoencephalitic), chronic granulomatous (tumorous form), and late inactive forms of nervous system involvement are seen. The CSF may be under increased pressure. The pleocytosis is primarily polymorphonuclear in acute forms and lymphocytic in more chronic forms. Eosinophils are occasionally present, and large numbers of red blood cells are occasionally seen in the acute cases. The protein content and gamma globulins are usually increased. The glucose content may be decreased. Diagnosis is most often made by detecting ova in the sputum and stool. Peripheral anemia, eosinophilia, leukocytosis, and elevated erythrocyte sedimentation rate and gamma globulins may occur. Serologic and skin tests are available. CT scanning may also be of assistance in diagnosis, revealing ventricular dilatation and intracranial calcifications including the characteristic "soap bubble" calcifications. During the early progressive course, mortality may reach 5 to 10%. The later chronic granulomatous state tends to be benign. Therapy includes the use of the drugs praziquantel or bithionol for the acute to subacute meningoencephalitis and surgical treatment for the chronic tumorous form.

OTHER HELMINTHS

Visceral larva migrans (toxocariasis) is a syndrome of pulmonary symptoms, hepatomegaly, and chronic eosinophilia caused by the larvae of the dog and cat ascarids (roundworms) Toxocara canis and T. cati. Eggs may be ingested, especially by children playing with infected dogs or contaminated soil. Although visceral larva migrans is uncommon and nervous system involvement is rare, the disease is always a potential threat due to the ubiquitous infections of domestic animals. Neurologic signs are manifested by focal deficits, especially hemiparesis. Eosinophils are infrequently seen in the CSF. Ocular involvement is more common than CNS disease. Serology is helpful for diagnosis, and hypergammaglobulinemia is common. Larvae may be identified in the sputum or in tissue granulomas from biopsy. Thiabendazole and diethylcarbamazine are the drugs of choice. An association of toxocariasis with pica and lead encephalopathy has been noted. Another ascarid, Ascaris lumbricoides, has been reported to cause a similar neurologic syndrome.

STRONGYLOIDIASIS

Strongyloidiasis is an intestinal infection of humans caused by the nematode Strongyloides stercoralis. This infection occurs in tropical and subtropical regions throughout the world, but has also been reported in most areas of the United States. In the usual infec-

tion, the CNS is spared. However, disseminated strongyloidiasis is not an infrequent complication in the immunosuppressed or immunodeficient host. CNS involvement occurs as part of this disseminated infection. Neurologic signs include meningitis, altered mental states (encephalopathy to coma), and focal deficits from mass lesions or infarction. CSF abnormalities are nonspecific and eosinophilia is infrequent. Diagnosis is usually made by finding the larvae in stool, sputum, or duodenal aspirates. Peripheral eosinophilia is not always present. Another clue to the diagnosis is the occurrence in the immunocompromised patient of an unexplained gram-negative bacteremia and meningitis, which is a frequent accompaniment of disseminated strongyloidiasis. Thiabendazole is the drug of choice.

Protozoan Infection

TOXOPLASMOSIS

Toxoplasmosis is the term used to describe infection in the human by the protozoan organism, Toxoplasma gondii. The infection, which has a predilection for the CNS and the eye, may be congenital with encephalitis and chorioretinitis. Toxoplasmosis is also an important opportunistic infection of immunocompromised patients, especially those with the acquired immunodeficiency syndrome (AIDS).

Etiology and Pathology. The toxoplasma are minute, about 2×3 µm, oval, pyriform, rounded, or elongated protoplasmic masses, with a central nucleus. One important host for this organism is the cat. Infection is acquired by ingestion of oocysts from cat feces or contaminated soil. Infection may also occur by eating unwashed vegetables or undercooked meat. The organisms invade the walls of blood vessels in the nervous system and produce an inflammatory reaction. Miliary granulomas are formed. They may become calcified or undergo necrosis. The granulomatous lesions are scattered throughout the CNS and may be found in the meninges and ependyma. Hydrocephalus may develop from occlusion of the aqueduct of Sylvius by the resulting ependymitis. The microorganisms are present in the epithelioid cells of the granulomas (Fig. 22–2); they may also be found in the endothelial cells of blood vessels and in the nerve cells. Lesions in the retina are common; occasionally, they are also present in the lungs, kidneys, liver, spleen, or skin.

Symptoms. In the congenital form, the symptoms are evident in the first few days of life. The common manifestations are inanition, microcephaly, seizures, mental retardation, spasticity, opisthotonos, chorioretinitis, microphthalmus, or other congenital defects in development of the eye. Optic atrophy is common, and there may be an internal hydrocephalus. The liver and spleen may be enlarged with elevated bilirubin. Fever, rash, and pneumonitis may also be present. The presence of calcified nodules in the brain can be demonstrated by CT or radiographs of the skull. Symptoms in the infantile form are similar to those of the congenital form, but may not make their appearance until the third or fifth year of life. Cerebral calcifications are not found in postnatally acquired infections.

Acquired toxoplasmosis is most often asymptomatic in the normal host. An infectious mononucleosis-like picture may be seen with lymphadenopathy. Although atypical lymphocytes may be present in the peripheral blood, serologic tests for Epstein-Barr virus are negative. Severe infection is more likely to occur in immunocompromised patients. Some of the infections in the immunocompromised host may be due to reactivation rather than to newly acquired infection. Manifestations may include pneumonitis, myocarditis, myositis, and choreoretinitis. Neuro-logic involvement in the acquired infections may take one of several forms. There may be an encephalopathic picture with confusion, delirium, obtundation, and coma, which is occasionally accompanied by seizures. Another presentation may be one of meningoencephalitis with headache, nuchal rigidity, and focal or generalized seizures leading to status epilepticus and coma. A third type of presentation, and probably the most common, is that of focal signs due to single or multiple mass lesions (toxoplasmic abscess). A combination of these three types of neurologic involvement is often seen.

Toxoplasmosis as a complication of neoplastic disease is relatively infrequent. However, toxoplasmosis is the most frequent CNS opportunistic infection of AIDS patients, accounting for about one third of all CNS complications.

Laboratory Data. A moderate or severe anemia and a mild leukocytosis or leukopenia may be present. The CSF may be under increased pressure. The protein content is generally increased, and there is an inconstant pleocytosis. Cell counts as high as several thousand/mm^3, mostly lymphocytes, have been recorded. The CSF glucose is normal or mildly reduced. CT may reveal calcifications, especially in congenital infections. Low-density focal lesions may be seen. With contrast enhancement (especially double-dose), these lesions may show ring enhancement similar to a brain abscess or diffuse enhancement.

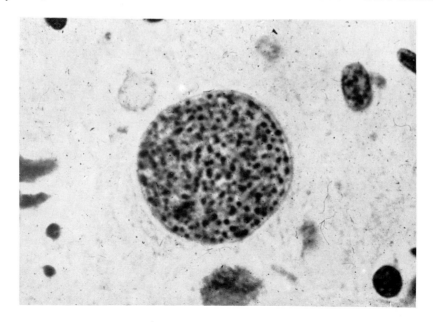

Fig. 22–2. Toxoplasma parasites within epithelioid cell. (Courtesy of Dr. Abner Wolf.)

Diagnosis. The diagnosis of congenital toxoplasmosis is usually considered in the newborn with choreoretinitis, microcephaly, seizures, mental retardation, cerebral calcifications, and evidence of systemic infection. The diagnosis is more difficult to make in older children and adults with either acquired disease or reactivation of a latent infection. Toxoplasma can be demonstrated in CSF sediment with Wright or Giemsa stain. The organism can be cultivated from CSF sediment by inoculation of laboratory mice. Despite the fact that a definite diagnosis can only be made by isolation of the organism from biopsy of brain or other tissues, a presumptive diagnosis can be made by using readily available serologic tests. Serologic tests include the Sabin-Feldman dye, indirect fluorescent antibody, complement fixation, agglutination, indirect hemagglutination, and ELISA tests. Demonstration of IgM antibodies by immunofluorescence is particularly helpful.

In AIDS patients, serum IgG antibody is usually positive, although a fourfold rise is infrequent. Serum IgM antibody is not usually detected. Preliminary studies suggest that a fourfold antibody rise is likely to be detected in the CSF of these patients.

Course, Prognosis, and Treatment. Prognosis is poor in the congenital form; more than 50% of affected infants die within a few weeks after birth. Mental and neurologic defects are present in the infants who survive. The mortality rate is also high in the infantile form of encephalitis. Most acquired infections in the immunocompetent patient are self-limited and do not require treatment. The severe, acquired or reactivated infections, which occur more commonly in immunocompromised patients, frequently result in death. These severe infections can at times be treated successfully with pyrimethamine and sulfadiazine. In AIDS patients, if a tissue diagnosis cannot be made but serum IgG titers are positive, empirical therapy should be considered. Indefinite suppression therapy is required for AIDS patients.

CEREBRAL MALARIA

Malaria is the most common human parasitic disease, with 250 to 300 million infected individuals in the world and 1 million deaths each year. This disease is endemic in tropical and subtropical areas of Africa, Asia, and Central and South America. However, the disease can be seen almost anywhere as a result of international travel. Malaria is transmitted by mosquitos.

Involvement of the nervous system occurs in about 2% of affected patients and is most common in infections of the malignant tertian form, almost always caused by Plasmodium-falciparum.

Pathology and Pathogenesis. The neurologic symptoms are due to occlusion of capillaries with pigment-laden cells and parasites (Fig. 22–3), and to the presence of multiple petechial hemorrhages. Lymphocytic and mononuclear perivascular inflammation and a microglial cell response may be seen. Areas of softening as a result of thrombotic occlusion of vessels are rare. It is probable that the pathologic changes in the nervous system are reversible.

Symptoms and Signs. The symptoms and signs are primarily those of an acute diffuse encephalopathy. Spinal cord lesions and a polyneuritis of the Guillain-Barré type have rarely been seen. The neurologic symptoms usually appear in the second or third week of the illness, but they may be the initial manifestation. The onset of cerebral symptoms has no relationship to the height of the fever. Headache, photophobia, vertigo, convulsions, confusion, delirium, and coma are the most common symptoms. There may be neck stiffness. Focal signs such as transient hemiparesis, aphasia, hemianopia, and cerebellar ataxia are uncommon. Myoclonus, chorea, and intention tremors have been observed. Cranial nerve palsies and papilledema are rarely seen, although retinal hemorrhages are common. Psychic manifestations such as delirium, disorientation, amnesia, or combativeness are present in a large percentage of the patients.

Laboratory Data. The laboratory findings include anemia and the presence in the red blood cells of great numbers of parasites. The CSF pressure may be elevated. The CSF may be slightly xanthochromic and may contain a small or moderate number of lymphocytes. The CSF protein content may be moderately increased. The CSF sugar content is normal. However, in most cases, the CSF is entirely normal.

Diagnosis. Cerebral malaria is diagnosed from the appearance of cerebral symptoms and the findings of the organisms of P. falciparum in the blood. Delirium, convulsions, or coma may occur as symptoms of general infection in patients with P. vivax in the absence of cerebral involvement. The symptoms

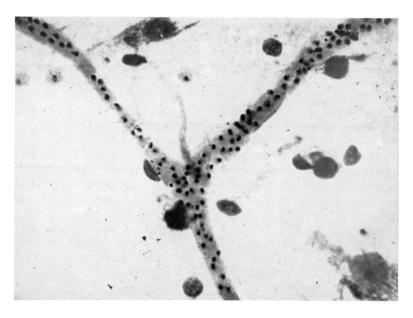

Fig. 22–3. Cerebral malaria. Cortical vessels congested with plasmodia. (Courtesy of Dr. Abner Wolf.)

in these cases are transient and respond readily to antimalarial therapy.

Prognosis. The mortality rate is 20 to 40% in all cases of cerebral malaria. It is highest (80%) when there is a combination of coma and convulsions. There are few or no residua in the patients who recover.

Treatment. Cerebral malaria is a true medical emergency. In critically ill patients, treatment includes chloroquine, usually given by intramuscular injection, and quinine given intravenously. If infection originated in an endemic area of chloroquine-resistant falciparum malaria, then quinine plus oral pyrimethaminosulfadoxine (Fansidar) should be used. For strains resistant to Fansidar, quinine plus tetracycline or clindamycin is indicated. Recent studies indicate that quinidine may be effective for chloroquine- and quinine-resistant falciparum malaria. Anticonvulsants should be given to control seizures. Transfusions of whole blood or plasma may be required. Other supportive measures include reduction of fever, fluid replacement, and respiratory support. Sedation may be necessary in excited or delirious patients. In a well-controlled, double-blind trial, Warrell and co-workers demonstrated that the use of dexamethasone is deleterious in the treatment of cerebral malaria.

TRYPANOSOMIASIS

Two distinct varieties of infection with trypanosomes are recognized: the African form (sleeping sickness), which is due to infection with Trypanosoma brucei, and the South American form (Chagas disease), which is endemic in South America, Central America, and Mexico, and is due to infection by T. cruzi.

Etiology and Pathology. In the African form of the disease, the organisms retain their trypanosome form and multiply by longitudinal fission. They are transmitted from person to person by the tsetse fly, occasionally by other flies or insects, and by mechanical contact. There are two variants of the species: T. brucei gambiense (mid- and west Africa) and T. brucei rhodesiense (east Africa). The pathologic changes are those of a chronic meningoencephalitis.

The organisms of South American trypanosomiasis, when found in the blood, have an ordinary trypanoform structure. They do not, however, reproduce in the blood, but invade tissues and are transformed into typical leishmania parasites. These may later assume the trypanosome form and re-enter the blood. The infection is transmitted from an animal host (e.g., rodents, cats, opossum, armadillo) to humans by a blood-sucking reduviid bug known as the "kissing bug."

The pathologic lesions in the nervous system consist of miliary granulomas composed of proliferated microglial cells. The organisms are present in glial and nerve cells. The lesions are diffusely scattered throughout the nervous system and are accompanied by a patchy reaction in the meninges and parenchyma.

Symptoms. African trypanosomiasis (sleeping sickness) passes through two indistinct stages: febrile and lethargic. The incubation period is variable. In some cases, symptoms may have their onset within two weeks of the infection. In others, it may be delayed for months or years. The first stage of the disease is characterized by a remitting fever, exanthems, lymphadenitis, splenomegaly, arthralgia, myalgia, and asthenia. During this period, which may last for several months or years, the organisms are present in the blood. The first stage passes imperceptibly into the second, in which the previous symptoms are exaggerated and involvement of the nervous system is evident in the form of tremors, incoordination, convulsions, paralysis, confusion, headaches, apathy, somnolence, and finally, coma. There is progressive weakness with loss of weight. If the condition is untreated, death usually ensues within a year after the appearance of cerebral symptoms. Death from intercurrent infection is common.

In South American trypanosomiasis, the acute stage generally lasts about one month and is characterized by fever, conjunctivitis, palpebral and facial edema, and enlargement of the lymph nodes, liver, and spleen. During this stage, trypanosomes are present in the blood, and the leishmaniform bodies are seen in the tissue. The secondary stage is characterized by evidence of involvement of the viscera, particularly the thyroid, heart, skeletal muscle, adrenal, and the CNS. Neurologic signs include hemiplegia, diplegia, aphasia, choreoathetosis, and mental alterations. Cranial nerve palsies and convulsions may occur. The disease is slowly progressive, with occasional acute exacerbations associated with fever. Death usually ensues within a few months or years.

Laboratory Data. Some degree of anemia is common in all forms of trypanosomiasis. The erythrocyte sedimentation rate, liver function tests, serum globulin reaction, and serum IgM may be increased. There is a lymphocytic pleocytosis in the CSF, increased protein content, increased gamma globulin fraction, and increased IgM.

Diagnosis. The diagnosis depends on the development of characteristic symptoms in residents of regions in which forms of the disease are endemic. The diagnosis is established by the demonstration of organisms in the blood or CSF, in material obtained from puncture of an enlarged node, or by the inoculation of these substances into susceptible animals (i.e., mice, guinea pigs, rabbits, monkeys). Serologic tests are also available.

Treatment. Melarsoprol, an organic arsenical, is of value in the treatment of T. brucei infections of the nervous system. No drug treatment is established as safe and effective in chronic Chagas disease. Nifurtimox is usually effective, however, in the acute stage of infection.

PRIMARY AMEBIC MENINGOENCEPHALITIS

It has been known for many years that amebae (Entamoeba histolytica) may rarely invade the brain and produce circumscribed abscesses. In recent years, however, there have been numerous reports of the findings of free-living amebae (Naegleria) in the CSF of patients with acute meningoencephalitis. Another free-living ameba (Acanthamoeba) has been recognized as a human pathogen and as the cause of both acute and granulomatous meningoencephalitis. Amebic meningoencephalitis is rare, but probably has a worldwide distribution. Most cases in the United States are reported from the Southeast.

Naegleria Infections. These infections usually occur in children or young adults who have been swimming in freshwater lakes or ponds. Inhalation of dust-borne cysts may also occur in arid regions. Interestingly, the organism apparently invades the nervous system through the olfactory nerves and does not cause a systemic infection. The incubation period is several days to a week. The onset of symptoms of meningoencephalitis is abrupt. Mild symptoms of an upper respiratory infection may occur. Fever, headache, and neck stiffness are followed within one or two days by nausea and vomiting, lethargy, disorientation, seizures, increased intracranial pressure, coma, and then death.

The CSF is purulent with several hundred to thousands of white blood cells/mm^3, primarily neutrophils. Red blood cells are usually present, often up to several thousand. The CSF is under increased pressure with an elevated protein content and decreased glucose. Trophozoites may be recognized in a wet preparation of uncentrifuged CSF. Amebae may also be seen with Wright's or Giemsa stains. No organisms are demonstrated on Gram stain or routine culture. The organism can be cultured on special media or by mouse inoculation. Serologic tests are available at the Centers for Disease Control. The disease is rapidly fatal, but recovery with treatment has been reported. Amphotericin B has been used effectively alone or in combination with several drugs.

Acanthamoeba Infections. Acanthamoeba is a ubiquitous organism that can cause a subacute or chronic granulomatous amebic encephalitis as an opportunistic infection in alcoholics and immunocompromised patients. The organism probably causes a systemic infection through the respiratory tract and then seeds the brain by hematogenous spread. The meningoencephalitis may present with chronic fever and headache, followed by the gradual onset of focal neurologic signs (e.g., hemiparesis, aphasia, seizures with focal signature, ataxia) and abnormalities of mentation. Other signs include skin lesions, corneal ulcerations, uveitis, and pneumonitis.

There is CSF pleocytosis that is more often lymphocytic than polymorphonuclear. The protein is usually elevated and the glucose is normal or slightly decreased. Organisms may occasionally be recognized on wet preparations, but have never been cultured from CSF. Experimental infections with Acanthamoeba are sensitive to sulfadiazine. Several cases of acute meningoencephalitis, similar to those caused by Naegleria, have been reported.

References

General

Anonymous. Drugs for parasitic infections. Med Lett 1988; 30:15–24.

Bia FJ, Barry M. Parasitic infections of the central nervous system. Neurol Clin 1986; 4:171–206.

Braunwald E, Isselbacher KJ, Petersdorf RG, Wilson JD, Martin JB, Fauci AS, eds. Harrison's Principles of Internal Medicine, 11th ed. New York: McGraw-Hill, 1987.

Brown WJ, Voge M. Neuropathology of Parasitic Infections. Oxford: Oxford University Press, 1982.

Manson-Bahr PEC, Apted FIC, eds. Manson's Tropical Diseases, 18th ed. London: Bailliere-Tindall, 1982.

Strickland GT. Hunter's Tropical Medicine, 6th ed. Philadelphia: WB Saunders Co., 1984.

Trelles JO. Parasitic disease and tropical neurology. In: Vinken PJ, Bruyn GW, Klawans HL, eds. Handbook of Clinical Neurology, vol 35. New York: Elsevier-North Holland, 1978:1–23.

Warren KS, Mahmound AAF, eds. Tropical and Geographic Medicine. New York: McGraw-Hill, 1984.

Helminthic Infection

Trichinosis

Dalessio D, Wolff HG. Trichinella spiralis infection of the central nervous system. Arch Neurol 1961; 4:407–417.

Ellrodt A, Lalfon P, LeBras P, et al. Multifocal central nervous system lesions in three patients with trichinosis. Arch Neurol 1987; 44:432–434.

Kramer MD, Aita JF. Trichinosis. In: Vinken PJ, Bruyn GW, Klawans HL, eds. Handbook of Clinical Neurology, vol 35. New York: Elsevier-North Holland, 1978: 267–290.

Merritt HH, Rosenbaum M. Involvement of the nervous system in trichinosis. JAMA 1936; 106:1646–1649.

Ochoa J, Pallis C. Trichinella thrives in both oxidative and glycolytic human muscle fibers. J Neurol Neurosurg Psychiatry 1980; 43:281–282.

Schistosomiasis

Bird AV. Schistosomiasis of the central nervous system. In: Vinken PJ, Bruyn GW, Klawans HL, eds. Handbook of Clinical Neurology, vol 35. New York: Elsevier-North Holland, 1978: 231–241.

Capron A, Dessaint JP, Capron M, Ouma JH, Butterworth AE. Immunity to schistosomes: progress toward vaccine. Science 1987; 238:1065–1072.

Kane CA, Most H. Schistosomiasis of central nervous system: experiences in World War II. Arch Neurol Psychiatry 1948; 59:141–183.

Lechtenberg R, Vaida GA. Schistosomiasis of the spinal cord. Neurology 1977; 27:55–59.

Marcial-Rojas RA, Fiol RE. Neurologic complications of schistosomiasis. Ann Intern Med 1963; 59:215–230.

Scrimgeour EM, Gajdusek DC. Involvement of the central nervous system in Schistosoma mansoni and S. haematobium infection. Brain 1985; 108:1023–1038.

Tillman AJB. Schistosomiasis japonica with cerebral manifestations. Arch Intern Med 1947; 79:36–61.

Watt G, Adapon B, Long GW, Fernando MT, Ranoa CP, Cross JH. Praziquantel in treatment of cerebral schistosomiasis. Lancet 1986; 2:529–532.

Echinococcus

Anderson M, Bickerstaff ER, Hamilton JC. Cerebral hydatid cysts in Britain. J Neurol Neurosurg Psychiatry 1975; 38:1104–1108.

Arana-Iniquez R. Echinococcus. In: Vinken PJ, Bruyn GW, Klawans HL, eds. Handbook of Clinical Neurology, vol 35. New York: Elsevier-North Holland, 1978: 175–208.

Ayres CM, Davey LM, German WJ. Cerebral hydatidosis. J Neurosurg 1963; 20:371–377.

Fiennes A, Thomas D. Combined medical and surgical treatment of spinal hydatid disease: a case report. J Neurol Neurosurg Psychiatry 1982; 45:927–931.

Hamza R, Touibi S, Jamoussi M, Bardi-Bellagha I, Chtiovi R. Intracranial and orbital hydatid cysts. Neuroradiology 1982; 22:211–214.

Pamir MN, Akalon N, Ozgen T, Erbengi A. Spinal hydatid cysts. Surg Neurol 1984; 21:53–57.

Cysticercosis

Bickerstaff ER, Cloake PC, Hughes B, Smith WT. The racemose form of cerebral cysticercosis. Brain 1952; 75:1–18.

Del Brutto OH, Sotelo J. Neurocysticercosis: an update. Rev Infect Dis 1988; 10:1075–1087.

Dixon HFB, Lipscomb FM. Cysticercosis: an analysis and follow-up of 450 cases. Medical Research Council Special Report Series No. 299. London: Her Majesty's Stationery Office, 1961.

Firemark H. Spinal cysticercosis. Arch Neurol 1978; 35:250–251.

Flisser A, Willms K, Laclette JP, Larralde C, Ridaura C, Beltran F, eds. Cysticercosis: present state of knowledge and perspectives. New York: Academic Press, 1982.

Grisolia JS, Wiederholt WC. CNS cysticercosis. Arch Neurol 1982; 39:540–544.

Loo L, Braude A. Cerebral cysticercosis in San Diego: a report of 23 cases and a review of the literature. Medicine 1982; 61:341–359.

McCormick GF, Zee C-S, Heiden J. Cysticercosis cerebri: review of 127 cases. Arch Neurol 1982; 39:534–539.

Scharf D. Neurocysticercosis. Arch Neurol 1988; 45:777–780.

Sotelo J, Escobedo F, Penagos P. Albendazole vs praziquantel for neurocysticercosis: a controlled trial. Arch Neurol 1988; 45:532–534.

Trelles JO, Trelles L. Cysticercosis of the nervous system. In: Vinken PJ, Bruyn GW. Klawans HL, eds. Handbook of Clinical Neurology vol 35. New York: Elsevier-North Holland, 1978: 291–320.

Wadia N, Desai S, Bhatt M. Disseminated cysticercosis: new observations, including CT scan findings and experience with treatment by praziquantel. Brain 1988; 111:597–614.

Eosinophilic Meningitis

Arseni C, Chimon D. Angiostrongylus cantonensis (eosinophilic meningitis). In: Vinken PJ, Bruyn GW, Klawans HL, eds. Handbook of Clinical Neurology, vol 35. New York: Elsevier-North Holland, 1978: 321–342.

Koo J, Pien F, Kliks MM. Angiostrongylus (Parastrongylus) eosinophilic meningitis. Rev Infect Dis 1988; 10:1155–1162.

Kuberski T, Wallace GD. Clinical manifestations of eosinophilic meningitis due to *Angiostrongylus cantonensis*. Neurology 1979; 29:1566–1570.

Nye SW, Tangchai P, Sudarakiti S, Punyagupta S. Lesions of the brain in eosinophilic meningitis. Arch Pathol 1970; 89:9–19.

Punyagupta S, Juttijudata P, Bunnag T. Eosinophilic meningitis in Thailand: clinical studies of 484 typical cases probably caused by *Angiostrongylus cantonensis*. Am J Trop Med Hyg 1975; 24:921–931.

Schmutzhard E, Boongird P, Vejjajiva A. Eosinophilic meningitis and radiculomyelitis in Thailand, caused by CNS invasion of Gnathostoma spinigerum and Angiostrongylus cantonensis. J of Neurol, Neurosurg, and Psychiatry 1988; 51:80–87.

Paragonimiasis

Brenes Madrigal R, Rodriguez-Ortiz B, Vargas Solano G, Ocampo Obdano E, Ruiz Sotela PJ. Cerebral hemorrhagic lesions produced by *Paragonimus mexicanus*. Am J Trop Med Hyg 1982; 31:522–526.

Miyazaki I, Nishimura K. Cerebral paragonimiasis. In: Hornabrook RW, ed. Topics on Tropical Neurology. Philadelphia: FA Davis, 1975: 109–132.

Oh SJ. Paragonimiasis in the central nervous system. In: Vinken PJ, Bruyn GW, Klawans, HL, eds. Handbook of Clinical Neurology, vol 35. New York: Elsevier-North Holland, 1978: 243–266.

Yoshida M, Moritaka K, Kuga S, Anegawa S. CT findings of cerebral paragonimiasis in the chronic state. J Comput Assist Tomogr 1982; 6:195–196.

Other Helminths

Garcia-Maldonado E, Gonzalez JE, Cespedes G. Helminthiasis of the nervous system (general features, epidemiology and pathogenesis). In: Vinken PJ, Bruyn GW, Klawans HL, eds. Handbook of Clinical Neurology, vol 35. New York: Elsevier-North Holland, 1978: 209–229.

Glickman LT, Schantz PM. Epidemiology and pathogenesis of zoonotic toxocariasis. Epidemiol Rev 1981; 3:230–250.

Gould IM, Newell S, Green SH, George RH. Toxocariasis and eosinophilic meningitis. Br Med J 1985; 291:1239–1240.

King TD, Moncrief JA, Vingiello R. Hemiparesis and Ascaris lumbricoides infection. J La State Med Soc 1979; 131:5–7.

Masdeu JC, Tantulavanich S, Gorelick PP, Maliwan N, Heredia S, Martinez-Lage JM, Rubino FA, Ross E, Mamdani M. Brain abscess caused by *Strongyloides stercoralis*. Arch Neurol 1982; 39:62–63.

Scowden EB, Schaffner W, Stone WJ. Overwhelming strongyloidiasis: an unappreciated opportunistic infection. Medicine 1978; 57:527–544.

Thomson AF. Other helminthous infections (Echinococcus, ascariasis and hookworm). In: Vinken PJ, Bruyn GW, Klawans HL, eds. Handbook of Clinical Neurology, vol 35. New York: Elsevier-North Holland, 1978: 343–370.

Wachter RM, Burke AM, MacGregor RR. *Strongyloides stercoralis* hyperinfection masquerading as cerebral vasculitis. Arch Neurol 1984; 41:1213–1216.

Protozoan Infection

Toxoplasmosis

Couvreur J, Desmonts G. Toxoplasmosis. In: Vinken PJ, Bruyn GW, Klawans HL, eds. Handbook of Clinical Neurology, vol 35. New York: Elsevier-North Holland, 1978: 115–141.

Cowen D, Wolf A, Paige BH. Toxoplasmic encephalomyelitis. Arch Neurol Psychiatry 1942; 48:689–739.

Ghatak NR, Poon TP, Zimmerman HM. Toxoplasmosis of the central nervous system in adults. Arch Pathol 1970; 89:337–348.

Luft BJ, Remington JS. Toxoplasmic encephalitis. J. Infect Dis 1988; 157:1–6.

McCabe R, Remington JS. Toxoplasmosis: the time has come. N Engl J Med 1988; 318:313–315.

Navia BA, Petito CK, Gold JWM, Cho E-S, Jordan BD, Price RW. Cerebral toxoplasmosis complicating the acquired immune deficiency syndrome: clinical and neuropathological findings in 27 patients. Ann Neurol 1986; 19:224–238.

Rowland LP, Greer M. Toxoplasmic polymyositis. Neurology 1961; 11:367–370.

Sabin AB. Toxoplasmic encephalitis in children. JAMA 1941; 116:801–807.

Townsend JJ, Wolinsky JS, Baringer JR, Johnson PC. Acquired toxoplasmosis: a neglected cause of treatable nervous system disease. Arch Neurol 1975; 32:335–343.

Wilson CB, Remington JS, Stagno S, Reynolds DW. Development of adverse sequelae in children born with subclinical congenital toxoplasma infection. Pediatrics 1980; 66:767–774.

Cerebral Malaria

Daroff RB, Deller JJ Jr., Kastl AJ Jr., Blocker WW Jr. Cerebral malaria. JAMA 1967; 202:679–682.

Hill GJ II, Knight V, Coaney GR, Lawless DK. Vivax malaria complicated by aphasia and hemiparesis. Arch Intern Med 1963; 112:863–868.

Marsden PD, Bruce-Chwatt LJ. Cerebral malaria. In: Hornabrook RW, ed. Topics on tropical neurology. Philadelphia: FA Davis, 1975: 29–44.

Oo MM, Aikawa M, Than T, Aye TM, Myint PT, Igarashi I, Schoene WC. Human cerebral malaria: a pathological study. J Neuropathol Exp Neurol 1987; 46:223–231.

Vietze G. Malaria and other protozoal diseases. In: Vinken PJ, Bruyn GW, Klawans HL, eds. Handbook of Clinical Neurology, vol 35. New York: Elsevier-North Holland, 1978: 143–160.

Warrell DA, Looareesuwan S, Warrell MJ, et al. Dexamethasone proves deleterious in cerebral malaria: a double-blind trial in 100 comatose patients. N Engl J Med 1982; 306:313–319.

White NJ, Looareesuwan S, Phillips RE, Chanthavanich P, Warrell DA. Single dose phenabarbitone prevents convulsions in cerebral malaria. Lancet 1988; 2:64–66.

Wyler DJ. Steroids are out in the treatment of cerebral malaria: What's next? J Infect Dis 1988; 158:320–324.

Trypanosomiasis

Dumas M, Girard PL. Human African trypanosomiasis (sleeping sickness). In: Vinken PJ, Bruyn GW, Klawans HL, eds. Handbook of Clinical Neurology, vol 35. New York: Elsevier-North Holland, 1978: 67–83.

Greenwood BM, Whittle HC. The pathogenesis of sleeping sickness. Trans R Soc Trop Med Hyg 1980; 74:716–725.

Haller L, Adams H, Merouze F, Dago A. Clinical and pathological aspects of human African trypanosomiasis (T. b. gambiense) with particular reference to reactive arsenical encephalopathy. Am J Trop Med Hyg 1986; 35:94–99.

Newton BA, ed. Trypanosomiasis. Br Med Bull 1985; 41:103–199.

Shafii A. Chagas' disease with cardiopathy and hemiplegia. NY State J Med 1977; 77:418–419.

Spencer HC Jr, Gibson JJ, Brodsky RE, Schultz MG. Imported African trypanosomiasis in the United States. Ann Intern Med 1975; 82:633–638.

Spina-Franca A, Mattosinho-Franca LC. American trypanosomiasis (Chagas' disease). In: Vinken PJ, Bruyn GW, Klawans HL, eds. Handbook of Clinical Neurology, vol 35. New York: Elsevier-North Holland, 1978: 85–114.

Primary Amebic Meningoencephalitis

Anonymous. Primary amebic meningoencephalitis—United States. MMWR 1980; 29:405–407.

Darby CP, Conradi SE, Holbrook TW, Chatellier C. Primary amebic meningoencephalitis. Am J Dis Child 1979; 133:1025–1027.

Duma RJ. Amoebic infections of the nervous system. In: Vinken PJ, Bruyn GW, Klawans HL, eds. Handbook of Clinical Neurology, vol 35. New York: Elsevier-North Holland 1978: 25–65.

Duma RJ, Helwig WB, Martinez J. Meningoencephalitis and brain abscess due to a free-living amoeba. Ann Intern Med 1978; 88:468–473.

Grunnert ML, Cannon GH, Kushner JP. Fulminant amebic meningoencephalitis due to *Acanthamoeba*. Neurology 1981; 31:174–177.

Martinez AJ. Is *Acanthamoeba* encephalitis an opportunistic infection? Neurology 1980; 30:567–574.

Rothrock JF, Buchsbaum HW. Primary amebic meningoencephalitis. JAMA 1980; 243:2329–2330.

Seidel JS, Harmatz P, Visvesvara GS, Cohen A, Edwards J, Turner J. Successful treatment of primary amebic meningoencephalitis. N Engl J Med 1982; 306:346–348.

23. BACTERIAL TOXINS
William A. Sibley

The toxins elaborated by several of the pathogenic bacteria have a special predilection for the nervous system. The exotoxin of the diphtheria bacillus affects chiefly the peripheral nerves; tetanus affects the activity of the neurons in the CNS; and botulism interferes with conduction at the myoneural junction.

Diphtheria

The mode of action of the exotoxin of Corynebacterium diphtheriae on the peripheral nerves is unknown. It has been suggested that the toxin interferes with the synthesis of cytochrome B or related enzymes, but direct proof for this theory is lacking. The toxin spreads from the site of infection into the blood and CSF. It has a predilection for the sensory and motor nerves of the limbs and, to a lesser extent, the ciliary muscle or nerve. The frequency of palatal and pharyngo-laryngo-esophageal involvement is possibly a result in part of local action of toxin; the incidence of involvement of these structures is lower in cutaneous diphtheria than in faucial diphtheria. The resistance of other cranial nerves and the brain is unexplained because they are all susceptible to an adequate dose.

The symptoms and course of diphtheritic neuritis are considered in Section 108, Acquired Neuropathies.

Tetanus

Tetanus (lockjaw) is an infectious disease that causes localized or generalized spasm of muscle due to the toxin produced by the causative organism, Clostridium tetani.

Etiology. Clostridium tetani is present in the excreta of humans and most animals, and is present in dirt and putrefying liquids. It is especially prevalent in fertilized or contaminated soil. The organisms usually gain entrance to the human body through puncture wounds, compound fractures, or wounds from blank cartridges and fireworks. Infection has been reported from contamination of operative wounds, burns, parenteral injections (particularly in heroin addicts), and through the umbilicus of the newborn. The mere deposition of spores of the organism is not sufficient for infection. Necrotic tissue and an associated pyogenic infection are necessary for growth of the organism and production of the toxin.

The symptoms are due to a toxin elaborated by the organism. The toxin has a local effect at the site of inoculation and travels through the blood and the perineural connective tissue. When the toxin spreads through the nerves, the symptoms are those of localized tetanus. The toxin acts on the muscles or motor nerve endings as well as on the spinal cord and brain stem.

Pathology. No pathologic changes occur in the central or peripheral nervous system.

Incidence. The disease is found in all portions of the world. In the United States, it is most commonly due to infection of puncture wounds of the extremities by nails or splinters contaminated by human or animal excreta, or by infections of wounds inflicted by cap pistols and fireworks. The incidence of infection in soldiers by wounds received in combat was high until the introduction of active immunization of all recruits and passive immunization of all wounded soldiers. In the United States, the infection is most common in narcotic addicts. This finding may occur because the narcotic is "cut" by admixing with quinine, which favors the growth of the organisms at the site of the injection.

Symptoms. The incubation period is usually between 5 and 10 days. Occasionally, it may be as short as three days or as long as three weeks. As a rule, the severity of the disease is greater when the incubation period is short.

The symptoms may be localized or generalized. In the localized form, the muscular spasms and contractions are confined to the injured limbs. This form is relatively rare and is most commonly seen in patients who have been partially protected by prophylactic doses of antitetanic serum. When the portal of entrance is in the head (e.g., face, ear, tonsils), the symptoms may be localized to that region (cephalic tetanus). Trismus, facial paralysis, and ophthalmoplegia are characteristic of this rare form of tetanus.

In the generalized form, the presenting symptom is usually stiffness of the jaw (trismus). This condition is followed by stiffness of the neck, irritability, and restlessness. As the disease progresses, stiffness of the muscles becomes generalized. Rigidity of the back muscles may become so extreme that the patient assumes the position of opisthotonos. Rigidity of the facial muscles gives a characteristic facial expression, the so-called risus sardonicus. Added to the stiffness of the muscles are paroxysmal tonic spasms or generalized convulsions. These may occur spontaneously or may be precipitated by an external stimulus. Dysphagia may develop from spasm of the pharyngeal muscles; cyanosis and asphyxia may result from spasm of the glottis or respiratory muscles. Consciousness is preserved except during convulsions. The pulse and respiratory rates are elevated. The temperature may be normal, but more commonly it is elevated to 101° to 103° F.

Laboratory Data. No specific changes occur in blood, urine, or CSF.

Diagnosis. The diagnosis of tetanus is made on the appearance of the characteristic signs of the disease (i.e., trismus, risus sardonicus, tonic spasms, and generalized convulsions) in a patient who has received a wound of the skin and deeper tissues. The symptoms of strychnine poisoning differ from those of tetanus in that the muscles are relaxed between spasms and the jaw muscles are rarely involved.

Course and Prognosis. The outlook is grave in all cases of tetanus. The mortality rate is over 50%. Prognosis is best when the incubation period is long or when generalized convulsive seizures are either absent or do not develop until several days after the onset. The mortality rate is reduced by the prompt administration of serum. In fatal cases, death usually occurs in 3 to 10 days. Death is most commonly due to paralysis of respiration. In the patients who recover, there is a gradual reduction in the frequency of seizures and in the severity of muscular contractions.

Treatment. The patient should be treated in a special care unit. The wound should be surgically cleaned. Antiserum does not neutralize toxins that have been fixed in the nervous system, but it is administered on the chance that it will neutralize toxin that has not yet entered the nervous system. It is customary to administer human tetanus immune globulin (HTIG) in a dose of 3,000 to 6,000 units intramuscularly as soon as the diagnosis is made. On the basis of a controlled study, Gupta and colleagues reported a marked reduction in mortality rate (to 2% from 21%) with the early use of 250 international units of HTIG injected intrathecally; their patients all had mild tetanus (trismus, dysphagia, local spasm, but no generalized rigidity or spasms) when this treatment was given. It is postulated that intrathecally administered HTIG is more efficient than intramuscular injections in preventing toxin binding to neurons.

Penicillin G is the most effective antibiotic for inhibiting further growth of the organisms; dirty wounds should be debrided and cleaned. Tracheostomy should be performed to assure adequate ventilation. Sedatives, muscular relaxants, and anticonvulsants are given to combat the generalized spasms and convulsions. Paraldehyde, phenytoin, and diazepam should be given in sufficient dosage to prevent muscular spasms and convulsions. In severe cases, curarization may be necessary with use of a positive pressure respirator. Anticoagulation with heparin should then be considered because the risk of pulmonary embolism is high in curarized patients.

In prophylactic treatment, tetanus toxoid or 1,500 units of HTIG should be injected in all patients with perforating or contaminated wounds. Children, farmers, and all military personnel should be actively immunized by the injection of toxoid.

Botulism

Botulism is a poisoning by a toxin elaborated by Clostridium botulinum, an organism widely distributed in soil. Botulinum toxin impairs release of acetylcholine at all peripheral synapses, with resultant weakness of striated and smooth muscles.

Etiology and Pathology. The growth of botulinum organisms is inhibited by other more common bacteria. Methods of processing canned food, which kill common bacteria, but not the more resistant Clostridium spores, favor the germination and growth of botulinum organisms. Classic botulism is caused by toxin ingested after being produced in inadequately sterilized canned food. Infantile botulism, however, is caused by toxin that is produced by organisms growing in the intestine. It is believed that the bacterial flora in the intestinal tracts of some infants less than one year of age do not inhibit the growth of the organisms as effectively as the flora of older children and adults.

Six immunologic types of Clostridium botulinum have been identified. Human botulism usually results from toxin produced by types A, B, and E. Types A and B botulism follow the eating of inadequately processed vegetables or meat; the same types have been implicated in infantile botulism. Type E is associated with fish and marine mammal products.

The toxin is thermolabile and is easily destroyed by heat. Classic botulism occurs when the preserved food is served uncooked and the rancid taste obscured by acid dressings.

No significant pathologic changes occur in the nervous system; there is no good evidence that the toxin can cross the blood-brain barrier. It acts at all peripheral cholinergic synapses and, in high doses, at peripheral adrenergic synapses as well.

Symptoms and Signs. The symptoms of poisoning by the toxin appear 12 to 48 hours after the ingestion of contaminated food and may or may not be preceded by nausea, vomiting, or diarrhea. The initial symptom is usually difficulty in convergence of the eyes. This is soon followed by ptosis and paralysis of the extraocular muscles. The pupils are dilated and may not react to light. The ocular symptoms are followed by weakness of the jaw muscles, dysphagia, and dysarthria. The weakness spreads to involve muscles of the trunk and limbs. The smooth muscle of the intestines and bladder is occasionally affected, with resulting constipation and retention of urine. Mental faculties are usually preserved, but convulsions and coma may develop terminally. The results of the examination of the blood and CSF are normal. In the severe cases, the presenting symptoms may be those of cardiac and respiratory failure.

Infantile botulism occurs in the first year of life, with a peak incidence at two to four months of age. A period of constipation of about three days is followed by the acute onset of hypotonia, weakness, dysphagia, poor sucking, and ptosis. It is estimated that 5% of cases of sudden infant death syndrome are due to botulism, although the true frequency in unknown.

Diagnosis. The diagnosis is not difficult when several members of one household are affected or if samples of the contaminated food can be obtained for testing. Bulbar palsy in acute anterior poliomyelitis can be excluded by the normal CSF. Myasthenia gravis may be simulated, especially if the pupils are not clearly affected in a sporadic case of botulism. In myasthenia gravis, there is a decremental EMG response to repetitive stimulation of nerve, but in botulism there is an increasing response that resembles the Eaton-Lambert syndrome.

Course. The course depends on the amount of toxin absorbed from the gut. The symptoms are mild and recovery is complete if only a small amount is absorbed. When large amounts are absorbed, death usually occurs within four to eight days from circulatory failure, respiratory paralysis, or the development of pulmonary complications.

Treatment. Classic botulism can be prevented by taking proper precautions in the preparation of canned foods and discarding (without sampling) any canned food with a rancid odor in which gas has formed. The toxin is destroyed by cooking. There are no established means of preventing infant botulism, although the ingestion of honey occurred in about 30% of recorded cases prior to the onset of symptoms.

Patients who have been poisoned by botulinum toxin should be given botulinum antitoxin in dosage of 20,000 to 40,000 units two or three times daily. The antitoxin commercially available in this country is bivalent (type A and B). Attempts should be made to obtain type E or a trivalent antitoxin if fish is suspected as the source of the toxin. The stomach should be washed and the gastrointestinal tract cleansed as thoroughly as possible by enemas and cathartics not containing magnesium. The patient should be given artificial respiration if there is any embarrassment of respiration. Feedings should be given through a nasal tube. Although the symptoms of botulism are similar to those of myasthenia gravis, neostigmine is of no value in the treatment of botulism. Some beneficial results have been reported with the use of guanidine hydrochloride, but the evidence is conflicting and guanidine is hazardous.

References

Arnon SS. Infant botulism. Annu Rev Med 1980; 31:541–560.

Brown LW: Differential diagnosis of infant botulism. Rev Inf Dis 1979; 1:625–630.

Cherington M. Botulism: 10-year experience. Arch Neurol 1974; 30:432–437.

Cole L. Treatment of tetanus. Lancet 1969; 1:1017–1019.

Cornblath DR, Sladky JT. Sumner AJ. Clinical electrophysiology of infantile botulism. Muscle Nerve 1983; 6:448–452.

Gupta PA, Kapoor R, Goyal S, Batra VK, Jain BK. Intrathecal human immune tetanus immunoglobulin in early tetanus. Lancet 1980; 2:439–440.

La Force FM, Young LS, Bennett JV. Tetanus in the United States (1965–1966). Epidemiological and clinical features. N Engl J Med 1969; 280:569–574.

Sanchez-Longo LP, Schlezinger NS. Cephalic tetanus. Neurology 1955; 5:381–389.

Sellin LC. Botulism—an update. Milit Med 1984; 149:12–16.

24. REYE SYNDROME
Darryl C. DeVivo

In 1963, Reye and co-workers reported clinical and pathologic observations in 21 children with encephalopathy and fatty changes in the viscera. Since then, the number of reported cases has increased all over the world. The disorder also affects infants and adults, although rarely. White children in suburban or rural environments seem to be more susceptible than urban black children.

Reye syndrome is usually associated with influenza B epidemics or sporadic cases of influenza A and varicella. Characteristically, the encephalopathy develops 4 to 7 days after the onset of the viral illness. It is invariably heralded by recurrent vomiting, and often followed by somnolence, confusion, delirium, or coma. These children have frequently been treated with antiemetics, aspirin, or acetaminophen. Epidemiologic studies have shown a statistical association between the ingestion of aspirin-containing compounds and the development of Reye syndrome. These studies, however, do not prove a causal relationship.

Pathologic and metabolic observations suggest a primary injury to mitochondria throughout the body with prominent involvement of the liver and brain. The primary injury may be compounded by many associated insults including hyperpyrexia, hypoglycemia, hypoxia, hyperammonemia, free fatty acidemia, systemic hypotension, and intracranial hypertension. An appropriate clinical history, characteristic neurologic findings, absence of any other explanation for the encephalopathy, and distinctive laboratory abnormalities are usually sufficient for establishing the diagnosis. Important laboratory abnormalities include elevations of blood ammonia, lactate, and serum transaminases, and prolongation of the prothrombin time. CSF examination and CT scans are normal. The EEG is diffusely abnormal, occasionally displaying paroxysmal epileptiform activity in the more severely ill patients.

Many other conditions can present a similar clinical picture. The differential diagnosis includes bacterial meningitis, viral encephalitis, drug intoxication (e.g., aspirin, valproic acid, and amphetamines), and other metabolic disorders (e.g., inherited defects of fatty acid oxidation, branched-chain amino acid metabolism, and the Krebs-Henseleit urea cycle). Recurrent attacks of a Reye-like syndrome imply an underlying metabolic disorder. The current mainstay of treatment is intensive supportive care. Most patients recover completely within a week after onset.

References

Arcinue EL, Mitchell RA, Sarnaik AP, et al: The metabolic course of Reye's syndrome: distinction between survivors and nonsurvivors. Neurology 1986; 36:435–438.

Brown RE, Forman DT: The biochemistry of Reye's syndrome. CRC Crit Rev Clin Lab Sci 1982; 17:247–297.

Consensus Conference. Diagnosis and treatment of Reye's syndrome. JAMA 1981; 246:2441–2444.

Corey L, Rubin RJ, Hattwick MAW, Noble GR, Cassidy E. A nationwide outbreak of Reye's syndrome. Its epidemiologic relationship of influenza B. Am J Med 1976; 61:615–625.

DeVivo DC. How common is Reye's syndrome? N Engl J Med 1983; 309:179–180.

DeVivo DC, Keating JP. Reye's syndrome. Adv Pediatr 1976; 22:175–229.

Haymond MW, Karl I, Keating JP, De Vivo DC. Metabolic response to hypertonic glucose administration in Reye syndrome. Ann Neurol 1978; 3:207–215.

Heubi JE, Daughterty CC, Partin JS, et al: Grade I Reye's syndrome outcome and predictors of progression to deeper coma grades. N Engl J Med 1984; 311:1539–1542.

Hurwitz ES, Barrett MJ, Bregman D, et al: Public health service study on Reye's syndrome and medications: report of the pilot phase. N Engl J Med 1985; 313:849–857.

Huttenlocher PR. Reye's syndrome: relation of outcome to therapy. J. Pediatr 1972; 80:845–850.

Huttenlocher PR, Trauner DA. Reye's syndrome in infancy. Pediatrics 1978; 62:84–90.

Lyon G, Dodge PR, Adams RD. The acute encephalopathies of obscure origin in infants and children. Brain 1961; 84:680–708.

Partin JS, McAdams AJ, Partin JC, Schubert WK, McLaurin RL. Brain ultrastructure in Reye's disease. II. Acute injury and recovery process in three children. J Neuropathol Exp Neurol 1978; 37:796–819.

Partin JC, Schubert WK, Partin JS. Mitochondrial ultrastructure in Reye's syndrome (encephalopathy and fatty degeneration of the viscera). N Engl J Med 1971; 285:1339–1343.

Pranzatelli MR, De Vivo DC: The pharmacology of Reye syndrome. Clinical Neuropharmacology 1987; 10:96–125.

Reye BDK, Morgan G, Baral J. Encephalopathy and fatty degeneration of the viscera: a disease entity in childhood. Lancet 1963; 2:749–752.

Shaywitz SE, Cohen PM, Cohen DJ, Mikkelson E, Morowitz G, Shaywitz BA. Long-term consequences of Reye's syndrome: A sibling-matched, controlled study of neurologic, cognitive, academic, and psychiatric function. J Pediatr 1982; 100:41–46.

Stanley CA, Hale DE, Coates MP, et al: Medium-chain acyl-CoA dehydrogenase deficiency in children with nonketotic hypoglycemia and low carnitine levels. Pediatr Res 1983; 17:877–884.

Sullivan-Bolyai, Corey L. Epidemiology of Reye's syndrome. Epidemiol Rev 1981; 3:1–26.

Trauner DA, Stockard JJ, Sweetman L. EEG correlations with biochemical abnormalities in Reye syndrome. Arch Neurol 1977; 34:116–118.

Chapter III

Vascular Diseases

25. ETIOLOGY AND PATHOGENESIS
James F. Toole

The 1500 g of neurons and glia that constitute the adult brain require an uninterrupted supply of about 150 g of glucose and 72 L of oxygen every 24 hours. The brain does not store these substances and can function for only a few minutes if either the oxygen or glucose content is reduced below critical levels. The arterial blood supplies these and other nutrients; the venous blood removes heat and waste products (especially CO_2 and lactate) and serves as a transport system for neurohormones. In the resting state, each cardiac contraction thrusts about 70 mL of blood into the ascending aorta; 10 to 15 mL is allocated to the brain. Every minute, about 350 mL flows through each internal carotid artery and about 100 to 200 mL through the vertebral-basilar system.

Vascular disease affecting the brain may originate in any part of this system (e.g., heart, aortocervical or intracranial arteries, microcirculation, veins, or in the blood itself).

Anatomy

Each cerebral hemisphere is supplied by one internal carotid artery, which originates from the common carotid artery, usually behind the angle of the jaw, and ascends posterolaterally to the pharynx to enter the cranium through the carotid canal. The artery then travels intradurally beside the sella turcica and within the cavernous sinus. Above the sella, the ophthalmic and anterior choroidal arteries arise before the carotid terminates by dividing into the anterior and middle cerebral arteries. The carotid system therefore supplies the optic nerves and retina plus the anterior portion of the cerebral hemisphere, which comprises the frontal, parietal, and anterior temporal lobes. In nearly 5% of adults,

the posterior cerebral artery also arises directly from the internal carotid artery so that the entire cerebral hemisphere (including the occipital lobe) is supplied by the internal carotid artery.

The two internal carotid systems function independently; however, they are connected by the anterior communicating artery. In contrast, the vertebral-basilar system functions as a unit. Each vertebral artery arises in the supraclavicular space from the subclavian artery and ascends in a bony canal in the cervical vertebrae to enter the skull through the foramen magnum. There, each gives off the posterior inferior cerebellar artery and the anterior and posterior spinal arteries. At the pontomedullary junction, the two vertebral arteries join to form the basilar artery, which has three groups of branches: paramedian, short, and long circumferential arteries (Fig. 25–1). At the midbrain level, the basilar artery ends by dividing into the two posterior cerebral arteries. The vertebral-basilar system normally nourishes the cervical cord, brain stem, cerebellum, thalamus, auditory and vestibular functions of the inner ear, and usually the medial temporal and occipital lobes of the cerebral hemisphere.

Three types of anastomoses between the carotid and vertebral-basilar systems help to ensure an even distribution of blood. The first connects the external carotid with the vertebral arteries; the second is external to the internal carotid through the orbit; and the third is entirely intracranial and consists of the circle of Willis, which connects the two carotid systems through the anterior communicating artery and the vertebral-basilar and carotid systems through the posterior communicating arteries. Pial anastomoses over the surface of the brain and choroidal collateral arteries in the ventricles complete the network of collateral circulation.

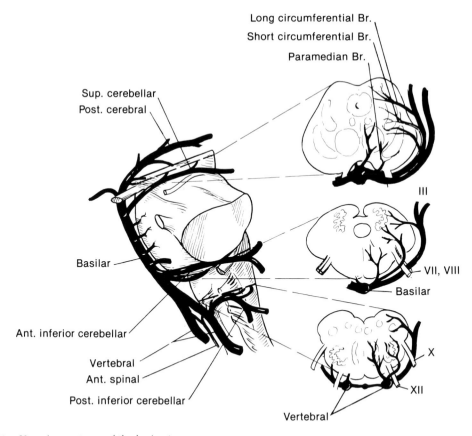

Long circumferential Br.
Short circumferential Br.
Paramedian Br.

Sup. cerebellar
Post. cerebral

III

Basilar

VII, VIII

Basilar

Ant. inferior cerebellar

X

Vertebral
Ant. spinal

XII

Post. inferior cerebellar

Vertebral

Fig. 25–1. Vascular anatomy of the brain stem.

As a group, these rich anastomotic networks protect the brain by providing alternate routes to circumvent obstructions in the main arteries: obstruction of the internal carotid artery in the neck may be bypassed by a collateral path from the external carotid to the ophthalmic to the internal carotid circulation; segmental obstruction of a vertebral artery can be bypassed by interconnections between the external carotid and distal vertebral anastomoses; occlusion of a branch of a middle cerebral artery may be symptomless if there are adequate interconnections with branches of the posterior and anterior cerebral arteries. On the other hand, the small arteries and arterioles (100 μm or less in diameter) that spring from the surface arteries and penetrate the brain parenchyma have few interconnections and therefore function as end arteries; obstruction of one of these small vessels causes tissue ischemia or infarction.

A well-developed muscular coat gives the major cerebral arteries the capacity to constrict in response to increased blood pressure and to dilate with hypotension, helping to assure constant perfusion pressure and blood flow through the capillary networks. In chronic hypertension, however, this muscular coat thickens and arteriolar caliber becomes fixed, resulting in loss of autoregulation.

The capillaries are near the cell bodies of neurons and are joined to the nerve cells by protoplasmic astrocytes that are interposed between the two structures, with one extension wrapped around the capillary and another applied to the neuron. Astrocytes regulate the flow of nutrients and metabolites between the cell body and capillary blood.

In this vascular system only the arterioles, which are exquisitely sensitive to changes in Pa_{CO_2} and Pa_{O_2}, respond to pharmacologic agents. When the partial pressure of CO_2 increases, the arterioles dilate and cerebral blood flow increases. When CO_2 tension is reduced, the arterioles constrict and blood flow is reduced. Changes in the partial pressure of O_2 have the opposite effect. Focal cerebral activity, such as occurs in moving a limb, is accompanied by accelerated metabolism in the appropriate region, which is accommodated by an increase in the local blood flow. In cerebrosvascular disease, this compensatory mechanism may be destroyed.

Etiology and Pathology

ISCHEMIA AND INFARCTION

When blood supply is interrupted for 30 seconds, brain metabolism is altered. After 1 minute, neuronal function may cease. After 5 minutes, anoxia initiates a chain of events that may culminate in cerebral infarction; however, if oxygenated blood flow is restored quickly enough, the damage may be reversible.

Whether a permanent vascular lesion actually causes symptoms and signs depends on its location and the collateral arteries with which a person is born or that develop over time to circumvent it. Their adequacy depends on many factors, especially the rate of development of the obstruction.

Ischemia has many causes, including arterial occlusion by atherosclerosis, thrombus or embolus, systemic hypotension, or by constituents of the blood that are too viscous to be propelled through the system (as in polycythemia, dysproteinemia, or thrombocytosis).

Meningitis or arteritis caused by tuberculosis, syphilis, fibromuscular dysplasia, polyarteritis nodosa, and occlusion of the veins that drain the brain may also cause cerebral infarction. Aortocranial arteries may be occluded by dissecting hematoma, and the vertebral arteries may be compressed by arthritis of the cervical spine. Cerebral arterial spasm is a debated cause of ischemia but is incriminated in migraine and may be a major complication of subarachnoid hemorrhage.

The most common causes of infarction are

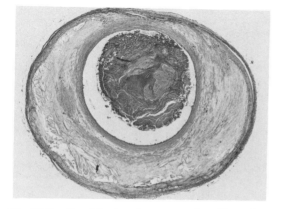

Fig. 25–2. Carotid artery in cross section. Note atherosclerotic changes and intraluminal thrombus.

the end stages of atherosclerosis and hypertension. Atherothrombosis is presumed to be due to clotting at the site of an ulcerated plaque in the vessel wall (Fig. 25–2). The clot propagates until it occludes the lumen or sheds microemboli that plug distal arteries. In one autopsy series of 142 patients who died soon after cerebral infarction, Moossy found only 78 (55%) with intracranial thrombosis consistent with the clinical picture; the others were presumably due to emboli that had fragmented and lysed before death. Arteriosclerotic plaques may develop at any point along the carotid artery and the vertebral-basilar system, but the most common sites are those with a predilection to atherosclerosis (e.g., the bifurcation of the common carotid artery into the external and internal carotid arteries, the origins of the middle and anterior cerebral arteries, and the origins of the vertebral from the subclavian arteries).

Of 161 white patients with TIAs, only 14% had normal arteriograms, 8% had primarily intracranial lesions, and 78% primarily extracranial atherosclerotic plaques. The proportion of extra- and intracranial vascular pathologic conditions causing stroke varies among racial groups. In white people, extracranial lesions are frequent; in blacks and Asians, intracranial lesions are common and extracranial lesions are infrequent. The relationship of blood pressure, occupation, diet, and socioeconomic factors in causing these differences has yet to be adequately explained.

Pathology. The following steps occur in the evolution of an infarct: (1) local vasodilatation and (2) stasis of the blood column with segmentation of the red cells are followed by (3) edema, and (4) necrosis of brain tissue (Fig. 25–3). Although most infarcts are pale, a "red infarct" is occasionally caused by local hemorrhage into the necrotic tissue. Gray matter tends to have petechial hemorrhages and white matter tends to have pale (ischemic) infarction. Hemorrhagic infarct probably occurs when the occluding clot or embolus breaks up and migrates, restoring flow through the infarcted area. If the interruption is sufficiently prolonged and infarction results, the brain tissue first softens, then liquefies; a cavity finally forms when the debris is removed by the phagocytic microglia. In attempts to fill the defect, astroglia in the surrounding brain proliferate and invade the softened area, and new capillaries are formed. If the area is large, the cavity may collapse or become the site for the formation of small

Table 25–1.   Atherosclerosis in Cervicocranial Arteries of 161 White Patients with TIAs

Artery Involved	Percentage of Patients		
	Stenosis	Occlusion	Both
Brachiocephalic	1		
One carotid	31	6	
Two carotids	11	1	
One vertebral	5	3	
Two vertebrals			2
One subclavian	3	2	
Carotid and vertebral	2	16	
Carotid and subclavian	0	2	
Three-artery disease			10
Four-artery disease			5

Fourteen percent had normal findings. Atherosclerosis was primarily extracranial in 78% and primarily intracranial in 8%. (From Janeway R, Toole J. Trans Am Neurol Assoc 1972; 97:137.)

multilocular cysts that are filled with clear fluid.

Some patients have multiple infarcts that may cause dementia. Small cystic infarcts, or lacunas, are the most common form of infarction. They usually occur in the basal ganglia, internal capsule, and basis pontis, and less commonly in the centrum semiovale or cerebellum (Fig. 25–4). Lacunas result from occlusions of perforating arteries damaged by long-standing hypertension or diabetes mellitus.

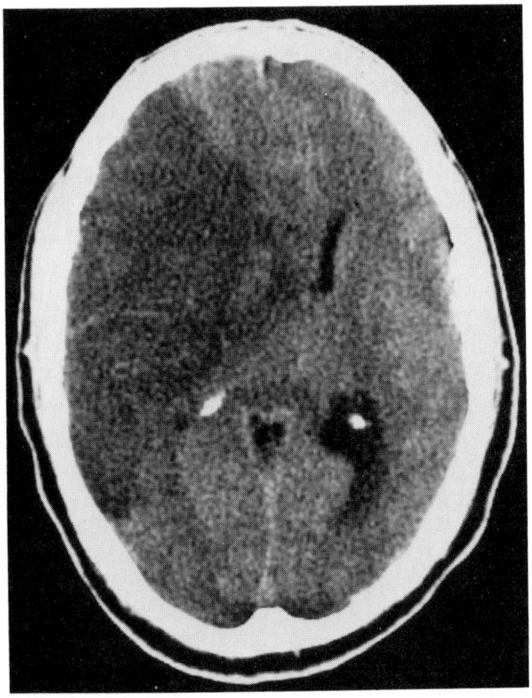

EMBOLISM

The term cerebral embolism describes occlusion of an artery by a fragment of clotted blood, neoplasm, fat, air, or other foreign

Fig. 25–3. Acute infarct, right MCA distribution. Non-contrast axial CT shows right frontal and temporal hypodensity including cortex as well as edema producing ventricular effacement and midline shift. Right ACA and PCA territories are spared. Similar appearance could result from occlusion of right internal carotid artery with competent circle of Willis. (Courtesy of Drs. J.A. Bello and S.K. Hilal.)

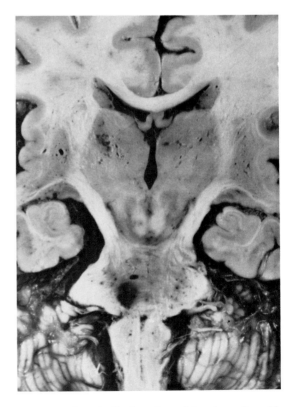

Fig. 25–4. Longitudinal cut through basal ganglia, midbrain pons, and brain stem, showing multiple lacunar infarctions and a small pontine hemorrhage.

substance. The course of the disorder is similar to that described for infarction, except that an element of vasospasm may be superimposed. Most emboli are sterile, but some may contain bacteria if emboli arise secondary to subacute or acute bacterial endocarditis or if there is a lung infection. Infected emboli may result in arteritis with or without mycotic aneurysm formation, brain abscess, localized encephalitis, or meningitis.

Air embolism usually follows injuries or surgical procedures involving the lungs, the dural sinuses, or jugular veins. It may also be caused by the release of nitrogen bubbles into the general circulation after a rapid reduction in barometric pressure. Fat embolism is rare and almost always arises from a bone fracture.

In children, cerebral emboli are commonly associated with valvular heart disease (rheumatic or congenital) and superimposed endocarditis. In adults, atrial fibrillation or myocardial infarction is the usual cause. Thrombi in the left atrium may dislodge during fibrillation or after cardioversion has restored more forceful and rhythmic contractions. After myocardial infarction, a part of the clot that forms on the necrotic endocardium may break off. Emboli may be asymptomatic or may cause TIAs or stroke, depending on how rapidly blood flow is reconstituted. Emboli from the heart are often multiple and one to the brain may be preceded or followed by others that lodge in other arteries of the body.

Recurrent emboli in the lungs may cause pulmonary hypertension with a resultant inversion of the pressure gradient across the foramen ovale. As a consequence, subsequent emboli may traverse the foramen to the left side of the heart and then to the brain—a "paradoxical" embolus. Other rare causes of cerebral embolism are atrial myxoma, marantic endocarditis, and prolapse of the mitral valve.

The most common symptom of cerebral embolism is a TIA, which results from microemboli from atherosclerotic plaques on the aortocranial arteries. These plaques form a nidus for clots and may break off or ulcerate, discharging their contents of cholesterol and calcium into the bloodstream (Fig. 25–5).

Pathology. The arterial bed in which the embolus lodges constricts and may go into spasm. Tissue becomes ischemic, resulting in infarction unless the embolus fragments and migrates further. If the embolus lyses, blood flow is restored and a hemorrhagic infarction

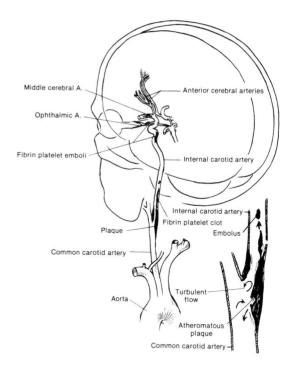

Fig. 25–5. Atheromatous plaques at the carotid bifurcation may be a source of retinal and cerebral microemboli.

may follow. Except when an embolus contains bacteria, the pathologic changes in the brain are the same as those of infarcts due to atherothrombosis. Cerebral emboli are often multiple and may be associated with emboli from the heart to other parts of the body.

INTRACEREBRAL HEMORRHAGE

Hemorrhage may result from rupture of a vessel anywhere within the cranial cavity. Intracranial hemorrhages are classified according to location (e.g., extradural, subdural, subarachnoid, parenchymatous, intraventricular), according to the nature of the ruptured vessel or vessels (e.g., arterial, capillary, venous), or according to cause (e.g., traumatic, coagulation defect, degeneration, hypertension, infection). Laceration of the middle meningeal artery or vein causes extradural hematoma, and many subdural hematomas result from traumatic rupture of veins that traverse the subdural space. The most frequent ruptures in hypertensive patients result from aneurysmal dilatations of intracerebral arterioles. These microaneurysms are most commonly found in the basal ganglia, particularly the putamen and thalamus.

Hemorrhage is also caused by arteriovenous malformations, amyloid angiopathy, blood dyscrasias, coagulation disorders, neoplasms, or infections that damage cerebral vessels, toxins, or therapeutic administration of anticoagulants. In blood dyscrasias (e.g., acute leukemia, aplastic anemia, polycythemia, thrombocytopenic purpura, scurvy), the hemorrhages may be multiple and of varied size.

Rupture of a vessel may follow softening of the surrounding brain tissue. Moreover, it is probable that changes in blood pressure in the vessels (from exertion, emotional excitement, or a valsalva maneuver) can be contributory factors.

Pathology. About half of hypertensive intracerebral hemorrhages are fatal. At autopsy, it is found that the blood has destroyed or displaced brain tissue. If the hemorrhage is large, it is often impossible to find the ruptured vessel. The most common site for a single hemorrhage is the basal ganglia; such hemorrhages usually originate in the thalamus or the lenticular nucleus and extend to involve the internal capsule (Fig. 25–6). The hemorrhage sometimes ruptures into the lateral ventricle and spreads through the ventricular system into the subarachnoid space; these are almost always fatal. Bleeding into one lobe of the cerebral hemisphere or cerebellum usually remains confined within brain parenchyma.

If the patient survives an intracerebral hemorrhage, blood and necrotic brain tissue are removed by phagocytes. The destroyed brain tissue is partially replaced by connective tissue, glia, and newly formed blood vessels, leaving a shrunken, fluid-filled cavity. Less frequently, the blood clot is treated as a foreign body, calcifies, and is surrounded by a thick glial membrane.

Of 113 autopsied cases of hypertensive cerebral hemorrhage, Aring and Merritt found only five that showed two or more hemorrhages; in the remaining cases, a single hemorrhage was present in the following locations: basal ganglia, 70; lobes of the cerebral hemisphere, 32; brain stem, four; and cerebellum, two. These figures are similar to those reported by other authors, except that cerebellar hemorrhages have occurred in up to 10% of patients in some series. In only seven of the 113 cases was there evidence of a previous cerebral vascular lesion. In these, the old lesions appeared softened due to infarction.

The advent of CT revolutionized the diagnosis and management of cerebral hemorrhage. It is extraordinarily accurate in pin-

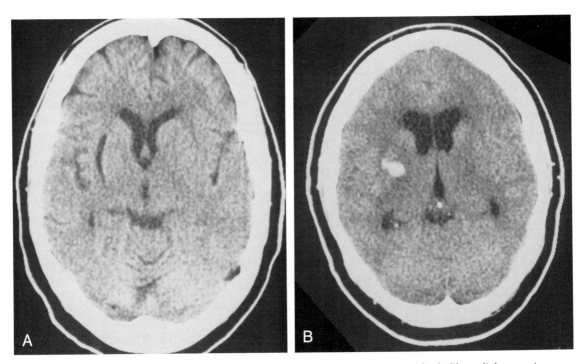

Fig. 25–6. *A.* Hypertensive hemorrhage, chronic phase. Noncontrast axial CT reveals slit-like radiolucency in area of right putamen. *B.* Acute hypertensive basal ganglia hemorrhage. Axial noncontrast CT shows region of hyperdensity within right putamen. (Courtesy of Drs. J.A. Bello and S.K. Hilal.)

pointing the location of a hemorrhage because of the increased density of fresh blood.

SUBARACHNOID HEMORRHAGE

Subarachnoid hemorrhage occurs when blood leaks into the subarachnoid space. It is considered "primary" when the ruptured vessel normally traverses the subarachnoid space, such as arterial aneurysms of the circle of Willis. Secondary subarachnoid hemorrhage occurs when a hemorrhage of brain parenchyma ruptures through the subarachnoid space.

Clinical Considerations

Cerebrovascular disease is the most common neurologic disorder of adults in the United States. Stroke is overwhelmingly the result of atherosclerosis, hypertension, or both, and it kills 175,000 and disables 200,000 people in the United States each year. At any one time, 2 million Americans are estimated to be victims of stroke, and about 25% of these are younger than 65. Cerebral arteriosclerosis and associated neurologic disability are responsible for about 15% of admissions to institutions for chronic care in the United States.

The frequency of symptomatic cerebrovascular disease depends in part on age, gender, and geographic location and whether the data were gathered clinically, by CT, or at autopsy. It is therefore misleading to be too specific about the incidence of the several forms. In the prospective Framingham study of 35,000 people, 59% of strokes were due to atherothrombosis, 15% to hemorrhage, and 14% to embolism. TIAs accounted for 0.9% of strokes and other causes accounted for 3%. The mix of different forms of cerebrovascular disease in a hospital differs from that in a general population because hospital data depend on the population served and whether it is a general or referral hospital.

Although cerebrovascular disorders may occur at any age, at any time, in either sex, and in all races, each factor affects the incidence and prevalence of the various types of cerebrovascular disease. Except for embolic causes, stroke is uncommon before age 40. The incidence of cerebral infarction is greatest between ages 60 and 80. Cerebral hemorrhage occurs most frequently among people between the ages of 40 and 60. The incidence of cerebral embolism and primary subarachnoid hemorrhage is more evenly spread, but

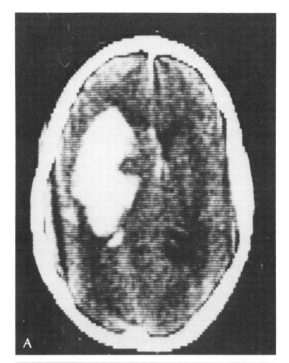

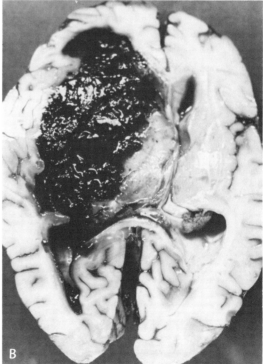

Fig. 25–7. Hypertensive basal ganglia hemorrhage. *A.* On CT the hemorrhage has ruptured into and compresses the ipsilateral ventricle (slit-like white area medial to the hemorrhage). *B.* Cut brain of same patient.

is highest in the fifth and sixth decades of life (Fig. 25–8).

THE STROKE-PRONE PROFILE

Cerebral infarction is not an accidental occurrence as the commonly used but poorly chosen term "cerebral vascular accident" implies; rather it is the end result of a chain of events set in motion decades before. Epidemiologic investigations are now identifying susceptible persons and the factors that predispose them to stroke. Known components of the stroke-prone profile are the following:

Age. Stroke more than doubles in incidence in each successive decade after age 55. Because the elderly population is enlarging, there will likely be increased prevalence of stroke. However, even with advances in detection and prevention of stroke, almost 25% occur before age 65. In children the incidence is 2.3 cases per 100,000 population/year. Further, the probable etiology of stroke changes with the age of the patient (Fig. 25–8).

Gender. Brain infarcts and stroke occur some 30% more frequently in men than women; the gender differential is even greater before age 65.

Race. In the United States, stroke is the third most frequent cause of death after heart disease and cancer. Most often strokes are caused by atherosclerotic changes rather than by hemorrhage. An exception occurs in middle aged black women, in whom hemorrhage leads the list. In Japan, stroke is the leading cause of death in adults and hemorrhage is more common than atherothrombosis.

Transient Ischemic Attack. TIAs precede cerebral infarction in about half or fewer cases. After a single TIA or amaurosis fugax, some 10 to 20% of individuals have a cerebral infarct within the year, most within a month.

Hypertension. Elevated systolic or diastolic blood pressure (or both) accelerate the progression of atherosclerosis and thereby predispose to atherothrombotic infarction. Further, sustained hypertension affects the cerebral arterioles, predisposing to parenchymatous hemorrhage.

Cardiovascular Disease. This includes congenital anomalies and valvular disease, which can be a nidus for cerebral embolism, cardiomyopathies, and myocardial infarction. The latter may cause pump failure or thrombus adherent to the damaged left ventricle, which can embolize. Coronary artery disease, with or without angina pectoris, signals more generalized atherosclerosis. There is increasing evidence that preclinical or symptomatic disease in coronary vessels and in carotid circulation or the legs is often accompanied by atherosclerosis in another site. Some manifestations of coronary artery disease are EKG change, angina pectoris, myocardial infarction, and, in the legs, intermittent claudication or Leriche syndrome.

Cardiac Dysrhythmia. Atrial fibrillation, with or without valvular disease, is associated with increased risk of cerebral embolism.

Other accepted risk factors are:
Impaired glucose utilization
Elevated blood lipids
Tobacco abuse
Alcohol abuse
Street drug abuse
Erythrocytosis
Personality type with chronic stress

PREMONITORY AND INITIAL SYMPTOMS

Although the several types of cerebrovascular disease differ in mode of onset, symptoms, and course, clinical data alone often fail to identify the origin in an individual patient. Thus, the symptoms of the various underlying causes of stroke will be discussed together.

Patients with cerebrovascular disease are usually asymptomatic until the disorder reaches an advanced stage. Premonitory symptoms are infrequent. When they occur, they may be so nonspecific that they are not

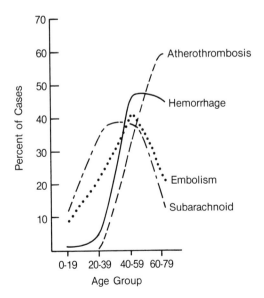

Fig. 25–8. Cerebrovascular disorders by age groups. (Modified from Aring CD, Merritt HH. Arch Intern Med 1935; 46:435, and McDonald CA, Korb M. Arch Neurol Psychiatr 1939; 42:298.)

recognized as signs of an impending stroke. Headache, dizziness, drowsiness, and confusion may be present for minutes or hours before the ictus.

Focal premonitory symptoms, when present, usually presage infarction rather than hemorrhage. In about 20% of cases, TIAs precede the permanent deficit. In most, these transient attacks are probably due to microemboli from an atherothrombotic plaque in the carotid or vertebral-basilar arteries. An aneurysm is a cul-de-sac in which blood can stagnate to form a clot that may embolize. Also, the aneurysm may enlarge to compress adjacent structures such as cranial nerves. Emboli may originate from a clot in the stump of an occluded artery, such as an internal carotid artery in the neck, then course through the external carotid circulation to the eye; they may go from the intracranial end of an occluded internal carotid artery to its distal branches.

The following list outlines the signs and symptoms of stroke:

I. CAROTID ARTERY DISEASE
   1. Contralateral weakness or numbness
   2. Dysphasia, dyspraxia, and confusion, if the dominant hemisphere is involved
   3. Transient blurring of vision or blindness in the ipsilateral eye (amaurosis fugax)
   4. Homonymous visual field loss
   5. Ipsilateral headache

II. VERTEBRAL-BASILAR ARTERY DISEASE
   1. With involvement of the upper spinal cord and lower brain stem (anterior spinal and vertebral arteries)
      a. Weakness or paralysis of the legs or of all four extremities (drop attacks) with preservation of consciousness
      b. Vertigo
      c. Ataxia (unsteady gait or clumsy limb movements)
      d. Dysarthria and dysphagia
      e. Unilateral or bilateral loss of sensation
      f. Occipital headache
   2. With involvement of the labyrinth and cochlea (internal auditory artery):
      a. Vertigo, nausea, and vomiting
      b. Tinnitus
      c. Acute onset of unilateral deafness

   3. With involvement of the pons and midbrain (basilar artery):
      a. Occipital headache
      b. Light-headedness or syncope
      c. Mental confusion or coma
      d. Diplopia
      e. Unilateral or bilateral numbness or weakness
   4. With involvement of the cerebral hemispheres, occipital lobes, and temporoparietal areas (posterior cerebral artery):
      a. Homonymous visual field loss
      b. Blindness, cortical type
      c. Temporal lobe seizures
      d. Transient global amnesia

In all cases, the following information should be obtained by asking specific questions of the patient or the patient's family. This helps to identify premonitory events or risk factors:

   1. *Seizures.* If known, a detailed history and description of the attacks must be obtained.
   2. *Cardiac irregularities.* Does the heart beat irregularly or slowly during attacks (suggesting Stokes-Adams' syndrome)? Has the patient had palpitations or syncope? Does the patient's face turn pale during the episode, suggesting hypotension?
   3. *Headaches.* What are their duration, frequency, type, severity, site, and radiation? What aggravates or relieves them?
   4. *Visual disturbances.* Are they unilateral or bilateral, transient or persistent? Is visual loss partial or total? does the patient have diplopia, visual hallucinations, or scotomata?
   5. *Auditory disturbances.* Does the patient have deafness or tinnitus?
   6. *Mental changes.* Have members of the family noted changes in the patient's cerebration, emotional reactions, or memory?
   7. *Precipitating factors.* Are any of the symptoms affected by a change in head position or body posture, or by arm exercise? Is there a history of head injury, suggesting the possibility of a subdural hematoma?
   8. *Predisposing factors.* Does the patient have hypertension, heart disease, or diabetes? Does the patient smoke? Is the patient using any medication that

could contribute to the problem (especially oral contraceptives, hypotensive drugs, anticoagulants, or alcohol)?

9. *Past history.* Have there been similar attacks in the past, especially minor or transient neurologic disturbances that cleared spontaneously?

10. *Family history.* Have blood relatives had strokes, seizures, hypertension, or heart attacks?

ONSET

The word "stroke" is appropriate because the initiation of a cerebrovascular episode is almost always sudden. Because the neurologic symptoms and signs are related to the site of the lesion, they are discussed later in connection with the syndromes of specific cerebral arteries.

There are only two types of stroke, hemorrhage and infarction. However, each of these generic categories has a myriad of causes. Rarely, cerebral infarction or hemorrhage may occur without apparent manifestations (perhaps because patient and family are unaware of minor symptoms or because a so-called "silent area" of brain has been affected). However, the cardinal feature of stroke is the sudden onset of neurologic symptoms. The abrupt development of neurologic abnormality marks it as a probable vascular event. Although the symptoms and signs are related to the location of the lesion, they give no clue to its cause. Thus, the classic evidence of stroke is rapid onset of loss of normal function, reaching maximum severity within an hour. Gradual evolution of symptoms, from a few days to weeks, indicates that the etiology (except for subdural hematoma) is probably not vascular and other causes should be considered.

RESOLUTION

All forms of stroke have characteristically rapid onset, providing few clues to etiology. When headache, vomiting, convulsions, or coma occur, the most likely causes are intracerebral or subarachnoid hemorrhage (Fig. 25–9).

When symptoms subside completely within 24 hours, the episode is considered a transient ischemic attack. This rapid resolution is also characteristic of embolism, which many believe is the etiology of most TIAs. For symptoms that exceed 24 hours, another category, reversible ischemic neurologic deficit

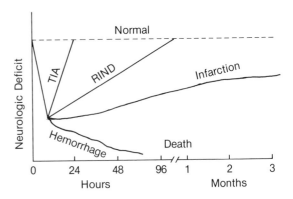

Fig. 25–9. Temporal profiles of signs and symptoms. TIA = transient ischemic attack. RIND = reversible ischemic neurologic deficit.

(RIND), has been proposed to account for protracted symptoms that eventually resolve completely. However, even after TIA or RIND with complete restitution of clinical function, CT or magnetic resonance imaging (MRI) may show a cerebral infarct, leading to a third category called cerebral infarction with transient symptoms (CITS).

Cerebral infarction is recognized clinically when neurologic disorders of sudden onset persist indefinitely and when a nonhemorrhagic lesion is shown by MRI or CT. With increasing use of CT, hemorrhages with clinical phenomena identical to those of ischemia and infarction have been found with some frequency. Because of these CT-identified exceptions to the recognized clinical manifestations and course of cerebrovascular lesions, the nosology of stroke is in a state of flux.

References

Ad Hoc Committee NINCDS. A classification and outline of cerebrovascular diseases. II. Stroke 1975; 6:564.

Aring C, Merritt HH. Differential diagnosis between cerebral hemorrhage and cerebral thrombosis, Arch Intern Med 1935; 56:435–456.

Becker C et al: Community hospital-based stroke programs: North Carolina, Oregon and New York. II: Description of study population. Stroke 1986; 17:285–293.

Davis PH, Dambrosia JM, Schoenberg BS, et al. Risk factors for ischemic stroke. Ann Neurol 1987; 22:319–327.

Homer D, Whisnant JP, Schoenberg BS. Trends in the incidence rates of stroke. Ann Neurol 1987; 22:245–251.

Moossy J. Cerebral atherosclerosis, intracranial and extracranial lesions. In: Minkler J, ed. Pathology of the Nervous System, vol 2. New York: McGraw-Hill, 1971.

Purves MJ. The Physiology of the Cerebral Circulation. New York: Cambridge University Press, 1972.

Toole JF. Cerebrovascular disorders, 3rd ed. New York: Raven Press, 1984.

Waxman SG, Toole JF. Temporal profile resembling TIA in the setting of cerebral infarction. Stroke 1983; 14:433–437.

Weinfeld FD, ed. The National Survey of Stroke. Am Heart Assoc Monograph 75, Stroke 1981; 12.

Whisnant JP. The role of the neurologist in the decline of stroke. Ann Neurol 1983; 14:1–7.

Wolf PA, Dawber TR, Kannel WB. Heart disease as a precursor of stroke. Adv Neurol 1978; 19:567–577.

Wolf PA, Kannel WB, Dawber TR. Prospective investigations: The Framingham study and the epidemiology of stroke. Adv Neurol 1978; 19:107–120.

Yatsu FM, et al. Community hospital-based stroke programs: North Carolina, Oregon and New York. I: Goals, objectives, and data collection procedures. Stroke 1986; 17:276–284.

26. EXAMINATION OF THE PATIENT

James F. Toole

The patient's head and ears must be examined for evidence of injury. The size and reactions of the pupils must be noted and the optic discs and retinal vessels must be examined. Breath odor, character of respiration, stiffness of the neck, temperature, heart rate, and blood pressure should be recorded.

If the hemorrhage is small or if a nonstrategic artery is occluded, there may be no change in vital signs. With a large hemorrhage, however, there may be fever or tachycardia, which, together with rapid respiration, indicate that the vasomotor and thermoregulating centers have been affected.

Because arteriosclerosis and hypertension are the most frequent causes of both intracerebral hemorrhage and intracerebral infarction, it is not surprising that cardiac abnormalities, increased blood pressure, and evidence of sclerosis in peripheral or retinal vessels are common findings. Blood pressure is usually within normal limits in patients with cerebral embolism, but is elevated in most with cerebral hemorrhage or infarction; nevertheless, either disorder may occur in people with normal blood pressure. The average systolic and diastolic pressures are slightly higher in patients with hemorrhage. Hypertension and cardiac enlargement are common in patients with primary subarachnoid hemorrhage after age 40. Atrial fibrillation or clinical signs of cardiac enlargement are present in more than 90% of patients with a cerebral embolus. Cardiac conduction defects and dysrhythmias or acute pulmonary edema occur in some patients with subarachnoid hemorrhage, presumably because of the effects of blood in the subarachnoid space or a sudden surge in intracranial pressure as a direct result of the trauma to the cardioregulation centers.

NEUROLOGIC EXAMINATION

It is of paramount importance to determine whether hemiplegia is present. In a noncooperative patient, this can usually be ascertained by observation of the face and limbs. When one cheek puffs out with each expiration, that side of the face is paralyzed. Paralysis of the limbs can be determined by lifting each one and allowing it to fall; the paralyzed limb falls heavily, while the normal one gradually sinks to the bed. If a patient is in deep coma, however, all limbs may fall heavily. Vigorous stimulation of the soles of the feet by a blunt stick or key causes withdrawal from the stimulus, but a paralyzed limb remains inert unless there is a reflex withdrawal with a Babinski sign.

The type and frequency of pupillary abnormalities after stroke depend on the stage of the disorder, the age of the patient, and other complicating factors, including the instillation of eye drops. If the lesion is in the cortex, the pupils may be of unequal size, the larger one usually being on the side opposite the cortical lesion. A homolateral, dilated, and fixed pupil is seen when a massive infarction or intracerebral hemorrhage has caused impaction of the temporal lobe into the incisura, compressing the third cranial nerve. Gaze palsy or conjugate deviation of the head and eyes together, or of the eyes alone, often follows large cerebral lesions. The gaze deviation is toward the destructive lesion in a hemisphere and away from a brainstem lesion. In irritative lesions, the opposite sequence of events occurs. Deviation of the head and eyes tends to disappear as the general condition of the patient improves.

Stiffness of the neck is common after intracerebral or primary subarachnoid hemorrhage and is related to the presence of blood in the CSF. Because nuchal rigidity also suggests the possibility of impending herniation of the cerebellar tonsils through the foramen magnum, CT should be performed before lumbar puncture.

Changes in tendon reflexes and plantar responses can usually be explained by the location of a focal lesion. All tendon reflexes may be lost in the comatose state that immediately follows a stroke; more commonly, however, the reflexes are hyperactive on the side opposite the cerebral lesion. When the lesion is unilateral, the plantar response may be extensor on both sides if cerebral edema has caused compression of the midbrain with impaction into the incisura.

Neurovascular Examination

After the general neurologic examination, neurovascular tests should be performed when stroke is suspected.

Neck Flexion. Both resistance and pain on neck flexion can be indicative of meningeal irritation, which might be due to blood in the subarachnoid space.

Palpation. The possibility of occlusive disease in a large artery can be quickly assessed by simultaneous bilateral palpation of the major arteries in the following order: the superficial temporal arteries; the carotids at their bifurcations and low in the neck; the subclavian arteries, above and below the clavicles; the brachial and radial arteries; the abdominal aorta; and the femoral artery or its branches in the legs. If any pulses are diminished or absent, more detailed evaluation is required.

Diminished pulsation in one superficial temporal artery suggests disease of the external or common carotid artery on that side; increased pulsation sometimes indicates stenosis or occlusion of the internal carotid, with collateral flow through the external carotid system. If the pulse beat in one radial artery follows the other asynchronously, "subclavian steal" is the likely explanation.

Auscultation. After auscultation of the heart, the stethoscope should be used to listen for bruits above the aortic and pulmonary areas and along the course of the subclavian arteries below and above the clavicle. The stethoscope should then be applied along the course of the vertebral and carotid arteries (particularly at the bifurcation of the carotid artery behind the angle of the mandible), at the subclavian-vertebral junction, and over the mastoid processes. Last, the stethoscope should be applied to the orbit.

Bruit is one of the few clinical signs of atherosclerosis and is present in the region of the carotid bifurcation in about 4% of Americans older than 45. Bruits at the carotid bifurcation suggest disease of the common, internal, or external carotid artery; bruits at the subclavian-vertebral junction suggest abnormality of the vertebral artery. If properly used, auscultation can give excellent clues about the degree of arterial stenosis and, in the case of carotid-bifurcation murmurs, which of the three is involved.

All arterial murmurs begin in systole, but only when disease involves more than 80% of the cross-sectional area of the lumen do they extend into diastole. Further, the intensity of arterial murmurs increases until the area is reduced by two-thirds, at which point the murmur becomes softer and, finally, inaudible. Lastly, the pitch increases as the lumen becomes smaller. Therefore the most highly stenotic arteries are those in which the murmur is soft and high pitched, extending into diastole. Common- and internal-carotid-artery flow continues in reduced volume through diastole, whereas the blood flow in the external carotid ceases; carotid-bifurcation murmurs with a diastolic component therefore originate in the internal or common carotid.

References

Barnett HJM, Mohr JP, Stein BM, Yatsu F. Stroke—Pathophysiology, Diagnosis and Management. New York, Churchill Livingstone, 1986.

Caplan LR, Hier DB, D'Cruz I. Cerebral embolism in the Michael Reese stroke registry. Stroke 1983; 14:530–537.

DiMarco JP, Garan H, Ruskin JN. Approach to the patient with recurrent syncope of unknown cause. Mod Concepts Cardiovasc Dis 1983; 52:11–17.

Harrison M, Dyken M (eds). Cerebral Vascular Disease. Neurology, vol. 3. London, Butterworth International Medical Reviews, 1983.

Millikan CH, McDowell F, Easton JD (eds). Stroke. Lea & Febiger, Philadelphia, 1987.

Norris JW, Hachinski VC. Misdiagnosis of stroke. Lancet 1982; 1:328–331.

Sage JI, Van Uitert RL. Risk of recurrent stroke in patients with atrial filbrillation and non-valvular heart disease. Stroke 1983; 14:537–540.

Toole JF. Cerebrovascular Diseases. New York: Raven Press, 1984.

Warlow C, Morris P (eds). Transient Ischemic Attacks. New York: Marcel Dekker, 1982.

27. LABORATORY STUDIES IN STROKE
J.P. Mohr
J.A. Bello

In few fields is the technology changing as rapidly as that which measures alterations of blood flow and brain tissue after stroke. Because equipment tends to be expensive, dissemination of new techniques occurs slowly, forcing physicians to maintain a range of expertise to keep current. Present techniques include conventional radiology of the head and neck; routine and digital subtraction arteriography with radiopaque contrast material injected into arteries or veins; computer-processed ultrasonic Doppler insonation of blood flowing in the extra- and intracranial arteries and veins; computed tomography (CT) of the head and neck, with or without contrast enhancement; magnetic resonance imaging (MRI) with or without spectroscopy; and computer-processed imaging of single photon or positron emission by agents that assess specific chemical reactions in the brain. Of these, conventional radiology provides limited differentiation of tissues based on different x-ray attenuation by air, fat, soft tissue and calcification. CT allows greater differentiation of the normal soft tissues, particularly after intravenous administration of iodinated contrast agents. Within the brain, abnormal enhancement requires breakdown of the blood-brain barrier to demonstrate a lesion. MRI may be limited in identifying calcification but is more sensitive than CT to parenchymal abnormalities independent of changes in the blood-brain barrier.

Plain Radiography. Plain films of the skull and neck are of little value in studying stroke, but are widely available. Radiographs can show extra- or intracranial arteries that are heavily calcified and occasionally calcified arteriovenous malformations. Unfortunately, neither are of special prognostic significance (Fig. 27–1). In massive strokes with edema and major mass effect, the pineal gland, if calcified, may be shifted from the midline position. *Pneumoencephalography,* an outdated technique, once was used to document focal brain atrophy long after a large infarct.

Computed Tomography. CT became the preferred method for imaging the tissue damage from stroke after 1973. In CT, a fan beam of x-rays emitted from a single source passes through the head to a corresponding array of detectors. The x-ray source rotates around the patient's head, measuring the x-ray attenuation through the section plane, which is divided into compartments called pixels. From about 800,000 attenuation measurements, the computer assigns a number to each pixel in a 512 × 512 matrix and, using a gray scale, reconstructs an image that is displayed on a monitor. Iodinated water-soluble contrast agents have been developed which, after intravenous administration, enhance differences of tissue density. Technical advances in both imaging and processing have dramatically decreased the time required for data acquisition and image reconstruction and have increased spatial resolution to 1 to 2 mm. Modern CT scans permit differentiation of white and gray matter, the main divisions of the basal ganglia and thalamus, and, after

contrast infusion, even the major arteries. The scanner gantry, which houses the x-ray source and detectors, can be tilted so that scans can be performed at standard angles. Scan time may be limited to 2 seconds to minimize motion artifact, an advantage in an acute setting with a restless patient. The major limitation to this technique is in the posterior fossa. Here, lucent linear artifacts due to attenuation of the x-ray beam by the thick osseous structures at the skull base often project across the brainstem, obscuring a diagnosis of infarction.

Acute hematomas have a characteristic high-density appearance on CT in the first week, making CT a reliable method of differentiating the low-attenuation lesion typical of bland infarction from the high attenuation from hematoma and grossly hemorrhagic infarction (Figs. 27–2, 27–3). The volume of an acute hematoma can be estimated accurately by CT. As the high signal of fresh blood is lost in days or weeks due to chemical changes in the blood, the CT appearance evolves from initial hyperdensity though an isodense (subacute) phase to hypodensity in the chronic state (Fig. 27–4A–D). In the subacute phase, contrast administration may result in ring enhancement around the hemorrhage (Fig. 27–5), a pattern different from the gyral enhancement that is typical of infarction (Fig. 27–2). In the chronic state, a hematoma is usually reduced to a slit-like cavity; many disappear into isodense tissue. Subarachnoid hemorrhage is even more transient and may not be visible unless particularly dense; lumbar puncture is useful to enable the diagnosis in those with normal CT scans.

With nonhemorrhagic infarction, CT may appear normal for several days. When there is collateral supply to the region, CT is usually positive within 24 hours, showing hypodensity due to edema. Ischemic infarcts with little collateral flow or edema may remain isodense or may not enhance for days or weeks, later appearing only as focal atrophy. While CT may overestimate the size of deep lesions, it better approximates the volume of discrete surface infarcts, especially after several months when the acute effects of edema and necrotic tissue reabsorption have subsided (Fig. 27–6). Contrast-enhanced infarction is usually seen within a week and may persist for 2 weeks to 2 months.

Standard CT techniques do not distinguish ischemia from actual infarction. In the early

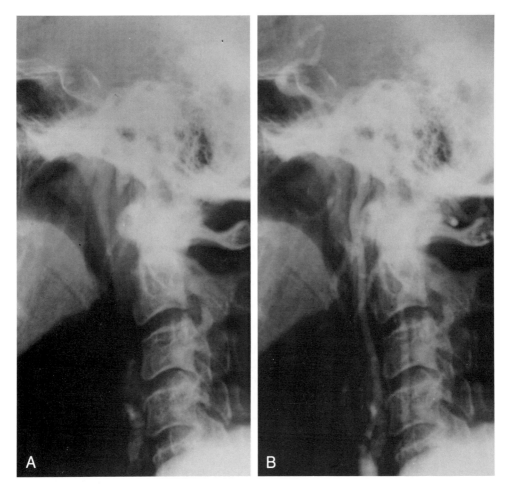

Fig. 27–1. Carotid calcification. *A.* Lateral angiographic "scout" film (before contrast) demonstrates calcification anterior to C_3-C_4 and C_4-C_5 in a typical location for carotid bifurcation. *B.* This is confirmed by contrast injection in the common carotid artery. There is evidence of significant narrowing of internal carotid artery by atherosclerotic plaque at the bifurcation. (External carotid is less severely involved.) (Courtesy of Drs. J.A. Bello and S.K. Hilal.)

stages, the physician may be frustrated by the difficulty in determining how much tissue is viable and how much damage is permanent. Stable xenon-enhanced CT, discussed below, may be useful.

Magnetic Resonance Imaging. MRI is rapidly overtaking CT in both hemorrhagic and ischemic stroke imaging. MRI is based on the interaction in body tissues between radio waves and nuclei of interest, usually hydrogen, within a powerful magnetic field that makes tissues susceptible to excitation by a radiofrequency pulse. Once excitation occurs, the absorbed energy is released at a rate that is easily measured. When the scanned tissue completely reemits the absorbed energy, it is in a state of relaxation, and two tissue-specific relaxation constants, T_1 and T_2, can be measured. Images are reconstructed from the signals obtained. In clinical practice, three types of images are generated: T_1-dependent, in which spinal fluid has decreased signal intensity relative to the brain and fat has increased signal; T_2-dependent, in which cerebrospinal fluid has increased signal relative to brain; and a "balanced" image in which the signals from brain and spinal fluid are comparable.

Multiplanar imaging is more easily achieved by MR than by CT. Selection of pulse sequence and plane of imaging is necessary to achieve the maximum utility of the technique. To diagnose and date hemorrhage, T_1 and T_2 images are necessary (Figs. 27–4, 27–7); however, to diagnose small infarcts, heavily weighted T_2 images are preferred. Balanced imaging is less useful for stroke. The changes in tissue water that accompany infarction are easily documented by MR, making it useful in following an infarct.

The lack of signal from bone gives MR an

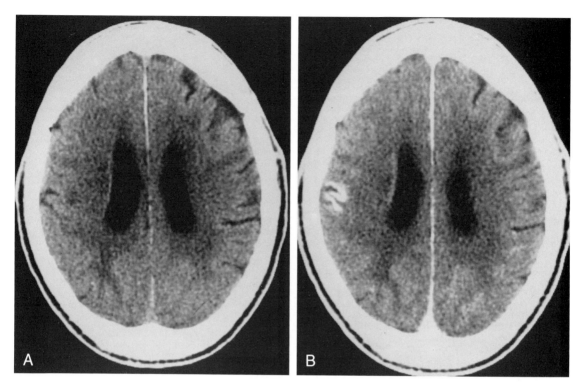

Fig. 27–2. Subacute cortical infarct. *A.* Precontrast axial CT scan. *B,* Postcontrast scan. Note gyral enhancement due to recent cortical infarction in vascular distribution of distal right MCA branch. (Courtesy of Drs. J.A. Bello and S.K. Hilal.)

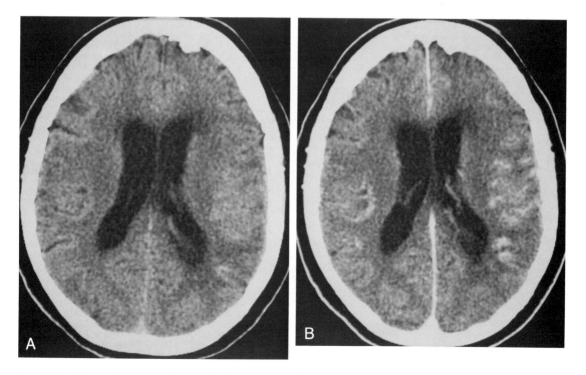

Fig. 27–3. Hemorrhagic infarction. *A.* Axial precontrast CT scan shows focal left parietal gyral density consistent with hemorrhagic infarction. Note edema and sulcal effacement in left frontoparietal cortical region. *B.* Postcontrast there is enhancement in area of recent hemorrhagic infarction. (Courtesy of Drs. J.A. Bello and S.K. Hilal.)

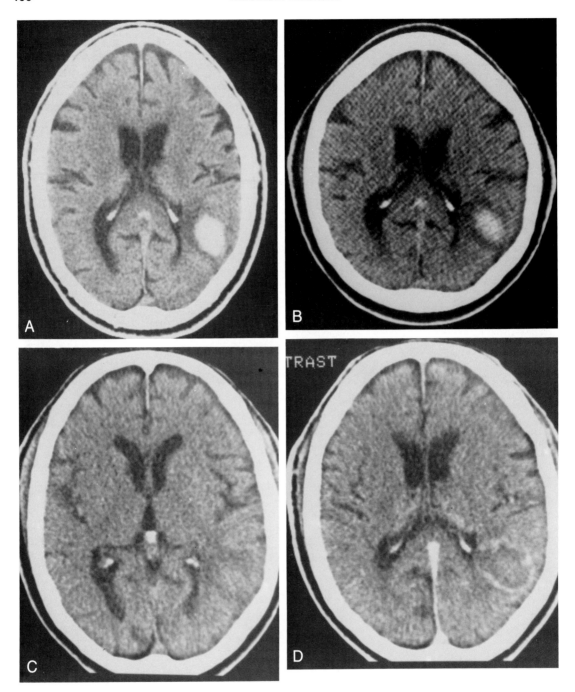

Fig. 27–4. Acute intracerebral hemorrhage with resorption over 6 weeks. *A.* Noncontrast axial CT scan in acute phase shows left parietal hyperdensity with mild mass effect and mild sulcal and ventricular effacement. *B.* Follow-up noncontrast axial CT scan 1 week later. Note decrease in density of hemorrhage. Surrounding lucency is due to edema with persistent mass effect. *C.* Noncontrast and *(D)* contrast-enhanced axial CT scans 3 weeks post-hemorrhage show further decrease in density of hemorrhage, which appears isodense in this phase with less surrounding lucency and mass effect. D. Peripheral ring enhancement postcontrast. (Courtesy of Drs. J.A. Bello and S.K. Hilal.)

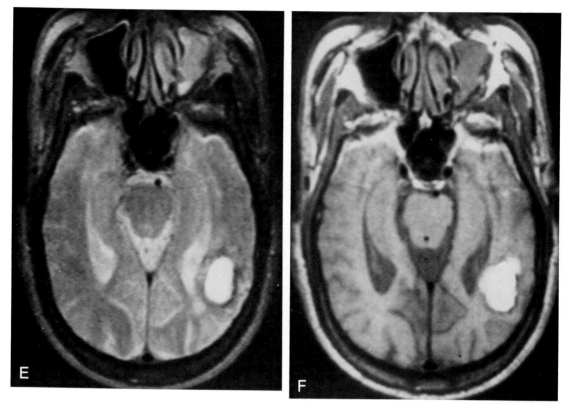

Fig. 27–4. *E.* T$_2$-weighted and *(F)* T$_1$-weighted axial MR scans 6 weeks posthemorrhage demonstrate near complete resolution of mass effect. In this subacute phase, hemorrhage appears typically hyperintense on both T$_2$ and T$_1$ pulse sequences, surrounded by a hypointense hemosiderin ring. (Courtesy of Drs. J.A. Bello and S.K. Hilal.)

advantage over CT for imaging infarcts in the brainstem (Fig. 27–8). Signal void is also characteristic of flowing blood, which moves out of a section plane before giving up its signal. High-resolution scans free of artifact allow inferences regarding vascular patency; a practical MR angiography technology is being developed. The paramagnetic effect of naturally occurring substances such as methemoglobin and hemosiderin enable dating of hematomas and their separation from hemorrhagic infarction. Paramagnetic agents to enhance MR imaging are being evaluated. With improved magnet design (1.5 Tesla and beyond) and computer programming, superb images may soon be possible.

MRI has no known direct biologic danger; however, the magnetic fields are so strong that ferromagnetic metallic implants, such as cardiac pacemakers, are contraindications. The technology is expensive and requires considerable expertise with cooling systems and computers, but is becoming more widely available as equipment becomes standard-

ized. The higher field magnets permit tissue spectroscopy, allowing measures of actual tissue chemical activity and opening the way to studying tissue viability and responses to stimulation.

Positron Emission Tomography (PET). PET also generates axial images using a technique similar to CT but the agents that are injected or inhaled are short-lived isotopes. Regional brain chemical activity is reflected in the emitted metabolic end products of such important substrates as oxygen and glucose. Few institutions have PET capabilities because an on-site or nearby cyclotron is needed to supply the isotopes.

Regional Cerebral Blood Flow. Several techniques have been developed to study regional cerebral blood flow (rCBF). In the most common, radiolabeled xenon is administered by inhalation or, less often, by injection into the carotid artery. An array of detectors over the head relates the proportion of accumulated radioactive xenon to rCBF. The study is a sen-

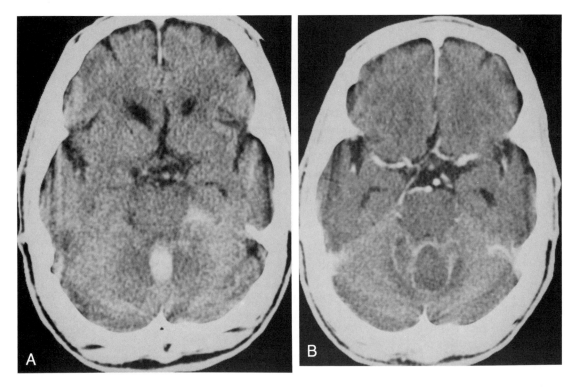

Fig. 27–5. Cerebellar hemorrhage, acute and subacute phases. *A.* Axial noncontrast CT scan depicts increased density within vermis due to acute hemorrhage. *B.* Follow-up contrast-enhanced scan 3.5 weeks later demonstrates interval decrease in hemorrhage density in addition to ring enhancement. (Courtesy of Drs. J.A. Bello and S.K. Hilal.)

sitive guide to perfusion over the cerebral surface but is less sensitive to changes in the deeper areas of the brain. This test method allows challenges of the cerebral vasoreactivity, hyperventilation with room air in the mixture normally produces vasoconstriction. Thus, regional failure of this effect suggests loss of vasoreactivity as may occur after acute infarction. Hyperventilation with an air mixture containing small amounts of CO_2 normally causes vasodilation, so failure of this effect indicates the circulation in the region is already dilated. This finding is a sign of increased collateral formation, which often occurs in occlusion or hemodynamic stenosis of the extracranial carotid.

Stable-Xenon CT. A separate test, stable-xenon CT, uses CT to measure changes in tissue density over a period when stable xenon gas (used as a contrast agent) is inhaled, circulates, and diffuses across the normal blood-brain barrier. The observed incremental changes in tissue density correspond to rates of cerebral blood flow. The values are calculated by a computer and displayed on a gray scale as a flow map corresponding to the axial

CT slice of interest. This method accurately measures flow in both deep and surface structures.

Single Photon Emission Tomography. In this technique, a gamma camera counts the density of signals emitted from an injected agent minutes after it is given intravenously. The injected agent circulates through the vasculature, making its relative local concentrations an index of vessel patency. The emitted signals are assigned to pixels and displayed in slice form similar to most CT images. The technique is sensitive and inexpensive, showing regional flow abnormalities from occlusions of individual branches and perfusion disturbances that are larger than the areas of tissue damage.

Angiography. With advances in brain imaging, angiography, the former mainstay of stroke diagnosis, has steadily lost ground. In this technique, water-soluble iodinated contrast media is selectively injected intraarterially, and the opacification of the extra- and intracranial arteries is filmed by either conventional radiographic or digital subtraction technique. Angiography remains unsur-

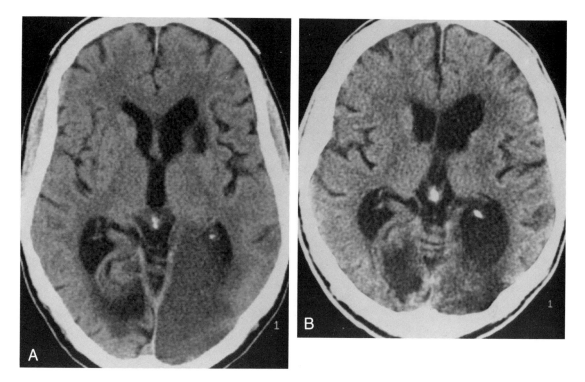

Fig. 27–6. Cerebral infarction, acute and chronic phases. *A.* Axial noncontrast CT scan reveals focal regions of discrete lucency in left basal ganglia and right occipital regions without mass effect, suggesting nonacute infarcts. A "fainter," less well defined left occipital lucency is also noted, with effacement of cortical sulci and the atrium of the ventricle, suggesting more recent infarction. *B.* Follow-up noncontrast scan 2 months later demonstrates interval demarcation of the left occipital infarct with evidence of focal atrophy, "negative mass effect" on the atrium, which appears larger. Similar change is noted in left frontal horn. (Courtesy of Drs. J.A. Bello and S.K. Hilal.)

passed in demonstrating occlusion, recanalization, ulceration, and dissection of large arteries and stenosis of small arteries (Fig. 27–9). It is relied on for study of aneurysms and arteriovenous malformations.

Because angiography does not reliably image vessels below 0.5 mm diameter, it usually is not helpful in diagnosing the cause of deep infarctions of the lacunar type. Before the availability of the direct brain imaging methods previously described, angiography was used to outline intra- and extraaxial hematomas, evaluate vasospasm after ruptured aneurysms, and estimate degree of extracranial arterial stenosis. However, the procedure may cause discomfort and is not without risk. Angiography remains an alternate technique to confirm a diagnosis. It is often undertaken only once in the course of a stroke, and thus requires appropriate forethought to maximize the information to be gained. For a diagnosis of embolism, angiography should be undertaken within hours of the ictus because the embolic particle may fragment early, chang-ing the appearance of the affected vessel from occlusion to one indistinguishable from arterial stenosis or arteritis and subsequently to patency with a normal lumen. When atheromatous stenosis of large arteries is suspected, preangiographic studies of central retinal artery pressure or Doppler ultrasound (see below) help to tailor the angiographic study and enable the angiographer to concentrate on the major territories thought to be affected.

Retinal Arterial Pressure Measurements. Before the development of Doppler techniques to measure central retinal arterial pressure, *ophthalmodynomometry* and *pneumoplethysmography* were used to measure the pressure required to start the central retinal artery pulsating. In ophthalmodynomometry a small foot plate is attached to a strain gauge, which is pressed against the sclera, and the number of grams of pressure is read off the scale. In pneumoplethysmography, a suction cup is placed on the sclera. These techniques require low-cost equipment and are easily

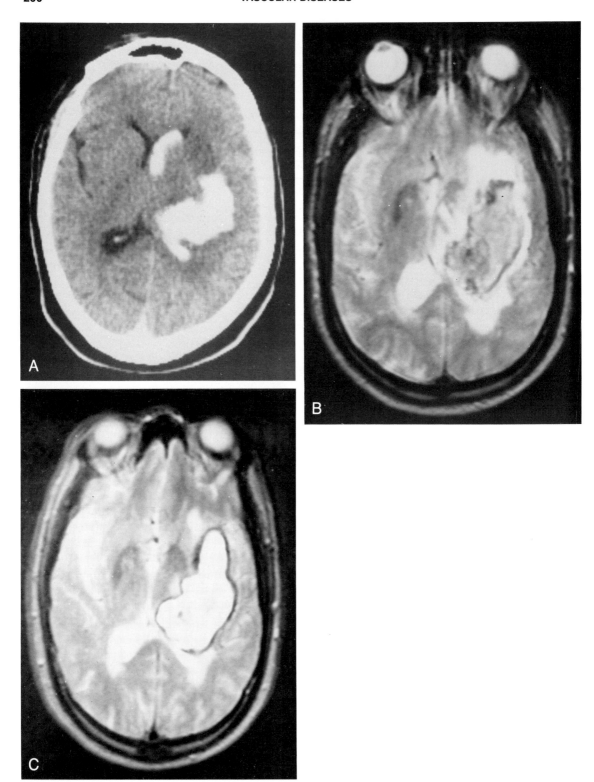

Fig. 27–7. Intracerebral hemorrhage, acute and subacute phases. *A*. Noncontrast axial CT scan shows acute (hyper-dense) hemorrhage involving left thalamus and putamen with left lateral intraventricular components. (On MR signal from this hemorrhage would be *hypo*intense on T_2-weighted scan.) *B*. T_2-weighted axial MR scan 1 week later reveals signal to be roughly *iso*intense to cerebral parenchyma. *C*. 3 weeks after initial hemorrhage axial T_2-weighted MR image signal is *hyper*intense surrounded by ring of *hypo*intensity related to hemosiderin. (Courtesy of Drs. J.A. Bello and S.K. Hilal.)

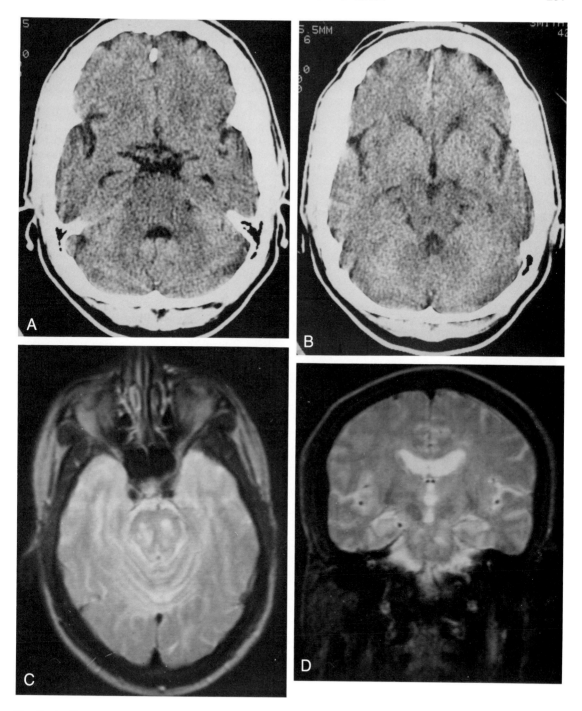

Fig. 27–8. Brainstem infarction. *A* and *B*. Noncontrast axial CT scans reveal possible infarcts in left brachium pontis in *(A)* and right midbrain *(B)*. *C.* Axial, and *(D)* coronal T$_2$-weighted MR scans of same patient clearly show these and additional small infarcts not well seen on CT. (Courtesy of Drs. J.A. Bello and S.K. Hilal.)

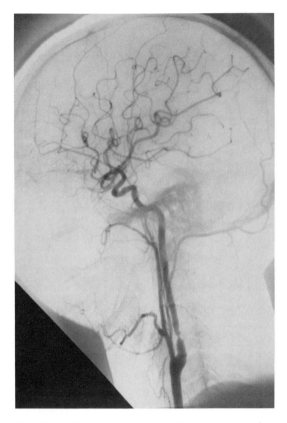

Fig. 27–9. Proximal internal carotid stenosis. Lateral arteriogram of common carotid shows ulcerated plaque of proximal internal carotid with hemodynamically significant stenosis. Anterior circulation failed to fill and cross-filled from contralateral side. (Courtesy of Drs. J.A. Bello and S.K. Hilal.)

learned. The findings give an accurate estimate of the central retinal arterial pressure, although they fail to disclose the cause of the decreased pressure and no inferences are possible about the intracranial circulation cephalad to the carotid siphon.

Doppler Measurements. The simplest Doppler devices pass a high frequency continuous wave sound signal over the tissues in the neck, receive the reflected signal, and process them through a small speaker. The user of such a *continuous wave Doppler* listens for the pitch of the sound and makes a rough judgment of the degree of the Doppler shift to infer whether the blood moving through the artery beneath the probe is normal, decreased, or increased and, if increased, is smooth or turbulent flow. Little experience is required to separate the high-frequency arterial signal from the low-frequency venous and to hear the extremely high frequencies

typical of severe stenosis. More effort is required to quantitate the signal to permit its comparison with the same test at a later date. Because the Doppler shift equation depends on the cosine of the beam versus the flowing blood within the artery, casual angulation of the probe can have major effects on signal production.

To assist in proper probe angulation, modern *duplex Doppler* devices have two crystals, one atop the other, in a single probe head; one crystal handles the Doppler shift for spectral analysis, the other the B-mode image of the vessel walls. Improvements in crystal designs are steadily reducing the size of the probe but it remains so bulky that it is difficult to image and insonate the carotid artery high up under the mandible. The Doppler shift crystal in modern units has an adjustable range gate to permit analysis of flow signals from specific depths in the tissues, eliminating conflicting signals where arteries and veins overlie one another. Some even have two range gates, allowing an adjustable "volume" or "window" to insonate the moving blood column in an artery at volumes as small as 0.6 mm, the size of the tightest stenosis. The capacity to interrogate the flow pattern from wall to wall across the lumen has made this technique useful for detecting, measuring, and monitoring degrees of stenosis (Fig. 27–10). Because duplex Doppler is sensitive to cross-sectional area and not to wall anatomy, if used before angiography, frequently it warns the angiographer to seek stenotic lesions that might be missed on a survey angiogram. Unfortunately, B-mode vessel imaging remains disappointingly insensitive to most minor ulcerations, which are better seen by conventional angiography. Although duplex Doppler methods were developed to insonate the carotid, they can assess the extracranial vertebral artery through the intervertebral foramina.

Using a probe with great tissue penetration properties, it is possible to insonate the major vessels of the circle of Willis, the vertebrals, and the basilar. Current transcranial Doppler devices are range gated but not (yet) duplex (Fig. 27–11). The signals accurately document the direction and velocity of the arterial flow insonated by the narrow probe beam. Spectrum analysis of the signal allows estimation of the degree of stenosis as does extracranial duplex Doppler. Hemodynamically important extracranial stenosis may damp the waveform in the ipsilateral arteries above, allowing the

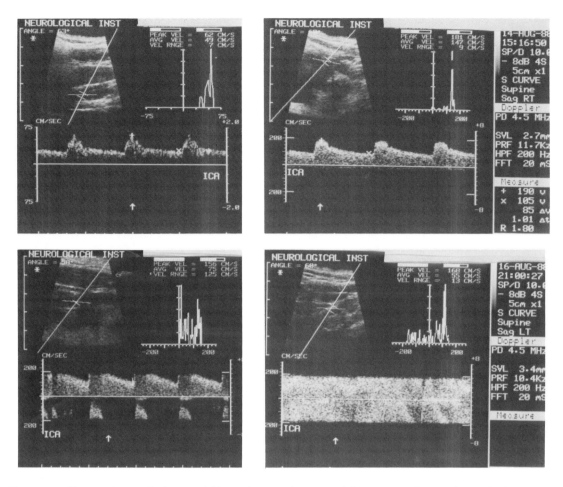

Fig. 27–10. Four studies, each showing different degrees of stenosis of the extracranial internal carotid. The studies, obtained with the Diasonics DRF 400 instrument, image the carotid by B-mode ultrasound (upper left hand corner of each of the four pictures) by passing the ultrasound beam through the tissues (angled line) and sampling the flow velocity at a point within the lumen of the vessel (horizontal bracketed line). From this sample the device displays the waveforms representing the velocity profile calculated from the Doppler shift (waveforms shown with velocity in cm/sec in each picture). The mean velocities are then calculated from a sample taken near the peak of each waveform (small arrow under each of waveform line) and the spectrum of velocities (i.e., degree of turbulence) is displayed as "peak vel" (i.e., velocity), "mean vel" and "vel rnge" (shown in graphic form in the upper right hand corner of each picture). Examples of varying degrees of stenosis are shown: normal flow, left upper corner; moderate (60 to 80%) stenosis with moderate turbulence, right upper corner; severe (80 to 90%) stenosis with marked turbulence, left lower corner; extremely severe (90 to 99%) stenosis with extreme turbulence, right lower corner.

effect of the extracranial disease to be measured and followed serially. A challenge test of contralateral compression can be done to determine whether the effects of unilateral extracranial stenosis are compensated or lack anatomic collaterals. Care must be taken to assess which artery is being insonated; the middle cerebral and posterior cerebral are often misinsonated. The technique is user sensitive, requiring patience to detect the signal and then find the best angle for insonation at a given depth. Minor anatomic variations can cause misleading changes in signal strength. Because the procedure is safe, fast, and uses a probe and microprocessor of table-top size,

the device can be taken to the bedside even in an intensive care unit and used to diagnose developing vasospasm, collateral flow above occlusions, recanalization of an embolized artery, and the presence of important basilar or cerebral artery stenosis. When combined with high-field MR imaging, it is possible to diagnose basilar and middle cerebral stem stenosis noninvasively.

References

Baron JC, Bousser MG, Rey A, et al. Reversal of focal "misery-perfusion syndrome" by extra-intracranial arterial bypass in hemodynamic cerebral ischemia. Stroke 1981: 12:454.

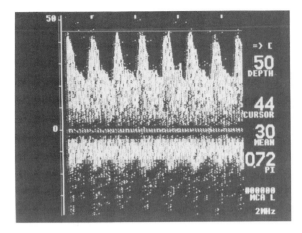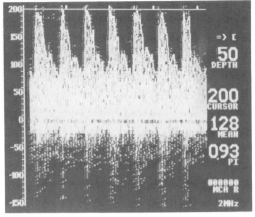

Fig. 27–11. Two examples of transcranial Doppler insonations of the middle cerebral artery, obtained at a depth of 50 mm from the side of the head overlying the temporal bone, using the Carolina Medical Electronics TC-64B device. The velocity profile of the Doppler shift is insonated at this depth from the blood in the middle cerebral artery flowing toward the probe (upper arrow directed to the right in each picture). The left picture shows a normal peak (cursor 44 [cm/sec], left picture) mean (30) and pulsatility index (0.72 PI, i.e., the difference between the peak systolic velocity and the end diastolic velocity divided by the mean velocity). In the right picture, the peak (200 cursor) and mean (128 mean) velocities and the pulsatility index (0.93) are higher, consistent with local stenosis at this point in the course of the middle cerebral artery.

Bradley WG Jr, Schmidt PG. Effects of methemoglobin formation on the MR appearance of subarachnoid hemorrhage. Radiology 1985; 156:99–103.

Damasio H. A computed tomographic guide to the identification of cerebral vascular territories. Arch Neurol 1985; 40:138–142.

Delal PM, Shah PM, Aiyar RR. Arteriographic study of cerebral embolism. Lancet 1965; 2:358.

DeWitt LD. Clinical use of NMR imaging in stroke. Stroke 1986; 17:328–331.

DeWitt LD, Wechsler LR. Transcranial doppler. Stroke 1988; 19:674–680.

Dion J, et al. Clinical events following neuroangiography. Stroke 1987; 18:997–1004.

Frackowiak RSJ, Wise RJS. Positron tomography in ischemic cerebrovascular disease. Neurol Clin N Am 1983; 1:183.

Furlan AJ, Weinstein MA, Little JR, Modic MT. Digital subtraction angiography in the evaluation of cerebrovascular disease. Neurol Clin N Am 1983; 1:55.

Gomori JM, Grossman RI, Goldberg HI, Zimmerman RA, Bilaniuk LT. Intracranial hematomas: Imaging by high-field MR. Radiology 1985; 157:87–93.

Heiss W-D, ed. Functional Mapping of the Brain in Vascular Disorders. Berlin: Springer-Verlag, 1985.

Heiss W-D, Herholz K, Boecher-Schwarz HG, et al. PET, CT, and MR imaging in cerebrovascular disease. J Compt Tomogr 1986; 10:903–911.

Hilal SK, Maudsley AA, Simon HE, et al. *In vivo* imaging of sodium-23 in the human head. J Comput Asst Tomog 1985; 9:1.

Irino T, Tandea M, Minami T. Aniographic manifestations in postrecanalized cerebral infarction. Neurology 1977; 27:471.

Kelcz F, Hilal SK, Hartwell P, Joseph PM. CT measurement of the xenon blood-brain partition coefficient and implications for RCBF. A preliminary report. Radiology 1978; 127:385.

Lassen N, Ingvar DH, Skinhoj EL. Brain function and blood flow. Sci Am 1978; 239:62–71.

Marshall VG, Bradley WG, Jr, Marshall CE, Bhoopat T, Rhodes RH. Deep white matter infarction: Correlation of MR imaging and histopathologic findings. Radiology 1988; 167:517–522.

Maudsley A, Hilal SK, Perman W, Simon H. Spatially resolved high resolution spectroscopy by "four dimensional" NMR. J Magnetic Resonance 1983; 51:147.

McNamara MT, Brant-Zawadzki M, Berry I, et al. Acute experimental cerebral ischemia: MR enhancement using Gd-DTPA. Radiology 1986; 158:701–705.

Norrving B, Nilsson B, Olsson J. Progression of carotid disease after endarterectomy: A Doppler ultrasound study. Ann Neurol 1982; 12:548.

Pessin MS, Hinton RC, Davis KR, et al. Mechanisms of acute carotid stroke: A clinicoangiographic study. Ann Neurol 1979; 6:245.

Schwartz A, Hennerici M. Noninvasive transcranial Doppler ultrasound in intracranial angiomas. Neurology 1986; 36:626–635.

Shinar D, Mohr JP, Kunitz S, et al. Interobserver variation in the clinical diagnosis of stroke. Arch Neurol 1986; 44:413–425.

Sipponen JT, Kaste M, Ketonen L. Serial nuclear magnetic resonance (NMR) imaging in patients with cerebral infarction. Comput Assist Tomogr 1983; 7:585–589.

Stillman MJ, et al. Cerebral infarction; shortcomings of angiography in evaluation. Medicine 1987; 18:257–263.

28. BLOOD AND CSF IN CEREBROVASCULAR DISEASE
Lewis P. Rowland

Routine laboratory data have less diagnostic importance since the advent of CT and MRI but are still important in individual cases.

Evaluation of the heart and kidneys is important in all patients, especially in young adults and in patients with hypertension. *Thrombocytopenia* may be responsible for cerebral or subarachnoid hemorrhage. Other hemorrhagic syndromes may be due to natural or iatrogenic coagulopathy, as indicated by prolonged *prothrombin time.* On the other hand, polycythemia or high platelet counts *(thrombocythemia)* may predispose to cerebral infarcts in adults. In children, cerebral infarction may be due to lack of serum *protein C* or *protein S* (naturally occurring anticoagulants that regulate the coagulation system by inhibiting activated factors V and VIII); these syndromes may be due to either arterial or venous thrombosis.

The white blood cell count in the peripheral blood is usually normal in patients with infarction, but may increase to 20,000 cells/mm³ after intracerebral or subarachnoid hemorrhage or septic embolus. An abnormally high ESR should cause the physician to suspect endocarditis or temporal arteritis. Focal abnormalities are found in the EEG of most patients with vascular lesions of the cerebral hemispheres. Transient hyperglycemia and glycosuria may follow hemorrhage.

Lumbar puncture is no longer done routinely in cases of stroke, but is reserved for diagnostic problems, especially if there is any question of neurosyphilis or meningitis. The CSF pressure is usually normal after cerebral embolus or infarction. Pressures between 200 and 300 mm H₂O are present in a few cases, but CSF pressures greater than 300 mm H₂O are rarely seen. In contrast, the pressure is greater than 200 mm H₂O in most patients with intracerebral or subarachnoid hemorrhage.

The CSF is bloody in all cases of primary subarachnoid hemorrhage, in 85% of the cases of cerebral hemorrhage, and in only 15% of those with cerebral embolism. The fluid is clear in most cases of infarction, although there may be a slight xanthochromic tinge; a few red blood cells are seen on microscopic examination.

The white blood cell count of the CSF is usually normal in patients with cerebral infarction, although a slight pleocytosis (up to 50 cells) may occasionally be seen. The cell count is usually normal in cases of aseptic cerebral embolism; however, when the embolus is from a septic focus, a moderate or severe pleocytosis (up to 4000 cells/mm³) is the rule. In most cases, this increase in white

cells is due to an aseptic meningeal reaction to the septic embolus, which is shown by a normal sugar content of the CSF and the absence of organisms.

In most patients with an intracerebral or subarachnoid hemorrhage, the white-cell count of the CSF is usually directly proportional to the amount of blood in the CSF. In rare cases of intracerebral hemorrhage, the CSF may contain 500 to 4000 white cells/mm³ and no red cells. This is attributed to an aseptic meningeal reaction secondary to hemorrhagic necrosis of the ventricular wall that has spread to the ventricles but has not ruptured into them.

When lumbar puncture is performed within 24 hours after the onset of a cerebral infarction, the protein content is usually normal if the CSF is clear. A slight elevation in CSF protein content (up to 75 mg/100 ml) is present in about 30% of such cases; however, values higher than 100 mg/100 ml are rare. The protein content of bloody CSF is directly proportional to the amount of blood present.

When the CSF is clear, serologic tests for syphilis are negative, unless the CNS is infected. If the CSF is bloody, the presence of syphilitic reagin may cause a false-positive reaction. The lumbar puncture should be repeated and the CSF retested after enough time has elapsed for the blood to clear.

Reference

Israels SJ, Seshia SS. Childhood stroke associated with protein C or S deficiency. J Pediat 1987; 111:562–4.

29. TRANSIENT ISCHEMIC ATTACKS
J.P. Mohr

As the name indicates, transient ischemic attacks (TIAs) are thought to result from ischemia too brief to cause infarction. TIAs and infarction are caused by the same mechanisms as embolism or thrombus, and the syndromes are essentially the same except for duration.

TIAs have been defined as syndromes that last less than 24 hours; usually, they last only minutes. In the typical TIA, the deficit usually lasts about 10 minutes and never more than an hour. These attacks show a low frequency of intracranial arterial branch occlusions attributable to embolism, and a high frequency (about 50%) of severe stenosis or occlusion of major arteries. The other type of clinically short-lived stroke, often also classified as TIA, lasts longer than an hour and is more often associated with angiographically demonstrable intracranial embolism. These attacks have a low frequency of severe stenosis or occlusion of major arteries. Although both types of ischemic episodes imply increased risk of stroke, it is mainly the brief attacks that are associated with atherosclerotic occlusive disease.

Two types of TIA syndromes occur in the carotid artery region. The first is *transient monocular blindness* (TMB), or amaurosis fugax. In over 95% of cases, it develops within seconds as a sudden painless darkness or blurring that affects vision uniformly or from above downward in window-shade fashion. Vision is restored after a few minutes, like the clearing of atmospheric fog. Variants of TMB are rare enough to question whether they are really signs of arterial stenosis. In cases where repeated TMBs occur, the clinical syndrome is almost always the same.

The second type of carotid territory TIA is the *transient hemisphere attack* (THA), which affects the region of the middle cerebral artery: combinations of focal motor or sensory deficits occur, most often involving the fingers, hand, or forearm, and sometimes distorting language or behavior. The syndrome begins suddenly, is usually maximal at the moment of onset, and subsides slowly in several minutes. Nonfocal symptoms such as headache, lightheadedness, dizziness, forgetfulness, seizures, or behavior are not correctly diagnosed as carotid territory TIAs. TMB and THA almost never occur simultaneously, and only occasionally occur at separate times in the same patient; when TIAs are multiple, the clinical symptoms usually remain of the same type in the same patient.

Severe ipsilateral internal carotid stenosis or occlusion is present in 50% of patients with either TMB or THA that last less than an hour. The frequency is slightly higher if both types of TIA occur in the same patient. TMB rarely lasts longer than 10 minutes. THA may last hours. When it does, it is more likely to be due to an embolus than to significant extracranial carotid stenosis.

In *vertebrobasilar TIAs*, the variety of symptoms is too large to list, but the most diagnostically reliable are diplopia, circumoral numbness, dysarthria, and ataxia. Dizziness, hemiparesis, or hemisensory syndromes may affect one or both sides, but these symptoms are more difficult to classify as vertebrobasilar in origin when they occur alone.

There is a smooth clinical continuum from transient ischemia to infarction. At one end is infarction, caused by a persisting arterial occlusion when collateral vessels fail to spare the endangered arterial region distal to the occlusion. At the other end is ischemia, which is caused by the same severe stenosis or occlusion but is either rapidly relieved or adequately collateralized. Some clinical improvement is the rule in almost all symptomatic arterial occlusions; but even when function returns to normal, the attack should not be regarded as a TIA if it lasts longer than 24 hours because there usually is an infarct due to embolism or thrombosis. If the ischemic attack lasts more than 24 hours, it should be diagnosed as an ischemic stroke. The term *reversible ischemic neurologic deficit* (RIND) has been applied to syndromes that improve within 24 hours but leave some minor neurologic abnormality; these are also properly regarded as minor ischemic strokes.

References

Araki G. Small infarctions in the basal ganglia with special references to transient ischemic attacks. Excerpta Medica Int Congr Series 1979; 469:161–162.

Barnett HJM. Progress toward stroke prevention. Neurology 1980; 30:1212–1225.

Caplan LR. TIAs. Neurology 1988; 38:791–793.

Heyman A, Wilkinson WE, Heyden S, et al. Risk of stroke in asymptomatic persons with cervical arterial bruits. N Engl J Med 1980; 302:838–841.

Kistler JP, Lees RS, Friedman J, et al. The bruit of carotid stenosis versus radiated basal heart murmurs: differentiation by phonoangiography. Circulation 1978; 57:375–381.

Pessin MS, Duncan GW, Mohr JP, Poskanzer DC. Clinical and angiographic features of carotid transient ischemic attacks. N Engl J Med 1977; 296:358–362.

Rothrock JF. Crescendo TIAs: clinical and angiographic correlations. Neurology 1988; 38:198–201.

Werdelin L, Juhler M. The course of TIAs. Neurology 1988; 38:677–680.

Wiebers DO, Whisnant JP, O'Fallon WM. Reversible ischemic neurologic deficit (RIND) in a community: Rochester, Minnesota, 1955–1974. Neurology 1982; 32:459–465.

Wolf PA, Kannel WB, Sorlie P, McNamara P. Asymptomatic carotid bruit and the risk of stroke. JAMA 1981; 245:1442–1445.

30. CEREBRAL INFARCTION

John C.M. Brust

Ischemic syndromes of specific vessels depend not only on the site of the occlusion but on previous brain damage, collateral circulation, and variations in the region supplied by a particular artery, including aberrations in the circle of Willis (e.g., if both anterior cerebral arteries arise from a common trunk, carotid artery occlusion may cause bilateral leg weakness; if one or both posterior cerebral arteries arise from the internal carotid, occlusion of the basilar artery is less likely to cause visual symptoms). Syndromes of specific vessels do not always define the site or the nature of the occlusion (e.g., infarction in the region of the middle cerebral artery is often the result of thrombotic occlusion of the internal carotid artery; occlusion of the middle cerebral artery or its branches is usually embolic). Nonetheless, knowledge of individual artery syndromes helps the clinician to localize a lesion and to determine whether it is vascular (Figs. 30–1 to 30–4 and Table 30–1).

Specific Vessel Occlusions

MIDDLE CEREBRAL ARTERY

Infarction in the region of the middle cerebral artery causes contralateral weakness, sensory loss, homonymous hemianopia, and depending on the hemisphere involved, either language disturbance or impaired spatial perception. If the artery's main trunk is occluded, infarction affects the cerebral convexity and deep structures, including not only the motor and sensory cortices over the cerebral convexity but also the posterior limb of the internal capsule; the face, arm, and leg are equally affected by weakness and sensory loss. If infarction spares the diencephalon after occlusion of the upper division, weakness and sensory loss are greater in the face and arm than in the leg. When infarction is limited to the region of the rolandic branch, such weakness and sensory loss may be the only signs. A small infarct or lacune in the internal capsule (from occlusion of a penetrating lenticulostriate branch of the proximal middle cerebral artery) may cause a syndrome of pure hemiparesis with no other symptoms.

With cerebral lesions, motor and sensory loss tend to be greatest distally, perhaps because the proximal limbs and the trunk are more likely to be represented in both hemispheres. Paraspinal muscles, for example, are rarely weak in unilateral cerebral disease, which also spares muscles of the forehead, pharynx, and jaw. Tongue weakness is variable. If weakness is severe, muscle tone usually decreases initially, then gradually increases in days or weeks to spasticity with hyperactive tendon reflexes. A Babinski sign is usually present from the outset. When weakness is mild, or during recovery, there is more clumsiness and incoordination than loss of strength.

There is often paresis of contralateral conjugate gaze after an acute lesion in the so-called "frontal gaze center" anterior to the prerolandic motor cortex; the gaze palsy usu-

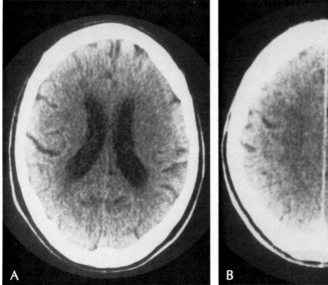
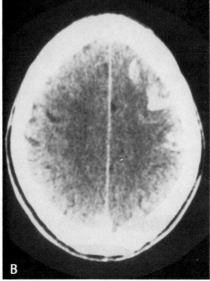

Fig. 30–1. Cerebral infarction, 1 week after stroke. *A.* Before injection of contrast material, CT was normal. *B.* After injection of contrast material, there was gyral enhancement in a pattern conforming to the distribution of the middle cerebral artery. (Courtesy of Drs. S.K. Hilal and S.R. Ganti.)

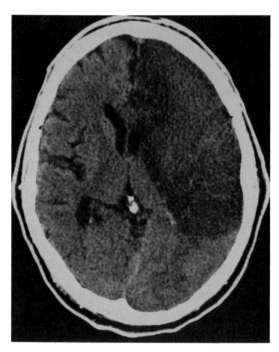

Fig. 30–2. Subacute infarct, ACA and MCA distributions. Noncontrast axial CT scan demonstrates radiolucency in left basal ganglia and frontal and temporal opercula extending through cortex. Note sulcal effacement and mild shift due to recent infarction involving left ACA and MCA territories; left PCA territory is spared. (Courtesy of Drs. J.A. Bello and S.K. Hilal.)

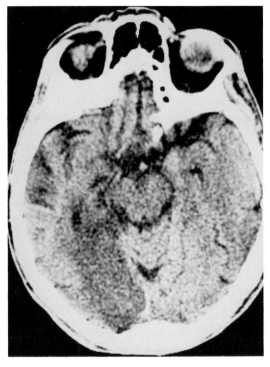

Fig. 30–3. Acute posterior cerebral infarct. Noncontrast axial CT scan shows right occipital lucency, corresponding to posterior cerebral vascular distribution with mild mass effect (sulcal effacement) due to acute infarction and edema. (Courtesy of Drs. J.A. Bello and S.K. Hilal.)

ally lasts only 1 or 2 days, even when other signs remain severe. Sensory loss tends to involve discriminative and proprioceptive modalities. Pain and temperature sensation may be impaired but are seldom lost. Joint position sense, however, may be severely disturbed, causing limb ataxia or *pseudoathetosis,* and there may be loss of two-point discrimination, astereognosis, or failure to appreciate a touch stimulus if another is delivered simultaneously to the normal side of the body ("extinction"). Homonymous hemianopia is the result of damage to the optic radiations. If the lesion is primarily parietal, the field cut may be an inferior quadrantanopia; with temporal lesions, quadrantanopia is superior.

A lesion of the left opercular (perisylvian) cortex is likely to cause aphasia; when damage is widespread, the aphasia is global, causing muteness or nonfluent and amelodic speech and severe impairment of speech-comprehension, writing, and reading abilities. Restricted damage from branch occlusions can cause an aphasic syndrome. Frontal opercular lesions tend to cause *Broca's aphasia,* with impaired speaking and writing ability,

but with relative preservation of comprehension. With posterior periopercular lesions, fluency and prosody are preserved but paraphasia can reduce speech output to jargon; there may be impairment of speech comprehension and naming, repetition, reading, and writing abilities in different combinations. When aphasia is severe, there is usually some impairment of nonlanguage cognitive functions; when aphasia is global, dementia is obvious. With Broca's or global aphasia, hemiparesis is usually severe. When aphasia is the result of a restricted posterior lesion, hemiparesis is mild. Aphasia in left-handed patients, regardless of the hemisphere involved, tends to be milder and resolves more rapidly than in right-handed patients with left hemisphere injury.

Left hemisphere convexity lesions, especially parietal, may cause bilateral *ideomotor apraxia,* in which the patient cannot perform learned motor acts on command, but can describe the act and perform it when the setting is altered (e.g., after the examiner has given the patient an object the use of which the patient could not imitate). Buccolingual

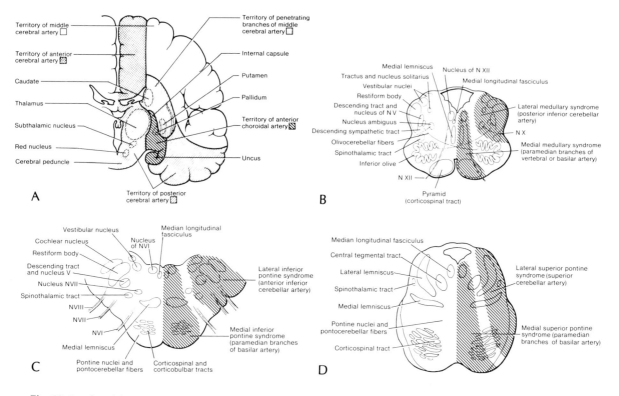

Fig. 30–4. Arterial territories of the cerebrum *(A)*, of the medulla *(B)*, of the lower pons *(C)*, and of the upper pons *(D)*.

apraxia often accompanies Broca aphasia. *Ideational apraxia* (loss of understanding of the purpose of actions and difficulty manipulating objects) follows bilateral hemisphere damage and associated dementia. Infarction of the angular or supramarginal gyri of the dominant hemisphere can cause one *Gerstmann syndrome* (i.e., agraphia, acalculia, left-right confusion, and finger agnosia).

Right-hemisphere convexity infarction, especially parietal, causes disturbances of spatial perception; the patient has difficulty copying simple pictures or diagrams *(constructional apraxia, or apractognosia)*, interpreting maps, maintaining physical orientation (topographagnosia), or putting on clothing *(dressing apraxia)*. Difficulty recognizing faces *(prosopagnosia)* is attributed to bilateral temporo-occipital lesions. The patient's extero- and proprioception contralateral to the lesion may be affected; this *"hemineglect"* may follow lesions restricted to either the frontal or parietal lobes (or, rarely, the diencephalon). The patient may not recognize the hemiplegia *(anosognosia)*, or his arm *(asomatognosia)*, or any external object to the left of his own midline. These phenomena may occur without visual field defects in patients who are otherwise men-

tally intact. Patients with right hemisphere convexity damage may have difficulty expressing or recognizing nonpropositional aspects of speech ("pragmatics") such as emotional tone, sarcasm, or jokes. Right hemisphere lesions may also produce an acute confusional state.

ANTERIOR CEREBRAL ARTERY

Infarction in the area of the anterior cerebral artery causes weakness, clumsiness, and sensory loss affecting mainly the distal contralateral leg. There may be urinary incontinence. Damage to the so-called "supplementary motor cortex" may cause a speech disturbance that is considered aphasic by some physicians and a kind of motor inertia by others. Involvement of the anterior corpus callosum may cause tactile anomia or ideomotor apraxia of the left limbs, which is attributed to the disconnection of the left language-dominant hemisphere from the right motor or sensory cortex. If the damage includes the territory supplied by the diencephalon branch (recurrent artery of Heubner), the anterior limb of the internal capsule is affected and the face and arm are also weak.

Bilateral infarction in the anterior cerebral

Table 30–1.   Syndromes of Cerebral Infarction

Artery Occluded	Syndrome
Common carotid	Asymptomatic
Internal carotid	Ipsilateral blindness
	Contralateral hemiparesis and hemianesthesia
	Hemianopia
	Aphasia or denial and hemineglect
Middle cerebral	
Main trunk	Hemiplegia
	Hemianesthesia
	Hemianopia
	Aphasia or denial and hemineglect
Upper division	Hemiparesis and sensory loss (arm and face more affected than leg)
	Broca aphasia or denial and hemineglect
Lower division	Wernicke aphasia or nondominant behavior disorder without hemiparesis
Penetrating artery	Pure motor hemiparesis
Anterior cerebral	Hemiparesis and sensory loss affect leg more than arm
	Impaired responsiveness ("abulia" or "akinetic mutism"), especially if bilateral infarction
	Left-sided ideomotor apraxia or tactile anomia
Posterior cerebral	Cortical, unilateral: isolated hemianopia (or quadrantic field cut); alexia or color anomia
	Cortical, bilateral: cerebral blindness, with or without macular sparing
	Thalamic: pure sensory stroke; may leave anesthesia dolorosa with "spontaneous pain"
	Subthalamic nucleus: hemiballism
	Bilateral inferior temporal lobe: amnesia
	Midbrain: oculomotor palsy and other eye-movement abnormalities

artery region can cause a severe behavior disturbance, with apathy (abulia), motor inertia, muteness, incontinence, suck and grasp reflexes, and diffuse rigidity (Gegenhalten), or total unresponsiveness with open eyes (akinetic mutism). Symptoms and signs are attributed to destruction of the orbitofrontal cortex, deep limbic structures, supplementary motor cortex, or cingulate gyri.

POSTERIOR CEREBRAL ARTERY

Occlusion of the posterior cerebral artery most often causes contralateral homonymous hemianopia by destroying the calcarine cortex. Macular (central) vision tends to be spared because the occipital pole receives a collateral blood supply from the middle cerebral artery.

In contrast to lesions of the optic radiations, a decrease in the visual field caused by an occipital lobe infarction is usually associated with preserved opticokinetic nystagmus; there may be partial preservation of vision, visual perseveration (palinopsia), or release hallucinations in the blind field.

If the lesion affects the dominant hemisphere and includes the posterior corpus callosum, there may be alexia (without aphasia or agraphia) attributed to disconnection of the right occipital cortex (vision) from the left hemisphere (language). Such patients often have anomia for colors.

When infarction is bilateral, there may be cortical blindness and sometimes the patient does not recognize or admit the loss of vision (*Anton syndrome*). Macular sparing, on the other hand, may produce tunnel vision. Other unusual phenomena of bilateral occipital injury are simultanagnosia (inability to synthesize the parts of what is seen into a whole), poor eye-hand coordination, difficulty coordinating gaze, metamorphopsia (distortion of what is seen, associated especially with occipitotemporal lesions), and visual agnosia.

Whether unilateral infarction in the posterior cerebral artery's supply to the inferior temporal lobe causes memory disturbance is controversial. When bilateral, such lesions may cause severe and lasting amnesia resembling Korsakoff syndrome. TIAs that affect these areas may account for transient global amnesia, but this vascular theory is also controversial. Patients with bilateral lesions affecting both the occipital and temporal lobes may present with agitated delirium.

If posterior cerebral artery occlusion is proximal, the lesions may include the thalamus or midbrain which are supplied by interpeduncular, paramedian, thalamoperforating, and thalamogeniculate branches. Infarction of the ventral posterior nucleus may cause severe loss of all sensory modalities on the opposite side or, sometimes, dissociated sensory loss with relative preservation of touch, proprioception, and discriminative modalities or, conversely, of pain and temperature sensation. As sensation returns, there may be intractable, persistent pain and hyperpathia on the affected side (*"thalamic pain," "analgesia dolorosa,"* or *Roussy-Dejerine syndrome*). A lesion of the subthalamic nucleus causes contralateral hemiballism. Whether lesions of the ventral anterior or ventral lateral thalamus cause hemichorea, ataxia, or other movement disorders is less certain.

Several abnormal eye signs may be found when posterior cerebral artery disease affects the midbrain: bilateral (or, less often, unilateral) loss of vertical gaze, convergence spasm, retractatory nystagmus, lid retraction (Collier sign), oculomotor palsy, internuclear ophthalmoplegia, decreased pupillary reactivity, and corectopia (eccentrically positioned pupil). Lethargy or coma may follow damage to the reticular activating system. *Peduncular hallucinosis* consists of hallucinations, often formed and vivid, that usually occur in somnolent patients with presumed mesencephalic lesions, but the symptoms probably arise from thalamic or occipitotemporal lesions rather than the midbrain itself. Posterior cerebral artery occlusion can sometimes cause contralateral hemiparesis by damaging the midbrain peduncle; it may also cause contralateral ataxia by affecting the superior cerebellar outflow above its decussation.

ANTERIOR CHOROIDAL ARTERY

Infarction in the area of the anterior choroidal artery produces inconsistent deficits. Usually these are in varying combinations of contralateral hemiplegia, sensory loss, and homonymous hemianopia (sometimes with striking sparing of a beak-like zone horizontally). Causes are involvement of the midbrain peduncle or posterior limb of the internal capsule and the lateral geniculate body or early optic radiations. Symptoms are often incomplete and temporary.

INTERNAL CAROTID ARTERY

Internal carotid occlusion may be clinically silent or it may cause massive cerebral infarction. Damage occurs most often in the territory of the middle cerebral artery or, depending on collateral circulation, of one of its branches, with syndromes of varying severity. When the anterior communicating artery is not present, infarction may include the territory of the anterior cerebral artery. Internal carotid artery occlusion (or abrupt hypotension in someone with tight stenosis) can also cause infarction in the border zones ("watersheds") between the middle, anterior, and posterior cerebral arteries; syncope at onset, focal seizures, and transcortical aphasia (relatively preserved repetition) are often seen with such lesions. When the posterior cerebral artery arises directly from the internal carotid, there may be symptoms referable to the visual cortex, thalamus, inferior temporal lobe, or upper brain stem. Infrequently, carotid artery disease can cause vertebrobasilar TIAs.

Emboli dislodged from atherosclerotic plaques in the internal carotid artery reach the retina through the ophthalmic and central retinal arteries to cause partial or complete visual loss. Platelet-fibrin or cholesterol emboli can sometimes be seen ophthalmoscopically in retinal artery branches. When transient, these attacks are called *amaurosis fugax*.

VERTEBROBASILAR ARTERIES

Several eponyms have been applied to brain-stem syndromes, but except for the lateral medullary syndrome of Wallenberg, most of the original descriptions concerned patients with neoplasms. Brain-stem infarction is more often the result of occlusion of the vertebral or basilar arteries than their paramedian or lateral branches; classic medial or lateral brain-stem syndromes are encountered less often than incomplete or mixed clinical pictures (see Table 30–1). That an infarct involves posterior fossa structures is suggested by: (1) bilateral long-tract (motor or sensory) signs; (2) crossed (e.g., left face and right limb) motor or sensory signs; (3) dissociated sensory loss on one half of the body, with pain and temperature sensation more involved than proprioception; (4) cerebellar signs; (5) stupor or coma; (6) dysconjugate eye movements or nystagmus, including internuclear ophthalmoplegia; (7) Horner syndrome; and (8) involvement of cranial nerves not usually affected by single hemispheric infarcts (e.g., unilateral deafness or pharyngeal weakness). Brain-stem infarction may cause only unilateral weakness indistinguishable from that seen with lacunes in the internal capsule.

Syndromes of Infarction

LATERAL MEDULLARY INFARCTION

This infarction usually follows occlusion of the vertebral or, less often, the posterior inferior cerebellar artery. Manifestations include vertigo, nausea, vomiting, and nystagmus (from involvement of the vestibular nuclei); gait and ipsilateral limb ataxia (cerebellum or inferior cerebellar peduncle); impaired pain and temperature sensation on the ipsilateral face (descending tract and nucleus of the trigeminal nerve) and the contralateral body (spinothalamic tract); dysphagia, hoarseness, and ipsilateral weakness of the palate and vocal cords and decrease of the gag reflex (nucleus ambiguus, or ninth and tenth nerve outflow tracts); and ipsilateral Horner syndrome (descending sympathetic fibers). There may be hiccup and, if the nucleus or tractus solitarius is affected, ipsilateral loss of taste (Table 30–2).

INFARCTION OF MEDIAL MEDULLA

An infarction of the medial medulla usually follows an occlusion of a vertebral artery or a branch of the lower basilar artery and involves the pyramidal tract, medial lemniscus, and hypoglossal nucleus or outflow tract. There is ipsilateral tongue weakness (with deviation toward the paretic side) and contralateral hemiparesis and impaired proprioception, but cutaneous sensation is spared.

LATERAL PONTINE INFARCTION

This may affect caudal structures when there is occlusion of the anterior inferior cerebellar artery or rostral structures after occlusion of the superior cerebellar artery. The caudal syndrome resembles that of lateral medullary infarction, with vertigo, nystagmus, ataxia, Horner syndrome, crossed face-and-body pain, and temperature loss. There is ipsilateral deafness and tinnitus (from involvement of the cochlear nuclei); if damage includes more medial structures, there may be ipsilateral gaze paresis or facial weakness. Rostral lateral pontine infarction causes the same constellation of symptoms except that the seventh and eighth cranial nerves are

spared. There is ipsilateral paresis of the jaw muscles.

MEDIAL-PONTINE INFARCTION SYNDROMES

These syndromes occur after occlusion of paramedian branches of the basilar artery and depend on whether the lesion is caudal or rostral. A constant feature is contralateral hemiparesis. When the lesion includes the nucleus of the seventh nerve, there is ipsilateral facial weakness; when damage is more rostral, facial paresis is contralateral. There may also be ipsilateral gaze palsy (abducens nucleus or paramedian reticular formation), abducens palsy (sixth-nerve outflow tract), internuclear ophthalmoplegia, and limb or gait ataxia. Caudal lesions can cause contralateral loss of proprioception. Palatal myoclonus is attributed to involvement of the central tegmental tract and may be accompanied by rhythmic movements of the pharynx, larynx, face, eyes, or respiratory muscles.

ATAXIC HEMIPARESIS

This disorder is characterized by weakness and limb ataxia on the same side and can be caused by lacunar infarcts in the ventral pons, which affect the pyramidal tract, nuclei of the basis pontis, and crossing pontocerebellar fibers. Why the cerebellar signs should be entirely contralateral is unclear.

Symptoms resembling acute labyrinthitis, with vertigo, nausea, vomiting, and nystagmus, may accompany either infarction of the interior cerebellum or occlusion of the internal auditory artery, which arises from the basilar or anterior inferior cerebellar arteries, with resulting infarction of the inner ear. Large cerebellar infarcts may mimic cerebellar hemorrhage with headache, dizziness, ataxia, and, if there is brain-stem compression, abducens or gaze palsy and progression to coma and death.

Drop attacks are caused by fleeting loss of strength or muscle tone, without loss of consciousness; bilateral ischemia of the pontine or medullary pyramidal tract is the explanation in some cases. Infarction of the corticobulbar and corticospinal tracts in the basis pontis (sparing the tegmentum) causes the *"locked-in-syndrome,"* with paralysis of limbs and lower cranial nerves; communication by preserved eye movements reveals that consciousness is intact.

MIDBRAIN INFARCTION

This follows occlusion of the posterior cerebral artery, but the classic mesencephalic

Table 30–2.   Signs that Indicate the Level of Brain-Stem Vascular Syndromes

Syndrome	Artery Affected	Structure Involved	Manifestations
Medial syndromes			
Medulla	Paramedian branches	Emerging fibers of twelfth nerve	Ipsilateral hemiparalysis of tongue
Inferior pons	Paramedian branches	Pontine gaze center, near or in nucleus of sixth nerve	Paralysis of gaze to side of lesion
		Emerging fibers of sixth nerve	Ipsilateral abduction paralysis
Superior pons	Paramedian branches	Medial longitudinal fasciculus	Internuclear ophthalmoplegia
Lateral syndromes			
Medulla	Posterior inferior cerebellar	Emerging fibers of ninth and tenth nerves	Dysphagia, hoarseness, ipsilateral paralysis of vocal cord; ipsilateral loss of pharyngeal reflex
		Vestibular nuclei	Vertigo, nystagmus
		Descending tract and nucleus of fifth nerve	Ipsilateral facial analgesia
		Solitary nucleus and tract	Taste loss on ipsilateral half of tongue posteriorly
Inferior pons	Anterior inferior cerebellar	Emerging fibers of seventh nerve	Ipsilateral facial paralysis
		Solitary nucleus and tract	Taste loss on ipsilateral half of tongue anteriorly
		Cochlear nuclei	Deafness, tinnitus
Mid-pons		Motor nucleus of fifth nerve	Ipsilateral jaw weakness
		Emerging sensory fibers of fifth nerve	Ipsilateral facial numbness

(Modified from Rowland LP. In: Kandel ER, Schwartz JH, eds. Principles of Neural Science, 2nd ed. New York: Elsevier-North Holland, 1985.)

syndromes (oculomotor palsy with contralateral hemiparesis, the *Weber syndrome*: or crossed hemiataxia and chorea, the *Benedikt syndrome*) are infrequently the result of stroke.

BILATERAL UPPER BRAIN STEM INFARCTION

An infarction at this site causes coma by destroying the reticular activating system. When the level is pontine, signs mimic those caused by hemorrhage with reactive miotic pupils and loss of eye movements. When damage is mesencephalic, ophthalmoplegia is accompanied by midposition unreactive pupils. If there is only partial loss of consciousness, bilateral long-tract motor and sensory signs or cerebellar ataxia may be detected.

PSEUDOBULBAR PALSY

This is a syndrome that follows at least two major cerebral infarcts on different sides of the brain (which may occur at different times) or numerous lacunes on both sides. The bi-

lateral hemisphere lesions cause bilateral corticospinal reflex signs (with or without major bilateral hemiparesis), supranuclear dysarthria and dysphagia (with impaired volitional movements but exaggerated reflex movement of the soft palate and pharynx), and emotional incontinence with exaggerated crying (or less often, laughing) that is attributed to release of limbic functions. Other causes of pseudobulbar palsy are multiple sclerosis and amyotrophic lateral sclerosis (ALS).

MULTI-INFARCT DEMENTIA

Cerebral infarction can cause dementia either by affecting critical structures such as the inferomedial temporal lobes or by destroying a sufficient volume of brain, usually 100 cc. Clinical or radiographic evidence of stroke in a demented patient does not necessarily signify cause and effect; multi-infarct dementia is undoubtedly overdiagnosed.

References

Bogousslavsky J, Regli F. Unilateral watershed cerebral infarcts. Neurology 1986; 36:373–377.

Brust JCM. Dementia and cerebrovascular disease. In: Mayeux R, Rosen WG, eds. The Dementias. New York, Raven Press, 1983:131–147.

Brust JCM, Behrens MM. "Release hallucinations" as the major symptoms of posterior cerebral artery occlusion: a report of 2 cases. Ann Neurol 1977; 2:432–436.

Brust JCM, Plank C, Burke A, Guobadia MI, Healton EB. Language disorder in a right-hander after occlusion of the right anterior cerebral artery. Neurology 1982; 32:492–497.

Brust JCM, Plank CR, Healton EB, Sanchez GF. The pathology of drop attacks: a case report. Neurology 1979; 29:786–790.

Caplan LR. "Top of the basilar" syndrome. Neurology 1980; 30:72–79.

Caplan LR, DeWitt LD, Pessin MS, et al. Lateral thalamic infarcts. Arch Neurol 1988; 45:959–965.

Castaigne P, Lhermitte F, Buge A, Escourolle R, Hauw JJ, Lyon-Caen O. Paramedian thalamic and midbrain infarcts: Clinical and neuropathological study. Ann Neurol 1981; 10:127–148.

Damasio AR, Damasio H, Van Hoesen GW. Prosopagnosia: anatomic basis and behavioral mechanisms. Neurology 1982; 32:331–341.

Devinsky O, Beard D, Volpe BT. Confusional states following posterior cerebral artery infarction. Arch Neurol 1988; 45:160–163.

Duncan GW, Parker SW, Fisher CM. Acute cerebellar infarction in the PICA territory. Arch Neurol 1975; 32:364–368.

Fisher CM. Ataxic hemiparesis: a pathologic study. Arch Neurol 1978; 35:126–128.

Healton EB, Navarro C, Bressman S, Brust JCM. Subcortical neglect. Neurology 1982; 32:776–778.

Helgason C, Caplan LR, Goodwin J, Hedges T. Anterior choroidal artery-territory infarction. Report of cases and review. Arch Neurol 1986; 43:681–686.

Jones HR, Caplan LR, Come PC, Swinton NW, Breslin DJ. Cerebral emboli of paradoxical origin. Ann Neurol 1983; 13:314–319.

Kubik CS, Adams RD. Occlusion of the basilar artery—clinical and pathological study. Brain 1946; 69:73–121.

Lehrich JR, Winkler GF, Ojemann RG. Cerebellar infarction with brainstem compression. Arch Neurol 1970; 22:490–498.

Mehler MF. The neuro-ophthalmologic spectrum of the rostral basilar artery syndrome. Arch Neurol 1988; 45:966–972.

Mohr JP, Caplan LR, Melski JW, et al. The Harvard Cooperative Stroke Registry: a prospective registry. Neurology 1978; 28:754–762.

Mohr JP, Pessin MS, Finkelstein S, et al. Broca aphasia: pathologic and clinical aspects. Neurology 1978; 28:311–324.

Rowland LP. Clinical syndromes of the brain stem. In: Kandel ER, Schwartz JH, eds. Principles of Neural Science, 2nd ed. New York: Elsevier-North Holland, 1985:597–607.

Sacco RL, Bello JA, Traub R, Brust JCM: Selective proprioceptive loss from a thalamic lacunar stroke. Stroke 1987; 18:1160–1163.

31. CEREBRAL AND CEREBELLAR HEMORRHAGE

J.P. Mohr

Most hemorrhages in the brain parenchyma arise in the region of the small arteries that serve the basal ganglia, thalamus, and brain stem, and are caused by an arteriopathy of chronic hypertension. This disorder causes either occlusions with lacunar infarction or leakages that result in the characteristic syndromes of brain hemorrhage. A smaller number arise from *congophilic amyloid angiopathy*, a degenerative disorder affecting the media of the smaller arteries, mainly of the cerebral gray matter in elderly individuals. While hypertensive hemorrhages rarely recur in the same or other locations, congophilic angiopathy recurs frequently enough to be considered characteristic of this disorder. Brain tumors, sympathomimetic drugs, and small arteriovenous malformations round out the list of cerebral and cerebellar hemorrhages.

Because the hemorrhages arise from tiny vessels, the accumulation of the hematoma takes time, and determines the smooth onset of the clinical syndrome over minutes or hours. This smooth uninterrupted onset and the occurrence of frequent vomiting are major points that help differentiate hemorrhage from infarction. The hemorrhage usually stops spontaneously by 30 minutes, but may continue to the point of fatal brain disruption and compression. The *putamen* is the site most frequently affected. When the expanding hematoma involves the adjacent internal capsule there is a contralateral hemiparesis, usually with hemianesthesia and hemianopia and, in large hematomas, aphasia or impaired awareness of the disorder. When the hemorrhage arises in the *thalamus*, hemianesthesia precedes the hemiparesis; however, once contralateral motor, sensory, and visual field signs are established, the main points that distinguish the two syndromes are conjugate horizontal ocular deviation in putaminal hemorrhage and impaired upward gaze in thalamic hemorrhage.

Pontine hemorrhage usually plunges the patient into coma with quadriparesis and grossly dysconjugate ocular motility disorders, although small hemorrhages may mimic syndromes of infarction. When hemorrhages affect one or more cerebral lobes, the syndrome is difficult to distinguish clinically from infarction because smooth onset and vomiting are much less frequent; also, lobar hemorrhages often result from arteriovenous malformations, amyloid angiopathy, tumors, or other causes that rarely affect the basal ganglia, thalamus, and pons.

Cerebellar hemorrhage warrants separate description because the mode of onset differs from that of cerebral hemorrhage and because it is often reversible by surgical evacuation. The syndrome usually begins abruptly with vomiting and severe ataxia (which usually prevents standing and walking); it is occasionally accompanied by paralysis of conjugate lateral gaze to one side. These symptoms occur without changes in the level of consciousness and without any focal weakness or sensory loss. Enlargement of the mass does not change the clinical picture until there is enough brain-stem compression to precipitate coma, at which point it is too late for surgical evacuation of the hemorrhage to reverse the disorder. This small margin of time between an alert state and an irreversible coma makes it imperative to consider the diagnosis in all patients with this clinical syndrome; CT should be carried out promptly, and surgery should be performed within hours on all of the larger hemorrhages.

References

Aring CD, Merritt HH. Differential diagnosis between cerebral hemorrhage and cerebral thrombosis. Arch Intern Med 1935; 56:435–456.

Fieschi C et al. Changing prognosis of primary intracerebral hemorrhage. Stroke 1988; 19:192–195.

Hier DB, Davis KR, Richardson ER, Mohr JP. Hypertensive putaminal hemorrhage. Ann Neurol 1977; 1:152–159.

Kase CS. Intracerebral hemorrhage: Non-hypertensive causes. Stroke 1986; 17:590–595.

Macdonell RAL et al. Cerebellar infarction: natural history, prognosis, pathology. Stroke 1987; 18:849–855.

Ojemann RG, Heros RC. Progress in cerebrovascular disease: Spontaneous brain hemorrhage. Stroke 1983; 14:468–475.

Ojemann RG, Mohr JP. Hypertensive brain hemorrhage. Clin Neurosurg 1976; 23:220–244.

Okudera T et al. Primary pontine hemorrhage: Correlations of pathologic features with postmortem microangiographic and vertebral studies. Mt Sinai J Med 1978; 45:305–321.

Ott KH, Kase CS, Ojemann RG, Mohr JP. Cerebellar hemorrhage: Diagnosis and treatment. A review of 56 cases. Arch Neurol 1974; 31:160–167.

Vinters HV. Cerebral amyloid angiography. Critical review. Stroke 1988; 19:311–314.

32. OTHER CEREBROVASCULAR SYNDROMES
Frank M. Yatsu

Lacunar Strokes

Occlusion of small penetrating arterioles (150 μm diameter) usually follows sustained hypertension and leads to cystic cerebral degeneration or lacune formation. Although these small occlusions are frequently located in clinically silent areas, discrete and well-defined lacunar syndromes have been described. These include *pure motor hemiplegia, pure hemisensory stroke, sensorimotor pseudobulbar palsy, ipsilateral ataxia* and *hemiparesis*, and *dysarthria-clumsy hand syndrome.*

Pure motor hemiplegia usually involves the face, arm, and leg without sensory loss; the lacune disrupts the corticospinal tracts in the internal capsule or pons. As with other lacunar syndromes, diseases other than hypertension may cause identical symptoms; these include emboli and hemorrhage.

Pure hemisensory stroke without motor impairment is characterized clinically by numbness or paresthesias involving the face, arm, and leg. The impaired sensation can be explained by a lacune in the sensory nucleus of the thalamus. Pseudobulbar palsy results from multiple bilateral frontal lobe lacunes. CT may occasionally demonstrate lacunar hypodensities. When the lacunar syndrome can be explained adequately by hypertensive disease, no specific therapy other than hypertension control is indicated.

HYPERTENSIVE ENCEPHALOPATHY

In 1928, Oppenheimer and Fishberg introduced the term "hypertensive encephalopathy" to describe encephalopathic symptoms (e.g., headaches, confusion, drowsiness, blurring of vision, occasional seizures and infrequent focal signs) in association with an accelerated, malignant phase of hypertension. The diastolic pressures are greater than 140 mm Hg and the fundi usually demonstrate Grade IV changes with hemorrhages and edema. Because this constellation of clinical findings may be found with strokes and systemic disorders (e.g., uremia and electrolyte imbalance), the diagnosis of hypertensive encephalopathy is frequently erroneous. The term is now reserved for nonfocal symptoms of altered mental state, with or without generalized convulsion, that occur in patients with malignant hypertension; the symptoms are reversed when blood pressure is reduced and renal function does not change. The syndrome is attributed to generalized arteriolar dilatation when cerebral autoregulation is lost. It must be distinguished from stroke, uremia, and other metabolic encephalopathies. Because the sustained hypertension may be life-threatening, the clinically pragmatic, therapeutic approach has been to treat these patients with hypotensive agents (e.g., sodium nitroprusside, trimethaphan camsylate) as demand therapy, unless stroke or some other condition clearly explains the encephalopathic symptoms. If the symptoms do not improve, however, establishment of diagnosis is more difficult. With hypotensive therapy, care must be taken not to reduce the blood pressure excessively because "watershed" infarct is a possible complication.

Fibromuscular Hyperplasia

Fibromuscular bands of unknown origin form segmental narrowing in large arteries and may cause ischemic symptoms of the brain, including TIAs and infarcts, although they most frequently present as an asymptomatic carotid bruit. The common involvement of the renal arteries leads to hypertension. The clinical diagnosis of fibromuscular hyperplasia is suggested by the combination of carotid and renal artery bruits in the presence of systemic hypertension. Women are usually affected in middle age. The diagnosis is rarely suspected before the lesions are demonstrated by angiography (Fig. 32–1). Antiplatelet drugs, anticoagulation, bypass surgery, and surgical dilatation have all been reported to reduce the frequency of TIAs in this syndrome.

Multi-Infarct Dementia

This syndrome is discussed in Articles I and III, Delirium and Dementia and The Dementias, respectively.

Cerebral Amyloid Angiopathy

Cerebral amyloid angiopathy or "congophilic angiopathy" most commonly manifests as intracerebral hemorrhage, primarily after age 65. Amyloid deposits are found in medium and small cortical and leptomeningeal arteries and are not associated with systemic amyloidosis. Intracerebral hemorrhage, particularly when lobar in location, tends to recur within months or years and multiple hemorrhages may occur simultaneously. Progressive dementia occurs in some 30% of patients, and features of Alzheimer disease are seen pathologically in 50%.

The diagnosis of cerebral amyloid angiopathy should be considered in a normotensive elderly individual, commonly demented, with a lobar intracerebral hemorrhage. No therapy is known for the primary process; indications for hematoma evacuation are similar

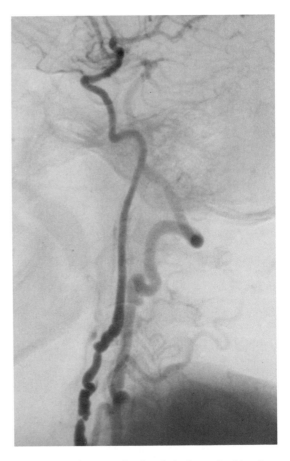

Fig. 32–1. Fibromuscular dysplasia. Lateral subtraction film from right carotid arteriogram shows reflux of the vertebral, occlusion of the ECA, and segmental stenoses of the CCA and ICA pattern typical of fibromuscular dysplasia. (Courtesy of Drs. J.A. Bello and S.K. Hilal.)

to those for other etiologies, namely, location, mass effect, and declining sensorium. Familial forms may be detected by the presence of gamma trace alkaline microprotein in serum.

Lupus Anticoagulants

Lupus anticoagulants, a misnomer because thrombosis is the usual clinical syndrome, are immunoglobulins, usually IgG, but occasionally IgM. They inhibit coagulation by interfering with phospholipid-dependent coagulation tests without inhibiting in vivo activity of coagulation factors. Lupus anticoagulants were first described in patients with systemic lupus erythematosus (SLE), but have been reported with drug-induced lupus, other autoimmune diseases, neoplasms, phenothiazines, and idiopathically. Lupus anticoagulants may prolong partial thromboplastin time (PTT), but are paradoxically associated with thrombosis rather than a bleeding diathesis. The condition may be associated with a false-positive VDRL test and mild thrombo-cytopenia. Most thrombotic episodes are venous, although cerebral TIAs and infarcts of the arterial system have been described. Treatment should be directed to the primary underlying condition, but reported therapies have been primarily anecdotal and include corticosteroids, antiplatelet drugs, and anticoagulation.

References

Lacunar Strokes

Bamford JM, Warlow CP. Evolution and testing of the lacunar hypothesis. Stroke 1988; 19:1074–1082.

Fisher CM. Lacunar strokes and infarcts: A review. Neurology 1982; 32:1–6.

Fisher CM. Pure sensory stroke and allied conditions. Stroke 1982; 13:434–447.

Mohr JP. Lacunes. Stroke 1982; 13:3–10.

Hypertensive Encephalopathy

Chester EM, Agamanolis DP, Banker BQ, Victor M. Hypertensive encephalopathy: A clinicopathologic study of 20 cases. Neurology 1978; 28:928–939.

Gifford RW Jr, Westbrook E. Hypertensive encephalopathy: Mechanisms, clinical features, and treatment. Prog Cardiovasc Dis 1974; 17:115–124.

Hauser RA, Lacey DM, Knight MR. Hypertensive Encephalopathy. Arch Neurol 1988; 45:1078–1083.

Healton EB, Brust JCM, Feinfeld DA, Thomson GE. Hypertensive encephalopathy and the neurologic manifestations of malignant hypertension. Neurology 1982; 32:127–132.

Meyer JS, Watz AG, Gotoh F. Pathogenesis of cerebral vasospasm in hypertensive encephalopathy. Neurology 1960; 10:734–744.

Oppenheimer BS, Fishberg AM. Hypertensive encephalopathy. Arch Intern Med 1928; 41:264–278.

Ziegler DK, Zosa A, Zileli T. Hypertensive encephalopathy. Arch Neurol 1965; 12:472–478.

Fibromuscular Hyperplasia

Mettinger KL, Ericson K. Fibromuscular dysplasias and the brain. Stroke 1982; 13:46–58.

Sandok BA. Fibromuscular dysplasia of the internal carotid artery. Neurol Clin 1983; 1:17–26.

Starr DS, Lawrie GM, Morris GC. Fibromuscular disease of carotid arteries: Long term results of graduated internal dilatation. Stroke 1981; 12:197–199.

Cerebral Amyloid Angiopathy

Gilbert JJ, Vinters HV. Cerebral amyloid angiopathy: Incidence and complications in the aging brain. I. Cerebral hemorrhage. Stroke 1983; 14:915–923.

Gilles C, Brucher JM, Khoubesserian P, Vanderhaeghen JJ: Cerebral amyloid angiopathy as a cause of multiple intracerebral hemorrhages. Neurology 1984; 34:730–735.

Grubb A et al. Abnormal metabolism of gamma-trace alkaline microprotein. The basic defect in hereditary cerebral hemorrhage. N Engl J Med 1984; 311:1547–1549.

Vinters HV. Cerebral amyloid angiopathy. Critical review. Stroke 1988; 19:311–324.

Lupus Anticoagulant

Hart RG, et al. Cerebral infarction associated with lupus anticoagulant. Preliminary report. Stroke 1984; 15:114.

Levine S, Welch KMA. Cerebrovascular ischemia and lupus anticoagulant. Stroke 1987; 18:257–263.

33. DIFFERENTIAL DIAGNOSIS OF STROKE
J.P. Mohr

The differential diagnosis of cerebral hemorrhage and cerebral infarction or embolus is important when determining the patient's prognosis and in deciding about the use of anticoagulants or surgery.

A diagnosis of *cerebral embolism* is suggested by a sudden onset and a syndrome of circumscribed focal deficit, attributable to cerebral surface infarction, such as in pure aphasia or pure hemianopia. The more complex the neurologic syndrome, the larger the arterial territory involved and the more the diagnosis of *thrombosis* must be considered. A diagnosis of embolism is important because the risk of recurrence is high. The source of the embolus may be found in acute or chronic endocarditis, atrial fibrillation, or recent myocardial infarction. The brain is the first site of symptoms in most cases of systemic embolism; clinically recognized embolization at other anatomic sites is rare. When the source of embolization is not obvious on hospital admission, useful procedures include routine blood cultures and EKG monitoring. The size of the embolic material sufficient to cause a focal stroke is often too small to make echocardiography helpful, and all too often eludes all efforts at diagnosis. A third or more of the cases fail to show the cause of the embolus, despite full use of laboratory investigations. Angiography within 48 hours of stroke usually demonstrates a pattern of arterial occlusion that is typical of embolus and permits diagnosis. If angiography is delayed, the results are usually normal. On the other hand, CT scans will appear positive for infarction for a week if the embolus is sufficiently large to cause a deficit that persists several days.

A diagnosis of thrombosis is considered first when the stroke has been preceded by TIAs. When the syndrome is of sudden onset, thrombus is clinically inseparable from embolus. No specific clinical syndrome separates the two mechanisms of infarction.

Hemorrhage has a characteristically smooth onset that is a helpful historical point in differential diagnosis. When the syndrome develops to an advanced stage within minutes or is halted at an early stage with only minor signs, the smooth evolution may not be apparent and the clinical picture may then be inseparable from that of infarction. Within a day of onset CT can separate the clinically inobvious hemorrhage from infarct and should be used whenever treatment with anticoagulants is planned. There are no reliable CT findings to distinguish hemorrhagic infarction and frank hematoma.

The suddenness of onset and the focal signs give these syndromes the popular term stroke and help to distinguish cerebrovascular disease from other neurologic disorders. Hypertension, arteriosclerosis, or other evidence of vascular disease are commonly present, but only the disappearance of symptoms within minutes or hours permits the separation of TIA from stroke. In the acute state, considerations of differential diagnosis apply equally to TIA and stroke.

Sudden onset also characterizes trauma, epilepsy, and migraine. External signs usually indicate trauma, but when they are absent, the diagnosis depends on a history that is not always easily obtained. The most frequent sites of brain contusions are the frontal and temporal poles, but these lesions neither produce an easily recognized clinical picture nor one often encountered in cases of stroke; however, epidural and subdural hematomas occur in a setting of trauma and may mimic a stroke. Although the trauma itself is sudden, the accumulation of the hematoma takes time: minutes or hours for epidural hemorrhage and as long as weeks for subdural hemorrhages.

Epidural hemorrhage is arterial in origin, and usually produces a blood mass large enough to displace the brain and cause coma within hours after the injury. Apart from slower evolution, the clinical picture is otherwise similar to that of putaminal hemorrhage. Radiographs of the skull may reveal a fracture line that passes through the groove of the middle meningeal artery, which is usually a laceration. CT is the most helpful radiologic test; it demonstrates the position of the hematoma in all cases and gives the diagnosis even in comatose patients, when the fine points of clinical examination cannot be used. Operation to evacuate the hematoma is usually appropriate even in cases with severe deficits, because the brain dysfunction is due primarily to compression, and the syndrome may be reversible when pressure from the hematoma has been relieved.

Subdural hematoma is typically venous in origin. The bleeding may be recurrent. The precipitating trauma may have been trivial or forgotten, and the blood may have been present long enough (over a week) to become isodense (radiographically inapparent) on CT. Fluctuating and false localizing signs are frequent. Further, a clot may be found on both sides. These common features often make subdural hematoma difficult to diagnose. Lumbar puncture shows a range of findings from normal to the extremes of xanthochromic CSF under high pressure with increased protein content. The most reliable diagnosis is by angiography, which shows displacement of the brain away from the inner table of the skull.

As a sign of acute stroke, *seizures* are rare, except in cases of lobar hemorrhage. The immediate postictal deficit mimics that caused by major stroke. Only the obtundation and amnestic state help suggest prior seizure. In a small percentage of cases seizures develop months or years after a large infarct or hemorrhage. In these, the postictal state often represents a relapse of the original stroke syndrome, which usually resolves toward the chronic preictal state after a few days. Without a proper history, it may be nearly impossible to rule out new stroke.

Migraine is increasingly appreciated as a major source of difficulty in the diagnosis of TIA. Migraine may begin in middle age; the aura alone, without headache, is commonly experienced by those who suffer chronic migraine. When symptoms are visual and a diagnosis of transient mononuclear blindness is considered, the differential diagnosis from migraine is the easiest: migraine typically produces a visual disorder that marches across the vision of both eyes as an advancing thin scintillating line that takes 5 to 15 minutes to pass out of vision. Subsequent unilateral pounding headache need not occur, but makes the diagnosis certain. It is difficult to diagnose migraine as a cause of symptoms of hemisphere dysfunction because the auras of classic migraine only rarely include motor, sensory, language, or behavioral elements. TIA rarely goes from one limb to another like the visual disorder of migraine. A diagnosis of migraine probably should not be seriously considered as an explanation for transient hemisphere attacks unless the patient is young, has repeated attacks, experiences classic visual migraine auras at other times, and has a pounding headache contralateral to the sensory or motor symptoms in the hours after the attack.

The differential diagnosis of stroke is important in any patient with a focal or lateralizing disturbance in cerebral function, but the history often suffices to eliminate stroke. Here the major possibilities include *neoplasm* and *abscess*. Both usually evolve in days or weeks, which is longer than stroke. Seizures often occur before focal signs are evident, a sequence that is rare in stroke. CT in tumor or abscess usually demonstrates an enhancing mass even when symptoms are mild. In contrast, CT in ischemic stroke is often negative in the first few days, contrast enhancement may not occur, and there are signs of a mass only when the syndrome is severe. In parenchymatous hemorrhage, the areas around the hematoma do not usually enhance with contrast, but contrast enhancement is common when hemorrhage has occurred into a tumor. If the CSF is examined, increased pressure and clear or slightly cloudy fluid are encountered equally in tumors, early abscesses, and large infarcts. The CSF usually shows mild or moderate pleocytosis in abscess, but the same findings may be present in large infarcts.

When coma is present, other diagnoses that must be considered include metabolic disturbances of glucose, renal function, electrolytes, alcohol, and drugs. The odor of acetone on the breath and the presence of sugar in the urine favor a diagnosis of diabetes mellitus. Transient mild glycosuria and hyperglycemia often follow cerebral hemorrhage or infarction, but do not approach the elevations seen in diabetic coma. In renal failure, high levels of BUN and creatinine often cause coma. Focal signs occasionally occur and then remit when the cause is reversed, often accompanying unrecognized infection or severe disturbances in electrolyte balance. An alcoholic odor to the breath, normal blood pressure, no evidence of hemiplegia, and a normal CSF are characteristic findings in cases of coma due to acute alcoholism. In barbiturate intoxication, the coma may feature total paralysis of ocular motility and flaccid paralysis of the limbs with preserved pupillary reactions, which is a rare combination in stroke. The CSF pressure may be slightly elevated (200–300 mm H_2O) in any form of coma, due to hypoventilation and CO_2 retention. Because alcoholics and drug abusers are prone

to head injuries, the diagnosis of subdural hematoma should always be considered.

References

Abdon NJ, Zettervall O, Carlson J, et al. Is occult atrial disorder a frequent cause of stroke? Long-term ECG in 86 patients. Stroke 1982; 13:832–837.

Barnett HJM. Peerless SJ, Kaufmann JCE. "Stump" of internal carotid artery. A source for further cerebral embolic ischemia. Stroke 1978; 9:448–456.

Caplan LR. "Top of the basilar" syndrome. Neurology 1980; 30:72–79.

Come PC, Riley MF, Bivas BA. Roles of echocardiography and arrhythmia monitoring in patients with suspected systemic embolism. Ann Neurol 1983; 13:527–531.

Furlan AJ, Cavalier SJ, Hobbs RE, Weinstein MA, Modic MT. Hemorrhage and anticoagulation after nonseptic embolic brain infarction. Neurology 1982; 32:280–282.

Halperin JL, Hart RG. Atrial fibrillations and stroke: new ideas, persisting dilemmas. Stroke 1988; 19:937–941.

Harrison MJG, Hampton JR. Neurologic presentation of bacterial endocarditis. Br Med J 1967; 2:148–151.

Hinton RC, Mohr JP, Ackerman RH, et al. Symptomatic middle cerebral artery stem stenosis. Ann Neurol 1979; 5:152–157.

Knopman DS, Anderson DC, Asinger RW, Good DC, et al. Indications for echocardiography in patients with ischemic stroke. Neurology 1982; 32:1005–1011.

Kooiker JC, MacLean JM, Sumi SM. Cerebral embolism, marantic endocarditis and cancer. Arch Neurol 1976; 33:260–264.

Mohr JP. Neurologic complications of cardiac valvular disease and cardiac surgery including systemic hypotension. In: Vinken PJ, Bruyn GW, Klawans HL, eds. Handbook of Clinical Neurology (vol 38). New York: Elsevier-North Holland, 1979; 143–171.

Rogers LR, et al. Cerebral infarction from non-bacterial thrombotic endocarditis. Am J Med 1987; 83:746–756.

Wolf PA, Dawber TR, Thomas HE, Kannel WB. Epidemiologic assessment of chronic atrial fibrillation and risk of stroke: The Framingham Study. Neurology 1978; 28:973–977.

34. STROKE IN CHILDREN
Arnold P. Gold

Children can no longer be considered as small adults for diagnostic purposes. Unlike adults, the brain of the fetus and child is rapidly changing in organization and chemical composition. There are changes in neurologic function with neurologic maturation. The nervous system in a nonverbal, relatively spastic newborn is different from that in a school-age child who has mastered language skills and has purposeful locomotion and prehension.

Strokes in children differ from those in adults in three important ways: predisposing factors, clinical evolution, and anatomic site of pathology.

Cyanotic heart disease is one of the most common childhood conditions that predisposes to cerebral arterial or venous thrombosis. Leukemia commonly leads to cerebral hemorrhage. In contrast, atherosclerosis and hypertension predispose to stroke in adults.

Most stroke-prone children do not die as a direct result of stroke; they often improve much more than an adult with a comparable lesion because of the abundant collateral circulation or because of the differences in response of the immature brain to the lesion. The infant or young child with a complicating hemiplegia usually recovers to the point of being able to walk. If a child less than 4 years of age has a stroke, speech is invariably recovered and permanent aphasia does not occur. Children, especially before age 2 years, are more prone to behavioral changes, intellectual deficits, and epilepsy.

The anatomic site of the stroke lesion also differs in children. For example, affected children commonly show occlusion of the intracranial portion of the internal carotid artery and its branches, whereas adults more frequently show extracranial occlusions of the internal carotid. Cerebral aneurysms in children usually occur at the peripheral bifurcations of cerebral arteries; in adults, cerebral aneurysms usually occur near the circle of Willis.

Incidence

Cerebrovascular disease in a well-defined pediatric population in Rochester, Minnesota, had an annual incidence of 2.52 cases/100,000 children or about 50% the incidence of primary intracranial neoplasm. This figure did not include conditions associated with birth, infection, or trauma, and there were few black children in the study. Cerebrovascular complications occur in 6% to 25% of patients with sickle cell disease; the untreated child has a 67% risk of a second stroke. Premature infants weighing less than 1500 g who require intensive care for more than 24 hours have a 50% incidence of complicating subependymal hemorrhage or intraventricular hemorrhage. Intracranial infections, viral or bacterial, may also precipitate vascular complications. Craniocerebral trauma occurs in 3% of children during the first 7 years of life and cerebrovascular complications are common. Sonography, MRI, and CT (Figs. 34–1 through 34–4) are changing our concepts of the incidence of these disorders in children.

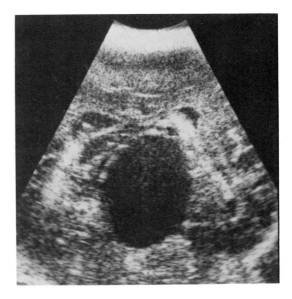

Fig. 34–1. Coronal cranial sonogram of newborn demonstrates aneurysmal dilatation of vein of Galen due to deep midline vascular malformation.

Etiology

A rigid classification of childhood stroke is not possible because a specific cause (e.g., sickle cell disease) may cause hemorrhage in one child and thrombosis in another. Nevertheless, the following list is a clinically useful classification and includes occlusive vascular disease caused by thrombus or embolus, congenital anomalies (especially aneurysm or vascular malformation), hemorrhage, blood dyscrasias, and disorders that alter the permeability of the vascular wall:

Dural sinus and cerebral venous thrombosis
  Infections—face, ears, paranasal sinuses, meninges
  Dehydration and debilitating states
  Blood dyscrasias—sickle cell, leukemia, thrombotic thrombocytopenia
  Neoplasms—neuroblastoma
  Sturge-Weber-Dimitri (trigeminal encephaloangiomatosis)
  Lead encephalopathy

Arterial thrombosis
  Idiopathic
  Dissecting cerebral aneurysm
  Arteriosclerosis—progeria
  Cyanotic heart disease
  Cerebral arteritis
  Collagen disease—lupus erythematosus, periarteritis nodosa, Takayasu, Kawasaki

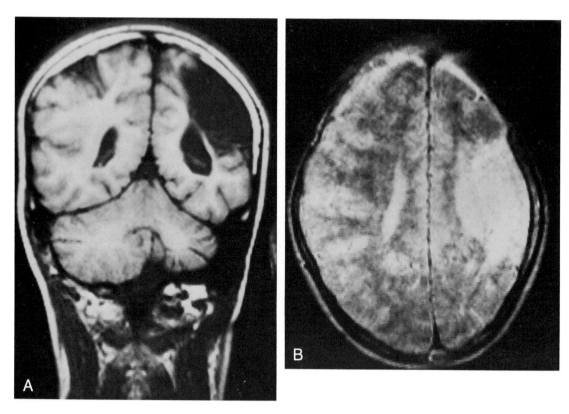

Fig. 34–2. MR scans of child with middle cerebral artery thrombosis and resultant hemiplegia with ischemic infarct. *A.* T_1 coronal image. *B.* Axial T_2 image of left MCA ischemic infarct.

Trauma to cervical carotid or cerebral arteries
Inflammatory bowel disease
Delayed radiation
Sickle-cell disease
Extra-arterial disorders—craniometaphyseal dysplasia, mucormycosis, tumors of the base of the skull
Metabolic (diabetes mellitus, hyperlipidemia, homocystinuria)
Oral contraceptives
Drug abuse

Arterial embolism
Air—complications of cardiac, neck, or thoracic surgery
Fat complications of long-bone fracture
Septic complications of endocarditis, pneumonia, lung abscess
Arrhythmias
Complications of umbilical vein catheterization

Intracranial hemorrhage
Neonatal
Premature—subependymal and intraventricular
Full term—subdural

Vascular malformation
Aneurysm
Blood dyscrasias
Trauma
Vitamin-deficiency syndromes
Hepatic disease
Hypertension
Complications of immunosuppressants and anticoagulants

Arterial Thrombosis

Cerebral arterial thrombosis in children usually involves the intracranial area of the internal carotid artery, although the cervical portion of the internal carotid artery or a spinal artery may be occluded. Neurologic manifestations vary according to the area involved.

As in adults, systemic diseases including collagen-vascular diseases and arteritis may cause cerebral thrombosis in children. Cerebral arteritis usually results from bacterial infections, but other infections may also involve cerebral arteries. Herpes zoster ophthalmias and rarely chickenpox, may have complicating vasculitis that cause delayed onset hemiparesis. Bacterial pharyngitis, cervical adenitis, sinusitis, or pneumonitis may lead to cerebral arteritides. Mucormycosis infection associated with uncontrolled diabetes may extend from the paranasal sinuses to the arteries in the frontal lobe. Both syphilis and tuberculosis may result in cerebral thrombosis in children and adults.

Extrinsic conditions may traumatize or compress the cerebral arteries. Most of these occlusions in children affect the anterior circulation. Vertebrobasilar occlusion may follow cervical dislocations and occlusion of the vertebral artery at the C2 level. Tumors of the base of the skull, craniometaphyseal dysplasia, and retropharyngeal abscesses may compress cerebral arteries.

Sickle-cell disease commonly causes thrombosis of large or small arteries; less commonly, it results in dural sinus thrombosis. Large cerebral artery thrombosis with telangiectasia. (i.e., *moyamoya disease*) results in acute hemiplegia or alternating hemiplegia. Small arterial thrombosis can produce an altered state of consciousness, convulsions, or visual disturbances. About 65% of untreated children have repeated thromboses with additional impairment of motor and intellectual functions. Cerebrovascular complications are less common in children with sickle hemoglobin C disease and rarely occur in sickle cell trait.

Inflammatory bowel disease may lead to a hypercoagulable state with or without thrombocytosis.

Delayed radiation vasculopathy, juvenile diabetes mellitus, homocystinuria, hyperlipidemias, drug abuse, and oral contraceptives result in acute hemiplegia.

Malignancies, most commonly lymphoreticular tumors, may be complicated by a cerebrovascular incident. Most often this is a complication of disseminated vascular occlusion or chemotherapy. Stroke may also result from direct metastatic spread or a complicating thrombocytopenia or fungal infection.

Many children with cerebral arterial thrombosis are healthy before the vascular occlusion occurs and there is no apparent predisposing factor. A dissecting aneurysm due to a congenital defect of the arterial wall has been implicated in some of these idiopathic cases.

Signs and Symptoms. Depending on the predisposing factor, the child with arterial thrombosis has specific clinical signs of the underlying disorder plus neurologic signs of the occluded cerebral artery that are usually found in the anterior circulation. A previously healthy child usually has an acute hemiplegia that is preceded by focal or generalized convulsions, fever, and altered consciousness; less commonly, a series of TIAs eventually results in a completed stroke. Acute hemiplegia is the typical neurologic finding, but hemisensory loss, visual field defects, and aphasia may be seen. The motor deficit maximally involves the hand; if it persists, the involved limbs are spastic, short, and atrophic. Seizures, focal or generalized, are often refractory to anticonvulsants.

The hemiplegia is usually an isolated episode. Bilateral carotid artery thrombosis with telangiectasia typically presents with headaches before the hemiplegia, and recurrences or alternating hemiplegia is characteristic.

Laboratory Data. Blood count, erythrocyte sedimentation rate (ESR), and urinalysis are normal at the time of thrombosis. The CSF is normal at first and a mild leukocyte pleocytosis may occur a few weeks later. The EEG often reveals a slow-wave focus over the involved area. Although skull radiographs are normal when thrombosis occurs, after several years they may show signs of cerebral atrophy with thickening of calvarium, enlargement of the frontal and ethmoid sinuses, and elevation of the petrous pyramid of the temporal bone on the involved side.

CT supplies information about the site and age of the infarct. Within 24 hours there is a nonhomogeneous, decreased-density lesion secondary to edema (Fig. 34–3). By the end

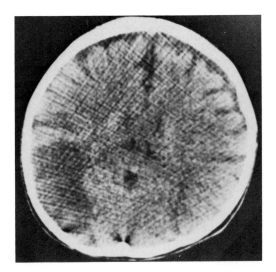

Fig. 34–3. Middle cerebral artery thrombosis of 24 hour duration. CT scan reveals inhomogeneous hypodensity with hazy margins in the parieto-occipital region (early scanner, right and left reversed).

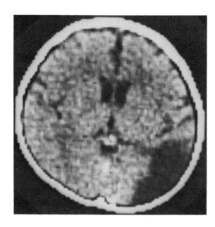

Fig. 34–4. Middle cerebral artery thrombosis, 3 week duration. CT scan (same child as in Fig. 34–1, but with different scanner) show homogeneous lucency with sharp, well-defined margins.

of the first week, liquefaction necrosis develops, and the infarct becomes homogeneous with defined margins (Fig. 34–4). At 3 months, the necrotic infarct is replaced by a cystic fluid-containing cavity, and the lesion with sharp margins has the homogeneous density of CSF.

Sonography is invaluable in defining cerebral anatomy and hemorrhagic complications in the infant, especially the premature (see Fig. 34–1). MRI has become an important diagnostic tool in the early diagnosis of ischemic lesions (see Fig. 34–2).

Arteriography, when performed early, may demonstrate the thrombosed cerebral artery; later there may be a recanalized vessel or evidence of collateral circulation. Cerebral angiography can usually be performed safely in children of all ages. The patency of other cerebral arteries and the ample collateral circulation in children contrast with the status of the cerebral arteries and collateral circulation in adult stroke patients. Children with sickle cell disease are at greater risk if the level of hemoglobin S is not maintained at a level below 20% by exchange transfusion.

The following practical angiographic classification was formulated by Hilal and his associates to supply diagnostic and prognostic information for the following patterns:

Extracranial Occlusion
 Trauma is the most common cause of thrombosis of the cervical portion of the internal carotid artery. Blunt trauma in the paratonsillar area of the oropharynx or direct impact of the carotid artery against the transverse process of the second cervical segment can cause occlusion. Characteristically, about 24 hours lapse between the traumatic incident and clinical manifestations. Nontraumatic conditions are usually infectious in origin.

Basal Occlusion Disease without Telangiectasia
 The thrombotic lesion involves the arteries of the base of the brain: supraclinoid area of the internal carotid artery, proximal segments of anterior or middle cerebral artery, or basilar artery. The condition is unilateral and does not recur.

Basal Occlusive Disease with Telangiectasia (Moyamoya)
 This condition involves the arteries at the base of the brain, is often bilateral, and is associated with prominent telangiectasia, especially in the region of the basal ganglia. Of varied etiology, it may complicate sickle-cell disease, bacterial or tuberculous meningitis, or neurofibromatosis; it may also complicate the treatment plans of radiotherapy. Recurrent episodes of thrombosis are common and may result in alternating hemiplegia, epilepsy, and learning disabilities.

Peripheral Leptomeningeal Artery Occlusions
 Branch occlusions of the distal leptomeningeal arteries may occur with diabetes mellitus, sickle-cell disease, trauma, infection, tumor encasement, or neurocutaneous syndromes. The excellent collateral circulation usually results in rapid recovery from the acute hemiplegia.

Perforating Artery Occlusion
 Involvement of the small perforating arteries, most commonly the striate arteries, is seen in children with homocystinuria or periarteritis nodosa. Episodes recur, causing a progressive neurologic deficit with alternating hemiparesis or quadriparesis, subarachnoid hemorrhage, or death.

Treatment. Therapeutic measures may include parenteral fluids, antibiotics when indicated, anticonvulsants, anticoagulants to prevent extension of the thrombus, and agents to control increased intracranial pressure.

Anticoagulants are rarely indicated except when a stroke is in progress. Rarely does arterial thrombosis result in sufficient increased pressure to require intracranial pressure monitoring or measures to reduce intracranial pressure. Bilateral cervical sympathectomies to increase regional blood flow and anastomosis of the external and internal carotid arteries have been of dubious value.

Sickle-cell disease is treated by repeated blood transfusions. The risk of future strokes is reduced by a chronic transfusion program to maintain hemoglobin S at a level below 20%.

Cerebral Embolism

In cerebral embolism, an artery can be occluded by air, fat, tumor, bacteria, parasites, foreign body, or a fragment from an organized thrombus. The middle cerebral artery or its branches is most commonly involved.

Cerebral embolism in childhood is usually cardiogenic, especially after cardiac catheterization or open heart surgery, but is also seen with cardiac arrhythmias due to cyanotic congenital heart disease or rheumatic valvular disease, bacterial endocarditis, or atrial myxoma. Septic embolism from pulmonary inflammatory disease or bacterial endocarditis may result in brain abscesses or mycotic aneurysms. Fat embolism is an unusual complication of long-bone fractures.

Signs and Symptoms. The focal neurologic signs vary according to the artery occluded; manifestations are complete within seconds or minutes. There are also signs and symptoms of the causal disorder: transient blindness with air embolism, petechiae and hematuria with septic emboli, cutaneous petechiae, urinary free fat, and fat in the retinal vessels with fat emboli due to long-bone fracture or intravenous fat infusions.

Fat embolism has a characteristic clinical picture. A lucid interval of 12 to 48 hours occurs after a long-bone fracture. The child then becomes febrile with pulmonary symptoms that include dyspnea, cyanosis, and blood-tinged sputum. Within a few hours there is an acute encephalopathy that may include focal neurologic signs, diabetes insipidus, seizures, delirium, stupor, or coma.

Laboratory Data. Routine laboratory studies after cerebral embolism are often normal, but a moderate polymorphonuclear leukocytosis may be present. The CSF is usually nor-

mal, but there may be a mild elevation of the protein content. Septic embolism in bacterial endocarditis may cause an elevated CSF protein content and pleocytosis. Atrial myxomas commonly show leukocytosis, anemia, and an elevated ESR. The EEG characteristically shows a slow-wave abnormality in the areas supplied by the occluded vessel.

CT is often characteristic in showing multiple infarcts, some of which are hemorrhagic (Fig. 34–5). The lesions become lucent with sharp margins 2 to 3 months later.

Cerebral angiography should be performed in all children with septic emboli. It delineates the occluded artery and may demonstrate mycotic aneurysm.

Treatment. Management of cerebral embolism is primarily symptomatic, including anticonvulsants for seizures. Anticoagulants are rarely used in children. Corticosteroids, in dosages used in the management of cerebral edema, are effective in reversing the pulmonary symptoms of fat embolism.

Intracranial Hemorrhage

Hemorrhagic stroke in children usually results from trauma or bleeding disorders. When these conditions are excluded, intracranial hemorrhage is caused by an arteriovenous malformation or aneurysm.

Signs and Symptoms. The child with subarachnoid hemorrhage usually presents with acute onset of headache, vomiting, stupor or coma, and convulsions. Findings include stiff neck and Brudzinski and Kernig signs. Extensor plantar responses and sub-

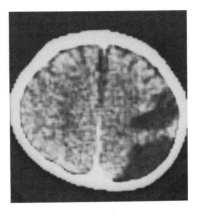

Fig. 34–5. Cerebral embolism. CT scan 3 months after cerebral embolism shows multiple infarcts. Sharp margins have density of CSF.

hyaloid hemorrhages on funduscopic examination are often noted early. Fever and systemic hypertension are nonspecific findings. Ruptured cerebral aneurysm frequently presents with a catastrophic clinical picture. Bleeding from an arteriovenous malformation is less dramatic and is often associated with focal signs.

Laboratory Data. Blood dyscrasias are identified by appropriate blood studies. Children with bleeding from other causes have polymorphonuclear leukocytosis, normal or moderately elevated ESR, and transient albuminuria and glycosuria.

CSF analysis and CT document subarachnoid hemorrhage. Sonography in the infant with an open fontanel and CT scan at any age are invaluable in the diagnosis of intracranial hemorrhage and its complications. CT may demonstrate arteriovenous malformation (Fig. 34–6) or giant cerebral arterial aneurysm. Cerebral angiography is the definitive diagnostic technique for these conditions.

Treatment. The management of intracranial hemorrhage varies with the cause of the hemorrhage. Repeated lumbar punctures, mannitol, and corticosteroids are often used, but their effectiveness is controversial. Ruptured intracranial aneurysms require good nursing care and, unless the child is comatose or there is a medical contraindication, surgical extirpation offers the best prognosis. Except in cases of mycotic aneurysms, the occurrence of a second hemorrhage shortly after the initial hemorrhage is uncommon in children. Arteriovenous malformations (AVMs) should be surgically removed whenever possible. Embolization may be used preoperatively to reduce the size of the malformation or to treat inaccessible lesions. Traumatic arteriovenous fistulas are treated by ligation of the fistula, embolization, or the implantation of detachable balloons.

References

Allan WC, Volpe JJ. Periventricular-intraventricular hemorrhage. Pediatr Clin North Am 1986; 36:47–63.

Carter S, Gold AP. Acute infantile hemiplegia. Pediatr Clin North Am 1964; 14:851–864.

Eeg-Olofsson O, Ringheim Y. Stroke in children. Clinical characteristics and prognosis. Acta Paediatr Scand 1983; 72:391–396.

Gold AP, Challenor YB, Gilles FH, Hilal SK, Leviton A, Rollins EI, et al. IX Strokes in children. Stroke 1973; 4:835–894, 1009–1052.

Gold AP, Ransohoff J, Carter S. Arteriovenous malformation of the vein of Galen in children. Acta Neurol Scand (suppl 11) 1964; 40:1–31.

Hilal SK, Solomon GE, Gold AP, Carter S. Primary cerebral arterial occlusive disease in children. II. Neurocutaneous syndromes. Radiology 1971; 99:71–87.

Kamholz J, Tremblay G. Chickenpox with delayed contralateral hemiparesis caused by cerebral angiitis. Ann Neurol 1985; 18:358–360.

Lacey DJ, Terplan K. Intraventricular hemorrhage in fullterm neonates. Dev Med Child Neurol 1982; 14:332–337.

Laxer RM, Dunn HG, Flodmark O. Acute hemiplegia in Kawasaki disease and infantile polyarteritis nodosa. Dev Med Child Neurol 1984; 26:814–821.

Levin S. Moyamoya disease. Dev Med Child Neurol 1982; 24:850–853.

Limbord TG, Ruderman RJ. Fat embolism in children. Clin Orthop 1978; 136:267–269.

Martinowitz U, Heim M, Tadmor R, Eldor A, et al. Intracranial hemorrhage in patients with hemophilia. Neurosurgery 1986; 18:538–540.

Natowicz M, Kelley RI. Mendelian etiologies of stroke. Ann Neurol 1987; 22:175–192.

Packer RJ, Rorke LB, Lange BJ, Siegel KR, et al. Cerebrovascular accidents in children with cancer. Pediatrics 1985; 76:194–201.

Paradis K, Bernstein ML, Adelson JW. Thrombosis as a complication of inflammatory bowel disease in children: A report of four cases. J Pediatr Gastroenterol Nutr 1985; 4:659–662.

Pavlakis S et al. Brain infarction in sickle cell anemia: MRI correlates. Ann Neurol 1988; 23:125–130.

Sandok BA, von Estorff I, Giuliani ER. CNS embolism due to atrial myxoma—clinical features and diagnosis. Arch Neurol 1980; 37:485–488.

Shields WD, Manger MN. Ultrasound evaluation of neo-

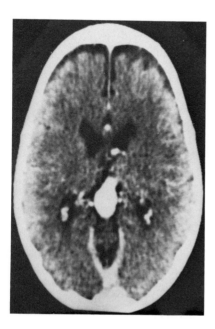

Fig. 34–6. Arteriovenous malformation. CT scan shows aneurysmal dilatation of vein of Galen due to large, deep malformation. Note enlargement of draining sinuses, and mild hydrocephalus with ventricular enlargement.

natal intraventricular hemorrhage. I. Anatomy. Perinatol Neonatol 1983; 75:19–25.

Shields WD, Manger MN. Ultrasound evaluation of neonatal intraventricular hemorrhage. II. Pathology. Perinatol Neonatol 1983; 76:28–35.

Solomon GE, Hilal SK, Gold AP, Carter S. Natural history of acute hemiplegia of childhood. Brain 1970; 93:107–120.

Stein BM, Wolpert SM. Arteriovenous malformations of the brain. Current concepts and treatment. Arch Neurol 1980; 37:1–5; 69–75.

van Hoff J, Ritchey AK, Shaywitz BA. Intracranial hemorrhage in children with sickle cell disease. Am J Dis Child 1985; 139:1120–1123.

Volpe JJ. Neonatal periventricular hemorrhage: past, present, and future. J Pediatr 1978; 92:693–696.

Wilimas J, Goff JR, Anderson HR, Langston JW, Thompson E. Efficacy of transfusion therapy for one to two years in patients with sickle cell disease and cerebrovascular accidents. J Pediatr 1980; 96:205–208.

Yoffe G, Buchanan GR. Intracranial hemorrhage in newborn and young infants with hemophillia. J Pediatr 1988; 113:333–336.

35. STROKE IN YOUNG ADULTS
Rosalie A. Burns

The annual incidence of initial strokes/100,000 persons under the age of 35 years is about 3.5; it increases to 30 to 50/100,000 persons between the ages of 35 and 44 and then doubles in each decade of life thereafter. There is a male preponderance in victims of initial strokes after age 45, but between ages 15 and 45, the incidence is equal, in part because of complications of pregnancy or oral contraception.

In contrast to older patients, the prognosis of young adults with ischemic stroke is better; nearly 75% of young adult survivors improve or recover completely. Mortality data are unreliable. The annual recurrence rate of 0.5% compares with 5% to 6% in older persons; cardiogenic cerebral embolus is the most frequent cause of stroke recurrence.

Classification

The causes of cerebral infarction in young adults can be defined in more than 50% of the cases. These differ from those in the elderly because the lesion is less often atherosclerotic and more often potentially treatable (Table 35–1). Hypertension, diabetes, and hyperlipidemia with presumed premature atherosclerosis are common in those strokes without otherwise defined cause. Thrombosis and embolus cause about 60% of first strokes in patients younger than 55; hemorrhagic stroke and subarachnoid hemorrhage account for the others. In some series, cardiogenic emboli account for nearly half of the identifiable causes of infarction in patients between the ages of 15 and 40. Other nonatherosclerotic causes of stroke in young adults include venous thrombosis, disorders associated with pregnancy or oral contraceptives, hematologic disturbances, migraine, arteritis, drug abuse, moyamoya syndrome, dissection of cerebral arteries, fibromuscular dysplasia, trauma, and homocystinuria. Among the causes of hemorrhagic stroke, subarachnoid hemorrhage arises from aneurysms or arteriovenous malformations. Parenchymal hemorrhage is due to hypertension, venous thrombosis, eclampsia, hematologic disorders, or hemorrhage into tumors.

Clinical and Pathologic Entities. Premature atherosclerotic cerebrovascular disease may develop in patients with hypertension, diabetes mellitus, or hyperlipidemia. Hypertension is common in young adults when there is no other obvious cause of stroke.

Most cardiogenic emboli are due to *rheumatic heart disease*, with or without atrial fibrillation; others follow *atrial fibrillation* alone, other arrhythmias, *subacute bacterial endocarditis*, or mural thrombi after *myocardial infarction*. Less common sources are mitral valve prolapse, atrial myxoma, and cardiomyopathies.

Mitral valve prolapse (MVP) is due to myxomatous degeneration of the valve. It is usually asymptomatic and occurs in 5 to 10% of the population, with a marked preponderance in women. Its frequency and the manner in which it causes cerebral ischemia are uncertain, but in one series of young stroke patients without other cause, 30% had MVP, which was 4.5 times more frequent than in the control group. Asymptomatic MVP is found by echocardiography. Patients may experience bouts of chest pain, palpitation, or dyspnea. Auscultation may reveal midsystolic clicks, a mid-, late, or pansystolic murmur at the apex, or cardiac arrhythmias. Cerebral symptoms may arise from nonseptic or septic emboli; paroxysmal arrhythmias may play a role. Diagnostic tests inlude two-dimensional echocardiography and left ventricular angiography.

Atrial myxomas are uncommon cardiac tumors of endothelial or subendothelial origin that arise most often from the left side of the atrial septum and are potential sources of cerebral emboli. They may also cause obstructive cardiac and general systemic symptoms that mimic collagen-vascular disease or arteritis.

Table 35–1. Causes of Brain Infarction in Young Adults: Aggregate from Literature

Causes	Aggregate	Range
Atherosclerosis	20%	7–48%
Embolism (recognized source)	20%	11–31%
Nonatherosclerotic arteropathy	10%	0–10%
Coagulopathy/systemic	10%	2–16%
Peripartum	5%	2–5%
Uncertain cause	35%	27–47%
Oral contraceptive use—28 of 54 women		
Idiopathic	15%	

(From Hart RG, Miller VT. Stroke 1983; 14:110–114.)

The sedimentation rate may be elevated. There may be fatigue, fever, weight loss, and rapidly developing heart failure. Any patient with cerebral emboli, normal sinus rhythm, and no evidence of bacterial endocarditis is a suspect for atrial myxoma. There may be a characteristic "tumor plop" on auscultation of the heart or other findings suggesting rheumatic mitral valve disease. Auscultatory findings may vary with change of the patient's position. Diagnostic tests include histologic examination of embolic material, echocardiography, and atrial angiography. Cerebral angiography may demonstrate emboli. Even after surgical removal of the tumor, long-term follow-up is necessary because there may be delayed aneurysmal dilatation or metastatic invasion of the embolized cerebral vessel wall. Cerebral emboli may arise from recurrent cardiac tumors.

Cardiomyopathies, idiopathic or associated with systemic diseases such as thyrotoxicosis and amyloidosis, may be sources of cerebral emboli, even when they are subclinical. Echocardiography may suggest a cardiomyopathy. Gingival or rectal biopsies with congored staining of the specimen should be done if amyloidosis is considered.

Occlusion of intracranial venous sinuses or cortical veins can cause infarction or hemorrhage. Since the introduction of antibiotics, venous occlusion is more commonly aseptic than septic and was the second most common cause of stroke in young women in some series. Thrombosis of cerebral veins has been associated with the puerperium, pregnancy, the use of oral contraceptives, ulcerative colitis, cardiac disease with congestive heart failure, diabetes mellitus, dehydration, sepsis, and hematologic diseases such as sickle cell anemia, hemolytic anemia, thrombocytopenia, paroxysmal nocturnal hemoglobinuria, cryofibrinogenemia, disseminated intravascular coagulation, and polycythemia. Cerebral venous thrombosis occurring in association with oral contraceptive usage occurs most often during the first year of use. The development of severe headache and seizures, often focal, in the early postpartum period or in a patient recently using oral contraceptives should suggest venous thrombosis.

About 65% of the nonhemorrhagic hemiplegias of pregnancy, however, are due to arterial rather than venous occlusion. In one series, 35% of young women with carotid territory infarcts were pregnant or puerperial when the stroke occurred. Alterations of clotting factors during pregnancy and in the postpartum period (e.g., a decrease in fibrinolysins and an increase in fibrinogen) lead to a hypercoagulable state. The risk of ischemic stroke is higher during pregnancy than in women taking oral contraceptives.

Other disorders leading to *stroke during pregnancy or puerperium* include internal carotid artery dissection, emboli from mural thrombi of peripartum cardiomyopathy, and amniotic-fluid or air emboli. Hemorrhage during pregnancy or in the postpartum period may follow rupture of a berry aneurysm or arteriovenous malformation; subarachnoid hemorrhage ranked third among nonobstetric causes of maternal death in one study. Other causes of hemorrhage in pregnancy are eclampsia, thrombotic thrombocytopenic purpura, leukemia, metastatic choriocarcinoma, and other brain tumors. Consumptive coagulopathies of the peripartum period are associated with amniotic-fluid embolism, premature separation of the placenta, septic abortion, hydatidiform mole, intrauterine fetal death, and uterine rupture.

The risk of stroke with the use of oral contraceptives is increased five- to nine-fold for thrombosis, and perhaps two-fold for hemorrhage. The risks are increased with increasing age, cigarette smoking, and hypertension. Oral contraceptives may predispose to vascular disease by elevating blood pressure, causing endothelial proliferation, or altering blood coagulability.

Spontaneous *carotid-cavernous sinus fistulas,* in which shunts develop between the meningeal branches of the internal carotid artery and the cavernous sinus, almost always occur in persons younger than 40, with a 3:1 predilection for women. Some 25% develop in the second half of pregnancy or at childbirth. Symptoms and signs include unilateral frontal headache, ipsilateral conjunctival erythema, mild proptosis, decreased monocular vision, and diplopia. Cerebral angiography demonstrates the fistula. This is not a life-threatening disorder, and may be corrected surgically.

Hematologic disorders associated with stroke include hyperviscosity syndromes, sickle cell anemia, polycythemia, paroxysmal nocturnal hemoglobinuria, and disorders of platelets or blood coagulation.

The hyperviscosity syndrome is most often associated with increased amounts of IgM in Waldenström macroglobulinemia, carcinomas, lymphomas, and rheumatoid arthritis. Multiple myeloma with an IgA or IgG paraprotein can also cause hyperviscosity, small vessel occlusion, and multiple areas of infarction or hemorrhage. Signs may be diffuse or focal.

Sickle-cell disease can cause ischemic or hemorrhagic infarction, intracerebral hemorrhage, venous sinus and cortical vein thrombosis, and subarachnoid hemorrhage. The overall incidence of stroke in sickle cell disease is 6 to 15%; the risk of cerebral infarction is greatest in children with sickle cell anemia. Stroke occurs infrequently in sickle cell patients older than 20 and in those with sickle cell trait. Hemorrhagic complications are more common in adults. In addition to small vessel occlusion from intravascular sickling, endothelial proliferation affects small arteries and arterioles, and angiopathy may involve the anterior part of the circle of Willis. Diagnostic tests include the sickle cell preparation and hemoglobin electrophoresis. Stroke recurrence is common in sickle cell anemia, and may be avoided by periodic exchange transfusions aimed at keeping hemoglobin-S levels below 20%.

In polycythemia, there is a predisposition to both arterial and venous thrombosis and retinal vein occlusion. Intracerebral and subarachnoid hemorrhages may occur occasionally. Diagnostic testing beyond the basic hematocrit and hemoglobin should include a determination of red cell mass, which is increased in polycythemia vera. Phlebotomy can cause a rise of cerebral blood flow and may play a preventive role.

Paroxysmal nocturnal hemoglobinuria may result in cerebral venous thrombosis and is suspected in patients with chronic hemolytic anemia, unexplained pain, and multiple episodes of venous thrombosis at different systemic sites. Laboratory evaluation demonstrates the ready hemolysis of red blood cells by activated complement through the Ham test or the sucrose lysis test. In addition to symptomatic treatment of anemia with androgens or transfusion, and of hemolysis with prednisone, anticoagulants are indicated in patients who have thrombotic episodes.

Among the *platelet and coagulation disorders* resulting in stroke are chronic idiopathic (autoimmune) *thrombocytopenic purpura* (ITP), *thrombotic thrombocytopenic purpura* (TTP), and *disseminated intravascular coagulation* (DIC). Chronic ITP is three to four times more common in women than in men and may occasionally result in intracerebral hemorrhage. The triad of TTP includes thrombocytopenic purpura, hemolytic anemia, and focal cerebral signs; seizures are also common. This disorder may start in the second half of pregnancy, simulating eclampsia. The small cerebral vessels demonstrate hyperplasia and platelet thrombi. There is no known satisfactory treatment. DIC may lead to either cerebral hemorrhage or thrombosis. It involves the consumption of coagulation factors and platelets and may be associated with carcinoma, disorders of the peripartum and postpartum period, and sepsis.

In *idiopathic thrombosis,* recurrent cerebral hemorrhage, thrombosis, or both are associated with an elevated platelet count, megakaryocytic hyperplasia of the bone marrow, and sometimes splenomegaly. *Chronic inflammatory bowel diseases* such as ulcerative colitis and regional enteritis have been associated with a hypercoagulable state and thrombocytosis, predisposing to recurrent retinal artery branch occlusions, carotid thromboembolism, and cerebral venous and arterial thromboses. Isolated reports of occlusive cerebrovascular disease have appeared in association with elevation of plasma factor VIII and deficiency of factor XII. Platelet hyperaggregability and occlusive cerebral vascular disease may occur with the use of estrogens or in patients with migraine.

Arteritis may be due to collagen-vascular disease, infection, drugs, or irradiation. The collagen disorder most frequently causing stroke is *lupus erythematosus.* Fibrinoid changes in small arterioles and capillaries may cause diffuse microinfarction and small hemorrhages. Emboli may arise from the vegetations of Libman-Sacks endocarditis, and there may be an increased risk of thrombosis in patients with an immunoglobulin called the "lupus anticoagulant." The incidence of stroke is less in *polyarteritis nodosa,* with 13% reportedly experiencing cerebral infarction or hemorrhage; stroke is infrequent in scleroderma or rheumatoid arthritis.

Granulomatous arteritis, a rare and presumably autoimmune giant cell disorder of small cerebral vessels, may occur at any age but is more common in the fifth to eighth decades of life. Screening diagnostic tests for patients with possible arteritis include sedimentation rate, antinuclear antibody (ANA) determinations, and serum protein electrophoresis. In granulomatous arteritis, CSF shows a moderate mononuclear pleocytosis and elevation of total protein, frequently exceeding 100 mg/dl. Leptomeningeal biopsy should be considered if the diagnosis is obscure because treatment with steroids may be effective.

Takayasu arteritis (pulseless disease, or aortic-arch syndrome) is a giant cell arteritis that may cause narrowing and thrombosis of the large branches of the aortic arch at their origins and aneurysmal formation. This disorder has a sporadic worldwide distribution with a predilection for young women of Asian or Mexican descent. Increased frequency of HLA antigen Bw52 in the Japanese and two β-cell alloantigens in North Americans suggest a genetic predisposition. Signs of ischemia of the head and arms include cataracts, retinal and optic atrophy, transient monocular blindness (amaurosis fugax), focal cerebral symptoms, hypertension in the legs with intermittent claudication in the arms (reversed coarctation), and other signs of tissue ischemia in the distribution of the extracranial cerebral and subclavian arteries. There may be a low-grade fever. The sedimentation rate is always increased. Angiography shows narrowing of the aortic arch branches at their origins. The disorder is poorly responsive to steroids; other immunosuppressive agents and surgical repair, including bypass techniques, may be tried.

Stroke of otherwise unknown cause has been described in young adults, predominantly men, with *heterozygous deficiency of the C2 component of complement.* Vasculitis has not been demonstrated although C2 deficiency may be found in other connective tissue or immunologic disorders.

Meningeal infection can result in cerebral infarction through the development of inflammatory changes in vessel walls. In meningovascular syphilis, this is attended by CSF pleocytosis and elevated total protein content. Serologic testing for syphilis should be included in the laboratory evaluation of all young adults with stroke. Mucormycosis is another infection that may cause cerebral arteritis. The fungus obtains access to the brain through the nose and sinuses in debilitated diabetics, patients with blood dyscrasias, and in immunosuppressed patients; it causes cerebral thrombosis by invasion of the internal carotid artery. Hyphae proliferate in small- and medium-size arteries and may be detected in mucosal biopsies. Because of acute onset with pain, proptosis, and ophthalmoplegia, cavernous sinus thrombosis must be considered in the differential diagnosis. Treatment is by extensive surgical debridement and the use of amphotericin B. Pyogenic and tubercular arteritides occur infrequently. Other rare causes of cerebral infarction are typhus, schistosomiasis, falciparum malaria, and trichinosis.

Drugs, alcohol use, and cigarette smoking are all stroke risk factors for young adults.

Drugs that have been associated with stroke include the methamphetamines, lysergic acid diethylamide (LSD), heroin and cocaine. The amphetamines induce a necrotizing vasculitis that may result in either diffuse petechial (or larger) intracerebral, subdural, and subarachnoid hemorrhages. In experimental animals given intravenous methamphetamines, focal areas of ischemia and infarction, diffuse cerebral edema, and petechial hemorrhages have been described. An angiographic appearance compatible with arteriospasm has been reported in a patient who ingested LSD, which is an ergot alkaloid derivative. Heroin, or the substances used to adulterate it, may produce allergic vascular hypersensitivity leading to infarction. Illicit use of intravenous agents may lead to either septic or nonseptic embolism.

Subarachnoid hemorrhage and *cerebral infarction* have been reported after the intranasal or parenteral use of cocaine. Cocaine prevents the uptake of sympathomimetic neurotransmitters by nerve terminals and leads to vasoconstriction. Also, increased risk of cerebral infarction and subarachnoid hemorrhage has been associated with alcohol abuse in young adults. Mechanisms by which ethanol may produce stroke include effects on blood pressure, platelets, plasma osmolarity, hematocrit, and red blood cells; also, alcohol-induced cardiomyopathy, arrhythmias, or changes in cerebral blood flow and autoregulation. Rebound thrombocytosis may occur after abrupt alcohol withdrawal. Cigarette smoking, studied primarily in men, carries a risk of thromboembolic or hemorrhagic stroke more than three times that in nonsmokers. Smoking may lead to stroke by promoting vasoconstriction, platelet aggregation, increased blood levels of fibrinogen or other clotting factors, increased blood viscosity, and possibly by arterial weakening and transient increases in blood pressure.

Moyamoya disease is a syndrome of stenosis of the vessels in and around the circle of Willis, with profusion of telangiectatic collateral vessels at the base of the brain that angiographically appear like a puff of smoke. First described in the Japanese, it has been seen in other nationalities. Meningeal collaterals are called a "rete mirabile." Microaneurysms may develop, and either infarction or subarachnoid hemorrhage may result. A similar angiographic appearance may be seen in other causes of stenosis near the circle of Willis, including sickle cell anemia and tuberculous meningitis, and after radiotherapy for optic gliomas.

Dissection of arteries supplying the brain may account for 5% of ischemic strokes in young adults. Dissection of intracranial cerebral arteries most often affects the middle cerebral or basilar arteries with clinical syndromes of acute infarction. These subintimal dissections of unknown cause develop in otherwise healthy individuals with a mean age of 25 years. Dissection of the major extracranial cerebral arteries may be spontaneous or due to trauma and occurs most often in patients younger than 50. Dissection of the internal carotid artery causes ipsilateral head and face pain and often neck pain; there may be a Horner syndrome and focal cerebral signs of ischemia. Cervical vertebral artery dissection also causes headache, usually high in the neck and often with signs of the lateral medullary syndrome. When obstruction of the extracranial cerebral arteries follows dissection of the proximal aorta, it is seen most often in hypertensive men older than 50.

Fibromuscular dysplasia is a nonatheromatous vascular disorder in which there is intimal and medial fibroplasia of the extracranial internal carotid artery and other large systemic vessels. The intracranial arteries are usually spared. On cerebral angiography, vessels have a beaded appearance with segmental sections of narrowing, alternating with areas of dilatation. The disorder is far more common in women. It is most often discovered as an incidental angiographic abnormality; the cause is not understood. Symptoms of cerebral ischemia are managed in the usual way.

Homocystinuria homozygous form predisposes to cerebral arterial or, less often, venous thromboses and to thromboemboli in other organs. The estimated risk of stroke at a young age is 10 to 16%. This diagnosis is usually made in childhood because of other stigmata such as the Marfan-like appearance, malar flush, dislocated ocular lens, bony deformities, mental retardation, and seizures. Many young patients with premature cerebral occlusive and peripheral vascular disease show biochemical evidence of heterozygosity for homocystinuria.

Laboratory Data

Investigations for a cardiac source of emboli include two-dimensional echocardiography, 24-hour Holter cardiac monitoring for rhythm disorders, and, if indicated, angiocardiography. A contrast echocardiogram with the Valsalva maneuver should be requested if paradoxical embolism is suspected. In cases of atrial myxoma, histologic examination of embolic material may be diagnostic. Gum or rectal biopsy is stained for amyloid if amyloid cardiomyopathy is considered. An elevated sedimentation rate suggests systemic lupus erythematosus (SLE), subacute bacterial endocarditis (SBE), Takayasu arteritis, or atrial myxoma. Tests for antinuclear antibodies and serologic tests for syphilis should be obtained.

In addition to differentiating hemorrhage from infarction, CT may suggest venous thrombosis. Multiple infarctions on CT could be compatible with emboli or arteritis. In addition to delineating these same disorders, angiography shows the characteristic features of Takayasu disease, moyamoya syndrome, spontaneous carotid-cavernous sinus fistula, arteriovenous malformation, fibromuscular dysplasia, and dissection of cerebral arteries.

Hematologic studies include sickle cell preparations, hemoglobin and serum protein electrophoresis, Ham test, sucrose lysis test, antithrombin III level, partial thromboplastin time (PPT), serum lipids, serum viscosity, platelet count, fibrinogen levels, red cell mass, and bone marrow evaluation, when warranted by earlier studies. CSF should be examined if meningeal infection or arteritis is possible. Leptomeningeal biopsy may be indicated for evaluation of giant cell arteritis. Homocystinuria is evaluated by the cyanide nitroprusside test for increased urinary homocystine or by finding a low level of cystathionine synthetase in cultures of fibroblasts or liver biopsy.

References

Abbott RD et al. Risk of stroke in male cigarette smokers. N Engl J Med 1986; 315:717–720.

Adams RJ, Nichols FT, McKie V, et al. Cerebral infarction in sickle cell anemia. Neurology 1988; 38:1012–1017.

Barnett HJM, Boughner DR, Taylor DW, Cooper PE, Kostuk WJ, Nichol PM. Further evidence relating mitral-valve prolapse to cerebral ischemic events. N Engl J Med 1980; 302:139–144.

Biller J, et al. Echocardiographic evaluation of young adults with nonhemorrhagic cerebral infarction. Stroke 1986; 17:608–612.

Boers GHJ, et al. Heterozygosity for homocystinuria in premature peripheral and cerebral occlusive arterial disease. N Engl J Med 1985; 313:709–715.

Collaborative Group for the Study of Stroke in Young Women. Oral contraception and increased risk of cerebral ischemia or thrombosis. N Engl J Med 1973; 288:871–878.

Cross JN, Castro PO, Jennett WB. Cerebral strokes associated with pregnancy and the puerperium. Br. Med J 1968; 3:214–218.

Donaldson JA. The neurology of pregnancy. Philadelphia: WB Saunders, 1978:115–156.

Dorfman LJ, Marshall WH, Enzmann DR. Cerebral infarction and migraine: Clinical and radiologic correlations. Neurology 1979; 29:317–322.

Gill JS et al. Stroke and alcohol consumption. N Engl J Med 1986; 315:1041–1046.

Golbe LI, Merkin MD. Cerebral infarction in a user of free-base cocaine ("crack"). Neurology 1986; 36:1602–1604.

Grindal AB, Cohen RJ, Saul RF, Taylor JR. Cerebral infarction in young adults. Stroke 1978; 9:39–42.

Hart RG, Easton JD. Dissections. Editorial. Stroke 1985; 16:925–927.

Hart RG, Miller VT. Cerebral infarction in young adults: a practical approach. Stroke 1983; 14:110–114.

Humphrey PRD, Du Boulay GH, Marshall J, et al. Cerebral blood-flow and viscosity in relative polycythaemia. Lancet 1979; 2:873–876.

Jennett WB, Cross JN. Influence of pregnancy and oral contraception on the incidence of strokes in women of childbearing age. Lancet 1967; 1:1019–1023.

Marshall J. Case series of stroke in children and young adults. Adv Neurol 1979; 25:325–328.

Mizutani T, Goldberg H, Parr J, Harper C, Thompson CJ. Cerebral dissecting aneurysm and intimal fibroelastic thickening of cerebral arteries. J Neurosurg 1982; 56:571–576.

Mody CK, Miller Bl, McIntryre HB, et al. Neurologic complications of cocaine abuse. Neurology 1988; 38:1189–1193.

Moore PM, Cupps TR. Neurological complications of vasculitis. Ann Neurol 1983; 14:155–167.

Petitti DB, Wingord J, Pellegrin F, Ramcharan S. Risk of vascular disease in women; smoking, oral contraceptives, noncontraceptive estrogen, and other factors. JAMA 1979; 242:1150–1154.

Powars D, Wilson B, Imbus C, Pegelow C, Allen J. The natural history of stroke in sickle cell disease. Am J Med 1978; 65:461–471.

Rice GPA, Ebers GC, Newland F, Wysocki GP. Recurrent cerebral embolism in cardiac amyloidosis. Neurology 1981; 31:904–906.

Robins M, Baum HM. Incidence. In: Weinfeld FD, ed. The National Survey of Stroke. Stroke 1981; 12(suppl 1):45–55.

Roeltgen DP, Weimer GR, Patterson LF. Delayed neurologic complications of left atrial myxoma. Neurology 1981; 31:8–13.

Simard D, Parent C, Mathieu JP. Stroke in young adults with C_2 deficiency. Abstracts of the 7th joint meeting on stroke and cerebral circulation. Stroke 1982; 13:14.

Snyder BD, Ramirez-Lassepas M. Cerebral infarction in young adults; Long-term prognosis. Stroke 1980; 11:149–153.

Stadel BV. Oral contraceptives and cardiovascular disease. N Engl J Med 1981; 305:672–677.

Volkman DJ, Mann DL, Fauci AS. Association between Takayasu's arteritis and a B-cell alloantigen in North Americans. N Engl J Med 1982; 306:464–465.

Werner MH, Burger PC, Heinz ER, et al. Intracranial atherosclerosis following radiotherapy. Neurology 1988; 38:1158–1160.

White HH, Rowland LP, Araki S, Thompson HL, Cowen D. Homocystinuria. Arch Neurol 1965; 13:455–470.

Wolf PA, Kannel WB, McGee DL. Epidemiology of stroke in North America. In: Barnett HJM, Mohr JP, Stein BM, Yatsu FM, eds. Stroke, Pathophysiology, Diagnosis, and Management (vol 1). New York: Churchill Livingstone, 1986:19–29.

36. TREATMENT AND PREVENTION OF STROKE

Frank M. Yatsu

Treatment of Strokes

Medical therapy of stroke is designed: (1) to mimimize or avert ischemic brain infarction, (2) to prevent stroke recurrence, and (3) to maximize functional recovery. Specific therapies depend upon the stroke syndrome as discussed below.

THROMBOTIC STROKES OR ATHEROTHROMBOTIC BRAIN INFARCTION OR THROMBOEMBOLIC STROKES DUE TO ATHEROSCLEROSIS OF INTRACRANIAL AND EXTRACRANIAL ARTERIES

Atherothrombotic brain infarction and artery-to-artery thromboembolic strokes are interchangeable terms for this most common stroke syndrome. They refer to a clinical continuum from transient ischemic attacks (TIAs) to completed stroke, with fixed neurologic signs. Intermediate manifestations of thrombotic strokes are *RINDs (reversible ischemic neurologic deficits)* and *progressing strokes or strokes-in-evolution.*

Transient Ischemic Attacks. TIAs are brief attacks with neurologic symptoms, such as amaurosis fugax, hemiparesis, or aphasia in the carotid circulation. Usually they last from 5 to 10 minutes to several hours. By convention, symptoms and signs may persist for 24 hours; those beyond this period are termed RINDs, a distinction with little clinical meaning because the pathophysiologic mechanisms must be similar. Both TIAs and RINDs are attributed to platelet aggregates that form on atheromatous plaques and embolize distally to occlude, temporarily, a distal arteriole. The resulting focal ischemia in brain or retina causes neurologic symptoms and signs. Because similar symptoms of ischemia can be caused by hemodynamic factors due to reduced regional cerebral or retinal blood flow and by compressive lesions of brain, the transient symptoms alone cannot securely identify the underlying pathology. For example, transient neurologic symptoms may occur with emboli or cardiac origin, thrombocytosis, polycythemia vera, arteritis or, rarely, with mass lesions such as meningiomas or subdural hematomas.

With vertebrobasilar TIAs, frequent symptoms are tinnitus and vertigo, often accompanied by focal symptoms such as diplopia, ataxia, hemiparesis, and bilateral visual impairment. Symptoms may be simulated by hemodynamic causes of reduced blood flow in the vertebrobasilar circulation such as decreased cardiac output. Because cardiac arrhythmias may cause these conditions, Holter monitoring is a necessary diagnostic test.

Carotid endarterectomy is commonly prescribed for carotid TIAs in suitable operative candidates with stenotic or ulcerating atheromas at the carotid bifurcation. However, the value of endarterectomy in averting thrombotic strokes is still controversial; the results may depend, in part, on the operative skills of the surgeon. Extracranial-intracranial bypass surgery and angioplasty, the dilatation of stenotic extracranial arteries, are of no value in averting strokes after TIAs.

Medical therapy of TIA includes antiplatelet drugs, particularly aspirin and anticoagulation, although, unlike aspirin, anticoagulants have not been proven of benefit in prospective randomized studies. Aspirin reduces by half the expected 5% annual rate of thrombotic strokes appropriate to the carotid TIA; benefit was found with either low or high doses, i.e., with one or four aspirin tablets daily (0.3 to 1.2 g).

Progressing Strokes. The gradual (or stuttering) increase in neurologic signs over hours suggests this diagnosis, if mass lesions such as hematoma or edema have been excluded. The progressive increment in symptoms is attributed to an enlarging intra-arterial thrombus and immediate anticoagulant therapy is indicated to halt progression; intravenous heparin is followed by warfarin for chronic anticoagulation. Chronic anticoagulation may be required for 6 months to 1 year.

Completed Strokes with Fixed Neurologic Signs. The rationale for acute therapy of completed stroke is based on critically reduced blood flow surrounding an infarct. Brain tissue in this "ischemic penumbra" is viable but impaired; timely delivery of blood theoretically could restore brain function. Also, the ischemia may be aggravated by intravascular platelet aggregation and coagulation and by brain edema.

Therapies to improve flow in the ischemic penumbra have been investigated, however, there is no reliable or predictable intervention. These therapies have included vasodilators such as carbon dioxide and papaverine, aminophylline, vasopressors, naloxone, hyperventilation, and prostacyclin. Reduction of viscosity to improve microcirculation is currently being investigated.

Although therapies aimed at reducing platelet aggregation and coagulation have not been of value, acute use of antiplatelet drugs (such as aspirin) is warranted because platelet aggregation is increased after acute thrombotic strokes. Efforts to dissolve intra-arterial thrombi with fibrinolytic agents have been unsuccessful; however, successful use of these agents in acute coronary thrombosis has led to evaluation of tissue plasminogen activator (TPA) and streptokinase in the treatment of acute stroke.

Substances that reduce brain edema, such as the dehydrating agents mannitol, glycerol, and urea, are of value in averting herniation syndromes but do not improve the microcirculation around an infarct. Corticosteroids do not benefit acute ischemic strokes.

Drugs that may protect brain pharmacologically from ischemia (e.g., barbiturates) have not been beneficial in acute ischemic strokes. However, pretreatment before open-heart bypass surgery reduces the incidence of persisting neurologic signs attributed to surgery-related emboli. Currently, calcium channel blockers are being investigated; seemingly they protect ischemic brain from irreversible damage. Experimental and organ transplant data suggest that "reperfusion" is associated with the formation of damaging "free radicals"; this process can be reduced with free radical scavengers, agents that have not yet been investigated systematically in ischemic stroke. Routine use of glucose infusions should be abandoned in acute ischemic strokes unless the patient is hypoglycemic; glucose-induced intracellular-lactic acidosis can provoke irreversible brain damage in ischemic tissues.

EMBOLIC STROKES OF CARDIAC ORIGIN

Specific therapy of cardiac emboli depends on the cardiac pathology. For example, an infected prosthetic valve may require replacement and myxomatous emboli necessitate surgical excision of the tumor. The more common causes of embolic stroke of cardiac origin are atrial fibrillation with or without mitral pathology and recent myocardial infarction, particularly large anterior or septal infarcts and those with akinetic segments detected by two-dimensional echocardiography. Before age 45, mitral valve prolapse may be a more frequent cause.

For emboli associated with atrial fibrillation or myocardial infarction, anticoagulation to reduce reembolization is indicated. However, to decrease the hazards of converting an ischemic infarct into a hemorrhagic one, heparinization is not recommended if the infarct is large (by CT or clinical signs). Lumbar puncture is not needed to exclude hemorrhage if CT studies are adequate. With atrial fibrillation, the estimated 5 to 6% annual incidence of embolization is considered an indication of the need for chronic anticoagulation therapy with warfarin. The risk of complications, such as intracerebral hemorrhage, with chronic anticoagulation is 1 to 2%/year. To treat emboli after an acute myocardial infarct, anticoagulation therapy to prevent reembolization can only be given for 2 to 4 weeks.

INTRACEREBRAL HEMORRHAGE

Medical management of this condition is supportive. For cerebellar hemorrhage and infarcts, surgical decompression is indicated if vital structures of the medulla are at risk as suggested by displacement of the fourth ventricle, ventricular enlargement, or declining level of consciousness. Surgical evacuation of a hematoma is considered for lobar or cortical white matter hemorrhages if there are signs of declining sensorium or herniation in an operative candidate. Surgery is of no proven benefit for hemorrhages in the other common sites, the putamen, thalamus, and pons. Lumbar puncture in the presence of intracerebral hemorrhage may precipitate herniation and is contraindicated.

SUBARACHNOID HEMORRHAGE DUE TO CONGENITAL OR BERRY ANEURYSMS

Surgical extirpation is the definitive therapy. After subarachnoid hemorrhage, sedation and a quiet environment are essential to prevent large surges of arterial pressure that may provoke rebleeding. The use of antifibrinolytic agents to minimize rebleeding is controversial; some experts prescribe epsilon aminocaproic acid (36 g/day).

A second complication of subarachnoid hemorrhage is vasospasm, which correlates with moderate amounts of blood in the subarachnoid space and is attributed to blood products, not yet defined. Calcium channel blockers, particularly the water soluble form of dihydropyridine compounds, may avert vasospasm but further studies are needed.

Stroke Rehabilitation

Physical rehabilitative measures to maximize functional recovery should begin as soon after stroke as possible. These activities are directed toward improving activities of daily living, muscle strength, ambulation, transfer, dressing, hygiene, avoidance of contractures, and such psychological factors as depression and motivation. Speech and occupational therapies also can assist in optimizing rehabilitation. The value of rehabilitation has not been evaluated in randomized studies but is generally considered beneficial.

Stroke Prevention

Stroke prevention is tailored to the underlying pathologic process causing the stroke syndrome.

Thrombotic or Atherothrombotic Brain Infarction. Treatment of hypertension is the most important preventive measure and has led to a 25% decrease in stroke incidence since 1960. Control of hypertension also reduces stroke recurrence. Measures against the other risk factors for atherosclerosis, the primary pathology in thrombotic strokes, is uncertain but should be considered. These include better control of blood glucose in diabetes, dietary and drug modification of blood lipid content (particularly cholesterol), and reduction of smoking, obesity, stress, and sedentary life-styles. Requiring investigation are the prophylactic use of aspirin and the dietary addition of fish oils, the so-called omega "3" or eicosapentaenoic acids. To reduce plasma cholesterol levels the American Heart Association recommends a diet low in cholesterol and fatty acids and high in unsaturated fats. Drugs such as the bile sequestrants (cholestyramine and colestipol) may be required to reduce blood cholesterol; drugs to inhibit cholesterol synthesis, such as compactin and mevinolin, may be necessary as secondary agents.

Asymptomatic Carotid Bruit or Stenosis. Blood turbulence resulting from carotid bifurcation stenosis is heard as a bruit. Blood flow may be reduced distally with "reversal of flow" through the orbits, but there is no increase in ipsilateral thrombotic strokes. No data support the value of prophylactic carotid endarterectomy to avert strokes, however, as investigations into the temporal and morphologic characteristics of carotid atheromas advance, it seems likely that a subset of plaques will be deemed highly thrombogenic. These may benefit from prophylactic endarterectomy or from therapies designed to provoke "atheroma regression."

Embolic Strokes of Cardiac Origin. While anticoagulation may reduce the incidence of reembolization associated with atrial fibrillation and postmyocardial infarction, caution must be exercised to avoid hemorrhagic transformation of a bland or ischemic infarct.

References

Treatment

Adams HP Jr. Antifibrinolytic therapy for prevention of recurrent aneurysmal subarachnoid hemorrhage. Semin Neurol 1986; 5:309–315.

Antiplatelet Trialists Collaboration. Secondary prevention of vascular disease by prolonged antiplatelet treatment. BMJ 1988; 296:320–331.

Allen SG, Ahn HS, Preziosi TJ, et al. Cerebral arterial spasm—a controlled trial of nimodipine in patients with subarachnoid hemorrhage. N Engl J Med 1983; 308:619–624.

Barnett HJM, Gent M, Sackett DL, Taylor DW. A randomized trial of aspirin and sulfinpyrazine in threatened stroke: The Canadian Cooperative Study Group. N Engl J Med 1978; 299:53–59.

Del Zoppo GJ. Thrombolytic therapy in cerebrovascular disease. Stroke 1988; 19:1174–1179.

The EC/IC Bypass Study Group. Failure of extracranial-intracranial arterial bypass to reduce the risk of ischemic stroke. Results of an international randomized trial. N Engl J Med 1985; 313:1191–1200.

Ennix CL Jr, Lawrie GM, Morris GC Jr, et al. Improved results of carotid endarterectomy in patients with symptomatic coronary disease: an analysis of 1,546 consecutive carotid operations. Stroke 1979; 10:122–125.

Graf CJ, Nebbelink DW. Cooperative study of intracranial aneurysms and subarachnoid hemorrhage: report on a randomized treatment study. III. Intracranial surgery. Stroke 1974; 5:559–601.

Grotta JC. Medical and surgical therapy for cerebrovascular disease. N Engl J Med 1987; 315:1505–1516.

Miller VT, Hart RG. Heparin anticoagulation in acute brain ischemia. Stroke 1988; 19:403–406.

Synder DB, Tabbaa MA. Assessment and treatment of neurological dysfunction after cardiac arrest. Stroke 1988; 19:269–273.

Toole JF, Yuson CP, Janeway R, et al. Transient ischemic attacks: a prospective study of 225 patients. Neurology 1978; 28:746–753.

Whisnant JP, Cartlidge NEF, Elveback LR. Carotid and vertebral-basilar transient ischemic attacks: effect of anticoagulants, hypertension, and cardiac disorders on survival and stroke occurrence: a population study. Ann Neurol 1978; 3:107–115.

Yatsu FM. Pharmacologic basis of acute stroke therapy. Clin Neuropharmacol 1977; 2:113–150.

Yatsu FM, Grotta JC, Pettigrew LC. Asymptomatic carotid bruit and stenosis. Semin Neurol 1986; 6:262–266.

Yatsu FM, McKenzie J, Lockwood AH. Cardiopulmonary arrest and glucose infusion. Emergency Med 1987; 2:1–3.

Prevention

Asinger RW, Mikell FL, Elsperger J, Hodges M. Incidence of left-ventricular thrombosis after acute transmural myocardial infarction: serial evaluation by two-dimensional echocardiography. N Engl J Med 1981; 305:297–302.

Barnett HJM. Progress toward stroke prevention. Neurology 1980; 30:1212–1225.

Furlan AJ, Whisnant JP, Elveback LR. The decreasing incidence of primary intracerebral hemorrhage: a population study. Ann Neurol 1979; 5:367–373.

Hinton RC, Kistler JP, Fallon JT, Friedlich AL, Fisher CM. Influence of etiology of atrial fibrillation on incidence of systemic embolism. Am J Cardiol 1977; 40:509–512.

Lovett JL, Sandok BA, Giuliani ER, Nasser EN. Two-dimensional echocardiography in patients with focal cerebral ischemia. Ann Intern Med 1981; 95:1–4.

Noma A, Matsushita S, Komori T. High and low density lipoprotein cholesterol in myocardial and cerebral infarction. Atherosclerosis 1979; 32:327–331.

Nussmeier NA, Arlund C, Slogoff S. Neuropsychiatric complications after cardiopulmonary bypass: Cerebral protection by a barbiturate. Anesthesiology 1986; 64:165–170.

Wiebers DO, Whisnant JP, O'Fallon WM. The natural history of unruptured intracranial aneurysms. N Engl J Med 1981; 30:696–698.

The most common cause of bloody CSF is head trauma. Spontaneous subarachnoid bleeding frequently follows hypertensive intracerebral hemorrhage with ventricular rupture. The most frequent cause of primary subarachnoid hemorrhage is bleeding from a saccular arterial aneurysm. In the United States, about 26,000 subarachnoid hemorrhages each year cause about 10% of all stroke deaths; more than half affect patients under age 45.

Saccular aneurysms occur most often at the circle of Willis or its major branches, especially at bifurcations. They arise where the arterial elastic lamina (and, perhaps, the media) are defective, but the role of atherosclerosis and whether these defects are congenital or acquired remain uncertain. Saccular aneurysms are found in up to 4% of routine adult autopsies. They are rare in children. Saccular aneurysms may enlarge to the size of an orange (Fig. 37–1). Some lie entirely within the subarachnoid space; others are buried in the substance of the brain. Large aneurysms may be partially or completely filled with an organized clot, which occasionally is calcified.

Some 95% of single aneurysms are on the anterior circulation (Table 37–1, Fig. 37–1). On the internal carotid artery, the most common site is the junction with the posterior communicating artery. Aneurysms of the anterior cerebral artery are most often at the region of the anterior communicating artery; the aneurysms of the middle cerebral artery most frequently affect the first major branching in the sylvian fissure. Posterior aneurysms occur most often at the apical bifurcation of the basilar artery. Intracranial aneurysms are occasionally found at the origin of the ophthalmic artery, at the origin of the three cerebellar arteries, on the internal carotid artery at its bifurcation into the middle and anterior cerebral arteries, and in the cavernous sinus (where rupture causes a carotid-cavernous fistula rather than subarachnoid hemorrhage). In about 20% of cases, there are two or more aneurysms, which often are bilateral.

Hypertension may contribute to, but is not the only cause of, aneurysm formation and rupture; normal blood pressure in a middle-aged or older patient with a hemorrhagic stroke favors the diagnosis of saccular aneurysm. The association of berry (small saccular) aneurysms with polycystic kidney disease and with coarctation of the aorta is considered by some workers to be significant. The risk of subarachnoid hemorrhage is increased, independent of other risk factors, among alcohol drinkers, smokers, and women over age 35 taking oral contraceptives.

Symptoms and Signs. The symptoms and signs of an intracranial aneurysm result from compression of the cranial nerves or the brain, thrombosis in the aneurysm and dispersion of emboli to distal branches, or bleeding. Pressure on the optic tract, nerve, or chiasm in the region of the anterior communicating artery or at the origin of the ophthalmic artery may cause unilateral amblyopia, bitemporal hemianopia, or a homonymous or altitudinal field cut. Aneurysms at the internal-carotid–posterior-communicating-artery junction may compress the oculomotor nerve (almost always affecting the pupil) or optic tract. Aneurysms in the cavernous sinus may damage the third, fourth, fifth, or sixth cranial nerves, and vertebrobasilar aneurysms may cause lower cranial neuropathies. Less often, large aneurysms compress neighboring brain tissue or the pituitary, causing focal neurologic signs, seizures, neuroendocrinologic symptoms, or sellar enlargement.

Thrombosis within the aneurysmal sac occasionally sends emboli to the artery's distal territory, causing TIAs or infarction. Headache without hemorrhage or other signs is unusual in patients with aneurysms; more than 90% are asymptomatic until they rupture.

Aneurysmal bleeding may follow trauma or physical exertion (including coitus), but more often happens during normal daily activities; about 33% occur in sleep. The first symptom is usually sudden excruciating headache, which may be occipital, unilateral, or generalized. The pain is often described by the patient as "the worst headache of my life" and differs from any previously experienced headache pain. Some patients remain alert and lucid; others become confused, delirious, amnestic, lethargic, or comatose. Loss of consciousness occasionally occurs without preceding headache; massive aneurysmal hemorrhages, unlike other kinds of stroke, may cause sudden death. Consciousness may be regained in a few minutes, but generally, loss

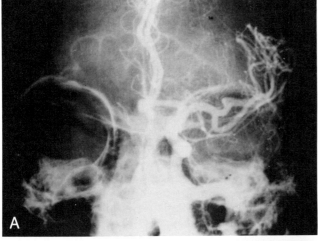
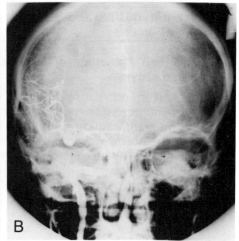
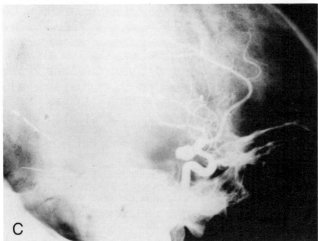

Fig. 37–1. Cerebral arteriograms demonstrating saccular aneurysms at the anterior communicating artery *(A)*, the middle cerebral artery *(B)*, and the junction of the internal carotid and posterior communicating arteries *(C)*. (A ventricular draining shunt for hydrocephalus is seen in *A*.) (Courtesy of Dr. Allan J. Schwartz.)

of consciousness at the outset implies a grave prognosis.

More than half of patients with acute aneurysmal rupture give a history of suspicious symptoms for days or weeks. Headaches of abrupt onset may last hours or days, and are sometimes associated with stiff neck, nausea, vomiting, syncope, disturbed vision, or motor and sensory symptoms. Sometimes head

or neck discomfort is vaguely described, yet in retrospect, probably signified a warning leak. When headache is of recent onset, lumbar puncture or CT must be considered.

Neck stiffness and the Kernig sign are hallmarks of subarachnoid hemorrhage; however, they are not invariably present, even in awake patients, and lower back pain is sometimes more prominent than headache. In adults, preretinal or subhyaloid hemorrhages—large, smooth-bordered, and on the retinal surface—are practically pathognomonic of subarachnoid hemorrhage. Fever is common.

Neurologic signs may point to the site of bleeding. Oculomotor palsy, especially in an awake patient (i.e., not attributable to transtentorial herniation) suggests an aneurysm at the internal-carotid–posterior-communicating-artery junction. Hemiparesis or aphasia suggests a middle cerebral artery aneurysm, and paraparesis or abulia suggests an aneu-

Table 37–1. Site Distribution of Single Aneurysms

	No. Cases	%
Middle cerebral	529	20.0
Internal carotid	1104	41.2
Anterior cerebral	895	33.5
Posterior cerebral	22	0.8
Basilar	77	2.9
Vertebral	25	0.9
Cerebral	20	0.7
Total	2672	100

rysm of the proximal anterior cerebral artery. Early focal signs may be due to an intraparenchymal or subdural hematoma that may call for emergency evacuation. Transient signs that occur within hours or even minutes of the hemorrhage are not understood.

Deterioration of consciousness, with or without focal signs, that occurs a few days after the hemorrhage may result from either rebleeding of the aneurysm or vasospasm. The latter can be widespread and cause frank cerebral infarction. (The term vasospasm may be a misnomer because affected vessels histologically show both inflammatory and proliferative changes; the primary vasculopathic event is uncertain.) Sudden worsening favors rebleeding whereas gradual deterioration favors vasospasm, but it is not always easy to distinguish them.

Laboratory Data. The CSF is usually uniformly grossly bloody with xanthochromic supernatant. The first evidence of xanthochromia or of the presence of even the red cells in the CSF may be delayed for hours. CSF pressure is nearly always high, the protein is elevated, and the glucose may be abnormally low. Initially, the proportion of CSF leukocytes to erythrocytes is that of the peripheral blood; later there may be reactive pleocytosis. Red blood cells and xanthochromia disappear in about 2 weeks unless hemorrhage recurs.

CT may show an intra- or extraparenchymal hematoma or, in severe hemorrhages, subarachnoid blood may appear in basal cisterns, the sylvian or interhemispheric fissures, or even over the cerebral convexities (Figs. 37–2A, 37–3). These findings may allow lumbar puncture to be deferred, especially when there is clinical suspicion of increased intracranial pressure. A normal CT scan, however, does not rule out subarachnoid hemorrhage. If initial CT scans show no abnormality, they may later detect cerebral infarction due to vasospasm or progressive hydrocephalus, which may be an indication for ventriculoatrial shunting. Acute subarachnoid hemorrhage is difficult to detect with magnetic resonance imaging.

Large aneurysms are occasionally demonstrated by CT, but cerebral arteriography is the definitive diagnostic procedure (Figs. 37–1, 37–2B). Cerebral arteriography reveals the aneurysm in about 90% of cases. Because there is often more than one aneurysm, the entire cerebral arterial system must be studied. Vasospasm sometimes masks an aneurysm; an initially negative arteriogram with vasospasm is therefore repeated 1 or 2 weeks later.

Nonspecific laboratory abnormalities include peripheral leukocytosis, albuminuria, glycosuria, and either diabetes insipidus or inappropriate secretion of antidiuretic hormone. EKG changes may suggest myocardial ischemia.

Course and Prognosis. The most reliable data on the natural history of ruptured intracranial aneurysms come from the Cooperative Study's Section on Randomized Treatment. Of patients treated only with bed rest and followed for 5 years, the cumulative mortality was 50%. (This figure would be higher if it included patients who died before reaching the hospital.) Some 30% of patients had recurrent hemorrhage in the first month, especially between the fifth and ninth days. Seven percent of patients rebled between the first and third months after hemorrhaging; 1% rebled between the third and sixth month. The hemorrhage occurred in 1% to 3% of the survivors each year between 6 months and 5 years after the original episode. Other reports have indicated a late mortality of up to 5% annually. For all aneurysm sites in the Cooperative Study, the cause of death was proven or suspected to be rebleeding in 39%; progressive deterioration after initial rupture was the cause of death in 8%. Prognosis was worse in older men with a poor initial neurologic or medical condition, middle cerebral artery aneurysm, high mean blood pressure, large aneurysm, or diffuse vasospasm; however, there is no way to reliably predict whether an individual aneurysm will rebleed.

More recent researchers have reported that the greatest risk of rebleeding is within the first 24 hours and is then spread rather evenly over the next 2 weeks. Clinical deterioration actually may result more often from vasospasm, which occurs from 3 to 21 days after subarachnoid hemorrhage, with a peak at about 1 week; its presence and severity correlate with the amount of cisternal blood seen on the initial CT scan. Angiographic vasospasm does not necessarily predict neurologic deficit, but when neurologic deficit is severe prognosis for functional recovery is poor. Patients with subarachnoid hemorrhage and normal arteriography have a much better prognosis than those with demonstrated aneurysms.

Treatment. The definitive treatment for saccular aneurysms is surgical. There is contro-

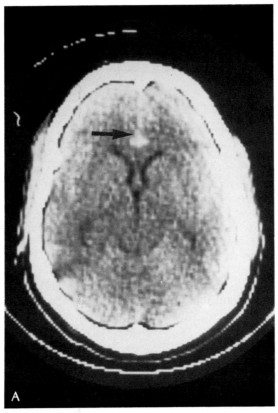

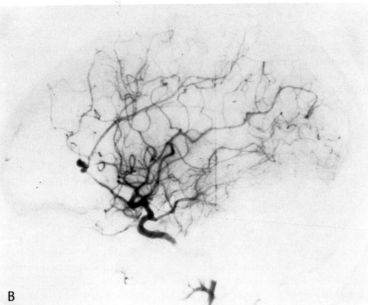

Fig. 37–2.   Subarachnoid hemorrhage. *A.* Noncontrast CT shows blood in interhemispheric fissure anterior to corpus callosum *(arrow). B.* Angiography shows lesion is an aneurysm of anterior cerebral artery. (Courtesy of Drs. S.K. Hilal and S.R. Ganti.)

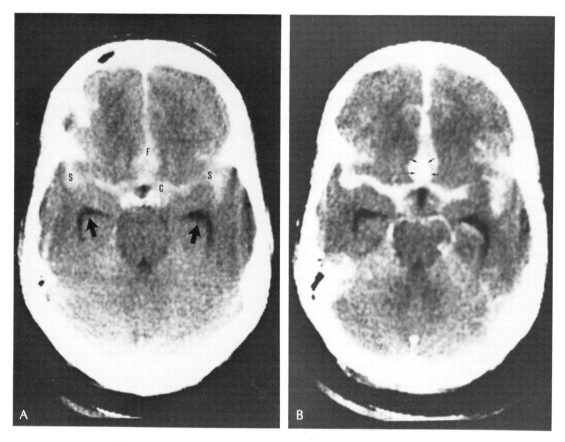

Fig. 37–3. *A.* Noncontrast CT demonstrating hyperdensity within the suprasellar cistern (C) and interhemispheric fissure (F). Note the hyperdensity of subarachnoid blood within both sylvian fissures (S). There is prominence of both temporal horns indicative of mild obstructive communicating hydrocephalus. *B.* A contrast CT scan was performed which demonstrates enhancement of an anterior communicating artery aneurysm observed within the interhemispheric fissure (arrows). (Courtesy of Dr. Richard S. Pinto.)

versy, however, over when it should be done and, if delayed, how to forestall rebleeding and prevent or treat vasospasm. Those who advocate deferring surgery for 1 or 2 weeks point to high mortality and morbidity after early operation, especially when there is evidence of unstable neurologic condition, vasospasm, or increased intracranial pressure. During the waiting period, patients are treated with strict bed rest, sedatives, analgesics, and laxatives. If hypertension is present, lowering of blood pressure theoretically would make aneurysmal rerupture less likely, but this consideration may be offset by the likelihood of causing cerebral infarction in patients with vasospasm. Prophylactic anticonvulsants or drugs that reduce coughing or vomiting are often indicated.

Although some neurosurgeons delay arteriography until just before surgery, most obtain it at an early elective time to confirm the diagnosis and location of an aneurysm. In the

Cooperative Study, unexpected deterioration occurred during or within 24 hours of arteriography in 10.8% of patients, and the mortality rate of the procedure was estimated to be 2.6%.

Antifibrinolytic agents such as epsilon aminocaproic acid (EACA) and tranexamic acid have been used to delay aneurysm clot lysis and thereby prevent rerupture. Controlled studies have demonstrated that they prevent rebleeding; unfortunately this advantage is offset by a higher incidence of vasospasm and hydrocephalus with no overall reduction in mortality or morbidity.

Vasoactive contituents of cisternal blood clots, including serotonin, catecholamines, prostaglandins, platelet derived growth factor, and peptides, have been implicated in the production of vasospasm. Accordingly, treatment has included reserpine, kanamycin, aminophylline, isoproterenol, prostacyclin, naloxone, lidocaine, dipyridamole, and thromboxane synthetase inhibitor. No clear benefit has been shown by any of these regimens. More promising is nimodipine, a calcium channel blocker, which reduces the incidence of persistent ischemic deficits after subarachnoid hemorrhage, although whether this benefit is the result of vasodilatation or of the drug's effect on calcium entry into ischemic neurons is unclear.

Increasingly popular, although not yet the subject of a scientific investigation, is induced hypertension with dopamine plus intravascular volume expansion and hematocrit lowering with colloid and blood. Such treatment requires intensive care and Swan-Ganz catheter monitoring and carries the potential hazard preoperatively of aneurysmal rerupture and postoperatively of hemorrhagic infarction.

Cerebral edema and increased intracranial pressure may be reduced with fluid restriction; such treatment has been associated with improved neurologic function and decreased mortality despite the theoretically increased risk of both rebleeding and cerebral ischemia. The combined use of mannitol (0.75 to 1.5 g/kg as bolus and then up to 10 g every 2 hours, depending on intracranial pressure monitoring and serum osmolality), controlled hyperventilation, and CSF drainage has been recommended when intracranial pressure exceeds 20 mm Hg. Whether corticosteroids, barbiturates, or body hypothermia are of benefit is uncertain.

Because of the difficulties in management, many neurosurgeons now advocate early surgery—within 72 hours of the subarachnoid hemorrhage—to flush clotted blood from the subarachnoid space and to clip the aneurysm. These workers believe that the higher operative mortality of early surgery is offset by prevention of both rebleeding and vasospasm. Moreover, if vasospasm subsequently occurs, hypertension and intravascular volume expansion can be instituted without fear of aneurysmal rerupture. A controlled study to test this hyopthesis has not been done.

Except for emergency evacuation of hematoma, shunt placement for hydrocephalus, or, more controversially, cisternal flushing, the aim of surgery is to prevent rebleeding, preferably by clipping the neck of the aneurysm. In experienced hands, operative mortality should be less than 5% when surgery is performed 1 or 2 weeks after subarachnoid hemorrhage in patients in good medical and neurologic condition. If direct aneurysm clipping is technically impossible, alternative procedures include ligation of the common carotid artery; wrapping or coating of the aneurysm by fascia, muscle, or plastic; ligature trapping of the aneurysm; and ligation of a main feeding artery.

The management of asymptomatic unruptured aneurysms is controversial. Although some investigators have claimed that aneurysms less than 1 cm in diameter rarely rupture, over two thirds of ruptured aneurysm sacs in the Cooperative Study appeared angiographically to be less than 1 cm in diameter. Some neurosurgeons recommend surgery on aneurysms larger than 5 mm; others operate only on larger aneurysms.

Other Kinds of Macroscopic Aneurysm

Fusiform or diffuse aneurysms are circumferential vessel dilatations, usually of the carotid, basilar, or vertebral arteries. Atherosclerosis probably plays a role in their formation, but a developmental defect of the wall may be present in some. Fusiform aneurysms seldom become occluded with thrombus and rarely rupture.

Mycotic Aneurysms. Mycotic aneurysms are caused by septic emboli, which are most often formed by bacterial endocarditis. They are usually only a few millimeters in size and tend to occur on distal branches of pial vessels, especially those of the middle cerebral artery. Surgery is therefore often easier than with saccular aneurysms. Mycotic aneurysms have been reported in up to 10% of endocarditis patients, but arteriography is not performed routinely and the incidence is probably underestimated. Because rupture is fatal in 80% of patients with mycotic aneurysms, cerebral arteriography should be performed when endocarditis is accompanied by suspicious headaches, stiff neck, seizure, focal neurologic symptoms, or CSF pleocytosis. Although mycotic aneurysms occasionally disappear radiographically with antimicrobial therapy, the outcome cannot be predicted and the aneurysm should be treated surgically as soon as possible. Multiple mycotic aneurysms or those located at the base of the brain are treated conservatively and followed by serial arteriography to detect enlargement.

Vascular (Arteriovenous) Malformation. There are five types of vascular or arteriovenous malformations (AVM), and these account for less than 10% of all subarachnoid hemorrhage: telangiectasia, varix, cavernous malformation, arteriovenous fistula, and ve-

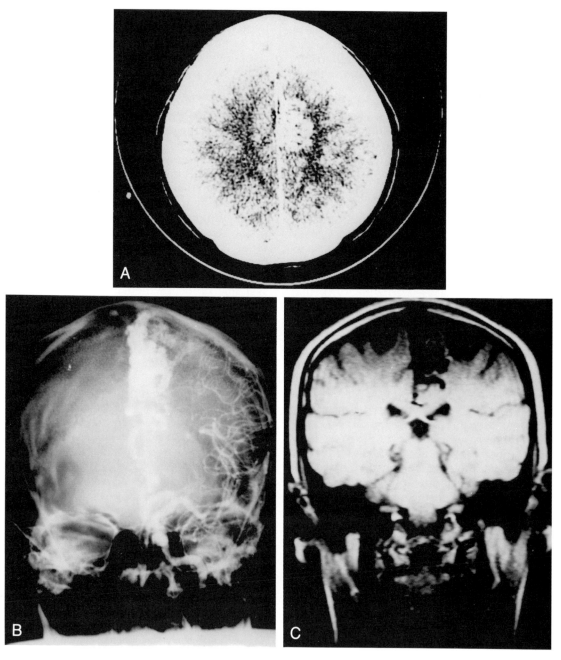

Fig. 37–4. AVM demonstrated by axial contrast-enhanced CT scan *(A)*, cerebral arteriography (AP view) *(B)*, and coronal T_1 weighted magnetic resonance imaging *(C)*.

nous malformation. Bleeding may occur in patients at any age, but is most likely to occur in patients under 30. They are occasionally familial and may coexist with saccular aneurysms.

Symptoms often appear in adolescence or become prominent during menstrual periods or pregnancy. Unruptured AVMs cause headache (which may resemble migraine), focal or generalized seizures, dizziness or syncope, fleeting neurologic symptoms resembling TIAs, and progressive neurologic disorders, including altered mental state (perhaps due to vascular steal and brain ischemia). AVMs are therefore more likely to be symptomatic without subarachnoid hemorrhage than are saccular aneurysms.

When bleeding occurs, reported initial mortality has ranged from 4 to 20%. Early rebleeding is far less likely than after aneurysm rupture, but recurrent hemorrhage, with higher mortality than with the initial bleed, occurs in about 2.5% of patients annually over the next two decades. For patients without hemorrhage, the risk of bleeding is 1.5%, if epilepsy is present, and less than 0.5% if the patient has only a focal neurologic deficit or is asymptomatic.

Most AVMs bleed into the brain, and lateralizing signs are usually present. A systolic bruit may be heard over the carotids, mastoids, or eyes. A systolic bruit may also be heard over a spinal AVM. Proptosis or a retinal AVM may be associated with AVMs that extend from the optic nerve into the orbit. Scalp or face veins may be enlarged.

Skull radiographs sometimes reveal calcification in the AVM or increased vascular markings in the overlying bone. Diagnosis, however, is made by CT and arteriography (Fig. 37–4). Small or thrombosed AVMs, especially in the brain stem, may be missed by arteriography but detected by CT; an arteriographically demonstrable AVM is only rarely missed by CT. Both studies are usually indicated. CT is a more sensitive screening procedure, but arteriography more accurately distinguishes AVM from neoplasm and delineates the blood supply. Magnetic resonance imaging also is higly sensitive in detecting vascular malformations (Fig. 37–4C). Spinal cord AVM should be kept in mind in patients with radiographically unexplained subarachnoid hemorrhage.

Treatment depends on the location of the AVM and the condition of the patient. If surgical resection is not feasible, alternative procedures include ligation of the carotid artery or other feeding vessels, embolization with plastic beads or resins to occlude the abnormal vessels, or irradiation. The long-term value of these treatments is unclear; embolization appears to be more effective in relieving symptoms than in preventing recurrent hemorrhage. Embolization may be most useful in shrinking the malformation before surgery.

Galen-vein malformation occurs when a branch of the carotid or vertebrobasilar artery communicates directly with this vein. Cyanosis and respiratory distress are the most common neonatal symptoms, seizures and hydrocephalus predominate in infancy, and headache and subarachnoid hemorrhage become increasingly frequent in older children and adults.

Other Causes of Subarachnoid Hemorrhage

Unusual causes of spontaneous subarachnoid hemorrhage include intradural arterial dissection, blood dyscrasias (e.g., leukemia, sickle cell anemia, polycythemia vera, hemophilia, thrombocytopenic purpura, anticoagulation therapy); primary or metastatic neoplasms (e.g., glioblastoma, pinealoma, pituitary adenoma, melanoma, choriocarcinoma, renal carcinoma); infection (e.g., bacterial or tuberculous meningitis, syphilis, herpes encephalitis); and arterial or venous hemorrhagic infarction, and vasculitis (e.g., systemic lupus erythematosus, polyarteritis nodosa, Henoch-Schönlein syndrome). In most such cases, bleeding is intraparenchymal. Some subarachnoid hemorrhages remain undiagnosed, even at autopsy.

References

Adams HP Jr, Jergenson DD, Kassell NF, Sahs AL. Pitfalls in the recognition of subarachnoid hemorrhage. JAMA 1980; 244:794–796.

Allen GS et al. Cerebral artery spasm: A controlled trial of nimodipine in subarachnoid hemorrhage patients. N Engl J Med 1983; 308:619–624.

Angtuaco EJC, Binet EF. High resolution computed tomography in intracranial aneurysms. CRC Crit Rev Diagn Imaging 1986; 25:113–158.

Beck DW. Combination of aminocaproic acid and nicardipine in treatment of aneurysmal subarachnoid hemorrhage. Stroke 1988; 19:63–67.

Biller J, Godersky JC, Adams HP. Management of aneurysmal subarachnoid hemorrhage. Stroke 1988; 19:1300–1305.

Crawford PM, West CR, Chadwick DW, Shaw MDM. Arteriovenous malformations of the brain: Natural history in unoperated patients. J Neurol Neurosurg Psychiatry 1986; 49:1–10.

de la Monte SM, Moore GW, Monk MA, Hutchins GM. Risk factors for the development and rupture of intracranial berry aneurysms. Am J Med 1985; 78:957–964.

Drake CG. Management of cerebral aneurysm. Stroke 1981; 12:273–283.

Frazee JG, Cahan LD, Winter J. Bacterial intracranial aneurysms. J Neurosurg 1980; 53:633–641.

Jane JA, Kassell NF, Tonern JC, Winn HR. The natural history of aneurysms and arteriovenous malformations. J Neurosurg 1985; 62:321–323.

Kassell NF, Sasaki T, Colohan ART, Nazar G. Cerebral vasospasm following aneurysmal subarachnoid hemorrhage. Stroke 1985; 16:562–572.

Kassell NJ et al. Treatment of ischemic deficits from vasospasm with intravascular volume expansion and induced arterial hypertension. Neurosurgery 1982; 11:337–341.

Longstreth WT, Koepsell TD, Yerby MS, van Belle G.

Risk factors for subarachnoid hemorrhage. Stroke 1985; 16:377–385.

Pakarinen S. Incidence, etiology and prognosis of primary subarachnoid hemorrhage. Acta Neurol Scand 1967; 43(suppl 29):1–27.

Pasqualin A et al. Intracranial hematomas following aneurysmal rupture: Experience with 309 cases. Surg Neurol 1986; 25:6–17.

Sahs AL, Nibbelink DW, Torner JC, eds. Aneurysmal Subarachnoid Hemorrhage: Report of the Cooperative Study. Baltimore: Urban & Schwartzenberg, 1981.

Sahs AL, Perret GE, Locksley HB, Nishioka H, eds. Intracranial Aneurysms and Subarachnoid Hemorrhage: A Cooperative Study. Philadelphia: JB Lippincott, 1969.

Solomon RA, Fink ME: Current strategies for the management of aneurysmal subarachnoid hemorrhage. Arch Neurol 1987; 44:769–774.

Solomon R, et al. Prophylactic volume expansion therapy for prevention of delayed cerebral ischemia after aneurysm surgery. Arch Neurol 1988; 45:325–332.

Vermeulen M et al. Antifibrinolytic treatment in subarachnoid hemorrhage. N Engl J Med 1984; 311:432–437.

Wilson CB, Stein BM (eds.) Intracranial Arteriovenous Malformations. Baltimore, Williams & Wilkins, 1984.

Winn HR, Richardson AE, Jane JA. The long-term prognosis in untreated cerebral aneurysm. I. The incidence of late hemorrhage in cerebral aneurysm: A 10-year evaluation of 364 patients. Ann Neurol 1977; 1:358–370.

38. CEREBRAL VEINS AND SINUSES
Robert A. Fishman

Occlusion of the cerebral veins and sinuses occurs due to thrombus, thrombophlebitis, or tumors. Occlusion of the cortical and subcortical veins may cause focal neurologic symptoms and signs. The dural sinuses that are most frequently thrombosed are the lateral, cavernous, and superior sagittal sinuses. Less frequently affected are the straight sinus and the vein of Galen. The following is a list of the predisposing factors and associated disorders:

Primary idiopathic thrombosis

Secondary thrombosis
  Pregnancy
  Postpartum
  Birth-control pills
  Trauma—after open or closed head injury
  Tumors
    Meningioma
    Metastatic tumors
  Malnutrition and dehydration (marantic thrombosis)
  Infection—sinus thrombophlebitis, bacterial, fungal

Hematologic disorders
  Polycythemia
  Cryofibrinogenemia
  Sickle cell anemia
  Leukemia
  Disseminated intravascular coagulation
Paraneoplastic syndrome

Lateral Sinus

Thrombosis of the lateral sinus is usually secondary to otitis media and mastoiditis. Lateral sinus thrombosis is now a clinical rarity. Infants and children are most commonly affected. The thrombosis may occur coincidental with the acute attack of otitis and mastoiditis or it may be delayed to the chronic stage of the infection.

Symptoms and Signs. Involvement of the sinus is usually heralded by septic fever and chills, however, occasionally the thrombosis is not accompanied by a febrile reaction. Septicemia occurs most commonly with hemolytic streptococcus and is present in about half the cases. Petechiae in the skin and mucous membranes and septic embolism of the lungs, joints, and muscles are infrequent complications of the septicemia.

The classic symptoms of lateral sinus thrombosis are fever, headache, nausea, and vomiting. The latter signs are due to increased intracranial pressure and are most apt to occur when the right sinus is occluded; in most individuals, the right sinus drains the greater portion of blood from the brain. Local signs of thrombosis of the sinus are usually absent, but occasionally there is swelling over the mastoid region with distention of the superficial veins and tenderness over the jugular vein in the neck.

Because of increased intracranial pressure, papilledema develops in about half the cases. This is usually bilateral, but occasionally may be on only one side, possibly the result of asymmetric extension of the process to the cavernous sinuses. Increased intracranial pressure may cause separation of the sutures or bulging of the fontanelles in infants.

Drowsiness and coma are not uncommon symptoms. Convulsive seizures may also occur, however, focal neurologic symptoms are rare. A few cases have been reported with jacksonian convulsive seizures followed by hemiplegia, possibly due to extension of infection into the veins draining the lateral surface of the hemisphere. These signs, however, usually indicate an abscess in the cerebral hemisphere. Diplopia may result from injury to the sixth cranial nerve by increased intracranial pressure or from involvement of the nerve by extension of the infection in the petrous bone. The combination of sixth nerve palsy (lateral rectus weakness) and pain in the face as the result of damage to the fifth nerve is the *Gradenigo syndrome.* There may occasionally be signs of damage of the ninth, tenth, and eleventh nerves. These are attributed to pressure on these nerves as they pass through the jugular foramen by the distended jugular vein. It seems more probable that they are caused by extension of the infection into the bone (osteomyelitis) surrounding these structures.

Laboratory Data. There is a leukocytosis in the blood and, as previously noted, the organism may be recovered from the blood in half the cases. The CSF shows the changes characteristic of an aseptic meningeal reaction. The pressure is increased. The fluid is usually slightly turbid or cloudy and contains several to many hundred leukocytes. The sugar content of the fluid is normal and cultures are sterile unless an actual bacterial meningitis has developed.

Diagnosis. The diagnosis of lateral sinus thrombosis is made on the basis of signs of increased intracranial pressure in a patient with an acute or chronic otitis and mastoiditis. The only other diagnosis that may cause difficulty is abscess of the temporal lobe or other parts of the cerebral hemisphere. The development of a hemiplegia, aphasia, or hemianopia is in favor of the latter diagnosis and the possibility of an intracerebral abscess should be excluded by CT or magnetic resonance imaging (MRI), if necessary, in all cases with these focal signs.

Course and Prognosis. The mortality rate is high in untreated cases of lateral sinus thrombosis. The infected thrombus may occasionally heal by complete organization, but more commonly death results from septicemia, meningitis, extension of the infection to the cavernous or longitudinal sinus or abscess of the brain.

When patients recover, intracranial pressure may continue to be elevated for some months, especially if the jugular vein on the right side is ligated.

Treatment. The occurrence of a thrombosis of the lateral sinus should be prevented by the prompt treatment of infections of the middle ear. Treatment of a thrombosis is by antibiotics and surgical drainage. Infected bone should be removed, the sinus should be exposed and drained, and the jugular vein should be ligated if necessary.

Cavernous Sinus

Cavernous sinus thrombosis usually originates in suppurative processes of the orbit, nasal sinuses, or upper half of the face. The infection commonly involves only one sinus at the onset but rapidly spreads through the circular sinus to the opposite side. One or both may be secondarily involved by extension of infection from one of the other dural sinuses. Nonseptic thrombosis of the cavernous sinus is rare. The sinus may be partially or totally occluded by tumor masses, trauma, or arteriovenous aneurysms.

Symptoms and Signs. The onset of symptoms of a septic thrombosis is usually sudden and dramatic. The patient appears acutely ill and there is a septic type of fever. There is pain in the eyes and the orbits are painful to pressure. The bulbs are proptosed and there is edema and chemosis of the conjunctivae and eyelids. Diplopia follows involvement of the oculomotor nerves. Ptosis may be present and obscured by the exophthalmos. The optic discs are swollen and there are numerous small or large hemorrhages around the disc when the orbital veins are occluded. The corneas are cloudy and ulcers may develop. The pupils may be dilated or small. The pupillary reactions are preserved in some cases and lost in others. Visual acuity may be normal or moderately impaired.

The described signs are present when the infection spreads to the sinus from the face or nasal sinuses, but subject to some modification when the infection originates in the throat, sphenoids, or ear. In these cases, the evolution of symptoms is subacute and there is less engorgement of the orbit.

Laboratory Data. The laboratory findings in patients with cavernous sinus thrombosis are similar to those in patients with lateral sinus thrombosis.

Diagnosis. Cavernous sinus thrombosis must be distinguished from other conditions that produce exophthalmos and congestion in the orbit. These include orbital tumors, meningiomas and other tumors in the region of the sphenoid, malignant exophthalmos, and arteriovenous aneurysms. The evolution of symptoms is slow in all of the latter conditions except arteriovenous aneurysms. Arteriovenous aneurysm can be differentiated by the pulsating exophthalmos, the presence of a bruit, and recession of the exophthalmos when the carotid artery is occluded by digital pressure. Computed tomography, MRI, and carotid angiography are valuable in establishing the diagnosis.

Treatment. Until recent years, septic thrombosis of the cavernous sinus was almost invariably fatal because of the development of an acute meningitis. Cures have been effected with antibiotics with or without anticoagulants.

Superior Sagittal Sinus

The superior sagittal sinus is less commonly the site of an infective thrombosis than either the lateral or cavernous sinus. Infections may reach the superior sagittal sinus from the nasal cavities or as secondary extensions from the lateral or cavernous sinuses. The superior sagittal sinus may also be occluded by the extension of infection from osteomyelitis or from epidural or subdural infection.

The superior sagittal sinus is the most common site of nonseptic sinus thrombosis associated with dehydration and marasmus in infancy. It may also be occluded by trauma or by tumors (meningiomas). Sagittal sinus thrombosis has also been associated with the use of oral contraceptives, pregnancy, hemolytic anemia, sickle cell trait, thrombocytopenia, ulcerative colitis, diabetes, and other diseases. Nonseptic thrombosis of the sinus may occasionally occur in adults without any obvious cause.

Symptoms and Signs. The general signs are prostration, fever, headache, and papilledema. Local signs include edema of the forehead and anterior part of the scalp, and engorgement of the veins in the area of the anterior or posterior fontanelles, with the formation of a caput medusae.

Focal neurologic signs and symptoms may be entirely absent in nonseptic thrombosis with increased intracranial pressure as the only presenting sign. Extension of the clot into the larger cerebral veins is, however, almost always accompanied by the onset of dramatic signs caused by hemorrhage into the cortical white and gray matter. Extension into these veins is common in septic thrombosis and in a high percentage of the nonseptic type. Convulsive seizures (often unilateral), hemiplegia, aphasia, or hemianopia may occur.

Laboratory Data. The laboratory findings with septic thrombosis of the superior sagittal sinus are similar to those in patients with lateral sinus thrombosis. In the nonseptic type, the CSF is under increased pressure but there is no evidence of an aseptic meningeal reaction in the fluid such as pleocytosis. Occasionally the CSF is bloody or xanthochromic as the result of cortical and meningeal hemorrhage.

Diagnosis. The diagnosis of superior longitudinal sinus thrombosis should be considered in all patients with a septic focus in the head when there are jacksonian convulsive seizures and focal neurologic signs. The diagnosis of nonseptic thrombosis should be considered in all infants who develop signs of increased intracranial pressure and cerebral symptoms during the course of severe nutritional disturbances and cachexia. The diagnosis can be established by angiography. CT may show multiple lesions, some hemorrhagic, others radiolucent, which are often bilateral (Fig. 38–1). The *"cord" sign* is a linear area of increased density that is related to clot in veins or sinus. The *"empty delta sign"* appears after injection of contrast material, which outlines the periphery of the sinus where blood still flows, leaving the central area of the clot dark; there may also be enhancement of the gyri or tentorium. Ventricles may be large or small. Cerebral angiography is definitive, showing the venous block or collateral flow.

Prognosis. The prognosis is poor in patients with a septic thrombosis. Death usually results from meningitis or hemorrhagic lesions in the brain. Occasionally, cases in which the diagnosis seemed fairly well-established have survived, some with residuals in the form of hemiplegia, mental deficiency, and recurrent convulsive seizures.

The prognosis is less grave in patients with nonseptic thrombosis. Symptoms may recede after several months after recanalization of the sinus or development of collateral circulation.

Treatment. Antibiotics should be administered to patients with septic thrombosis. Craniotomy with evacuation of subdural or epidural abscess should be performed when these are present. There is no satisfactory treatment of nonseptic thrombosis. The hazards of hemorrhagic venous infarction are considered contraindications to the use of anticoagulants in most cases.

Other Dural Sinuses

Thrombosis of the inferior longitudinal sinus, the straight sinus, the petrosals, or the vein of Galen rarely occurs alone. They are

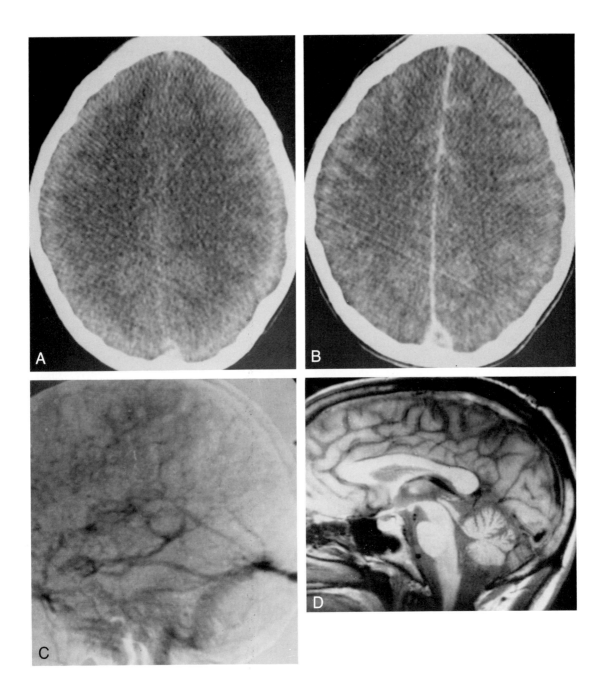

Fig. 38–1. Sinus thrombosis, hemorrhagic venous infarction. *A.* Axial CT scan, without contrast, demonstrates density in sagittal sinus posteriorly. *B.* At same level, postcontrast, "delta sign" is noted in affected sinus. Thrombus density caused central filling defect within sinus. Triangular enhancement at periphery is related to collateral venous channels within dura. *C.* Lateral digital subtraction arteriogram confirms sagittal sinus occlusion. *D.* Superior sagittal sinus occlusion (in a different patient). Sagittal T_1 MRI demonstrates high signal within the superior sagittal sinus. (Normally the sinus demonstrates signal void, due to flow.) (Courtesy of Drs. S.K. Hilal and J.A. Bello.)

usually involved by secondary extension of a septic or nonseptic thrombosis of the lateral, superior sagittal, or cavernous sinuses. Any signs or symptoms that may be produced by thrombosis of the inferior longitudinal, straight, or petrosal sinuses are usually masked by those resulting from involvement of the more important sinuses. Thrombosis of the great vein of Galen may cause hemorrhages in the central white matter of the hemispheres or in the basal ganglia and lateral ventricles.

DURAL ARTERIOVENOUS MALFORMATIONS

Dural arteriovenous malformations are more common in women than men and are more likely located in the posterior fossa than above the tentorium. They present with peripheral cranial nerve involvement (third, seventh, eighth, and twelfth most commonly) or central nervous system manifestations. The latter are attributed to intracranial venous hypertension, decreased CSF absorption, venous sinus thrombosis, or minimal subarachnoid bleeding. Seizures, motor weakness, brain stem and cerebellar syndromes have been observed depending on the region involved. Some cases present as idiopathic pseudotumor with papilledema and headache only. Diagnosis requires detailed cerebral angiography including selective injection of the external carotid and both vertebral arteries. Therapy with selective embolization using silicone or other agents may be beneficial as well as direct surgical excision. Spontaneous thrombosis of the dural arteriovenous malformation with remission of symptoms is often observed; many lesions have a benign prognosis.

References

Anderson SC, et al. Congested deep subcortical veins as a sign of dural venous thrombosis: MR and CT correlations. J Comput Assist Tomogr 1987; 11:1059–1061.

Averback P. Primary cerebral venous thrombosis in young adults: The diverse manifestations of an underrecognized disease. Ann Neurol 1978; 3:81–86.

Estanol B et al. Intracranial venous thrombosis in young women. Stroke 1979; 10:680–684.

Gates PC, Barnett HJM. Venous disease: Cortical veins and sinuses. In: Stroke: Pathophysiology, Diagnosis, and Management. New York, Churchill-Livingstone, 1986: 731–743.

Hanley DF, et al. Treatment of sagittal sinus thrombosis with cerebral hemorrhage and intracranial hypertension. Stroke 1988; 19:903–909.

Kalbag RM, Woolf AL. Cerebral Venous Thrombosis. London: Oxford University Press, 1967.

Lasjaunias P, Chiu M, Brugge K, et al. Neurological man-

ifestations of intracranial dural arteriovenous malformations. J Neurosurg 1986; 64:724–730.

Rao KC, Knipp HC, Wagner EJ. Computed tomographic findings in cerebral sinus and venous thrombosis. Radiology 1981; 140:391–398.

Sigsbee B, Deck MDF, Posner JB. Non-metastatic superior sagittal sinus thrombosis complicating systemic cancer. Neurology 1979; 29:139–146.

Towbin A. The syndrome of latent cerebral venous thrombosis: Its frequency and relation to age and congestive heart failure. Stroke 1973: 4:419–430.

Vinuela F, Fox AJ, Pelz DM, Drake CG. Unusual clinical manifestations of dural arteriovenous malformations. J Neurosurg 1986; 64:554–558.

39. VASCULAR DISEASE OF THE SPINAL CORD
Leon A. Weisberg

Blood supply to the spinal cord and nerve roots originates in the vertebral, thyrocervical, costocervical, intercostal, and lumbar arteries; these major arterial trunks give rise to radicular and medullary arteries. The segmental radicular arteries supply the nerve roots; they originate near the vertebral foramina. The six to nine large medullary arteries come from the vertebral, subclavian, or iliac arteries, and the aorta (Fig. 39–1). Branches of the medullary arteries form a single anterior median spinal artery and two posterior spinal arteries that perfuse the spinal cord. The anterior median spinal artery arises from a branch of each vertebral artery and it runs along the entire length of the cord. The pial arteriolar plexus and posterior spinal arteries supply the dorsal aspect.

In the cervical region, the anterior median artery is reinforced at several levels by unpaired medullary arteries from the vertebral and subclavian arteries; the blood supply is rich in collateral branches. In the thoracic region, the anterior median spinal artery is joined by only a few branches of the thoracic aorta and the blood supply is relatively sparse. The midthoracic spinal cord is supplied by terminal vessels that descend from the subclavian-vertebral arteries or ascend from the abdominal aorta; this watershed is particularly vulnerable to vascular insufficiency, and spinal cord infarction is most likely to occur at T4. Lumbar and sacral spinal areas are supplied by the largest and most constant of the medullary arteries, the "great anterior radicular artery" of Adamkiewicz, which is usually found at L1 or L2 (occasionally as high as T12 or as low as L4). This artery, paired or single, travels through the ver-

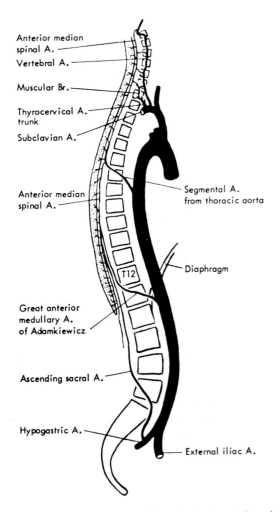

Fig. 39–1. The anterior median spinal artery is joined at the various levels by arteries that arise from vertebral and subclavian arteries, the aorta, and iliac arteries.

tebral foramen and anastomoses with the anterior medial spinal artery; the largest branch supplies the lumbosacral spinal cord and the conus medullaris. The conus and cauda equina are also supplied by sacral branches that ascend from the iliac arteries.

The central (sulcal) arteries originate in the anterior spinal artery to supply the anterior two thirds and central area of the spinal cord. Penetrating branches from the pial arterial plexus supply the periphery and posterior third of the cord. Within the spinal cord, these arterial feeders anastomose in their most distal parts, creating border zones similar to those in the brain. These vascular border zones may explain the incomplete or partial syndromes that are seen after some spinal cord infarctions (see Fig. 39–1).

The plexiform venous system interconnects freely with the radicular arteries within the subarachnoid space. The radicular veins empty into the epidural venous plexus, which in turn communicates with the inferior vena cava and the azygos system through the perivertebral plexus.

Infarction of the Spinal Cord

Softening or infarction of the spinal cord (myelomalacia) results from occlusion of major vessels. Anterior spinal artery infarction is much more common than the posterior spinal artery syndrome because of the difference in collateral supply.

Etiology. Spinal cord infarction is most often caused by atheromata involving the aorta. Although atherosclerosis of the aorta is common, clinical evidence of spinal artery infarction is rare. Less common causes of spinal cord infarction include collagen vascular disease, syphilitic angiitis, dissecting aortic aneurysm, embolism, pregnancy, sickle-cell disease, neurotoxic effects of iodinated contrast material used in angiography, compression of spinal arteries by tumor, systemic arterial hypotension after cardiac arrest, aortic surgery, and decompression sickness. Paraplegia may follow surgical repair of an aortic aneurysm when the cross-clamp time is longer than 25 minutes; the risk may be lessened by avoiding systemic arterial hypotension, placing a shunt around the cross-clamp, and using thiopental anesthesia.

Symptoms and Signs. The symptoms of spinal infarction usually appear within a few minutes or a few hours of the onset of the infarction. The first symptom may be local or radicular back pain that is lancinating or burning and usually transient. There may be diffuse, deep, aching pain in both legs, or a burning dysesthetic pain may start in the feet and rapidly ascend to calves, thighs, and abdomen. These sensory symptoms are followed by rapid onset of weakness of the legs; the patient is soon unable to walk. At first, the weakness is flaccid and tendon reflexes are absent. The pattern of this neurologic disorder depends on the site of the lesion and the collateral circulation.

Occlusion of the cervical part of the anterior spinal artery is followed by tetraplegia, incontinence of urine and feces, and sensory impairment below the level of the lesion. Proprioception and vibration sensations are spared because the posterior columns are supplied by the posterior arterial plexus. If proprioception and vibration sensation are impaired, the lesion is not an anterior spinal artery infarction. Focal atrophy and weakness of the arms and hands signify ischemia of the anterior horn cells. Spastic weakness in the legs results from lesions of the lateral corticospinal tract. Sometimes, signs are restricted to those of either upper or lower motor neurons (or both), causing a pattern similar to that of amyotrophic lateral sclerosis, but differing in mode of onset.

Most clinical spinal cord strokes affect the midthoracic region with paraplegia, urinary incontinence, and loss of pain and temperature sensation below the lesion. There may be sacral sparing of cutaneous sensation and normal proprioception and vibration sensation. The weakness is flaccid at first, but Babinski signs are seen and spasticity and hyperreflexia usually develop in a few weeks.

Arterial insufficiency of the lumbar region causes paraplegia, sphincter symptoms, and loss of cutaneous sensation with sacral sparing. The weakness is more likely to remain flaccid because the anterior horn cells are affected.

TIAs of the spinal cord and cauda equina may occur; but there is no way to confirm this clinical impression. These attacks may precede spinal artery infarction and may be in patients with spinal vascular malformations or lumbar spondylosis and stenosis. Symptoms of spinal claudication include paresthesias of the feet, difficulty walking, loss of tendon reflexes, and the appearance of Babinski signs. The episodes occur during exercise, presumably because blood is shunted away from the spinal cord and into the muscles. The symptoms may be exacerbated by postural change in patients with lumbar stenosis. In cervical spondylosis, the role of arterial compression is uncertain.

Diagnosis. Plain radiography, myelography, CT, and magnetic resonance imaging are needed to rule out abnormalities due to spinal cord neoplasm or cervical spondylosis. Lumbar puncture excludes hemorrhagic or infectious disorders. In spinal cord infarction, CSF may show a slight elevation of the protein content, but the gamma globulin content is normal. Two conditions that may simulate spinal infarction are multiple sclerosis and cord neoplasm. In multiple sclerosis or transverse myelitis, the CSF frequently shows an elevated gamma globulin content. Neoplasms are more likely to increase CSF protein content to values of several hundred mg/dl. In spinal cord infarction, myelography is usually normal; however, edema may cause signs of an intramedullary mass and subarachnoid block. Spinal angiography may cause cord infarction and is contraindicated unless a spinal vascular malformation is deemed likely for other reasons. Electromyography may show denervation potentials in muscle with normal nerve conduction velocities at the level of the lesion, which is the pattern of anterior horn cell lesions. In patients who undergo thoracic or abdominal aneurysm surgery, somatosensory potential monitoring is not helpful in predicting spinal cord ischemia when the aorta is clamped.

Treatment and Prognosis. Treatment of the specific disease responsible for the spinal cord infarction is indicated. The general principles of care for a patient with quadriplegia or paraplegia are followed, with attention to bladder and skin care, plus physical therapy. There may be some return of function but there is usually little improvement of paraplegia or incontinence. Naloxone and calcium channel blockers have been used experimentally to treat spinal cord ischemia. However, trials with humans have yet to be undertaken.

Venous Disease

Venous disorders of the spinal cord are even less common than arterial lesions. The *Foix-Alajouanine syndrome* is characterized by spinal cord necrosis and evidence of enlarged, tortuous, and thrombosed veins. Although this necrotic myelitis is attributed to venous thrombosis, usually there is no angiographic evidence of venous thrombosis or vascular spinal cord malformation. There is occasional pathologic evidence of vascular malformations that are thought to have undergone spontaneous thrombosis. Pathologically, the major destruction involves the corticospinal tract, sparing anterior horn cells.

Clinically, there is usually progressive worsening of the condition for several weeks. Symptoms include weakness of the legs, incontinence, and sensory loss. Findings usually include spastic paraparesis, hyperreflexia, bilateral Babinski signs, and a sensory level below the lesion. CSF may show an elevated protein content, leukocytic pleocytosis, and red blood cells. Treatment with anticoagulants or corticosteroids has not been effective. Because some venous infarctions of the spinal cord are hemorrhagic, anticoagulation may be potentially dangerous.

Spinal Cord Hemorrhage

Hemorrhage in the spinal cord may be epidural, subdural, subarachnoid, or intramedullary in location. Hematomyelia (hemorrhage into the substance of the spinal cord) usually results from trauma, and usually immediately follows a spinal injury; however, this may be delayed for hours or days. Nontraumatic causes of spinal cord hemorrhage include blood dyscrasias, anticoagulation therapy, arteriovenous malformation, and venous spinal cord infarction.

Pathology. At first, the spinal cord is swollen because of the intramedullary central blood clot. The blood dissects longitudinally for several segments below and above the hemorrhage, most severely affecting the gray matter and contiguous white matter. The clot is usually surrounded by a rim of normal nervous tissue. If the patient survives, the blood is liquefied and removed by phagocytes. Glial replacement is usually incomplete, resulting in a syrinx-like cavity that extends over several cord segments.

Signs and Symptoms. There is sudden onset of severe localized back or radicular pain. If the hemorrhage is small, there may be only spastic weakness associated with hyperreflexia in the legs and bladder dysfunction. If the hemorrhage is large, signs of transection of the cord include flaccid paralysis, complete sensory loss below the lesion, absent reflexes, Babinski signs, and loss of sphincter control. Autonomic disturbance and vasomotor instability may result in shock. If the patient survives, the hematoma is reabsorbed and symptoms may improve, but the outcome is uncertain.

Diagnosis. The CSF is bloody or xanthochromic and protein content is increased. Myelography shows evidence of an intradural intramedullary mass with subarachnoid block. Spinal angiography may be indicated in nontraumatic cases if spinal vascular malformation is suspected.

Spinal epidural or subdural hemorrhage may cause a mass effect that rapidly compresses the cord. This may follow spinal trauma even without evidence of bone fracture; other etiologies include anticoagulation, blood dyscrasias, and cases without obvious etiology. Epidural hemorrhage may follow lumbar puncture in patients with a coagulation disorder. The symptoms of epidural and subdural spinal hematoma are similar. Symptoms of epidural hemorrhage appear rapidly, with back pain, sensory loss, and sphincter impairment. The diagnosis is established by myelography, which shows evidence of cord compression by an extradural mass. Spinal subarachnoid hemorrhage may be due to vascular malformation, spinal neoplasm (most commonly ependymoma), blood dyscrasia, or periarteritis nodosa, which is characterized by sudden, severe back pain at the level of the lesion. Symptoms may be due to blood in the subarachnoid space or to blood dissecting into the spinal cord or along the nerve-root sheaths. CSF is bloody and xanthochromic. Myelography and spinal angiography are necessary to establish the etiology. Ruptured intracranial aneurysm may occasionally present with severe back pain rather than with the more characteristic headache and stiff neck; in these cases, cerebral angiography is necessary.

Treatment. Treatment of spinal cord hemorrhage depends on the cause and location of the hemorrhage. For subdural and epidural hemorrhage, surgery is necessary; however, prognosis is poor if paraplegia appears rapidly and there is delay in surgical intervention. Patients with spinal cord hematomas caused by anticoagulant therapy should receive fresh whole blood and vitamin K. Angiography is indicated only when spinal cord hemorrhage is spontaneous. When hematomyelia is due to vascular malformation, treatment is nonsurgical. In hematomyelia, physical therapy is important because partial or complete recovery is more likely than in cases of spinal cord infarction.

References

Garland H, Greenberg J, Harriman DGF. Infarction of the spinal cord. Brain 1966; 89:645–662.

Gillilan LA. Arterial and venous anatomy of the spinal cord. In: Moossy J, Janeway R, eds. Cerebral Vascular Diseases, Transactions of the Seventh Princeton Conference. New York: Grune & Stratton, 1971:3–9.

Henson RA, Parson M. Ischemic lesions in the spinal cord: An illustrated review. QJ Med 1967; 36:205–222.

Hogan EL, Romanul F. Spinal cord infarction occurring during insertion of aortic graft. Neurology 1966; 16:67–74.

Kim RC, Smith HR, Henbest ML. Nonhemorrhagic venous infarction of the spinal cord. Ann Neurol 1984; 15:379–385.

Mair WCP, Folkerts JF. Necrosis of spinal cord due to thrombophlebitis (subacute necrotic myelitis). Brain 1953; 76:536–572.

Margolis G. Circulation dynamics of the spinal cord. In: Moossy J, Janeway R, eds. Cerebral Vascular Diseases, Transactions of the Seventh Princeton Conference. New York: Grune & Stratton, 1971:10–17.

Russel NA, Benoit BG. Spinal subdural hematoma. A review. Surg Neurol 1983; 20:133–137.

Satran R. Spinal cord infarction. Stroke 1988; 19:529–532.

Silver JR, Buxton PH. Spinal stroke. Brain 1974; 97:539–550.

Zull D, Cydulka R. Acute paraplegia and aortic dissection. Am J Med 1988; 84:765–770.

Chapter IV

Disorders of Cerebrospinal and Brain Fluids

40. HYBROCEPHALUS

Leon D. Prockop
Chunilal P. Shah

Hydrocephalus is characterized by increased CSF volume and dilation of the cerebral ventricles. The following list shows the classification of the types of hydrocephalus:

Obstructive Hydrocephalus
    Congenital malformations
    Postinflammatory or posthemorrhagic
    Mass lesions

Normal Pressure Hydrocephalus

Communicating Hydrocephalus
    Overproduction of CSF
    Defective absorption of CSF
    Venous drainage insufficiency

Hydrocephalus Ex Vacuo

When there are no clinical signs or symptoms of intracranial hypertension, hydrocephalus is *occult*. It is *active* when the disease is progressive and there is increased intracranial pressure; hydrocephalus is *arrested* when ventricular enlargement has ceased. Dandy and Blackfan introduced the terms *communicating* and *noncommunicating* hydrocephalus to describe the flow of CSF. They injected a tracer dye into one lateral ventricle. If the dye appeared in lumbar CSF, the hydrocephalus was termed communicating; if the dye did not appear in the lumbar CSF, the hydrocephalus was termed noncommunicating. This functional classification was widely accepted because it proved useful in surgical shunt placement; however, by this definition, noncommunicating hydrocephalus refers only to that caused by obstruction within the ventricular system. We now use the term *obstructive hydrocephalus* to describe conditions after obstruction of either intraventricular or extraventricular pathways. In communicating

hydrocephalus, no obstruction can be demonstrated by standard tests. *Normal pressure hydrocephalus* (NPH) warrants separate classification and discussion. These forms of hydrocephalus are distinguished from *hydrocephalus ex vacuo*, in which CSF volume increases without change in CSF pressure because brain tissue has been lost, as in Alzheimer disease (Fig. 40–1).

Obstructive Hydrocephalus

Obstructive hydrocephalus is the best characterized and most common form of hydrocephalus. It follows obstruction of either the intraventricular or extraventricular pathways. In the former, the obstruction site determines proximal dilatation, with preservation of normal ventricular size distal to the block. Obstruction may occur at the foramen of Monro, the third ventricle, the aqueduct of Sylvius, the fourth ventricle, or the outflow of the foramina of Luschka and Magendie. In obstruction of extraventricular CSF pathways, absolute or relative reduction of flow may occur in the subarachnoid spaces at the base of the brain, at the tentorial level, and over the hemispheric convexities. Because of the limitations of the clinical tests discussed later, the precise location of the obstruction or absorptive block cannot always be determined.

Obstructive hydrocephalus is caused by congenital malformations or developmental lesions, postinflammatory or posthemorrhagic fibrosis, or mass lesion.

Congenital Malformation or Developmental Lesions. Congenital hydrocephalus occurs with an incidence of 0.5 to 1.8/1,000 births and may result from either genetic or nongenetic causes. Common nongenetic causes include intrauterine infection, intracranial hemorrhage secondary to birth trauma or prematurity, and meningitis. Genetically, an X-linked hydrocephalus has been described. In

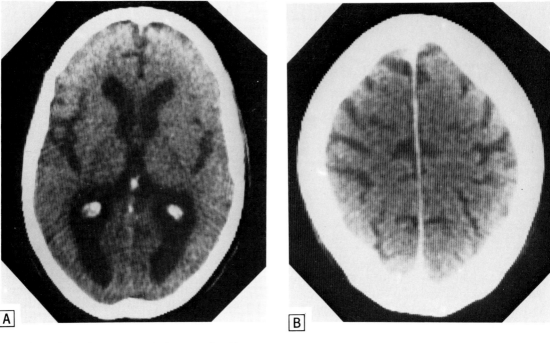

Fig. 40–1. Brain CT scans. Marked ventricular dilatation *(A)* and widening of cortical sulci *(B)* indicative of hydrocephalus ex vacuo in a 64-year-old woman with dementia.

most of these cases, aqueductal stenosis has been documented radiographically, by MRI, or at postmortem examination. In some families, the occurrence of aqueductal stenosis, hydrocephalus of undetermined anatomic type, and the Dandy-Walker syndrome in siblings of both sexes has suggested alternate modes of inheritance. In the Dandy-Walker syndrome, there is expansion of the fourth ventricle and of the posterior fossa with obstruction of the foramina of Luschka and Magendie (Fig. 40–2). It is not clear whether aqueductal lesions (e.g., gliosis or fibrosis) occur developmentally or whether they are the residue of prior viral inflammatory disease contracted in utero or in early life (Fig. 40–3). The Arnold-Chiari malformation may be associated with hydrocephalus at birth or it may develop later.

POSTINFLAMMATORY OR POSTHEMORRHAGIC HYDROCEPHALUS

Posthemorrhagic hydrocephalus is a major complication of cerebral intraventricular hemorrhage in low-birth-weight infants, with an incidence from 26 to 70%, depending on the severity of hemorrhage. Hydrocephalus results from obstruction of CSF flow by a clot within the ventricular system or by obliterative basilar or transcortical arachnoiditis. Af-

ter subarachnoid hemorrhage, the arachnoid villi are distended with packed red cells, suggesting an absorptive defect. Consequently, fibrotic impairment of extraventricular CSF pathways after intracranial hemorrhage may be complicated by dysfunction of arachnoid villi.

Likewise, intramedullary and/or intraventricular hemorrhage in adults causes hydrocephalus, especially if there are clots in the ventricles (Fig. 40–4A). Hydrocephalus also occurs in adults after subarachnoid bleeding due to head trauma or aneurysmal rupture (Fig. 40–4B). In some patients, the obstruction of CSF flow is transient; intracranial pressure increases and hydrocephalus appears, but then disappears spontaneously. Other patients exhibit progressive hydrocephalus. This form of obstructive hydrocephalus is due to extraventricular obstruction to CSF flow and may be a form of, or may cause, NPH (Fig. 40–5).

Among infectious diseases, tuberculous and luetic meningitis may cause hydrocephalus secondary to basal arachnoiditis. CT has demonstrated that hydrocephalus may also follow other forms of meningitis (e.g., bacterial, fungal, viral, carcinomatous—Figs. 40–6, 40–7).

Mass Lesions. Intracranial neoplasms may

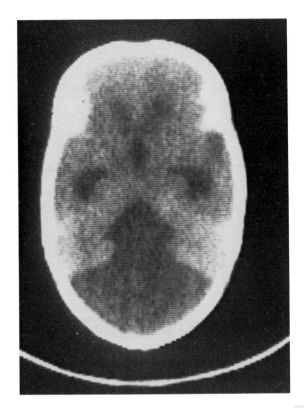

Fig. 40–2. Brain CT scan. Hydrocephalus associated with Dandy-Walker malformation in a 4-month-old child with increasing head circumference and bulging fontanelles.

cause obstructive hydrocephalus (Figs. 40–8, 40–9). Other mass lesions, such as cerebellar infarction or hemorrhage, may lead to acute hydrocephalus. Basilar artery ectasia and other vascular abnormalities (e.g., vein of Galen malformation) have been associated with hydrocephalus.

Communicating Hydrocephalus

When impairment of neither intraventricular nor extraventricular CSF flow can be documented, three other mechanisms may cause hydrocephalus: oversecretion of CSF, venous insufficiency, or impaired absorption of CSF by arachnoid villi.

When oversecretion occurs, the absorptive capacity of the subarachnoid space is about three times the normal CSF formation rate of 0.35 ml/minute; formation rates greater than 1.0 ml/minute may produce hydrocephalus. Clinically, *choroid plexus papilloma* is the only known cause of oversecretion hydrocephalus.

Otitic hydrocephalus is a condition that occurs in children after chronic otitis media or mastoiditis with lateral sinus thrombosis; oth-erwise, impaired cerebral venous drainage (e.g., thrombosis of cortical veins or intracranial venous sinuses) rarely causes hydrocephalus. Hydrocephalus due to extracranial venous drainage impairment only rarely follows radical neck dissection or obstruction of the superior vena cava.

Communicating hydrocephalus has been attributed to *congenital agenesis of the arachnoid villi* and the consequently impaired CSF absorption (Fig. 40–10). Because detailed pathologic study of the number of villi and their structural characteristics is difficult and rarely performed, this defect may be more common than statistics indicate. Likewise, dysfunction of arachnoid villi without obstruction of basilar or transcortical CSF pathways cannot be assessed easily.

Hydrocephalus has also been described when CSF protein content exceeds 500 mg/dl in cases of polyneuritis or spinal cord tumor. The protein may interfere with CSF absorption. Ependymoma, the most common spinal cord tumor associated with hydrocephalus, may be due to tumor seeding of the arachnoid villi.

Normal Pressure Hydrocephalus

As a potentially treatable cause of dementia, NPH has captured wide attention. The syndrome was first delineated in 1964 as an occult form of hydrocephalus. The absence of papilledema with normal CSF pressure at lumbar puncture led to the term *normal pressure hydrocephalus;* however, intracranial hypertension probably occurs prior to diagnosis. Intermittent intracranial hypertension has been noted during monitoring of suspected cases. Often the syndrome follows head trauma, subarachnoid hemorrhage, or meningitis or is associated with occult mass lesion.

There is considerable speculation about the pathophysiology of NPH. Obliteration or insufficiency of the transcortical subarachnoid space may occur alone or with an impaired absorption defect at the arachnoid villi, leading to reduced conductance to CSF outflow.

General Clinical Data

Signs and Symptoms. In children, before the cranial sutures fuse, hydrocephalus causes skull enlargement and widened fontanels. The face, although of normal size, appears small relative to the enlarged head. Exophthalmos and scleral prominence result from downward displacement of the orbits. Severe intracranial hypertension produces

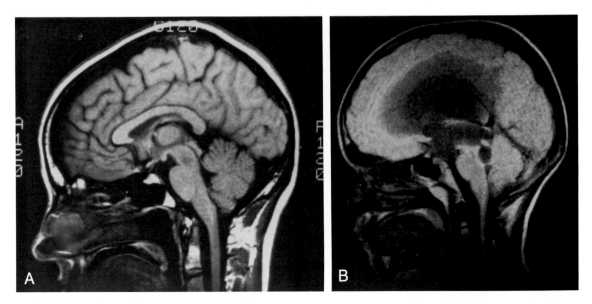

Fig. 40–3. *A.* Normal midsagittal brain anatomy demonstrated by T-1 weighted MRI. *B.* On a similar scan of a child, abnormal membranous structures within the 4th ventricle and aqueduct of Sylvius caused dilation of the upper 4th, 3rd, and lateral ventricles. (Courtesy of Dr. Reed Murtagh.)

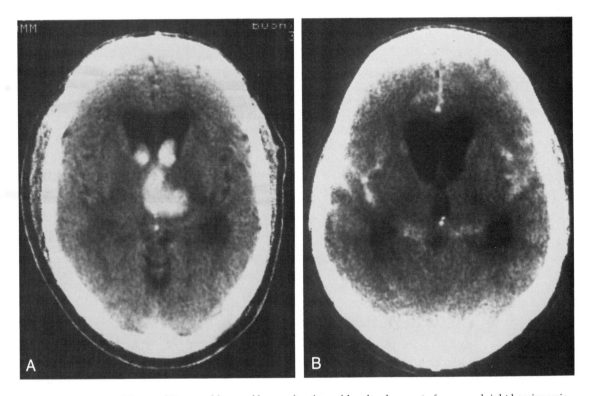

Fig. 40–4. *A.* Brain CT scan of 58-year-old several hours after the sudden development of coma and right hemiparesis. Blood in the left thalamus and within the 3rd and lateral ventricles is associated with hydrocephalus. *B.* Similar scan of adult 24 hours after the sudden onset of severe headache and meningism. Acute hydrocephalus with subarachnoid space blood is seen.

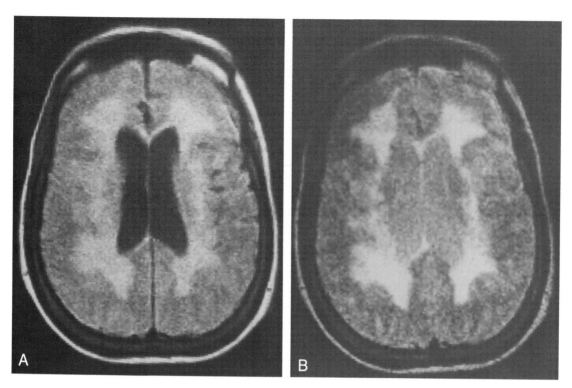

Fig. 40–5. *A.* Axial T-1 weighted MRI brain scan showing lateral ventricular dilatation in a 42 year old woman with dementia, ataxia, and urinary incontinence 3 months after subarachnoid hemorrhage. *B.* A more T-2 axial weighted image in this woman demonstrated periventricular increased signal intensity consistent with transependymal migration of CSF. She improved after CSF shunting.

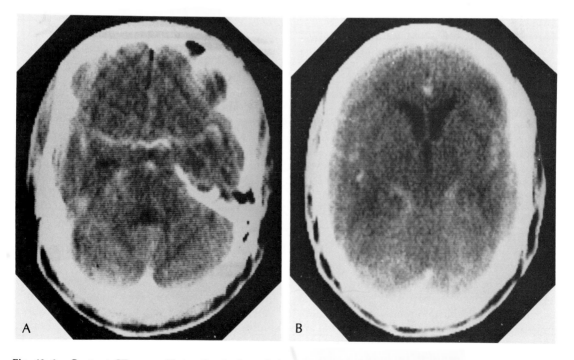

Fig. 40–6. Contrast CT scans. Obstructive hydrocephalus in a 22-year-old man who suffered a second episode of streptococcal meningitis. Early ventricular dilatation as well as obliteration of basilar cisterns with patchy enhancement of basilar meninges are noted.

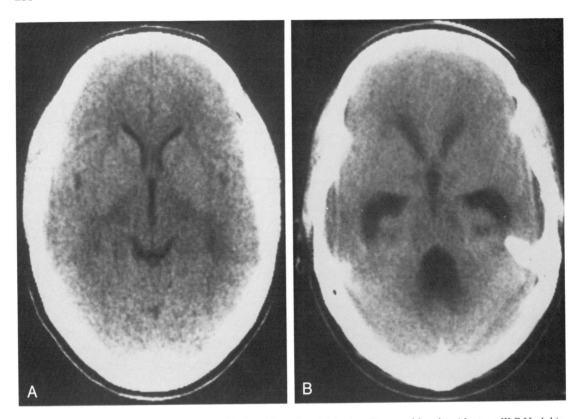

Fig. 40–7. Noncontrast CT scans. *A.* Normal 3rd and lateral ventricles in a 25-year-old male with stage III-B Hodgkin disease. *B.* Four years later, his scan showed dilation of the 4th, 3rd, and lateral ventricles. CSF findings were those of carcinomatous meningitis.

sluggish pupillary reaction, absence of upward gaze, impaired lateral gaze, paralysis or spasm of conversion, nystagmus, retractions, and absence of visual fixation or response to visible threat. Untreated hydrocephalic infants fail to thrive and show retardation of motor and intellectual development. Limb movements, particularly of the legs, show progressive weakness and spasticity. Seizures are common. Prominent skull veins are evident and a sound similar to that made by a cracked pot is noted on percussion. There is wasting of trunk and limb muscles, with spasticity, increased tendon reflexes, and Babinski signs. With progression, the child is unable to lift the enlarged head. Visual loss is followed by optic atrophy. Scalp necrosis may lead to CSF leakage, infection, and death.

In otitic hydrocephalus the child may be febrile and listless. Eardrum perforation and purulent otic discharge usually occur. Ipsilateral sixth nerve paralysis and papilledema are often noted.

In adults, symptoms include headache, lethargy, malaise, incoordination, and weakness. Seizures are uncommon. Findings may include dementia, altered consciousness, ocular nerve palsies, papilledema, ataxia, or corticospinal tract signs. Ventricular enlargement is not usually a uniform process and frequently occurs at the expense of periventricular white matter, but with relative preservation of gray matter. Therefore, significant degrees of hydrocephalus may remain occult. Severe hydrocephalus, uncomplicated by brain tumor or other etiologic factors, may be noted by CT in adults with preserved mental alertness and neurologic findings that suggest only pyramidal tract or cerebellar dysfunction.

NPH is characterized by insidious onset and gradual development for weeks or months of the triad of dementia, ataxia of gait, and urinary incontinence (Fig. 40–11). Headache and signs of increased intracranial pressure do not occur. Symptoms may begin weeks after head trauma or subarachnoid hemorrhage. In advanced disease, there may be frontal release signs, hyperactive and pathologic reflexes, and spasticity.

Laboratory Data. In infants, hydrocephalus must be distinguished from other forms

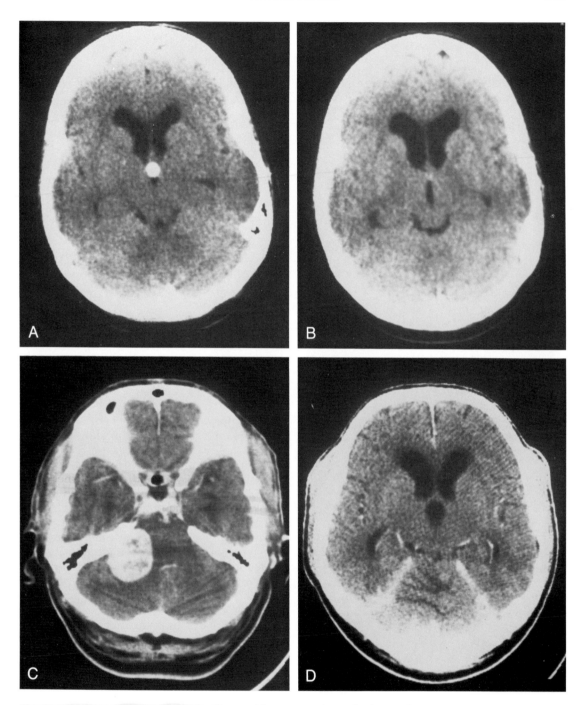

Fig. 40–8. Noncontrast CT scans of a 53-year-old woman with a colloid cyst of the 3rd ventricle (A) and lateral ventricular dilation (B). Contrast-enhanced CT scan of a 65-year-old man showing acoustic neurinoma with mass effect on the 4th ventricle (C) resulting in enlargement of the 3rd and lateral ventricles (D).

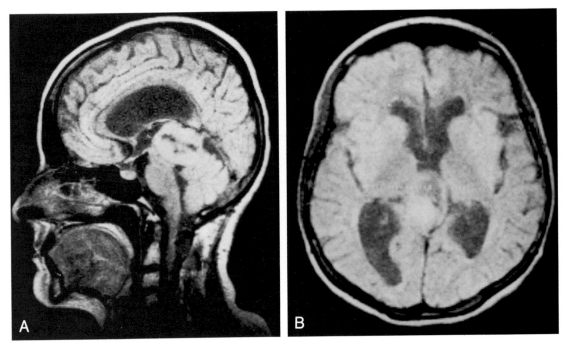

Fig. 40–9. *A.* Midsagittal T-1 weighted MRI of a 42-year-old woman demonstrated a pinealoma causing lateral ventricular dilation with a normal 4th ventricle. *B.* T$_1$ axial image demonstrated the pineal region tumor and dilation of the proximal 3rd and lateral ventricles.

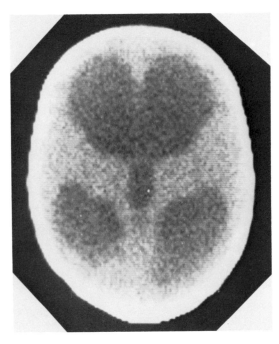

Fig. 40–10. Noncontrast CT scan. Communicating hydrocephalus in a 7-month-old child whose 4th ventricle was also prominent. (Courtesy of Dr. C.P. Shah)

of macrocephaly, such as subdural hematoma. Skull transillumination should be performed. Plain skull radiographs and skull measurements are useful to follow the course. Nonetheless, CT and MRI are the best diagnostic tools for all forms of hydrocephalus and have replaced pneumoencephalography.

Lumbar puncture is sometimes indicated to measure CSF pressure and to determine the presence of blood or signs of inflammatory or infectious disease. Continuous monitoring of intraventricular pressure may differentiate arrested from progressive disease in patients in whom lumbar sac CSF pressure is normal or in whom the CSF pressure may not accurately reflect intraventricular pressure. Likewise, CSF pulse-wave analysis may be more reliable than CSF pressure alone in diagnosis of hydrocephalus. Ultrasonography is useful in evaluating subependymal and intraventricular hemorrhage in high-risk premature infants and in following these infants for the development of progressive hydrocephalus. Results correlate well with CT. As a bedside procedure, ultrasound requires minimal manipulation of critically ill infants.

In adult-onset NPH, some clinicians believe that the best results are achieved in patients who have the typical clinical triad or who improve when 30 to 50 ml of CSF are removed

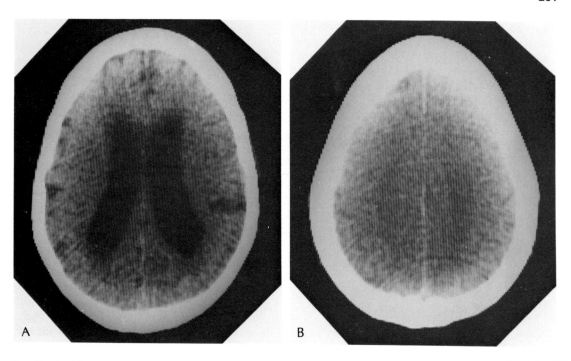

Fig. 40–11. Noncontrast CT scans. Ventricular dilatation with obliteration of cortical gyri consistent with NPH is noted in a 72-year-old man whose dementia, urinary incontinence, and ataxia improved after CSF shunting.

by lumbar puncture. Several diagnostic procedures help to predict shunt responsiveness in NPH. CT and MRI are best because they determine whether there is diffuse cortical atrophy, obliteration of the transcortical subarachnoid space, and transependymal CSF migration. Other tests help to assess whether there is a delay in normal transcortical CSF clearance and whether there is reflux of CSF from the subarachnoid space to the lateral ventricles, reversing the normal flow. Delay of CSF clearance and intraventricular transependymal penetration often, but not always, predict shunt responsiveness. These tests include: CSF compartment infusion or perfusion tests, and lumbar isotope cisternography; however, none of these tests is absolutely reliable. Cerebral angiography is occasionally indicated in diagnostic problems of hydrocephalus due to intracranial mass lesions. Visual, auditory, and brain-stem-evoked potentials, EEG, and psychometric analysis may provide auxiliary diagnostic and prognostic data and aid in following patients after shunts.

Prognosis and Treatment. Prognosis is sometimes related to an underlying disease (such as cerebral neoplasms), and treatment of hydrocephalus is palliative if it is given. In other cases, there may be spontaneous arrest,

as in benign communicating hydrocephalus of infants. In untreated progressive infantile hydrocephalus, the mortality rate is 50% at 1 year of age, and 75% at 10 years of age. After intracranial hemorrhage of high-risk premature infants, the outcome in hydrocephalus is usually related to factors (e.g., asphyxia) other than shunt responsiveness.

Pharmacologic therapy is of limited value; there have been a few favorable reports of acetazolamide, furosemide, and isosorbide use, with or without repeated lumbar punctures. The major therapeutic approach is surgical, including choroid plexectomy for papilloma. Numerous CSF shunting procedures have been advocated to effect CSF removal from one portion of the craniospinal space to another (ventriculocisternal shunting) or from the craniospinal space to an extracranial reservoir (ventriculopleural shunt). Results vary with the procedures used, operative techniques, patient status, cause and duration of hydrocephalus, and incidence of complications such as infection, subdural hematoma, shunt failure, or seizures.

Ventricular enlargement begins immediately and is grossly evident within three hours of experimental obstruction of the fourth ventricle in monkeys. After three weeks damage is irreversible. If these experimental results apply to humans, early intervention is indicated. Even when management of progressive infantile hydrocephalus is optimal, the survival rate is 50% after 15 years of age with 15% incidence of mental retardation. In NPH, the success rate is best in patients with recent progression of mild dementia, gait disorder, and urinary incontinence. Under those circumstances, 60% of the patients may improve, but a complication rate of 35% is not uncommon.

References

Bradley WE Jr. "Hydrocephalus and Atrophy" in Magnetic Resonance Imaging (Stark D, Bradley WG Jr. eds). St. Louis: CV Mosby, 1988.

Borgesen SE, Gjerris F. Relationship between intracranial pressure, ventricular size and resistance to CSF outflow. J Neurosurg 1987; 67:535–537.

Callen PW, Hashimoto BE, Newton TH. Sonographic evaluation of cerebral cortical mantal thickness in the fetus and neonate with hydrocephalus. J Ultrasound Med 1986; 5:251–255.

Chervenak FA, Berkowitz RL, Tortora M, Hobbins JC. The management of fetal hydrocephalus. Am J Obstet Gynecol 1985; 151:933–942.

El Gammal T, Allen MD Jr, Brooks BS, Mark EK. MRI evaluation of hydrocephalus. AJR 1987; 149:807–813.

Fishman RA. Cerebrospinal Fluid in Diseases of the Nervous System. Philadelphia: WB Saunders Co, 1980.

Gradin WC, Taylon C, Fruin AH. Choroid plexus papilloma of the third ventricle: case report and review of the literature. Neurosurgery 1983; 12:217–220.

Hakim S, Adams RD. The special clinical problem of symptomatic hydrocephalus with normal cerebrospinal fluid pressure. J Neurol Sci 1965; 2:307–327.

Hochwald GM. Animal models of hydrocephalus: recent developments. Proc Soc Exp Biol Med 1985; 178:1–11.

Jack CR, Jr, Mokri B, Laws ER, Jr, Houser OW, Baker HL, Jr, Petersen RC. MR findings in normal-pressure hydrocephalus: Significance and comparison with other forms of dementia. J Comput Assist Tomogr 1987; 2:923–931.

Jansen J, Jorgensen M. Prognostic significance of signs and symptoms in hydrocephalus. Analysis of survival. Acta Neurol Scand 1986; 73:55–65.

McLone DG, Naidich TP. The investigation of hydrocephalus by computed tomography. Clin Neurosurg 1985; 32:527–539.

Miller JD. ICP Monitoring—Current status and future directions. Acta Neurochir 1987; 85:80–86.

Shapiro K, Marmarou A, Portnoy H. Hydrocephalus. New York: Raven Press, 1984.

Skinner S, Gammon K, Bergman E, Epstein M, Freeman J. Management of hydrocephalus in infancy: use of acetazolamide and furosemide to avoid cerebrospinal fluid shunts. J Pediatr 1985; 107:31–37.

Spanu G, Karussos G, Adinolfi D, Bonfanti N. An analysis of cerebrospinal fluid shunt infection in adults. A clinical experience of twelve years. Acta Neurochir 1986; 80:79–82.

Thomsen AM, Borgesen SE, Bruhn P, Gjerris F. Prognosis of dementia in normal-pressure hydrocephalus after a shunt operation. Ann Neurol 1986; 20:304–310.

Th J, Tang J, Poorvlict DCJ. Reduction of ventricular size

after shunting for normal pressure hydrocephalus related to CSF dynamics before shunting. J Neurol Neurosurg Psychiatry 1988; 51:521–525.

Wikkelso C, Anderson H, Blomstrand C, Lindqvist G, Svendsen P. Normal pressure hydrocephalus; predictive value of the cerebrospinal fluid tap-test. Acta Neurol Scand 1986; 73:566–573.

41. BRAIN EDEMA AND DISORDERS OF INTRACRANIAL PRESSURE

Robert A. Fishman

Brain Edema

Brain edema accompanies a wide variety of pathologic processes and contributes to the morbidity and mortality of many neurologic diseases. It plays a major role in head injury, stroke, and brain tumor, as well as in cerebral infections, including brain abscess, encephalitis and meningitis, lead encephalopathy, hypoxia, hypo-osmolality, the disequilibrium syndromes associated with dialysis and diabetic ketoacidosis, Reye syndrome, and the various forms of obstructive hydrocephalus. Brain edema occurs in several different forms; clearly it is not a single pathologic or clinical entity.

Brain edema is defined best as an increase in brain volume due to an increase in water and sodium content. Brain edema, when well localized or mild in degree, is associated with little or no clinical evidence of brain dysfunction; however, when it is severe it causes focal or generalized signs of brain dysfunction, including various forms of brain herniation and medullary failure of respiration and circulation. The major forms of herniation are uncal, cerebellar tonsillar, upward cerebellar, cingulate, and transcalvarial herniation.

Brain edema and brain engorgement are different processes. *Brain engorgement* is an increase in the blood volume of the brain caused by obstruction of the cerebral veins and venous sinuses, or by arterial vasodilatation such as that caused by hypercapnia. Brain engorgement may result in a major increase in brain volume during craniotomy because of the absence of the rigid restriction of the bone skull; such vasodilatation may coexist with brain edema. Intracranial hypertension and brain edema commonly occur together. Focal or generalized brain edema results in intracranial hypertension when severe enough to exceed the compensatory mechanisms for the modulation of the intracranial pressure.

Brain edema has been classified into three

major categories: vasogenic, cellular (cytotoxic), and interstitial (hydrocephalic). The features of the three forms of cerebral edema are summarized in terms of pathogenesis, location and composition of the edema fluid, and changes in capillary permeability in Table 41–1.

VASOGENIC EDEMA

Vasogenic edema is characterized by increased permeability of brain capillary endothelial cells to macromolecules, such as the plasma proteins and various other molecules, whose entry is limited by the capillary endothelial cells. The increase in permeability is visualized when contrast enhancement is observed with CT. Increased CSF protein levels are also indicative of increased endothelial permeability. MRI is more sensitive than CT in demonstrating the increased brain water

and increased extracellular volume that characterize vasogenic edema.

Vasogenic edema is characteristic of clinical disorders in which there is frequently a positive contrast-enhanced CT or increased signal intensity with MRI, including brain tumor, abscess, hemorrhage, infarction, and contusion. It also occurs with lead encephalopathy or purulent meningitis. The functional manifestations of vasogenic edema include focal neurologic deficits, focal EEG slowing, disturbances of consciousness, and severe intracranial hypertension. In patients with brain tumor, whether primary or metastatic, the clinical signs are often caused more by the surrounding edema than by the tumor mass itself.

CELLULAR (CYTOTOXIC) EDEMA

Cellular edema is characterized by swelling of all the cellular elements of the brain (neu-

Table 41–1. Classification of Brain Edema

	Vasogenic	Cytotoxic	Interstitial (Hydrocephalic)
Pathogenesis	Increased capillary permeability	Cellular swelling (glial, neuronal, endothelial)	Increased brain fluid due to block of CSF absorption
Location of edema	Chiefly white matter	Gray and white matter	Chiefly periventricular white matter in hydrocephalus
Edema fluid composition	Plasma filtrate including plasma proteins	Increased intracellular water and sodium	CSF
Extracellular fluid volume	Increased	Decreased	Increased
Capillary permeability to large molecules (RISA, inulin)	Increased	Normal	Normal
Clinical Disorders Syndromes	Brain tumor, abscess, infarction, trauma, hemorrhage, lead encephalopathy Ischemia Purulent meningitis (granulocytic edema)	Hypoxia, hypo-osmolality (e.g., water intoxication). Disequilibrium syndromes Ischemia Purulent meningitis (granulocytic edema) Reye's syndrome	Obstructive hydrocephalus, pseudotumor (benign intracranial hypertension) Purulent meningitis (granulocytic edema)
EEG changes	Focal slowing common	Generalized slowing	EEG often normal
Therapeutic Effects Steroids	Beneficial in brain tumor, abscess	Not effective (? Reye's syndrome)	Uncertain effectiveness (? pseudotumor, ? meningitis)
Osmotherapy	Reduces volume of normal brain tissue only, *acutely*	Reduces brain volume *acutely* in hypo-osmolality	Rarely useful
Acetazolamide	? Effect	No effect	Minor usefulness
Furosemide	? Effect	No effect	Minor usefulness

(Adapted from Fishman RA. Cerebrospinal Fluid in Diseases of the Nervous System. Philadelphia: WB Saunders Co., 1980.)

rons, glia, and endothelial cells), with a concomitant reduction in the volume of the extracellular fluid space of the brain. Capillary permeability is not usually affected in the various cellular edemas; patients so affected have a normal CSF protein and isotopic brain scan. CT does not reveal enhancement with contrast, and MRI is normal.

There are several causes of cellular edema: *hypoxia, acute hypo-osmolality of the plasma,* and *osmotic disequilibrium* syndromes. Hypoxia after cardiac arrest or asphyxia results in cerebral energy depletion. The cellular swelling is osmotically determined by the appearance of increased intracellular osmoles (especially sodium, lactate, and hydrogen ions) that induce the rapid entry of water into cells. Acute hypo-osmolality of the plasma and extracellular fluid is caused by acute dilutional hyponatremia, inappropriate secretion of antidiuretic hormone, or acute sodium depletion. The brain adapts to hyponatremia by losing intracellular osmoles, chiefly potassium, thereby preserving cellular volume. Osmotic disequilibrium syndromes occur with hemodialysis or diabetic ketoacidosis, in which excessive brain intracellular solutes result in excessive cellular hydration when the plasma osmolality is rapidly reduced with therapy. The precise composition of the osmotically active intracellular solutes responsible for cellular swelling in the disequilibrium syndromes that are associated with hemodialysis and diabetic ketoacidosis is not known.

In uremia, the intracellular solutes presumably include a number of organic acids, which have been recovered in the dialysis bath. In diabetic ketoacidosis, the intracellular solutes include glucose and ketone bodies; however, there are also unidentified, osmotically active, intracellular solutes, termed *idiogenic osmoles,* that favor cellular swelling. Increased intracellular osmolality in excess of the plasma level not only causes cellular swelling but also is responsible for complex changes in brain metabolism affecting the concentrations of the neurotransmitter amino acids, ammonia, and other metabolites, which in turn have profound effects on brain function.

Major changes in cerebral function occur with the cellular edemas, including stupor, coma, EEG changes and asterixis, myoclonus, and focal or generalized seizures. The encephalopathy is often severe with acute hypo-osmolality but, in more chronic states of hypo-osmolality of the same severity, neurologic function may be spared. Acute hy-

poxia causes cellular edema, which is followed by vasogenic edema as infarction develops. Vasogenic edema increases progressively for several days after an acute arterial occlusion. The delay in obtaining contrast enhancement with CT following an ischemic stroke illustrates the passage of time that is needed for defects in endothelial cell function to develop and mature.

ISCHEMIC BRAIN EDEMA

Most patients with arterial occlusion have a combination of first cellular and then vasogenic edema, together termed *ischemic brain edema.* The cellular phase takes place after acute ischemia over minutes to hours and may be reversible. The vasogenic phase takes place over hours to days and results in infarction, a largely irreversible process, although the increased endothelial cell permeability usually reverts to normal within weeks. The factors that determine the reversibility of ischemic edema at the cellular level are poorly understood.

BRAIN EDEMA IN REYE SYNDROME

Reye syndrome, a neurologic disorder of children, is characterized by fulminant hepatic failure, a rapidly progressive encephalopathy, and severe intracranial hypertension, with brain edema as a major and often fatal complication. The brain has features of cellular edema and the CSF protein is characteristically normal. There are electron microscope findings of astrocytic swelling and intralamellar blebs in the myelin.

INTERSTITIAL (HYDROCEPHALIC) EDEMA

Interstitial edema is the third type of edema, best characterized in obstructive hydrocephalus, in which the water and sodium content of the periventricular white matter is increased because of the movement of CSF across the ventricular walls. Obstruction of the circulation of the CSF results in the transependymal movement of CSF and thereby an absolute increase in the volume of the extracellular fluid of the brain. This is observed in obstructive hydrocephalus with CT. Low-density changes are observed at the angles of the lateral ventricles. The chemical changes are those of edema, with one exception: the volume of periventricular white matter is rapidly reduced rather than increased. After successful shunting of CSF, interstitial edema is reduced and the thickness of the mantle is restored.

Functional manifestations of interstitial edema are usually relatively minor in chronic hydrocephalus unless the changes are advanced, when dementia and gait disorder become prominent. The EEG is often normal in interstitial edema. This finding indicates that the accumulation of CSF in the periventricular extracellular fluid space is much better tolerated than is the presence of plasma in the extracellular fluid space, as seen with vasogenic edema, which is characterized by focal neurologic signs and EEG slowing.

The pathophysiology of the syndromes associated with benign intracranial hypertension (pseudotumor cerebri) is discussed later.

GRANULOCYTIC BRAIN EDEMA

Severe brain edema occurs with brain abscess and purulent meningitis due to collections of pus, which are often sterile as a result of antibiotic treatment. Such edema, associated with membranous products of granulocytes (pus), has been termed *granulocytic brain edema*. The features of cellular and vasogenic edema occur concurrently in purulent meningitis, and in severe cases interstitial edema also develops, so that granulocytic brain edema may include the features of all three types of brain edema.

THERAPEUTIC CONSIDERATIONS

The therapy of brain edema depends on the cause. Appropriate and early treatment of intracranial infection is essential. Surgical therapy is directed toward alleviating the cause by excision or decompression of intracranial mass lesions, as well as by a variety of shunting procedures. A patent airway, maintenance of an adequate blood pressure, and the avoidance of hypoxia are fundamental requirements in the care of these patients.

The administration of appropriate parenteral fluids to meet the needs of the patient is also essential. Caution is necessary in the choice of isotonic parenteral fluids. Administration of salt-free fluids should be avoided. Intravenous infusion of a 5% glucose solution results in a significant increase in intracranial pressure, which may be avoided with use of normal saline or 5% glucose in saline. If the excessive administration of salt is to be avoided, the use of 2.5% or 5% glucose in half-normal saline is satisfactory. In patients with cerebral edema, serum hypo-osmolality has deleterious effects and should be avoided.

The pharmacologic treatment of brain edema is based on the use of glucocorticoids, osmotherapy, and drugs that reduce CSF formation. Hyperventilation, hypothermia, and barbiturate therapy have also been tested experimentally and in clinical practice.

Glucocorticoids. The rationale for the use of steroids is largely empirical. There is widespread conviction that glucocorticoids dramatically and rapidly (in hours) begin to reduce the focal and general signs of brain edema around tumors. The major mechanism suggested to explain their usefulness in vasogenic brain edema is a direct effect on endothelial cell function that restores normal permeability.

The biochemical basis of the changes in membrane integrity that underlie vasogenic and cellular edema is now under study. Attention has focused on the role of free radicals (i.e., superoxide ions, hydroxyl radicals, and singlet oxygen) and on the effects of polyunsaturated fatty acids, most notably arachidonic acid, in the peroxidation of membrane phospholipids. The ability of adrenal glucocorticoids to inhibit the release of arachidonic acid from cell membranes may explain their beneficial effects in vasogenic edema; however, steroids have not been shown to be therapeutically useful in the brain edema of hypoxia or ischemia. Cellular damage is more important than brain edema in these conditions.

Long-acting, high-potency glucocorticoids have been used most widely. The usual dosage of dexamethasone is a starting dose of 10 mg followed by 4 mg administered 4 times a day thereafter—a dose equivalent in potency to 400 mg of cortisol daily. These large doses are about 20 times the normal rate of human endogenous cortisol production. Even larger dosages are sometimes used. Insufficient data are available to establish a formal dose-response curve for steroids in the treatment of brain edema; dosage schedules remain empirical.

Although any of the usual complications of steroid therapy are to be expected, gastric hemorrhage is usually the most troublesome. Fortunately, convulsive seizures apparently have not been increased in frequency by high dosages of the glucocorticoids. The risks of increased wound infection and impaired wound healing appear to be outweighed by the therapeutic effects in most patients receiving short-term therapy.

Although published data indicate that dexamethasone has therapeutic value in the treatment of vasogenic edema associated with mass lesions, its effectiveness with acute cerebral infarction has not been established. The literature recommending its use in stroke has, in general, been poorly documented and is controversial. Steroids may be useful in the treatment of intracerebral hematoma with extensive vasogenic edema due to the mass effect of the clot. In head injury, steroid therapy has been used frequently. Although some effectiveness following trauma has been documented, reduction in morbidity and mortality attributable to steroids is not great.

There are no convincing data, clinical or experimental, that glucocorticoids have beneficial effects in the cellular edema associated with hypo-osmolality, asphyxia, or hypoxia in the absence of infarction with mass effects. There is little basis for recommending steroids in the treatment of the cerebral edema associated with cardiac arrest or asphyxia.

The use of steroids in the management of Reye syndrome is controversial. Steroid therapy benefits chiefly the vasogenic edemas and would not be expected to be useful in the management of Reye syndrome; however, there are no controlled data regarding this conclusion.

When intracranial hypertension and obstructive hydrocephalus occur because of inflammatory changes in the subarachnoid space or at the arachnoid villi, whether attributable to leukocytes or to blood, there is a reasonable rationale for the use of steroids. However, despite the frequent use of steroids in purulent or tuberculous meningitis, few data are available to document the effectiveness of steroids against the brain edema of the acute disease. There are conflicting reports about the efficacy of steroids in acute bacterial meningitis or tuberculous meningitis. The use of steroids has not been shown to affect the subsequent incidence of chronic sequelae such as obstructive hydrocephalus or seizures. Steroids appear useful in the management of other conditions characterized by an inflammatory CSF, such as chemical meningitis following intrathecal radioiodinated serum albumin (RISA), meningeal sarcoidosis, or cysticercosis.

Osmotherapy. Hypertonic solutions (including urea, mannitol, and glycerol) have been used to treat the intracranial hypertension associated with brain edema. The several solutes have been difficult to compare because a large variety of laboratory models, dosages, time intervals, and pathologic processes have been used.

A few principles seem certain. First, brain volume falls only as long as there is an osmotic gradient between blood and brain. Second, osmotic gradients obtained with hypertonic parenteral fluids are short-lived because each of the solutes reaches an equilibrium concentration in the brain after a delay of only a few hours. Third, the parts of the brain most likely to "shrink" are normal areas; thus, with focal vasogenic edema, the normal regions of the hemisphere shrink but edematous regions with increased capillary permeability do not. Fourth, a rebound in the severity of the edema may follow use of any hypertonic solution because the solute is not excluded from the edematous tissue; if tissue osmolality rises, the tissue water is increased. Finally, there is scant rationale for chronic use of hypertonic fluids, either orally or parenterally, because the brain adapts to sustained hyperosmolality with an increase in intracellular osmolality due to the solute and to idiogenic osmoles.

There is some uncertainty about the size of an increase in plasma osmolality that causes a therapeutically significant decrease in brain volume and intracranial pressure in humans. Acute increases as small as 10 mOsm/L may be therapeutically effective. It should be emphasized that accurate dose-response relationships in different clinical situations have not been well defined with any of the hypertonic agents.

Other Therapeutic Measures. Hyperventilation, hypothermia, and barbiturates have been used in the management of intracranial hypertension, but none is established and the extensive literature is not reviewed here. Acetazolamide and furosemide reduce CSF formation in animals but have limited usefulness in the management of interstitial edema.

Benign Intracranial Hypertension

Benign intracranial hypertension (BIH) describes a heterogeneous group of disorders that are characterized by increased intracranial pressure when intracranial mass lesions, obstructive hydrocephalus, intracranial infection, and hypertensive encephalopathy have been excluded. BIH is also termed *pseudotumor cerebri.* In the past the terms "serous meningitis" and "otitic hydrocephalus" were used. The term "benign" has also been used because spontaneous recovery is characteristic, but serious threats to vision make accurate diagnosis and therapeutic intervention a necessity.

The following is a list of a variety of pathologic conditions that are associated with BIH, although in most cases the pathogenesis of these syndromes is poorly understood:

1. Endocrine and metabolic disorders
   Obesity and menstrual irregularities
   Pregnancy and postpartum (without sinus thrombosis)
   Menarche
   Female sex hormones
   Addison disease
   Adrenal steroid withdrawal
   Hyperadrenalism
   Hypoparathyroidism
2. Intracranial venous-sinus thrombosis
   Mastoiditis and lateral sinus thrombosis
   After head trauma
   Pregnancy and postpartum
   Oral progestational drugs
   "Marantic" sinus thrombosis
   Cryofibrinogenemia
   Primary (idiopathic) sinus thrombosis
3. Drugs and toxins
   Vitamin A
   Tetracycline
   Nalidixic acid
   Chlordecone
   Amiodarone
   Lithium carbonate
4. Hematologic and connective tissue disorders
   Iron deficiency anemia
   Infectious mononucleosis
   Wiskott-Aldrich syndrome
   Lupus erythematosus
5. High CSF protein content
   Spinal cord tumors
   Polyneuritis
6. "Meningism" with systemic bacterial or viral infections
7. Empty-sella syndrome
8. Miscellaneous
   Sydenham chorea
   Familial syndromes
   Rapid growth in infancy
9. Idiopathic conditions

Symptomatic intracranial hypertension without localizing signs may simulate BIH. Such conditions include obstructive hydrocephalus, chronic meningitis (sarcoid, fungal, or neoplastic), hypertensive encephalopathy, pulmonary encephalopathy due to paralytic hypoventilation, obstructive pulmonary disease, or pickwickian syndrome (morbid obesity). High-altitude cerebral edema is an unusual manifestation of hypoxia.

Clinical Manifestations. The presenting symptoms are headache and impaired vision. The headache may be worse on awakening and aggravated by coughing and straining. It is often mild or may be entirely absent. The most common ocular complaint is visual blurring, a manifestation of papilledema. Some patients complain of brief, fleeting movements of dimming or complete loss of vision, occurring many times during the day (amaurosis fugax), at times accentuated or precipitated by coughing and straining. This ominous symptom indicates that vision is in jeopardy. Visual loss may be minimal despite severe chronic papilledema, including retinal hemorrhages; however, blindness may occasionally develop rapidly (i.e., in less than 24 hours). Visual fields characteristically show enlargement of the blind spots, and may show constriction of the peripheral fields and central or paracentral scotoma. Diplopia caused by unilateral or bilateral sixth-nerve palsy may develop as a result of increased intracranial pressure. The neurologic examination is otherwise normal. A major clinical point is that patients with BIH usually look well; their apparent well-being belies the ominous appearance of the papilledema. Although the disorder most often lasts for months, it may persist for years without serious sequelae. Remissions may be followed by one or more recurrences in 5 to 10% of cases. In some patients, BIH may be responsible for development of the *empty-sella syndrome,* in which radiographic enlargement of the sella turcica simulates a pituitary tumor. CT reveals that the enlarged sella is filled with CSF due to a defect of its diaphragm.

Pathophysiology. Several mechanisms have been considered as possible explanations for the pathophysiology of BIH. These include: an increased rate of CSF formation, a sustained increase in intracranial venous pressure, a decreased rate of CSF absorption by arachnoid villi apart from venous occlusive disease, and an increase in brain volume due to an increase in blood volume or extravascular-fluid volume, simulating a form of brain edema.

No data are available regarding the rate of CSF formation in BIH because the only reliable method for measurement (ventriculocisternal perfusion) is not applicable to these patients. The only condition in which increased CSF formation has been demonstrated is choroid plexus papilloma. Increased CSF production might explain the pathophysiology in some of the diverse conditions associated with BIH, but this mechanism remains unproved. A sustained increase in intracranial venous pressure associated with decreased CSF absorption readily explains the pathophysiology of BIH associated with venous-sinus thrombosis. Increased venous-sinus pressures are readily transmitted to the CSF and would also interfere with CSF absorption. Decreased CSF absorption (in the absence of venous occlusion) due to altered function of the arachnoid villi would explain the occurrence of BIH in some cases; this reasonable hypothesis is also unproved. The fact that BIH is associated with normal or small ventricles rather than hydrocephalus is consonant with such a mechanism. Abnormal spinal infusion tests do not differentiate between impairment of CSF absorption and decreased intracranial compliance. The occurrence of BIH in patients with polyneuritis or spinal cord tumors appears to support the hypothesis that defective CSF absorption may be the basis for the syndrome. This is not directly correlated with the degree of CSF-protein elevation; it is presumed to depend upon an alteration of the function of the arachnoid villi.

The hypothesis that BIH might be due to an increase in brain volume (a special form of brain edema) secondary to an increase in blood or extracellular fluid volume is supported by the presence of small ventricles. An increase in brain volume would be expected if the extracellular space of the brain were expanded; this might occur if there were an excessive amount of CSF in the brain due to either increased formation or decreased absorption.

Any theory of the pathogenesis of BIH must be consonant with the rapid therapeutic response of BIH to shunting of CSF by a lumbar-peritoneal shunt. Impaired CSF absorption or increased CSF formation would explain the occurrence of BIH in most cases; however, the limited data available do not allow any firm conclusions.

ENDOCRINE AND METABOLIC DISORDERS

BIH is most commonly seen in healthy women with a history of menstrual dysfunction. The women are frequently moderately or markedly overweight (without evidence of alveolar hypoventilation). Menstrual irregularity or amenorrhea is common. Galactorrhea is an unusual associated symptom. The histories often emphasize excessive premenstrual weight gain. Endocrine studies have not revealed specific abnormalities of urinary gonadotropins or estrogens, and the pathogenesis is unknown. BIH has a complex relationship to adrenal hormones. Rarely is BIH a complication of Addison disease or Cushing disease. Improvement occurs after restoration of a normal adrenal state; the mechanism in either circumstance is unknown.

BIH has also occurred in patients treated with adrenal corticosteroids for prolonged periods. Many of the patients had allergic skin disorders or asthma during childhood; BIH generally occurred when the steroid dosage was reduced, but evidence of hyperadrenalism persisted. Hypoparathyroidism may also present with increased intracranial pressure; hypocalcemic seizures or cerebral calcifications may further complicate the clinical picture. BIH has been reported in women taking oral progestational drugs when angiography has excluded sinus thrombosis.

INTRACRANIAL VENOUS-SINUS THROMBOSIS

Intracranial hypertension occurs secondary to occlusion of the intracranial venous sinuses as a consequence of acute or chronic otitis media with extension of the infection into the petrous bone and lateral sinus. The sixth cranial nerve may also be involved, giving rise to diplopia on lateral gaze. Thrombosis of the superior longitudinal sinus may occur after mild closed head injury, giving rise to BIH. (Occlusion of this sinus, which drains both cerebral hemispheres, is more likely to result in hemorrhagic infarction of the cerebrum as the thrombosis extends into the cerebral veins, giving rise to bilateral signs. In such cases, the course is frequently fulminant and the prognosis guarded, although occasionally complete recovery may occur.) Aseptic or primary thrombosis of the superior longitudinal sinus may also be responsible for a pseudotumor syndrome, especially as a complication of pregnancy; it has been reported in the first two to three weeks postpartum as well as at the end of the first trimester of pregnancy. Sinus thrombosis has been reported with the use of oral progestational drugs. A disorder of blood clotting is suggested as the basis for these events, although this has not been substantiated. Sinus thrombosis occurs as a complication of dehydration and cachexia ("marantic" thrombosis), and in association with cryofibrinogenemia.

DRUGS AND TOXINS

BIH has been reported in otherwise healthy adolescents taking huge doses of vitamin A for the treatment of acne. Oral doses as low as 25,000 units daily may cause headache and papilledema with rapid improvement after cessation of the therapy. The syndrome is said to have occurred in Arctic explorers who consumed polar-bear liver, a great source of vitamin A. Some cases of BIH, manifested by bulging fontanelle and papilledema, have been reported in children given tetracycline or nalidixic acid. The mechanisms involved are obscure. Spontaneous, rapid recovery occurs when the drugs are stopped. Chlordecone (an insecticide) intoxication has also been reported to cause BIH, as well as amiodarone and lithium carbonate.

HEMATOLOGIC AND CONNECTIVE TISSUE DISORDERS

Papilledema and increased intracranial pressure have been attributed to severe iron deficiency anemia, with striking improvement after treatment of the anemia. The mechanism presumably reflects in part the marked increase in cerebral blood flow that accompanies profound anemia. BIH has been reported with infectious mononucleosis and the Wiskott-Aldrich syndrome, but the mechanism is not known. BIH has also been observed as the major manifestation of systemic lupus erythematosus.

PULMONARY ENCEPHALOPATHY

BIH can be a major complication of chronic hypoxic hypercapnia caused by paralytic states such as muscular dystrophy and cervical myelopathy, as well as of obstructive pulmonary disease and the pickwickian syndrome. There is a chronic increase of cerebral blood flow because of the anoxemia and carbon dioxide retention. These patients usually appear mentally dull and encephalopathic, and thus differ from most patients with BIH.

SPINAL CORD DISEASES

BIH occurs rarely with tumors of the spinal cord or cauda equina, or with polyneuritis. Papilledema and headache disappear with treatment of the spinal lesion or regression of the polyneuropathy. The mechanism may involve the effects of an elevated CSF protein on CSF absorption at the arachnoid villi in both cranial and spinal subarachnoid spaces. However, occurrence of this syndrome does not correlate with the degree of protein elevation.

Meningism is an old term that is applied to patients with stiff neck, increased intracranial pressure (usually 200 to 300 mm), but an otherwise normal CSF. This syndrome occurs in patients with acute systemic viral infections such as influenza. The mechanism of the intracranial hypertension is unknown.

One of the more common forms of BIH appears in otherwise healthy subjects in the absence of any of the aforementioned etiologic factors. Both sexes are affected and the occurrence is most often between the ages of 10 and 50 years. This is the idiopathic form of BIH; its pathogenesis is a mystery. There have been rare case reports of BIH with roseola infantum and Sydenham chorea.

Diagnosis. The patient with headache and papilledema without other neurologic signs must be considered to have symptomatic intracranial hypertension due to intracranial mass, ventricular obstruction, or intracranial infection until proved otherwise. This is true in about 35% of these cases. Although the diagnosis of BIH may be suspected by the appearance of apparent well-being and by the history of some of the associated etiologic features listed previously, the diagnosis is essentially one of exclusion and is dependent upon ruling out the more common causes of increased intracranial pressure. Brain tumor, particularly when located in relatively silent areas such as the frontal lobes or right temporal lobe, or when obstructing the ventricular system, may be manifested only by headache and papilledema. Patients with chronic subdural hematoma, without history of significant trauma, may have the same symptoms.

Diagnostic evaluation depends upon CT, which has negated the need for angiography in most cases. Lumbar puncture should be deferred until CT indicates that the ventricular system is normal in size and location. Diagnostic lumbar puncture is mandatory to establish the diagnosis of BIH. In obesity, the normal upper limit of CSF pressure is 250 mm. In BIH, the CSF pressure is elevated, usually between 250 and 600 mm, but the fluid is otherwise normal. The protein content is often in the lower range of normal, and lumbar CSF protein levels of 10 to 20 mg/dl are common. A CSF protein content greater than 50 mg/dl, decreased CSF glucose, or increased cell count throw doubt on the diagnosis of idiopathic BIH and are indications of another disease. The EEG is normal in BIH.

Pseudopapilledema may be a source of diagnostic confusion. In this developmental anomaly of the fundus, the ophthalmologic appearance may be indistinguishable from true papilledema; there is elevation of the optic disc, although exudates and hemorrhages are absent. Visual acuity is normal but visual fields may show enlargement of the blind spots. The unchanging appearance of the fundus in subsequent examinations favors the diagnosis of pseudopapilledema, as does the finding of normal CSF pressure on lumbar puncture. Optic neuritis is differentiated from BIH by visual loss and normal CSF pressure.

Treatment. The idiopathic form of BIH and its occurrence in patients with menstrual disorders and obesity require individualized management. This syndrome is self-limited in most cases and, after some weeks or months, spontaneous remissions occur, making evaluation of therapy difficult. Recurrent episodes have been noted in about 5 to 10% of patients, and the illness seldom lasts for years. In the very obese, weight reduction is recommended. The use of daily lumbar punctures has been advocated to lower CSF pressure to normal levels by removing sufficient fluid; 15 to 30 ml of fluid may be removed, but the value of this procedure is dubious. A CSF shunting procedure, such as a lumbar-peritoneal shunt, is the procedure of choice in patients with intractable headache and particularly in those with progressive visual impairment. It may dramatically relieve symptoms. Optic nerve decompression has its advocates to preserve vision, but it does not treat increased intracranial pressure. The use of dexamethasone has been advocated empirically because it minimizes cerebral edema of diverse causes and it seems effective in some patients. However, use of steroids should be avoided unless acetazolamide and furosemide fail because hyperadrenocorticism may precipitate BIH. Acetazolamide has been used because this carbonic anhydrase inhibitor reduces CSF formation. Furosemide also reduces CSF formation in animals and may be useful. Hypertonic intravenous solutions (25% mannitol) to lower intracranial pressure can be used in acute situations when there is rapidly failing vision and neurosurgical intervention is awaited; however, prolonged dehydration therapy is deleterious. The use of oral glycerol has the disadvantage of high caloric intake for obese patients. Sub-

temporal decompression was widely used in the past, but its efficacy has been questioned. This procedure may be necessary for patients with serious threat to vision when drug therapy and lumbar peritoneal shunts have failed.

In patients with lateral sinus thrombosis caused by chronic infection in the petrous bone, surgical decompression is often indicated. When the pseudotumor syndrome is a manifestation of hypoadrenalism or hypoparathyroidism, replacement therapy is indicated. Vitamin A intoxication disappears when administration of the vitamin is stopped. Anticoagulation therapy has been recommended for patients with dural-sinus thrombosis; however, for patients with extension of the clot into cerebral veins and infarction of tissue, anticoaglation is hazardous because it increases the likelihood of hemorrhagic infarction.

Intracranial Hypotension

The normal lumbar CSF pressure is 70 to 200 mm H_2O (or 5 to 15 mm Hg). Symptoms of intracranial hypotension may occur with pressures between 50 and 90 mm H_2O or lower. The CSF pressure is usually not measurable, and the fluid can be obtained only by aspiration with a syringe. The symptoms of intracranial hypotension include severe headaches precipitated by the erect position and relieved by the horizontal position. It is aggravated by cough or strain. There may also be nausea, vomiting, and dizziness precipitated by similar postural changes. A unilateral or bilateral sixth nerve palsy may accompany low-pressure syndromes.

The most common cause is previous lumbar puncture with persistent CSF leakage into the subdural or epidural spaces. Low-pressure syndromes also occur with CSF rhinorrhea, which may be spontaneus or post-traumatic, or may arise because of a pituitary tumor. Bacterial meningitis may complicate such cases. Traumatic avulsion of spinal roots may also result in a CSF leak. Spinal arachnoid cysts may also be associated with such leaks. Severe dehydration results in intracranial hypotension, as exemplified by the sunken fontanelle observed in dehydrated infants. An erroneously low CSF pressure may be recorded in the presence of spinal block or when it is technically difficult to place the needle in the subarachnoid space. A rare syndrome of idiopathic CSF hypotension has been observed as a benign self-limited disorder.

Symptomatic intracranial hypotension after lumbar puncture usually responds to bed rest with the head flat. The common practice of forcing fluids or parenteral hydration has not been shown to have advantages over bed rest alone. Injection of 10 to 20 ml of the patient's own blood into the epidural space (a "blood patch") is a highly effective treatment when simple bed rest fails. Multiple blood patches are occasionally needed. Surgical closure of a persistent dural hole in the lumbar region is seldom necessary. Location of the dural hole may be visualized by combined injection of metrizamide using CT and of radiolabelled albumin using a scintillation camera. (A cervical injection is preferred because it avoids passage of contrast material into the lumbar extradural region due to a lumbar puncture.) The patient is placed in a sitting or erect position for an hour to allow diffusion of the contrast agent to the lumbar region. Metrizamide may successfully identify the site of the leak when the isotopic scan fails, or vice versa.

References

Brain Edema

Cervos-Navarro J, Ferszt R, eds. Brain edema: pathology, diagnosis and therapy. Adv Neurol 1980; 28:1–501.

Fishman RA. Brain edema. In: Cerebrospinal Fluid in Diseases of the Nervous System. Philadelphia: WB Saunders Co., 1980:107–28.

Fishman RA. Steroids in the treatment of brain edema. N Engl J Med 1982; 302:352–360.

Hamilton AJ, Cymmerman A, Black PMcl. High altitude cerebral edema. Neurosurgery 1986; 19:841–849.

Inaba Y, Klatzo I, Spatz M. Brain Edema. Berlin: Springer-Verlag, 1985:1–682.

James HE, Langfitt TW, Kumar VS, et al. Treatment of intracranial hypertension: analysis of 105 consecutive recordings of intracranial pressure. Acta Neurochir 1977; 36:189–200.

Benign Intracranial Hypertension

Britton C, Boshill C, Brust JCM, et al. Pseudotumor cerebri, empty sella syndrome, and adrenal adenoma. Neurology 1980; 30:292–296.

Corbett JJ. Problems in the diagnosis and treatment of pseudotumor cerebri. Can J Neurol Sci 1983; 10:221–229.

Duncan FJ, Corbett JJ, Wall M. The incidence of pseudotumor cerebri. Arch Neurol 1988; 45:875–877.

Fishman RA. Benign intracranial hypertension. In: Cerebrospinal Fluid in Diseases of the Nervous System. Philadelphia: WB Saunders, 1980: 128–139.

Johnston I, Paterson A, Besser M. The treatment of benign intracranial hypertension: a review of 134 cases. Surg Neurol 1981; 16:3, 218–224.

Knight RSG, Fielder AR, Firth JL. Benign intracranial hypertension: visual loss and optic nerve sheath fenestration. J Neurol Neurosurg Psychiatry 1986; 49:243–250.

Ridsdale L, Moseley I. Thoracolumbar intraspinal tumors presenting features of raised intracranial pressure. J Neurol Neurosurg Psychiatry 1978; 41:737–745.

Saul RF, Hamburger HA, Selhorst JB. Pseudotumor cerebri secondary to lithium carbonate. JAMA 1985; 253:2869–2870.

Wall M, George M. Visual loss in pseudotumor cerebri. Arch Neurol 1987; 44:170–179.

Intracranial Hypotension

Abouleish E, de la Vega S, Blendinger, et al. Long-term follow up of epidural blood patch. Anesth Analg 1975; 54:459–463.

Bell WE, Joynt RJ, Saks AL. Low spinal fluid pressure syndrome. Neurology 1960; 10:512–521.

Murros, K, Fogelholm R. Spontaneous intracranial hypotension with slit ventricles. J Neurol Neurosurg Psychiatry 1983; 46:1149–1151.

42. HYPEROSMOLAR HYPERGLYCEMIC NONKETOTIC DIABETIC COMA
Leon D. Prockop

Encephalopathy may be caused by hyperosmolarity. In general, these reactions may be classified as those due to hypernatremia and those seen with hyperglycemia.

In the hypernatremic states, the serum sodium level is elevated and total body sodium is also usually increased. In hyperglycemic states, usually seen with dehydration, serum sodium levels are in the normal range or slightly low and total body sodium is low.

The most common and serious of these conditions is a medical emergency, hyperosmolar hyperglycemic nonketotic (HHNK) diabetic coma. Another category of hyperosmolar hyperglycemic nonketotic coma is not associated with diabetes but follows burns, steroid and immunosuppressive therapy, or dialysis therapy. Some of these patients may have a type of the HHNK diabetic coma, so we will consider only the major category, HHNK diabetic coma.

HHNK diabetic coma may occur in patients with mild or occult diabetes without acidosis recognized preceding hyperglycemia. The earliest description was probably given by Dreschfeld in 1886. In 1923, soon after the discovery of insulin, a report to the British Medical Research Council on the first seven cases of diabetic coma referred to "three cases of coma in not very serious diabetics. The blood sugar was very high. Air hunger, and dyspnea were not conspicuous features; little acetone in the breath and not much acetoacetic acid in the urine." Modern awareness of the syndrome is generally ascribed to descriptions published in 1956 and 1957. By 1968 the focal neurologic symptoms and signs that include seizures and severe metabolic encephalopathy were well recognized. The serious nature of the disorder was documented in a 1970 report of 34 deaths in 84 patients.

The average age of patients with HHNK diabetic coma is 60 years with equal frequency in men and women. The syndrome is rarely seen in children or juvenile diabetics, although the age range is 1.5 to 87 years. Many patients have no previous history of diabetes mellitus. Of those known to be diabetic, most do not have insulin-dependent disease, and most had been easily controlled in the past, with no prior episodes of ketoacidosis. In many, the admitting diagnosis was "probable stroke."

In half of the reported cases, the onset of acute symptoms was traced to a specific condition such as infection, acute enteritis, surgery, pancreatitis, or ingestion of drugs that may complicate diabetic control, including thiazide diuretics, adrenocorticosteroids, or phenytoin. Other reported causes include Down syndrome, brain tumor, ingestion of a concentrated carbohydrate drink, or propranolol therapy.

In most patients there is insidious onset of polyuria, polydipsia, and polyphagia. Because there is no ketosis, the precoma phase is often much longer than typically seen in diabetic ketoacidosis. Half of the patients have had polyuria for a week or more. Even though intensely thirsty, the patient becomes dehydrated.

Upon admission to the hospital, almost all patients are clinically dehydrated and one third are febrile and in shock. Unlike diabetic ketoacidosis, respiration is not of the Kussmaul type and there is no characteristic odor to the breath. Seizures occur in 25% of patients. Other clinical features include hallucinations, myoclonic twitches, nystagmus, photophobia, pupillary reflex abnormalities, hyporeflexia, asymmetric caloric responses, and tonic deviation of the eyes. Focal signs include homonymous hemianopia, hemiparesis, hemisensory loss, unilateral hyperreflexia, and unilateral Babinski signs.

The diagnosis can be made in the laboratory. Delay in instituting therapy can be avoided by analyzing the blood of any comatose patient for glucose content. The hallmarks of laboratory diagnosis are: (1) extreme hyperglycemia, (2) 3+ or 4+ glycosuria without acetonuria, and (3) absence of ketoacidosis. The average blood glucose level in these patients is about 1,000 mg/dl. Although common, hyperosmolarity is not an absolute

requirement. Plasma osmolarity averages 353 mOsm/kg H_2O (normal is 289 to 301) with a range of 268 to 364.

Other laboratory abnormalities are those commonly seen in severe dehydration: hemoconcentration with increased blood levels of hemoglobin, hematocrit, and plasma proteins; leukocytosis; and azotemia out of proportion to the increase in creatinine concentration. The BUN:creatinine ratio is 30:1, compared to the usual 10:1. This disproportionate elevation in BUN is attributed to the prerenal azotemia due to depletion of extracellular fluid volume. Some patients develop parenchymal renal damage with acute polyuric renal failure. Several have required renal dialysis. Initial hyperkalemia is uncommon. Serum sodium concentrations in 70 of 84 patients in one series were 119 to 188, with an average value of 144 meq/L. This average value may be deceiving because the patients are also dehydrated and the total body sodium may be severely depressed.

The pathogenesis of HHNK diabetic coma has been discussed extensively in the literature. Three main factors seem to be involved: hyperglycemia, hyponatremia, and the effect of hyperglycemia on the polyol pathway. Hyperglycemia is undoubtedly the primary element in the pathophysiology. The other two may play contributory roles.

The treatment of HHNK diabetic coma has attracted considerable discussion, stimulated by the 40 to 80% mortality rate. There is controversy about the amount of insulin required and the type of fluid to be administered in attempts to achieve the goal of correcting the hyperglycemia and repairing the fluid loss. In general, the patients, usually in shock, first need rapid repair of the marked sodium depletion, and then a rapid but incomplete repair of water loss. In a third, more cautious phase, fluid volume and composition are slowly returned to normal. The first priority is to reestablish the intravascular volume to reduce the risk of heart attack, stroke, thrombophlebitis, and metabolic complications that might result from hypoperfusion. Although these patients need replacement of free water, isotonic saline solution should be given first through a large-bore needle (1 to 2 liters in the first three hours). Thereafter, hypotonic saline solution may be needed. Total fluid requirements vary considerably, but most survivors have received at least 5 liters in the first 12 hours of treatment. The maximal initial insulin dose should not exceed 50 units or 25 units/hour until the blood pressure is stable. Commonly, 10 units of insulin are given initially and then as a continuous infusion at a rate of 5 to 10 units/hour until the blood sugar is stable between 250 and 300 mg/dl. Then, glucose is added to the infusion. Attention must be paid to serum potassium and to any underlying medical illness that may have precipitated the syndrome.

References

Arieff A, Carroll HJ. Non-ketotic hyperosmolar coma with hyperglycemia: clinical features, pathophysiology, renal function, acid-base balance, plasma-cerebrospinal fluid equilibrium and the effects of therapy on 37 cases. Medicine 1972; 51:73–96.

Asplund K, Eriksson S, Hagg F, Lithner T, Strand T, Wester PO. Hyperosmolar non-ketotic coma in diabetic stroke patients. Acta Med Scand 1982; 212:407–411.

British Medical Research Council. Some clinical results of the use of insulin. Br Med J 1923; 1:737–742.

Dreschfeld J. The Bradshaw Lecture on diabetic coma. Br Med J 1886; 18:603–618.

McCurdy DK. Hyperosmolar hyperglycemic non-ketotic diabetic coma. Med Clin N Am 1970; 54:683–699.

Maccario M. Neurological dysfunction associated with nonketotic hyperglycemia. Arch Neurol 1968; 19:525–534.

Prockop LD. Hyperglycemia: effects on the nervous system. In: Vinken PJ and Bruyn GW, eds. Metabolic and Deficiency Diseases of the Nervous System, Handbook of Clinical Neurology, vol 27. Amsterdam: North-Holland, 1976:79–98.

Prockop LD. Hyperglycemia, polyol accumulation and increased intracranial pressure. Arch Neurol 1971; 25:126–140.

Rosenthal NR, Barrett EJ. An assessment of insulin action in hyperosmolar hyperglycemic non-ketotic diabetic patients. J Clin Endocrinol Metab 1985; 60:607–610.

Seki S. Clinical features of hyperosmolar hyperglycemic non-ketotic diabetic coma associated with cardiac operations. J Thorac Cardiovasc Surg 1986; 91:867–873.

Singh BM, Strobos RJ. Epilepsia partialis continua associated with non-ketotic hyperglycemia: clinical and biochemical profile of 21 patients. Ann Neurol 1980; 8:155–160.

Vernon DD, Postellon DC. Non-ketotic hyperosmolar diabetic coma in a child: management with low-dose insulin infusion and intracranial pressure monitoring. Pediatrics 1986; 77:770–777.

Wegierko J. Typical syndrome of clinical manifestations in coma with fatal termination in coma without ketotic acidemia; so-called third coma. Pol Tyg Lek 1956; 11:2020–2023.

West ML, Marsden PA, Singer GG, Halperin ML. Quantitative analysis of glucose loss during acute therapy for hyperglycemia hyperosmolar syndrome. Diabetes Care 1986; 9:465–471.

Chapter V

Tumors

43. GENERAL CONSIDERATIONS
Michael R. Fetell
Bennett M. Stein

The term *intracranial tumor* is used here to refer to all neoplasms arising from the skull, meninges, blood vessels, pituitary and pineal glands, cranial nerves, brain tissue or congenital rests, as well as metastatic tumors, parasitic cysts, granulomas, and lymphomas.

Intracranial tumors may be divided into nine subdivisions as follows:

1. Tumors of the skull and cranial nerves
   Hyperostosis
   Osteomas
   Hemangiomas
   Metastatic
   Granulomas
   Involvement of the skull in systemic diseases
   Xanthomatosis
   Osteitis deformans
2. Tumors of the meninges
   Meningiomas
   Gliomatosis
   Sarcomatosis
   Metastatic
3. Tumors of the supportive tissue (gliomas)
4. Tumors of the pineal region
5. Tumors of the pituitary gland
6. Congenital tumors
   Craniopharyngiomas
   Cholesteatomas
   Chordomas
   Teratomas and dermoids
   Cysts
7. Blood vessel tumors
   Hemangioblastomas
   Angiomas
8. Metastatic tumors and granulomas
9. Multiple tumors of the cranial nerves

Tumors involving the spinal cord are divided by location into three major groups: intramedullary, extramedullary, and extradural.

Pathology. The symptoms that develop with various types of intracranial tumors are related to the nature of the tumor and to its location. These are dependent in part upon the destructive nature of the growth and in part upon the secondary effects of increased intracranial pressure. Details of the pathologic changes are considered in the discussion of the various types of tumors.

Pathogenesis. Meningiomas and malignant mesenchymal tumors have sometimes followed irradiation of the head. Brain tumors have been produced in animals by chemical carcinogens, such as anthracine derivatives and N-nitroso compounds, and by viruses. In recent years, chromosomal abnormalities, gene rearrangements, and the presence of oncogenes have been discovered with increased frequency in CNS tumors.

Epidemiology. Using 300,000,000 population, it can be estimated that 24,000 primary brain tumors are diagnosed in the United States each year; about 75% of them are pathologically verified. An equal number of metastatic brain tumors occur each year, but only 20% of these are pathologically verified. For the pre-CT years 1973 and 1974, estimated age-adjusted rates for primary brain tumors ranged from 5.9 per 100,000 in the Connecticut Tumor Registry to 12.6 per 100,000 population in Rochester, Minnesota. In Rochester, both case ascertainment and autopsy rates are higher than elsewhere, and many asymptomatic tumors, particularly meningiomas, are diagnosed at autopsy. The overall estimated frequency of primary brain neoplasms in the United States was 8.2 per 100,000 per year in 1973–1974 (Table 43–1). It is possible that earlier diagnosis of brain tumors by CT and MRI will result in higher yearly rates.

The frequency of brain tumors is high in children (1 to 5 per 100,000 per year) because

Table 43–1. Estimated Annual Number of Primary Intracranial Neoplasms and Incidence Rates Per 100,000 Population by Age and Sex, United States, 1973–1974

Age Group	Number			Incidence Rate per 100,000		
	Total	Male	Female	Total	Male	Female
All ages	17,030	8,250	8,780	8.2	8.2 (8.5)*	8.1 (7.9)*
Under 5	410	240	170	2.5	2.9	2.1
5–14	830	460	370	2.1	2.3	2.0
15–24	1,170	540	630	3.1	2.9	3.3
25–34	1,290	270	1,020	4.5	1.9	6.9
35–44	1,280	490	790	5.7	4.5	6.8
45–54	4,110	2,050	2,060	17.3	17.9	16.7
55–64	3,950	2,160	1,780	20.4	23.6	17.4
65–74	2,750	1,510	1,240	20.4	26.0	16.2
75 and over	1,250	530	720	15.4	17.3	14.2

*Rates in parentheses are age-adjusted using the direct method.
Adapted and used with permission from Walker AE, Robins M, Weinfeld FD: Epidemiology of brain tumors: The national survey of intracranial neoplasms. Neurology 1985; 35:219–226.

of the occurrence of cerebellar astrocytomas and medulloblastomas. The frequency drops slightly in the mid teens and then rises steadily to a peak in the sixth decade, followed by a slight decline above age 70 (Table 43–1). Gliomas are the most common primary intracranial tumor, followed by meningiomas (Table 43–2).

Although a few general statements may be made concerning the age incidence of the various subtypes of tumors, there are numerous exceptions. In children younger than 16, tumors of the CNS are second only to leukemia in frequency and account for 15 to 20% of all tumors. Two thirds of the tumors in this age group are in the posterior fossa.

The common tumors of childhood in the first two decades of life are gliomas of the cerebellum, brain stem, and optic nerve, pineal tumors, craniopharyngiomas, teratomas, granulomas and primitive neuroectodermal tumors (PNETs) such as medulloblastoma. Tumors of adult life and early middle age include meningiomas, neurofibromas, gliomas of the cerebral hemisphere (particularly glioblastoma multiforme), and pituitary tumors. Metastatic tumors are most frequent in late middle life (Table 43–3).

Intracranial tumors in general are slightly more common in men. Cerebellar medulloblastomas, cerebral astrocytomas, and glioblastomas are more commonly seen in men than in women, whereas the reverse is true of meningiomas and acoustic neuromas.

Symptoms. The signs and symptoms of intracranial tumors are customarily divided into two groups. The first, or general, symptoms include a wide variety of manifestations presumably due to a disturbance of cerebral function resulting from edema, increased intracranial pressure, and other unknown factors. The second group comprises special symptoms and signs that can be attributed to localized destruction or compression of nervous tissue.

Because there is no significant difference between the special symptoms of intracranial tumors and those of other types of lesions, they are not discussed in detail here. Constellations of symptoms that may occur with a particular type of tumor or with tumors that have a predilection for certain localities are discussed in the appropriate section.

Table 43–2. Average Annual Estimated Number of Pathologically Confirmed* Intracranial Neoplasms by Histologic Diagnosis in the United States, 1973–1974

Histologic Diagnosis	No.	%
Glioma	7,940	57.8
Glioblastoma	2,740	20.0
Medulloblastoma	300	2.2
Cerebellar astrocytoma	120	0.9
Other astrocytomas and gliomas	4,780	34.8
Meningioma	2,680	19.5
Neurinoma	940	6.9
Adenoma*	1,970	14.4
Total	13,720	100.0

*Includes 1,110 unconfirmed cases of pituitary neoplasms assumed to be adenoma.
Adapted and used with permission from Walker AE, Robins M, Weinfeld FD: Epidemiology of brain tumors: The national survey of intracranial neoplasms. Neurology 1985; 35:219–226.

Table 43–3. Distribution of Major Brain Tumors by Age and Location

Location	Infancy and Adolescence (0–20 yr)		Middle Age (20–60 yr)		Old Age (>60 yr)	
	Tumor Type	% of All Tumors	Tumor Type	% of All Tumors	Tumor Types	% of All Tumors
Supratentorial	Glioma of cerebral hemisphere	10–14	Glioblastoma	25	Glioblastoma	35
	Craniopharyngioma	5–13	Meningioma	14	Meningioma	20
	Ependymoma	3–5	Astrocytoma	13	Metastases	10
	Choroid plexus papilloma	2–3	Metastases	10		
	Pineal tumors	1.5–3	Pituitary tumors	5		
	Optic glioma	1–3.5				
Infratentorial	Cerebellar Astrocytoma	15–20	Metastases	5	Acoustic neuroma	20
	Medulloblastoma	14–18	Acoustic neuroma	3	Metastases	5
	Brain stem glioma	9–12	Meningioma	1	Meningioma	5
	Ependymoma	4–8				

(From Butler AB, Brooks WH, Netsky MG. Classification and Biology of Brain Tumors. In: Youmans JR ed. Neurological Surgery. Philadelphia: WB Saunders Co., 1982.)

No constellation of symptoms is pathognomonic of an intracranial tumor. Headache, vomiting, and papilledema, the triad of symptoms commonly considered characteristic of brain tumors, may appear early in the course of some cases, in others not until the terminal stages and, in some, never at all. Other general symptoms and signs of intracranial tumors are convulsive seizures, abnormal states of consciousness, mental symptoms, and diplopia or blurred vision. Vasomotor phenomena, cardiac arrhythmias, or bradycardia may appear as terminal symptoms.

The *headaches* of patients with intracranial tumors cannot be differentiated by either their nature or their location from headaches due to other causes. Severe recurrent headaches in a person previously free of them should put the physician on guard. The headache may be localized, but more commonly it is generalized or more intense in the frontal or occipital region, regardless of the location of the tumor. Localized tenderness of the scalp or the underlying skull is not of absolute localizing value, but it is occasionally found in close relationship to the tumor. The headaches of intracranial tumors are usually intermittent, occurring at irregular intervals and lasting for several minutes or hours. They may be increased by change of posture, coughing, or straining. With progress of the growth they tend to become more frequent and of longer duration. The frequency of headaches in patients with brain tumors is high (estimated at 90% by some researchers), but their absence, especially when there are few other generalized symptoms, cannot be taken as evidence that a tumor is not present. The cause of the headaches is not known. They are not directly related to the level of intracranial pressure, and it is probable that pressure on or traction of pain-producing structures (e.g., dura, blood vessels, nerves) plays a role.

Nausea and vomiting are much less frequent than headache. Projectile vomiting without nausea or headache is rare and it usually occurs as a symptom of a cerebellar tumor in childhood.

Swelling of the head of the optic nerve with engorgement of the retinal veins and hemorrhages into the nerve and adjacent retina *(papilledema)* is a common finding in patients with intracranial tumors, but absence of these changes in the optic nerve cannot be taken as evidence against the diagnosis. The incidence of papilledema is variously estimated as between 50% and 90% of the cases, depending to a great extent upon the stage of the disease at which the examination is made. The nature and location of the tumor are also important factors in the development of papilledema. In general, papilledema appears early in all patients with intracranial tumors of whatever nature if the tumor is located so that it interferes with the circulation of the CSF and produces internal hydrocephalus. Thus, tumors that occlude the third ventricle, the cerebral aqueduct, fourth ventricle, or the foramina of exit of the fluid in the posterior fossa are more likely to produce papilledema. Examples of such tumors are gliomas of the thalamus, cysts of the third ventricle, pineal tumors, and posterior fossa tumors in general (e.g., cerebellopontine angle tumors, medulloblastomas, and cerebellar astrocytomas and hemangioblastomas). On the other hand, large tumors can invade and entirely destroy one cerebral hemisphere without producing papilledema. Tumors confined to the cerebral hemisphere do not cause papilledema until they grow large enough to cause increased intracranial pressure. Intracranial tumors with a low incidence of papilledema are pituitary adenomas, slowly growing cerebral astrocytomas, and small meningiomas on the convexities of the cerebral hemispheres.

The pathologic physiology of papilledema is generally assumed to be due to increased intracranial pressure that is transmitted in the vaginal sheaths of the optic nerves with resultant stagnation of the venous return from the retina and nerve head. Papilledema in patients with brain tumor is usually accompanied by other evidence of increased intracranial pressure. On the other hand, even in the presence of a high degree of increased intracranial pressure, the optic discs may be normal. In patients with a tumor compressing the optic chiasm or optic nerve, the optic disc may be atrophied without any evidence of papilledema. If a tumor compressing one optic nerve grows to a size sufficient to produce a generalized increase in intracranial pressure, there may be optic atrophy in one eye and papilledema in the other *(Foster Kennedy syndrome)*. In these cases, the tumor is on the side opposite the choked disc. With this exception, an unequal degree of swelling in the two optic discs has no localizing value and is possibly related to a difference in the intraocular tension in the two eyes. Papilledema is rarely seen in patents with a high degree of myopia, or with pre-existing optic atrophy.

It is not always possible to differentiate with certainty between the papilledema due to intracranial tumor and swelling of the nerve head associated with multiple sclerosis, other demyelinating diseases, or arterial disease of the retina. As a rule in papilledema, the swelling of the nerve head is greater than in the optic neuritis of multiple sclerosis. The hemorrhages in the retina in papilledema are usually confined to the nerve head or the adjacent retina, whereas in arterial disease of the retina, hemorrhagic areas are often found at a distance from the nerve head. Characteristic of the latter condition, also, are changes in the caliber and silver wire appearance of the arteries.

Visual acuity is normal in the early stages of papilledema, but enlargement of the blind spot is proportional to the degree of swelling of the nerve head. These findings are so characteristic of papilledema that they serve as a fairly accurate differential between papilledema and optic neuritis. In optic neuritis, visual acuity is usually greatly diminished, and there may be central or paracentral scotomas, with or without enlargement of the blind spots.

When swelling of the optic disc persists for weeks or months, a secondary type of atrophy develops in the optic nerve. The peripheral fields are constricted (Fig. 43–1) and a gradual failure of central vision sometimes progresses to complete amblyopia. As the atrophy of the nerve head advances, the degree of papilledema usually decreases.

Convulsive seizures of a focal or generalized nature are common in patients with tumors in the cerebral hemispheres (Table 43–4); they are rare with tumors in the brain stem or posterior fossa. The focal seizures of brain tumor do not differ in any way from those that occur with organic lesions in the brain from other causes, such as birth injury or head injury. Nor do the generalized seizures differ from those of so-called idiopathic epilepsy, except that rarely, if ever, does one find the classic petit mal attacks with their characteristic 3-per-second spike and wave EEG. Prolonged coma after a generalized seizure or transient hemiparesis *(Todd paralysis)* after a jacksonian, focal, or generalized seizure is more common in patients with a tumor than in those having convulsive seizures caused by other conditions.

Seizures are not infrequently the first symptom of an intracranial tumor, and this diagnosis must be considered in all patients with seizures, especially if the first attack occurs after age 20. Seizures may be the predominating or only symptom of slowly growing tumors for several or many years.

Because tumors in any portion of the cerebral hemispheres may cause generalized convulsive seizures, this symptom in itself has no localizing value. Jacksonian or focal sensory seizures localize the lesion to the motor-sensory strip of the opposite hemisphere. Seizures preceded by or consisting mainly of

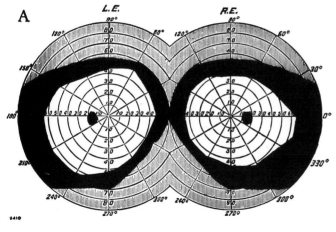

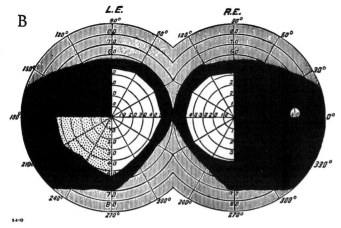

Fig. 43–1. Visual-field defects in intracranial tumors. *A,* Enlargement of blind spots and constriction of peripheral fields with increased intracranial pressure. *B,* Bitemporal hemianopia with pituitary adenoma. (From Merritt H, Mettler FA, Putnam TJ. Fundamentals of Clinical Neurology. New York: Blakiston Co., 1947.)

olfactory or gustatory hallucinations (uncinate fits) localize the lesion to the temporal lobe or orbital frontal cortex, but do not indicate the site of the lesion. Visual phenomena preceding or accompanying a convulsive seizure localize the lesion to either the temporal or occipital lobe, but these symptoms usually have no lateralizing value. As a rule, hallucinations of formed images with or without an auditory accompaniment occur with lesions in the temporal lobe, and unformed images (flashes of light) occur with lesions in

the occipital lobe. Hemianopic visual field defects indicate that the tumor is in the opposite temporal or occipital lobe. Partial complex seizures may occur with tumors in any portion of the cerebrum, but they are more commonly associated with lesions in the temporal lobe.

The *mental symptoms* of intracranial tumors include lethargy, drowsiness, changes in personality, disorders of conduct, impairment of the mental faculties, and psychotic episodes. Any or all of these symptoms may occur with any of the intracranial tumors, and although they have no localizing value, they are more common with tumors in the anterior portions of the cerebral hemisphere. Urinary incontinence, or rather an indifference to the propriety of the act of voiding, is a rare symptom and is usually associated with a tumor of the frontal lobe.

Diagnosis of Intracranial Tumors

The diagnosis of an intracranial tumor and its exact location are determined from the history, physical findings, and laboratory ex-

Table 43–4. Frequency of Convulsions in Cerebral, Cerebellar, and Pituitary Tumors

Location of Tumor	No. of Cases	Cases with Seizures	
		Number	%
Cerebrum	397	138	35
Cerebellum	247	12	5
Pituitary	79	0	0
Total	723	150	21

aminations: radiographs of the skull, CT, EEG, MRI, and angiography.

HISTORY

The diagnosis of an intracranial tumor should be entertained whenever focal neurologic symptoms develop slowly and gradually increase in severity. Although occasionally symptoms of brain tumor may have a sudden and dramatic onset, they more commonly evolve over weeks, months, or years. The occurrence of convulsive seizures, headaches, dizziness, or mental symptoms, or the slow development of focal neurologic symptoms always leads to concern regarding the possibility of an intracranial tumor.

PHYSICAL EXAMINATION

Significant findings on examination that point to the diagnosis of an intracranial tumor are papilledema and signs of focal damage to the nervous system. Although an intracranial tumor may be present without either of these findings, the diagnosis can rarely be made in the absence of both. It must be kept in mind, however, that these symptoms may also appear in conditions other than intracranial tumors.

When focal neurologic signs are present, the localization of intracranial tumors can be made from their nature. Careful examination of visual fields and speech functions should never be neglected. If the condition of the patient does not permit an accurate perimetric examination, a simple confrontation test may give valuable information. If there are no abnormal findings on neurologic examination, localization of the tumor depends on the results of other examinations.

False localizing signs may occur when there is a high degree of increased intracranial pressure or distortion of the intracranial structures. Unilateral or bilateral weakness of the external rectus muscles may result from compression of one or both sixth cranial nerves against the floor of the skull. Less common false localizing signs include: hemiplegia on the same side as the tumor, presumably caused by distortion of the brain and compression of the opposite cerebral peduncle against the incisura of the tentorium; homonymous hemianopia on the same side as the tumor due to distortion of the brain and compression of the opposite posterior cerebral artery; paralysis of the third nerve accompanied by a fixed dilated pupil on the same side as the tumor, resulting from a downward her-

niation of the hippocampus through the tentorium; and changes in the visual fields due to compression of the optic chiasm or tracts by a dilated third ventricle.

LABORATORY EXAMINATION

Roentgenography. With the advent of CT, plain radiographs have become less important; nevertheless, examination of the skull with conventional radiologic techniques may suggest the diagnosis of intracranial tumor by showing changes such as displacement of a calcified pineal gland, resorptive changes in the bones of the skull due to increased intracranial pressure (increase in the convolution markings on the skull, erosion of the dorsum sellae and, in children, separation of sutures), or calcification within the substance of the tumor, which is frequently seen in craniopharyngiomas and in about 12% of the gliomas, particularly astrocytomas and oligodendrogliomas. Approximately 50% of the meningiomas cause bone changes, mostly hyperostosis of the adjacent bone, and sometimes an enlargement of the vascular channels. Pituitary tumors may cause erosion of the walls of the sella turcica; in the smaller microadenomas of the pituitary gland, an asymmetric depression of the floor of the sella is often present. Acoustic neuromas may manifest by erosion of the petrous ridge and dilatation of the internal auditory meatus. Gliomas of the optic nerve sometimes produce enlargement of the optic foramen.

Electroencephalography. EEG is of value in localizing tumors of the cerebral hemisphere that are near the surface. Perhaps more important is a changing EEG pattern in the follow-up of long-standing seizure disorder. Focal abnormalities in the electrical activity (Fig. 43–2) are helpful in indicating the site of a lesion, but their character does not make possible an absolute differential diagnosis between a tumor and other lesions of the cortex. An increase in the degree of abnormality on repeated testing is in favor of the diagnosis of a tumor. Deep-seated tumors of the hemispheres or tumors of the posterior fossa may be accompanied by diffuse slowing of the electrical activity of the cerebral cortex.

Examination of the Cerebrospinal Fluid. Lumbar puncture is rarely indicated as a first step in the diagnosis of brain tumors and is usually unnecessary when CT is available. Lumbar puncture may be dangerous in the presence of increased intracranial pressure. It is of great importance, however, when tumor

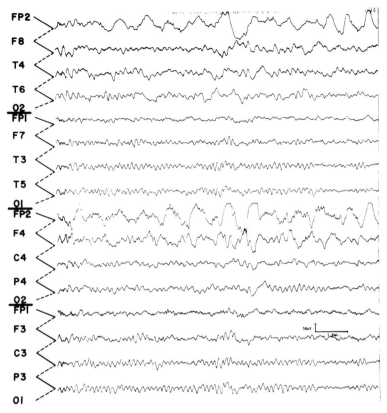

Fig. 43–2. Slow-wave focus in a brain tumor. The EEG shows rhythmic and arrhythmic slowing in the frontal areas (FP2) with extension of the irregular slowing into the lateral frontal and temporal areas (F8, T4, and T6).

dissemination in the subarachnoid spaces is suspected. This occurs not only with gliomas, medulloblastomas, ependymomas, and some pineal tumors, but also with metastatic tumors. The presence of abnormal cells, which is frequently associated with an increase in the protein content and a decrease in the glucose value, is of diagnostic value. Tumor cells in the CSF may be identified by special cytologic techniques. (See discussion of neoplastic meningitis.)

Computerized Tomography. CT should be performed whenever the diagnosis of brain tumor is entertained. The accuracy of the CT is increased by intravenous injection of contrast material and by the use of sections in different planes.

CT gives an accurate localization of the lesion and frequently helps in the diagnosis of the histologic type. Cysts, calcification, areas of necrosis or hemorrhage, edema, or associated hydrocephalus are readily appreciated. CT also demonstrates changes in the calvarium such as hyperostosis, erosion, or enlargement of the foramina.

In the diagnosis of tumors of the posterior fossa, or of the sellar and suprasellar region, this test has replaced invasive techniques such as ventriculography and pneumonencephalography. The test is also helpful in he investigation of primary or secondary tumors of the orbit.

Another area in which CT has made a great contribution is in the follow-up of patients with brain tumors not only in the immediate postoperative period, but also to determine the response to therapy and to detect recurrence.

Magnetic Resonance Imaging. MRI (Fig. 43–3) now complements CT scan and frequently replaces the CT. The advantages include (1) excellent visualization of most intracranial and spinal tumors, (2) clear representation of anatomy distorted by tumors, (3) the ability to obtain virtually three-dimensional representation of disease through multiple views, and (4) lack of radiation. In spite of the great utility of MRI in neurodiagnosis, the technique has some drawbacks: slowness of imaging, obscurity of some tumors, in particular meningiomas, and lack of readily available contrast technique. To compensate for these, CT scan may be used as an adjuvant. The development of par-

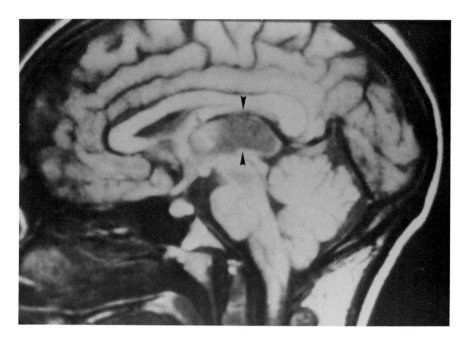

Fig. 43–3. Sagittal T₁ MRI demonstrating large partially cystic pineal region tumor (arrows).

amagnetic compounds that are injected intravenously and enhance the signal of tumor tissue will probably soon overcome these deficiencies.

Angiography. Although CT and MRI are now the most important tests in the diagnosis of brain tumor, cerebral angiography is still

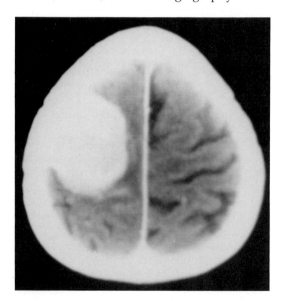

Fig. 43–4. Convexity meningioma. An axial CT scan with contrast demonstrates homogeneous enhancement of the dural-based right frontoparietal tumor, and sulcal effacement. (Courtesy of Drs. T.L. Chi, J.A. Bello, and S.K. Hilal.)

of value in the differential diagnosis of mass lesions and in the determination of relation to vascular structures (Figs. 43–4, 43–5, 43–6). It should be performed through selective catheterization of the major arteries (including the external carotid artery). Magnification and subtraction views are also of great help. The different histologic types often have characteristic angiographic pictures. For instance, meningiomas are usually fed by branches of the external carotid artery, and have a blush that appears relatively late in the series. In contrast, an early blush with an early filling vein is more consistent with a malignant glioma.

Other Tests. Ventriculography and pneumoencephalography have largely been replaced by CT and MRI. They may still be of help in outlining small tumors in the ventricles or suprasellar region.

Radioisotope scanning with technetium-99 was often helpful in patients allergic to intravenously administered contrast agents, but it has been largely supplanted by MRI. Lesions in the cerebral hemispheres can be localized by an abnormal concentration of the isotope. The technique is most valuable for vascular tumors that are more than 2 cm in diameter, but only rarely shows a tumor that is not seen in CT.

DIFFERENTIAL DIAGNOSIS

Intracranial tumors must be differentiated from other conditions accompanied by focal

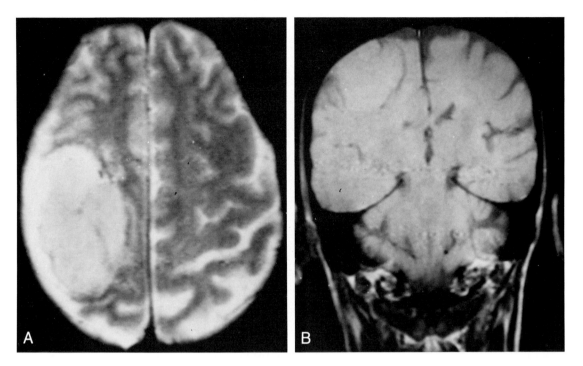

Fig. 43–5. Convexity meningioma (same patient as Fig. 43–4). Axial T_2 weighted *(A)* and *(B)* coronal T_1 weighted MR images demonstrate the extra-axial lesion without associated edema but with mass effect on the right lateral ventricle. The signal from this tumor is typically less intense than that from other tumors using T_2 imaging, and is isointense to the brain parenchyma on the T_1 scan in *B*. (Courtesy of Drs. T.L. Chi, J.A. Bello, and S.K. Hilal.)

neurologic signs or signs of increased intracranial pressure. As this obviously encompasses the whole field of neurology, it is necessary to limit discussion to the more common diseases with symptoms that may mimic intracranial tumors. These conditions include strokes, infections, degenerative diseases, and subdural hematoma. With the diagnostic methods now available, errors in the diagnosis of intracranial tumors are rare.

Cerebrovascular Disease. Strokes are differentiated from intracranial tumors by the sudden onset of symptoms and lack of progression of focal signs, but the symptoms of an intracranial tumor may also have a sudden onset, and there may be a progressive increase in the severity of the neurologic signs in patients with cerebrovascular lesions. The presence or absence of arteriosclerosis and hypertension is not of absolute diagnostic sig-

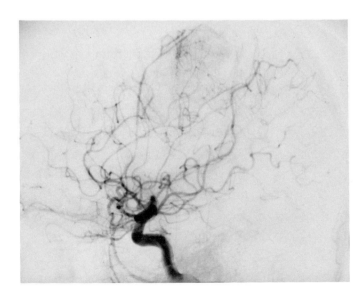

Fig. 43–6. Convexity meningioma (same patient as Figs. 43–4 and 5). A lateral view of a right common carotid arteriogram demonstrates a tumor stain supplied by the middle meningeal artery diagnostic of a meningioma. These extra-axial tumors are typically more striking on CT and angiogram than MRI, because of their relatively low signal intensity (attributed to calcification). (Courtesy of Drs. T.L. Chi, J.A. Bello, and S.K. Hilal.)

nificance because intracranial tumors are common in the age group that is subject to arteriosclerosis; moreover, cerebrovascular disease may occur without hypertension or other signs of arteriosclerosis.

The establishment of the correct diagnosis may be difficult in patients with cerebrovascular disease accompanied by changes in the optic disc simulating the papilledema of increased intracranial pressure. Papilledema may occur in patients with an intracranial hemorrhage who survive for days or weeks. If the CSF is bloody immediately after the onset of symptoms, the diagnosis of an intracerebral hemorrhage is probable. Hemorrhage within brain tumors is, however, not rare. Glioblastomas and certain metastatic tumors, such as melanoma, choriocarcinoma, and renal carcinoma, are the ones most frequently implicated.

Intracranial aneurysms, particularly giant aneurysms, may mimic an intracranial tumor. CT, MRI, and angiography are, however, usually diagnostic.

Infections of the Nervous System. Patients with acute infections of the meninges with symptoms simulating those of brain tumors are readily diagnosed by CT and examination of the CSF. The same is true of the subacute infections of the meninges with tuberculosis, syphilis, or the yeast organisms. Localized granulomatous lesions due to these organisms cannot be differentiated from other intracranial tumors unless there is accompanying meningitis.

Angiography may be necessary, however, to document the obstruction of a major venous channel. The differential diagnosis with an intracranial abscess is usually based on the clinical presentation and the radiographic (CT) picture, but occasionally direct surgical intervention is the only way to make a firm diagnosis.

Viral infections of the CNS are diagnosed by their clinical course and by the changes in the CSF.

Demyelinating Disease. Multiple sclerosis is characterized by a multiplicity of symptoms and signs and by a remitting course. Occasionally in multiple sclerosis and more frequently in Schilder disease, the signs and symptoms may be progressive and localized to one region of the cortex or the brain stem. Changes in the CSF, CT, and evoked potential responses are usually diagnostic.

Degenerative Disease. The degenerative diseases that may simulate intracranial tumors by the slow progression of mental symptoms or focal neurologic signs, particularly aphasia, are Pick and Alzheimer diseases. The diagnosis of tumor can be excluded with certainty by CT and MRI.

Subdural Hematoma. Acute subdural hematomas are readily differentiated from intracranial neoplasms by the history of recent head injury. CT may be necessary to exclude chronic subdural hematoma in cases where the initial head injury was so mild that it was forgotten, or in chronic alcoholics who may have injured their head in an unremembered alcoholic debauch.

CLINICAL COURSE AND TREATMENT

The clinical course of patients with intracranial tumors is closely related to the type of tumor. For this reason, it is more appropriate to discuss this subject in more detail in connection with the various types of tumors. In general, the symptoms and signs of intracranial tumors are usually of slow onset (Table 43–5) and they progress in most instances until they are removed or cause the death of the patient. Remissions are relatively infrequent, but may occur even in the most malignant tumor.

The treatment of brain tumors is surgical

Table 43–5. Comparison of the Duration of Symptoms before Admission to the Hospital in the Various Types of Intracranial Tumors

Type of Tumor	No. of Cases	Duration of Symptoms (in months)				
		Less than 1	1 to 4	4 to 12	12 to 36	More than 36
Glioma	47	13	20	6	4	4
Meningioma	21	1	4	8	5	3
Metastatic	14	2	10	1	—	1
Neurofibroma	7	—	—	—	4	3
Pituitary adenoma	6	—	1	—	—	5
Miscellaneous	5	1	1	1	1	1
Total	100	17	36	16	14	17

extirpation, when possible, followed by radiation therapy when indicated. If the tumor cannot be completely removed, partial removal followed by radiation therapy may appreciably lengthen the period of useful life. In general, patients with meningiomas, acoustic neuromas, cystic astrocytomas of the cerebellum, colloid cysts of the third ventricle, lipomas, angiomatous malformations, and some of the granulomas and congenital tumors can be cured by surgical removal of the tumor. The infiltrating gliomas cannot be entirely extirpated. In these cases, biopsy for the establishment of the diagnosis, partial removal when clinically feasible, and radiation therapy are the accepted treatment.

Corticosteroids are effective in reducing peritumoral edema, and symptoms of increased intracranial pressure and local mass effect both respond to high doses (16–60 mg/day) of dexamethasone.

References

Epidemiology of Brain Tumors

Schoenberg BS, Christine BW, Whisnant JP: The resolution of discrepancies in the reported incidence of primary brain tumors. Neurology 1978; 28:817–823.
Annegers JH, Schoenberg BS, Okazaki H, Kurland LT: Epidemiologic study of primary intracranial neoplasms. Arch Neurol 1981; 38:217–219.
Walker AE, Robins M, Weinfeld FD: Epidemiology of brain tumors: the national survey of intracranial neoplasms. Neurology 1985: 35:219–226.

44. TUMORS OF THE SKULL AND CRANIAL NERVES

Michael R. Fetell
Bennett M. Stein

Hyperostoses

Local overgrowth of the bones of the skull may be secondary to intracranial tumors, particularly meningiomas, or it may occur independently of the presence of such tumors. The present discussion is confined to the latter group.

Hyperostoses may involve either the outer or inner tables of the skull. Those involving the outer table are of no importance except for the disfigurement they produce when they become large. Those involving the inner table rarely grow to sufficient size to compress the intracranial content. Hyperostosis of the inner table of the frontal bone is a common incidental finding in routine radiographs of the skull, especially in middle-aged or elderly women. Attempts have been made to associate these changes in the skull with headaches and other somatic symptoms common at the time of the menopause. The frequency of hyperostosis of the frontal bone in patients without symptoms makes it unlikely, however, that overgrowth of the inner table of the frontal bone (*hyperostosis frontalis interna*) is related to dysfunction of the endocrine glands or that it is the cause of any symptoms.

Osteomas

Osteomas of the skull may arise in the paranasal sinuses, particularly the frontal and ethmoidal ones or from other areas of the calvarium. They are circumscribed lesions growing from either the outer or inner table of the skull. They appear radiographically as well defined homogeneous bone densities.

Osteomas of the nasal and frontal sinuses may cause local pain or headaches. They may grow into the orbit and cause deviation of the globe, or into the anterior fossa; they seldom erode through the dura to cause CSF rhinorrhea. When growing into the frontal sinuses, they may be associated with mucoceles. Tumors of the calvarium frequently present as hard, painless, localized masses. They rarely have intracranial extensions of sufficient size to cause symptoms.

The diagnosis is usually based on the radiographic appearance of the lesion. CT is helpful. Angiography is indicated for an unusually large tumor. The treatment of choice is surgical excision followed by cranioplasty.

Hemangiomas

Hemangiomas are vascular tumors that may involve the skull or spine. They vary in size from small, solitary lesions to huge lesions that receive blood from the scalp or meningeal vessels. They may cause headaches that are probably due to involvement of the periosteum. They present radiographically as areas of decreased density with a trabecular appearance. On tangential views, the diploë is usually expanded, but the inner table is well preserved. Surgical excision is usually curative. Radiotherapy has been advised, particularly for large lesions or multiple tumors of the spine.

Metastases to the Base of the Skull

The cranial nerves that exit through the bony foramina are vulnerable to entrapment and compression by tumor extending from osseous metastasis. The typical clinical syndrome is seen in patients with breast, lung, prostate, and head and neck tumors, or lymphoma. Localized cranial or facial pain occurs at the site of tumor invasion, and there are signs of cranial neuropathy. The pain is usually progressive, but the cranial neuropathy may appear in one day.

Typical clinical syndromes have been reviewed by Greenberg et al., and may be defined as the (1) orbital syndrome (proptosis, diplopia, fifth nerve sensory loss), (2) parasellar syndrome (diplopia, fifth nerve sensory loss), (3) middle fossa or gasserian ganglion syndrome (facial pain, trigeminal sensory loss, trigeminal neuralgia), (4) jugular foramen syndrome (hoarseness, dysphagia, and glossopharyngeal neuralgia), and (5) occipital condyle or hypoglossal canal syndrome (dysarthria, hypoglossal palsy, accessory nerve palsy). These syndromes, or minor variations thereof, carry eponymic designations such as Vernet (jugular foramen), Collet-Sicard (occipital condyle), Villaret (Collet-Sicard plus Horner syndrome), Foix-Jefferson (cavernous sinus), and Jacod-Rolet (apex of orbit), but anatomic descriptions seem preferable.

Pain is supraorbital or frontal in the orbital and parasellar syndromes, facial (cheek or jaw) in the middle fossa syndrome, retroauricular in the jugular foramen, and occipitonuchal (and worse with head motion) in the occipital condyle syndrome. In addition, trigeminal neuralgia occurs with the middle fossa syndrome and glossopharyngeal neuralgia with the jugular foramen syndrome. CT has largely replaced plain radiographs and linear tomography for diagnosis. Appropriate adjustment of window width and mean window level is necessary to visualize bony structures, and both axial and coronal scans may be necessary (see Fig. 51–6). Because erosion is not always seen, only about one half of cases can be verified radiographically, and it is often necessary to recommend treatment when the clinical picture is clear and the symptoms are progressive. Biopsy is difficult and hazardous, even with a stereotactic needle approach.

The most important differential diagnosis is meningeal carcinomatosis, and all patients should have examination of CSF cytology. In meningeal carcinomatosis, pain is usually less prominent, and other sites of involvement such as spinal cord or nerve roots are present. Occasionally, meningeal carcinomatosis may be found with metastases to the base of the brain.

Treatment for metastases to the base of the brain is palliative. Radiotherapy dosages of at least 3,000 rads should be given to the affected areas in 300-rad fractions. Overall success with palliation of symptoms is fairly good (86%). Early treatment (within one month of onset of symptoms) is effective in 92% of patients; after one month, treatment is effective in 78%.

The base of the skull may also be involved by direct extension of a carcinoma of the nasal sinuses or nasopharynx. These tumors usually cause pain and involvement of the cranial nerves. Erosion of the base of the skull or the presence of soft tissue masses may be detected in plain radiographs of the skull, tomograms, or CT. The primary growth may be discovered by careful examination of the nasopharynx, and a local biopsy is often diagnostic. The prognosis is usually poor. Radiotherapy and wide surgical excisions have been advocated.

Tumors of the glomus jugulare arise from the chromaffin cells in the region of the jugular bulb and invade the neighboring temporal or occipital bones. They cause tinnitus, an audible bruit, deafness, and involvement of the lower cranial nerves. Larger tumors cause cerebellar and brain stem symptoms. Not infrequently, however, they may be discovered as small, vascular masses that protrude into the middle ear cavity. These are vascular tumors, and complete angiographic evaluation is mandatory before a direct surgical approach is considered. Artificial embolization is useful in the management of these lesions, and radiotherapy may be beneficial.

Mental Neuropathy (The Numb Chin Syndrome)

This unique syndrome is due to mandibular metastasis in the region of the mental nerve foramen or inferior alveolar nerve. In some patients it may follow dental treatment of tooth abscess, and has been reported in sickle crisis, presumably due to infarction of nerve, bone, or marrow hyperplasia.

When progressive numbness of one or both sides of the chin, with or without pain, is reported by a patient with systemic cancer, mandibular metastasis should be suspected. Lymphoma or leukemia is responsible for 50% of cases; other common tumors include metastatic breast, lung, prostate, and myeloma. Sensory loss in the mental nerve (or alveolar nerve distribution) can be documented on physical examination and local tenderness may be present near the mental nerve foramen, but neurologic examination is otherwise normal. Radiographs may show osteolytic lesions (40%) (Fig. 44–1), but are not necessary for diagnosis. The high incidence (perhaps 30%) of coexistent meningeal carcinomatosis emphasizes the need for examination of CSF cytology in all patients with systemic tumors and numb chin syndrome.

Paresthesias and sensory loss may be relieved with chemotherapy, or radiotherapy delivered focally to the mandible. More important than the usually minor or trivial discomfort of the numb chin syndrome is the fact that it may be the presenting symptom of systemic malignant tumor (47% in Massey's series), or may herald relapse of systemic tumor in a patient thought to be in remission.

Involvement of the Skull in Systemic Diseases

The bones of the skull may be involved in xanthomatosis (Hand-Schüller-Christian disease), multiple myeloma, osteitis deformans (Paget disease), and osteitis fibrosa cystica. The symptoms and signs of these conditions are considered in detail elsewhere.

Other Tumors of the Skull

Epidermoid and dermoid tumors are relatively frequent and involve mostly the frontal and temporal areas, and may have intracranial extensions. They have a characteristic radiographic appearance with rounded or lobulated lytic lesions, with sharp sclerotic margins involving all three layers of the bone. The rarer benign tumors include chondromas, fibromas, ossifying fibromas, giant-cell tumors, and aneurysmal bone cysts.

Among the less common malignant tumors of the skull are the osteogenic sarcomas (sometimes associated with Paget disease), chondrosarcomas, and fibrosarcomas.

The skull may also be involved by other disorders that may simulate tumors such as leptomeningeal cysts (growing skull fractures), sinus pericranii, metabolic disease such as hyperparathyroidism and acromegaly, infections, sarcoidosis, Paget disease, and hysticytosis X. Fibrous dysplasia and the neuroectodermal dysplasias commonly involve the cranial bones.

Neurofibromas of the Fifth Cranial Nerve

Neurofibromas of the gasserian ganglion or of the fifth nerve in the middle or posterior fossa are rare. When the tumor is confined to the gasserian ganglion and middle fossa, the signs are usually limited to sensory loss (with or without spontaneous pain) in the face, and paralysis and atrophy of the muscles of mastication. With growth of the tumor into the posterior fossa there are signs and symptoms of involvement of the lower cranial nerves, medulla, and cerebellum. Radiographs of the base may show erosion of the foramen ovale or of the foramen rotundum.

Acoustic neuromas and involvement of the fifth nerve by metastatic tumor or carcinoma of the nasopharynx should be considered in

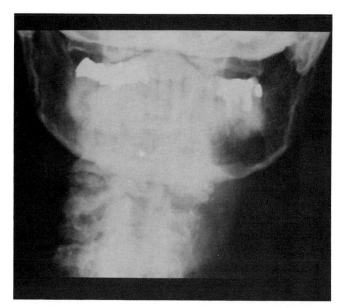

Fig. 44–1. Mental neuropathy. AP radiograph of patient with multiple myeloma who complained of numbness of his left chin. Note large osteolytic lesion involving mental nerve foramen and body of left mandible. (Courtesy of Dr. S. Fox.)

Table 44–1.   Laboratory Tests in Patients with Acoustic Neuroma

Test	No. of Patients Studied	% Abnormal
Pure tone hearing loss (more than 10 db)	66	97
Speech discrimination (less than 90%)	66	92
Tone decay	38	52
Acoustic reflex and decay	35	86
Brain stem auditory evoked response	26	96
Caloric responses	57	86
Petrous bone tomography	64	80
CT	76	89
Contrast rhombencephalography	19	100
Arteriography	16	88

(From Harner SG, Laws ER Jr. Neurosurgery 1981; 9:373–379.)

the differential diagnosis. Treatment is by surgical removal.

Acoustic Neuroma

Acoustic neuromas (acoustic neurinoma, acoustic neurofibroma) represent 5 to 10% of all intracranial tumors and about 80 to 90% of all tumors in the cerebellopontine angle. They occur more often in patients between the ages of 20 and 50. When present in younger patients, and particularly if the tumor is bilateral, the acoustic neuroma is usually associated with neurofibromatosis.

These tumors develop from Schwann cells of the vestibular branch, usually at the level of the porus acusticus, growing into both the internal auditory meatus and the cerebellopontine angle, where they displace the adjacent neural structures, cerebellum, pons, and cranial nerves. As a rule, acoustic neuromas grow slowly, may be large and even cystic before they become symptomatic. Macroscopically, they are usually yellowish, sometimes with areas of cystic degeneration; the tumor stretches the adjacent cranial nerves, particularly the seventh nerve. Microscopically, they follow two main patterns: the Antoni A type, with cells forming compact bands of elongated elements, often simulating a palisade effect, and the Antoni B type, with a looser pattern of stellate cells with long irregular processes.

With the increased clinical awareness and more sophisticated radiographic techniques, especially MRI, that allow detection of smaller

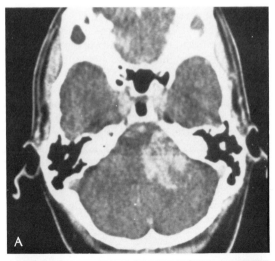

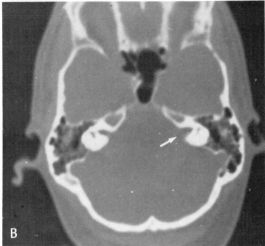

Fig. 44–2.   Acoustic neuroma. *A.* The large tumor in the posterior fossa is seen on contrast-enhanced CT. *B.* Bone window films show the widened internal auditory canal *(arrow).* (Courtesy of Drs. S.K. Hilal and S.R. Ganti.)

tumors, the clinical presentation of these tumors has changed in the last decade (Tables 44–1 and 44–2). Otologic symptoms may have been present for many years before the patient comes to consultation because of unilateral hearing loss (95% of the cases), tinnitus (70%), or unsteadiness of gait (70%). Less frequently, the patients may complain of vertigo, but typical Meniere syndrome is rare. Specific neurologic symptoms usually result from compression of the other cranial nerves and include numbness of the face and, less often, facial weakness, loss of taste, and otalgia. Paroxysmal pain in the trigeminal distribution is rare. Large tumors may cause headaches, nausea, vomiting, diplopia, and ataxia,

Table 44–2.   Symptoms and Signs in 76 Patients wth Surgically Confirmed Acoustic Neuroma

	%		%
Hearing loss	97	Decreased corneal reflex	37
Dysequilibrium	70	Nystagmus	34
Tinnitus	70	Facial hypesthesia	29
Headache	38	Abnormal eye movement	14
Facial numbness	33	Facial weakness	13
Nausea	13	Papilledema	12
Otalgia	11	Babinski sign	8
Diplopia	9		
Facial palsy	9		
Loss of taste	9		

From Harner SG, Laws ER Jr. Neurosurgery 1981; 9:373–379.)

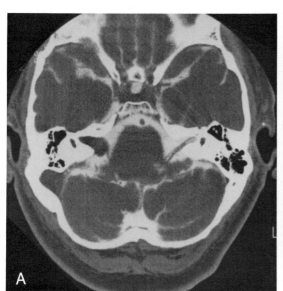

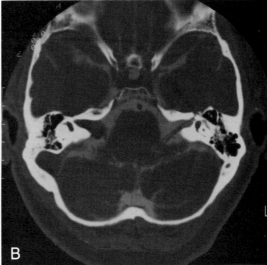

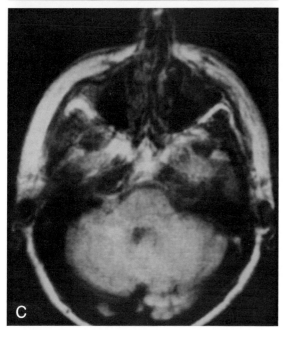

Fig. 44–3. Acoustic neuroma. *A,* An axial CT cisternogram using water-soluble iodinated contrast shows cranial nerves VII and VIII entering the left internal auditory canal (IAC), which is filled with contrast. Intracanalicular soft tissue protruding into the CP angle cistern on the right prevents contrast from filling the IAC. *B,* "Bone windows" taken of the same image accentuate the bony canal asymmetry, with flaring noted on the right. *C,* An axial T_1 weighted MRI on this patient demonstrates extra-axial soft tissue within the right CP angle cistern, enlarging it slightly. (Courtesy of Drs. J.A. Bello and S.K. Hilal.)

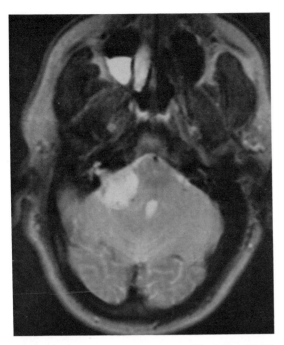

Fig. 44–4. Acoustic neuroma. An axial T_2 weighted MRI demonstrates a mixed signal intensity lesion in the right CP angle cistern admixed with CSF, which is hyperintense on this sequence. (Compare with the signal intensity of the slightly displaced fourth ventricle.) Note flaring of the internal auditory canal on the right. (Acute sinusitis is incidentally noted, with an air-fluid level in the right maxillary antrum.) (Courtesy of Drs. J.A. Bello, T.L. Chi, and S.K. Hilal.)

or symptoms of increased intracranial pressure and hydrocephalus.

In patients with small tumors, decreased hearing and tinnitus are the main signs. Other signs include nystagmus, facial weakness, decreased sensation over the trigeminal area with a decreased corneal reflex. With larger tumors, there may be a disturbance of eye movements, cerebellar and pyramidal signs, papilledema, or compromise of the lower cranial nerves.

With the addition of MRI and cisternography, preoperative diagnosis approaches 100%. Acoustic neuromas growing in the internal auditory canal or meatus cause erosion of the superior margin of the canal or asymmetric widening of the canal. These changes can be appreciated by plain radiographs, and even better by conventional tomography. CT is a most useful technique and demonstrates the tumor (particularly if it is larger than 2 cm) as a contrast-enhanced lesion (Fig. 44–2). Other signs include widening of the ipsilateral pontine cistern, deviation of the fourth ventricle, or hydrocephalus. CT cisternogra-

phy and MRI are the most useful studies (Figs. 44–3, 44–4). Angiography is now rarely used.

Caloric testing and electronystagmography are abnormal in a high percentage of the cases of acoustic neuroma. Audiometry usually shows pure tone abnormalities, with a high-frequency hearing loss. Speech discrimination is also frequently impaired. More sensitive tests are the acoustic reflex, brain stem auditory-evoked response (BAER).

The clinical presentation of an acoustic neuroma can be simulated by any mass growing in the cerebellopontine angle. These include neuromas of the fifth or other cranial nerves, meningiomas, cholesteatomas, choroid plexus papillomas, gliomas, cysts, and aneurysms.

The treatment of choice is surgical excision with microsurgical techniques. The tumors can often be removed totally with preservation of the facial nerve and, in small tumors, preservation of functional hearing. For larger tumors, a two-stage operation or a more simple intracapsular removal is sometimes indicated.

References

Abramson M, Stein BM, Emerson RG, Pedley TA, Wazen JJ. Intraoperative BAER monitoring and hearing preservation in the treatment of acoustic neuromas. Laryngoscope 1985; 95:1318–1322.

Adornato BT, Eil C, Head GL, Loriaux DL. Cerebellar involvement in multifocal eosinophilic granulomas: demonstration by computerized tomographic scanning. Ann Neurol 1980; 7:125–129.

Arseni C, Dumitrescu L, Constantinescu A. Neurinomas of the trigeminal nerve. Surg Neurol 1975; 4:497–503.

Berkman YM, Blatt ES. Cranial and intracranial cartilaginous tumors. Clin Radiol 1968; 9:327–333.

Caille JM, Constant P, Renaud-Salis JL, Dop A. CT studies of tumors of the skull base, facial skeleton and nasopharynx. J Comput Tomogr 1977; 1:217–224.

Calverley JR, Mohnac AM. Syndrome of the numb chin. Arch Intern Med 1963; 112:819–821.

Chang CH, Housepian EM, eds. Tumors of the Central Nervous System: Modern Radiotherapy in Multidisciplinary Management. New York: Masson, 1982.

Chin HW, Hazel JJ, Kim TH, et al. Oligodendrogliomas. I. A clinical study of cerebral oligodendrogliomas. Cancer 1980; 45:1458–1466.

Cushing H. Tumors of the Nervus Acusticus and the Syndrome of the Cerebellopontine Angle. Philadelphia: WB Saunders Co., 1917.

Cushing H. Intracranial Tumors: Notes upon a Series of 2000 Verified Cases with Surgical-Mortality Percentages Pertaining Thereto. Springfield: Charles C Thomas, 1932.

Dandy WE. Ventriculography following the injection of air into the cerebral ventricles. Ann Surg 1918; 68:5–11.

Dandy WE. Roentgenography of brain after injection of air into spinal canal. Ann Surg 1919; 70:397–403.

Enzmann DR, O'Donohue J. Optimizing MR imaging for detecting small tumors in the cerebellopontine angle and internal auditory canal. Am J Neuroradiol 1987; 8:99–106.

Fadul C. Morbidity and mortality of craniotomy for excision of supratentorial gliomas. Neurology 1988; 38:1374–1379.

Gardner G, Cocke EW Jr, Robertson JT, et al. Combined approach surgery for removal of glomus jugulare tumors. Laryngoscope 1977; 87:665–688.

Grant FC. A study of the results of surgical treatment of 2,326 consecutive patients with brain tumors. J Neurosurg 1956; 13:479–488.

Greenberg H, Deck MDF, Vikram B, Chu FCH, Posner JB. Metastases to the base of the skull: clinical findings in 43 cases. Neurology 1981; 31:530–537.

Greenberger JS, Cassady JR, Jaffe N, Vawter G, Crocker AC. Radiation therapy in patients with histiocytosis: management of diabetes insipidus and bone lesions. Int J Radiat Oncol Biol Phys 1979; 5:1749–1755.

Greenberger JS, Crocker AC, Vawter G, Jaffe N, Cassady JR. Results of treatment of 127 patients with systemic histiocytosis (Letterer-Siwe syndrome, Schuller-Christian syndrome and multifocal eosinophilic granuloma). Medicine 1981; 60:311–338.

Harner SG, Daube JR, Ebersold MJ, et al. Improved preservation of facial nerve function with use of electrical monitoring during removal of acoustic neuromas. Mayo Clin Proc 1987; 62:92–102.

Harner SG, Laws ER Jr. Clinical findings in patients with acoustic neurinoma. Mayo Clin Proc 1983; 58:721–728.

Hart RG, Gardner DP, Howieson J. Acoustic tumors: atypical features and recent diagnostic tests. Neurology 1983; 33:211–221.

Horton J, Means ED, Cunningham TJ, et al. The numb chin in breast cancer. J Neurol Neurosurg Psychiatry 1973; 36:211–216.

Jelsma R. Primary tumors of the calvaria. Springfield: Charles C Thomas, 1959.

Kasantikul V, Netsky MG, Glasscock ME, Hays JW. Acoustic neurilemmoma. Clinicoanatomical study of 103 patients. J Neurosurg 1980; 52:28–35.

Kirson LE, Tomaro AJ. Mental nerve paresthesia secondary to sickle-cell crisis. Oral Surg 1979; 48:509–512.

Kramer W. Glomus jugulare tumors. In: Vinken PJ, Bruyn GW, eds. Handbook of Clinical Neurology, vol 18. New York: Elsevier-North Holland, 1975: 435–455.

Lawson W. Glomus bodies and tumors. NY State J Med 1980; 80:1567–1575.

Leuinthal R, Bentson JR. Detection of small trigeminal neurinomas. J Neurosurg 1976; 45:568–575.

McIntosh N. Medulloblastoma—A changing prognosis? Arch Dis Child 1979; 54:200–203.

Martuza RL, Ojemann RG. Bilateral acoustic neuromas: clinical aspects, pathogenesis and treatment. Neurosurgery 1982; 10:1–12.

Massey EW, Moore J, Schold SC. Mental neuropathy from systemic cancer. Neurology 1981; 31:1277–1281.

Matson DD. Neurosurgery of Infancy and Childhood, 2nd ed. Springfield: Charles C Thomas, 1969.

Merritt HH. The cerebrospinal fluid in cases of tumors of the brain. Arch Neurol Psychiatry 1935; 34:1175–1187.

Mikhael MA, Ciric IS, Wolff AP. MR diagnosis of acoustic neuromas. J Comput Assist Tomogr 1987; 11:232–235.

Mork SJ, Loken AC. Ependymoma: a follow-up study of 101 cases. Cancer 1977; 40:907–915.

Nesbit ME, Perez CA, Tefft M, et al. The immune system and the histiocytosis syndromes. Am J Pediatr Hematol Oncol 1981; 3:141–149.

Nezelof C, Faileux-Herbert F, Cronier-Sachot J. Disseminated histiocytosis X: analysis of prognostic factors based on a retrospective study of 50 cases. Cancer 1979; 44:1824–1838.

Nobler MP: Mental nerve palsy in malignant lymphoma. Cancer 1969; 24:122–127.

Pereslegin IA, Ustinova VF, Podlyashok EL. Radiotherapy for eosinophilic granuloma of bone. Int J Radiat Oncol Biol Phys 1981; 7:317–321.

Pool JL, Pava A, Greenfield E. Acoustic Nerve Tumors, Early Diagnosis and Treatment, 2nd ed. Springfield: Charles C Thomas, 1970.

Rhoton AL, Jr. Microsurgical removal of acoustic neuromas. Surg Neurol 1976; 6:211–219.

Seitz W, Olarte M. Antunes JL. Ossifying fibroma of the parietal bone. Neurosurgery 1980; 7:513–516.

Stack JP et al. Gadolinium-DPTA as contrast agent in MRI of the brain. J Comput Assist Tomogr 1988; 12:698–701.

Suit HD, Goitein M, Munzenrider J, et al. Definitive radiation therapy for chordoma and chondrosarcoma of base of skull and cervical spine. J Neurosurg 1982; 56:377–385.

Svien HJ, Baker HL, Rivers MH: Jugular foramen syndrome and allied syndromes. Neurology 1963; 13:797–809.

Thomas JE, Yoss RE: The parasellar syndrome: problems in determining etiology. Mayo Clin Proc 1970; 45:617–623.

Vikram B, Chu FCH: Radiation therapy for metastases to the base of the skull. Radiology 1979; 130:465–468.

Winston K, Gilles FH, Leviton A, et al. Cerebellar gliomas in children. Natl Cancer Inst Monogr 1977; 58:833–838.

Yonas H, Jannetta PJ. Neurinoma of the trigeminal root and atypical trigeminal neuralgia: their commonality. Neurosurgery 1980; 6:273–277.

Young JL. Miller RW. Incidence of malignant tumors in U.S. children. J Pediatr 1975; 86:254–258.

Zinkham WH. Multifocal eosinophilic granuloma: natural history, etiology and management. Am J Med 1976; 60:457–463.

45. TUMORS OF THE MENINGES
Michael R. Fetell
Bennett M. Stein

Meningeal fibroblastomas, leptomeningiomas, arachnoid fibroblastomas, and dural endotheliomas all arise from the arachnoid cell clusters associated with the arachnoid villi or points of entry and exit of blood vessels and the cranial nerves through the dura. These tumors are discrete; they vary in size from that of a small pea to that of an orange, and are rarely multiple except in patients with von Recklinghausen's syndrome. They cause symptoms by compression. There is often a long history of seizures, with progressive neurologic symptoms and evidence of raised intracranial pressure. Meningiomas may invade the skull to cause hyperostosis, but only rarely violate the pia and invade the cortex. Recent cytogenetic studies show abnormalities of chromosome 22 meningioma tumor cells.

Pathology. Meningiomas are commonly round or nodular and well circumscribed, compressing and displacing adjacent portions of the nervous system. Occasionally, they form a diffuse sheet *(meningioma en plaque)*. Meningiomas are usually firm but may be soft or, rarely, cystic. The following characteristics are of clinical and surgical importance: they are encapsulated and may be nodular or smooth; they firmly attach to the adjacent dura and may involve bone; vascularity varies greatly as does the degree of edema around the tumor. Edema may be massive in some cases, although the tumor is small; the blood supply commonly arises from the dura and rarely comes from cerebral arteries. These tumors recur at a rate of 10%.

Tumor cells may be present within bone, but there is often no evidence of tumor cells within the hyperostotic area. The most common site of hyperostosis is in association with the parasagittal or sphenoid ridge meningiomas.

According to the microscopic characteristics of these tumors, five categories of meningioma may be designated: syncytial, transitional, fibrous, angioblastic, and malignant. Malignant tumors are defined by frequency of mitosis, invasion of the cortex, and distant metastases. The transitional form, composed of the characteristic whorls and psammoma bodies, may be combined with the syncytial type (composed of sheets of polygonal cells) to form the most common group of meningiomas. The angioblastic variety, histologically identical to the hemangioblastoma, has a higher rate of recurrence than other meningiomas. Because of this feature, it has been recommended that these meningiomas be radiated postoperatively.

Prevalence. Meningiomas account for approximately 15% of all intracranial tumors. They may occur at any age, but predominate in adults with a peak incidence among patients who are around age 45. They are more common (about 60% of all meningiomas) in women, and are rare in children, accounting for 1% of the intracranial tumors in patients younger than 20. In children, meningiomas usually occur in the posterior fossa and in-

Table 45–1. The Anatomic Distribution of Meningiomas

Site of Tumor	%
Parasagittal and falx	25
Convexity	20
Sphenoidal ridge	20
Olfactory groove	10
Suprasellar	10
Posterior fossa	10
Middle fossa	3
Intraventricular	2
Total	100

traventricular sites. In adults, most intracranial meningiomas are located in the parasagittal-falx region (Table 45–1 and Fig. 45–1). The convexity of the cerebral hemispheres (Fig. 45–2) and the sphenoid ridge are the next most common sites; the olfactory groove, suprasellar, posterior fossa, middle fossa, and intraventricular locations are of lesser frequency. Multiple meningiomas occur in fewer than 1% of cases; they usually occur in relation to other intracranial tumors or the von Recklinghausen syndrome.

Symptoms and Signs. The symptoms of meningiomas are similar to those of other intracranial tumors, but owing to the predilection for certain regions and the tendency to produce hyperostosis of the skull, they present special features that make it possible to diagnose their presence before operation.

Diagnosis. Despite the widespread use of CT, careful evaluation of the plain skull radiograph is still rewarding. These may show calcification within the tumor, hyperostosis, or blistering of the adjacent skull. Enlargement of the vascular channels over the vault of the skull is characteristic of convexity meningiomas, which are heavily supplied by the meningeal arteries. In 50 to 60% of the patients, the diagnosis may be suspected from the changes on plain skull radiographs. These tumors are radiographically calcified in about 10% of the cases.

CT is useful in identifying these tumors in the early stages or when the tumor has attained large size with minimal symptoms (Fig. 45–3). CT will almost certainly identify these tumors. They present as homogeneous, contrast-enhanced tumors with well-defined borders and often striking cerebral edema of the adjacent brain. Arteriography often precisely identifies the tumor as a meningioma because of the characteristic extracerebral arterial blood supply and a prolonged homo-

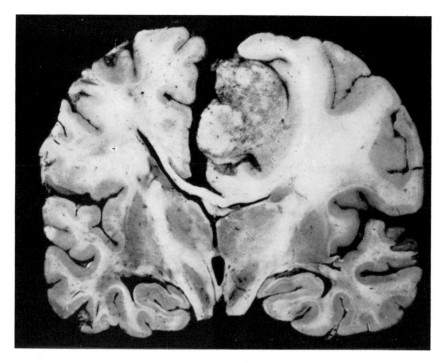

Fig. 45–1. Parasagittal meningioma. (Courtesy of Dr. Philip Duffy.)

geneous vascular stain that is seen well into the venous phase (Figs. 45–4 and 45–5). Because their water content is similar to that of brain, they may be difficult to identify with MRI scan, although their mass effect and displacement of brain provide a clue.

Clinical Course and Treatment. Although meningiomas may grow slowly, they grow at an inexorable pace and eventually attain large size and lead to death of the patient by compression of the cerebral tissue; nevertheless, small tumors may be found unexpectedly at autopsy. The enigma of these tumors is that, although they are benign and potentially curable, location and involvement of vital structures may make total removal impossible without unacceptable destruction of normal structures. Because of complicating factors such as location, involvement of vital structures, and extreme vascularity, the operative mortality may be as high as 5%. Attempts to reduce the vascularity of the tumor by ligation or direct embolization of feeding arteries has simplified surgical removal in some cases. Radiotherapy has been advocated for angioblastic or sarcomatous meningiomas and for those incompletely removed or persistently recurring meningiomas that spread or invade locally.

The overall percentage of recurrence of presumably removed tumors is approximately 10%; when the dural attachment is cauterized but not removed, 15%; and when a definite portion of the tumor remains, 39%. Despite these qualifications, the average interval for recurrence is five years. Surgical treatment of meningiomas is more uniformly successful than surgical treatment of any other brain tumor.

Sites of Meningiomas

Parasagittal Falx. This is the most common location for meningiomas. Hyperostosis frequently accompanies these tumors, but presents no major problem in surgical resection of the tumor. Falx tumors may be bilateral, but are usually asymmetric. These tumors frequently involve the sagittal sinus and the important cortical veins that drain into this sinus. Involvement of the sagittal sinus and its venous tributaries is the most important feature of these tumors. The middle and posterior thirds of the sinus, if involved but patent, cannot be sacrificed without severe neurologic sequelae; therefore, total resection of these tumors is often impossible and the recurrence rate from residual fragments is high.

Convexity. These tumors are usually concentrated around the coronal suture. Epilepsy and focal neurologic signs are common, whereas hyperostosis is uncommon. These

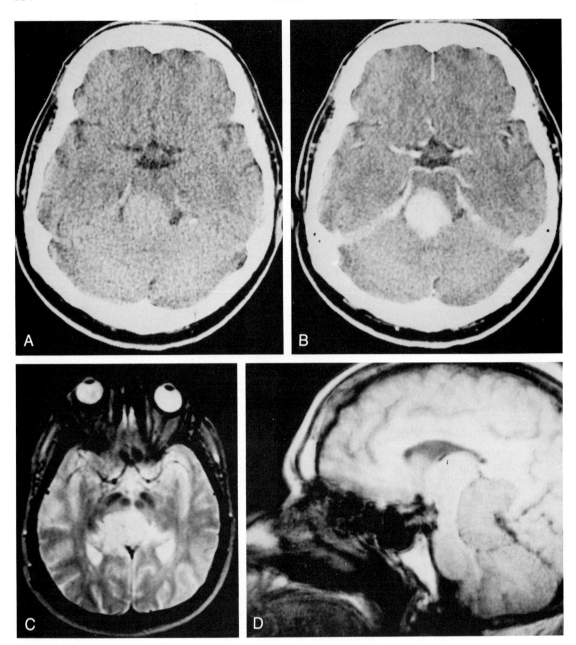

Fig. 45–2. Tentorial meningioma. *A,* Noncontrast and *B,* contrast-enhanced axial CT scans demonstrate a slightly dense mass precontrast with marked homogeneous enhancement. *C,* Axial T₂ weighted and *D,* sagittal T₁ weighted MRI scans depict its origin from the right tentorial incisura and demonstrate extra-axial mass effect on the midbrain. (Courtesy of Drs. J.A. Bello, T.L. Chi, and S.K. Hilal.)

tumors, although large, present little problem in removal.

Sphenoid Ridge. Tumors of this region have been divided into two categories: outer sphenoid ridge tumors and inner sphenoid ridge tumors. The outer sphenoid ridge (pterional type) tumor may be of the globoid or the en plaque variety. Outer sphenoid ridge tumors of the en plaque variety are seen most frequently in women. This location is associated with hyperostosis, seizures, unilateral exophthalmos, and extraocular movement disorders (if the superior orbital fissure is involved). These tumors are relatively easy to remove provided the infiltrated dura can be surgically resected.

Tumors of the inner sphenoid ridge (clinoidal type) create blistering or hyperostosis of the anterior clinoid and adjacent sphenoid wing. The optic nerve is often compressed or

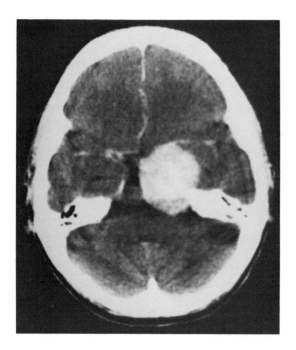

Fig. 45–3. CT scan showing a large tentorial meningioma with extension above and below the tentorium. Other than mild recent-memory loss, this patient was asymptomatic. The tumor was totally removed. (Courtesy of Dr. Bennett M. Stein.)

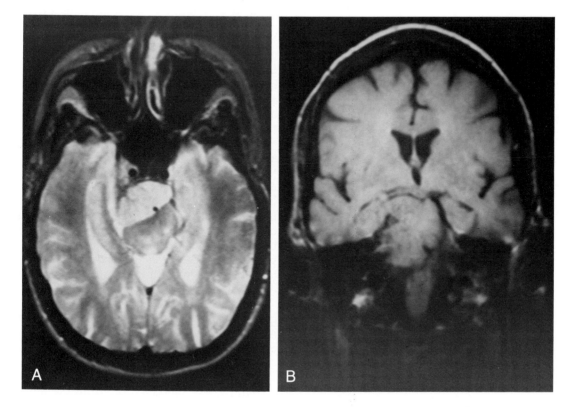

Fig. 45–4. Foramen magnum meningioma. A, An axial T_2-weighted MRI scan demonstrates a slightly hyperintense extra-axial lesion anterior to the brain stem and basilar artery, which are displaced posteriorly and to the left. B, A T_1-weighted coronal MRI scan again shows extra-axial mass effect on the brain stem and basilar artery. (Courtesy of Drs. T.L. Chi, J.A. Bello, and S.K. Hilal.)

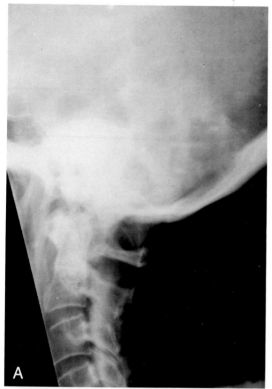

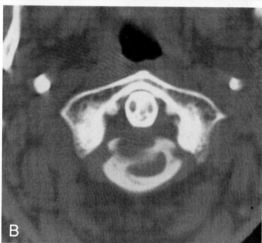

Fig. 45–5. Foramen magnum meningioma (different patient from Figure 45–4.) *A,* A lateral myelographic film shows widening of the gutter anterior to the upper cervical cord, which is displaced posteriorly at the C_1 level. *B,* An axial CT scan at the C_1-C_2 level demonstrates a dural-based intradural mass anterior to the cord, with cord displacement posteriorly and cord impingement, especially on the right. (Courtesy of Drs. T.L. Chi, J.A. Bello, and S.K. Hilal.)

surrounded early in the growth of these tumors, leading to unilateral visual failure and primary optic atrophy. Other symptoms and signs include unilateral exophthalmos, visual field defects, and oculomotor palsies if the superior orbital fissure is involved. Involvement of the ophthalmic branch of the trigeminal nerve may cause hypesthesia of the forehead. Encasement of the internal carotid artery is not only a major difficulty for the surgeon to overcome in resecting these tumors, but may lead to contralateral hemiparesis and other indirect effects by vascular compromise. If the tumor is large, ipsilateral optic atrophy may be associated with contralateral papilledema (Foster Kennedy syndrome). Because of the involvement of critical structures, total removal of these tumors may be impossible.

Olfactory Groove. These tumors arise from the cribriform and ethmoid regions. They may produce hyperostosis and may grow to a large size resulting in anosmia and visual loss due to involvement of both optic nerves and the chiasm. The Foster Kennedy syndrome may also be seen, and dementia may result from compression of the anterior cerebral arteries and frontal lobes.

Suprasellar. These tumors arise from the tuberculum sellae (which may be hyperostotic) or the diaphragm of the sella. The tuberculum origin gives rise to the characteristic arteriographic finding of enlarged penetrating branches of the ophthalmic artery that supply the base of the tumor. Vision fails early, with a classic bitemporal hemianopia that may be asymmetric. They are often mistaken for pituitary tumors or giant carotid artery aneurysms. It is difficult to preserve or improve the vision by the removal of these tumors because of the intimate involvement of the optic nerves. Involvement of the pituitary stalk may lead to diabetes insipidus pre- or postoperatively. In these tumors, arteriography is most important in differential diagnosis.

Posterior Fossa. These tumors arise frequently from the posterior surface of the petrous bone, clivus, the undersurface of the tentorium, the foramen magnum, or the convexity of the cerebellar hemispheres. When they arise from the tentorium, there is a characteristic blood supply from the tentorial arteries (i.e., branches of the internal carotid artery). Tentorial or convexity lesions may produce hydrocephalus and signs of raised intracranial pressure with or without indications of cerebellar dysfunction. Tentorial lesions also cause contralateral hemianopia. Tumors that arise from the petrous bone may involve the cranial nerves; in the cerebellopontine angle, they mimic acoustic nerve tumors. Those arising from the lowest portion of the clivus are the foramen magnum meningiomas, which cause a characteristic syndrome of cervical-occipital pain and signs of high spinal cord involvement with less obvious symptoms related to the lower cranial nerves and medulla. Meningiomas that arise from the base of the skull in the posterior fossa are extremely difficult to remove while sparing the cranial nerves and vertebral arteries that are often encased by these tumors. These tumors may go unrecognized for years because radiographic changes are minimal; the tumors may be large and extend over broad areas. They may also cause cerebellopontine angle syndromes, tic douloureux, or hemifacial spasm. Many tentorial meningiomas grow both above and below the tentorium to varying extent in either direction. The resulting signs include disorders of the midbrain, of the third, fourth, fifth, and sixth cranial nerves, and of the cerebellum. Total removal is achieved with difficulty and may require a transtentorial approach.

Intraventricular. These tumors arise wholly within the brain substance from the tela choroidea or choroid plexus of the cerebral fissures. The choroid plexus of the third and lateral ventricle is associated with a cerebral fissure and tela choroidea that contains arachnoidal membrane and, presumably, arachnoid cluster cells. These tumors occur most commonly in the atrium of the lateral ventricle, posterior third ventricle, and fourth ventricle. They are associated with longstanding intracranial pressure, focal ventricular dilatation and, occasionally, hemorrhage.

Primarily Intraorbital. These tumors are rare but critically important because they ensheath the optic nerve and are difficult to remove while preserving vision. They may also cause proptosis.

Extracranial or extradural meningiomas are rare. These apparently arise without dural attachment, and may be located in such uncharacteristic sites as the paranasal sinuses, temporal bones, and spinal region.

References

Adegbite AB, Khan MI, Paine KWE, Tan LK. The recurrence of intracranial meningiomas after surgical treatment. J Neurosurg 1983; 58:51–56.

Alvarez F, Roda JM, Perez-Romero M, et al. Malignant and atypical meningiomas: a reappraisal of clinical, histological, and computed tomographic features. Neurosurgery 1987; 20:688–694.

Barbaro NM, Gutin PH, Wilson CB, et al. Radiation therapy in the treatment of partially resected meningiomas. Neurosurgery 1987; 20:525–528.

Barrows HS, Harter DH. Tentorial meningiomas. J Neurol Neurosurg Psychiatry 1962; 25:40–44.

Castellano F, Ruggiero G. Meningiomas of the posterior fossa. Acta Radiol (Suppl) 1953; 104:1–177.

Crompton MR, Gautier-Smith PC. The prediction of recurrence in meningiomas. J Neurol Neurosurg Psychiatry 1970; 33:80–87.

Crouse SK, Berg BO. Intracranial meningiomas in childhood and adolescence. Neurology (Minneap.) 1972; 22:135–141.

Cushing H. The meningiomas arising from the olfactory groove and their removal by the aid of electrosurgery. Lancet 1927; 1:1329–1343.

DeBusshcher J, Van Renynghe de Voxrie G, Hoffman G. Meningiomas of the lateral recess. Acta Neurol Psychiat Belg 1957; 57:67–84.

Ellenberger C Jr. Perioptic meningiomas. Syndrome of long-standing visual loss, pale disk edema, and optociliary veins. Arch Neurol 1976; 33:671–674.

Guyer DR, Miller NR, Long DM, Allen GS. Visual function following optic canal decompression via craniotomy. J Neurosurg 1985; 62:631–638.

Hoessly GF, Olivercrona H. Report on 280 cases of verified parasagittal meningioma. J Neurosurg 1955; 12:614–626.

Kupersmith MJ, Warren FA, Newall J, et al. Irradiation of meningiomas of the intracranial anterior visual pathway. Ann Neurol 1987; 21:131–137.

Lisch KP, Gross S. Estrogen receptor immunoreactivity in meningiomas. Comparison with the binding activity of estrogen, progesterone, and androgen receptors. J Neurosurg 1987; 67:237–243.

Pitkethly DT, Hardman JM, Kempe LG, Earle KM. Angioblastic meningiomas: clinicopathologic study of 81 cases. J Neurosurg 1970; 32:539–544.

Quest DO. Meningiomas: An update. Neurosurgery 1978; 3:219–225.

Rosenstein J, Symon L. Surgical management of suprasellar meningioma. Part 2: prognosis for visual function following craniotomy. J Neurosurg 1984; 61:642–648.

Russell DS, Rubinstein LJ. Pathology of Tumours of the Nervous System, 3rd ed. Baltimore: Williams & Wilkins, 1972:48–73.

Sakaki S, Nakagawa K, Kimura H, et al. Intracranial meningiomas in infancy. Surg Neurol 1987; 28:51–57.

Seizinger BR, de la Monte S, Atkins L, et al. Molecular genetic approach to human meningioma: loss of genes on chromosome 22. Proc Natl Acad Sci USA 1987; 84:5419–5423.

Stein BM, Leeds NE, Taveras JM, Pool JL. Meningiomas of the foramen magnum. J Neurosurg 1963; 20:740–751.

Wara WM, Sheline GE, Newman H, Townsend JJ, Boldrey EB. Radiation therapy of meningiomas. AJR 1975; 123:453–458.

Wood MW, White RJ, Kernohan JW. One hundred intracranial meningiomas found incidentally at necropsy. J Neuropathol Exp Neurol 1957; 16:337–340.

46. GLIOMAS AND LYMPHOMAS
Michael R. Fetell

Gliomas

Gliomas arise from primitive forms of the glial cells and constitute nearly 60% of all intracranial tumors (Table 43–2).

There is considerable difference in the gross appearance of the various forms of gliomas. The slowly growing astrocytomas may appear firmer than the surrounding brain tissue, whereas the rapidly growing glioblastoma is soft, necrotic, and often hemorrhagic in appearance. In all forms of gliomas, there is usually no sharp dividing line between the tumor and the neighboring brain tissue. The tumor growth tends to follow fiber pathways and may spread through one entire hemisphere and across the corpus callosum into the other hemisphere. Necrosis with cyst formation is not rare. Small hemorrhages are common in the more malignant types, but large hemorrhages are rare.

A brief discussion of the more common forms of gliomas follows. It must be remembered that these tumors do not always occur in pure culture and that mixed or transitional forms are frequent.

Glioblastoma Multiforme and Other Malignant Gliomas

Between 11,000 and 17,000 new primary brain tumors are diagnosed each year in the United States. Of these, approximately half are malignant gliomas, tumors with a remarkably predictable but dismal prognosis. Despite improvements in diagnosis, surgery, radiotherapy, and chemotherapy, the prognosis has improved only slightly over the past two decades.

Tumor Biology. Tissue culture studies of malignant gliomas have routinely shown that these tumors are among the most heterogeneous of all human tumors. Furthermore, cell lines may show different cytogenetic abnormalities at different times. Most consistent abnormalities consist of changes on chromosomes 7, 10, and 22, but do not seem to carry prognostic significance. The *erb-b* oncogene that codes for the epidermal growth factor (EGF) receptor has been mapped to chromosome 7, and is amplified in one third of malignant gliomas. Similarly, the oncogene *sis* is located on chromosome 22 and codes for the platelet derived growth factor receptor (PDGF receptor). A recently described onco-gene, *gli*, has been identified in glioblastoma, and is localized on chromosome 12.

Attempts to use in vitro assays to predict chemosensitivity of malignant gliomas have been hampered by hetereogeneity in cell responsiveness. Tissue culture assays show 100% correlation with clinical resistance, but only 50 to 70% correlation with clinical sensitivity.

Classification. There are several classification schemes for malignant gliomas. The one advanced by Kernohan in 1949, rates gliomas from grade I to grade IV based upon pathologic findings of cellular anaplasia. Usually pathologists utilize a modification of this system that also considers necrosis and secondary changes of endothelial hyperplasia. Grade I and II gliomas are sometimes called "benign," a misnomer discussed under the section on Low-Grade Gliomas.

Glioblastomas (grade III and IV tumors in Kernohan's classification) are highly malignant tumors that generally occur in the cerebral hemispheres but may occur anywhere in the brain or spinal cord and may arise in the cerebellum, brain stem, or even optic chiasm. The classification scheme preferred by many neuropathologists today grades gliomas on a three-tiered scale with grade 1 representing a well-differentiated astrocytoma, grade 3 a glioblastoma, and grade 2 an intermediate tumor called an anaplastic astrocytoma. These two classification systems are *not* interchangeable, and a grade 2 glioma in this classification is closer to a grade III Kernohan tumor than to a grade II. The current trend is toward the three-tiered classification scheme because there is little prognostic distinction between grade III and IV tumors in Kernohan's scheme.

Regardless of the classification scheme, the presence of necrosis best predicts prognosis. Gliomas are often heterogeneous, and contain areas of varied pathologic grade, but prognosis is determined by the most malignant components. Surgical specimens, therefore, may not be representative of the true grade and spectrum of tumor malignancy. For example, the diagnosis of a grade I or II glioma in a patient with a rapidly growing neoplasm probably represents an error of sampling. Special staining techniques applied to small stereotactic needle biopsy specimens may permit identification of individual malignant cells, and suggest that the lucent region seen on CT surrounding the enhancing ring of a glioblastoma often contains malignant cells.

Clinical and Radiographic Features. The initial symptoms of a glioblastoma range from those as trivial as mild headache to the ominous signs of seizures, progressive hemiparesis, or aphasia. CT usually reveals a cerebral mass lesion with a zone of central lucency that represents necrosis, surrounded by variable degrees of edema (Fig. 46–1). Rarely, there may be little or no enhancement. MRI is more sensitive, but less specific, and does not differentiate tumor from peritumoral edema.

Treatment. Glioblastomas are rapidly growing tumors that recur despite all attempts at treatment, and eventually prove rapidly fatal. Numerous cooperative studies have shown that patients fare better when their age is 40 years or less, performance status (Karnofsky score) is good, and gross total resection of tumor has been performed. Overall, the survival of patients with glioblastoma with surgery alone is 14 weeks. With surgery plus radiotherapy, median survival increases to 40 weeks, justifying the time and effort involved in administering radiotherapy. Recent studies have shown that recurrence of tumor in almost all cases is within 2 cm of the original

tumor margins. These studies have permitted reduction in the total dose of whole brain radiation: 4,000 cGy is now given to the whole brain and 1,500 to 2,000 cGy to an extended local field of the tumor.

Adjuvant chemotherapy has been of modest benefit in increasing survival. In large cooperative trials of the Brain Tumor Cooperative Group (BTCG), median survival was minimally improved with nitrosoureas. An increase in 18-month survivors in the chemotherapy arm suggested that a subgroup of patients benefited from the nitrosoureas. Most recently, the BTCG compared intravenous 1,3-bis (2-chlorethyl)-1-nitrosourea (BCNU) with intra-arterial BCNU. The intra-arterial arm of the study was abandoned after it became apparent that survival was worse than in the intravenous arm, with several cases of irreversible encephalopathy and ipsilateral visual loss (retinal toxicity).

Disappointment with chemotherapy has led to newer strategies that include biologic modifiers such as interferons, interleukin-2, and the intracerebral administration of lymphokine-activated killer cells (LAK cells). Small tumors may be treated by implantation of high-energy radioactive seeds of iodine 125

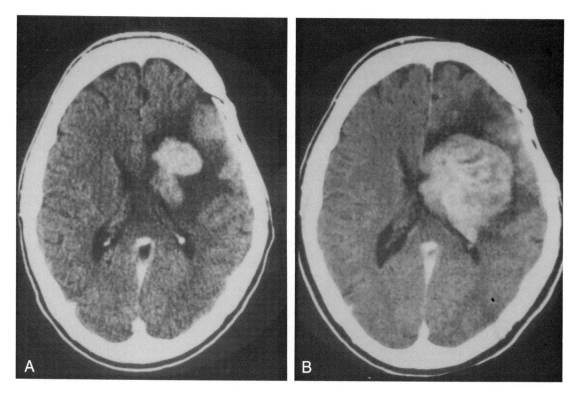

Fig. 46–1. Glioblastoma. Contrast-enhanced CT scans (*A* and *B*) of a patient with an extremely rapidly recurring left fronto-temporal glioblastoma. Note dramatic interval increase in tumor size from scan *A* to scan *B*, 8 weeks later.

or iridium 192, a procedure called interstitial brachytherapy. Hyperfractionation, the delivery of multiple doses of radiation per day, theoretically permits higher total tumor doses to be given without additional risk to normal tissue.

Meningeal Gliomatosis and Gliomatosis Cerebri

Meningeal gliomatosis refers to the dissemination of glial neoplasms throughout the CSF pathways in a pattern similar to that of meningeal carcinomatosis. In 1931, Cairns and Russell called attention to the high incidence of spinal seeding in cerebral gliomas at post mortem: 8 of 22 consecutive cases. The incidence of meningeal gliomatosis in patients with cerebral gliomas is not accurately known; estimates based upon clinical data are 5 to 10%. With CT and MRI, the detection rate may approach the figure of 20% seen at autopsy. Gliomatosis cerebri is sometimes used interchangeably with meningeal gliomatosis, but more accurately describes the rare syndrome of dramatic and diffuse white matter spread of glioma over wide areas of the cerebral hemispheres.

The clinical syndrome of meningeal gliomatosis is similar to that of meningeal carcinomatosis, with cranial neuropathies, radiculopathies, myelopathy, dementia, and hydrocephalus. The diagnosis should be considered when a patient with a cerebral glioma develops obstructive hydrocephalus or periependymal lesions on CT (Fig. 46–2C). Meningeal gliomatosis has been reported most often with hemispheric tumors, but also occurs with brain stem and spinal cord gliomas, and may rarely occur without an obvious parenchymal focus. Glioblastomas, oligodendrogliomas, and ependymomas may spread in this fashion. Diagnosis rests on recovery of malignant cells from CSF, and is accomplished in about two thirds of cases, less often than in meningeal carcinomatosis. The CSF formula may mimic inflammatory meningitis, but the most typical abnormality is an elevation of protein content, sometimes to more than 1.0 g/dl. Hypoglycorrhachia and pleocytosis are less common than in meningeal carcinomatosis, and malignant glial cells are difficult to identify on cytologic examination of CSF. Immunoperoxidase staining of CSF cytology specimens for glial fibrillary acidic protein (GFAP) permits identification of glial cells, but poorly differentiated tumors are less likely to produce GFAP, and detection of glial cells in CSF is not proof of malignant seeding.

There is no effective treatment for meningeal gliomatosis, and survival from time of diagnosis is usually only a few months. Palliative therapy includes radiotherapy to previously untreated sites of symptomatic disease. Intrathecal chemotherapy (methotrexate or cytosine arabinoside) has been tried in a few patients without apparent benefit.

Low-Grade Gliomas

Grade I and grade II gliomas in Kernohan's classification are considered low-grade tumors because they lack the malignant features of cellular anaplasia, mitosis, necrosis, and endothelial proliferation that characterize malignant gliomas. Sometimes "benign glioma" has been used to describe these tumors, but this term is misleading because, with few exceptions, low-grade gliomas eventually are fatal neoplasms.

Low-grade gliomas constitute one fourth to one third of all gliomas but, unlike malignant gliomas, their natural history is unknown. There is not a single prospective study from which one can obtain data on morbidity, mortality, incidence of malignant degeneration, or responsiveness to therapy (surgery or radiation). From retrospective studies (Laws, et al.), several prognostic factors have emerged: age is by far the most important variable with five-year survival of 83% for patients less than 20 years of age, 35% for those 20 to 49 years of age, and 12% for those older than 50 years of age. These data strongly support the concept that low-grade gliomas are tumors of childhood or, at the latest, young adulthood. Other factors that predict a better prognosis are total surgical resection (61% vs. 32% five-year survival) and lack of postoperative neurologic deficit or personality change (38 to 42% vs. 9 to 16% five-year survival). Combining favorable factors, one can find a subgroup with an 87% likelihood of surviving five years vs. 16% in the average case.

Several studies have addressed the issue of whether radiotherapy improves survival, but thus far the data are based upon retrospective analyses and the question is not settled. Tentative recommendations include high-dose radiation (5,500 to 6,000 cGy) for older patients, particularly when total resection is not achieved. Given the slow growth rate of low-grade gliomas, chemotherapy is not likely to be of benefit and is not advocated.

In contrast to low-grade gliomas of the cer-

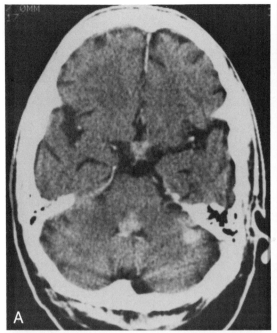

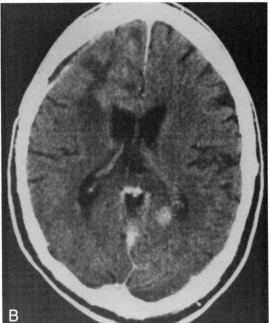

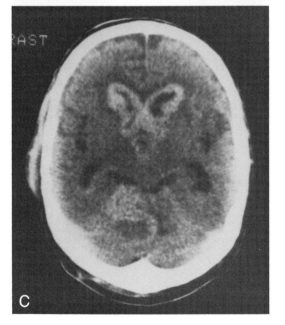

Fig. 46–2. Glioblastoma, meningeal seeding. *A,* An axial contrast-enhanced CT scan demonstrates abnormal enhancement in the suprasellar cistern, along the left tentorium and subependymal region of the fourth ventricle due to CSF seeding of tumor. *B,* A higher scan section from the same exam demonstrates persistent abnormal enhancement and mild mass effect at the primary site (right frontal), where a chronic postoperative extraaxial collection is also seen. Further subependymal seeding is evidenced by abnormal enhancement in the periatrial regions, especially on the left. *C.* In another patient, with a cerebellar glioblastoma, meningeal gliomatosis is demonstrated by contrast enhancement outlining the frontal horns and the right tentorium.

ebral hemispheres, those that occur in the cerebellum, particularly in childhood, have a favorable prognosis, and do not seem to require postoperative radiotherapy. They are often cystic with a mural nodule, but they may be solid, and they arise from either the vermis or the hemispheres. Astrocytomas that involve the wall of the third ventricle and hypothalamus are usually of the so-called "pilocytic" type and give rise to *hypothalamic syndromes* such as the one originally described

by *Fröhlich* (i.e., failure of sexual maturation and obesity), alterations of the sleep-wake cycle, poikilothermia, or autonomic disorders. The *diencephalic syndrome* is a distinct clinical entity that usually affects children who eat normally but become emaciated; they are usually alert and hyperactive, and endocrine studies are unrevealing. Patients with this syndrome who survive to adult years may become obese. Patients with tuberous sclerosis may develop a special variety of astrocytoma called *subependymal giant-cell astrocytoma*, which usually arises from the wall of the lateral ventricles and obstructs the foramen of Monro.

Treatment of these tumors includes a wide and, if possible, total surgical removal. This goal can be achieved in the majority of cerebellar tumors with a well-defined mural nodule and a cyst, permitting total excision.

Astrocytomas are also common in the optic nerve and brain stem. In these sites, the nuclei of the cells are likely to be elongated and arranged in parallel lines giving a palisade-like appearance (piloid astrocytoma).

Brain Stem Glioma

Infiltration of the brain stem by astrocytomas or other forms of glioma is most commonly seen in children or young adults, although it is not rare in middle-aged patients (Fig. 46–3). Brain stem gliomas account for about 16% of all brain tumors, and about 75% of all brain-stem tumors occur in patients younger than 20. Multiple cranial nerve palsies and signs of involvement of the long tracts in the brain stem are the characteristic clinical features. Increased intracranial pressure and papilledema develop when the aqueduct of Sylvius is occluded by the tumor or when the brain stem enlarges to a size sufficient to interfere with the drainage of the CSF. This stage is usually a late development and death may ensue before papilledema develops.

Any of the cranial nerve nuclei may be af-

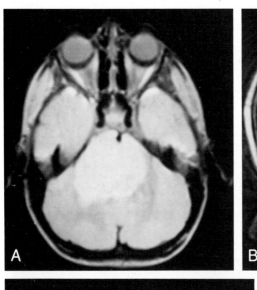

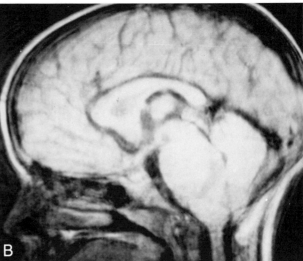

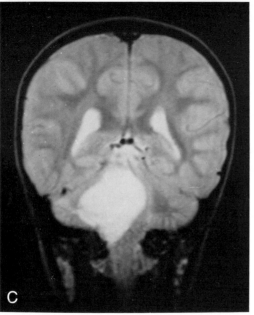

Fig. 46–3. Brain stem glioma. Axial *(A)* and sagittal *(B)* T_1 weighted MRI scans clearly demonstrate the intra-axial brain stem lesion with displacement of and slight mass effect on the fourth ventricle, but no evidence of hydrocephalus. *C,* On a coronal T_2 weighted image, the lesion has increased signal intensity, characteristic of glioma. (Courtesy of Drs. J.A. Bello and S.K. Hilal.)

fected, but unilateral or bilateral sixth nerve paralysis is the most common sign. Paralysis of the facial nerve, deafness, and palatal weakness (all usually unilateral) are the next most common symptoms. With growth of the tumor, there may be signs of involvement of the corticospinal tract, cerebellar peduncles, and spinal lemniscus. Gliomas may infiltrate the pons and destroy some nuclei and fiber paths while leaving others unaffected.

It is important to differentiate between gliomas of the brain stem and extramedullary tumors in the posterior fossa (e.g., neurofibromas, meningiomas, cysts), which are amenable to therapy. Some clinical points that are of value in localizing the lesion within the brain stem are: (1) the young age of the patient; (2) paralysis of conjugate gaze rather than simple paralysis of one external rectus muscle; (3) signs of injury to the long tracts before the appearance of papilledema; and (4) signs that rarely result from compression of the brain stem (i.e., Horner syndrome, vertical nystagmus, singultus). The diagnosis of intrapontine glioma can usually be established by demonstration of enlargement of the pons in CT.

Surgery is not indicated for these tumors, except for the rare cystic or exophytic tumor or for confirmation of the diagnosis. Radiation therapy has a palliatve effect, with a median survival period ranging from 5 to 47 months in different series. The role of chemotherapy in the management of these tumors is still unclear.

Oligodendrogliomas

Oligodendrogliomas are tumors derived from the oligodendroglia. They represent about 5% of all gliomas, and are found chiefly in the cerebral hemisphere (particularly in the frontal lobes) of young adults. They are firm in consistency and may appear well circumscribed. Areas of hemorrhage and cystic degeneration are uncommon; however, calcification is present in more than 50% of the patients. Microscopically, the tumor consists of many cells that are uniform in size and shape, evenly spaced, or in a loose meshwork. Cells have large rounded nuclei that are rich in chromatin with a faint halo of cytoplasm.

The effect of these tumors is somewhat unpredictable, and does not always correlate with the histologic appearance. It is not unusual for patients to have clinical symptoms, particularly seizures, for many years before the presence of a mass lesion becomes obvious. In contrast, these tumors may have a malignant course, with local or even systemic dissemination. Surgical excision followed by radiotherapy is the treatment of choice.

Gliomas of the Optic Nerve

Gliomas of the optic nerve constitute about 2% of all intracranial gliomas in adults, and about 7% of all intracranial gliomas in children. Patients with neurofibromatosis have a 25% incidence of these tumors. The tumor usually involves a single nerve. In about 70% of the patients without neurofibromatosis, the tumor involves the optic chiasm. More rarely, optic nerve gliomas have a multicentric origin, which is usually associated with neurofibromatosis. Histologically, optic nerve gliomas are highly differentiated astrocytomas. They seldom have malignant characteristics, invading the hypothalamus and causing hydrocephalus.

Clinically, these tumors cause impairment of vision either as monocular loss of vision or, when the chiasm is involved, as a depression or a scotoma of the central fields. Gliosis of the head of the optic nerve and proptosis are common findings. In young children, strabismus or oscillatory nystagmus is a frequent initial manifestation. These tumors may also grow into the suprasellar region, causing neuroendocrine dysfunction and hydrocephalus.

The radiographic diagnosis is based on the demonstration of an enlarged and rounded

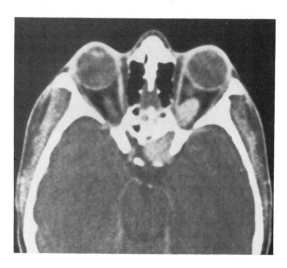

Fig. 46–4. Contrast CT. Optic nerve glioma is seen as an enhancing lesion that extends from the orbit, through the optic foramen, and into the suprasellar space. (Courtesy of Drs. S.K. Hilal and S.R. Ganti.)

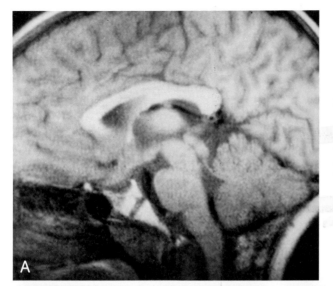

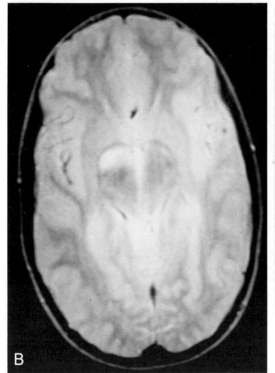

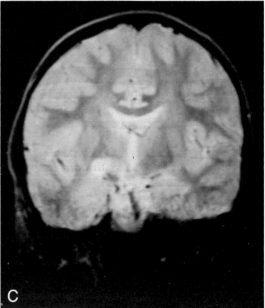

Fig. 46–5. *A,* Optic chiasm and optic tract glioma. Sagittal T_1 weighted MRI demonstrates soft tissue infiltration of the optic chiasm extending back along the right optic tract, representing extension of the tumor. Axial *(B)* and coronal *(C)* T_2 weighted MRI scans demonstrate extension of the chiasm lesion along the right optic tract. (Courtesy of Drs. T.L. Chi, J.A. Bello, and S.K. Hilal.)

optic foramen (Fig. 46–4), and occasional deformity of the sella turcica (Fig. 46–5). CT and MRI are the crucial diagnostic techniques.

In patients with visual impairment and disfiguring proptosis, surgical excision from the globe to the chiasm is the treatment of choice. When the chiasm is involved, radiotherapy is indicated.

Medulloblastomas

Medulloblastomas constitute 5 to 10% of intracranial gliomas, and 25 to 40% of all posterior fossa tumors. In 75% of the cases, the patients are under 16 years of age. These primitive tumors arise from the neuroepithelial roof of the fourth ventricle, which later forms the fetal external granular layer. In children, they are more commonly located in the midline, arising from the posterior vermis, occupying the fourth ventricle and invading adjacent structures. In adults, these tumors are frequently seen in the cerebellar hemispheres, sometimes reaching the surface.

Macroscopically, they are usually soft, reddish or grayish, sometimes with areas of necrosis, hemorrhage, or cystic degeneration. The hemispheric lesions are tougher in consistency, and may appear to be well circumscribed. Microscopically, they are cellular tumors. The cells have an ill-defined cytoplasm and hyperchromatic nucleus, and are arranged in the so-called "pseudorosettes." When the tumor reaches the leptomeninges, it usually stimulates proliferation of connective tissue. This desmoplastic variety of medulloblastomas has been called a cerebellar sarcoma. In addition, these tumors frequently disseminate through the CSF pathways, both around the brain and spinal cord or, rarely, outside the neuraxis (particularly in the bone marrow).

Medulloblastomas present clinically with a combination of signs and symptoms of increased intracranial pressure and cerebellar dysfunction, particularly ataxia. CT has become crucial for diagnosis of these tumors, which appear as hyperdense, usually homogeneous masses that enhance with contrast.

The treatment of choice is wide resection followed by radiotherapy, which should include the whole brain and spinal axis, with an added booster dose to the posterior fossa. The five-year-survival rate is now about 60%. In patients with advanced tumors (particularly with metastatic spread), chemotherapy (usually a combination of procarbazine, CCNU, and vincristine) may be of help. CSF shunting procedures are sometimes necessary for treatment of the hydrocephalus often associated with these lesions; however, these procedures may also lead to the dissemination of the tumor. In long-term survivors, the deleterious effects of comprehensive radiotherapy are unfortunately evident in a large proportion of patients. This finding has stimulated a search for better programs of chemotherapy as primary treatment, especially in patients five years of age and younger.

Ependymoma

Ependymomas derive from the ependymal glia and occur near the walls of the ventricles. They represent about 3% of all gliomas and 10% of all intracranial neoplasms in children. They are more commonly seen in the fourth ventricle, frequently arising from the floor and compressing the dorsum of the medulla. Ependymomas are grayish, granular, and moderately vascular, sometimes with small areas of calcification or cystic degeneration

(Fig. 46–6). Microscopically, they are composed of polyhedral or fusiform cells arranged in typical rosettes. The cells frequently contain cilia and blepharoplasts. Tumors that originate in the filum terminale sometimes have a distinct histologic appearance (i.e., myxopapillary ependymomas). In 15% of the cases, these tumors have more malignant characteristics and are called "ependymoblastomas." Spreading through the CSF pathways is not uncommon. The clinical presentation of ependymomas of the fourth ventricle is similar to that of the medulloblastomas. They frequently obstruct the CSF pathways and may cause focal symptoms.

The treatment of choice is surgical excision followed by radiotherapy. The five-year-survival rate is between 30% and 40%.

Primary and Secondary Lymphomas of the Central Nervous System

Lymphoma usually affects the nervous system by metastatic spread, but may (rarely) originate in the brain, spinal cord, or meninges. There are six major pathologic classification schemes for lymphomas, and an attempt to reconcile these has led to the Working Formulation. On histologic grounds, most CNS lymphomas seem to be diffuse, undifferentiated, large-cell, or immunoblastic, according to the individual classification scheme used. Analysis of lymphocyte surface immunoglobulins has led to a more functional classification. In addition, through DNA hybridization techniques, it is possible to determine whether a population of lymphocytes is mono- or polyclonal to distinguish a lymphoma from a reactive process. These CNS tumors are rare and it is difficult to obtain fresh tissue for analysis, so surface markers and DNA analysis are still lacking for CNS lymphomas.

The clinical signs and symptoms of primary and metastatic CNS lymphomas are identical. They resemble those of other space-occupying lesions, namely headache, vomiting, mental changes, papilledema, and hemiparesis. However, seizures are conspicuously less frequent than in patients with glial tumors. An important syndrome that may call attention to a primary CNS lymphoma (PCNSL) is uveitis, which results from contiguous spread of tumor directly from the brain along the uveal tract into the eye. In those cases diagnosis can be made by vitreous biopsy.

The radiographic appearance of CNS lym-

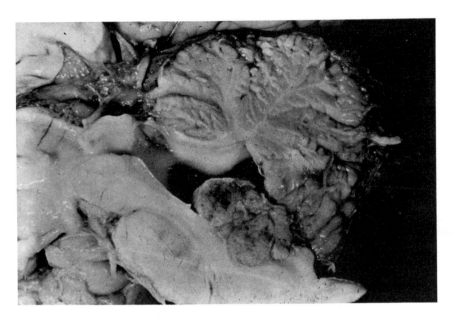

Fig. 46–6. Ependymoma of the fourth ventricle. (Courtesy of Dr. J. Kepes.)

phoma is not specific, but may be suggested by CT features. The tumor most often is hypodense, but may be iso- or hyperdense (Fig. 46–7A). Usually located in the white matter near the ventricles, PCNSL almost always enhances in contrast studies (Figs. 46–7B and C). The frontal lobes and vermis of the cerebellum are sites of predilection. The tumor may show evidence of spread through the white matter tracts such as the corpus callosum, or through the CSF pathways with diffuse periependymal or intraventricular enhancement. A pattern of mirror-image bilateral enhancing lesions of the basal ganglia is said to be pathognomonic. The border of the tumor with adjacent brain is fuzzy, rather than sharp as with metastatic tumors, and peritumor edema and mass effect are less prominent.

Angiography generally reveals an avascular mass; subtraction films are needed to demonstrate a blush that is never prominent. MRI may disclose more extensive tumor spread or multifocal lesions, but is not more specific than CT.

Spinal seeding, when present, is best visualized by myelography and may be difficult to diagnose because lymphocytic tumor cells are often interpreted as being "reactive." Proof of malignancy may be obtained by analysis of lymphocyte surface immunoglobulin or CSF electrophoresis. Patients with primary or metastatic CNS lymphomas are at risk for opportunistic infections, and it is critical to differentiate lymphomatous from infectious meningitis. A monoclonal population of B cells in CSF in a patient with lymphoma and proven cryptococcal meningitis implies that the patient has coexistent meningeal lymphoma. In contrast, reactive pleocytosis is characterized by polyclonal increase in lymphocytes with predominantly T cells. A monoclonal CSF immunoglobulin spike, seen in less than 50% of cases, is diagnostic of CNS lymphoma. Beta$_2$ microglobulin, a protein elevated in the serum of most patients with lymphoma, is usually elevated in the CSF in meningeal lymphoma, but this is a nonspecific marker and it may be falsely elevated in infectious meningitis.

SYSTEMIC LYMPHOMA

Overall, spread to the CNS occurs in about 10% of patients with systemic lymphoma, and is present at the time of original diagnosis in about 1%. In most cases, metastatic non-Hodgkin lymphoma (NHL) takes the form of meningeal lymphoma (45%) or epidural spinal cord compression (40%). Parenchymal brain metastases are less common but are found in 15% of patients with NHL.

In Hodgkin disease (HD), the pattern is different. Both epidural cord compression and meningeal lymphoma occur commonly, but intracerebral metastasis is rare, affecting 0.5% of patients (42 documented cases in the literature). Thus, an intracerebral CT-enhanc-

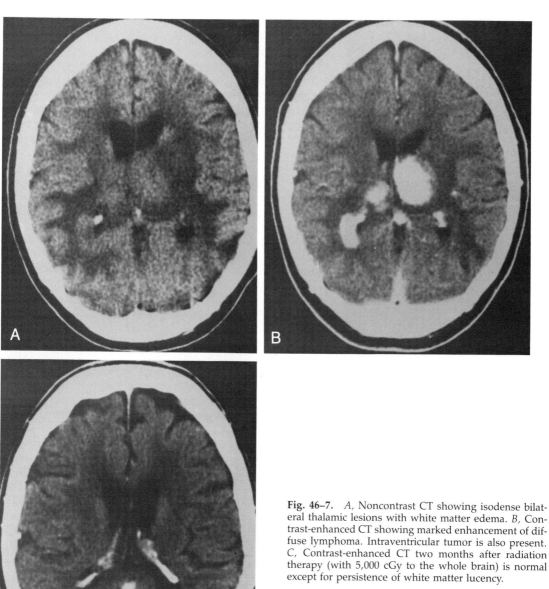

Fig. 46–7. *A,* Noncontrast CT showing isodense bilateral thalamic lesions with white matter edema. *B,* Contrast-enhanced CT showing marked enhancement of diffuse lymphoma. Intraventricular tumor is also present. *C,* Contrast-enhanced CT two months after radiation therapy (with 5,000 cGy to the whole brain) is normal except for persistence of white matter lucency.

ing lesion in a patient with HD is more likely to be infection than tumor.

Nervous system involvement in lymphomas in 95% of cases occurs with uncontrolled or relapsing systemic disease. Bone marrow lymphoma is a strong predisposing factor for CNS spread; lymphoma cells are found in

bone marrow in 66% of cases during life and 100% at autopsy. Diffuse histologic types of NHL carry increased risk, and nodular lymphomas usually convert to diffuse histology before the CNS is involved. Because of the high incidence of meningeal involvement in acute T-cell lymphoma (40%) and Burkitt lymphoma (50%), treatment includes prophylactic intrathecal chemotherapy with cytosine arabinoside or methotrexate.

PRIMARY CNS LYMPHOMA (PCNSL)

Primary CNS lymphomas constitute fewer than 1% of all intracranial tumors, 0.7% of all malignant lymphomas, and 1.6% of extranodal malignant lymphomas. These unusual tumors apparently arise in the CNS. Most cases affect the cerebral hemispheres, but some are found in the cerebellum, brain stem, spinal cord, or even meninges. In 1929, Bailey originated the term *perithelial small cell sarcoma*, and subsequent terminology has included *microglioma* and *reticulum cell sarcoma*, to reflect the suspected cell of origin. Current pathologic data point to a lymphocyte origin. Typically, the tumor is classified as a diffuse histiocytic lymphoma under the Rappaport scheme or as a large cell or immunoblastic lymphoma under the Working Formulation. Marker studies have identified many primary CNS lymphomas as B cell in origin based on surface or intracytoplasmic immunoglobulins. The male/female ratio is 1.5/1 and the peak incidence is in the fifth and sixth decades. Although CSF pleocytosis is seen in 50% of cases, seeding is documented in fewer than 25%. Extraneural dissemination, usually after a prolonged CNS illness, occurs in 11 to 27% of patients.

PRIMARY CNS LYMPHOMA AND IMMUNODEFICIENCY STATES

Nodal and, especially, extranodal lymphomas are often found in states of immunosuppression. In the general population, 3 to 4% of all malignant tumors are lymphomas. In contrast, lymphomas have accounted for 29% of all tumors seen by the Denver Transplant Tumor Registry, and 58% of tumors in patients with 14 types of naturally occurring immunodeficiency studied by the Immunodeficiency Cancer Registry. Most of these are NHL, but ataxia telangiectasia is associated with HD as well as NHL. HD is rare in allograft recipients.

Fewer than 2% of naturally occurring lymphomas involve the CNS, but in the Denver Transplant Tumor Registry, 28% were primary CNS lymphomas. One to two percent of renal transplant patients develop PCNSL, an estimated risk *100 times* that of the general population. In addition to renal allograft recipients, liver and cardiac transplant patients show increased susceptibility as do patients with immune deficiency associated with ataxia telangiectasia, Wiskott-Aldrich syndrome, agammaglobulinemia, or iatrogenic immunosuppression. In patients with AIDS, the risk is not clearly defined, but is estimated to be at least 1.5%. Patients receiving immunosuppressive therapy for autoimmune disease and patients receiving chemotherapy are at increased risk of systemic malignancy (particularly leukemia), but not PCNSL.

Malignant lymphomas in transplant patients have been attributed to infection with Epstein-Barr virus (EBV). EBV infection causes polyclonal proliferation of lymphocytes, and DNA hybridization studies in transplant recipients indicate that they begin as multiclonal, not monoclonal, lymphoid proliferation. Regression of systemic lymphomas in transplant recipients may follow reduction in immunosuppressive therapy or addition of antiviral therapy such as acyclovir administration. Through use of an EBV DNA probe, one primary CNS lymphoma in a patient with AIDS was found to contain 30 to 100 copies of the EBV genome per cell, suggesting an etiologic role in the genesis of that neoplasm. Several nonimmunosuppressed patients with primary CNS lymphomas showed high titers of serum antibody to EBV, and an increased number of copies of the EBV DNA was found in the tumor of one patient, suggesting that EBV may play an etiologic role even in non-immunosuppressed cases. Immunosuppression may lead to undue susceptibility to EBV infection that, in turn, results in a state of chronic lymphocyte stimulation and the induction of proliferating lymphocyte clones. Presumably, one or more clones eventually becomes autonomous.

The predilection for extranodal sites and, particularly, the CNS is unexplained, although the immunologic "sanctuary" status of the CNS may play a role. The incidence of Burkitt lymphoma, a malignant tumor clearly linked to EBV infection in Africans, is also increased in patients with AIDS. Burkitt lymphoma shows the highest predilection for CNS spread of any lymphoma; up to 50% of patients are affected. In addition to HIV, another virus, human B-lymphotropic virus (HBLV), has been implicated in the causation of B-cell lymphomas.

In 1986, for the first time, CNS lymphomas in patients with iatrogenic or acquired immunosuppression exceeded sporadic cases. Although radiographically and pathologically identical, tumors associated with immunosuppression are more aggressive and less likely to respond to therapy. In one series, all patients died within two months of diagnosis. Toxoplasma gondii brain abscess simulates CNS lymphoma on CT and is the most important differential diagnosis in patients with AIDS. Toxoplasmosis usually responds to appropriate antibiotic therapy and, when biopsy is impracticable, an empiric trial of therapy with pyremethamine and sulfonamides is warranted.

Treatment. There is no justification to perform subtotal or "total" resection of a CNS tumor known to be a lymphoma; stereotactic biopsy suffices in most cases. The margins of the tumor are ill-defined and there is no evidence that radical resection improves survival. Treatment of parenchymal lesions of malignant lymphoma, primary or metastatic, includes radiotherapy. A good case can be made for whole-brain radiotherapy because of the high incidence of multicentric lesions and seeding. Doses larger than 5,000 cGy have improved survival. Use of spinal radiotherapy is debatable because it suppresses bone marrow and reduces subsequent tolerance to chemotherapy. In all cases, CSF should be examined for evidence of spinal seeding, and patients with spinal symptoms should have a myelogram. If bulky spinal metastases are documented, spinal radiotherapy is added to the regimen.

Systemic chemotherapy with high-dose methotrexate or cytosine arabinoside may induce remissions in nonimmunosuppressed patients. However, experience with chemotherapy is limited to anecdotal reports or small uncontrolled series. In immunosuppressed patients, a reduction in dosage of immunosuppressive drugs may also be beneficial.

Although most primary CNS lymphomas respond to radiation, the tumors recur. Overall survival is only slightly better than in glioblastoma, with a mean survival of 13.5 months. Some patients survive (8% live more than three years, 3% live more than five years), but no criteria identify these patients in advance. Even in the long-term survivors, the incidence of relapse approaches 50%. Survival of patients with metastatic CNS lymphoma is closely linked to their overall status; 80% of patients die with progressive systemic disease.

Meningeal lymphoma is treated with intrathecal chemotherapy, either methotrexate or cytosine arabinoside, optimally adminis-

tered with an intraventricular Ommaya reservoir. Survival from time of diagnosis varies from several weeks to over one year, and some patients (e.g., those with childhood Burkitt lymphoma) may be cured.

INTRAVASCULAR LYMPHOMA (MALIGNANT ANGIOENDOTHELIOMATOSIS)

The origin of this unique and unusual disorder has only recently been clarified. Initially, the syndrome was thought to arise from tumor emboli diffusely distributed throughout the vascular system with a predilection for the cerebral vessels. The typical presentation is a middle-aged patient with multiple embolic strokes or rapidly progressive dementia. Half of the patients with this acute and fatal form of the disorder have cutaneous involvement. Many patients have systemic symptoms of fever and weight loss, and the ESR may be elevated, simulating subacute bacterial endocarditis or systemic vasculitis. CT reveals multiple cerebral infarctions, and CSF protein may be elevated with a modest mononuclear pleocytosis. The bone marrow is normal. Survival averages less than one year (the longest survival has been 22 months) despite all forms of therapy. One patient responded transiently to corticosteroids, and one remitted spontaneously. A mild self-limited, chronic, cutaneous form of the disorder has also been described.

Pathologically there is plugging of blood vessels by abnormal neoplastic cells that originally appeared to be of endothelial origin because of their light and electron microscopic features and positive immunoperoxidase staining for factor VIII. However, on closer examination the neoplastic cells more closely resemble activated or transformed lymphocytes, and the syndrome is now believed to be caused by an angiotropic large cell lymphoma. Positive factor VIII immunostaining is probably spurious, owing to reactive hyperplasia of adjacent endothelial cells, because staining of the intraluminal neoplastic cells is negative. Furthermore, in a few cases analysis of surface antigens has shown that the neoplastic lymphocytes express B- or T-cell antigens and are strongly positive for common leukocyte antigen. This form of lymphoma may have particular surface features that promote binding to endothelium, because the usual sites of involvement by lymphoma, lymph nodes, and bone marrow are spared, whereas skin and central nervous system are preferentially involved.

Primitive Neuroectodermal Tumors

The term primitive neuroectodermal tumor (PNET) was originally used by Hart and Earle to describe a highly malignant cerebral hemisphere tumor with undifferentiated cells occurring in children and young adults. The tumor, composed of cells with high mitotic activity, spreads in the CSF and (less often) extraneurally, and has a poor prognosis. Survival, even with surgery, radiation, and chemotherapy, is approximately 24 months. Approximately 50 such cases have been recognized.

More recently, PNET has been used in a generic sense to refer to CNS tumors with common pathologic features that suggest origin from primitive neuroectodermal cells. Differentiation may occur along glial or neuronal lines. Medulloblastoma, retinoblastoma, pineoblastoma, neuroblastoma, olfactory neuroblastoma, medulloepithelioma, ependymoblastoma, and polar spongioblastoma are included in this category. Rorke advocates abandoning these names and describing all tumors according to their location and type of differentiation. However, the names are so well known and recognizable that they remain useful. The hemispheric PNET of Hart and Earle would be classified as an undifferentiated PNET of the cerebrum.

Retinoblastoma is a PNET of childhood that may occur in families as a bilateral retinal tumor, sometimes associated with a pineal tumor as well. The predisposition for retinoblastoma has been mapped to a single locus on chromosome 13. Elegant molecular biological studies suggest that the defective gene leads to loss of function of an "antioncogene" or "tumor-suppressing" gene.

PNETs are distinguished by the uniform undifferentiated microscopic appearance of the tumor. More than 90% of the cells are small and darkly staining without characteristic features. Fetal neuroepithelial cells or matrix cells give rise to neurons, neuroglia, and subependymal and ependymal cells, and the matrix cells aggregate and proliferate in the subependymal plate region of the cerebellum. This location is the presumed site of origin of meulloblastomas.

Clinically, almost all PNETs, except those with gangliogliomatous differentiation, and the esthesioneuroblastoma, behave in a similar fashion. They are highly malignant tumors of presumed embryonal origin. Collin's rule, that patients surviving for a period of time equal to age at diagnosis plus nine months can be considered cured, was originally formulated for Wilms tumors, but seems to be valid for medulloblastoma as well. Only 2% of reported cases violate the rule. These tumors spread diffusely in the brain, and cannot be totally resected. PNETs respond to high doses of radiotherapy (5,000+ cGy), but tend to recur at the primary site. Seeding of the CSF is common with all PNETs and may be present at the time of initial diagnosis. Extraneural metastases occur more commonly than with any other primary CNS tumor, with bone, lymph nodes, liver, and lung the principal target sites. Chemotherapy is essential for patients with extraneural metastases, recurrent primary tumors, and higher-stage lesions. Numerous chemotherapeutic regimens have been effective in inducing remission in recurrent disease, but the remissions are not durable.

Predictors of a good prognosis are: limited local disease, gross total resection, surgical management without permanent shunt, negative postoperative evaluation for metastases, and irradiation with at least 5,000 cGy.

MEDULLOBLASTOMA

Medulloblastoma, the most common PNET, accounts for more than 25% of all childhood brain tumors. It is considered an undifferentiated PNET arising from the matrix cell layer of the cerebellum in the roof of the fourth ventricle. This hypothesis is in good accord with the observation that childhood medulloblastomas occur in the midline, and that more laterally placed tumors occur with increased age of onset. The pathogenesis of PNETs is unknown, and the significance of neuronal or astrocytic differentiation noted in some medulloblastomas remains debatable; it does not seem to alter prognosis.

Pineoblastoma is discussed in Section 47, Pineal Tumors.

References

Allen JC, Epstein F. Medulloblastoma and other primary malignant neuroectodermal tumors of the CNS. J Neurosurg 1982; 57:446–451.

Alvord EC, Jr, Lofton S. Gliomas of the optic nerve or chiasm. J Neurosurg 1988; 68:85–98.

Andrews AA, Enriques L, Renaudin J, et al. Spinal intramedullary glioblastoma with intracranial seeding. Arch Neurol 1978; 35:244–245.

Awad I, Bay JW, Rogers L. Leptomeningeal metastasis from supratentorial malignant gliomas. Neurosurgery 1986; 19:247–251.

Bader JL, Meadows AT, Zimmerman LE, et al. Bilateral retinoblastoma with ectopic intracranial retinoblastoma: trilateral retinoblastoma. Cancer Genet Cytogenet 1982; 5:203–213.

Bailey P, Cushing H. A Classification of the Tumors of the Glioma Group on a Histogenetic Basis with a Correlated Study of Prognosis. Philadelphia: JB Lippincott, 1926.

Bailey P, Robitaille Y. Primary diffuse leptomeningeal gliomatosis. Can J Neurol Sci 1985; 12:278–281.

Barone BM, Elvidge AR. Ependymomas. A clinical survey. J Neurosurg 1970; 33:428–438.

Bebin J, Tytus JS. Gliomatosis cerebri. Case report. Neurology 1956; 6:815–822.

Becker LE, Hinton K. Primitive neuroectodermal tumors of the central nervous system. Hum Pathol 1983; 14:538–550.

Berger PC, Dubois PJ, Schold SC, Smith KR, Odom GL, Crafts, DC, Giangaspero F. Computerized tomographic and pathologic studies of the untreated, quiescent, and recurrent glioblastoma multiforme. J Neurosurg 1983; 58:159–169.

Bernat JL. Glioblastoma multiforme and the meningeal syndrome. Neurology 1976; 26:1071–1074.

Berry MP, Jenkin RD, Keen CW, et al. Radiation therapy for medulloblastoma. J Neurosurg 1981; 55:43–51.

Bucy PC, Thieman PW. Astrocytomas of the cerebellum. Arch Neurol 1968; 18:14–19.

Burger PC. Malignant astrocytic neoplasms: classification, pathology, anatomy, and response to treatment. Semin Oncol 1986; 13:16–25.

Burger PC, Dubois PJ, Schold C Jr, et al. Computerized tomographic and pathologic studies of the untreated, quiescent, and recurrent glioblastoma multiforme. J Neurosurg 1983; 58:159–169.

Cairns H, Russell DS: Intracranial and spinal metastases in gliomas of the brain. Brain 1931; 54:377–419.

Carmel PW. Surgical syndromes of the hypothalamus. Clin Neurosurg 1980; 27:133–159.

Chang CH, Housepian EM. Tumors of the Central Nervous System: Modern Radiotherapy in Multidisciplinary Management. New York: Masson, 1982.

Chin HW, Hazel JJ, Kim TH, Webster JH. Oligodendrogliomas. I. A clinical study of cerebral oligodendrogliomas. Cancer 1980; 45:1458–1466.

Chutorian AM, Schwarz JF, Evans RA, Carter S. Optic gliomas in children. Neurology 1964; 14:83–95.

Civitello LA, Packer RJ, Roke LR, et al. Leptomeningeal dissemination of low-grade gliomas in childhood. Neurology 1988; 38:562–566.

Couch JR, Weiss SA. Gliomatosis cerebri. Neurology 1974; 24:504–511.

Daumas-Duport C, Scheithauer BW, Kelly PJ. A histologic and cytologic method for the spatial definition of gliomas. Mayo Clin Proc 1987; 62:435–449.

De La Monte, SM, Moore GW, Hutchins GM: Nonrandom distribution of metastases in neuroblastic tumors. Cancer 1983; 52:915–925.

Dohrmann GJ, Farwell JR, Flannery JT. Ependymomas and ependymoblastomas in children. J Neurosurg 1976; 45:273–283.

Duffner PK, Cohen ME, Heffner RR, et al. Primitive neuroectodermal tumors of childhood. J Neurosurg. 1981; 55:376–381.

Erlich SS, Davis RL. Spinal subarachnoid metastasis from primary intracranial glioblastoma multiforme. Cancer 1978; 42:2854–2864.

Farwell JR, Dohrmann GJ, Flannery JT. Medulloblastoma in childhood: an epidemiological study. J Neurosurg 1984; 61:657–664.

Friend SH, Dryja TP, Weinberg R: Oncogenes and tumor-suppressing genes. NEJM 1988; 318:618–622.

Fulton DS, Levin VA, Wara WM, Edwards MS, Wilson CB. Chemotherapy of pediatric brain-stem tumors. J Neurosurg 1981; 54:721–725.

Glasauer FE, Yuan RHP. Intracranial tumors with extracranial metastases. J Neurosurg 1963; 20:474–493.

Gutin PH, Phillips TL, Hosobuchi Y, et al. Permanent and removable implants for the brachytherapy of brain tumors. Int J Radiat Oncol Biol Phys 1981; 7:1371–1381.

Gutin PH, Phillips TL, Wara WM, et al. Brachytherapy of recurrent malignant brain tumors with removable high-activity iodine-125 sources. J Neurosurg 1984; 60:61–68.

Hart MN, Earle KM. Primitive neuroectodermal tumors of the central nervous system in children. Cancer 1973; 32:890–897.

Hinshaw DB Jr, Ashwal S, Thompson JR, Hasso AN. Neuroradioloy of primitive neuroectodermal tumors. Neuroradiology 1983; 25:87–92.

Ho K-L, Hoschner JA, Wolfe DE. Primary leptomeningeal gliomatosis. Symptoms suggestive of meningitis. Arch Neurol 1981; 38:662–666.

Hochberg F, Pruitt A. Assumptions in the radiotherapy of glioblastoma. Neurology 1980; 30:907–911.

Hoffmann HJ, Becker L, Craven MA. A clinically and pathologically distinct group of benign brain-stem gliomas. Neurosurgery 1980; 7:243–248.

Housepian EM. Current concepts in the diagnosis and treatment of optic glioma. Contemp Neurosurg 1981; 3:1–5.

Hoyt WF, Meshel LG, Lessell S, Schatz NJ, Suckling RD. Malignant optic gliomas of adulthood. Brain 1973; 96:121–132.

Imes RK, Hoyt WF. Childhood chiasmal gliomas: Update on the fate of patients in the 1969 San Francisco study. Br J Ophthalmol 1986; 70:179–182.

Ingraham FD, Bailey OT, Barker WF. Medulloblastoma cerebelli. N Engl J Med 1948; 238:171–174.

Jacobs SK, Wilson DJ, Kornblith RL, et al. Interleukin-2 and autologous lymphokine-activated killer cells in the treatment of malignant glioma. J Neurosurg 1986; 64:743–749.

Jereb B, Reid A, Ahuja RK. Patterns of failure in patients with medulloblastoma. Cancer 1982; 50:2941–2947.

Kelly PJ, Daumas-Duport C, Scheithauer BW, et al. Stereotactic histologic correlations of computed tomography and magnetic resonance imaging—defined abnormalities in patients with glial neoplasms. Mayo Clin Proc 1987; 62:450–459.

Kernohan JW, Mabon RF, Svien HS, et al. A simplified classification of the gliomas. Proc Staff Meetings Mayo Clin 1949; 24:71–75.

Kimmel DW, Shapiro JR, Shapiro WR. In vitro drug sensitivity testing in human gliomas. J Neurosurg 1987; 66:161–171.

Kinzler KW, Bigner SH, Bigner DD, et al. Identification of an amplified, highly expressed gene in a human glioma. Science 1987; 236:70–73.

Kleinman GM, Hochberg FH, Richardson EP Jr. Systemic metastases from medulloblastoma: report of two cases and review of the literature. Cancer 1981; 48:2296–2309.

Kopelson G, Lingood RM, Kleinman GM. Medulloblastoma. The identification of prognostic subgroups and implications for multimodality management. Cancer 1983; 51:312–319.

Kornblith PL, Smith BH, Leonard L. Response of cultured human brain tumors in nitrosoureas: correlation with clinical data. Cancer 1981; 47:255–265.

Kornblith PL, Walker M. Chemotherapy for malignant gliomas. J Neurosurg 1988; 68:1–17.

Kricheff II, Becker M, Schneck SA, Taveras JM. Intracranial ependymomas. A study of survival in 65 cases treated by surgery and irradiation. AJR 1964; 91:167–175.

Latchaw JP, Hahn JF, Moylan DJ, et al. Medulloblastoma. Period of risk reviewed. Cancer 1985; 55:186–189.

Laws ER Jr, Taylor WF, Bergstralh EJ, et al. The neurosurgical management of low-grade astrocytoma. Clin Neurosurg 1985; 33:575–588.

Laws ER Jr, Taylor WF, Clifton MB, et al. Neurosurgical management of low-grade astrocytoma of the cerebral hemispheres. J Neurosurg 1984; 62:665–673.

Leibel SA, Sheline GE. Radiation therapy for neoplasms of brain. J Neurosurg 1987; 66:1–22.

Levin VA, Rodriguez LA, Edwards MSB, et al. Treatment of medulloblastoma with procarbazine, hydroxyurea, and reduced radiation doses to the whole brain and spine. J Neurosurg 1988; 68:383–387.

Libermann TA, Nusbaum HP, Razon N, et al. Amplification, enhanced expression and possible rearrangement of EGF receptor gene in primary human brain tumors of glial origin. Nature 1985; 313:144–147.

Mahaley MS Jr, Urso MB, Whaley RA, et al. Immunobiology of primary intracranial tumors. Part 10: therapeutic efficacy of interferon in the treatment of recurrent gliomas. J Neurosurg 1985; 63:719–725.

Mantravadi RVP, Phatak R, Bellur S, Liebner EJ, Haas R. Brain stem gliomas. An autopsy study of 25 cases. Cancer 1982; 49:1294–1296.

McGinnis BD, Brady TJ, New PFJ, et al. Nuclear magnetic resonance (NMR) imaging of tumors in the posterior fossa. J Comp Assist Tomogr 1983; 7:575–584.

Mercuri S, Russo A, Palma L. Hemispheric supratentorial astrocytomas in children. Long-term results in 29 cases. J Neurosurg 1981; 55:170–173.

Nelson JS, Tsukada Y, Shoenfeld D, et al. Necrosis as a prognostic criterion in malignant supratentorial, astrocytic gliomas. Cancer 1983; 52:550–554.

Packer RJ, Allen J, Nielsen S, et al. Brainstem glioma: clinical manifestations of meningeal gliomatosis. Ann Neurol 1983; 14:177–182.

Park TS, Hoffman JH, Henrick EB, Humphreys RP, Becker LE. Medulloblastoma—clinical presentation and management—experience at the Hospital-For-Sick-Children. J Neurosurg 1983; 58:543–552.

Piepmeier J. Observations on the current treatment of low-grade astrocytic tumors of the cerebral hemispheres. J Neurosurg 1987; 67:177–181.

Punt JP, Pritchard J, Pincott JR, et al. Neuroblastoma: a review of 21 cases presenting with spinal cord compression. Cancer 1980; 45:3095–3101.

Quest DO. Medulloblastoma: biological characteristics and therapy. Contemp Neurosurg 1980; 2:1–6.

Roberts M, German WJ. A long-term study of patients with oligodendrogliomas. J Neurosurg 1966; 24:697–700.

Rorke LB. Cerebellar medulloblastoma and its relationship to primitive neuroectodermal tumors. J Neuropathol Exp Neurol 1983; 42:1–15.

Rubinstein LJ. Cytogenesis and differentiation of primitive central neuroepithelial tumors. J Neurol Exper Neuropathol 1972; 31:7–26.

Russell A. A diencephalic syndrome of emaciation in infancy and childhood. Arch Dis Child 1951; 26:274.

Salcman M. Glioblastoma multiforme. Am J Med Sci 1980; 279:84–93.

Schaumburg HH, Plank CR, Adams RD. The reticulum-cell sarcoma-microglioma group of brain tumours: A consideration of their clinical features and therapy. Brain 1972; 95:199–212.

Schmidek HH. The molecular genetics of nervous system tumors. J Neurosurg 1987; 67:1–16.

Shapiro JR. Biology of gliomas: heterogeneity, oncogenes, growth factors. Semin Oncol 1986; 13:4–15.

Shapiro WR, Shapiro JR. Principles of brain tumor chemotherapy. Semin Oncol 1986; 13:55–69.

Sheline GE. The role of radiation in the treatment of low-grade gliomas. Clin Neurosurg 1985; 33:563–574.

Stern J, DiGiacinto GV, Housepian EM. Neurofibromatosis and optic glioma: clinical and morphological correlations. Neurosurgery 1979; 4:524–528.

Tenny RT, Laws ER Jr, Younge BR, Rush JA. The neurosurgical management of optic glioma. J Neurosurg 1982; 57:452–458.

Tomita T, McLone DG. Medulloblastoma in childhood: results of radical resection and low-dose neuraxis radiation therapy. J Neurosurg 1986; 64:238–242.

Torrey EF, Uyeda CI. The Diencephalic Syndrome of Infancy. Am J Dis Child 1965; 110:689–696.

Trojanowski JQ, Lee V, Pillsbury N, et al. Neuronal origin of human esthesioneuroblastoma demonstrated with anti-neurofilament monoclonal antibodies. N Engl J Med 1982; 307:159–161.

Valavanis A, Imhof HG, Klaiber R, Dabir K. The diagnosis of solitary primary reticulum cell sarcoma of the posterior fossa with computed tomography. Neuroradiology 1981; 21:213–217.

Walker MD, Alexander E Jr, Hunt WE, et al. Evaluation of BCNU and/or radiotherapy in the treatment of anaplastic gliomas: a cooperative clinical trial. J Neurosurg 1978; 49:333–343.

Walker MD, Green SB, Byar DP, et al. Randomized comparisons of radiotherapy and nitrosureas for the treatment of malignant glioma after surgery. N Engl J Med 1980; 303:1323–1330.

Wechsler LR, Gross RA, Miller DC. Meningeal gliomatosis with "negative" CSF cytology: the value of GFAP staining. Neurology 1984; 34:1611–1615.

Wilson CB. Brain tumors. N Engl J Med 1979; 300: 1469–1471.

Winston K, Gilles FH, Leviton A, et al. Cerebellar gliomas in children. Natl Cancer Inst Monogr 1977; 58:833–838.

Yung WA, Horten BC, Shapiro WR. Meningeal gliomatosis: a review of 12 cases. Ann Neurol 1979; 8:605–608.

Lymphomatous CNS Metastases

Bunn PA Jr, Schein PS, Banks PM, et al. Central nervous system complications in patients with diffuse histiocytic and undifferentiated lymphoma: leukemia revisited. Blood 1976; 47:3–10.

Cuttner J, Meyer R, Huang VP. Intracerebral involvement in Hodgkin's disease. Cancer 1979; 43:1497–1506.

Ernerudh J, Olsson T, Berlin G, et al. Cell surface markers for diagnosis of central nervous system involvement in lymphoproliferative diseases. Ann Neurol 1986; 20:610–615.

Goodson JD, Strauss GM. Diagnosis of lymphomatous leptomeningitis by cerebrospinal fluid lymphocyte cell surface markers. Am J Med 1979; 66:1057–1059.

Griffin JW, Thompson RW, Mitchinson MJ, et al. Lymphomatous leptomeningitis. Am J Med 1971; 51:200–208.

Jellinger K, Radaszkiewicz TH. Involvement of the central nervous system in malignant lymphomas. Virchows Arch A Path Anat Histol 1976; 370:345–362.

Levitt LJ, Dawson DM, Rosenthal DS, et al. CNS involvement in the non-Hodgkin's lymphomas. Cancer 1980; 45:545–552.

Litam JP, Cabanillas F, Smith TL, et al. Central nervous system relapse in malignant lymphomas: risk factors and implications for prophylaxis. Blood 1979; 54:1249–1257.

Lokich J, Galbo C. Leptomeningeal lymphoma: perspectives on management. Cancer Treat Rev 1981; 8:103–110.

Mackintosh FR, Colby TV, Podolsky WJ, et al. Central nervous system involvement in non-Hodgkin's lymphoma: an analysis of 105 cases. Cancer 1982; 45:586–595.

Magrath IT, Janus C, Edwards BK, et al. An effective therapy for both undifferentiated (including Burkitt's) lymphomas and lymphoblastic lymphomas in children and young adults. Blood 1984; 63:1102–1111.

Mavligit GM, Studkey SE, Cabanillas FF, et al. Diagnosis of leukemia of lymphoma in the central nervous system by beta$_2$-microglobulin determination. N Engl J Med 1980; 303:718–722.

Recht L, et al. CNS metastases from Non-Hodgkin's lymphoma: Treatment and prophylaxis. Am J Med 1988; 84:425–435.

Sapozink MD, Kaplan HS. Intracranial Hodgkin's disease. A report of 12 cases and review of the literature. Cancer 1983; 52:1301–1307.

Sariban E, Edwards B, Janus C, et al. Central nervous system involvement in American Burkitt's lymphoma. J Clin Oncol 1983; 1:677–681.

Streuli RA, Kaneko Y, Variakojis D, et al. Lymphoblastic lymphoma in adults. Cancer 1981; 47:2510–2516.

The Non-Hodgkin's Lymphoma Pathologic Classification Project: National Cancer Institute sponsored study of classifications of non-Hodgkin's lymphoma. Summary and description of a working formulation for clinical usage. Cancer 1982; 49:2112–2135.

Primary CNS Lymphoma

Appen RE. Posterior uveitis and primary cerebral reticulum cell sarcoma. Arch Ophthalmol 1975; 93:123–124.

Ervin T, Canellos GP. Successful treatment of recurrent primary central nervous system lymphoma with high-dose methotrexate. Cancer 1980; 45:1556–1557.

Hautzer NW, Aiyesimoju A, Robitaille Y. "Primary" spinal intramedullary lymphomas: a review. Ann Neurol 1983; 14:62–66.

Helle TL, Britt RH, Colby TV. Primary lymphoma of the central nervous system. J Neurosurg 1984; 60:94–103.

Henry JM, Heffner RR Jr, Dillard SH. Primary malignant lymphomas of the central nervous system. Cancer 1974; 34:1293–1302.

Hochberg FH, Miller DC. Primary central nervous system lymphoma. J Neurosurg 1988; 68:835–853.

Hochberg FH, Miller G, Schooley RT, et al. Central nervous system lymphoma related to Epstein-Barr virus. N Engl J Med 1983; 309:745–748.

Jellinger K, Radaskiewicz TH, Slowik F. Primary malignant lymphomas of the central nervous system in man. Acta Neuropathol (Berl) 1975; Suppl VI:95–102.

Jiddabe M, Nicoll F, Diaz P, et al. Intracranial malignant lymphoma. J Neurosurg 1986; 65:592–599.

Jones GR, Mason WH, Fishman LS, et al. Primary central nervous system lymphoma without intracranial mass in a child. Diagnosis by documentation of monoclonality. Cancer 1985; 56:2804–2808.

Kawakami Y, Tabuchi K, Ohnishi R, et al. Primary central nervous system lymphoma. J Neurosurg 1985; 62:522–527.

Littman P, Wang CC. Reticulum cell sarcoma of the brain. A review of the literature and a study of 19 cases. Cancer 1975; 35:1412–1420.

Loeffler JS, Ervin TJ, Mauch P, et al. Primary lymphomas of the central nervous system: patterns of failure and factors that influence survival. J Clin Oncol 1985; 3:490–494.

Marsh WL Jr, Stevenson DR, Long HJ. Primary leptomeningeal presentation of T-cell lymphoma. Cancer 1983; 51:1125–1131.

Minckler DS, Font RL, Zimmerman LE. Uveitis and reticulum cell sarcoma of brain with bilateral neoplastic seeding of vitreous without retinal or uveal involvement. Am J Ophthalmol 1975; 80:433–439.

Murray K, Kun L, Cox J. Primary malignant lymphoma of the central nervous system. Results of treatment of 11 cases and review of the literature. J Neurosurg 1986; 65:600–607.

O'Neill BP, Kelly PJ, Earle JD, et al. Computer-assisted stereotaxic biopsy for the diagnosis of primary central nervous system lymphoma. Neurology 1987; 37:1160–1164.

Slager UT, Kaufman RL, Cohen KL, et al. Primary lymphoma of the spinal cord. J Neuropathol Exp Neurol 1982; 41:437–445.

Spillane JA, Kendall BE, Moseley IF. Cerebral lymphoma: clinical radiological correlation. J Neurol Neurosurg Psychiatry 1982; 45:199–208.

Immunosuppression and Lymphoma

Baumgartner JE, Rachlin JR, Levy TM, Rosenblum ML. AIDS associated primary CNS lymphoma (PCL) Proc ASCO 1988; 7:33.

Case Records Case #42-1986. N Engl J Med 1986; 315:1079–1086.

Cleary ML, Sklar J. Lymphoproliferative disorders in cardiac transplant recipients are multiclonal lymphomas. Lancet 1984; 2:489–493.

Epstein LG, et al. Primary lymphoma of the CNS in children with AIDS. Pediatrics 1988; 82:355–363.

Levy RM, Pons VG, Rosenblum ML. Central nervous system mass lesion in the acquired immunodeficiency syndrome (AIDS). J Neurosurg 1984; 61:9–16.

Payan MJ, Gambarelli D, Routy JP, et al. Primary lymphoma of the brain associated with AIDS. Acta Neuropathol (Berl) 1984; 64:78–80.

Penn I: Depressed immunity and the development of cancer. Clin Exp Immunol 1981; 46:459–474.

Rosenberg NL, Hochberg FH, Miller G, et al. Primary central nervous system lymphoma related to Epstein-Barr virus in a patient with acquired immune deficiency syndrome. Ann Neurol 1986; 20:98–102.

Salahuddin SZ, Ablashi DV, Markham PD, et al. Isolation of a new virus, HBLV, in patients with lymphoproliferative disorders. Science 1986; 234:596–601.

So YT, Becksteadd JH, Davis RL. Primary central nervous system lymphoma in acquired immune deficiency syndrome: a clinical and pathological study. Ann Neurol 1986; 20:566–572.

Starzl TE, Porter KA, Iwatsuki S, et al. Reversibility of

lymphomas and lymphoproliferative lesions developing under cyclosporin-steroid therapy. Lancet 1984; 1:583–587.

Ziegler JL, Becktead JA, Volberding PA, et al. Non-Hodgkin's lymphoma in 90 homosexual men. Relation to generalized lymphadenopathy and the acquired immunodeficiency syndrome. N Engl J Med 1984; 311:565–570.

Intravascular Lymphoma (Malignant Angioendotheliomatosis)

Ansell J, Bhawan J, Cohen S, et al. Histiocytic lymphoma and malignant angioendotheliomatosis. One disease or two? Cancer 1982; 50:1506–1512.

Bhawan J. Wolff SM, Ucci AA, et al. Malignant lymphoma and malignant angioendotheliomatosis: One disease. Cancer 1985; 55:570–576.

Bots GThAM. Angioendotheliomatosis of the central nervous system. Acta Neuropathol (Berl) 1974; 28:75–78.

Case Records: Case #39-1986. N Engl J Med 1986; 315:874–885.

Dolamn CL, Sweeney VP, Magli A. Neoplastic angioendotheliomatosis. The case of the missed primary? Arch Neurol 1979; 36:5–7.

Fulling KH, Gersell DJ. Neoplastic angioendotheliomatosis. Histologic, Immunohistochemical, and ultrastructural findings in two cases. Cancer 1983; 51:1107–1118.

LeWitt PA, Forno LS, Brant-Zawadzki M. Neoplastic angioendotheliomatosis: A case with spontaneous regression and radiographic appearance of cerebral arteritis. Neurology 1983; 33:39–44.

Petito CK, Gottlieb GJ, Dougherty JH, et al. Neoplastic angioendotheliomatosis: ultrastructural study and review of the literature. Ann Neurol 1978; 3:393–399.

Sheibani K, Battifora H, Winberg CD, et al. Further evidence that ''malignant angioendotheliomatosis'' is an angiotropic large-cell lymphoma. N Engl J Med 1986; 314:943–948.

---

47. PINEAL REGION TUMORS

Bennett M. Stein
Michael R. Fetell

The widest variety of pathologic types of CNS tumors occurs in the region of the pineal gland and posterior third ventricle. This finding is due to the presence in the pineal gland of glandular tissue, glia, and sympathetic nerve terminals. Pineocytomas and pineoblastomas are thought to arise from pineal glandular elements, astrocytomas and oligodendrogliomas from glial cells, and chemodectomas from sympathetic nerve cells. Nearby are arachnoid cells in the reflections of the tela choroidea that give rise to meningiomas. Ependymal cells in the third ventricle give rise to ependymomas. It is presumed that rests of germinal tissue give rise to the vast and complex array of germ cell tumors.

In the United States, pineal tumors consti-

Table 47–1. Pathologically Verified Pineal Tumors (New York Neurological Institute) (1978–1985)

Type	%
Germ cell	32
Glioma	31
Pineal cell	20
Meningioma	7
Metastatic	3
Miscellaneous	7
Total	100

tute approximately 1% of all intracranial tumors (Table 47–1). In Asia, all germ cell neoplasms are more common, and pineal cell tumors constitute 4 to 7% of all intracranial tumors.

Germ Cell Tumors

Germ cell tumors (GCTs) account for 32% of pineal tumors and include the germinoma, embryonal carcinoma, endodermal sinus tumor (or yolk sac tumor), choriocarcinoma, and teratoma (Fig. 47–1). Gonadal and extragonadal GCTs have similar pathologic features but, in general, extragonadal GCTs (including the CNS) have a poorer prognosis.

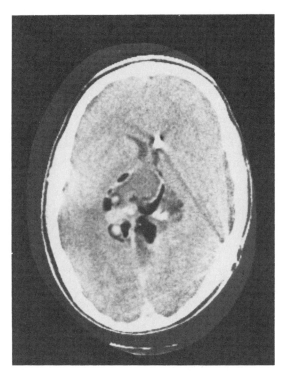

Fig. 47–1. Contrast-enhanced CT scan demonstrating a large teratoma of the pineal, with shunted hydrocephalus. This benign tumor was completely removed without neurologic complications.

Germinoma is a malignant tumor of primordial germ cells that occurs in the gonads and in midline sites in the nervous system (pineal and suprasellar region) or body (mediastinum and sacrococcygeal region). Germinomas are pathologically identical regardless of the organ or site of origin but, by convention, germinomas in the testes are called *seminomas* and, in the ovary, *dysgerminomas.*

Unlike suprasellar germ cell tumors, which show no sexual predisposition, germ cell tumors of the pineal region occur predominantly in males. Germinomas most often affect boys in the first or second decade and are malignant tumors, sensitive to both radiotherapy and chemotherapy, with a propensity to seed the CSF pathways.

Embryonal carcinomas, choriocarcinomas, and *endodermal sinus tumors* are rare malignant tumors that often occur in the pineal or suprasellar regions, but are generally more difficult to treat than the gonad counterparts. They are highly malignant and, like germinomas, often metastasize through the CSF. Choriocarcinoma contains cyto- and syncytiotrophoblastic cells that produce beta human chorionic gonadotropin (βHCG). Endodermal sinus tumors contain yolk sac elements that produce alpha-fetoprotein (AFP). βHCG and AFP may be used as reliable markers of germ cell tumors (Table 47–2), more reliable in CSF than in serum.

Accurate diagnosis of tumor type is impeded because 40% of germ cell tumors in the pineal region are mixed, containing elements of more than one cell type (Table 47–3). It is essential, therefore, to examine the pathologic specimen thoroughly, particularly if markers suggest the presence of malignant GCT elements. "Falsely elevated" CSF levels of AFP in germinomas are attributed to a mixed GCT with foci of embryonal carcinoma or endodermal sinus tumor that were overlooked.

Teratomas are well-differentiated neoplasms

Table 47–2. Biologic Markers in Germ Cell Tumors

Tumors	HCG	AFP
Teratoma	−	−
Germinoma	−	−
Germinoma with syncytiotrophoblastic cells	−	+
Embryonal carcinoma	±	±
Choriocarcinoma	+	−
Endodermal sinus tumor	−	+

Table 47–3. Pure vs. Mixed Germ Cell Tumors (N.Y. Neurological Institute, 1978–1985)

Tumor Type	Number
Pure Germ Cell Tumors	
Embryonal Ca	1
Germinoma	7
Dermoid	2
Teratoma	2
Total	12
Mixed Germ Cell Tumors	
Embryonal Ca/germinoma	3
Chorio Ca/germinoma	1
Chorio Ca/teratoma	1
Germinoma/teratoma	2
Epidermoid/teratoma	1
Dermoid/teratoma	1
Total	9

composed of tissue from all three germ cell lines (endo, ecto, and mesoderm). They are generally slowly growing tumors, but sometimes a so-called immature teratoma may grow rapidly and behave in a malignant fashion.

Pineal Cell Tumors

Although *pineocytoma* is considered a well-differentiated neoplasm arising from pineal parenchymal epithelium, and *pineoblastoma* is classified as a primitive neuroectodermal tumor, both may behave in a malignant fashion, recurring at the primary site and spreading through the CSF. Pineal cell tumors occur in children and young adults before age 40, with no sex predominance. Both are radiosensitive; their chemosensitivity is largely unknown because few have been treated with chemotherapy.

Gliomas

Gliomas are almost as frequent in the pineal region as germ cell tumors. Two thirds are invasive and malignant, but about one third are low-grade, cystic, and surgically removable. Oligodendrogliomas and ependymomas may also be seen in the pineal region.

Meningiomas

Middle-aged patients with pineal tumors are unlikely to have a germ cell or pineal cell tumor, and are more likely to have a glioma or meningioma (Fig. 47–2). The latter are removable surgically.

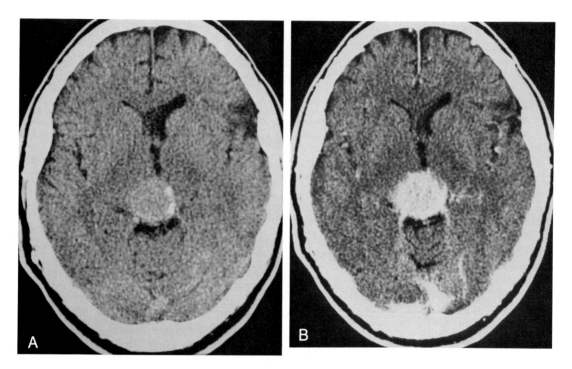

Fig. 47–2. Pineal region meningioma. *A,* A noncontrast axial CT scan shows a dense calcified lesion in the region of the pineal. *B,* Homogeneous enhancement is noted postcontrast consistent with a meningioma, documented at surgery. (Courtesy of Drs. T.L. Chi, J.A. Bello, and S.K. Hilal.)

Metastases and Other Miscellaneous Tumors

The pineal gland does not have a blood-brain barrier and, like the pituitary gland, may be under-recognized as a predilected site for CNS metastases of systemic tumors. Miscellaneous tumors include sarcomas, hemangioblastomas, choroid plexus papillomas, and chemodectomas.

Symptoms. Virtually all patients with pineal region tumors have hydrocephalus due to aqueductal obstruction by the tumor. Papilledema, gait disorder, vomiting, lethargy, and memory disturbance are the principal manifestations of the ventricular obstruction. Additionally, the tumor may cause disorders of ocular movement such as *Parinaud syndrome* (paralysis of upgaze, convergence or retraction nystagmus, and light-near pupillary disassociation or the *sylvian aqueduct syndrome* (paralysis of downgaze or horizontal gaze superimposed upon Parinaud syndrome). Either direct pressure on the tectum by the tumor or dilatation of the proximal aqueduct may cause the gaze disorders. Reversibility is a clue to pathogenesis: eye signs due to hydrocephalus recede promptly after ventricular shunting.

Diabetes insipidus is uncommon, occurring in fewer than 5% of pineal tumors, usually in germinomas. Its presence is evidence that the tumor has seeded the hypothalamic region even if CT does not document this. *Precocious puberty* is actually precocious *pseudopuberty* because the hypothalamic-gonadal axis is not mature. It occurs strictly in boys with choriocarcinomas or germinomas with syncytiotrophoblastic cells and is caused by ectopic secretion of βHCG. In males the luteinizing hormone (LH)-like effects of βHCG suffice to stimulate Leydig cells to produce androgens that induce development of secondary sexual characteristics and a state of pseudopuberty. Precocious puberty does not occur in girls with pineal region tumors for two reasons: the first is epidemiologic, i.e., pineal region GCTs rarely occur in females; the second is endocrinologic. To trigger ovarian estrogen production in females, both LH and follicle-stimulating hormone (FSH) are necessary.

Meningeal seeding may lead to symptoms of root compression or myelopathy, best detected by examination of CSF cytology and by myelography with CT.

Diagnosis. CT is the principal diagnostic test for pineal region tumors. MRI is useful for assessing tumors that infiltrate the brain

Table 47–4.   Pineal Tumors: Benign vs. Malignant (N.Y. Neurological Institute, 1978–1985)

Tumor Type	Benign	Malignant	Total
Germ cell tumors	5	16	21
Pineal cell tumors	1	13	14
Glial tumors	6	12	18
Meningiomas	5	0	5
Metastases	0	2	2
Others	3	3	6
	20 (30%)	46 (70%)	66 (100%)

stem, such as gliomas and ependymomas, and the sagittal view of the MRI is most useful in assessing the relationship of the tumor to the aqueduct and quadrigeminal plate. Despite improved imaging and CSF markers, a definitive histologic diagnosis cannot be made without pathologic examination of tumor tissue. Furthermore, because of the high incidence of mixed GCTs, pathologic verification of the tumor is mandatory. If the histology of the tumor appears benign, but the βHCG or AFP level in CSF is elevated, malignant components must be assumed to be present (Table 47–4).

Therapy. Surgery. Operative exposure, usually by the infratentorial-supracerebellar route, is preferred for benign tumors. With this approach, approximately 25% of tumors may be removed and cured without additional therapy. Surgical identification of malignant tumors itself affords a partial resection and may increase the effectiveness of radiotherapy or chemotherapy. It may also alert the physician to meningeal seeding. The operative mortality is 2%. For patients with known systemic malignant tumor and a mass in the pineal region, stereotactic biopsy can confirm the presence of metastasis, but stereotactic biopsy provides insufficient tissue for accurate diagnosis of germ cell tumors.

Postoperative Staging. A thorough search for evidence of CSF seeding is mandatory after surgery. This search includes myelography (with CT of lumbar region), serum and CSF marker assays, and CSF cytology. Asymptomatic seeding of the lumbar region occurs in up to 30% of germinomas and pineal cell tumors (Fig. 47–3).

Radiation and Medical Therapy. Radiotherapy of malignant pineal tumors usually consists of 4,000 cGy delivered to the entire brain, and an additional 1,500 cGy to the tumor area and third ventricular region. In the absence of documented spinal seeding following myelography and CSF cytology examinations, it is debatable whether spinal radiotherapy is

needed. The five-year survival of patients with pineal region tumors treated with radiotherapy is 60 to 80%, but the other malignant GCTs (embryonal, carcinoma, endodermal sinus tumor, and choriocarcinoma) are never cured with radiation therapy alone. Chemotherapy with combinations of cisplatin, vinblastine, bleomycin, or cisplatin and VP 16

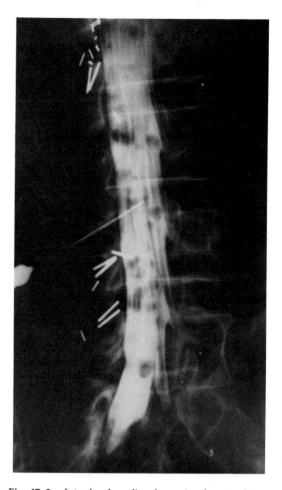

Fig. 47–3.   Intradural seeding from pineal tumor. Lumbar myelography, oblique view, demonstrates intradural filling defects studding the lumbar nerve roots. These represent "dropped" metastases. (Courtesy of Drs. J.A. Bello and S.K. Hilal.)

(etoposide) has been effective in controlling metastatic testicular carcinoma and has also been effective in isolated cases of recurrent germinomas or nongerminomatous malignant GCTs. We advocate a multimodality approach, consisting of surgical debulking followed by irradiation and chemotherapy. However, fewer than 5% of patients with malignant nongerminomatous GCTs survive for two years. Both pineocytomas and pineoblastomas respond to radiotherapy. Experience with chemotherapy for these tumors is limited. Malignant glial tumors of the pineal regions, like glioblastomas of the cerebral hemisphere, should be treated with radiotherapy.

References

Abray EO II, Laws ER Jr, Grado GL, Bruckman JE, Forbes GS, Gomez MR, Scott H. Pineal tumors in children and adolescents. J Neurosurg 1981; 55:889–895.

Allen JC, Nisselbaum J, Epstein F, et al. Alphafetoprotein and human chorionic gonadotropin determination in cerebrospinal fluid: an aid to the diagnosis and management of intracranial germ-cell tumors. J Neurosurg 1979, 51:368–374.

Amendola BE, McClatchey K, Amendola MS. Pineal region tumors: analysis of treatment results. Int J Radiol Oncol Biol Phys 1984; 10:991–997.

Araki C, Matsumoto S. Statistical re-evaluation of pinealoma and related tumors in Japan. J Neurosurg 1969; 30:146–149.

Becker LE, Hinton D. Primitive neuroectodermal tumors of the central nervous system. Hum Pathol 1983; 14:538–550.

Bjornsson J, Scheithauer BW, Okazaki H, et al. Intracranial germ cell tumors: pathobiological and immunohistological aspects of 70 cases. J Neuropathol Exp Neurol 1985; 44:32–46.

Chan HSL, Humphreys RP, Hendrick EB, et al. Primary intracranial choriocarcinoma: a report of two cases and a review of the literature. Neurosurgery 1984; 14:540–545.

DeGirolami U, Schmidek H. Clinicopathological study of 53 tumors of the pineal region. J Neurosurg 1973; 39:455–462.

Dehner LP. Gonadal and extragonadal germ cell neoplasms of childhood. Hum Pathol 1983; 14:493–511.

Fetell MR, Stein BM. Neuroendocrine manifestations of pineal tumors. Neurol Clin 1986; 4:877–905.

Fetell MR, Stein BM. Therapy of pineal region tumors. Neurology 1984; 34(Suppl. 1):184–185.

Gindhart TD, Tsukahara YC. Cytologic diagnosis of pineal germinoma in cerebrospinal fluid and sputum. Acta Cytol 1979; 23:341–346.

Griffin BR, Griffin TW, Tong DYK, et al. Pineal region tumors: results of radiation therapy and indications for elective spinal irradiation. Am J Radiat Oncol Biol Phys 1981; 7:605–608.

Haase J, Nielsen K. Value of tumor markers in the treatment of endodermal sinus tumors and choriocarcinomas in the pineal region. Neurosurgery 1979; 5:485–488.

Herrick MK, Rubinstein LJ. The cytological differentiating potential of pineal parenchymal neoplasms (the

pinealomas): A clinicopathological study of 23 tumors. Brain 1982; 102:321–332.

Jennings MT, Gelman R, Hochberg F. Intracranial germ-cell tumors: Natural history and pathogenesis. J Neurosurg 1985; 63:155–167.

Jooma R, Kendall BE. Diagnosis and management of pineal tumors. J Neurosurg 1983; 58:654–665.

Kawakami Y, Yamada O, Tabuchi K, et al. Primary intracranial choriocarcinoma. J Neurosurg 1980; 53:369–374.

Neuwelt EA, Glasberg M, Frenkel E, Clark WK. Malignant pineal region tumors. J Neurosurg 1979; 51:597–607.

Rao YTR, Medini F, Haselow RD, et al. Pineal and ectopic pineal tumors: the role of radiation therapy. Cancer 1981; 48:708–713.

Sano K. Pineal region tumors: Problems in pathology and treatment. Clin Neurosurg 1982; 30:59–91.

Schmidek HH. Pineal Tumours. New York: Masson, 1977.

Stein BM. Supracerebellar-infratentorial approach to pineal tumors. Surg Neurol 1979; 11:331–337.

Stein BM. Surgical treatment of pineal tumors. Clin Neurosurg 1979; 26:490–510.

Stein BM, Fetell MR. Therapeutic modalities for pineal region tumors. Clin Neurosurg 1985; 32:445–455.

Sung DI, Harisiadis L, Chang CH. Midline pineal tumors and suprasellar germinomas: highly curable by irradiation. Radiology 1978; 128:745–751.

Teilum G. Special Tumors of the Ovary and Testes and Related Extragonadal Lesions. Philadelphia: J.B. Lippincott, 1976.

Wara WM. Radiation therapy for brain tumors. Cancer 1985; 55:2291–2295.

Yamagami T, Handa H, Takeuchi J, et al. Choriocarcinoma arising from the pituitary fossa with extracranial metastasis: a review of the literature. Surg Neurol 1983; 19:469–480.

48. TUMORS OF THE PITUITARY GLAND
Earl A. Zimmerman

Tumors of the pituitary gland have been classified into three types, according to classic histologic techniques: *chromophobe adenoma*, the most common type, *acidophilic adenoma*, which causes acromegaly and, the least common, *basophilic adenoma*, which is associated with Cushing disease. It has become apparent, particularly since the advent of specific and sensitive techniques for measuring the different pituitary hormones, that this classification is of limited usefulness. Indeed, most pituitary tumors that secrete growth hormone, prolactin, or ACTH are chromophobe adenomas. Therefore the concept that chromophobe tumors are essentially nonfunctioning had to be revised. With CT it has been found that many patients with pituitary dysfunction and different clinical pictures, such as amenorrhea-galactorrhea, have small secreting tumors (*microadenomas*) that cannot be detected by standard radiologic procedures. Although it is generally considered that pituitary adenomas represent about 10% of all intracranial tumors, the real incidence is probably much higher if we include the small secreting tumors that are not diagnosed because of the paucity of neurologic manifestations. In fact, small pituitary adenomas are an incidental finding in about 25% of all glands studied at autopsy.

A more satisfactory classification divides pituitary tumors into *secreting* and *nonsecreting* types. The former are subdivided according to the hormone that is produced in excess—growth hormone (GH), prolactin (PRL), adrenocorticotropin (ACTH), thyrotropin (TSH) or gonadotropins, luteinizing hormone (LH), and follicle-stimulating hormone (FSH). From a therapeutic viewpoint it is important to consider the size of the lesion, and the criteria proposed by Hardy are particularly useful. The term *enclosed adenomas* applies whenever the floor of the sella turcica is intact, whereas *invasive adenomas* erode the floor. Further qualification depends on whether the tumor remains *intrasellar* or whether there is an *extrasellar* (more frequently *suprasellar)* extension. The designation *microadenoma* applies to tumors smaller than 10 mm in diameter. Pituitary tumors are more frequent in the third and fourth decades, and they affect both sexes equally.

Pathology. The majority are, by standard histologic techniques, chromophobe tumors. Macroscopically some of these are encapsulated, whereas others behave more like focal hyperplasias. They are usually dark, soft, and not infrequently hemorrhagic, necrotic, or cystic. Microscopically the cells are arranged in a syncytial or sinusoidal pattern. Eosinophilic and basophilic tumors are usually smaller.

Through the use of specific immunocytochemical techniques, it has been demonstrated that a number of chromophobe tumors are actively secreting hormones, particularly PRL and GH, and occasionally both of these. The small secreting adenomas occupy different locations in the gland, following the normal distribution of cell types. Tumors that secrete GH are usually lateral and superficial, and PRL-secreting adenomas are also lateral, but deeper. ACTH-secreting tumors are deep and centrally placed. The rare TSH-producing adenomas are more superficial. An occasional tumor secretes LH or FSH, or both.

As the adenoma grows, it displaces and eventually destroys the adjacent functioning parenchyma, and enlarges the sella turcica; further expansion depends in part on the size of the aperture of the diaphragma sellae. Frequently the tumor extends upward, filling the suprasellar cisterns, impinging on the recesses of the third ventricle and, rarely, obstructing the foramina of Monro to cause hydrocephalus. They occasionally expand laterally into the cavernous sinus or the temporal fossa, grow forward under the frontal lobes or caudally into the interpeduncular cistern. Not infrequently they erode the floor of the sella and protrude into the sphenoid sinus.

Intracranial or extracranial metastases from pituitary adenomas are exceptional, and the term *pituitary carcinoma* is, on histologic grounds, rarely justified. Some cases, however, may show remarkable invasive characteristics, rapid growth, and anaplastic features.

Some families have a high incidence of hyperplasia, or tumors that involve multiple endocrine glands (including parathyroids, pituitary, pancreatic islets, thyroid, and adrenal cortex) and many of these are functional. This syndrome, *multiple endocrine adenomatosis* is inherited as an autosomal dominant trait with high penetrance.

Tumors of the posterior lobe (neurohypophysis) are rare and behave like hypothalamic gliomas. They are of two distinct morphologic types: gliomas (infundibulomas) and choristomas (myoblastomas or granular cell tumors).

Clinical Features. The clinical manifestations of pituitary adenomas depend on two factors: (1) local expansion with displacement and compression of the adjacent neural and vascular structures, and (2) the endocrine dysfunctions they produce (see Section 149, Endocrine Diseases). In this discussion, we consider these lesions as tumors.

Headaches, frequently frontal, are a common complaint, and they are usually attributed to pressure upon the diaphragma sellae and adjacent structures. Visual symptoms are also frequent, and are practically constant in patients with suprasellar extension. The patients may complain of progressive blurring and dimming of vision. When present, visual-field defects involve the temporal fields (bitemporal hemianopia) (Fig. 48–1), starting with the upper quadrants. With further growth of the tumor, the lower nasal quadrants and finally the upper nasal quadrants may be also compromised. In some cases, the

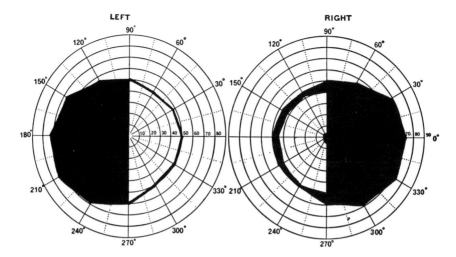

Fig. 48–1. Chromophobe adenoma. Bitemporal hemianopia; visual acuity O.D. 15/200, O.S. 15/30. (Courtesy of Dr. Max Chamlin.)

macular fibers of the chiasm are affected, giving rise to central hemianopic scotomas that may be missed unless the central fields are also examined. More rarely, loss of vision in one eye or a homonymous hemianopia are the presenting visual symptoms. Examination of the optic fundi frequently reveals pallor or atrophy of the optic discs; only exceptionally is there papilledema.

Involvement of other cranial nerves, particularly of the third, fourth, sixth cranial nerves, is present in 5 to 15% of the cases, and indicates lateral extension of the tumor. In these cases, facial hypesthesia is occasionally noticed.

Other neurologic manifestations depend on the direction of growth of the tumor. Thus some patients with large suprasellar extensions may present signs of hypothalamic dysfunction, including diabetes insipidus, or hydrocephalus. Tumors that insinuate under the frontal lobes may cause personality changes or dementia. Seizures or motor and sensory symptoms occasionally occur. CSF rhinorrhea may occur when the tumor has eroded the base of the skull.

Pituitary tumors only rarely affect children or adolescents. When present, they seem to have a higher incidence of extrasellar extensions, and obesity and extraocular palsies are more frequently seen than in adults (Table 48–1). Enlargement of adenomas during pregnancy has also been reported. This is of particular importance in women with amenorrhea and infertility in whom pregnancy was induced in the presence of an unrecognized pituitary tumor.

About 5% of patients with pituitary tumors suffer *pituitary apoplexy*, which frequently simulates subarachnoid hemorrhage, with sudden onset of severe headache, nausea, vomiting, alteration of consciousness, diplopia and, sometimes, rapid and progressive visual loss. Facial paresthesias, seizures, or focal signs seldom occur. The diagnosis is made by CT, which shows hemorrhagic infarction of an adenoma.

Diagnosis. Careful evaluation by radiologic and imaging techniques is important in the differential diagnosis of sellar and parasellar lesions, and in determining the extent of the lesion. This is obviously crucial for adequate planning of the treatment. Plain radiographs of the skull and polytomography have been useful over the years in evaluating the intrasellar growth of the lesion. Most pituitary tumors (Fig. 48–2) enlarge the sella and modify the contour—"ballooning"—thinning the dorsum, floor and, sometimes the clinoid processes. Microadenomas do not increase the volume of the sella, but almost always cause an asymmetric depression of the floor ("double floor"). Erosion of the floor of the sella and extension into the sphenoid sinus can also be appreciated.

In most cases, high-resolution CT and MR imaging have now replaced the need for polytomography and contrast studies in the evaluation of these lesions. In addition to bony changes, CT demonstrates the presence and size of pituitary adenomas. These are better seen with contrast material (Fig. 48–3). MR also provides excellent images of sellar lesions (Fig. 48–4).

Table 48–1. Manifestations of Pituitary Tumors

	Men		Women
	PRL-Secreting	*Nonsecreting*	*PRL-Secreting*
Number of patients	10	10	20
Mean age at onset	46	55	27
Percentage Showing Abnormality			
Amenorrhea	—	—	94
Impotence or decreased libido	90	90	—
Headache	40	30	60
Visual-field defect	50	50	15
Obesity	30	0	0
Diabetes mellitus	30	0	0
Galactorrhea	10	0	100
Gynecomastia	30	10	—
Abnormal plain radiographs	100	100	—
Suprasellar extension (CT)	60	70	20
Gonadotrophin deficiency	86	60	100
Panhypopituitarism	11	30	0

(From Post KD, Jackson JMD, Reichlin S, eds. The Pituitary Adenoma. New York: Plenum Medical Book Co, 1980.)

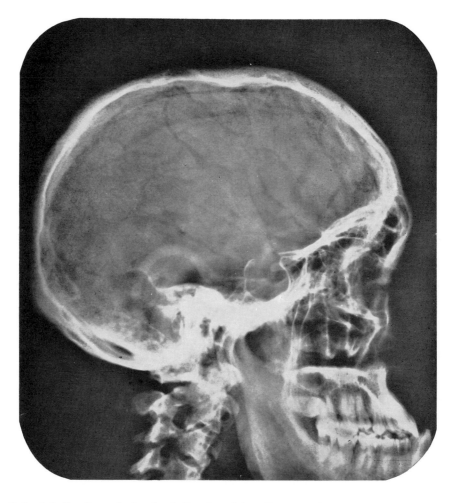

Fig. 48–2. Lateral skull radiograph showing ballooning of the sella turcica due to a pituitary tumor, prognathism, and enlargement of the bones of the skull. (Courtesy of Dr. Juan Taveras.)

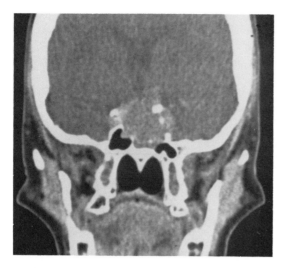

Fig. 48–3. Pituitary adenoma. Coronal CT scan demonstrates an intrasellar tumor with suprasellar and cavernous sinus extension as well as invasion of the sphenoid sinus inferiorly. (Courtesy of Drs. S.K. Hilal and S.R. Ganti.)

Lateral displacement of the intracavernous portion of the internal carotid artery and elevation of the initial segments of the anterior cerebral arteries are the characteristic angiographic findings. MR now provides most of the information previously provided by angiography (Figs. 48–5, 48–6). A tumor blush may be seen with appropriate techniques. Angiography may be important in excluding an intracranial aneurysm, which sometimes simulates pituitary adenoma.

In patients with acromegaly, other abnormal features can be demonstrated with simple radiologic techniques. These include enlargement of the paranasal sinus, increase in thickness of the cranial bones, enlargement of the mandible, and separation of the teeth. Hypertrophy of the hands, enlargement of the ungual tufts of the terminal phalanges (see Fig. 149–1) and hypertrophy of the soft tissues of the pad of the heel are also typical. Radiographs of the spine reveal an increase in anteroposterior diameter of the vertebral bodies and progressive kyphosis.

Differential Diagnosis. The diagnosis of pituitary tumors depends on a thorough radiologic and endocrine evaluation (see Section 149, Endocrine Diseases). Other sellar or parasellar lesions can, however, simulate the clinical and sometimes radiographic features of a pituitary adenoma (Table 48–2). These include tumors such as craniopharyngiomas, which usually manifest at an earlier age and are frequently calcified, meningiomas, optic gliomas, chordomas, atypical teratomas, dermoid tumors, metastasis, and invasive nasopharyngeal carcinomas. Intrasellar or parasellar aneurysms can be diagnosed by CT or angiography. Mucoceles of the sphenoid sinus may occasionally be difficult to distinguish from an invasive adenoma. Chronically increased intracranial pressure may cause enlargement of the sella turcica and visual symptoms.

In the *empty-sella syndrome*, the subarachnoid space extends into the sella through an incompetent diaphragm, flattening the gland against the floor (Figs. 48–7, 48–8). These cases are sometimes found after incidental

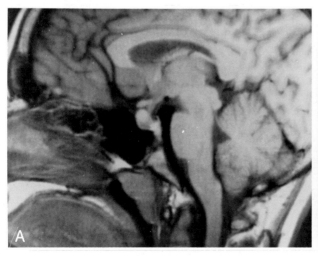

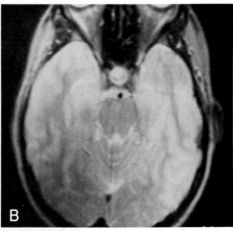

Fig. 48–4. Pituitary adenoma. This intrasellar lesion is isointense on *A,* a sagittal T_1 weighted MR image and hyperintense on *B,* an axial T_2 weighted image. Note the optic chiasm in its normal position. (Courtesy of Drs. J.A. Bello and S.K. Hilal.)

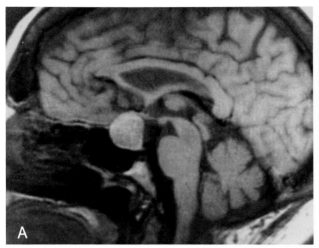
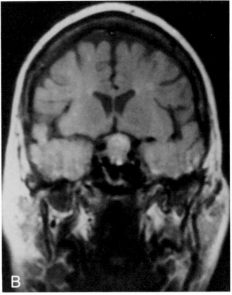

Fig. 48–5. Large pituitary adenoma. *A*, Sagittal and *B*, axial T₁ weighted MR scans demonstrate suprasellar mass effect with elevation of the chiasm in *A*, and elevation of the A₁ segments of the anterior cerebral arteries in *B*. (Courtesy of Drs. J.A. Bello and S.K. Hilal.)

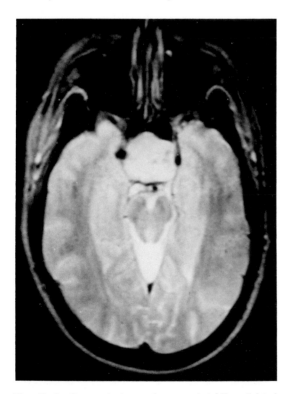

Fig. 48–6. Large pituitary adenoma. Axial T₂ weighted MR imaging shows a large intrasellar lesion with lateral displacement of both cavernous internal carotids, seen in cross section as circular structures of signal void due to flow. (Courtesy of Drs. J.A. Bello and S.K. Hilal.)

discovery of a large sella, or during a workup for headaches. In some cases, pseudotumor cerebri was present and increased intracranial pressure may have caused the empty sella. CSF rhinorrhea has also been described in this situation. Endocrine abnormalities, when present, are usually mild. The diagnosis is made by CT. An acquired empty sella occasionally follows surgical procedures.

Treatment. The first steps in the treatment of pituitary adenomas are the correction of any electrolyte imbalance and, if needed, institution of replacement therapy, particularly thyroid and adrenal hormones. These should be started if hypopituitarism is suspected, and immediately after blood specimens are taken for the endocrine evaluation. Adequate adrenal steroid coverage must be provided for surgical procedures.

The goals of treatment are different for the secreting tumors, especially microadenomas, and the nonsecreting lesions, usually chromophobe adenomas present with visual compromise. In the first case, a biologic cure is to be attained, correcting the hypersecreting status and preserving the normally functioning gland. This can often be achieved by selectively removing the tumor. In the latter cases, a more radical tumor excision, decompression of the optic pathways, and prevention of recurrence are the main objectives.

Not all pituitary tumors require immediate

Table 48–2.   Evaluation of the Enlarged Sella Turcica: Useful Features in Differential Diagnosis

	Nonsecreting Adenoma	Empty Sella	Cranio-pharyngioma	Other
Hypopituitarism	+ +	+	+ +	+ +
Diabetes insipidus	±	−	+ +	+
Abnormal visual fields	+ +	±	+ +	+ +
Ballooned sella, no erosion	−	+ +	−	−
Supasellar extension (CT)	+	−	+ +	+ +
Calcification	+	−	+ + +	+

Symbols: −, never seen; ±, rarely seen; +, sometimes seen; + +, common; + + +, characteristic
(From Post KD, Jackson JMD, Reichlin S, eds. The Pituitary Adenoma. New York: Plenum Medical Book Co, 1980.)

treatment. In some cases an enlarged sella turcica is found without any neurologic or endocrine manifestations. These patients should be closely watched and treatment may be deferred, although progression of the lesion may occur. The same attitude seems justified in patients with acromegalic features but without chemical evidence of active disease.

Radiotherapy and surgery are two basic and frequently complementary modalities of treatment. New medical approaches to therapy for secretory adenomas are discussed in Section 149.

Radiotherapy. Conventional irradiation using external beams and total doses of about 5,000 rad is indicated as the initial treatment for patients who are poor operative risks, or those with small, nonsecreting tumors with minimal or no visual involvement. If visual deterioration occurs, surgical decompression is indicated. Radiotherapy should also be

given after surgery whenever only subtotal removal of the tumor was possible because it reduces the incidence of recurrences. If these occur, surgical decompression through a subfrontal or transsphenoidal approach is usually preferred to a second course of radiotherapy. Radiotherapy is contraindicated in cases of pituitary apoplexy, or when there has been rapidly progressive visual loss.

In secreting tumors, conventional radiotherapy decreases the abnormal hormonal levels, but only infrequently to normal values and often only after several months. Radiotherapy is not without complications such as radiation necrosis of the brain, or, rarely, visual deterioration.

New irradiation techniques have also been proposed to achieve a better rate of cure of hypersecreting adenomas. These include proton-beam and heavy-particle irradiation and implantation inside the sella of radioactive isotopes like yttrium (^{90}Y) and gold (^{198}Au). These treatments are more effective in reducing abnormal hormonal levels, but have undesirable side effects, including a high incidence of post-treatment hypopituitarism.

Surgical Treatment. Surgical approaches to the pituitary gland changed with the introduction of antibiotics and steroids, and then with the development of microsurgical techniques. The transsphenoidal approach was used by Hirsch and Cushing, became less popular than the transcranial subfrontal approach, and has regained favor so that both methods are now used, depending on the specific case.

Transsphenoidal removal of a pituitary tumor is indicated for secreting microadenomas because it allows selective removal of the tumor, with preservation of the remaining gland. In these cases, radiotherapy is usually deferred, except when biologic cure was not

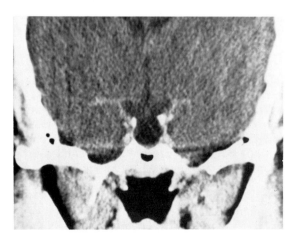

Fig. 48–7.   Empty-sella syndrome. Coronal contrast-enhanced CT section demonstrates subarachnoid space extending into the sella turcica without evidence of pituitary tissue. (Courtesy of Drs. S.K. Hilal and M. Mawad.)

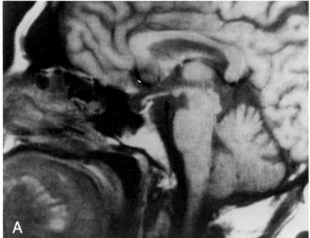

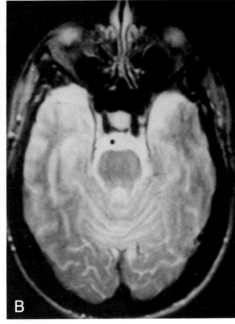

Fig. 48–8. Empty sella. *A*, Sagittal T_1 weighted MR image demonstrates low-intensity intrasellar signal representing CSF (compare to signal within the fourth ventricle). *B*, Axial T_2 weighted MR image on a different patient shows increased signal within the sella representing CSF on this pulse sequence (compare to signal from incidentally noted anterior temporal arachnoid cysts). (Courtesy of Drs. J.A. Bello and S.K. Hilal.)

achieved. In general, however, there is rapid reduction of the abnormal hormonal levels. The transsphenoidal approach is also the method of choice for tumors that invade the sphenoid sinus, in patients who are poor surgical risks, or for pituitary apoplexy.

In individuals with suprasellar extensions and an enlarged sella, either functioning or nonfunctioning, either or both transsphenoidal and subfrontal approaches can be used. Intracapsular removal of the tumor and decompression of the optic pathways are attempted, and radiotherapy should follow surgery.

A transcranial approach is indicated in patients with suprasellar lesions and a small sella, or for extrasellar extension into the anterior or temporal fossas. Again, radiotherapy should also be given.

Mortality of the transsphenoidal approach is 1 to 2%, and with the transcranial procedure, 3 to 5%. Other less commonly used forms of treatment include stereotactic radiofrequency lesions and cryohypophysectomy.

References

Barrow DL, Mizuno J, Tindall GT. Management of prolactinomas associated with very high serum prolactin levels. J Neurosurg 1988; 68:554–59.

Bonneville JF, Poulignot D, Cattin F, Couturier M, Mollet E, Dietemann JL. Computed tomographic demonstration of the effects of bromocriptine on pituitary microadenoma size. Radiology 1982; 143:451–455.

Cohen AR, Cooper PR, Kupersmith MJ, Flamm ES, Ransohoff J. Visual recovery after transsphenoidal removal of pituitary adenomas. Neurosurgery 1985; 17:446–452.

Ebersold MJ, Laws ER, Scheithauer BW, Randall RV. Pituitary apoplexy treated by transsphenoidal surgery. A clinicopathological and immunocytochemical study. J Neurosurg 1983; 58:315–320.

Harris JR, Levene MB. Visual complications following irradiation for pituitary adenomas and craniopharyngiomas. Radiology 1976; 120:167–171.

MacPherson P, Anderson DE. Radiological differentiation of intrasellar aneurysms from pituitary tumors. Neuroradiology 1981; 21:177–183.

McDonald WI. The symptomatology of tumors of the anterior visual pathways. Can J Neurol Sci 1982; 9:381–390.

Murphy FY, et al. Giant invasive prolactinomas. Am J Med 1987; 83:995–1002.

Post KD, Muraszko K. Management of pituitary tumors. In: Zimmerman EA, Abrams GM, eds. Neuroendocrinology and Brain Peptides. Philadelphia: WB Saunders, Co., 1986:801–831.

Serri O, Rasio E, Beauregard H, Hardy J, Somma M. Recurrence of hyperprolactinemia after selective transsphenoidal adenectomy in women with prolactinoma. N Engl J Med 1983; 309:280–283.

Serri O, Somma M, Comtois R, Rasio E, Beauregard H, Jilwan H, Hardy J. Acromegaly: biochemical assessment of cure after long-term follow-up of transsphenoidal selective adenectomy. J Clin Endocrinol Metab 1985; 61:1185–1189.

Weisberg LA, Numuguchi Y. Neuroimaging in neuroendocrine diseases. In: Zimmerman EA, Abrams GM, eds. Neuroendocrinology and Brain Peptides. Philadelphia: WB Saunders, Co., 1986:783–800.

49. CONGENITAL TUMORS

Earl A. Zimmerman

Craniopharyngiomas

Craniopharyngiomas (Rathke pouch tumors, hypophyseal duct tumors, adamantinomas) arise from remnants of the hypophyseal duct and constitute approximately 4% of all intracranial tumors. Owing to their location, they produce a syndrome similar to that of pituitary adenomas or other tumors in the suprasellar region. They vary from small, solid, well-circumscribed nodules to huge multilocular cysts that invade the sella turcica and displace neighboring cerebral structures (Fig. 49–1). The cysts are filled with a turbid fluid that may contain cholesterin crystals. There are three histologic types of craniopharyngioma: (1) mucoid epithelial cysts lined with ciliated columnar and mucus-secreting cells; (2) squamous epitheliomas composed of islands of squamous epithelium with cystic degeneration; and (3) adamantinomas, consisting of epithelial masses forming a reticulum resembling enamel pulp of developing teeth. Teratomas occasionally arise from epithelial remnants of the hypophyseal stalk. Craniopharyngiomas occur predominantly in infancy or childhood, with onset of symptoms before the age of 15 in 50% of cases, but symptoms may begin at any age, not infrequently after the age of 50 or 60.

The development of symptoms is usually slow, but occasionally they are of rapid or sudden onset. In most cases, the initial signs and symptoms are those of pituitary hypofunction. These are followed by evidence of involvement of the optic chiasm, optic tract, or one optic nerve. Diabetes insipidus is not infrequently seen. Because these tumors tend to invade the third ventricle, papilledema and other signs of increased intracranial pressure are more common than in pituitary adenomas.

The diagnosis of craniopharyngioma can usually be made from the age of the patient and CT or MRI (Fig. 49–2). Calcification in the suprasellar region is present in 80% of the patients. Although the sella turcica may be eroded, it is uncommon for it to be ballooned

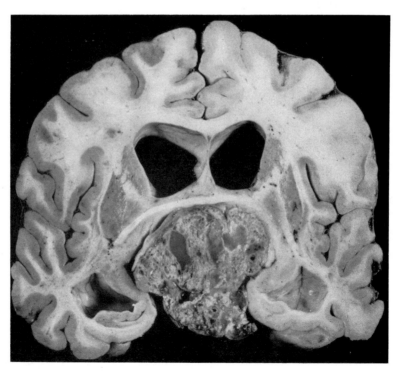

Fig. 49–1. Craniopharyngioma. Large tumor obstructing the third ventricle, causing hydrocephalus. (Courtesy of Dr. Abner Wolf.)

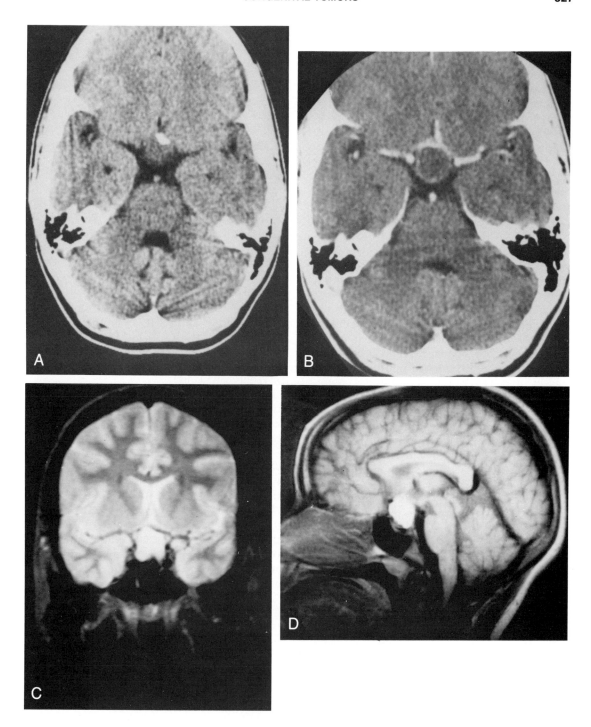

Fig. 49–2. Craniopharyngioma. *A,* Axial CT scanning demonstrates a soft tissue mass in the suprasellar cistern precontrast with calcification. *B,* Rim enhancement noted postcontrast typical of a craniopharyngioma. *C,* A coronal T_2 weighted MR scan demonstrates the cystic nature of the lesion, which elevates the anterior cerebral artery A_1 segments. Note signal void in the vascular structures due to flow. *D,* A sagittal T_1 weighted MR scan demonstrates the craniopharyngioma; typical hyperintensity on the T_1 image is attributed to the cyst contents. (Courtesy of Drs. J.A. Bello and S.K. Hilal.)

as in pituitary adenomas. These tumors occasionally arise within the sella. When the onset of symptoms is delayed until adult life and there is no calcification in the tumor, the diagnosis may not be established before operation.

The treatment of craniopharyngiomas is total removal of all of the solid tumor, evacuation of the cyst, removal of the cyst wall, and then radiation therapy. This regimen has resulted in a cure in a high percentage of the cases now that adequate endocrine therapy is available.

Cholesteatomas

Cholesteatomas (pearly tumors, epidermoids) are rare. They arise within the tables of the skull or in relationship to the dura. They occur in any portion of the cranial cavity. The most common sites (Table 49–1) are the cerebellopontine angle, suprasellar region, fourth ventricle, pineal recess, and over the convexity of the hemispheres. Cholesteatomas vary in size from small nodules to large masses that cover almost an entire hemisphere. They are usually sharply demarcated and completely encapsulated and have a pearly appearance. They may occasionally burrow into the cerebrum or brain stem. Microscopically, the tumor is divided into four layers: stratum durum, granulosum, fibrosum, and cellulosum.

Cholesteatomas may occur in patients at any age, but are most common in young adults. The signs and symptoms are related to the site of the tumor. Large cholesteatomas may overlie the cerebral hemisphere without symptoms. The diagnosis of cholesteatomas in the suprasellar region or in the posterior fossa is rarely made before operation. Those that underlie the cranial vault can be recognized from the characteristic shadow in the radiographs, a large evenly calcified area with sharp margins.

Cholesteatomas grow slowly, and the rate of progression of symptoms is related to the site of the tumor. Rapid advancement of symptoms is the rule when the tumor is in the fourth ventricle or cerebellopontine angle. Those over the cerebral hemisphere may be present for 10, 20, or more years without symptoms.

Treatment consists of surgical removal of the entire tumor with its capsule.

Chordomas

Chordomas develop from remnants of the notochord. Forty to sixty percent arise at the upper end of the notochord at the clivus Blumenbachii (Fig. 49–3), or at the junction of the sphenoid and occipital bones; 30 to 50% are in the sacrococcygeal region, and 10% occur elsewhere along the spine. These tumors have a smooth nodular surface of a milky-white color. The cut surface resembles cartilage but is often of jelly-like consistency. There may be cystic areas filled with slimy mucus. The characteristic feature of the histologic structure is the presence of large masses of spherical, oval, or polygonal cells, arranged in groups or cords, with large vacuoles that contain mucin in the cytoplasm (physaliferous cells).

Intracranial chordomas are highly invasive. They spread along the floor of the posterior fossa, damaging cranial nerves and compressing the brain stem. They may grow forward to cause bitemporal hemianopia as a result of involvement of the optic chiasm. They also invade the nasopharynx or the intracranial sinuses and may extend into the neck.

Chordomas that arise from the lower end of the notochord compress the roots of the cauda equina. Those that arise along other portions of the spinal cord compress and sometimes invade the substance of the spinal cord.

The diagnosis of intracranial chordoma can be made with certainty before operation only when the tumor invades the nasopharynx or neck and histologic identification is possible. It should be suspected whenever there are multiple cranial nerve palsies or when erosion of the floor of the skull in the region of the clivus Blumenbachii can be demonstrated in radiographs or CT. Treatment is by operation followed by radiation therapy. Complete removal is rarely possible, but growth of the tumor is inhibited by radiation.

Dermoids and Teratomas

Dermoids and teratomas that involve the CNS do not differ from similar tumors in other portions of the body. They tend to occur along the central axis, involving the regions

Table 49–1. The Location of Intracranial Cholesteatomas

Site of Tumor	No. of Cases	%
Suprasellar	44	39
Parapontine	53	47
Fourth ventricle	15	14

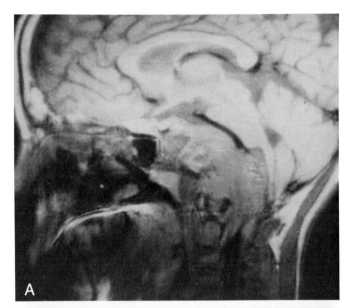

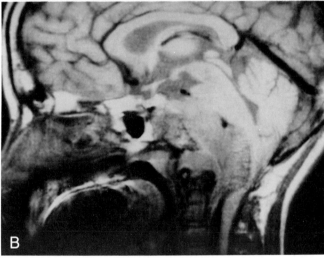

Fig. 49–3. Clival chordoma. *A, B,* Sagittal T_1 weighted MR scans demonstrate an exophytic lesion involving the clivus with extra-axial mass effect, posterior displacement of the basilar artery in *A,* and of the brain stem at the pontomedullary junction in *B.* Note also in *B,* mass effect on the fourth ventricle and definition of normal structures: optic chiasm, pituitary stalk, mamillary body, collicular plate, pineal gland, internal cerebral veins, vein of Galen, and straight sinus. (Courtesy of Drs. T.L. Chi, J.A. Bello, and S.K. Hilal.)

of the pituitary and pineal glands, the fourth ventricle, or the distal end of the spinal cord. Dermoids and teratomas vary greatly in size and are composed of several tissues, including elements of any of the three germ layers. Cystic degeneration is common. Although these tumors are present from birth, the onset of symptoms may be delayed for many years. More commonly, symptoms develop in the first decade of life. Ingraham and Bailey reported that teratomas constitute 4% of all intracranial tumors and 18% of all spinal tumors in childhood.

The signs and symptoms of teratomas are similar to those of other tumors. Calcification in the tumor may be seen in radiographs or CT, but the diagnosis can rarely be made before operative exposure of the tumor.

The result of the surgical removal of a teratoma depends on the degree of malignancy and invasiveness of the tumor. The results in 15 cases reported by Ingraham and Bailey were as follows: two patients lived more than five years after the operation without evidence of recurrence; five lived less than five years after operation without recurrence; the tumor recurred in two; six died.

Colloid Cysts of the Third Ventricle

Cystic degeneration may occur in many of the various types of intracranial tumors previously described. A large cyst with a mural nodule is most frequently seen in astrocytomas, particularly those in the cerebellar hemispheres, and in hemangioblastomas. A rare type of cystic tumor occurs within the cavity

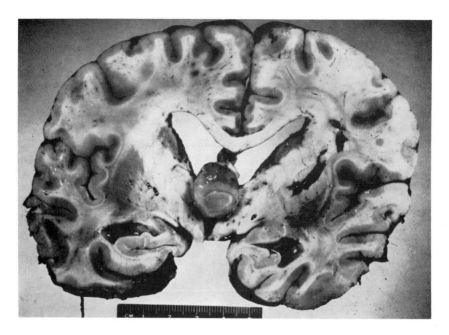

Fig. 49–4.   Colloid cyst of the third ventricle. (Courtesy of Dr. Philip Duffy.)

of the third ventricle and is known as a colloid cyst. This tumor presumably arises from the anlage of the paraphysis. It is located in the anterior superior part of the third ventricle (Fig. 49–4) and has the gross appearance of a small white ball. The cyst wall is composed of a layer of cuboidal and columnar ciliated cells and a layer of connective tissue. The cyst is filled with a homogeneous gelatinous material that becomes rubbery on fixation with formalin. In 1933, Dandy collected 16 cases from the literature and reported five additional cases. The age of the patients at the time of onset of symptoms varied between 10 and 60; most were in the third to fifth decades. Mental symptoms are common. Intermittent attacks of headache, dizziness, or weakness and numbness of the extremities, sometimes related to changes in posture, are attributed to acute hydrocephalus produced by a shift of the tumor so that it blocks the foramina of Monro. This train of symptoms may occur, however, on change of posture with a tumor anywhere in the cranial cavity. Colloid cyst of the third ventricle can be diagnosed from the CT appearance of the characteristic defect in the third ventricle (Fig. 49–5). Colloid cysts must be differentiated from other tumors that invade the third ventricle, such as gliomas, papillomas of the choroid plexus, craniopharyngiomas, pineal tumors, and pituitary adenomas. The differential diagnosis betwen colloid cyst and other tumors in the third ven-

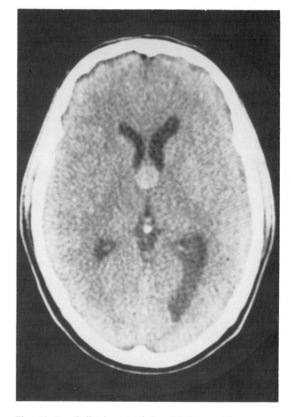

Fig. 49–5.   Colloid cyst of the third ventricle appears dense on noncontrast axial CT scan. (Courtesy of Drs. S.K. Hilal and S.R. Ganti.)

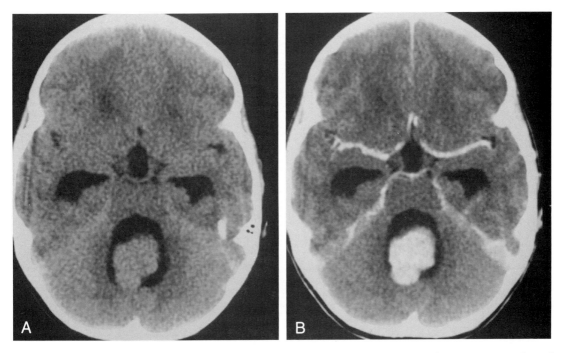

Fig. 49–6. Choroid plexus papilloma. *A,* An axial noncontrast CT scan shows posterior fossa intraventricular soft tissue. Fourth ventricle outlet obstruction is evidenced by prominent temporal horns and bulging lateral contours of the third ventricle. *B,* Marked postcontrast enhancement is typical of choroid plexus papilloma, a highly vascular tumor. (Courtesy of Drs. J.A. Bello and S.K. Hilal.)

tricle cannot always be made before operation, unless signs and symptoms characteristic of the various other types of tumors are present or unless the colloid cyst can be clearly visualized by CT. The treatment of colloid cysts is complete surgical removal through the foramen of Monro after frontal craniotomy.

Papillomas of the Choroid Plexus

Papillomas of the choroid plexus may be found in the lateral or third ventricles, but are more commonly found in the fourth ventricle (Fig. 49–6). Grossly, they are tufted, reddened, mulberry-like growths that may grow to a large size and may undergo cystic degeneration. Microscopically, the tumor is composed of papillae that have a central core of connective tissue and are covered by cuboidal choroidal epithelium. Papilloma of the choroid plexus is rare. Matson and Crofton collected 83 cases from the literature and Cushing found 12 in his series of 2,000 cases of verified intracranial tumors. They may occur at any age, but are common in children and young adults. Papillomas of the choroid plexus located in the lateral recess of the medulla may be accompanied by excessive formation of CSF. No signs or symptoms are

characteristic of papillomas of the choroid plexus. The diagnosis of an intraventricular tumor, but not the histologic type, can be ascertained by CT.

Arteriovenous Aneurysm

Direct connection between an artery and a vein in the brain with the exception of carotid-cavernous sinus fistula, is almost always the result of a congenital defect in the development of these vessels. Although any vessel may be affected, the vein of Galen is most frequently involved. Only a small number of patients with arteriovenous aneurysm have been reported. The symptoms and signs, which usually develop in infancy or early childhood, include headache, convulsive seizures, hydrocephalus, and cardiac failure. Death usually results from cardiac failure or cerebral decompression. A few patients have been cured by surgical ligation of the arterial feeders from the posterior and middle cerebral arteries and plication of the aneurysm.

Embolization of the malformation with elastic shears has symptomatically improved the condition of a number of patients with arteriovenous aneurysm by reducing the risk of hemorrhage, lessening headache pain, and reversing cardiac failure.

References

Craniopharyngiomas

Burns EC, Tanner JM, Preece MA, Gameron N. Growth hormone treatment in children with craniopharyngioma: final growth status. Clin Endocrinol 1981; 14:587–595.

Carmel PW, Antunes JL, Chang CH. Craniopharyngiomas in children. Neurosurgery 1982; 11:382–389.

Freeman MP, et al. Craniopharyngioma: CT and MRI in nine cases. J Comput Assist Tomogr 1987; 11:810–814.

Johnson LN, Helper RS, Yee RD, Frazee JB, Simons KB. Magnetic resonance imaging of craniopharyngioma. Am J Ophthalmol 1986; 102:242–244.

Krueger DW, Larson EB. Recurrent fever of unknown origin and meningiomas due to leaking craniopharyngioma. Am J Med 1988; 84:543–545.

Manaka S, Teramoto A, Takakura K. The efficacy of radiotherapy for craniopharyngioma. J Neurosurg 1985; 62:648–656.

Sorva R, Jääskinen J, Heiskanen O, Perheentupa J. Postoperative computed tomographic control of 38 patients with craniopharyngioma. Surg Neurol 1988; 29:115–119.

Thomsett MJ, Conte FA, Kaplan SL, Grumbach MM. Endocrine and neurologic outcome in childhood craniopharyngioma: review of effect of treatment in 42 patients. J Pediatr 1980; 97:728–735.

Till K. Craniopharyngioma. Childs Brain 1982; 9:179–187.

Chordomas

Brooks LJ, Afshani E, Hidalgo C, Fisher J. Clivus chordoma with pulmonary metastases appearing as failure to thrive. Am J Dis Child 1981; 135:713–715.

Grossman RI, Davis KR. Cranial computed tomographic appearance of chondrosarcoma of the base of the skull. Radiology 1981; 141:403–408.

Kendall BE, Lee BCP. Cranial chordomas. Br J Radiol 1977; 50:687–698.

Occhipinti E, Mastrostefano R, Pompili A, et al. Spinal chordomas in infancy. Report of a case and analysis of the literature. Childs Brain 1981; 8:198–206.

O'Neil P, Bell BA, Miller JD, Jacobson I, Guthrie W. Fifty years experience with chordomas in southeast Scotland. Neurosurgery 1985; 16:166–170.

Shallat RF, Taekman MS, Nagle RC. Unusual presentation of cervical chordoma wih long-term survival. J Neurosurg 1982; 57:716–718.

Singh W, Kaur A. Nasopharyngeal chordoma presenting with metastases. Case report and review of the literature. J Laryngol Otol 1987; 101:1198–1202.

Suit HD, Goitein M, Munzenrider J, et al. Definitive radiation therapy for chordoma and chondrosarcoma of base of skull and cervical spine. J Neurosurg 1982; 56:377–385.

Sundaresan N, Galicich JH, Chu FCH, Huvos AG. Spinal chordomas. J Neurosurg 1979; 50:312–319.

Tan WS, Spigos D, Khnie N. Chordoma of the sellar region. J Comput Assist Tomogr 1982; 6:154–158.

Yuh WT, Flickinger FW, Barloon TJ, Montgomery WJ. MR imaging of unusual chordomas. J Comput Assist Tomogr 1988; 12:30–35.

Dermoids and Teratomas

Abou-Samra M, Marlin AE, Story JL, Brown WE, Jr. Cranial epidermoid tumor associated with subacute extradural hematoma. Case report. J Neurosurg 1980; 53:574–575.

Arseni C, Canaila L, Constantinescu AI, Carp N, Decu P. Cerebral dermoid tumors. Neurochirurgia 1976; 19:104–114.

Chambers AA, Lukin RR, Tomsick TA. Cranial epidermoid tumors: diagosis by computerized tomography. Neurosurgery 1977; 1:276–280.

Gutin PH, Boehm J, Bank WO, Edwards MS, Rosegae H. Cerebral convexity epidermoid tumor subsequent to multiple percutaneous subdural aspirations. J Neurosurg 1980; 52:574–577.

Mikhael MA, Mattar AG. Intracranial pearly tumors: the roles of computed tomography, angiography and pneumoencephalography. J Comput Assist Tomogr 1978; 2:421–429.

Nosaka Y, Nagao S, Tabuchi K, Nishimoto A. Primary intracranial epidermoid carcinoma. J Neurosurg 1979; 50:830–839.

Schwartz JF, Balentine JD. Recurrent meningitis due to an intracranial epidermoid. Neurology 1978; 28:124–129.

Takeuchi J, Mori K, Moritake K, Tani F, Waga S, Handa H. Teratomas in the suprasellar region. Report of five cases. Surg Neurol 1975; 3:247–255.

Toglia JU, Netsky MG, Alexander E Jr. Epithelial (epidermoid) tumors of the cranium: their common nature and pathogenesis. J Neurosurg 1965; 23:384–393.

Valdiserri RO, Yunis EJ. Sacrococcygeal teratomas: a review of 68 cases. Cancer 1981; 48:217–221.

Zimmerman RA, Bilaniuk LT, Dolinskas C. Cranial computed tomography of epidermoid and congenital fatty tumors of maldevelopment origin. CT 1979; 3:40–50.

Cysts

Bosch DA, Rahn T, Backlund EO. Treatment of colloid cysts of the third ventricle by stereotactic aspiration. Surg Neurol 1978; 9:15–18.

Brunette JRR, Walsh FB. Neurophthalmological aspects of tumors of the third ventricle. Can Med Assoc J 1968; 98:1184–1192.

Cairns H, Mosberg WH Jr. Colloid cyst of the third ventricle. Surg Gynecol Obstet 1951; 92:545–570.

Dandy WE. Benign Tumors in the Third Ventricle of the Brain. Springfield: Charles C Thomas, 1933.

Ghatak NR, Kassoff I, Alexander E Jr. Further observation on the fine structures of a colloid cyst of the third ventricle. Acta Neuropathol 1977; 39:101–107.

Michels LG, Rutz D. Colloid cysts of the third ventricle. A radiologic-pathologic correlation. Arch Neurol 1982; 39:640–643.

Papillomas

Fortuna A, Celli P, Ferrante L, Turano C. A review of papillomas of the third ventricle. J Neurosurg Sci 1979; 23:61–76.

Gudeman SK, Sullivan H, Rosner M, Becker D. Surgical removal of bilateral papillomas of the choroid plexus of the lateral ventricles with resolution of hydrocephalus. J Neurosurg 1979; 50:677–681.

Hawkin JC III. Treatment of choroid plexus papillomas in children: a brief analysis of twenty years experience. Neurosurgery 1980; 6:380–384.

Milhorat TH, Hammock MK, Davis DA, Fenstermacker JD. Choroid plexus papilloma: I. Proof of cerebrospinal fluid overproduction. Childs Brain 1976; 2:273–289.

Sahar A, Feinsod M, Beller AJ. Choroid plexus papilloma: hydrocephalus and cerebrospinal fluid dynamics. Surg Neurol 1980; 13:476–478.

Zimmerman RA, Bienniuk LT. Computed tomography of choroid plexus lesions. CT 1979; 3:93–103.

Arteriovenous Aneurysm

Gold AP, Ranohoff J, Carter S. Vein of Galen malformation. Acta Neurol (Scand) 1964; 40(Suppl 11):5–31.

Gomez MR, et al. Aneurysmal malformation of the great vein of Galen causing heart failure in early infancy: A report of five cases. Pediatrics 1963, 31:400–411.

50. VASCULAR TUMORS AND MALFORMATIONS
Bennett M. Stein

The heterogeneous group of vascular lesions discussed here includes one category that represents neoplasms and another that represents malformations as indicated by the following list:

Vascular Tumors
Angioblastic meningiomas
Hemangiopericytomas
Hemangioblastomas
Vascular Malformations
Arteriovenous malformations
Venus malformations
Cavernous malformations
Telangiectases
Sturge-Weber disorder
Sinus pericranii

Vascular Tumors

The literature is replete with controversy as to whether the three neoplasms discussed in the group of neoplastic lesions listed above represent variations of the same tumor. By light microscopy they are indistinguishable; however, the hemangioblastoma is confined to the posterior fossa and is without dural attachment. The angioblastic meningioma is grossly identical to other meningiomas, having a significant dural attachment and being located either above or below the tentorium. The hemangiopericytoma originates in other areas of the body, presumably from blood vessel elements.

ANGIOBLASTIC MENINGIOMAS

These tumors are included here primarily because they are histologically similar to the other tumors discussed in this section.

HEMANGIOPERICYTOMAS

Whether this tumor deserves separate categorization is yet to be decided. The hemangiopericytoma arises from the endothelial elements of blood vessels and is recognized elsewhere in the body. It is histologically similar to the angioblastic meningioma and the hemangioblastoma, especially when the vascular spaces are separated more widely and the stroma cells are collected about the vascular spaces. It may be that the pial and endothelial cells are interconvertible, an assumption that is thus far unsupported.

HEMANGIOBLASTOMAS

Hemangioblastomas are rare tumors that are composed of primitive vascular elements. Their incidence ranges from 1 to 2% of all intracranial neoplasms. They occur in patients at all ages, but young and middle-aged adults are more frequently afflicted. In children, they are almost as common in the posterior fossa as meningiomas. The average age at onset is 33 and the symptoms are generally present for approximately a year before the diagnosis is made. Male incidence predominates. *Von Hippel-Lindau disease* is defined by the coexistence of hemangioblastoma and multiple angiomatoses of the retina, cysts of the kidney and pancreas and, occasionally, renal cell carcinomas and capillary nevi of the skin. There is a familial incidence in 20% of the cases. However, only 10 to 20% of the hemangioblastomas are associated with the Lindau syndrome. All gradations of clinical expression between the full syndrome and incomplete manifestations may be seen in the same family.

Other associations of hemangioblastomas are with pheochromocytoma and syringomyelia, especially when the hemangioblastoma is in the spinal cord. Polycythemia appears to disappear after resection of the neoplasm, but returns with recurrence; an erythropoietic substance from the cystic fluid has been identified. These tumors almost always occur in the cerebellum and are often associated with large cysts that are surrounded by a glial wall and that contain yellow proteinaceous fluid, which is the result of secretion and hemorrhage from the tumor. This tumor resembles the cyst and mural nodule of the cystic cerebellar astrocytoma. However, it has a distinctive vascular appearance on an angiogram. The cerebellar hemangioblastoma may be multiple, in which case difficulty in achieving a cure or total removal of the lesion may be encountered. These tumors have no dural attachment and rarely occur in the supratentorial area, where they may be confused with angioblastic meningiomas.

The most common site of the hemangioblastoma is in the paramedian cerebellar hemispheric area. The second most common site is the spinal cord. Hemangioblastomas also occur in the medulla, where they arise from the area postrema.

Clinical features of the hemangioblastoma of the cerebellum include headache, papilledema, and ataxia. When the tumor is located in one cerebellar hemisphere, the ataxia is ipsilateral. When multiple, these lesions may involve the brain stem and upper cervical cord, as well as the cerebellum. Hemangioblastoma of the cerebellum can be diagnosed without difficulty from the CT scan and posterior fossa angiogram. The diagnosis is even more certain when the tumor is associated with angiomas of the retina and polycythemia. These tumors are much less common than other tumors of the cerebellum such as the astrocytoma, medulloblastoma, and metastatic tumors.

Treatment is surgery with evacuation of the cyst and removal of the mural nodule; 85% of all patients who undergo this treatment are alive and well 5 to 20 years after surgery. However, there is a high incidence of recurrence if the tumor is partially removed or is associated with multiple tumors.

Vascular Malformations

Vascular malformations of the brain are discussed in detail below. These have been confused with vascular neoplasms because their clinical course may be progressive and their angiographic picture is sometimes indistinguishable from neoplasms of blood vessels. However, vascular malformations are congenital lesions without evidence of neoplasia.

ARTERIOVENOUS MALFORMATIONS

Arteriovenous malformations (AVM) may be limited to the brain or dura or may involve both of these structures. The AVMs confined to the brain are more common. Approximately 10% of these have varying degrees of blood supply from the dura. These malformations are congenital, do not grow except in rare circumstances, and therefore do not enlarge out of proportion to the growth of the brain. They do tend to acquire collateral circulation, especially when major feeding arteries to the malformation are compromised by natural or therapeutic means. These lesions consist of a tangle of abnormal arteries and veins with interposed sinuses consisting of cavernous vascular channels that are identified neither as arteries nor veins. The lesions may be discrete or may cover broad areas of the brain. They are related frequently to cerebral hemorrhage and, over the course of decades, may produce a progressive neurologic abnormality leading to severe disability or death in approximately 50% of young patients. They are most commonly seen in the middle decades of life. In addition to producing hemorrhage, they may be the cause of seizures, headaches, and progressive neurologic deficit without hemorrhage (Figs. 50–1, 50–2).

CT or MRI scan is accurate in indicating the presence of these lesions (Figs. 50–3, 50–4), but their anatomy is best defined by arteriography.

Because of the threat of neurologic catastrophe, AVM should be treated aggressively. Radiographic techniques such as embolization have been developed to lower the operative risk and to reduce the size and pressure within the malformation prior to surgery. The only certain means of eliminating them as a threat to the patient is surgical resection. The risk of these operations has been minimized by contemporary neurosurgical techniques.

AVMs that are strictly confined to the dura are difficult to manage because they receive a more complex arterial supply than the cerebral lesions and therefore are difficult to obliterate by radiographic or surgical techniques. These lesions produce abnormal shunts as well as intracranial bruits and severe intractable headaches. They may be the cause of subarachnoid hemorrhage or subdural hematomas. The ones that lie in the anterior meningeal region, especially around the anterior fossa and chiasm, have a high incidence of spontaneous regression and thrombosis. The surgical treatment of these lesions should not be taken lightly because they involve broad areas of the dura and may not be totally resectable without damage to major venous sinuses and cerebral structures.

The vein of Galen malformation is a special AVM associated with the deep venous system, often with marked aneurysmal dilatation of the vein of Galen region. The arterial supply may be complex and difficult to occlude by intravascular or surgical techniques. These lesions present in childhood, usually with severe shunting leading to cardiac failure and compression of the midbrain, which leads to hydrocephalus. The currently accepted treat-

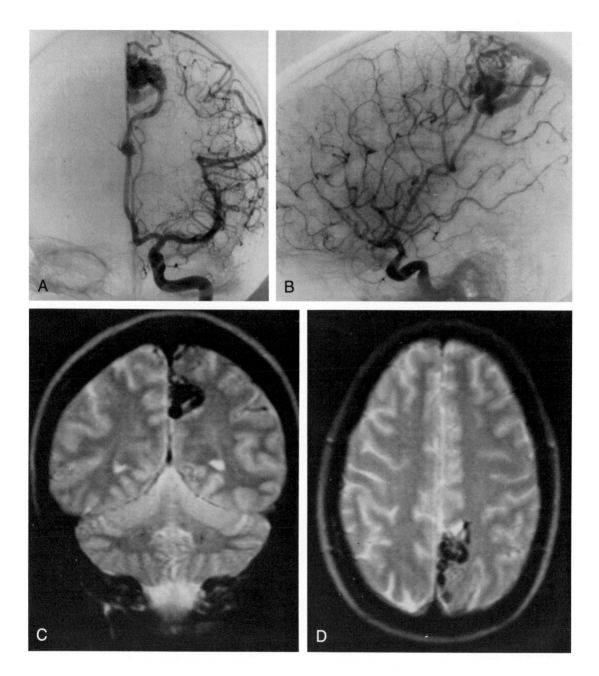

Fig. 50–1. Left parietal AVM. *A,* AP and *B,* lateral subtraction films in the arterial phase of a left internal carotid injection show the ACA supply and early superficial venous drainage of a left parietal AVM. *C,* Coronal and *D,* axial T_2 weighted MR images on the same patient show a serpiginous pattern of signal void representing flow in vascular structures. (Courtesy of Drs. J.A. Bello and S.K. Hilal.)

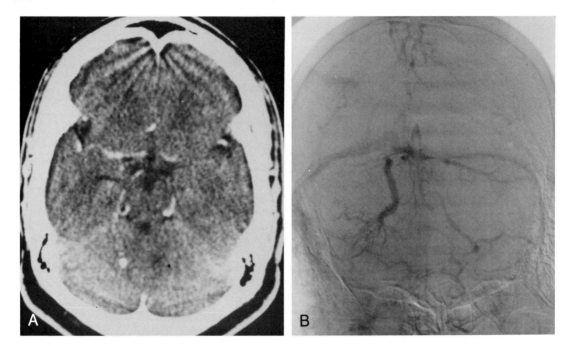

Fig. 50–2. Venous angioma. *A,* Post contrast CT scanning demonstrates a round enhancing structure in the right cerebellar hemisphere, seen on contiguous axial sections as well, and therefore consistent with a single prominent vessel, "end-on." This is the typical CT appearance of a venous angioma. *B,* An AP subtraction film in the venous phase of a vertebral angiogram shows medullary veins in the right cerebellar hemisphere converging toward a single vertically oriented draining vein, which corresponds to the vessel seen in cross section on CT. (The arterial phase was typically normal.) (Courtesy of Drs. J.A. Bello and S.K. Hilal.)

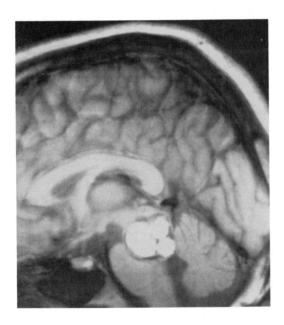

Fig. 50–3. Cavernous malformation, brain stem. Sagittal T₁ weighted MRI demonstrates a loculated appearing midbrain lesion of increased signal intensity surrounded by ring of decreased signal intensity which is characteristic of a subacute hemorrhage surrounded by a ring of hemosiderin. Cavernous vascular malformations typically show evidence of previous hemorrhage. (Courtesy of Drs. J.A. Bello and S.K. Hilal.)

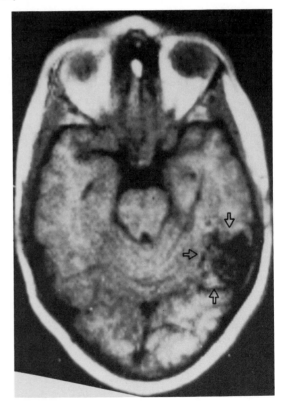

Fig. 50–4. An axial MRI scan demonstrating a left posterior temporal AVM (arrows).

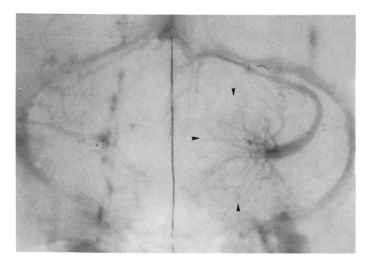

Fig. 50–5. Subtraction posterior fossa angiogram, venous phase. In this AP view the characteristic venous malformation is demonstrated (arrows).

ment of these lesions is embolization, occasionally followed by surgery.

VENOUS MALFORMATIONS

Venous malformations are lesions that were alluded to in the past but have only recently been identified for their true nature—that of a truly venous malformation without apparent arterial supply—as a result of CT scanning and precise angiography. These lesions may present with headaches, seizures and, rarely, with hemorrhage. They are identified by large venous channels that may be seen on a prolonged high-volume contrast angiogram (Fig. 50–5). They are easily recognized using CT because of their contrast enhancement. These lesions generally lie in the deep white matter, portions of the brain stem, and cerebellum. They are often diffuse and ill-defined and therefore are not amenable to surgical resection. They generally follow a benign course. The symptoms produced by the lesion should be treated individually. Only under extenuating circumstances should surgical resection be considered.

CAVERNOUS MALFORMATION

Similar to the venous malformation is the cavernous malformation, which presents with seizures, headaches, and vague neurologic symptoms. Hemorrhage from this lesion is rare. A cavernous malformation is clearly depicted by CT scan. Because of calcium content, it is visible without contrast and enhances moderately with contrast. It may be mistaken for a vascular tumor, however, without displacement of the surrounding structure. MRI scan is characterized by a "target" appearance (Fig. 50–6). A cavernous malformation generally does not appear on arteriographs because it has no artery-to-vein shunts. The diagnosis may be made by the typical histologic findings and because of the deep location of the cavernous malformation. It is advisable to remove the lesion if it is accessible. These lesions may occur in any portion of the CNS including brain stem and spinal cord.

TELANGIECTASIA

Telangiectases are collections of engorged capillaries or cavernous spaces separated by relatively normal brain tissue. They are usually small and poorly circumscribed, and may be found in any portion of the CNS. Telangiectases have a propensity for the white matter. They may be associated with telangiectasia of the skin, mucous membranes, and the respiratory, gastrointestinal, and genitourinary tracts, as in the *Rendu-Osler syndrome*. These lesions occasionally lead to gross hemorrhage and fatality. For the most part, these are neurologic curiosities; they cannot be identified on arteriography or CT and have no surgical significance. They are usually recognized only at autopsy.

STURGE-WEBER DISEASE (KRABBE-WEBER-DIMITRI DISEASE)

The two cardinal features of Sturge-Weber disease are a localized atrophy and calcification of the cerebral cortex associated with an ipsilateral port-wine-colored facial nevus, usually in the distribution of the first division of the trigeminal nerve. Angiomatous malformation in the meninges, ipsilateral exophthalmos, glaucoma, buphthalmos, angiomas of the retina, optic atrophy, and dilated ves-

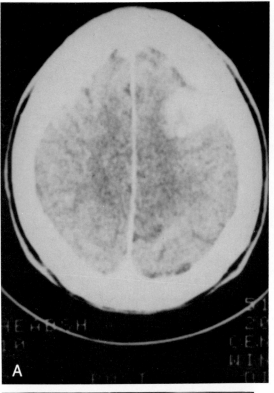

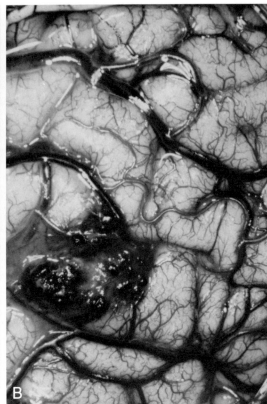

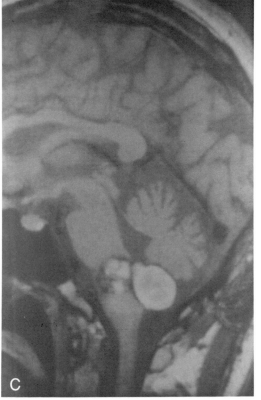

Fig. 50–6. *A,* Axial CT scan demonstrates a cavernous malformation extending deep from the cortical surface. *B,* Operative exposure of cavernous malformation showing the cortical component of this lesion. *C,* MRI showing the characteristic variegated appearance of a cavernous malformation of the brain stem in a different patient.

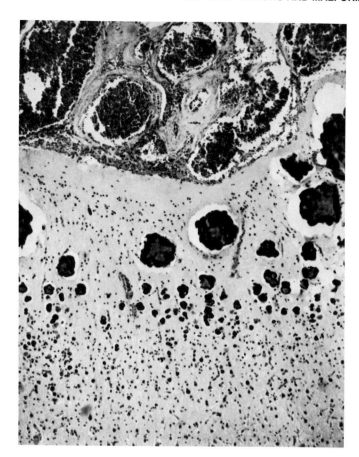

Fig. 50–7. Sturge-Weber syndrome. Angiomatous malformation in meninges and calcification in cortex. H&E stain. (Courtesy of Dr. Philip Duffy.)

sels in the sclera may also be present. Any portion of the cerebral cortex may be affected by the atrophic process, but the occipital and parietal regions are most commonly involved.

In the atrophic cortical areas there is a loss of nerve cells and axons and a proliferation of the fibrous glia. The small vessels are thickened and calcified, particularly in the second and third cortical layers. Small calcium deposits are also present in the cerebral substance (Fig. 50–7), and rarely are there large calcified nodules. When an angioma is present, it is limited to the meninges overlying the area of shrunken cortex. It is now generally agreed that the atrophy and calcification of the cortex are not secondary to the angiomatous malformations of the leptomeninges.

Sturge-Weber syndrome is probably more common than would be concluded from the relatively small number of cases that are recorded in the literature. Yakovlev and Guthrie, for example, found six cases in the clinical material of the Epileptic Colony at Monson, Massachusetts. It is possible for the combination of a port-wine facial nevus and local-ized cortical atrophy to exist without clinical symptoms but, in most patients, convulsive seizures are present from infancy. Mental retardation, contralateral hemiplegia (Fig. 50–8), or hemianopia are also present in most cases.

Sturge-Weber disease can be diagnosed without difficulty from the clinical syndrome. The presence of the cortical lesion can be demonstrated in most cases by the appearance of characteristic shadows in the radiographs (Fig. 50–9). The calcified area in the cortex appears as a sinous shadow with a double contour, showing both the gyri and sulci of the affected cerebral convolutions. The lesions in the occipital or parietal lobes are usually more definitely calcified than those that occur in the frontal lobe.

The treatment of patients with Sturge-Weber disease is essentially symptomatic. Anticonvulsive drugs should be given for the seizures. Radiation therapy has been recommended, but there is no evidence that it is of any benefit. Hemispherectomy may be of benefit in the control of the convulsive seizures, but is avoided because of a significant complication rate.

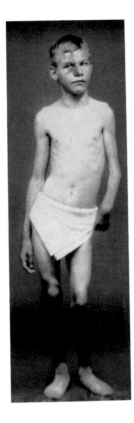

Fig. 50–8. Sturge-Weber disease. Right facial nevus in patient with convulsions and left hemiparesis. (Courtesy of Dr. P.I. Yakovlev.)

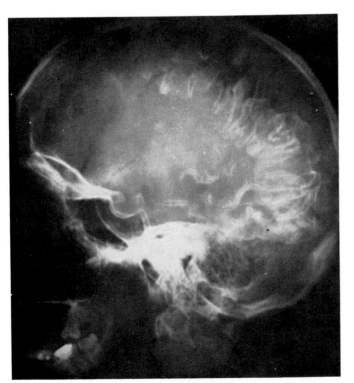

Fig. 50–9. Radiograph showing the intracerebral calcification in Sturge-Weber disease. (Courtesy of Dr. P.I. Yakovlev.)

SINUS PERICRANII

Sinus pericranii is composed of thin-walled vascular spaces interconnected by numerous anastomoses that protrude from the skull and communicate with the superior longitudinal sinus. The malformation appears early in life and is soft and compressible; it increases in size when the venous pressure in the head is raised by coughing, straining, or lowering the head. It may enlarge slowly over a period of years. The external protuberance may be seen at any portion of the midline of the skull, including the occiput, but is most often found in the midportion of the forehead. Except for the external swelling, there are usually no symptoms. There may occasionally be a pulsating tinnitus, increased intracranial pressure, or a variety of cerebral symptoms. Radiographs show a defect of the underlying bone, through which the lesion communicates with the longitudinal sinus.

References

Atuk NO, McDonald T, Wood T, et al. Familial pheochromocytoma, hypercalcemia, and von Hippel-Lindau disease. A ten year study of a large family. Medicine 1979; 58:209–218.

Baleriaux-Waha D, Retif J, Noterman J, et al. CT scanning for the diagnosis of the cerebellar and spinal lesions of von Hippel-Lindau's disease. Neuroradiology 1978; 14:241–244.

Bell, BA, Kendall BE, Symon L. Angiographically occult arteriovenous malformations of the brain. J Neurol Neurosurg Psychiatry 1978; 41:1057–1064.

Chao DH. Congenital neurocutanenous syndromes of childhood. III. Sturge-Weber disease. J Pediatr 1959; 55:635.

Cushing H, Bailey P. Tumors Arising from the Blood Vessels of the Brain. Springfield: Charles C Thomas, 1928.

Di Trapani G, Di Rocco C, Abbamondi AL, Caldarelli M, Pochhiari M. Light microscopy and ultrastructural studies of Sturge-Weber. Childs Brain 1982; 9:23–36.

Farrell DF, Forno LS. Symptomatic capillary telangiectasis of the brainstem without hemorrhage. Report of an unusual case. Neurology 1970; 20:341–346.

Gold AP, Ransohoff J, Carter S. Vein of Galen malformation. Acta Neurol Scand 1964; 40(Suppl 2).

Hoffman HJ, Hendrick EB, Dennis M, Armstrong D. Hemispherectomy for Sturge-Weber syndrome. Childs Brain 1979; 5:233–248.

Hull MT, Roth LM, Glover JL, Walker PD. Metastatic carotid body paraganglioma in von Hippel-Lindau disease. An electron microscopic study. Arch Pathol Lab Med 1982; 106:235–239.

Jeffreys RV, Napier JA, Reynolds SH. Erythropoietin levels in posterior fossa haemangioblastoma. J Neurol Neurosurg Psychiatry 1982; 45:264–266.

Kollarits CR, Mehelas TJ, Shealy TR, Zahn JR. Von-Hippel tumors in siblings with retinitis pigmentosa. Ann Ophthalmol 1982; 14:256–259.

Kruse F Jr. Hemangiopericytomas of the meninges (angioblastic meningioma of Cushing and Eisenhardt).

Clinicopathologic aspects and follow-up studies in 8 cases. Neurology 1961; 11:771–777.

McCormick WF, Nofzinger JD. 'Cryptic' vascular malformations of the central nervous system. J Neurosurg 1966, 24:865–875.

Mangiardi JR, Epstein FJ. Brainstem hematomas: review of literature and presentation of 5 new cases. J Neurol Neurosurg Psychiatry 1988; 51:966–976.

Mohr JP, Tatemichi TK, Nichols FC, et al: Vascular Malformations of the Brain: Clinical Considerations. Barnett HJM, Mohr JP, Stein BM, Yatsu FM (eds.). Stroke: Pathophysiology, Diagnosis, and Management, 1986. Vol. 2, Chap. 32: 679–706.

Moritake K, Handa H, Mori K, Ishikawa M, Morimoto M, Takebe Y. Venous angiomas of the brain. Surg Neurol 1980; 14:95–105.

Pia HW, et al. Cerebral Angiomas, Advances in Diagnosis and Therapy. New York: Springer-Verlag, 1975.

Rigamonti D, et al. Cerebral cavernous malformations: incidence and familial occurrence. N Engl J Med 1988; 319:343–347.

Sarwar M, McCormick WF. Intracerebral venous angioma. Arch Neurol 1978; 35:323–325.

Schulz MD, Wang CC, Zinninger GF, Tefft M. Radiotherapy of intracranial neoplasms. In: Kreyenbuhl H, Maspes PE, Sweet WH, eds. Progress in Neurological Surgery, vol 2. Chicago: Year Book Medical Publishers, 1968: 318–370.

Seeger JF, Burke DP, Knake JE, Gabrielsen TO. Computed tomographic and angiographic evaluation of hemangioblastomas. Radiology 1981; 138:65–73.

Simard JM, Garcia-Bengochea F, Ballinger WE, Mickle JP, Quisling RG. Cavernous angioma: a review of 126 collected and 12 new clinical cases. Neurosurgery 1986; 18:162–172.

Stein BM: Surgical Decisions in Vascular Malformations of the Brain. Barnett HJM, Mohr JP, Stein BM, Yatsu FM (eds.). Stroke: Pathophysiology, Diagnosis, and Management. vol. 2, Chap. 56:1129–1172.

Stein BM, Wolpert SM. Arteriovenous malformations of the brain I and II: Current concepts and treatment. Arch Neurol 1980; 37:1–5, 69–75.

Sung DI, Thang CH, Harisiadis L. Cerebellar hemangioblastomas. Cancer 1982; 49:553–555.

Wendling LR, Moore JS, Kieffer SA, et al. Intracerebral venous angioma. Radiology 1976; 119:141–147.

Wilson CB, Hoi Sang U, Domingue J. Microsurgical treatment of intracranial vascular malformations. J Neurosurg 1979; 51:446–454.

Wilson CB, Stein BM, eds. Current Neurosurgical Practice. Intracranial Arteriovenous Malformations. Baltimore: Williams & Wilkins, 1984.

---

51. METASTATIC TUMORS AND GRANULOMAS
Michael R. Fetell

Brain Metastases

Twenty-five percent of patients with systemic cancer develop brain metastases to the dura, meninges, or brain parenchyma. Parenchymal metastases are most common in lung cancer, melanoma, breast cancer, renal cancer, and lymphoma (Table 51–1). Dural metastases occur in patients with prostate and

Table 51–1. Primary Sites of Metastatic Tumors of the Brain

Type and Site of Primary Tumor	No. of Cases	%
Carcinoma		
Lung	184	46
Upper respiratory tract	14	3
Breast	51	13
Gastrointestinal tract	34	9
Pancreas	8	2
Liver and gallbladder	5	1
Endocrine organs	7	2
Urinary tract	10	3
Reproductive organs	15	4
Melanoma	13	3
Other and unknown	17	4
Nonepithelial		
Leukemia	27	7
Sarcoma	12	3
Total	397	100

(Modified from Aronson SM, Garcia JH, Aronson BE. Cancer 1964; 17:558–563.)

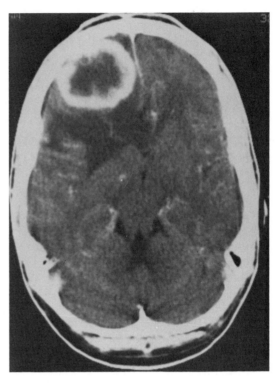

Fig. 51–1. Brain metastasis. Postcontrast CT shows large ring-enhancing metastasis of adenocarcinoma of lung, with significant edema.

breast carcinoma, and some sarcomas, but prostate carcinoma rarely metastasizes to brain parenchyma. The incidence of parenchymal brain metastases increases with increased survival, and the cumulative incidence is 60 to 80% in patients with small cell lung cancer who survive two years or more.

CT (Fig. 51–1) and MRI are the most efficient diagnostic procedures. One or both procedures should be performed in all patients with cerebral symptoms in the preoperative assessment of patients scheduled for resection of their primary tumor (Figs. 51–2, 51–3).

Rarely, brain metastases seem to respond to systemic chemotherapy, but far more often the blood-brain barrier has been blamed for the appearance of brain metastases in patients with systemic tumor controlled by chemotherapy. Because more than 50% of brain metastases are multiple, treatment consists of radiotherapy delivered to the whole brain. The standard treatment is palliative and consists of 3,000 cGy in 10 fractions of 300 cGy each. A boost of 1,550 to 2,000 cGy may also be given to the site of principal involvement if the primary tumor is well controlled. Treatment is effective in palliating symptoms in two thirds of the patients treated. The median survival is ≤9 months, however, with 68% of patients dying of neurologic disease, 16% of systemic disease, and 16% of combined neurologic and systemic disease.

Patients with solitary brain metastases (14 to 35%) who have surgical resection of tumor followed by radiotherapy fare much better than the group treated with radiotherapy alone. Most long-term survivors have undergone both surgery and radiation. However, there is marked selection bias in such retrospective series because patients referred for surgery are those with limited systemic disease and good performance status.

Prophylactic cranial irradiation (PCI) reduces the two-year cumulative incidence of brain metastases in patients with small cell carcinoma of lung from 47 to 10% and decreases concomitant neurologic morbidity, but it is debatable whether it improves survival. The high frequency of brain metastasis has led to trials of PCI in other lung carcinomas as well. However, a disturbing number of long-term survivors show a syndrome of leukoencephalopathy with dementia and ataxia. Larger fraction size predisposes to this complication, but it may also occur with standard radiotherapy fractionation, and has prompted reductions in both fraction size and total dosage. Another complication, spinal meningeal carcinomatosis, develops in about 22% of patients with small cell carcinoma treated with PCI. Its occurrence implies that

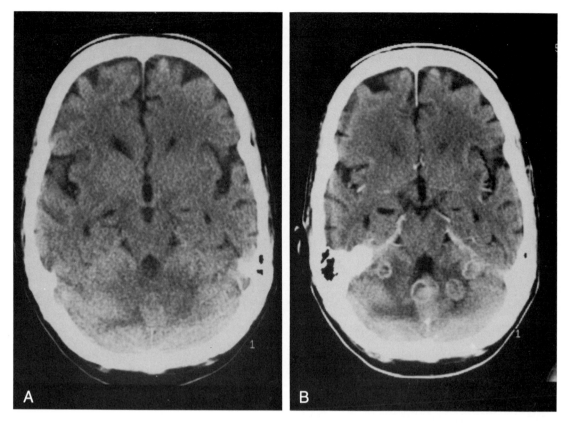

Fig. 51–2. Multiple brain metastases. Pre *(A)* and post *(B)* contrast CT scans of patient with adenocarcinoma of the lung showing multiple ring-enhancing lesions without surrounding edema. These cerebellar metastases would have been missed if contrast enhancement had been omitted. (Courtesy of Drs. J.A. Bello, S.K. Hilal, and M.R. Fetell.)

either spinal irradiation or intrathecal chemotherapy should be combined with PCI.

Meningeal Carcinomatosis

Diagnosis. When a patient with systemic cancer develops a cranial nerve palsy, strong suspicion of meningeal carcinomatosis is raised. This syndrome has been recognized with increased frequency as survival of patients with cancer has improved. Meningeal carcinomatosis is usually seen in patients with established systemic malignant tumors within six months to three years of initial diagnosis, but in about 6% of patients, causes the first symptoms. The signs of meningeal carcinomatosis parallel the course of systemic tumor; if meningeal carcinomatosis affects a patient in apparent clinical remission, evidence of recurrent tumor usually appears within weeks or months. Hematogenous metastasis to the meninges is rare, and spread of tumor presumably occurs by transgression of the dural barrier, either by direct extension of tumor from a vertebral or paravertebral focus, or from a cranial bony lesion (Fig. 51–4).

Meningeal carcinomatosis may also occur in patients with parenchymal brain metastasis when the lesion is close to the cortical or ventricular surface.

Some primary CNS tumors such as gliomas (meningeal gliomatosis), germinomas, and primitive neuroectodermal tumors develop secondary spread in the CSF that is called *meningeal seeding.* In such cases the clinical signs and symptoms resemble those seen with meningeal carcinomatosis, but are generally more leisurely in evolution.

There is usually a close correlation between meningeal carcinomatosis and evidence of osseous metastases. Other factors, such as ability of isolated cells to grow in CSF or cell surface receptors, may explain why some tumors show a propensity to seed the meninges (lung cancer, melanoma, breast cancer, lymphoma) whereas others, such as prostate carcinoma, do not affect the meninges even when widespread dissemination in bone occurs. Meningeal carcinomatosis may be the only evidence of relapse in patients with small cell cancer of lung who have received prophylactic cranial

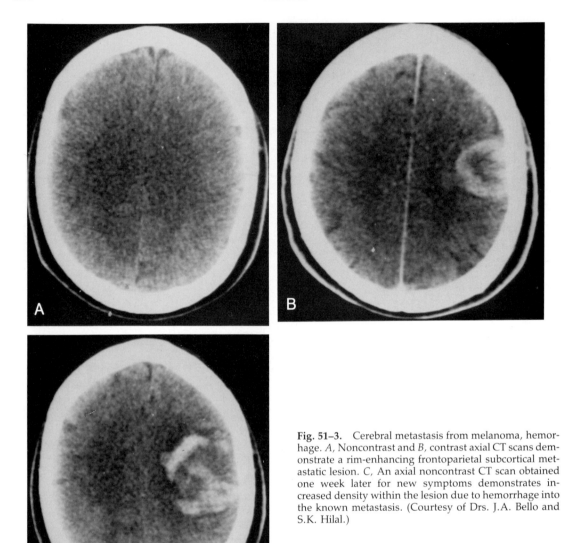

Fig. 51–3. Cerebral metastasis from melanoma, hemorrhage. *A,* Noncontrast and *B,* contrast axial CT scans demonstrate a rim-enhancing frontoparietal subcortical metastatic lesion. *C,* An axial noncontrast CT scan obtained one week later for new symptoms demonstrates increased density within the lesion due to hemorrhage into the known metastasis. (Courtesy of Drs. J.A. Bello and S.K. Hilal.)

irradiation. The spinal meninges may be a sanctuary for the tumor.

Once access to the subarachnoid space is gained, tumor cells spread throughout the neuraxis, forming colonies or nodules on roots, cranial nerves, spinal cord, brain stem, or cerebral cortex. There may be painful radiculopathies with multiple sensorimotor signs. Paraparesis or quadriparesis may result from spinal cord involvement. Cranial neuropathies are the most recognizable signposts of the syndrome, particularly if they are progressive. Headache and mental change arise when masses of tumor fill the subarachnoid

cisterns and sulci, or hydrocephalus may be due to obstruction of the aqueduct, incisura, or cerebral convexities.

Clinical diagnosis is straightforward when multiple levels of the CNS are affected. There may be headaches, seizures, mental change, visual disturbances, chiasmal syndromes, cranial neuropathies, radiculopathies, and myelopathies alone or in combinations. Untreated meningeal carcinomatosis is invariably progressive. Secondary transient ischemic attacks may follow infiltration of blood vessels. However, if signs such as cranial neuropathies develop subacutely and resolve

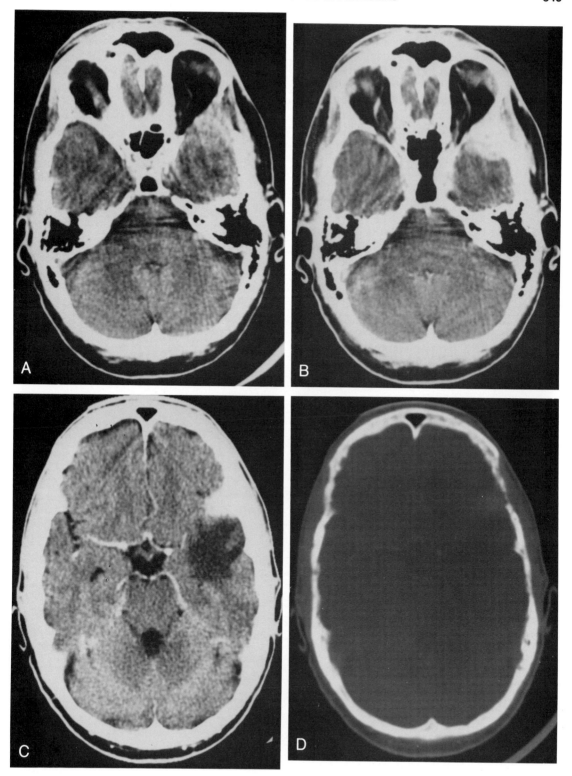

Fig. 51–4. Calvarial and epidural metastases. *A,* Pre and *B,* postcontrast axial CT scans demonstrate the anterior wall of the middle cranial fossa to be missing; it is replaced by an enhancing metastasis from breast carcinoma with an epidural component anterior to the left temporal lobe. The patient had left V_1 sensory loss. *C,* Higher postcontrast cut, and *D* bone window at the same level demonstrate extension of the epidural metastasis. Transdural involvement is suggested by the prominent white matter edema in the underlying temporal lobe, with effacement of the left sylvian fissure due to mass effect. Note the extensive calvarial involvement in *D.* Malignant cells were recovered from CSF, indicating coexistent meningeal carcinomatosis. (Courtesy of Drs. J.A. Bello and S.K. Hilal.)

spontaneously, the diagnosis of meningeal carcinomatosis should be questioned.

The sine qua non for diagnosis is recovery of malignant cells from CSF (Fig. 51–5), but this is not often achieved with the first lumbar puncture. Geographic variability of the lesions is common; if cranial nerve or cerebral signs predominate, CSF cytology yield is maximized by cisternal puncture, close to the meningeal infiltration. In about 50% of patients CSF cytology is abnormal on first examination, and abnormal cells are eventually found in 90%. The others are diagnosed at autopsy.

The most common CSF abnormality, seen in 73% of patients initially (and in 80% on subsequent examinations) is an elevated protein content. Less often there is a mononuclear pleocytosis (51% on initial exam, 65% subsequently). The CSF glucose is less than 40 mg/dl in about 28% initially (and subsequently in 37%). The CSF pressure may be elevated. However, a normal CSF profile does *not* exclude the diagnosis, and malignant cells

may be recovered from CSF by membrane filtration or centrifugation even when the CSF cell count is zero. Elevated CSF levels of tumor markers such as β-glucuronidase and carcinoembryonic antigen are not specific for meningeal carcinomatosis, but a decline in marker levels may be helpful in quantitating response to therapy. One problem is the differentiation of infection with reactive pleocytosis from meningeal carcinomatosis. Immunocytochemical techniques utilizing monoclonal antibodies applied to CSF cells may identify the malignant cells in CSF.

Other tests may provide inferential evidence of meningeal carcinomatosis, but are not proof of neoplastic invasion of meninges. CT may show hydrocephalus or enhancing tumor masses periependymally or in cisterns or sulci (Fig. 51–6). Filling defects on myelography (Fig. 51–7) are useful in detecting spinal involvement. A meningeal biopsy done for diagnostic purposes is a hit or miss

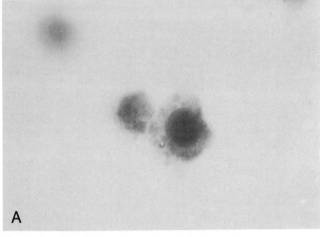

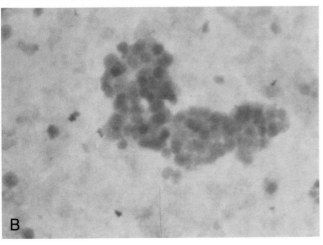

Fig. 51–5. Malignant cells in spinal fluid. Formalin-fixed millipore filtrates of lumbar CSF in two patients with meningeal spread of neoplasm. *A,* Isolated large cells with increased nuclear-to-cytoplasm ratio and fine clumps of cytoplasmic pigment in a patient with meningeal carcinomatosis due to malignant melanoma (Hematoxylin stain, ×450). *B,* A clump of cohesive cells in patient with a primitive neuroectodermal tumor and extensive meningeal seeding (Hematoxylin stain, ×180).

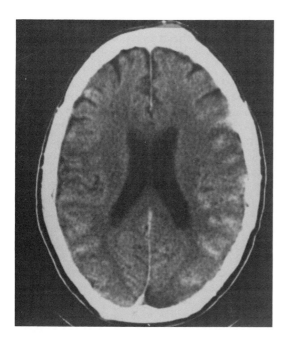

Fig. 51–6. Meningeal carcinomatosis. An axial contrast-enhanced CT scan demonstrates abnormal sulcal enhancement causing sulcal effacement in a patient with metastatic breast carcinoma.

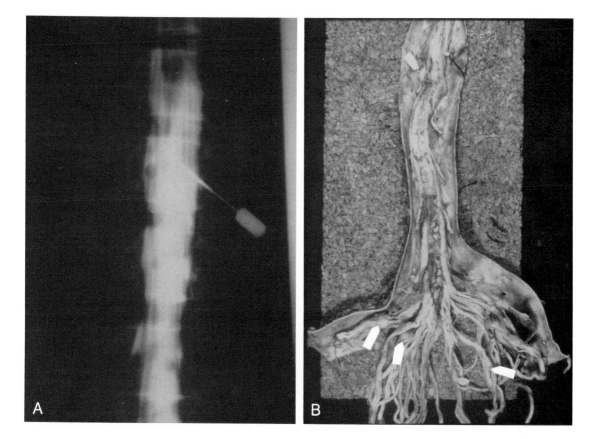

Fig. 51–7. Meningeal carcinomatosis. *A,* Myelogram and autopsy specimen of spinal cord from same patient with meningeal carcinomatosis. Note the intradural filling defects in the myelogram *(A),* that correspond to tumor nodules (arrows) seen on multiple nerve roots and thoracic spinal cord in pathologic specimen *(B).*

procedure because lesions are distributed irregularly.

Treatment. Although invariably fatal, the course of meningeal carcinomatosis may be slowed and the morbidity reduced by treatment. Most treatment protocols direct radiotherapy (2,400 to 3,000 cGy) to the sites of bulky disease, followed by chemotherapy delivered into the CSF. Only three agents have been safely administered in the CSF: methotrexate, cytosine arabinoside, and thiotepa. The best way to deliver chemotherapy is through an Ommaya reservoir placed in the lateral ventricle. This method assures entry of drug into the CSF. Diffusion throughout the CSF pathways is more uniform when the agent is given by this route than by lumbar puncture. The Ommaya reservoir also avoids pain and discomfort of repeated lumbar punctures. With each dose of chemotherapy, the CSF is sampled to assess response to therapy.

Half of the patients with meningeal carcinomatosis die of neurologic causes; the other half die of the systemic tumor. When symptoms begin in the cauda equina, the course may be more indolent, with survival for several years. In general, however, survival averages six months, longer for patients with tumors (such as breast cancer or lymphoma) that are sensitive to intrathecal medication, and shorter for such poorly responsive tumors as lung cancer and melanoma.

Granulomas

Granulomas are focal nodules of tissue with histologic signs of chronic inflammation. They may occur in the nervous system as a result of sarcoidosis or infections with syphilis, tuberculosis, fungi, or the larvae of intestinal parasites.

TUBERCULOMAS

Tuberculomas of the brain are always secondary to tuberculosis elsewhere in the body; the primary tuberculosis need not be clinically active. Small or microscopic tuberculomas are a frequent finding in patients with tuberculous meningitis, but in most cases there is no clinical evidence of these small tuberculomas. Tuberculomas of sufficient size to produce focal neurologic signs or an increase in intracranial pressure are now rare in the United States.

Solitary tuberculomas have been found in all portions of the nervous system. They may involve the dura, the arachnoid, or the substance of the nervous system. These CNS tuberculomas have a histologic appearance similar to that of tuberculomas elsewhere in the body. Although they may be found in patients of any age, they are most common in children or young adults.

The symptoms produced by tuberculomas are similar to those of any tumor, and it is rarely possible to diagnose a tuberculoma before operation in the absence of frank tuberculous meningitis. The clinical course is usually short, but remissions or complete healing with calcification may occur.

A presumptive diagnosis of tuberculoma can be made before operation when active tuberculosis is evident elsewhere in the body or when a positive tuberculin reaction is present in a child. The laboratory studies are not conclusive. The CSF is under increased pressure and may contain cells. The latter finding is not, however, rare in other types of intracranial tumors. The CSF sugar content is normal. Tubercle bacilli are not found unless there is diffuse tuberculous meningitis.

Treatment of tuberculomas is based on the use of chemotherapy. If the lesion is accessible and is causing significant mass effect, surgical excision can be performed.

CRYPTOCOCCAL GRANULOMAS

The central nervous system is involved in practically all patients in whom the meninges are affected by cryptococci. Usually, however, this condition takes the form of microscopic foci of necrosis filled with the organisms. Occasionally, however, large fibrous nodules may be present within the substance of the nervous system or they may invade it from the meninges. These granulomatous nodules may be present in the cerebral hemispheres, brain stem, cerebellum or, rarely, in the spinal cord. The diagnosis cannot be established unless the accompanying meningitis is of sufficient degree to produce a cellular reaction in the CSF; the organism can be cultured from the fluid. Surgical excision is rarely successful.

OTHER GRANULOMAS

Parasitic infestations may spread into the CNS and behave like mass lesions. Patients with AIDS are particularly susceptible to reactivation of parasitic disease, and CNS toxoplasmosis in particular is commonly seen on CT as multiple deep ring enhancing masses. Cysticercosis is due to infestation by the larva of the Taenia solium, and is being diagnosed with increasing frequency in the United

States. It is frequently accompanied by hydrocephalus. Other parasitic diseases are less common; they include: hydatid disease (echinococcosis), schistosomiasis, and paragonimiasis. Praziquantel is a new antibiotic that is extremely effective in the treatment of parasitic diseases, particularly cysticercosis.

Fungi may occasionally form granulomatous lesions that stimulate brain tumors. Aspergillosis, candidiasis, coccidioidosis, and cryptococcosis are the more frequent agents. Antibiotics are the treatment of choice, but surgery may play a role in the presence of a mass lesion.

Sarcoidosis is a multisystem granulomatous disease that affects the nervous system in about 5% of the patients. It rarely presents as a large solitary nodule, and sometimes causes hydrocephalus.

References

Brain Metastases

Aroney RS, Dalley DN, Chan WK, et al. Meningeal carcinomatosis in small cell carcinoma of the lung. Am J Med 1981; 71:26–32.

Baglan RJ, Marks JE. Comparison of symptomatic and prophylactic irradiation of brain metastases from oat cell carcinoma of the lung. Cancer 1981; 47:41–45.

Black P. Brain metastasis: current status and recommended guidelines for management. Neurosurgery 1979; 5:617–631.

Bullard DE, Cox EB, Seigler HF. Central nervous system metastases in malignant melanoma. Neurosurgery 1981; 8:26–30.

Cairncross JG, Kim J-H, Posner JB. Radiation therapy for brain metastases. Ann Neurol 1980; 7:529–541.

Cox JD, Stanley K, Petrovich Z, Paig C, Yesnar R. Cranial irradiation in cancer of the lung of all cell types. JAMA 1981; 245:469–472.

De Lattre JY, et al. Distribution of brain metastases. Arch Neurol 1988; 45:741–745.

Globus JH, Meltzer T. Metastatic tumors of the brain. Arch Neurol Psychiatry 1942; 163–226.

Holtas S, Cronqvist S. Cranial computed tomography of patients with malignant melanoma. Neuroradiology 1981; 22:123–127.

Komaki R. Prophylactic cranial irradiation for small cell carcinoma of the lung. Cancer Treat Symp 1985; 2:35–39.

Markesbery WR, Brooks WH, Gupta GD, Young AB. Treatment for patients with cerebral metastases. Arch Neurol 1978; 35:754–756.

Olson ME, Chernik NL, Posner JB: Infiltration of the leptomeninges by systemic cancer. Arch Neurol 1974; 30:122–137.

Palling MR, et al. Tumor invasion of the anterior skull base. Comparison of MRI nd CT. J Comput Assist Tomogr 1987; 11:824–830.

Patchell RA, Cirrincione C, Thaler HT, et al. Single brain metastases: surgery plus radiation or radiation alone. Neurology 1986; 36:447–453.

Rosen ST, Aisner J, Markuch RW, et al. Carcinomatous leptomeningitis in small cell lung cancer. Medicine 1982; 61:45–53.

Rosen ST, Makuch RW, Lichter AS, et al. Role of pro-
phylactic cranial irradiation in prevention of central nervous system metastases in small cell lung cancer. Potential benefit restricted to patients with complete response. Am J Med 1983; 74:615–624.

Rosner D, Nemoto T, Lane WW. Chemotherapy induces regression of brain metastases in breast carcinoma. Cancer 1986; 58:832–839.

So NK, O'Neill BP, Frytak S, et al. Delayed leukoencephalopathy in survivors with small cell lung cancer. Neurology 1987; 37:1198–1201.

Sundaresan N, Galicich JH, Beattie EJ. Surgical treatment of brain metastases from lung cancer. J Neurosurg 1983; 58:666–671.

Tarver RD, Richmond BD, Klatte EC. Cerebral metastases from lung carcinoma: neurological and CT correlation. Radiology 1984; 153:689–692.

Umsawasdi T, Valdivieso M, Chen TT, et al. Role of elective brain irradiation during combined chemotherapy for limited disease non-small cell lung cancer. J Neurooncol 1984; 2:253–259.

Van Hazel GA, Scott M, Eagan RT. The effect of CNS metastases on the survival of patients with small cell cancer of the lung. Cancer 1983; 51:933–937.

Weiss L, Gilbert HA, Posner JB. Brain Metastasis. Boston: GK Hall, 1979.

Zimm S, Wampler GL, Stablein D, Harza T, Young HF. Intracerebral metastases in solid tumor patients. Cancer 1981; 48:385–394.

Meningeal Carcinomatosis

Ascherl GF, Hilal SK, Brisman R. Computed tomography of disseminated meningeal and ependymal malignant neoplasms. Neurology 1981; 31:567–574.

Brereton H, O'Donnell J, Kent C, et al. Spinal meningeal carcinomatosis in small cell carcinoma of the lung. Ann Intern Med 1978; 88:517–519.

Coakham HB, Harper EI, Garson JA, et al. Carcinomatous meningitis diagnosed with monoclonal antibodies. Br Med J 1984; 288:28.

Giannone LF, Greco A, Hainsworth JD. Combination intraventricular chemotherapy for meningeal neoplasia. J Clin Oncol 1986; 4:68–73.

Grossman SA, Trump DL, Chen D, et al. Cerebrospinal fluid flow abnormalities in patients with neoplastic meningitis. Am J Med 1982; 73:641–647.

Hancock WW, Medley G. Monoclonal antibodies to identify tumor cells in the CSF. Lancet 1983; 2:739–740.

Kokkoris CP. Leptomeningeal carcinomatosis. How does cancer reach the pia-arachnoid? Cancer 1983; 51:154–160.

Murray JJ, Greco FA, Wolff SN, et al. Neoplastic meningitis. Marked variations of cerebrospinal fluid composition in the absence of extradural block. Am J Med 1983; 75:289–294.

Olson ME, Chernik NL, Posner JB. Infiltration of the leptomeninges by systemic cancer. Arch Neurol 1974; 30:122–137.

Ongerboer de Visser BW, Somers R, Nooyen WH, et al. Intraventricular methotrexate therapy of leptomeningeal metastasis from breast carcinoma. Neurology 1983; 33:1565–1572.

Oster MW, Fetell MR, Green PHA, et al. Meningeal carcinomatosis in small cell carcinoma of the lung. Med Pediatr Oncol 1982; 10:157–160.

Schold SC, Wasserstrom WR, Fleisher M, et al. Cerebrospinal fluid biochemical markers of central nervous system metastases. Ann Neurol 1980; 8:597–604.

Shapiro WR, Posner JB, Ushio Y, et al. Treatment of meningeal neoplasms. Cancer Treat Rep 1977; 61:733–743.

Ushio Y, Shimizu K, Aragaki Y, et al. Alteration of blood-CSF barrier by tumor invasion into the meninges. J Neurosurg 1981; 55:445–449.

Wasserstrom WR, Glass JP, Posner JB. Diagnosis and treatment of leptomeningeal metastases from solid tumors. Cancer 1982; 49:759–772.

Granulomas

Dastur HM, Desai AD. A comparative study of brain tuberculomas and gliomas based upon 107 case records of each. Brain 1965; 88:375–396.

Nash RE, Neva FA. Recent advances in the diagnosis and treatment of cerebral cysticercosis. N Engl J Med 1984; 311:1492–1496.

Obrador S. Intracranial tuberculomas: A review of 47 cases. Neurochirurgia 1959; 1:150–157.

Robles C, Sedano AM, Vargas-Tentori N, Galindo-Virgen S. Long-term results of praziquantel therapy in neurocysticercosis. J Neurosurg 1987; 66:359–363.

Rowe FA, Youmans JR, Lee HJ, Cabieses F. Parasitic and fungal diseases of the central nervous system. *In*: JR Youmans, ed. Neurological Surgery. Philadelphia: WB Saunders, 1982:3366–3440.

Sibley WA, O'Brien JL. Intracranial tuberculomas: A review of clinical features and treatment. Neurology 1956; 6:157–165.

Van Dyk A. CT of intracranial tuberuclomas with specific reference to the "target sign". Neuroradiology 1988; 30:329–336.

Table 52–1. Relative Frequency of Various Types of Spinal Tumor

Type	%
Neurofibromas	29
Meningiomas	26
Ependymomas	13
Sarcomas	12
Astrocytomas	7
Metastatic and other	13
Total	100

Table 52–2. The Location of Spinal Tumor with Reference to the Spinal Cord and Its Covering

	No. of Cases	%
Extradural	141	25
Extramedullary	334	59
Intramedullary	62	11
Cauda equina	30	5
Total	567*	100

*Data compiled from the literature

52. SPINAL TUMORS

Michael R. Fetell
Bennett M. Stein

Tumors that involve the spinal cord or nerve roots are similar to intracranial tumors in cellular type. They may arise from the parenchyma of the cord, nerve roots, meningeal coverings, intraspinal vascular network, sympathetic chain, or vertebral column. They may be metastases from tumors elsewhere in the body.

Spinal tumors are divided according to location into three major groups: intramedullary, extramedullary, and extradural. Occasionally, an extradural tumor extends through the intervertebral foramina, lying partially within and partially outside of the spinal canal (dumbbell or hourglass tumors).

Pathology. The histologic characteristics (Table 52–1) of the several types of primary and secondary tumors are similar to those of intracranial tumors and need not be repeated here in detail. Tumors of the substance of the spinal cord are rare and account for about 10% of all spinal tumors (Table 52–2). In contrast, the benign encapsulated tumors (Figs. 52–1 and 52–2), meningiomas, and neurofibromas constitute about 65% of all primary spinal tumors. As a rule, intramedullary tumors are more common in children and extramedullary tumors are more common in adults.

The leading primary sites of metastatic tumors to the spine in order are: lung, breast, and prostate.

Frequency. Tumors of the spinal cord are much less prevalent than intracranial tumors, the ratio being about 1:4. The incidence in the two sexes is approximately equal except that meningiomas are more common in women and ependymomas are more common in men. Spinal tumors occur predominantly in young or middle-aged adults, and are less common in childhood and old age (Tables 52–3 and 52–4). Although spinal tumors are more common in the thoracic region, when the actual length of the various portions of the spinal cord is taken into consideration, the distribution is relatively equal. Ependymomas may be either intra- or extramedullary; frequently originating at the conus, an ependymoma may be wholly or partially extramedullary at this site.

Symptoms. Extramedullary tumors cause symptoms by involving the nerve roots, compressing the spinal cord, or occluding the spinal blood vessels. The symptoms of intramedullary tumors result from direct interference with the intrinsic structures of the spinal cord.

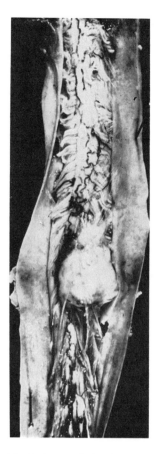

Fig. 52–1. Meningioma of the lower cervical spinal cord. (Courtesy of Dr. Abner Wolf.)

Extramedullary Tumors

This group includes both intradural and extradural tumors. They usually involve a few segments of the spinal cord and cause focal clinical signs by compressing nerve roots, especially the dorsal roots. Extramedullary tumors may progress to compromise the spinal cord, with complete loss of function below the level of the lesion. The initial symptoms, focal pain and paresthesias, signify involvement of the dorsal nerve roots; neurofibromas originate from these roots. This symptom pattern is soon followed by sensory loss, weakness, and muscular wasting in the distribution of the affected roots. Compression of the spinal cord first interrupts the functions of the pathways that lie at the periphery of the spinal cord. The early signs of cord compression include: (1) spastic weakness below the lesion; (2) impairment of cutaneous and proprioceptive sensation below the lesion; (3) impaired control of the bladder and, to a lesser extent, of the rectum; and (4) increased ten-

don reflexes, extensor plantar responses, and loss of appropriate superficial abdominal reflexes. If untreated, this syndrome may progress to signs and symptoms of complete transection of spinal cord, with wasting and atrophy of muscles at the level of the root lesion and, below the lesion, paraplegia or quadriplegia in flexion.

The severity and distribution of the motor weakness and sensory loss may vary considerably, depending to some degree on the location of the tumor in relation to the anterior, lateral, or posterior portion of the spinal cord. Eccentrically placed tumors may cause a typical Brown-Séquard syndrome: ipsilateral signs of posterior column and pyramidal tract dysfunction, with contralateral loss of pain and temperature due to involvement of the lateral spinothalamic tract. Usually, however, the modified Brown-Séquard features are incomplete.

Spinal vessels may be occluded by extradural tumors, particularly metastatic carcinoma, lymphoma, or abscesses. When the arteries destined for the spinal cord are occluded by tumor, myelomalacia results with signs and symptoms similar to those of severe intradural compression and necrosis of the spinal cord. Occlusion of major components of the anterior spinal artery, however, results in focal lower motor neuron signs at the appropriate level, loss of pain and temperature sensation on both sides of the body, and some involvement of both pyramidal systems with upper motor neuron signs below the lesion. The posterior columns are generally spared.

Spinal Metastases

EPIDURAL SPINAL CORD COMPRESSION

As patients with primary malignant tumors survive longer, the incidence of epidural spinal cord compression has increased to about 5 to 10% of all cancer patients. Treatment of cord compression does not prolong survival, but may relieve pain and may prevent neurologic disability.

Signs and symptoms of epidural spinal cord compression are easily overlooked in the patient with cancer, who is often wracked by asthenia and diffuse pain. However, the physician must respond to neck or back pain that is relentless and persists when the patient lies in bed, even if the pain is relieved by analgesics. Limb weakness, paresthesias in the distribution of a nerve root, and bowel or

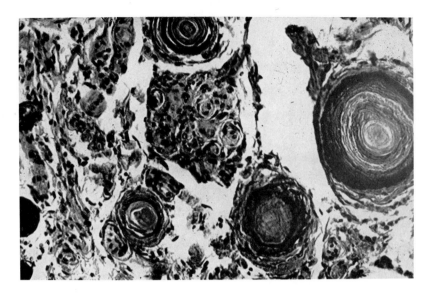

Fig. 52–2. Meningioma of the spinal cord with whorls.

Table 52–3.   Age Incidence of Spinal Tumors of all Types*

Age in Years	No. of Cases	%
0–9	19	2
10–19	98	10
20–29	156	16
30–39	177	18
40–49	238	25
50–59	186	19
Over 60	101	10
Total	975	100

*Data compiled from the literature

Table 52–4.   The Incidence of Tumors of the Spinal Cord in Childhood

Type	%
Astrocytomas	14
Ependymomas	12
Neuroblastomas	18
Dermoids	10
Metastatic	13
Teratoma	10
Lipomas	5
Neurofibromas	4
Meningiomas	2
Hemangioblastomas	2
Miscellaneous	10

(Modified from Matson DD. Neurosurgery of Infancy and Childhood, 2nd ed. Springfield: Charles C Thomas, 1969.)

bladder dysfuncton are symptoms of a neuro-oncologic emergency that require prompt evaluation and treatment. Rarely, the only manifestation of cord compression may be a gait disorder, most likely due to sensory ataxia, without overt evidence of weakness or cutaneous sensory loss. It may even be difficult to demonstrate impaired proprioception, and the deficits may be caused by compression of spinocerebellar pathways. The tumor in more than 50% of cases of epidural cord compression arises from lung or breast, and more than 80% of cases arise from primary tumors in lung, breast, gastrointestinal system, prostate, melanoma, or lymphoma.

Tumor spreads to the epidural space by (1) direct centripetal invasion from a paravertebral focus, entering through a nerve root foramen; (2) hematogenous metastases to the vertebrae with extension from bone into epidural space, or (3) retrograde spread along Batson's venous plexus. Hematogenous spread is the most common, and plain spine radiographs show lytic or blastic changes at the site of the lesion in 85% of patients. Osteoblastic changes are common with myeloma, prostate carcinoma, and Hodgkin disease, and occasionally are seen with breast cancer. Radioisotope bone scans (Fig. 52–3) show increased activity in the affected area of the spine in two thirds of patients, but are actually less specific in predicting cord compression than plain spine radiographs. CT of the spine may show osseous metastases that are not seen on plain films, but contrast myelography is required to resolve the question

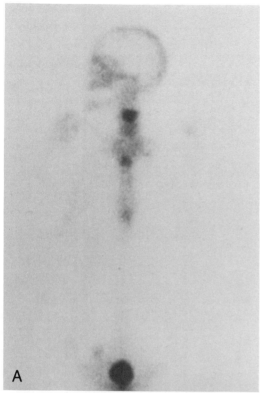

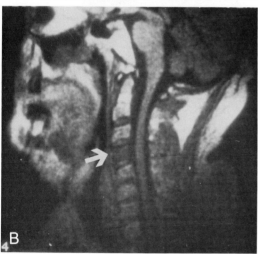

Fig. 52–3. Patient with neck pain and widespread osseous metastases from prostate cancer. *A,* Radioisotope bone scan shows increased radiotracer uptake throughout the skeleton, particularly in the cervical spine. *B,* T_1-weighted MRI shows low signal in the C_4 vertebral body (arrow) due to replacement of marrow by tumor. Epidural spinal cord compression is not present.

of spinal cord compression (Fig. 52–4). MRI is a sensitive technique for the detection of spinal osseous metastases and may soon replace myelography (Figs. 52–3B, 52–5).

Often, the site of cord compression is inapparent on clinical grounds, or with the help of plain radiographs, but the decision to perform a myelogram is frequently controversial. Indications for myelography include (1) the need to determine radiotherapy ports as precisely as possible; (2) identification of precompressive lesions at more than one spinal level; (3) identification of intramedullary metastasis or subarachnoid seeding; and (4) exclusion of patients with radiation myelopathy, peripheral neuropathy, or neuromuscular disorders that simulate myelopathy. Rodichok, et al. showed that myelography is normal in patients with back pain if there are no abnormalities on clinical neurologic examination or plain spine films, but showed epidural cord compression in almost 75% of patients if either spine radiographs or bone scan is positive. Myelography is therefore recommended for all cancer patients who show signs of myelopathy, cauda equina syndrome, or radiculopathy, and for patients who have back pain with no abnormality in neurologic examination, but who have positive radiographic studies.

CSF should be obtained at the time of myelography for chemical and cytologic analysis because meningeal carcinomatosis may coexist with epidural metastases. If there is complete myelographic block and the contrast material does not flow past the block, a C_{1-2} puncture is necessary to ascertain the rostral extent of the block and to exclude a second site of ESCC. When a myelogram fails to show compression at the expected site, CT or MRI should be performed to detect intramedullary metastasis or seeding.

Treatment. Radiotherapy (RT) has become the preferred form of therapy for most patients because RT alone is as effective as a posterior decompressive laminectomy followed by RT. The radiotherapy dose is generally 3,000 cGy in two weeks delivered in 10 fractions of 300 cGy each. The port should encompass at least one vertebral body above and below the lesion. Of patients diagnosed and treated early (while still ambulatory), 94% remain ambulatory until they die. The patient who walks into the hospital with epidural spinal cord compression, if diagnosed and treated promptly, will almost always walk out of the hospital. Loss of bowel and bladder

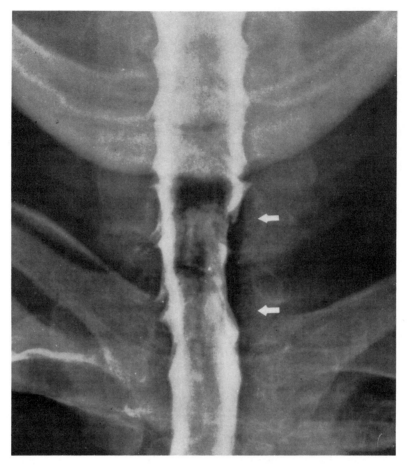

Fig. 52–4. Myelograph of an extradural metastatic carcinoma showing the smooth even impression on the lower cervical subarachnoid outline (arrows), obliteration of nerve-root shadows, and slight displacement of the spinal cord. (Courtesy of Dr. Ernest Wood.)

function, however, is an ominous prognostic sign, and is usually irreversible.

Posterior laminectomy can do little more than provide transient decompression converting a complete spinal block to an incomplete block. Postoperative radiotherapy is mandatory. Surgery is indicated in patients with epidural cord compression who are not known to have a primary malignant tumor, for palliative treatment of patients who have received maximal radiotherapy to the affected area, and for primary tumors known to be resistant to radiation, such as melanoma.

Recently, there has been enthusiasm for an anterior decompressive approach to the spine that is far more effective in debulking tumor. Even patients with bowel or bladder dysfunction treated with this approach may improve. However, in patients with terminal cancer, the anterior decompressive approach is a major operation, usually requiring tho-

racotomy because the thoracic region is most commonly involved. Thus, anterior decompression is best suited for the few patients with limited systemic disease and long expected survival, or for patients with tumors that often metastasize in a solitary fashion such as renal cell carcinoma.

High-dose (100 mg daily) dexamethasone therapy has been used, but effectiveness is unproved except in steroid-responsive tumors such as lymphoma. Intravenous estrogen therapy may help patients with cord compression due to prostate cancer while radiotherapy is being delivered.

Intramedullary Metastases

Cancer patients with overt myelopathy, but a normal myelogram, should be suspected of having intramedullary spinal cord metastases. The most common tumors that cause intramedullary metastases are lung cancer or

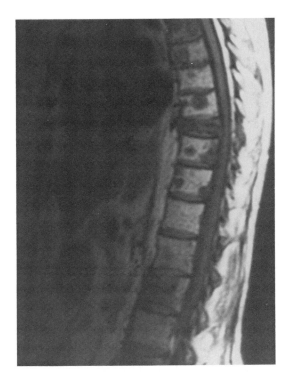

Fig. 52–5. Cord compression, vertebral metastases. A sagittal T_1 weighted MR scan shows pathologic compression of the T_8 vertebra with cord impingement. The multiple foci of low signal throughout the vertebrae replacing the normal signal of marrow represent bony metastases. (Courtesy of Drs. J.A. Bello and S.K. Hilal.)

breast cancer. In contrast to epidural cord compression, plain radiographs of the spine are positive in only 25% of these patients. In 42%, the myelogram is also normal; in the others the myelogram shows cord enlargement, confirmed by CT. Intramedullary metastases occur in patients with advanced metastatic disease, and 61% of patients with intramedullary metastases had multiple sites of cerebral or spinal lesions at autopsy. MRI may prove to be the best modality for detection of intramedullary metastases. Reversal or stabilization of neurologic signs depends upon early diagnosis, but survival is poor; 80% of patients in one series died within three months of diagnosis.

Intramedullary Tumors

Intramedullary tumors usually extend over many spinal cord segments, sometimes even the whole length of the spinal cord. For this reason the signs and symptoms of intramedullary tumors are more variable than those of extramedullary tumors (Fig. 52–6). If the tumor is restricted to one or two segments of the cord, the syndrome is similar to that of

an extramedullary tumor. However, the common scenario involves several segments, with patterns of disassociated sensory loss. Pain may be an early manifestation if the dorsal root entry zone is affected. The involvement of the crossing pain fibers in the central portion of the cord may cause a pattern of pain and temperature loss only in the affected segments. As the tumor spreads peripherally, the spinothalamic tracts may be affected; in the thoracic and cervical areas, pain and temperature fibers from the sacral area lie near the external surface of the cord and may be spared (sacral sparing). Involvement of the central gray matter leads to destruction of the anterior horn cells, with weakness and atrophy in the appropriate segments; however, pyramidal fibers may be spared. The clinical picture may be identical to that of syringomyelia.

Regional Syndromes

FORAMEN MAGNUM TUMORS

Tumors in the region of the foramen magnum may extend into the posterior fossa or caudally into the cervical region. The syndrome is typified by a conglomerate of signs and symptoms due to involvement of the lower cranial nerves—primarily the twelfth, eleventh, and rarely, the ninth and tenth cranial nerves. The most characteristic foramen magnum tumor, the ventrolateral meningioma, compresses the spinal cord at the cervicomedullary junction to cause posterior column deficits with loss of position, vibratory, and light touch sensation (more prominent in the arms than in the legs). Upper motor neuron signs affect all four limbs. There may be cutaneous sensory loss in distribution of C_2 or the occiput, with posterior cranial headache and high cervical pain. The progression of the sensory and motor symptoms may involve the limbs asymmetrically.

CERVICAL TUMORS

Involvement of the upper segments of the cervical cord is accompanied by pain or paresthesias in the occipital or cervical region, stiffness of the neck, and weakness and wasting of neck muscles. Below the lesion, there may be a spastic tetraplegia or hemiplegia and weakness of the ventrolateral region. Cutaneous sensation may be affected below the lesion, and the descending trigeminal nucleus may be involved. The characteristic findings that make it possible to localize the upper level of spinal tumors in the middle and lower cervical segments are outlined below.

> Fourth Cervical—Paralysis of the diaphragm.
> Fifth Cervical—Atrophic paralysis of the deltoid, biceps, supinator longus, rhomboid, and spinati muscles. The upper arms hang limp at the side. The sensory level extends to the outer surface of the arm. The biceps and supinator reflexes are lost.
> Sixth Cervical—Paralysis of triceps and wrist extensors. The forearm is held semiflexed and there is a partial wrist-drop. The triceps reflex is lost. Sensory impairment extends to a line running down the middle of the arm slightly to the radial side.
> Seventh Cervical—Paralysis of the flexors of the wrist and of the flexors and extensors of the fingers. Efforts to close the hands result in extension of the wrist and slight flexion of the fingers (preacher's hand). The sensory level is similar to that of the sixth cervical segment but slightly more to the ulnar side of the arm.
> Eighth Cervical—Atrophic paralysis of the small muscles of the hand with resulting clawhand (main-en-griffe). *Horner syndrome*, unilateral or bilateral, results from lesions at this level and is characterized by the triad of ptosis, small pupil (miosis), and loss of sweating on the face. Sensory loss extends to the inner aspect of the arm and involves the fourth and fifth fingers and the ulnar aspect of the middle finger.

Other signs of cervical tumors include nystagmus, especially with tumors in the upper segment. This condition is presumably due to damage to the descending portion of the median longitudinal fasciculus. Horner syndrome may be found with intramedullary lesions in any portion of the cervical cord if the descending sympathetic pathways are affected.

THORACIC TUMORS

Clinical localization of tumors in the thoracic region of the cord is usually made by the sensory level. It is difficult to determine the location of lesions in the upper half of the thoracic cord by testing the strength of intercostal muscles. Lesions that affect lower abdominal muscles but spare the upper ones can be localized by the *Beevor sign*, in which the umbilicus moves upward when the patient, in the supine position, attempts to flex the head on the chest against resistance. The abdominal skin reflexes are absent below the lesion.

LUMBAR TUMORS

Lesions in the lumbar region can be localized by the level of the sensory loss and motor weakness. Tumors that compress only the first and second lumbar segments cause loss of the cremasteric reflexes. The abdominal reflexes are preserved; knee and ankle jerks are increased.

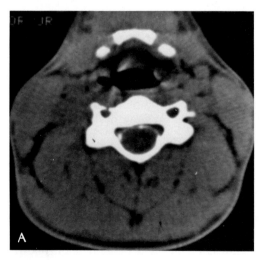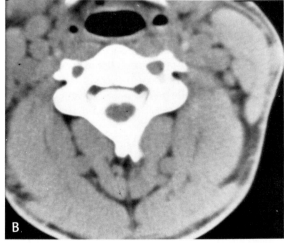

Fig. 52–6. Intramedullary spinal cord tumor. *A*, The lucent area in the center is a much enlarged and abnormally rounded spinal cord. The white ring surrounding the cord is the subarachnoid space, which is filled with contrast medium and much reduced in width. *B*, A normal spinal cord. Compare with *A*. (Courtesy of Drs. S.K. Hilal and M. Mawad.)

If the tumor affects the third and fourth segments of the lumbar cord and does not involve the roots of the cauda equina, there is weakness of the quadriceps, loss of the patellar reflexes, and hyperactive Achilles reflexes. More commonly, lesions at this level also involve the cauda equina to cause flaccid paralysis of the legs with loss of knee and ankle reflexes. If both the spinal cord and cauda equina are affected, there may be spastic paralysis of one leg with increased ankle reflex on that side and flaccid paralysis with loss of reflexes on the other side.

TUMORS OF THE CONUS AND CAUDA EQUINA

The initial symptom of tumors that involve the conus or cauda equina is pain in the back, rectal area, or both lower legs, often leading to a diagnosis of sciatica. Loss of bladder function and impotence are seen early. As the tumor grows, there may be flaccid paralysis of the legs, atrophy of the leg muscles, and foot drop. Fasciculation may be seen in the atrophied muscles. Sensory loss may affect the perianal or saddle area as well as the remaining sacral and lumbar dermatomes. This loss may be slight or it may be so severe that a trophic ulcer develops over the lumbosacral region, the buttocks, the hips, or heels.

Signs of raised intracranial pressure may be seen with ependymomas of this region if the CSF protein content is very high.

Diagnosis of Spinal Tumors

Tumors compressing the spinal cord or the cauda equina are characterized by radicular pain and the slow evolution of signs of an incomplete transverse lesion of the cord or signs of compression of the roots of the cauda equina. Extradural tumors that do not compress the spinal cord may produce symptoms by obstructing the blood supply to the cord; if this occurs, the symptoms are often of sudden onset and the tumor is either metastatic or a granuloma of the Hodgkin type.

The diagnosis of an intraspinal tumor can be established before operation with absolute certainty by CT, MRI, and myelography. Vascular malformations or vascular tumors may be visualized by spinal angiography. Examination of the CSF may also be helpful.

Radiography. In about 15% of spinal neoplasms, one or more of the following abnormalities are seen in plain radiographs.

1. Localized destruction of the vertebrae is manifested by scalloping of the posterior margin of the vertebral body or lucency of a portion of the vertebra or pedicle.

2. Changes occur in the contour of or separation of the pedicles (the interpediculate distance can be measured and compared with normal values). Localized enlargement of foramina is seen in the dumbbell neurofibroma. Localized enlargement of the spinal canal is usually diagnostic of an intraspinal tumor, but enlargement of many segments may be a developmental anomaly.

3. Paraspinal tissues are distorted by tumors (frequently neurofibromas) that extend through the intervertebral foramen or by tumors that originate in the paraspinal structures.

4. Proliferation of bone, which is rare except in osteomas and sarcomas, is also occasionally seen in hemangiomas of bone and meninges.

5. Calcium deposits are occasionally present in meningiomas or congenital tumors.

Myelography. Myelography (Figs. 52–4 and 52–7 to 52–9) with metrizamide is necessary to localize the level of compressive spinal lesions and to establish the diagnosis of tumors of the cauda equina. If the spinal block is complete or nearly complete and the progress of the dye upward is blocked by the tumor, instillation of more dye at the upper cervical region by a lateral cervical puncture under television control delineates the upper border of the tumor. Extradural tumors displace the dura toward the subarachnoid space and deform the contrast column on its outer aspect (see Fig. 52–4). An intradural extramedullary lesion, lying within the subarachnoid space, displaces the spinal cord away from the tumor; the tumor may be outlined by the contrast material. Intramedullary tumors cause enlargement of the cord shadow and displace the contrast column laterally (see Fig. 52–9B).

Computerized Tomography. Without the intrathecal instillation of a contrast agent, CT cannot be relied upon to demonstrate the soft tissue changes of intraspinal tumors; however, the extraspinal aspects, such as metastatic cancer, may be identified. With intrathecal injection of metrizamide, intraspinal tumors may usually be seen. The contrast material may leach into the cavity to establish the diagnosis of syringomyelia or septic tumor. CT-metrizamide studies are more time-consuming than standard myelography, but

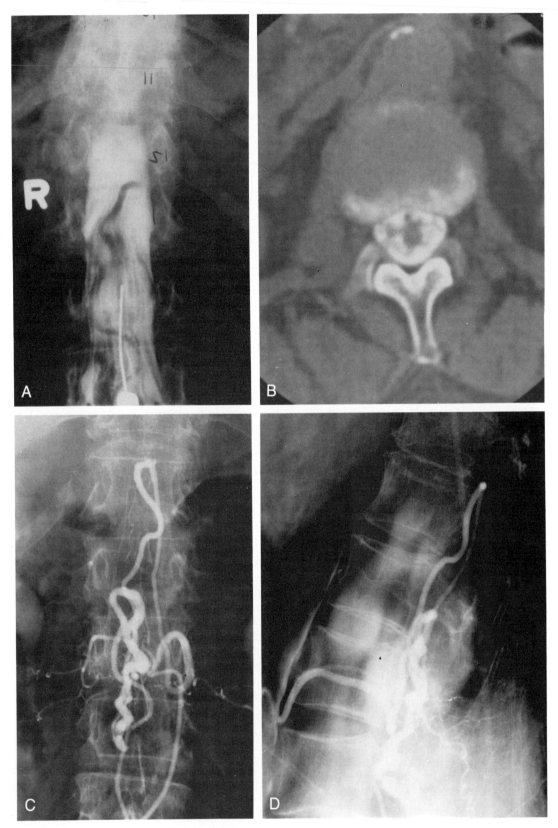

Fig. 52–7. Spinal AVM. *A,* Water-soluble contrast myelography at the thoracolumbar junction in an AP projection demonstrates serpiginous intradural filling defects at the T_{12}-L_1 level. *B,* An axial CT scan obtained after myelogram demonstrates a prominent anterior spinal artery at the level of the conus. AP *C,* and lateral *D* views from the spinal angiogram on this patient show anterior spinal artery supply to an AVM and serpiginous draining veins.

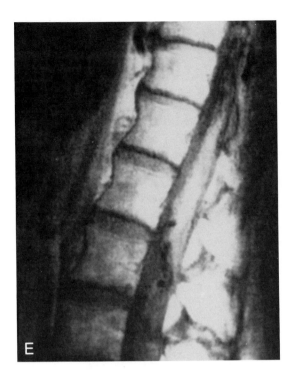

Fig. 52–7 (cont.). *E,* A sagittal T_1 weighted MRI scan demonstrates the draining veins as serpiginous structures of signal void (due to flow) anterior to the conus. The "loop" made by the anterior spinal artery supplying the lesion is slightly less well seen compared to *D.* (Courtesy of Drs. J.A. Bello, S.K. Hilal, and T.L. Chi.)

provide a more precise representation of the intraspinal disease.

Magnetic Resonance Imaging. As MRI gains acceptance and widespread use, it has been used primarily as an adjuvant to CT and myelography. The accuracy of MRI combined with its ability to do what CT and myelography cannot accomplish predicts that, in the future, it will be the single important examination of spinal tumors. With surface coils, the MRI is able to image the interior of the spinal cord, demonstrating cystic and solid tumor (Fig. 52–9A). Extramedullary tumors are disclosed with unequalled clarity.

Evaluation of Cerebrospinal Fluid. If an intraspinal tumor is suspected, CSF should be obtained at the time of, rather than before, myelography. This sequence avoids subdural injection of the contrast material and avoids displacement of tumor-spinal cord relations that might lead to neurologic deterioration.

When there is a complete subarachnoid block, the CSF is usually xanthochromic as a result of the high protein content. It may be only slightly yellow or colorless if the subar-achnoid block is incomplete. The cell count is usually normal, but a slight pleocytosis is found in about 30% of the patients. Cell counts between 25 and 100/mm³ are found in about 15% of the patients. The protein content is increased in over 95%. Values over 100 mg/dl are present in 60% of the patients and values over 1000 mg/dl are present in 5% (Table 52–5). The sugar content is normal unless tumor of the meninges is present. Cytologic evaluation of the CSF is useful when malignant tumors are suspected.

Differential Diagnosis. Spinal tumors must be differentiated from other disorders of the spinal cord, including transverse myelitis, multiple sclerosis, syringomyelia, combined system disease, syphilis, ALS, anomalies of the cervical spine and base of the skull, spondylosis, adhesive arachnoiditis, radiculitis of the cauda equina, hypertrophic arthritis, ruptured intervertebral discs, and vascular anomalies.

Multiple sclerosis, with a complete or incomplete transverse lesion of the cord, can usually be differentiated from spinal cord tumors by the remitting course, signs and symptoms or more than one lesion, evoked potential studies, cranial MRI, and presence of CSF oligoclonal bands. If the syndrome is focal and progressive, myelography is indicated. The lesions of multiple sclerosis may occasionally enlarge the cord to simulate an intramedullary tumor, but there is usually no myelographic abnormality.

The differential diagnosis between syringomyelia and intramedullary tumors is complicated because intramedullary cysts are commonly associated with these tumors. Extramedullary tumors in the cervical region may give rise to localized pains and muscular atrophy in conjunction with a Brown-Séquard syndrome, producing a clinical picture similar to that of syringomyelia. The diagnosis of syringomyelia is likely when trophic disturbances are present. The differential diagnosis can often be made by CT with subarachnoid metrizamide or the characteristic cord collapse on air myelogram in syringomyelia.

Combined system disease is diagnosed by the neurologic findings, vitamin B_{12} levels, Schilling test, and characteristic hematologic changes. Myelography is rarely necessary. Syphilis may produce signs and symptoms of a transverse lesion of the cord. The diagnosis of syphilis is established by the serologic findings in the CSF.

The combination of atrophy of hand mus-

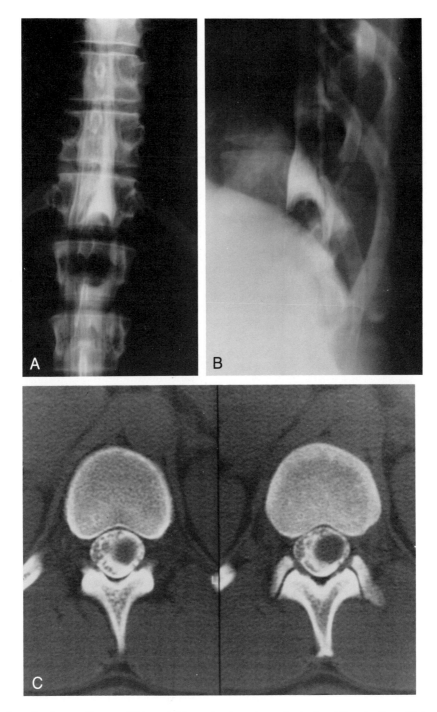

Fig. 52–8. Intradural neurofibroma. Water-soluble contrast myelography in the AP projection *(A)* demonstrates an intradural filling defect at the T_{12}-L_1 level with widening of the gutter on the left due to displacement of the neural structures to the right. *B,* Lateral projection shows typical "capping" of the contrast. *C,* Axial CT sections postmyelography demonstrate the large intradural myofibroma displacing the conus to the patient's right. (Courtesy of Drs. J.A. Bello and S.K. Hilal.)

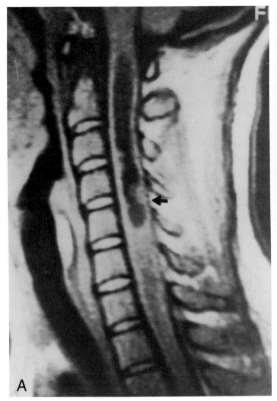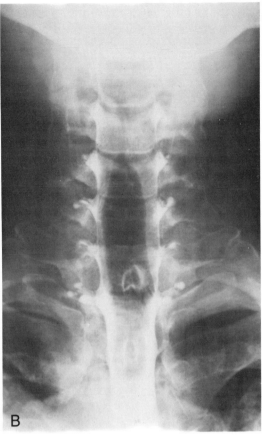

Fig. 52–9. *A,* Sagittal T$_1$ weighted MRI of cervical spinal cord demonstrating a large cystic intramedullary tumor with a mural nodule (arrow): a hemangioblastoma. *B,* Cervical myelogram of a different patient demonstrating the typical appearance of spinal cord widening due to an extensive cervical intramedullary ependymoma (air-filled trachea overlies the tumor).

Table 52–5. Protein Content of Cerebrospinal Fluid in 36 Patients with Spinal Tumors

Protein Content (mg/dl)	No. of Patients	%
Less than 45	5	14
45–100	7	19
100–1,000	22	61
More than 1,000	2	6
Total	36	100

cles and spastic weakness in the legs in ALS may suggest the diagnosis of a cervical cord tumor. Tumor is excluded by the normal sensory examination, the presence of fasciculation, or atrophy in leg muscles; sometimes, however, myelography is warranted.

Cervical spondylosis, with or without rupture of the intervertebral discs, may cause symptoms and signs of root irritation and compression of the spinal cord. The osteo-

arthritis can be diagnosed by findings in plain radiographs, but this is so common in asymptomatic people that myelography may be necessary to determine whether there is concomitant disease of the discs or whether an extramedullary tumor is also present.

Anomalies in the cervical region or at the base of the skull, such as platybasia or Klippel-Feil syndrome, are diagnosed by the characteristic radiographic findings.

The arachnoid may be thickened in patients with primary disease of the spinal cord such as syringomyelia, syphilis, or multiple sclerosis. In these cases, the thickening of the arachnoid may not play a significant role in the production of the cord symptoms, which are attributed to the intrinsic cord disease. However, the pia-arachnoid may also be thickened in the absence of intrinsic spinal cord disease following meningitis or subarachnoid hemorrhage, following injection of serum, iodinated contrast agents, spinal anesthetics, or other substances into the subarachnoid space, and after spinal surgery for tumors or herniated discs. Occasionally this *arachnoiditis* may interfere with the circulation in the cord, causing the signs and symptoms of a transverse lesion. The CSF protein content is moderately elevated. Diagnosis is made by complete or partial arrest of the contrast column on myelography or by fragmentation of the material into globules at the site of the lesion. Separation of the adhesions and removal of the thickened arachnoid by surgery have been of little benefit; the results of steroid therapy are not much better.

The signs and symptoms of a ruptured intervertebral disc in the lumbar region may be similar to those of a cauda equina tumor. Extensive sensory or motor loss is much more common in tumors, and the CSF protein content is usually greater than 100 mg/dl, whereas such values are rare with ruptured intervertebral disc. The differential diagnosis can usually be established by the size and position of the defect in the myelogram.

Course and Prognosis. Benign tumors of the spinal cord are characterized by a slowly progressing course for many years. If a neurofibroma arises from a dorsal root, there may be years of radicular pain before the tumor is evident from other manifestations of growth. Intramedullary tumors are generally benign and slow-growing; they may attain enormous size (over the course of six to eight years) before they are discovered.

Conversely, the sudden onset of a severe neurologic disorder, with or without pain, is usually indicative of a malignant extradural tumor such as metastatic carcinoma or Hodgkin disease.

Treatment. Once the diagnosis of an intraspinal tumor has been made, the treatment is surgical removal of the tumor whenever possible. When the neurologic disorder is severe or rapidly progressing, emergency surgery should be done. Through the use of microneurosurgery, the best results are obtained when the signs and symptoms are due solely to compression of the spinal cord by meningiomas, neurofibromas, or other benign encapsulated tumors. Some of these tumors, especially meningiomas, may lie anterior to the spinal cord and require the most delicate expertise of the neurosurgeon. Function may be completely restored even when severe spastic weakness has been present for years. However, the postoperative results are often predicated on the severity of preoperative neurologic disability, which is a strong point in favor of early diagnosis and surgery for these tumors. Radiotherapy is not indicated for most intradural extramedullary tumors, even when removal has been incomplete, because these tumors are usually benign.

The most common intramedullary tumors are ependymomas and astrocytomas. In almost all ependymomas, the tumor can be resected following a myelotomy and microsurgical approach (Fig. 52–10). Radiotherapy is not indicated after total removal and is rarely indicated after partial removal; the patient should be observed for recurrent mass effect. Additional operative procedures should be considered if they are indicated. Perhaps half of all intramedullary astrocytomas are resectable by microsurgical technique; again, postoperative radiotherapy is not indicated. When radiotherapy is given after incomplete removal of an astrocytoma, the results are discouraging. In the uncommon presence of other intramedullary tumors such as hemangioblastomas, teratomas, or dermoids, complete removal without adjuvant radiotherapy is the rule.

After radical and extensive surgery for these tumors, spinal deformities (which may have been present preoperatively) may appear or increase, requiring fixation. These deformities, if allowed to progress, may in turn create neurologic syndromes due to spinal cord compression. This condition is especially pertinent in children. Some surgeons have advocated replacement of the lamina after definitive surgery, rather than the standard laminectomy. The additional use of radiotherapy for intraspinal tumors in children may affect the growth of the spine, leading to or increasing preexisting deformities of the spine.

Extradural metastatic lesions require special consideration. These tumors may compress the spinal cord; however, cord damage more often results from obliteration of arterial blood supply. In these circumstances, surgical decompression does little more than relieve the mechanical distortion. Results of high-dose steroid therapy combined with emergency radiation are comparable or superior to surgical decompression of these malignant tumors. This form of treatment, however, should be used only when the nature of the metastatic tumor is known and when previous radiotherapy has not been given to the affected area of the spine. If malignancy is unconfirmed or only suspected, surgical de-

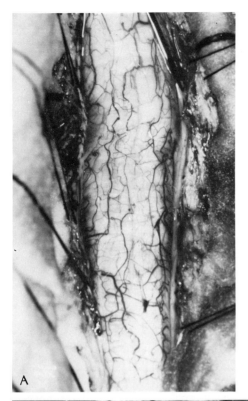

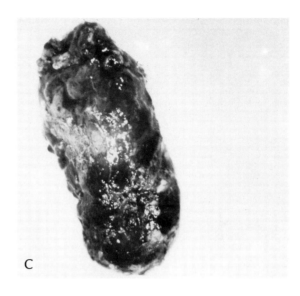

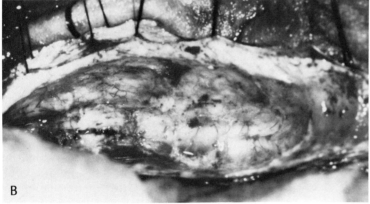

Fig. 52–10. *A,* Operative exposure of intramedullary tumor shown in Fig. 52–9*B.* The spinal cord shows diffuse widening over the entire cervical region without any visible evidence of the tumor on the dorsal surface. *B,* Spinal cord opening after total removal of intramedullary ependymoma. The patient made a progressive recovery following operative procedure. *C,* Complete gross specimen of intramedullary tumor removed in a single portion. The tumor was a benign ependymoma.

compression and biopsy may be necessary to confirm the diagnosis.

References

Ammerman BJ, Smith DR. Papilledema and spinal cord tumors. Surg Neurol 1975; 3:55–57.

Constans JP, Divitiis ED, Donzelli R, et al. Spinal metastases with neurological manifestations. J Neurosurg 1983; 59:111–118.

Costigan DA, Winkelman MD. Intramedullary spinal cord metastases. A clinicopathological study of 13 cases. J Neurosurg 1985; 62:227–233.

Doppman JL, DiChiro G, Dwyer AJ, Frank JL, Oldfield EH. MRI of spinal arteriovenous malformations. J Neurosurg 1987; 66:830–834.

Elsberg CA. Surgical Diseases of the Spinal Cord, Membranes and Nerve Roots. New York: Paul B Hoeber, 1941.

Epstein F, Epstein N. Surgical treatment of spinal cord astrocytomas of childhood. J Neurosurg 1982; 57:685–689.

Fischer G, Mansuy L. Total removal of intramedullary

ependymomas: follow-up study of 16 cases. Surg Neurol 1980; 14:243–249.

Gilbert RW, Kim JH, Posner JB. Epidural spinal cord compression from metastatic tumor: diagnosis and treatment. Ann Neurol 1978; 3:40–51.

Greenberg HS, Kim JH, Posner JB. Epidural spinal cord compression from metastatic tumor: results wth a new treatment protocol. Ann Neurol 1980; 8:361–366.

Grem JL, Burgess J, Trump DL. Clinical features and natural history of intramedullary spinal cord metastasis. Cancer 1985; 56:2305–2314.

Harrington KD. Anterior cord decompression and spinal stabilization for patients with metastatic lesion of the spine. J Neurosurg 1984; 61:107–117.

Ibrahim AW, Ibrahim EM, Mitry NM, Satir AA, Kupa A. Spinal cord compression due to intrathoracic extramedullary hematopoiesis in homozygous thalassemia. J Neurol Neurosurg Psychiatry 1983; 46:780–782.

Katzman H, Waugh T, Berdon W. Skeletal changes following irradiation of childhood tumors. J Bone Joint Surg 1969; 51-A:825–843.

Lee KS, Angelo JN, McWhorter JM, et al. Symptomatic subependymoma of the cervical spinal cord. J Neurosurg 1987; 67:128–131.

Martenson JA, Evans RG, Lie MR, et al. Treatment outcome and complications in patients treated for malignant epidural spinal cord compression. J Neurooncol 1985; 3:77–84.

Matson DD. Neurosurgery of Infancy and Childhood, 2nd ed. Springfield: Charles C Thomas, 1969.

Otenasek FJ, Silver ML. Spinal hemangioma (hemanglioblastoma) in Lindau's disease. Report of six cases in a single family. J Neurosurg 1961; 18:295–300.

Pickens JM, Wilson J, Garth GM, Grunnet ML. Teratoma of the spinal cord. Report of a case and review of the literature. Arch Pathol 1975; 99:446–448.

Rodichok LD, Ruckdeschel JC, Harper GR, et al. Early detection and treatment of spinal epidural metastases: the role of myelography. Ann Neurol 1986; 20:696–702.

Rosenquist H, Saltzman GF. Sacrococcygeal and vertebral chordomas and their treatment. Acta Radiol 1959; 52:177–193.

Schroth G, Thron A, Gutil L, et al. Magnetic resonance imaging of spinal meningiomas and neuromas. Improvement of imaging by paramagnetic contrast enhancement. J Neurosurg 1987; 66:695–700.

Scotti G, Scialfa G, Colombo N, et al. Magnetic resonance diagnosis of intramedullary tumors of the spinal cord. Neuroradiology 1987; 29:130–135.

Siegal T, Siegal T, Robin G, Korn IL, Fuks Z. Anterior decompression of the spine for metastatic epidural cord compression: a promising avenue of therapy. Ann Neurol 1982; 11:28–34.

Skalpe IO, Sortland O. Adhesive arachnoiditis in patients with spinal block. Neuroradiology 1982; 22:243–245.

Shapiro JH, Och M, Jacobson HG. Differential diagnosis of intradural (extramedullary) and extradural spinal canal tumors. Radiology 1961; 76:718–732.

Stein BM. Spinal Intradural Tumors. In: Wilkins RH, Rengachary SS, eds. New York, McGraw-Hill Book Company, 1985.

Stein BM. Surgery of intramedullary spinal cord tumors. Clin Neurosurg 1979; 26:529–542.

Stein BM, Leeds NE, Taveras JM, Pool JL. Meningiomas of the foramen magnum. J Neurosurgery 1963; 20:740–751.

Sundaresan N, Galicich JH, Lane JM, et al. Treatment of neoplastic epidural cord compression by vertebral body resection and stabilization. J Neurosurg 1985; 63:676–684.

Tachdjian MO, Matson DD. Orthopaedic aspects of intraspinal tumors in infants and children. J Bone Joint Surg 1965; 47A:223–248.

Thomas JE, Miller RH. Lipomatous tumors of the spinal canal: a study of their clinical range. Mayo Clin Proc 1973; 48:393–400.

Williams AL, Haughton VM, Pojunas KW, et al. Differentiation of intramedullary neoplasms and cysts by MR. Am J Radiol 1987; 149:159–164.

Winkleman MD, Adelstein DJ, Karlins NL. Intramedullary spinal cord metastasis. Diagnostic and therapeutic considerations. Arch Neurol 1987; 44:526–531.

Yasargil MG, Antic J, Laciga R, dePreux J, Fideler RW, Boone SC. The microsurgical removal of intramedullary spinal hemangioblastomas: report of twelve cases and a review of the literature. Surg Neurol 1976; 6:141–148.

Young RF, Post EM, King GA. Treatment of spinal epidural metastases. J Neurosurg 1980; 53:741–748.

53. MULTIPLE TUMORS OF THE CRANIAL NERVES

Michael R. Fetell
Bennett M. Stein

Solitary tumors (usually neurofibromas) may develop on any of the peripheral nerves, but more commonly these tumors are multiple and are a part of the syndrome of neurofibromatosis. The symptoms produced by tumors of peripheral nerves are similar to those produced by other lesions. They are discussed elsewhere in this chapter. This section is limited to consideration of cases with multiple tumors of the nerves.

Neurofibromatosis (von Recklinghausen disease) is an inherited disorder that is characterized by multiple tumors of the spinal or cranial nerves, tumors of the skin, and cutaneous pigmentation. Other manifestations of the condition are discussed in Section 100, Neurofibromatosis.

Etiology and Pathology. It is generally agreed that the manifestations are due to an abnormality in germ plasm that results in localized overgrowth of various mesodermal and ectodermal elements in the skin, peripheral nerves, CNS, and other organs of the body.

The pathologic manifestations are variable and widespread. Most characteristic are the tumors of the peripheral nerve, which may occur as nodules scattered along nerves in peripheral, intracranial, or intraspinal portions. They may occur on terminal nerve fibers in a widespread fashion (plexiform neuroma). Coincidental with the neuromas, there may be tumors of the meninges (meningiomas), tumors of the glial cells (astrocytomas, ependymomas, or glioblastomas), as well as small nodules of gliosis or glial proliferation within the CNS.

Changes in the skin, in addition to the plexiform neurofibromas, include pedunculated or sessile polypi, café-au-lait spots, and portwine or anemic nevi.

Other lesions include changes in the bones (osteitis fibrosa cystica) and local overgrowth of tissue causing hemihypertrophy of tongue, face, extremities, or viscera. Associated maldevelopments are not uncommon and the coincidence of neurofibromatosis and syringomyelia is not rare. Dysfunction of endocrine glands may also be conjoined. Pheochromocytoma or cystic lung disease has been reported.

Premature puberty, gynecomastia, and disorders of growth are uncommon features. Glaucoma, buphthalmos, glioma of the optic nerve, and involvement of the uveal coat are occasionally seen.

Incidence. Neurofibromatosis is rare in the fully developed form; abortive forms with only selected features of the disease are more common. It may be transmitted as a mendelian dominant genetic trait, appearing usually in the same form in successive generations. Skipping of one or more generations may occur or there may be abortive or partial forms. The disease is more common in men and may be transmitted by either parent.

The lesions in the nerves and skin may be present at birth, but more commonly appear at puberty and then grow slowly or rapidly.

Symptoms and Signs. For purposes of description, the symptoms and signs of neurofibromatosis are divided into those that pertain to the nervous system and those of other systems. Serious disability is usually due to tumors on nerves in the cranium or spinal cord or to the coincidence of meningeal or glial tumors of the nervous system.

Patients with von Recklinghausen disease may be divided into three groups according to whether the tumor formation occurs only on the peripheral portion of the nerve (peripheral type), on the nerve root (central type), or on both (mixed type). In the peripheral form, nodules appear on the nerves of the somatic or autonomic nervous system. These are most common on the nerve trunks of the extremities, but may also be found on the nerves of the head, neck, and body (Fig. 53–1). The trunks and plexuses of the auto-

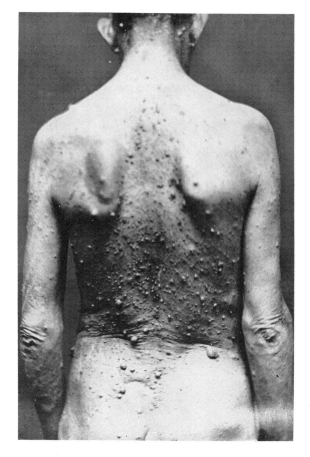

Fig. 53–1. Von Recklinghausen disease. Multiple subcutaneous nodules (neurofibromas) on the trunk and extremities. (Courtesy of Dr. P.I. Yakovlev.)

nomic system are sometimes affected. The number of nodules in individual cases varies from a few to many thousands, and their size varies from that of a small seed to that of an orange. The tumors often do not cause any symptoms except that they may be painful to pressure or may cause neuralgic or paresthetic pain. Only rarely is there weakness, atrophy, or sensory loss in the distribution of the affected nerve.

Neuroma formation in the terminal distribution of the nerve fibers (plexiform neuroma) may be accompanied by diffuse proliferation and fibrosis of the affected parts. The resulting picture has been described by the term *elephantiasis neuromatosa*. Overgrowth of all tissues of one extremity or localized overgrowth of the tissues of the head or trunk may occur. As a result, there may be elephantiasis of one extremity or hypertrophy of one half of the face, of the lips, or of the tongue. Overgrowth of the skin of the skull, neck, or other portions of the body may be of such an extent that the excess tissue falls in loose folds of enormous size over the eyes, shoulders, or trunk. Hypertrophy of the viscera has been reported in association with plexiform neuromas of the autonomic nervous system.

In the central or mixed form of neurofibromatosis, the symptoms and signs are those that are appropriate to tumors in the spinal cord or cranium. Small neurofibromas on the spinal roots and larger ones on the cauda equina may not cause any clinical symptoms. Large fibromas in the cervical or thoracic portion of the cord compress the spinal cord and produce a Brown-Séquard syndrome or the signs and symptoms of a transverse lesion of the spinal cord (Fig. 53–2).

Large fibromas on the roots of the cranial nerves may be accompanied by symptoms and signs of increased intracranial pressure and those due to compression of the brain stem. A form of central neurofibromatosis has been reported by Gardner and Frazier in which bilateral involvement of the eighth cranial nerve is the only manifestation. According to Thomson, however, the tenth and fifth cranial nerves are much more frequently involved than the eighth nerve (Table 53–1), in the usual form of neurofibromatosis.

Neurologic symptoms may also appear in patients with von Recklinghausen disease as the result of meningiomas, gliomas of the optic nerve, cerebrum, or spinal cord, or the coincidence of syringomyelia or other congenital defects.

The cutaneous manifestations, together with the overgrowth of skin and other tissues associated with plexiform neuromas, are the source of considerable suffering because of the unsightly deformities and disfigurements they produce.

Subperiosteal fibromas may cause rarefaction of any of the bones with the formation of bone cysts (osteitis fibrosa cystica). Spontaneous fractures of the spine or long bones may occur.

Laboratory Data. There are no significant

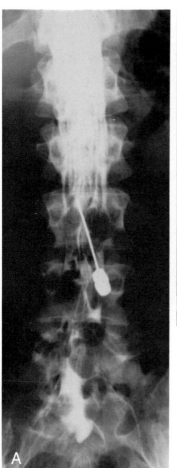
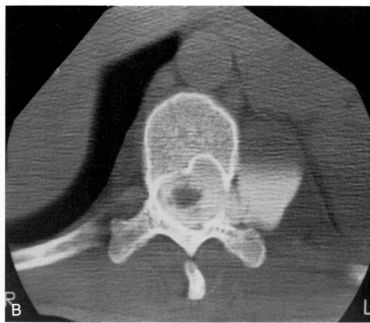

Fig. 53–2. Neurofibromatosis. *A,* Myelography in the AP projection shows multiple intradural lesions filling the lumbar thecal sac. *B,* A postmyelogram axial CT scan in the thoracic region demonstrates scalloping of the posterior aspect of the vertebral body on the left, erosion of the pedicle, and a contrast-fluid level in a lateral thoracic meningocele. (Courtesy of Drs. J.A. Bello and S.K. Hilal.)

Table 53–1. Frequency of Involvement of the Cranial Nerves in 45 Necropsy-Studied Cases of Neurofibromatosis

Nerve	No. of Cases
Vagus	29
Trigeminal	12
Hypoglossal	7
Facial	6
Spinal accessory	6
Oculomotor	6
Glossopharyngeal	4
Optic	4
Auditory	3
Abducens	3
Trochlear	3
Olfactory	1

(From Thomson A. On Neuroma and Neuro-fibromatosis. Edinburgh: Turnbull & Spears, 1900, p. 65.)

laboratory findings in patients with neurofibromatosis, except in the changes in the CSF and radiographic findings that may accompany large tumor masses in the skull or spinal cavity and the changes in the bone due to subperiosteal neurofibromas.

Diagnosis. The diagnosis is made without difficulty by the characteristic lesions of the skin and peripheral nerves. The pure central form of neurofibromatosis can be diagnosed only from the family history and the finding of neurofibromas at surgery. The changes in the bone can be differentiated from those of hyperparathyroidism by determination of the blood calcium content.

Course and Prognosis. The course is often relatively benign with no shortening of the life span. The lesions, when fully developed, may remain stationary for many years. Oc-

casional periods of unexplained rapid growth of the lesions may occur. The prognosis in the patients with lesions on the cranial nerves or spinal roots is poor because of the disabling nature of the symptoms they produce and because they are usually multiple. Sarcomatous degeneration sometimes occurs in the peripheral tumors and leads to a fatal outcome.

Treatment. There is no adequate treatment for neurofibromatosis. The peripheral tumors and hypertrophic folds of skin should be removed only when they interfere with normal activity or when they are disfiguring. Removal, however, may lead to an increase in the malignancy of the growths. Intraspinal and intracranial tumors should be removed when possible.

References

Crowe FW, Schull WJ, Neel JV. A Clinical, Pathological and Genetic Study of Multiple Neurofibromatosis. Springfield: Charles C Thomas, 1956.

Jacoby CG, Go RT, Beren RA. Cranial CT of neurofibromatosis. AJR 1980; 135:553–557.

Kanter WR, Eldridge R, Fabricant R, Allen JC, Koerber T. Central neurofibromatosis with bilateral acoustic neuroma: genetic, clinical, and biochemical distinctions from peripheral neurofibromatosis. Neurology 1980; 30:851–859.

Lusk MD, Kline DG, Garcia CA. Tumors of the brachial plexus. Neurosurgery 1987; 21:439–543.

Martuza RL, Eldridge R. Neurofibromatosis 2 (Bilateral acoustic neurofibromatosis). N Engl J Med 1988; 318:684–688.

Riccardi VM, Mulvihill JJ. Neurofibromatosis (von Recklinghausen disease) genetics, cell biology, and biochemistry. Adv Neurol 1981; 29:1–9.

Seizinger BR, Rouleau GR, Ozelius LJ, et al. Common pathogenetic mechanism for three tumor types in bilateral acoustic neurofibromatosis. Science 1987; 236:317–319.

Thomson A. On Neuroma and Neurofibromatosis. Edinburgh: Turnbul & Spears, 1900.

von Recklinghausen F. Ueber die multiplen Fibrome der Haut und ihre Beziehung zu den multiplen Neuromen. Berlin: A Hirschwald, 1882.

Chapter VI

Trauma

54. HEAD INJURY

Lewis P. Rowland
Daniel Sciarra

Epidemiology. Head injury is a modern scourge of industrialized society. It is a major cause of death, a leading cause of death in young adults, and a major cause of disability. The costs in human misery and dollars are exceeded by those of few other conditions.

Almost 10% of all deaths in the United States are caused by injury, and about half of traumatic deaths involve the brain. The annual incidence of brain injury in different areas of the United States is about 200/100,000 population.

Brain injuries occur at all ages but the peak is in young adults, between the ages of 15 and 24. Men are affected three or four times as often as women. The major cause of brain injury differs in different parts of the country but in all areas motor vehicle accidents are prominent. In metropolitan ghettos, however, personal violence is more prevalent (Table 54–1).

The costs to society of brain injury are difficult to determine. Kraus estimated, however, that in 1984 there were 70,000 deaths at the accident scene and 400,000 hospital admissions. It could thus be reasonably supposed that 74,000 people are disabled each year, a rate of 31 to 42/100,000. Methods are being developed to determine the exact number and the expenses incurred.

Craniocerebral Trauma

Craniocerebral trauma may be divided according to the nature of injury to the skull into three groups: closed head injuries, depressed fracture of the skull, and compound fracture of the skull. This division is important in deciding whether operative therapy is necessary for the patient. The prognosis is dependent more on the nature and severity of the damage to the brain than on the severity of the injury to the skull.

In *closed head injuries,* there is either no injury to the skull or only a linear fracture. These cases can be subdivided according to the severity of brain damage into two main groups: those with no significant degree of structural damage to the brain, usually designated by the term *concussion;* and those with destruction of brain tissue related to edema, contusion, laceration, or hemorrhage.

In simple *depressed fractures* of the skull the pericranium is intact but a fragment of fractured bone is depressed inward to compress or injure the underlying brain. These cases can be subdivided according to the severity of the damage to the cerebral substance.

The term "compound fracture" of the skull indicates that the pericranial tissues have been torn and that there is direct communication between the lacerated scalp and the cerebral substance through the depressed or comminuted fragments of bone and lacerated dura. With compound fractures of the skull there is less likelihood of simple concussion and the patient is more likely to have severe brain damage.

The complications of head injury include vascular lesions (e.g., hemorrhage, thrombosis, aneurysms), infections (e.g., osteomyelitis, meningitis, abscess), rhinorrhea, otorrhea, pneumocele, leptomeningeal cysts, injury to the cranial nerves, and focal cerebral lesions. The sequelae of head injury are convulsive seizures, psychosis and other psychiatric disorders, and the so-called "post-traumatic syndrome," which has no established pathologic basis.

Pathology.

Cerebral Concussion and Diffuse Brain Injury. Traditionally, the term "concussion" describes brief loss of consciousness after head

Table 54–1. Some Characteristics of Head Injury as a Cause of Death in the United States

| | Study Population and Study Years | | | |
Characteristic	Olmsted County, Minn. 1965– 1974	Bronx County, N.Y. 1980	Harris County, Tex. 1980	San Diego County, Calif. 1980
Total number of head injury deaths*	175	313	758	476
Head injury death rate per 100,000 population	22	27	32	25
Male/female mortality ratio	3.5	4.5	4.0	3.7
Age of peak head injury mortality	65–75 yr	25–34 yr	15–24 yr	15–24 yr
Mechanism of injury (%)†				
Traffic/transport	53	20	44	49
Assault (nonfirearm)	1	15	4	5
Fall	14	18	5	15
Gunshot	20	40	44	30
Place of death (%)				
Scene/DOA	Not reported	62	62	56
Emergency room	Not reported	12	12	10

*Under the 9th Revision ICDA a case was classified as a head injury death if one or more of the following codes applied: N800, N801, N803, N804, N850–854. These include skull fractures and intracranial injuries.
†Olmsted County percents are based on all head injury deaths in the period 1935–1974.
(From Frankowski RF, Annegers, JF, Whitman S. Epidemiological and descriptive studies. Part 1. The descriptive epidemiology of head trauma in the United States. In: Becker DP, Povlishock JT, eds. Central Nervous System Trauma Status Report—1985. Bethesda: National Institutes of Health, NINCDS, 1985:33–43.)

injury, with no immediate or delayed evidence of structural brain damage. The defining word is "brief," but this criterion is open to interpretation. Consciousness may be lost for only a few seconds, as in a boxing knockout or, after more severe injury, consciousness may be lost for hours or days.

Some investigators put the arbitrary division at 6 hours. If the patient recovers consciousness before that time concussion is the appropriate word, and the long-term outcome is excellent. The mechanism is uncertain but it is thought that there is a functional disconnection of the brain stem from the cerebral hemispheres. There is presumably no histologic change.

If coma lasts longer than 6 hours there is presumed to have been brain tissue injury. It is now believed that there is a continuum of diffuse brain injuries that are caused by the acceleration and deceleration of the head resulting in shearing or stretching of axons, or *diffuse axonal injury* (DAI). This term is used if coma lasts longer than 6 hours. Coma for 6 to 24 hours is deemed mild DAI; moderate or severe DAI depends on the duration of coma but more prolonged coma is likely to be associated with focal cerebral signs or evidence of cerebral edema, and has an unfavorable outcome.

DAI has been described in three forms: a focal lesion in the corpus callosum; a focal lesion in the dorsolateral quadrants of the rostral brain stem; or a diffuse lesion. Diffuse lesions are at first microscopic, manifested by axonal retraction bulbs throughout the white matter of the cerebral hemispheres. If the patient survives there may be later evidence of wallerian degeneration.

Brain Swelling. Brain swelling after head injury may be caused in part by cerebral edema, as described in Section 41. The formal definition of brain edema, however, implies an increase in the content of extravascular brain water. In post-traumatic brain swelling it is thought that there is also an increase in the intravascular volume of blood in the brain, an abnormal vasodilatation. The swelling may be diffuse or it may be focal, adjacent to contusion or hemorrhage.

Contusion and Laceration. In the simplest visible injury of the brain, a *contusion*, the pia-arachnoid is intact. These membranes are torn in a *laceration*. Both types of lesion are found primarily in the frontal and temporal poles and on the undersurfaces of these areas, where the brain comes into contact with bony protuberances (Fig. 54–1). If there is no DAI, brain swelling, or secondary hemorrhage, recovery from contusion may be excellent. Healed contusions are often found on autopsy examination of those with no clinical evidence of permanent brain damage.

Contusions may occur at the site of skull fractures but may also occur without fracture. They may be found at the site of the blow to the head or at a point opposite the impact *(contrecoup contusion)*. Whatever the site of injury, however, contusions are likely to be most severe in the frontal and temporal lobes. There are more frontal lesions after occipital injury than vice versa.

The degree of damage to the meninges and

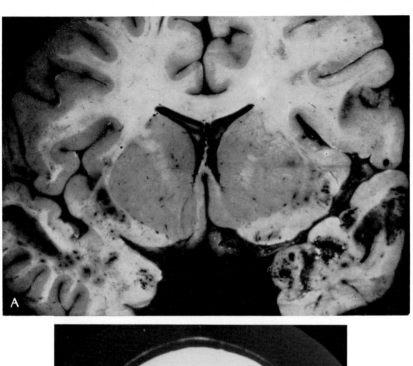

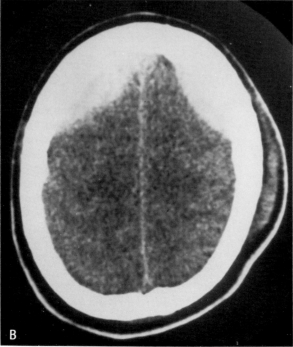

Fig. 54–1. Cerebral trauma. *A.* Contusion of temporal poles with fresh hemorrhages in temporal lobes. *B.* CT scan of bilateral acute epidural hematomas. Extracranial soft tissue swelling on the left.

cerebral substance is related to the force of the blow. With minor injuries there are petechial hemorrhages in the surface of the cortex and a mild degree of meningeal hemorrhage. With more severe injuries the meninges and cortical substances are torn and there may be extensive hemorrhagic necrosis of the cortex and subcortical white matter. There may also be small or large hemorrhages into the basal ganglia, brain stem, or other portions of the brain (Fig. 54–2) far removed from the site of injury. Laceration of the middle meningeal artery or the dural sinuses is followed by bleeding into the extradural spaces except in older patients, in whom bleeding may be in the subdural space.

Rupture of arachnoidal vessels causes hemorrhage into the subarachnoid space, which may extend into the subdural space. It is probable, however, that subdural hemorrhage is more commonly caused by rupture of the vessels that bridge the space between the arachnoid and the dura mater.

Depressed fractures of the skull may not be accompanied by any injury to the brain; the cerebral substance beneath the depressed fragment may be compressed, contused, or even lacerated. The superior longitudinal sinus may be torn or compressed and thrombosed by depressed fractures of the vertex.

Penetration of the skull and cerebral substance by bullets, bomb fragments, or other missiles causes laceration, necrosis, and hemorrhage around the track of the missile.

The evolution of the pathologic changes in the patient who recovers is related to the nature of the injury to the brain. Superficial lacerations of the meninges and cortex heal by gliosis, with the formation of small punched-out areas, denuded of their meningeal covering. These areas usually retain a yellowish color because of the presence of blood pigment. Larger areas of necrosis that extend deep into the cerebral substance heal by the formation of scar tissue that is composed of glia, fibroblasts, and meninges (meningocerebral cicatrix). The introduction of scalp or other infected tissues into the cranium may be followed by the development of an abscess or meningitis.

Symptoms and Signs. Disturbance of consciousness is the most common symptom of head injury. Coma or brief loss of contact with the environment is the characteristic feature of simple concussion. Coma may be more prolonged, lasting for several hours, days, or weeks when there is swelling, hemorrhage, DAI, or contusion or laceration of the cortex. The duration of the coma depends on the site and severity of the injury. Coma prolonged over several days or many weeks is not uncommon when the brain or brain stem has been severely contused or lacerated. Loss of consciousness in patients with perforating wounds of the skull and brain is related to the size of the missile and to the region of the brain injured. Penetration of the frontal or parietal lobes by small missiles may not cause loss of consciousness, whereas those that pass through the petrous bone into the cerebellum and posterior fossa commonly produce coma of several or many days' duration.

On recovering consciousness, the severity and nature of the symptoms are related to the degree of brain damage. Patients with a concussion may be normal within a few minutes. Others may be slightly dazed for a few minutes and complain of headaches for 12 hours or longer. The period of mental confusion is prolonged, roughly proportional to the degree of brain injury, whenever there is contusion or laceration of the cortex. Surgical shock may be present, particularly if there is injury to other portions of the body. Headaches and dizziness may be present after a head injury, regardless of the severity of brain damage. The presence of hemiplegia, aphasia, cranial nerve palsies, and other focal neu-

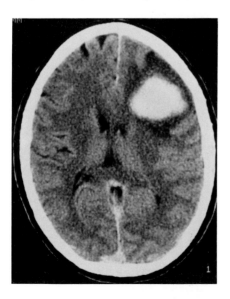

Fig. 54–2. Traumatic hemorrhage, frontal lobe. Axial noncontrast CT demonstrates left frontal lobe density (hemorrhage), surrounding lucency (edema) and mass effect (sulcal and ventricular effacement). (Courtesy of Drs. S.K. Hilal and J.A. Bello.)

rologic signs is dependent on the extent and site of the damage to intracranial structures.

Emergency Care and Evaluation. Diagnosis and management of head injury are inextricably linked from the outset. Immediate attention to the injured is linked to the organization of emergency services in a particular area. It is estimated that 60% of fatalities occur before patients can be admitted to a hospital—40% at the scene and 20% in the emergency room. Thus, improved care at the site of injury might reduce mortality rates.

Improved care has led to a reduction of mortality rates for military injuries, from 4.5/100 in World War II to 2.5/100 in Korea, and to less than 1/100 in Viet Nam. Although there have been many improvements, rapid evacuation is given much of the credit. In cases of civilian injuries the availability of helicopter transport has also lowered mortality rates. Trained teams of rescue workers who are not physicians are able to provide such services as intubation, treatment of shock, and other emergency measures.

On arrival in the hospital it is imperative to evaluate hypoxia, shock, and multiple injuries. A baseline neurologic evaluation is done while cardiopulmonary assessment is carried out. If there are no signs of external trauma the differential diagnosis may be that of coma, as described in Chapter 42.

The Glasgow Coma Scale (Table 54–2) has been widely accepted as a semiquantitative clinical measure of the severity of brain injury; it also provides a guide to prognosis (Table 54–3). The Glasgow score, however, is not valid for children or for patients in shock or those who are intoxicated, hypoxic, or postictal. Orbital and spine injuries may also invalidate the score.

In addition to evaluating the Glasgow score, the examiner assesses ocular movements, oculovestibular reflexes, and pupils, as described in the evaluation of coma (Chapter 42). Evidence of hemiparesis or third nerve palsy is usually contralateral to the side of injury but may be a false localizing sign if there is cerebral swelling and peduncular compression. Signs of *decorticate rigidity* (e.g., flexion of arms, extension of legs) or *decerebrate rigidity* (e.g., extension of legs and arms) are probably better described than named because the physiology is debated and there is doubt about the traditional teaching that decerebration implies injury in the rostral midbrain.

Early in the evaluation the head is exam-

Table 54–2. Glasgow Coma Scale

Activity	Score*
Verbal response	
None	1
Incomprehensible sounds	2
Inappropriate words	3
Confused	4
Oriented	5
Eye opening	
None	1
To pain	2
To speech	3
Spontaneously	4
Motor response	
None	1
Abnormal extensor	2
Abnormal flexor	3
Withdraws	4
Localizes	5
Obeys	6

*Total score = sum of the score for each of the three components. Score for a fully oriented alert patient = 15. Score for a mute immobile patient with no eye opening = 3.

(From Teasdale G, Jennett B. Assessment of coma and impaired consciousness. A practical scale. Lancet 1974; 2:81–83.)

ined for lesions of the scalp or skull. Seizures may have to be treated on the spot, as described in Chapter 145 for status epilepticus. Before any other radiographic studies are carried out it is necessary to ascertain that there is no injury of the cervical spine. Depending on the circumstances, radiographs of the cervical spine may be needed first.

The use of CT has replaced radiography for evaluation of the head injury itself if there has been any alteration of consciousness or if there are focal signs. Surgery may be needed if there is evidence of a depressed fracture or a mass lesion. If not, further management depends on the presence of a CSF leak or the appearance of signs of brain swelling or delayed intracranial hemorrhage. Intracranial pressure is monitored in many centers, and the device may have to be installed. CT is not necessary if there has been no loss of consciousness and no abnormality is found on neurologic examination, unless there is reason to suspect depressed fracture or CSF leak.

There has been intense debate about guidelines for taking routine skull films after mild head injury. The consensus is growing that this is not necessary for an alert patient with no neurologic abnormalities on examination unless there is evidence or suspicion of a de-

Table 54–3. Outcome Associated with Best Level of Clinical Function in First 24 Hours after Onset of Coma

		Outcome	
Clinical Feature	No. Patients	Dead or vegetative (%)	Moderate Disability or Good Recovery (%)
Coma response sum*			
>11	57	12	82
8/9/10	190	27	68
5/6/7	525	53	34
3/4	176	87	7
Pupils			
Reacting	748	39	50
Nonreacting	226	91	4
Eye movements			
Intact	463	33	56
Impaired	143	62	25
Absent or bad	186	90	5
Motor response pattern (any limb)			
Normal or weak	568	36	54
Abnormal	393	74	16
Motor response pattern (best limb)			
Obeys or localizes	395	31	58
Withdraws or reflexes	402	54	35
Extensor or nil	191	85	8

*Glasgow Coma Scale.
Eye opening (E): spontaneous (4), to speech (3), to pain (2), nil (1).
Best motor response (M): obeys (6); localizes (5); withdraws (4); abnormal flexion (3); extensor response (2); nil (1).
Verbal response (V): oriented (5); confused conversation (4); inappropriate words (3); incomprehensible words (3); incomprehensible sounds (2); nil (1).
Coma score = E + M + V = 3 to 15.
(From Jennett B, et al. J Neurol Neurosurg Psychiatry 1980; 43:289–295.)

pressed skull fracture. In one series more than 90% of patients who developed intracranial hematomas had an altered state of consciousness on admission, and almost all the others had some other reason for admission.

Admission to the Hospital. Any patient with a serious head injury is admitted to the hospital. If there has been no loss of consciousness and there are no abnormalities on examination, the patient may be sent home. There is a gray area for patients between these extremes, however—patients with minor head injury as defined by a Glasgow Coma Scale score of 13 to 15.

Patients may be admitted for any of the following abnormalities: loss of consciousness for 10 minutes or more (or doubt about the duration); focal signs on neurologic examination; post-traumatic seizure; depressed skull fracture or penetrating wounds; persistent alteration of consciousness; basal skull fracture or CSF leak; or doubt about any of these criteria.

Other Laboratory Studies. If CT is not available, recourse must be made to plain skull films, air encephalography, or arteriography. CT alone, however, provides information about skull fractures, cerebral swelling, contusion, and intracranial hemorrhage. MRI and PET studies may become important in the evaluation of late stages of recovery from head injury but are not likely to be important in acute care.

Lumbar puncture was once important in the evaluation of head injuries but has largely been replaced by the use of CT and intracranial monitoring. Examination of the CSF is important if there is any question of meningitis or other infection. Several different devices are available for monitoring intracranial pressure. The management of increased pressure by hyperventilation, administration of mannitol, and other measures varies in different centers.

EEG is not an emergency test but if it is taken at some convenient time after admission it may aid in prognosis. With head injury of any type there is usually suppression of the electrical activity of the cerebral cortex at the time of injury. With recovery the activity returns to normal, often going through a phase of generalized slowing and increased voltage. Areas of focal damage to the cortex may show evidence of abnormal activity (slowing and spike activity) for weeks or months after the injury. These abnormalities are important because of the possibility of later development of convulsive seizures. A common feature of the EEG in all patients with head injuries is an undue susceptibility of the cortical activity to overventilation. This may persist for many weeks.

Course and Prognosis. The prognosis of patients with head injury is related to the site and severity of the injury. The mortality rate is zero in patients with simple concussion and is less than 2% when there is a mild degree of cerebral edema and congestion. The mortality rate increases greatly when the cortex is contused (5%) or lacerated (41%). Death may result immediately after the injury or may be delayed for several weeks. Death may result from the direct effect of the injury or from the complications that ensue.

With concussion or with minor degrees of cerebral edema or contusion, patients recover from coma with no residual effects. There may be loss of memory for the events that occurred in the immediate period after recovery of consciousness (*post-traumatic amnesia*) and a similar amnesia for the events immediately preceding the injury (*pretraumatic amnesia*). The duration of pre- and post-traumatic amnesia is related to the severity of the brain damage. With a minor degree of concussion either one or both may be absent but, when there has been severe contusion and laceration or other injury of the brain, periods of amnesia may extend for days or weeks. In the weeks after recovery from the injury there is partial return of memory for events that occurred before and after the accident; there is also a reduction of the period of absolute memory loss.

Headaches, dizziness, or vertigo may be present in the immediate post-traumatic period. These symptoms usually disappear in a few weeks but may be prolonged for months. With severe injuries to the brain and prolonged coma there is usually a period of mental cloudiness and confusion before full consciousness is restored. Headaches, dizziness, vertigo, and other features of the post-traumatic syndrome may be present, as well as signs of cranial nerve injuries or focal damage to the brain. With the passage of time there is usually considerable improvement in the signs and symptoms of brain damage but permanent sequelae are not uncommon when there has been extensive damage to the brain. Attempts to make a firm prognosis in severe head injuries, especially in the early stages, are hazardous because the outcome depends on so many variables. Some indices, however, such as the Glasgow Coma Sale (Table 54–2), are valuable as prognostic indicators.

Treatment. Treatment of patients with craniocerebral injuries is operative or nonoperative. The operative therapy of the complications of head injuries is discussed below. Simple wounds of the scalp should be thoroughly cleaned and sutured. Compound fractures of the skull should be completely debrided. Operative treatment of compound fractures should be performed as soon as possible but may be delayed for 24 hours until the patient is transported to a hospital equipped for this purpose, or until the patient has recovered from surgical shock. Elevation of small depressed fractures need not be performed immediately, but the depressed fragments should be elevated before the patient is discharged from the hospital, particularly if the inner table of the skull is involved.

After admission nonoperative therapy is concerned chiefly with the general care of the patient and control of increased intracranial pressure. Severely injured patients are best treated in an intensive care unit. In many cities a single center is designated as the center for head injuries. In some hospitals head injuries are treated in a special neurologic or neurosurgical intensive care unit. Concerns include multiple injuries, pulmonary function and infection, bladder function, nutrition, and skin care.

The patient should be examined repeatedly and regularly to evaluate the state of awareness and the presence or absence of signs of injury to the cerebral substance or cranial nerves. Variations in the level of consciousness while the patient is under observation, or the appearance of hemiplegia or other focal neurologic signs should lead to the consideration of the diagnosis of an extradural or subdural hematoma. CT is repeated as needed.

If the patient remains comatose for more than 12 hours, nutrition can be administered by nasal tube or parenterally. The administration of sedative drugs should be avoided if possible. Restlessness may be combated by giving small doses of paraldehyde or other sedatives. The use of morphine is contraindicated because it depresses respiration. Excessive sedation with barbiturates or other drugs may prolong the period of mental confusion and restlessness. Anticonvulsant drugs can be used, but the value of prophylactic use of anticonvulsants early in the course of head injury is debatable. Meticulous attention should be given to pulmonary care. Serial determinations of blood gas values are necessary to assess pulmonary function in comatose or confused patients.

Lumbar puncture should be performed only for diagnostic problems. Increased intracranial pressure can be combated by the administration of steroids, particularly dexamethasone, or by the intravenous administration of hypertonic solutions of sucrose. Care should be taken to see that the patient is not dehydrated by such measures and fluid intake should be kept at an adequate level by parenteral injections, if necessary.

Patients with simple concussion should be kept under observation for 24 hours and allowed to return to their usual activities after another 24 to 48 hours. The period of bed rest and convalescence of patients with more severe head injuries must be determined by the response of the patient to the treatment administered. Care should be taken not to overemphasize the severity of the injury and unnecessarily prolong the period of invalidism. Patients should be allowed out of bed as soon as their condition permits. Activity should be gradually increased during the hospital stay. Convalescence should be continued at home with graduated exercises. Return to active work should be deferred for 2 to 3 months after discharge from the hospital whenever there has been a severe degree of brain injury. The use of alcohol is prohibited because of the decrease in the tolerance that occurs in patients with head injury.

Complications of Head Injuries

The vascular complications of head injury include subarachnoid hemorrhage, extradural hemorrhage, subdural hemorrhage, subdural hygroma, intracerebral hemorrhage, cerebral thrombosis, and arteriovenous aneurysms.

SUBARACHNOID HEMORRHAGE

Some extravasation of blood into the subarachnoid spaces is to be expected in any patient with an injury to the head. In most cases it is of little clinical importance except to indicate that the brain has been injured and to

warn the physician that serious damage to the brain or its coverings may have occurred. No specific treatment for simple subarachnoid bleeding is needed. Close observation, however, and repeated CT are used to exclude the possibility of additional intracranial loculated blood.

EXTRADURAL HEMORRHAGE

Hemorrhage into the extradural space is generally caused by a tear in the wall of one of the meningeal arteries, usually the middle meningeal artery, but in approximately 15% of patients the bleeding is from one of the dural sinuses. The dura is separated from the skull by the extravasated blood. The size of the clot increases until the ruptured vessel is occluded by the formation of a clot in its torn walls. The hematoma is usually large and is located over the convexity of the hemisphere in the middle fossa, but occasionally the hemorrhage may be confined to the anterior fossa, possibly as a result of tearing of an anterior meningeal artery. Extradural hemorrhage in the posterior fossa may occur when the torcula Herophili is torn. Bilateral extradural hemorrhages are extremely rare. In the vast majority of cases the hematoma is on the side of the head injury. Because the body has no mechanism for the absorption of an extradural hemorrhage the clotted blood remains in the epidural space as a tumor until it is removed by operation. Organization of the clot by the dura does not occur because hemorrhage into the epidural space usually causes death within a few days.

Incidence. Extradural hemorrhage is a relatively rare complication of head injury (Table 54–4). It is found in less than 1% of all cases of head injury in unselected series. The figure is higher in series of severe head injuries and in autopsy series, however, because this complication is so serious.

Extradural hematoma is primarily a prob-

Table 54–4.   Incidence of Different Types of Traumatic Hematomas*

	% of cases
Extradural only	11–24
Extradural and intradural	7–11
Subdural only	3–42
Subdural and intracerebral	23–58
Intracerebral (discrete)	6–20

*Data compiled from 2907 cases in the literature. (From Jennett B, Teasdale G. Management of Head Injuries. Philadelphia: FA Davis, 1981.)

lem of young adults. It is exceptional before the age of 2 and after the age of 60. In those in both groups the dura tends to adhere more to the inner table of the skull than in young adults.

Symptoms and Signs. The typical sequence of events in a patient with an extradural hemorrhage is as follows: loss of consciousness at the time of the injury, a lucid interval for several hours, and subsequent relapse into coma accompanied by the development of a hemiplegia. The initial coma is caused by concussion or cerebral trauma. The secondary loss of consciousness and hemiplegia are the result of compression of the brain by expansion of the hemorrhage. The relatively slow development of the symptoms of cerebral compression is explained by the close adherence of the dura to the skull.

The typical sequence of events described above is not present in as high a percentage of the cases as is commonly assumed. In some series the lucid interval was absent in over 50% of patients because the damage to the brain at the time of the injury was so severe that the immediate coma lasted long enough to merge with that resulting from compression of the brain by the hematoma. The hemiplegia is usually contralateral to the hematoma but is sometimes on the same side. Ipsilateral hemiplegia is attributed to compression of the opposite cerebral peduncle against the tentorium.

In the usual case the signs of brain compression, coma, and hemiplegia develop within a few hours after the accident. Occasionally they may be delayed for several days or as long as 3 weeks. The optic discs are usually normal in patients who develop signs of cerebral compression within a few hours of the injury but papilledema may develop in patients who live for 3 weeks after the injury. Convulsive seizures are rarely seen, but jacksonian or generalized seizures have been reported in a few cases. The presence of cerebellar signs, nuchal rigidity, and drowsiness, together with a fracture of the occipital bone, should lead to the suspicion of a clot in the posterior fossa.

A finding of value in the diagnosis and localization of an extradural hemorrhage is a dilated pupil that does not react to light or accommodation. This dilated fixed pupil, usually accompanied by other signs of paralysis of the third nerve, is always on the same side as the clot and is caused by compression of the third nerve by the hippocampal gyrus

when herniated over the free edge of the tentorium. Pupillary dilatation, however, may also be bilateral.

Diagnosis. The diagnosis of an extradural clot is made by CT (Figs. 54–3 and 54–4). Lumbar puncture is no longer used; formerly, the CSF pressure was found to be over 200 mm H_2O in about 65% of patients. The fluid was usually clear but could be bloody if there was contusion or laceration of the brain in addition to the extradural clot.

The use of EEG has also been superseded by that of CT as a diagnostic test for extradural hemorrhage. Although sometimes there are unilateral abnormalities the patterns are not consistent, and the EEG record might even be normal. EEG becomes important, however, if there are seizures.

The diagnosis of extradural hemorrhage can be made without difficulty in patients with the typical clinical history and CT evidence of hemorrhage or fracture through one of the meningeal arteries or large sinuses. Less obvious cases of extradural hemorrhage can be diagnosed if the variations in the clinical picture are kept in mind; diagnostic exploratory trephine openings in the skull are made if indicated by CT.

Course and Prognosis. Extradural hemorrhage is the most fatal complication of head injury. The mortality rate is nearly 100% in untreated patients and over 30% in treated patients. The high mortality rate in treated patients is partly a result of delay in establishing diagnosis and partly because of the severity of brain damage. In untreated patients death usually occurs within 12 to 72 hours after the injury, but the patient may live for 2 to 3 weeks. The clinical course in fatal cases is a gradual increase in the depth of the coma, with death ensuing as result of failure of the cardiac and respiratory centers with herniation. Secondary brain stem lesions are the usual cause of death.

Treatment. The treatment of extradural hemorrhage is removal of the clot through an enlargement of trephine openings in the skull. The bleeding point should be identified and either ligated or clipped if arterial, or closed with muscle if venous. Postoperative treatment includes transfusions and other methods to combat shock, and treatment of the cerebral edema. The operative results depend to a great extent on the degree of associated brain damage. If this is slight, complete recovery is the rule, with disappearance of the hemiplegia or other focal neurologic

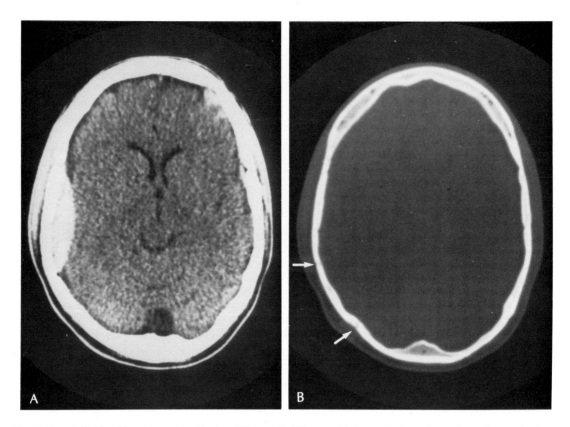

Fig. 54–3. *A.* Epidural hematoma is evident on CT scan. *B.* CT scan with bone windows shows two adjacent fractures *(arrows);* the anterior fracture is at the site of the groove for the middle meningeal artery.

signs. Occasionally a large clot may dislocate the brain so greatly that secondary hemorrhages occur in the brain stem. In such cases recovery may not be possible even though the original head injury had not produced any other serious change.

Sometimes the CT scan shows evidence of an extradural hematoma but there is no clinical indication of hazard. Under such circumstances some clinicians have treated the patient without surgery. If the patient is alert, however, the mortality rate is almost zero with surgical evacuation of the clot.

SUBDURAL HEMORRHAGE

A collection of blood between the dura and arachnoid in the subdural space is known as a *subdural hematoma.* It is practically always secondary to an injury to the head that is usually severe but sometimes mild and unnoticed; it may occur in connection with blood dyscrasias or cachexia in the absence of trauma. Subdural hematoma has been reported as the result of blast injury and has been found in the newborn and infants as a

complication of delivery and postnatal trauma. Organized subdural hemorrhages were formerly a common finding at necropsy in psychotic patients, especially those suffering with dementia paralytica. Such hematomas were described in the literature as pachymeningitis hemorrhagia interna, and were at times ascribed to a syphilitic origin. It is now recognized that syphilis plays no role in the production of these hematomas and that they are the result of head trauma in convulsive seizures or other blows to the head.

Pathology. The bleeding in the subdural space is practically always of venous origin except when the branches of the middle meningeal artery are lacerated by a fracture of the skull. In older patients the dura does not strip and the acute hemorrhage occurs in the subdural space with clinical symptoms of an epidural hematoma. The fluid in the subdural space may be admixed with CSF if the arachnoid is torn. When the fluid collection is composed mainly of CSF it is known as a *subdural hygroma.* The hemorrhage is usually over the convexity of the hemisphere in the region of

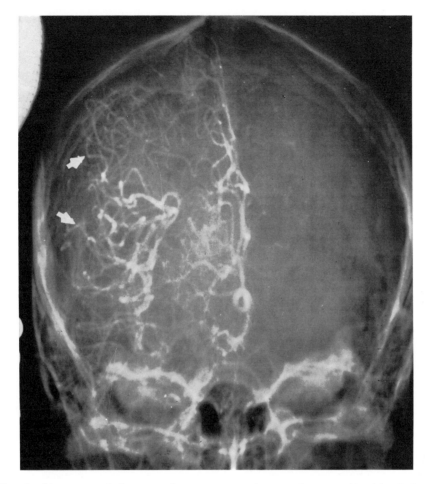

Fig. 54–4. Extradural hematoma. A clear avascular area is present between the inner table of the skull and the surface vessels of the brain in the angiogram. The vessels are displaced inward *(arrows)*, but there is relatively little shift of the anterior cerebral artery because of the rigidity of the dura mater between the hematoma and the brain. Compare with Figure 54–9.

the frontal and parietal lobes. It may occasionally be confined to the anterior or temporal fossa and, rarely, to the posterior fossa. The hematoma is bilateral in approximately 15% of patients.

Blood that is extravasated into the subdural space is not absorbed but is organized or encapsulated by the dura. Fibroblasts proliferate from the inner surface of the dura and invade the clot at all points where it is in contact with the dura. Newly formed capillaries enter the clot and gradually absorb the liquefied blood. If the clot is small it is completely organized by fibroblasts. When the clot is large fibroblasts not only invade the clot directly, but also grow along the undersurface of the clot to form new membranes on the inner surface of the clot, as well as on the surface adjacent to the dura. Thus the incompletely liquefied clot is encapsulated.

If death does not occur the end result of a small subdural hematoma is a thickening of the dura by the addition of the organized membrane. When the clot is large a subdural cyst with inner and outer membranes is formed and, in some cases, it may become calcified (Fig. 54–5).

The cerebral cortex is compressed and molded by the clot. The compression of the cortex may result in the herniation of the brain through the tentorium and damage to remote portions of the nervous system, producing false localizing signs. The opposite posterior cerebral artery may be compressed, producing a homolateral hemianopia, or the opposite cerebral peduncle may be caught against the tentorium, causing a homolateral hemiplegia. Paralysis of the oculomotor nerves or disorganization of gaze may result from hemorrhages in the brain stem as a result of com-

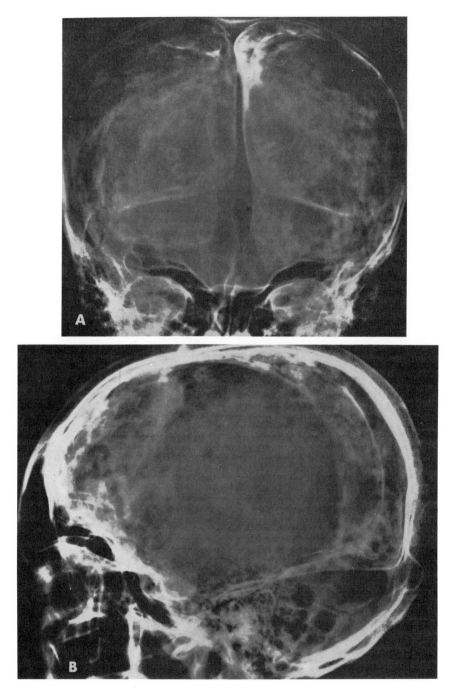

Fig. 54–5. Calcified subdural hematomas. *A.* In the frontal view, bilateral shell-like calcifications form a cast of the cerebral hemispheres. *B.* In the lateral view, the outer calcified membranes are near the bony skull and the inner membranes are separated from the outer by relatively clear zones.

pression of its vessels. Because subdural hematoma is caused by venous bleeding, the increase in intracranial pressure develops slowly. Herniation of the hippocampus through the free edge of the tentorium and compression of the third nerve with a dilated fixed pupil are not often seen as early signs but may occur as late signs.

Incidence. In some epidemiologic studies subdural hematomas are divided into acute and chronic types: this division depends on the definition of "acute," which sometimes means surgery within 24 hours of injury. In both types patients are more likely to be men than women and are generally older than patients with other types of head injury. Motor vehicle accidents are somewhat less likely to be the cause than falls or assaults. Acute subdural hemorrhage occurs in 1 to 5% of all head injury admissions and in 10 to 20% of serious head injuries.

Subacute subdural hematomas cause symptoms that appear between 3 and 20 days after injury. Those that occur in the first week are similar to acute hematomas; those that occur in the third week are similar to chronic subdural hematomas. The incidence of chronic subdural hematoma is about 1 to 2/100,000 population annually. In one series more than 75% of patients were older than 50, with an average age of 63 years. The incidence increases with age, from 0.13/100,000 for those in their twenties to 7.4/100,000 for those in their seventies.

In 25 to 50% of cases of chronic subdural hematoma there is no history of head injury. In some series, however, 50% of patients were thought to abuse alcohol, which may have affected recall of head injury. Other risk factors are seizure disorders, intracranial shunting procedures, and clotting disorders.

Current figures for the incidence of subdural hematoma in mental hospitals are unavailable but, from 1914 to 1934, Allen and colleagues found subdural hematomas in 8% of autopsies of psychotic patients. The clot seemed especially likely in patients who might have been subject to head injury—the elderly, epileptic, alcoholic, or paretic.

Subdural hematoma of infancy is discussed later in this section. The frequency of all types of intracranial hemorrhage in the newborn is estimated to be 2 to 3%. This figure is obviously too low. Subdural hematoma constitutes only a small portion of these, but the experience of pediatric neurosurgeons would indicate that subdural hematoma is more fre-

quent in infants than is commonly supposed. Ingraham and Matson reported an average of 17 cases per year at the Children's Hospital in Boston; the Hospital for Sick Children in Toronto reported an incidence of 5.2% in a series of 4465 cases admitted after injury to the head.

No characteristic symptoms differentiate an acute subdural hematoma from cerebral contusion or laceration or a chronic hematoma from an intracranial neoplasm. The symptoms of an acute subdural hematoma usually develop within the first few days after the injury. Headache is almost invariably present. The state of consciousness is variable and depends to some extent on the degree of concomitant cerebral damage. After recovery from the coma caused by the injury, the development of irritability, mental confusion, or varying degrees of coma is a common occurrence in patients with a subdural hematoma. Similarly, there may be fluctuations in the level of consciousness from day to day or during 1 day. Hemiplegia or central facial weakness is present in approximately 50% of patients. The paralysis is usually on the side opposite to the hematoma but may be on the same side. Convulsive seizures, usually generalized, occur in less than 5% of patients. Aphasia is uncommon and hemianopia does not occur unless the optic radiations have been contused or the opposite posterior cerebral artery has been compressed by dislocation of the cerebrum. In the latter case the hemianopia is ipsilateral to the hematoma.

The symptoms of a chronic subdural hematoma are similar to those of an acute hematoma. The symptoms usually date from the time of the injury. Intermittent headache, slight or severe impairment of the intellectual faculties, and hemiparesis are the most characteristic symptoms if the initial trauma was slight and not remembered. The symptoms are identical to those of any expanding intracranial lesion and are indistinguishable from those of a neoplasm.

Signs. The common signs of an acute subdural hematoma are fluctuations in the level of consciousness and hemiplegia. The hemiplegia, which may be present on recovery of consciousness or may develop in the next few days, is usually of the spastic type, with increases of tendon reflexes and Babinski sign. Changes in the vital signs are not present unless there is associated cerebral injury. Papilledema is rarely seen. The size of the pupils has no value in localizing the hematoma unless one pupil is large and does not react to light. This large nonreacting pupil, which is on the same side as the hematoma, is much less common in patients with subdural hematoma than in patients with extradural hemorrhage. Weakness of the extraocular muscles or disorganization of gaze may rarely be seen as a result of hemorrhages into the brain stem.

The signs of a chronic subdural hematoma are similar to those of an acute hematoma except that convulsive seizures and papilledema are more frequently seen.

The manifestations of chronic subdural hematoma are diverse, however, and the clot may be unsuspected before CT is carried out. Some patients are thought to be demented. Others are suspected of an intracranial tumor because of slow progression of focal signs. Sometimes symptoms begin abruptly, as in a stroke; there may be seizures, or symptoms similar to those of a transient ischemic attack may occur. (Figs. 54–6, 54–7, and 54–8).

Laboratory Data. The diagnosis is established by CT (Figs. 54–6, 54–7, and 54–8). There is usually evidence of a hyperdense lesion with a concave medial border, and there may be evidence of a shift of midline structures. If there are no pressure effects, an additional lesion on the other side may be suspected. Isodense hematomas may be difficult to discern. The role of MRI is yet to be elucidated but that procedure may be especially useful for detecting isodense lesions.

Lumbar puncture is no longer used; the CSF is usually bloody but may be clear. Similarly, plain skull films may show evidence of a linear fracture or displacement of the pineal gland and arteriograms may show evidence of the mass, but these techniques are rarely needed when CT is available. Carotid angiograms demonstrate inward displacement of the terminal branches of the middle cerebral artery (Fig. 54–9).

Because there are no characteristic symptoms for either an acute or chronic subdural hematoma, the diagnosis of subdural hemorrhage may be difficult. The hematoma is usually accompanied by cerebral contusion and laceration, and the situation is further complicated because subdural hemorrhage is frequent in patients who are addicted to alcohol and are admitted to a hospital in coma, unable to give a history of an accident. In these cases the erroneous diagnosis of spontaneous intracerebral or subarachnoid hemorrhage may be considered before CT examination. The diagnosis should be considered

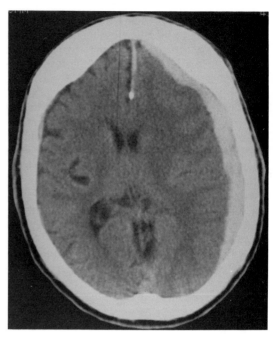

Fig. 54–6. Acute subdural hematoma. Noncontrast axial CT scan demonstrates a hyperdense crescent-shaped extra-axial collection showing mass effect (sulcal and ventricular effacement) and midline shift from left to right. (Courtesy of Drs. J.A. Bello and S.K. Hilal.)

in any patient who has suffered a head injury if there are fluctuations in level of consciousness, if focal neurologic signs develop, or if the patient does not respond satisfactorily to adequate treatment of a head injury.

Treatment. The treatment of subdural hematoma is evacuation of the clot and neomembrane through trephine openings or craniotomy. Subdural hematoma is frequently bilateral. In the presence of other serious medical illness or other severe injuries, especially in the elderly, or if the subdural hematoma is asymptomatic, a few patients with subdural hematomas may not be candidates for evacuation of the clot. With long-term monitoring and clinical observation, the hematoma may shrink and disappear without surgery.

SUBDURAL HEMORRHAGE IN INFANTS

Acute subdural hematoma was once considered to be the most common intracranial birth injury, but this syndrome seems to be disappearing with improved obstetric care. Seizures, pallor, and a tense anterior fontanelle are the manifestations of overt subdural hematoma in the neonatal period. The infants may be abnormal at birth, with no spontaneous respiration or with severe hypoten-

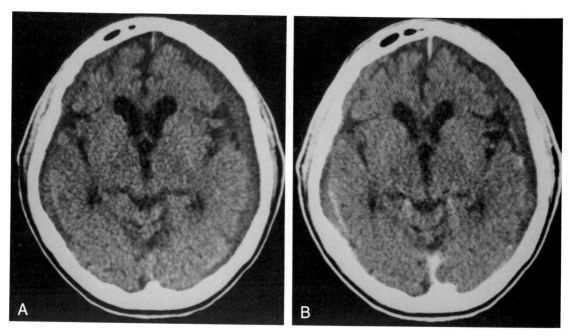

Fig. 54–7. Subacute subdural hematoma. *A.* Noncontrast axial CT scan shows bilateral isodense extra-axial collections, larger on the left. *B.* These are better demonstrated on the postcontrast scan, in which enhancing membranes, typical of the subacute phase, can be seen. (Courtesy of Drs. J.A. Bello and S.K. Hilal.)

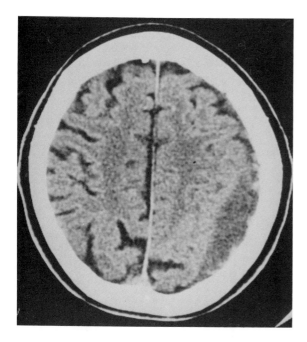

Fig. 54–8. Chronic subdural hematoma. Noncontrast axial CT scan shows an extra-axial collection of hypodensity with extra-axial mass effect—medial displacement of the white-gray junction on the left compared with the right. (Courtesy of Drs. J.A. Bello and S.K. Hilal.)

sion, seizures, and retinal hemorrhage. Diagnosis by subdural taps has been supplanted by the use of CT. Surgical evacuation is accomplished through a craniotomy rather than a burr hole.

Acute and chronic subdural hematomas are rarely seen in older children, except as a complication of shunt procedures or bleeding disorders. In infants the manifestations are macrocrania, tense anterior fontanelle, irritability, vomiting, and seizures. Diagnosis is made by CT. Skull films and skeletal surveys are carried out to evaluate the possibility of child abuse *(the battered child syndrome)*. The fluid collection can be treated by repeated subdural taps monitored by CT. If more than 10 taps are done, surgical treatment is needed. Removal of the subdural membranes was once considered to be important to avoid restriction of growth of the brain, but this no longer seems necessary. Normal later development is seen in 75% of these children, but 25% have some psychomotor retardation.

SUBDURAL HYGROMA

An excessive collection of CSF in the subdural space is known as *subdural hygroma*. There are three common causes. The first and most common is cranial trauma with tearing of the arachnoid and escape of CSF into the subdural space. In these patients the CSF is

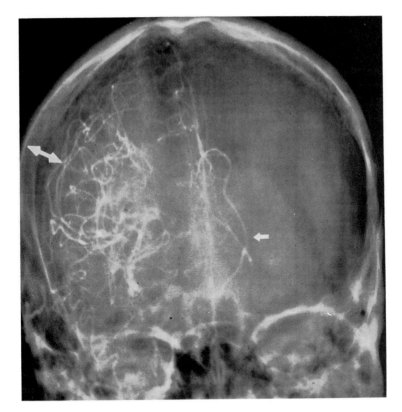

Fig. 54–9. Subdural hematoma. The pial vessels are separated from the inner table of the skull in this carotid angiogram *(double arrow).* The anterior cerebral artery *(single arrow)* is shifted from right to left. Compare with Figure 54–4.

usually admixed with blood due to coincident rupture of meningeal vessels. The second is a subdural effusion after infection of the meninges or skull, most commonly seen with influenzal meningitis or mastoiditis. The third cause of a subdural hygroma is the rupture of the arachnoid at the basal cistern in cases of communicating hydrocephalus.

The signs and symptoms of subdural hygroma after head injury are similar in character and in evolution to those of a subdural hematoma. The diagnosis, as with subdural hematoma, can be made by CT and, with certainty, only by trephine openings in the skull. Drainage of the CSF results in relief of the symptoms when there is a large collection of CSF and when there is no other associated pathologic condition. If satisfactory resorption does not occur shunting of the subdural space may be necessary.

TRAUMATIC INTRACEREBRAL HEMORRHAGE

The use of CT has transformed notions about the prevalence of intracerebral hemorrhage after head injury. Earlier, it had been estimated to occur in fewer than 1 to 2% of all patients, but CT shows intracerebral bleeding in 4 to 23%. The bleeding is attributed primarily to the effects of acceleration and deceleration. As described also for lacerations and contusions, hemorrhage is most common

in the frontal and temporal lobes. Occipital hemorrhages are rare. Unlike contusions, however, hemorrhage is almost always most prominent in white matter. The lesions are multiple in about 20% of patients, and linear skull fractures are found in 40 to 80%.

More than 50% of these patients are unconscious on impact. Some regain consciousness for a lucid interval, and about one-third

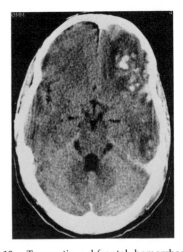

Fig. 54–10. Traumatic subfrontal hemorrhage. Axial noncontrast view demonstrates areas of contusion with small focal hemorrhages involving the lower poles of the left frontal and temporal lobes adjacent to the rough cranial vault. (Courtesy of Drs. S.K. Hilal, J.A. Bello, and T.L. Chi.)

have no loss of consciousness. The symptoms and signs of focal brain injury are similar to those of contusion or extradural collections. The diagnosis is made by CT (Fig. 54–10). The time from injury to clinical evidence of hemorrhage may be from minutes of injury to as long as 10 days later; 66% of operations are performed within 48 hours.

Delayed hemorrhage, which occurs in 1 to 7% of patients with severe head injuries, is diagnosed when the first CT scan shows no bleeding but a later one does. This phenomenon was known before the advent of CT but recognition of delayed hemorrhage now depends on CT, which is therefore mandatory for any patient with clinical evidence of deterioration.

Treatment is surgical evacuation of the hemorrhage through a craniotomy. The mortality rate has dropped from 72 to 25% but the outcome for comatose patients is still about 50%, and a satisfactory outcome is seen in about 25%.

CEREBRAL THROMBOSIS

Thrombosis of the contralateral posterior cerebral artery is a rare complication of distortion of the brain by an extradural or subdural hematoma. Injury to the wall of the carotid or other arteries may be followed by thrombosis of these vessels. Thrombosis of branches of the cerebral arteries occasionally develops several days or weeks after a head injury in elderly patients with cerebral arteriosclerosis. It is difficult to assess the role of the cerebral trauma in the production of these strokes.

CAROTID-CAVERNOUS FISTULAS

Trauma is a common cause of arteriovenous fistulas most commonly laceration of the internal carotid artery as it passes through the cavernous sinus by penetrating missiles or fracture of the sphenoid bone. No history of overt trauma, however, is noted in 20% or more of patients. The patient may be aware of a bruit that is synchronous with the pulse. Other symptoms are similar to those of cavernous sinus obstruction from other causes. Exophthalmos, distended orbital and periorbital veins, and paralysis of cranial nerves, most commonly the sixth, can all be traced to increased tension in the cavernous sinus caused by direct infusion of arterial blood (Fig. 54–11). The bruit and the exophthalmos may be reduced by manual occlusion of the carotid artery in the neck. CT is not usually

of diagnostic aid in these cases; the fistula must be demonstrated by arteriography (Fig. 54–12). If spontaneous regression does not occur ligation of the internal or common carotid artery may be necessary. If there is total diversion of the flow from the carotid artery into the fistula more extensive procedures may be necessary, with ligation of the internal carotid in the neck and the internal carotid and ophthalmic artery intracranially. There have been many attempts to occlude either the arteries or the veins by balloon techniques, and these seem to be more effective than direct surgical attack.

Sequelae of Head Injuries

INFECTIONS

Infections within the intracranial cavity following injury to the head may be extradural, subdural, subarachnoid (meningitis), or intracerebral (abscess).

Extradural Infections

These are usually accompanied by, and are secondary to, infection of the external wound or osteomyelitis of the skull and can be diagnosed by inspection of the wound and by CT. Treatment includes debridement of infected bone, evacuation of the abscess, and administration of antibiotics.

Subdural Abscess

This is one of the rarest suppurative lesions after head injury. It may be a complication of subdural hematoma. Symptoms are similar to those of subdural abscess from other causes and include localized headache, fever, neck stiffness, jacksonian seizures, and focal neurologic signs. The CSF is under increased pressure and shows an aseptic meningeal reaction (i.e., a pleocytosis and increased protein level with normal sugar concentration and negative culture). Treatment is similar to that for subdural abscess from other causes.

Meningitis

Meningitis may follow compound fractures, penetrating missiles, or linear fracture that extend into the nasal sinuses or the middle ear. Any of the pathogenic organisms may be the cause of the meningitis. The incidence of meningitis in civilian practice was estimated by Munro as less than 1% in patients with "closed head" injuries and approximately 6% in patients with compound fracture of the skull. The incidence of meningitis

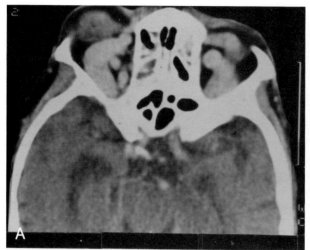

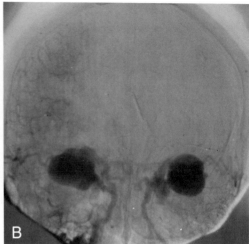

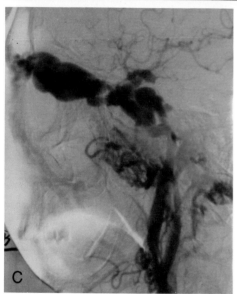

Fig. 54–11. Carotid cavernous fistula. *A.* Axial contrast-enhanced CT scan demonstrates prominent superior ophthalmic veins bilaterally. *B.* Anteroposterior and *C,* lateral subtraction, films from a right carotid arteriogram demonstrate bilateral carotid cavernous fistulae with drainage anterior into the superior ophthalmic veins. (Courtesy of Drs. T.L. Chi, J.A. Bello and S.K. Hilal.)

is affected by the degree of care in the treatment of the scalp and skull wound.

Meningitis commonly develops 2 to 8 days after injury but may be delayed for several or many months, particularly in patients with fractures through the mastoid or nasal sinuses. Recurrence of the meningitis with as many as seven or eight attacks has been reported. The presence of a CSF fistula with rhinorrhea or otorrhea favors the recurrence of meningitis. Treatment in such cases must include the closure of this fistula after the patient has recovered from the meningitis.

The treatment of post-traumatic meningitis follows the same principles as those outlined for the treatment of meningitis from other sources.

Brain Abscess

Intracerebral abscess may follow compound fractures of the skull and the entrance of penetrating missiles. This rare complication of head injury is usually related to infection of the scalp wound. The symptoms of the abscess commonly develop in the first few weeks after injury, but may be delayed. The symptoms, course, and treatment of cerebral abscess following head injury are the same as those of abscess from other causes, unless foreign material has accompanied the track infection and requires operative intervention.

CSF FISTULAS: RHINORRHEA AND OTORRHEA

CSF fistulas occur in about 3% of all patients with head injury, and in 5 to 10% of those with basal skull fractures. There is generally a fracture of the ethmoid or sphenoid bone or of the orbital plate of the frontal bone. The diagnosis is usually obvious because fluid drains from the nose within 48 hours of the injury. If there has been local bleeding the

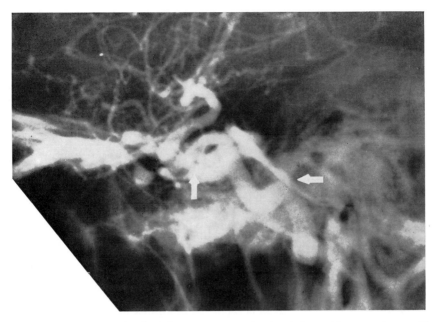

Fig. 54–12. Carotid cavernous sinus fistula. A large communication *(vertical arrow)* between the carotid artery *(above)* and the cavernous sinus can be seen in this carotid angiogram. In addition to the enlarged orbital veins that drain forward from the cavernous sinus, there is backward drainage through the petrosal sinus *(horizontal arrow)*.

presence of the CSF may be obscured, but nosebleeds usually stop in 1 or 2 days. If there is no admixture of blood CSF can be distinguished from nasal secretions because the CSF glucose concentration is 30 mg/dl or more, while lacrimal secretions and nasal mucus usually contain less than 5 mg/dl.

If there is a leak and the site of the fracture is not evident, CT-metrizamide studies have become the diagnostic method of choice. Most fistulas close spontaneously but operation should be considered if drainage persists for 2 weeks. Persistent rhinorrhea increases the risk of meningitis. Similar considerations guide the management of drainage of CSF from the ear after temporal bone fractures.

PNEUMOCELE

The presence of air in the cranial cavity is a rare complication of head injury. The air is usually in the frontal region in association with a fracture of one of the frontal sinuses, but cases have been reported with an occipital pneumocele following fracture through the mastoid. The air may not appear for several days after injury and then only after patients sneeze or blow their nose.

The pneumocele may be asymptomatic but headaches or mental symptoms may be present. Signs of increased intracranial pressure do not develop unless the pneumocele becomes infected or filled with CSF. The diagnosis of pneumocele is made by radiographs or CT. If spontaneous absorption of the air does not occur the opening in the frontal sinus should be covered with a strip of fascia lata through a transfrontal craniotomy to relieve whatever symptoms may be present and to prevent intracranial infection.

LEPTOMENINGEAL CYSTS

A rare complication of head injuries is the formation of a cyst in the space between the pia mater and the arachnoidal membrane. This complication may develop when there is a linear fracture of the skull with separation of the edges of the fracture and laceration of the dura; the arachnoid may be caught between the edges of the fracture. Pulsation of the brain forces CSF into the cyst and produces erosion of the skull. This complication is most commonly seen following fracture of the skull in infants and young children. Convulsive seizures, mental retardation, and increased intracranial pressure are the common signs and symptoms. The diagnosis is made from radiographic evidence of a circular or oval area of erosion of the skull in a patient who has had a previous fracture of the skull. Treatment consists of excision of the cyst and repair of the dural defect.

CRANIAL NERVE PALSIES

Injury to the cranial nerves is a frequent complication of fracture at the base of the skull. In addition, the cranial nerves, especially the olfactory, may be torn or bruised by the movement of the brain within the skull.

Cranial nerve palsies, when present, can usually be detected as soon as the patient's state of consciousness permits. Occasionally the paralysis may not be evident for several days. Facial paralysis, for example, may begin several days after head injury. Partial or complete recovery of function is the rule with traumatic injuries to the cranial nerves, with the excepton of the first or second nerves.

FOCAL CEREBRAL LESIONS

Focal brain lesions are much less common in the injuries of civilian life than in those of war. Hemiplegia and speech disturbance are the most common symptoms of focal brain damage in both civilian and war injuries. Symptoms of damage to the occipital lobe or cerebellum are found almost exclusively in war casualties.

Hemiplegia was found in 9% and disturbance of speech, aphasia, or dysphasia was found in 6% of those in one series. Complete or almost complete return of motor power and speech function is the rule when the injury is the result of compression of the brain by a hematoma, but a severe residual defect may be expected when there has been extensive laceration of the brain.

Injury to the hypothalamus of the pituitary gland is a rare complication of head injury. Transient or permanent diabetes insipidus has been reported in a few cases, probably as result of injury to the supraoptic-hypophyseal tract. Anosmia is usually also present in these cases as a result of injury to the olfactory bulb.

Acromegaly and other pituitary disorders have been reported as sequelae of head injury. Traumatic hemorrhage into the pituitary gland may be followed by the development of pituitary cachexia, but it is unlikely that acromegaly or other evidence of pituitary hyperfunction could result from trauma. Some cases of narcolepsy have been attributed to cerebral trauma but, because there is no known anatomic basis for narcolepsy, it is difficult to prove or disprove claims that it may be caused by a head injury.

Parkinsonism and other basal ganglia syndromes have been reported after a single episode of head trauma. In some of these cases the temporal relationship between the injury and the development of symptoms suggest that there may be a possible relationship between the symptoms and the trauma. In most cases, however, it is doubtful that the trauma played even a contributing role in the onset of the symptoms.

EPILEPSY

Convulsive seizures are an infrequent symptom of the acute phase of a head injury. They may occur immediately after or within the first few days of the injury. In these cases the seizures are related to the acute brain damage or to the presence of intracerebral hematomas or infection. In most patients, however, seizures do not develop until several months after the injury; 6 to 18 months is the most common interval. The seizures that follow head injury may be of any type except the classic absence seizure and, contrary to the usual impression, they are more often generalized than focal.

The exact incidence of seizures following head injury is unknown. Figures in the literature vary from 2.5 to 40%. The lower figure is probably correct if all types of head injury are included. As a rule, the more severe the injury, the greater the likelihood that seizures will develop. The incidence is as high as 50% when there has been penetration of the dura and laceration of the underlying cortex with formation of a cerebromeningeal scar. There is no evidence that the retention of a deeply situated foreign body predisposes to the development of seizures.

Little is known about the prophylaxis of seizures in patients with head injuries. A thorough debridement of a compound fracture, removal of all foreign material and necrotic cerebral tissue, and suturing of the dura should decrease the amount of scar formation and thus reduce the tendency toward seizures. Some evidence has been accumulated in regard to the prediction of later seizures. Persistence in the EEG of a focus of abnormal cortical activity beyond several months after injury suggests that seizures will develop. It has been recommended that all patients with severe head injuries receive anticonvulsant medication for 1 or 2 years after the injury, but the value of such treatment is unproven. Anticonvulsant medication may be given to patients with a persistent focus of abnormal electrical activity in the EEG.

The prognosis for remission of seizures is good if they occur in the first few days or weeks after injury. If seizures are a manifestation of acute brain injury, they rarely persist. There may be a remission of the seizures at any time.

The treatment of post-traumatic epilepsy is both medical and surgical. As a rule these patients do not respond as well to medical therapy as patients with so-called "idiopathic epilepsy," but surprisingly good results can be obtained in many cases. Medical treatment should be given a trial in all cases when indicated; surgery is reserved for the few who are not benefited by this form of therapy. Operative treatment should be carried out only in neurosurgical clinics in which there are adequate facilities for localizing the abnormal cortex that is presumably responsible for the seizures. This area may be removed with or without excision of the neighboring scar. Medical treatment should be given to patients for 2 to 3 years following the operation even if seizures seem to remit. The results of surgery are not always satisfactory, but about 50% of patients so treated are relieved of their attacks.

PSYCHOSIS AND MENTAL DISORDERS

Transient psychotic episodes and some permanent impairment of the mental faculties are not uncommon after injuries to the head, but long-continued psychotic episodes are rare.

Serious residual mental problems are found only after severe injury. Almost every patient with severe brain injury shows mental changes immediately after recovery of consciousness, and frequently the steps to complete recovery are semistupor, bewilderment, a Korsakoff-like phase, and euphoria. In patients who do not recover fully the clinical syndromes are usually classified as traumatic delirium, mental deterioration, and post-traumatic personality disorders. Focal neurologic signs and convulsive seizures are common in these patients. Less severe mental disturbances (e.g., impairment of memory or minor changes of personality) that do not make confinement in an institution necessary are frequent and can be expected in a high percentage of elderly patients. The relationship of head injury to the subsequent development of other types of psychoses is a medicolegal problem that has not been solved. It is reasonable to assume that a severe head injury may adversely influence pre-existing brain pathology and accentuate the symptoms and signs of other organic diseases, especially those leading to organic dementia. The problem is more complex in connection with schizophrenia and manic-depressive or other psychoses that do not have a definite structural pathology. It seems unlikely that head trauma could have any direct causal relationship to these conditions. An indirect relationship with chemical intermediaries may be postulated.

POST-TRAUMATIC SYNDROME

Approximately 35 to 40% of patients who sustain minor or severe injuries to the head complain of headache, dizziness, insomnia, irritability, restlessness, inability to concentrate, hyperhidrosis, depression, and other personality changes. This group of symptoms, which may be present for only a few weeks or may persist for years, has been described by the terms "postconcussional state" or "post-traumatic neurosis." Neither term is satisfactory because both imply that the symptoms are the direct result of injury to the brain or the psychologic reaction of the patient to the injury. Extensive physiologic and psychologic studies have not yielded any criteria that make it possible to define the role of either physiologic or psychologic factors. In some patients the symptoms appear to be related to the brain damage and in others they seem to be entirely psychologic in origin, but in most patients both factors play a contributing role.

There is no direct correlation between the severity of the injury and the development of post-traumatic symptoms. The symptoms may develop in patients who were only dazed by the injury, but they do occur in a higher percentage of patients who were rendered unconscious; the incidence of post-traumatic symptoms, however, is not related to the duration of retrograde amnesia, coma, or the post-traumatic amnesia. The symptoms that are commonly present in adults after head injury are rare in children, although behavioral disorders and personality changes may follow head injury in the young. MRI in patients with the post-traumatic syndrome suggest that there is an element of metabolic brain disturbance in some of these patients.

Post-traumatic symptoms may develop in patients who had previously shown a normal adjustment of life, but are more likely to occur in patients who had neurotic symptoms before the injury. Factors such as hazardous occupations, domestic or financial difficulties, and the desire to obtain compensation, financial or otherwise, tend to produce and may prolong the symptoms once they have developed.

Symptoms. Headaches usually begin with the return of consciousness but occasionally may not appear until the patient is ambulatory. At first the headache is severe and more or less constant. With time it decreases in severity and there are periods of relative freedom. As a rule, the periods in which the patient is free of headache become longer and, after 1 or 2 weeks, the headaches are paroxysmal. The headache is usually described as a dull aching, throbbing, or pressure sensation. Sometimes the headache is described as quite severe, "a bursting feeling." Occasionally the headache develops without apparent reason, waking the patient out of a sound sleep. More frequently it occurs with excitement or when the patient tries to concentrate. Headaches recur daily for years but, most often, the severity and frequency diminish. The headaches usually disappear entirely within 6 to 12 months.

Dizziness is a fairly constant symptom of the post-traumatic syndrome. As with the headaches, it usually appears soon after return of consciousness. Many patients report that the least movement in bed produces severe vertiginous attacks. In other instances, the dizziness first appears when patients begin to get on their feet. The dizziness, like headaches, after a time becomes paroxysmal and is produced by quick movements, turning about, or attempting to rise from a recumbent position; not infrequently, the attacks of dizziness are associated with headache. Some patients find that putting the head in certain positions precipitates vertigo. The dizziness is seldom associated with any nystagmus. Nausea and even vomiting occasionally accompany a dizzy attack, but this effect is usually short-lived. Labyrinthine tests generally throw little light on the mechanism, although sometimes these tests indicate disturbance of the vestibular connections and may indicate a previously undisclosed fracture at the base of the skull.

Insomnia is bothersome and real. When patients can sleep, they complain that it is a restless sleep in which they feel half awake and that it is broken by periods of wakefulness and interspersed with terrifying dreams, frequently in relation to the events of the accident. Disturbance of sleep usually continues as long as the other symptoms are relatively severe.

Irritability, restlessness, lack of ability to concentrate, change of personality, and depression all fall into one group of symptoms. Patients state that they cannot tolerate noises, are bothered by children, cannot enjoy themselves, find even the television unpleasant, have little control of their temper or emotions and, in general, are a burden to themselves and a great trial to their family. The reality of these changes is borne out by the accounts of family and friends, and frequently is obvious to the examiner.

Hyperhidrosis, although not as frequent as the other symptoms, may be present to such an extent that it leaves no doubt in the observer's mind that there is a marked vasomotor instability.

Prognosis. The prognosis in cases of so-called post-traumatic syndrome is uncertain. In general, progressive improvement may be expected. The duration of symptoms is not directly related to the severity of the injury. In some patients with only a mild injury symptoms continue for a long period, whereas patients with severe injuries may have only mild or transient symptoms. By and large, however, it is a matter of 2 to 6 months before the headache and dizziness as well as the more definite mental changes show much improvement. Slight residuals are to be expected and in those patients who develop convulsive seizures, it is often 6 to 18 months before the first attacks occur, so that there is no definite assurance that things are going to go entirely well until at least 1 or 2 years have transpired. Definitely functional or psychoneurotic symptoms are often added to the picture and the prognosis must then be modified by taking into account the life style of the patient.

Treatment. The general medical, surgical, and psychologic treatment of the patient immediately after injury is of great importance in preventing post-traumatic syndrome. To many patients the idea of an injury to the head is bound up with the fear of all sorts of disasters, including the idea that brain injury causes insanity or brain tumor. Not infrequently, the physician and lawyer may aggravate the anxiety by making too much of the injury, telling patients how near to death they may have been, being unduly concerned about later symptoms, keeping patients from reasonable activity, or intensifying other worries. As the weeks and months pass with continuance of symptoms, the patients' worst fears seem to be materializing. If, in addition, patients become economically handicapped and in dire financial straits, another cause for the development and continuance of symptoms is present. Legal activity induces a real complication in almost every case and prolongs the period of disability.

With the exception of surgery for the rare case of chronic subdural hematoma coupled with a post-traumatic syndrome, physiotherapy and re-education of neurologic defects, and the administration of anticonvulsive drugs, treatment is largely comprised of psychotherapy. Reassurance is important at all times. An adept examination and evaluation, followed by talks with the patient, in which the whole matter is explained in detail, are the first essentials. Constant attention must be given to relieve fears of serious outcome, always remembering that patients reflect the attitudes and anxieties of their physicians. It is wise to keep a patient quiet for a few days after any moderately severe head injury, but it is important to resume normal activity promptly.

Sedatives, tranquilizers, and analgesic drugs in moderation are helpful. Sedation and antihistamines for dizziness and analgesics for headache usually are helpful. Relief of financial difficulties and settlement of insurance or liability claims are also important. Most patients have insurance, industrial accident, or liability claims; when difficulty arises about the settlement of such claims, functional and even organic symptoms are prolonged.

THE NEUROLOGY OF PROFESSIONAL BOXING

The term *punch drunk* is ascribed to a 1928 paper by Martland, and another term is *dementia pugilistica*. The current nonpejorative term is *chronic traumatic encephalopathy*. Whatever the name, there seems to be little doubt that professional boxers are especially at risk for a syndrome that is dominated by parkinsonism and other extrapyramidal features— tremor, ataxia, cerebellar signs, and, in some cases, dementia. Behavioral abnormalities may include morbid jealousy and rage reactions. Pathologic studies have shown hypothalamic anomalies, degeneration of substantia nigra, widespread neurofibrillary changes, and scarring of cerebellar folia.

Although the syndrome is well known, few prospective studies have been done to determine precise risk factors, whether signs can be seen early enough to prevent the severe late syndrome, whether the syndrome could be prevented by offering protective guidelines for boxing matches (e.g., neurologic examination, including CT and MRI, better head protection, different gloves), and whether it is a progressive disorder after the boxer has ceased to fight. According to the early study of Critchley, manifestations begin from 6 to 40 years after starting a boxing career, with an average of 16 years.

Other sports involve the risk of serious injury, but only boxing includes the goal of deliberately injuring the brain of an opponent. The knockout is the prized achievement. Many neurologists have therefore urged the abolition of boxing, but this has not yet been achieved, and it may never be; many powerful social forces promote the sport in the United States and elsewhere. If boxing is not to be banned, physicians and other health care workers must take every opportunity to regulate the profession. Physicians must stop matches when there is evidence of brain injury. Better protection for boxers must be available during training as well as in the ring. Appropriate prospective epidemiologic studies are needed. Once the symptoms of chronic traumatic encephalopathy have become evident, no therapy is actually effective.

References

Craniocerebral Trauma

Clifton GL, McCormick WF, Grossman RG. Neuropathology of early and late deaths after head injury. Neurosurgery 1981; 8:309–314.

Cooper PR. Head Injury, 2nd Ed. Baltimore: Williams & Wilkins, 1987.

Frankowski RF, Annegers JF, Whitman S: Epidemiological and descriptive studies. Part 1. The descriptive epidemiology of head trauma in the United States. In: Becker DP, Povlishock JT, eds. Central Nervous System Trauma Status Report—1985. Bethesda: National Institutes of Health, NINCDS, 1985:33–43.

Grossman R, Gildenberg PL. Head Injury: Basic and Clinical Aspects. New York: Raven Press, 1982.

Hans JH, Kaufman B, Alfidi RJ, et al. Head injury evaluated by MRI and CT; a comparison. Radiology 1984; 150:71–77.

Hardman JM. The pathology of traumatic brain injuries. Adv Neurol 1979; 22:15–50.

Jane JA, Stewart D, Genarelli TA. Axonal degeneration induced by experimental non-invasive minor head injury. J Neurosurg 1985; 62:96–100.

Jennett B, Teasdale G. Management of Head Injuries. Philadelphia: FA Davis, 1981.

Jennett B, Teasdale G, Braakman R, Minderhoud J, Heiden J, Kurze T. Prognosis of patients with severe head injury. Neurosurgery 1979; 4:283–289.

Kraus JF. Epidemiology of head injury. In: Cooper PR. Head Injury, 2nd ed. Baltimore: Williams & Wilkins, 1987:1–19.

Lobato RD, Sarabia R, Cordobes F, Rivas JJ, Adrados A, Cabrera A, Gomez P, Madera A, Lamas E. Posttraumatic cerebral hemispheric swelling: analysis of 55 cases studied with computerized tomography. J Neurosurg 1988; 68:417–423.

Masters SJ, et al. Skull X-ray examinations after head trauma. N Engl J Med 1987; 316:84–91.

Merritt HH. Head injury. War Med 1943; 4:61–82.

Roberson FS, Kishore PRS, Miller JD, et al. The value of serial CT in the management of severe head injury. Surg Neurol 1979; 12:161–167.

Rosenblum WI, Greenberg RP, Seelig JM, Becker DP. Mid-brain lesions: frequent and significant prognostic features in closed head injury. Neurosurgery 1981; 9:613–620.

Russell WR. The traumatic amnesias. London: Oxford University Press, 1971.

Shalen PR, Handel SF. Diagnostic challenges in closed head trauma. Radiol Clin North Am 1981; 19:53–68.

Symonds C. Concussion and its sequelae. Lancet 1962; 1:1–5.

Teasdale G, Jennett B. Assessment of coma and impaired consciousness. A practical scale. Lancet 1974; 2:81–83.

Walker AE, Caveness WF, Critchley M. The Late Effects of Head Injury. Springfield, IL: Charles C Thomas, 1969.

Complications of Head Injuries

Extradural Hemorrhage

Bricolo AP, Pasut LM. Extradural hematoma; toward zero mortality. Neurosurgery 1984; 14:8–12.

Bullock R, Smith RM, van Dellen JR. Nonoperative management of extradural hematoma. Neurosurgery 1985; 16:602–606.

Cordobés F, Lobato RD, Rivas JJ, et al. Observations on 82 patients with extradural hematoma. Comparison of results before and after the advent of computerized tomography. J Neurosurg 1981; 54:179–186.

Dhellemmes P, Lejeune JP, Christiaens JL, Cambelles F. Traumatic extradural hematomas in infancy and childhood. J Neurosurg 1985; 62:861–865.

Garza-Mercado R. Extradural hematoma of the posterior cranial fossa; report of seven cases with survival. J Neurosurg 1983; 59:664–672.

Ingraham FD, Campbell JB, Cohen J. Extradural hematoma in infancy and childhood. JAMA 1949; 140:1010–1013.

Kushner MJ, Luken MG. Posterior fossa epidural hematoma; 3 cases with CT. Neuroradiology 1983; 24:169–172.

Ratcliffe PJ, Bell JI, Collins KJ, Frackowiak RS, Rudge P. Late onset post-traumatic hypothalamic hypothermia. J Neurol Neurosurg Psychiatry 1983; 46:72–77.

Subdural Hemorrhage

Allen AM, Moore M, Daly BB. Subdural hemorrhage in patients with mental diseases. N Engl J Med 1940; 223:324–329.

Bender MB. Recovery from subdural hematoma without surgery. Mt Sinai J Med 1960; 26:52–58.

Bruce DA, Alavi A, Bilaniuk L, et al. Diffuse cerebral swelling following head injuries in children. J Neurosurg 1981; 54:170–178.

Jacobson PL, Farmer TW. The hypernormal CT scan in dementia: Bilateral isodense subdural hematomas. Neurology 1979; 29:1522–1524.

Klun B, Fettich M. Factors influencing the outcome in acute subdural hematoma: 330 cases. Acta Neurochir 1984; 71:171–178.

Munro D, Merritt HH. Surgical pathology of subdural hematoma. Arch Neurol Psychiatry 1936; 35:64–78.

Shapiro K, ed. Pediatric Head Trauma. Mount Kisco, NY: Futura Publishing, 1983.

St. John JN, Dila C. Traumatic subdural hygroma in adults. Neurosurgery 1981; 9:621–626.

Traumatic Intracerebral Hemorrhage

Cordobés F, Fuente M, Lobato RD, et al. Intraventricular hemorrhage in severe head injury. J Neurosurg 1983; 58:217–221.

Jennett B, Teasdale G, Fry J, Brackman R, Minderhoud J, Heiden J, Kurze T. Treatment for severe head injury. J Neurol Neurosurg Psychiatry 1980; 43:289–295.

Lipper MH, Kishore PR, Girevendolis AK, Miller JD, Becker DP. Delayed intracranial hematoma in patients with severe head injury. Radiology 1979; 133:645–649.

Arteriovenous Fistulas

Chung JW, et al. Computed tomography of cavernous sinus diseases. Neuroradiology 1988; 30:319–328.

Davis JM, Zimmerman RA. Injury to the carotid and vertebral arteries. Neuroradiology 1983; 25:55–70.

Dott NM. Carotid-cavernous arteriovenous fistula. Clin Neurosurg 1969; 16:17–21.

Sequelae of Head Injuries

Annegers JF, Grabow JD, Groover RV, Laws ER Jr, Elveback LR, Kurland LT. Seizures after head trauma: a population study. Neurology 1980; 30:683–689.

Baron JB. Postural aspects of the post-concussional syndrome. Clin Otolaryngol 1980; 11:155–166.

Bongartz EB, Nau HE, Liesegang J. The cerebrospinal fluid fistula. Rhinorrhoea, otorrhoea and orbitorrhoea. Neurosurg Rev 1981; 4:195–200.

Brenner C, Friedman AP, Merritt HH, Denny-Brown DE. Post-traumatic headache. J Neurosurg 1944; 1:379–392.

Brooke OG. Delayed effects of head injuries in children. BMJ 1988; 296:948.

Dacey RG Jr, Alves WM, Rimel RW, Winn HR, Jane JA. Neurosurgical complications after apparently minor head injury. J Neurosurg 1987; 65:203–210.

Dikman S, Reitan RM, Temkin NR. Neuropsychological recovery in head injury. Arch Neurol 1983; 40:333–338.

Friedman AP, Merritt HH. Damage to cranial nerves resulting from head injury. Bull Los Angeles Neurol Soc 1944; 9:135–139.

Guthkelch AN. Post-traumatic amnesia, post-concussional symptoms and accident neurosis. Eur Neurol 1980; 19:91–102.

Jennett B. Post-traumatic epilepsy. Adv Neurol 1979; 29:137–147.

Jennett B. Epilepsy after Blunt Head Injuries, 2nd ed. London: William Heinemann, 1975.

Keshavan MS, Channabasavanna SM, Reddy GN. Post-traumatic psychiatric disturbances: Patterns and predictors of outcome. Br J Psychiatry 1981; 138:157–160.

Kishore PR, Liper MH, Domingues Da Silva AA, et al. Delayed sequelae of head injury. CT 1980; 4:287–295.

Kosteljanetz M, Jensen TS, Norgard B, Lunde I, Jensen PB, Johnsen SG. Sexual and hypothalamic dysfunction in the post-concussional syndrome. Acta Neurol Scand 1981; 63:169–180.

Lantz EJ, Forbes GS, Brown ML, Laws ER Jr. Radiology of cerebrospinal fluid rhinorrhea. AJR 1980; 135:1023–1030.

Laun A. Traumatic cerebrospinal fluid fistulas in the anterior and middle cranial fossae. Acta Neurochir 1982; 60:215–222.

Levin HS, Amparo E, Eisenberg HM, et al. MRI and CT in relation to the neurobehavioral sequelae of mild and moderate head injuries. J Neurosurg 1987; 66:706–713.

Levin HS, High WM, Goethe KE, et al. The neurobehavioral rating scale; assessment of behavioral sequelae of head injury by the clinician. J Neurol Neurosurg Psychiatry 1987; 50:183–193.

Manelfe C, Cellerier P, Sobel D, Prevost C, Bonafe A. Cerebrospinal fluid rhinorrhea: Evaluation with metrizamide cisternography. AJR 1982; 138:471–476.

Meirowsky AM, Caveness WF, Dillon JD, Rish BL. Mohr JP, Kistler JP, Weiss GH. Cerebrospinal fluid fistulas complicating missile wounds of the brain. J Neurosurg 1981; 54:44–48.

McKinlay WW, Brooks DN, Bond MR, Martinage DP, Marshall MM. The short-term outcome of severe blunt head injury as reported by relatives of the injured persons. J Neurol Neurosurg Psychiatry 1981; 44:527–533.

McMillan TM, Glucksman EE. The neuropsychology of moderate head injury. J Neurol Neurosurg Psychiatry 1987; 50:393–397.

Morgan MK, Besser M, Johnston I, Chaseling R. Intracranial carotid artery injury in closed head trauma. J Neurosurg 1987; 66:192–197.

Ratcliffe PJ, Bell JI, Collins KJ, Frackowiak RS, Rudge P. Late-onset post-traumatic hypothalamic hypothermia. J Neurol Neurosurg Psychiatry 1983; 46:72–77.

Savino PJ, Glaser JS, Schatz NJ. Traumatic chiasmal syndrome. Neurology 1980; 30:683–689.

Schoenhuber R, Gentilini M. Anxiety and depression after mild head injury: case control study. J Neurol Neurosurg Psychiatry 1988; 51:722–724.

Walker AE, Caveness WF, Critchley M, eds. The Late Effect of Head Injury. Springfield, IL: Charles C Thomas, 1969.

Weiss GH, Feeney DM, Caveness WF, et al. Prognostic factors for the occurrence of post-traumatic epilepsy. Arch Neurol 1983; 40:7–10.

Young B, Rapp RP, Norton JA, Haack D, Tibbs PA, Bean JR. Failure of prophylactically administered phenytoin to prevent post-traumatic seizures. J Neurosurg 1983; 58:231–241.

Zomeren AHV, Van Den Burg W. Residual complaints of patients two years after severe head injury. J Neurol Neurosurg Psychiatry 1985; 48:21–28.

Neurology of Boxing

Council Report. Brain injury in boxing. JAMA 1983; 249:254–257.

Critchley M: Medical aspects of boxing, particularly from a neurological standpoint. Br Med J 1957; 1:351–357.

Jordan BD. Neurologic aspects of boxing. Arch Neurol 1987; 44:453–459.

Martland HS. Punch drunk. JAMA 1928; 91:1103–1107.

Richards NG. Ban boxing. Neurology 1984; 34:1485–1486.

Ross RJ, Cole M, Thompson JS, Kim KH. Boxers—computed tomography, EEG, and neurological examination. JAMA 1983; 249:211–213.

55. SPINAL INJURY

Joseph T. Marotta

Trauma to the vertebral column may irreversibly damage the spinal cord and accompanying nerve roots. Spinal cord injury is acute and unexpected, dramatically changing the course of an individual's life. The social and economic consequences to patient, family, and society may be catastrophic.

The annual incidence of spinal cord injury is estimated at 30 to 40/1,000,000, with about 6,600 new cases per year. The prevalence is estimated at 906/1,000,000 with approximately 200,000 patients now in the United States.

Etiology. Of those suffering acute spinal cord trauma, 65% are younger than the age of 35. The greatest incidence occurs among people between the ages of 20 to 24. After age 35, there is a slightly increased incidence of spinal cord injury in those between the ages of 55 and 59. The male:female ratio is at least 3:1. The incidence of injury is highest during the summer months and on weekends.

Road accidents are the most common cause of traumatic tetraplegia and paraplegia. Patients in this group, which encompasses single and multiple motor vehicle accidents, motorcycle accidents, and injuries to pedestrians, accounts for 30 to 50% of all new cases of spinal cord injury. Other causes include industrial accidents, diving into shallow water, injuries sustained during participation in sports (e.g., hockey, football, water sports, such as water-skiing and surfing, tobogganing), stabbing, high-velocity missiles, gunshot wounds, and nonindustrial falls. Birth injuries, particularly in breech deliveries, may result in a stretched or compressed spinal cord, the result of traction and hyperextension of the cervical spine.

Mechanism of Injury. Indirect severe force applied to the vertebral column is the most frequent mechanism of spinal cord injury. Such a force, generated during sudden flexion, hyperextension, vertebral compression, or rotation of the vertebral column, may result in dislocation of facet joints, fracture of vertebral bodies, misalignment of the vertebral canal, herniation of disk material, and bone splintering. The spinal cord may consequently be contused, stretched, lacerated, or crushed. When there is associated cervical spondylosis or spinal stenosis a trivial injury may cause significant neurologic injury, even without fracture or dislocation.

Direct injury to the spinal cord may result from stabbing with a sharp object, such as a knife, if the object is directed away from the midline and at an angle. Under such circumstances the protection afforded by the laminae is bypassed. Indirect injury to the cord from comminuted bone, as well as direct injury from impact, may occur when bullets or high-velocity missiles are responsible for the injury.

Appreciation of the mechanism of injury provides insight into the potential stability or instability of spinal injuries. Sudden violent flexion, particularly in the cervical region, may cause anterior compression fractures of vertebral bodies and unilateral or bilateral facet joint dislocation, with locking and rupture of longitudinal and interspinous ligaments. Severe compression injuries, usually in the thoracolumbar area, may burst a vertebral body; bone splinters and disk material may then be pushed into the spinal canal. Rotational injuries may result in unilateral fracture dislocation with variable trauma to the cord. Hyperextension injuries, caused by a fall forward, result in fracture of the posterior elements of the vertebral bodies. Any combination of forces may occur in any single case. It is therefore important to recognize the mechanism of injury for assessing not only the nature and extent of underlying spinal cord injury but also the stability of the spinal column at the site of the injury.

Pathology. The type of spinal column injury determines the nature and extent of underlying cord damage. There may be extensive contusion and compression of the cord, with partial or complete laceration and gross spinal cord injury or, as with stab wounds, a discrete hemisection of the cord.

In the early stages after acute injury gross examination reveals a cord that is swollen, reddish, soft, and mushy. The subarachnoid and subdural spaces are obliterated. Subarachnoid hemorrhage is rare and any extradural hemorrhages are small. Cross-sectional investigation of the swollen cord most frequently reveals centrally placed hemorrhages and softening. Microscopic investigation reveals fragmented myelin sheaths, splayed myelin lamellae, broken axons, and eosinophilic neurons. In this acute phase the exudate consists of red cells, polymorphs, lymphocytes, and plasma cells. These changes extend several segments above and below the level of injury. The edema subsides within several weeks, hemorrhages are absorbed, and the acute exudate is replaced by macrophages, with the most prominent cell being the lipid phagocyte. This reparative stage may persist for up to 2 years, resulting in cavitation (often syrinx-like), gliosis, and fibrosis. In the later phase, 5 or more years after injury, the area becomes shrunken and the cord is replaced by fibrous tissue. Progressive prolif-eration of acellular connective tissue results in dense and chronic adhesive arachnoiditis.

In traumatic hematomyelia, hemorrhage occurs within the central gray matter. It is limited in extent and is eventually absorbed, leaving a centrally placed, smooth-walled cyst. It differs from the much more common hemorrhagic softening seen in contusion.

On rare occasions, after several years of neurologic stability, residual intramedullary cysts may become distended, leading to a progessive neurologic disorder. There is no explanation for the delayed myelopathy, sometimes classified as *traumatic syringomyelia*. The neurologic progression is invariably rostral to the original injury. Traumatic syringomyelia occurs most frequently in the cervical region.

Experimental impact injury to the cord in dogs has demonstrated the dynamic and progressive changes that occur after acute trauma, as follows: 30 minutes after injury, small hemorrhages in the central gray matter develop, the result of damage to and subsequent rupture of small vessels, usually venules. Within 2 hours the small hemorrhages may enlarge to produce hematomyelia and neuronal changes (loss of Nissl substance). At 4 hours there is visible necrosis of the central gray matter and contiguous white matter. At 24 hours, infarction of cord tissue is histologically identifiable. The central cord region is particularly susceptible to injury. The pathophysiology of cord injury has not been proven. Other factors, including a breakdown in the blood-cord barrier, axonal membrane injury, ischemia, and increased catecholamine levels locally, have all been suggested as mechanisms but remain unproven.

Once initiated, these acute changes are progressive and time-dependent. Various types of therapy have been directed toward reversing this autodestructive process.

Signs and Symptoms. Signs and symptoms are related to the level, type, and severity of injury. The following indicates the clinical patterns seen in spinal injury:

Cauda equina lesions
Conus medullaris lesions
Mixed cauda-conus lesions
Spinal cord injuries:
    Cord concussion
    Spinal shock
    Complete cord transection
    Incomplete cord transection:
        Brown-Sequard syndrome
        Central cervical cord syndrome

Anterior cord syndrome
Posterior cord syndrome

Damage to the roots of the cauda equina causes flaccid, areflexic paralysis and sensory loss in the area supplied by the affected roots, with paralysis of bladder and rectum. The findings may be symmetric or asymmetric. If only the conus is damaged there is urinary fecal incontinence, failure of erection and ejaculation in men, paralysis of the pelvic floor muscles, and sensory impairment, which is frequently dissociated, in the saddle region. In a pure conus lesion tendon reflexes are frequently preserved, but occasionally the ankle jerks are lost. A mixture of anatomically appropriate clinical signs is seen because conus and cauda injuries commonly occur together.

Spinal cord concussion is used to describe transient neurologic symptoms, with recovery in minutes or hours. Symptoms develop below the level of the blow. *Spinal shock* occurs after an abrupt, complete, or incomplete lesion of the spinal cord. There is immediate complete paralysis and anesthesia below the lesion, with hypotonia and areflexia. The plantar responses may be absent, extensor, or equivocal. The areflexic hypotonic state is gradually replaced by pyramidal signs, usually within 3 or 4 weeks. The evolution from an areflexic to hyperreflexic state may be delayed by urinary tract infection, infected bed sores, anemia, or malnutrition.

Chronic and complete transection of the cord, after the period of spinal shock, results in permanent motor, sensory, and autonomic paralysis below the level of the lesion. Chronic and incomplete transverse section results in different clinical pictures, depending on the pathways involved. In the *Brown-Sequard syndrome,* after hemisection of the spinal cord, the following signs are found, usually with the upper level one or two segments below that of the lesion: ipsilateral paresis, ipsilateral corticospinal signs, contrateral loss of pain and temperature sensation, and ipsilateral impairment of vibration and joint position sense. There is usually little loss of tactile sensation. There may be ipsilateral segmental loss of sensation or weakness appropriate to the level of the lesion.

The *central cervical cord syndrome* is characterized by weakness, which is more marked in the arms than the legs, urinary retention, and patchy sensory loss below the level of the lesion. The arms or hands may be paralyzed or moderately weak. In the legs there may be severe paresis or only minimal weakness, with overactive tendon reflexes and Babinski signs. Micturition may be normal. Complete cord transection may be diagnosed at first because there seems to be no cord function below the level of the lesion; careful testing, however, may reveal sacral sparing and therefore an incomplete lesion. If so, the potential for recovery without operative intervention is better and depends on the degree of central hemorrhage.

In the *anterior cervical cord syndrome,* immediate complete paralysis is associated with mild to moderate impairment of pinprick response and light touch below the injury, with preservation of position and vibration sense. This syndrome may be caused by an acutely ruptured disc, with or without fracture or fracture dislocation in the cervical region. The *posterior cord syndrome* (contusio cervicalis posterior) is characterized by pain and paresthesias in the neck, upper arms, and trunk. The paresthesias are usually symmetric and have a burning quality. The sensory manifestations may be combined with mild paresis of the arms and hands, but the long tracts are only slightly affected. The symptoms of both the anterior and posterior cord syndromes are reversible.

Clear demarcation of incomplete spinal cord syndromes may be clinically impossible. The clinical findings must be carefully recorded at the time of injury and repeatedly thereafter to provide the information necessary for proper treatment, management, and prognosis. Most patients with cervical and thoracolumbar injuries suffer complete spinal cord lesions, but lumbar spine injuries produce incomplete lesions.

Diagnosis. In addition to clinical observations, it is essential to obtain accurate and complete radiographs of the spinal column at the time of injury. In the cervical region a single lateral view is most significant but has two limitations that must be appreciated. An odontoid fracture may go unrecognized, and the lower cervical segment may not be adequately visualized. If these lesions are suspected clinically, an open-mouthed view of the odontoid and a "swimmer's" view of the lower cervical spine most be obtained to visualize the cervicothoracic junction.

Tetraplegia and paraplegia may be present clinically, with no radiographic evidence of fracture or fracture dislocation. This is especially true in children with flexible spinal columns, in adults with marked cervical spondylosis and spinal stenosis, or in those in whom dislocation may have been spontaneously corrected. Conversely, fracture dislocations or fracture may be seen with no clinical findings.

In the presence of unquestioned neurologic signs, plain films (anteroposterior and lateral) will be positive for fracture or dislocation in 90% of adults. Special views (obliques and tomography) increase the risk of further spinal cord damage, particularly in the presence of unstable fractures, and are seldom necessary. The use of CT has improved the radiologic assessment of spinal fractures, particularly in determining the degree of compression of the spinal cord. CT combined with myelography using metrizamide is indicated if neurologic signs deteriorate, if there is a neurologic disorder in the absence of radiologic abnormality, if penetrating injuries are present, or if an operable lesion (e.g., intradural compression) is suspected when other data are inconclusive. Traction must be maintained during myelography to minimize any further cord damage during the procedure. In the future MRI may replace the use of CT and CT-myelography for evaluation of spinal cord trauma. Because of risk of further damage to an injured spinal cord, spinal angiography is not advised.

Somatosensory evoked potentials (SEPs) are helpful in distinguishing complete or incomplete lesions. The test is brief, noninvasive, and repeatable. Absence of a normal evoked potential, using an averaging technique, suggests complete spinal cord injury. In cases of incomplete injury, changes in the configuration of the SEP precede clinical improvement. SEPs are considered to be helpful and reliable in determining the extent of spinal cord injury. Some feel that SEPs are more sensitive than clinical examination in detecting residual function in sensory pathways. Further investigation is required before SEPs can be used as a reliable and precise prognostic indicator. Shortly after acute spinal injury it was noted that the presence of an identifiable SEP suggests a better prognosis, but this has not yet been proven conclusively.

Course and Prognosis. It is estimated that 40% of all patients with spinal cord injury die within 24 hours of the accident. Long-term survival depends on the level and extent of the lesion, the age of the patients, and the availability of special treatment units, in which multidisciplinary personnel are available.

A long-term follow-up of survival in a large number (1501) of patients with spinal cord injury was presented by a Toronto group in a series of reports (1961, 1968, 1977, 1983). The follow-up extended from January 1, 1945 to December 31, 1980 and revealed the following: (1) spinal cord-injured patients had a higher mortality rate than those in the general population; (2) the mortality rate was highest for those with complete lesions particularly tetraplegia; (3) the mortality rate was significantly reduced over the length of the follow-up especially in complete lesions; (4) the mortality rate of incomplete lesions was closer to that of the general population; (5) there was a marked decrease in the number of deaths caused by renal disease in those with spinal cord injury; and (6) deaths from suicide remained high.

Therefore, the quality of life and long-term survival have been impressively enhanced. Improvements and advances have occurred in the prevention of renal failure caused by renal infection and amyloidosis, in the use of mechanical ventilation for high tetraplegics (phrenic nerve pacemakers), in the organization and development of specialized spinal cord injury centers, in the surgical treatment of pressure sores to prevent chronic osteomyelitis, and in social and psychologic rehabilitation. Although much progress has been made, however, much remains to be done. Independence in terms of eating, drinking, dressing and grooming, bladder and bowel control, transfer to and from a wheelchair, and ability to use a wheelchair are the goals of rehabilitation. In those with complete lesions, motor and sensory functions do not return, but in a few weeks the initial level may settle at one or two segments lower than was originally suspected. In those with high cervical cord lesions this change is significant.

Evolution of symptoms and signs in complete lesions depends on restoration of function in the isolated segment of the cord. Immediately after injury spinal shock with no neurologic function is noted. After recovery from spinal shock tendon reflexes return and frequently become brisk, with *reflex spasms* of the paralyzed limbs. These spasms, flexor or extensor, involve many or all of the paralyzed muscles. They may be evoked by different stimuli and may be painful. They are thought to result from the heightened sensitivity of the isolated segment of the cord that has been released from inhibitory control of higher centers. The classic reflex spasm is a withdrawal reflex or mass reflex, induced by the application of any noxious stimulus to the foot or lower leg; the touch of the bedclothes or even a slight draft is sometimes sufficient. There is dorsiflexion of the great toe and ankle and flexion of the knee and thigh toward the abdomen.

The prognosis of three specific functions in severe spinal cord injuries deserves comment. Bladder function is always markedly impaired and is manifested by complete retention, dribbling and incontinence, or periodic micturition. Bladder function can improve and, with training, automatic control is developed, except in cases in which there has been injury to the sacral outflow.

Bowel function is also disturbed. Two or three days after injury, there is often a transient ileus of the small bowel with abdominal distension that may compromise ventilation. In a few days small bowel function returns to normal, but large bowel and rectal function may be lost permanently.

Sexual function is impaired. In men, priapism is seen early, especially after high cord lesions. In the long term this is followed by reflex but no psychogenic erections or seminal emissions. In women, paraplegia and tetraplegia result in interruption of the menstrual cycle for months, but this returns with time. Conception and pregnancy are possible.

Treatment. Treatment of the spinal cord-injured patient encompasses five phases: (1) emergency treatment with attention to circulation, breathing, patent airway, appropriate immobilization of the spine, and transfer to a specialized center; (2) treatment of general medical problems (e.g., hypotension, poikilothermy, ileus); (3) spinal alignment; (4) surgical decompression of the spinal cord, if indicated; and (5) a well-structured rehabilitation program.

Of primary importance is the treatment of airway obstruction, hemorrhage, and shock. An adequate airway can be ensured by nasotracheal intubation, which should be done with particular care in those with suspected cervical spinal injuries.

Because cord injury may result in loss of sympathetic tone with peripheral vasodilatation, bradycardia, and hypotension, secondary ischemic damage may aggravate the spinal cord injury resulting from mechanical causes. Treatment of this potential hazard includes the judicious administration of intra-venous fluids to prevent fluid overload, alpha-agonists and, occasionally, intravenous atropine to counter unopposed parasympathetic activity. Vasomotor paralysis may also cause loss of thermal control, and lead to poikilothermy, which can usually be treated by the appropriate use of blankets.

Extrication of the patient from an automobile must be attempted only after the patient's head and back have been strapped in a neutral position on a firm base. There must be similar concern for head and neck stability in diving accidents. Rapid evacuation to a hospital is essential. It is estimated that 10% of patients suffer progressive cord or root damage between the time of diagnosis at the site of injury and the beginning of appropriate treatment by trained personnel in the hospital.

In the acute phase, intermittent bladder catheterization must be instituted to prevent permanent bladder atony that may result from urinary retention. The insertion of a nasogastric tube will control abdominal distension, reducing the risk of secondary respiratory impairment.

In the acute phase, use of steroids, mannitol, hyperbaric oxygen, cord cooling, catecholamine antagonists, dimethyl sulfoxide, and microsurgical myelotomy have yet to be of proven value. Despite the lack of confirmation of the effectiveness of steroids and mannitol, these agents are used in many spinal cord injury units during the acute phase.

After control of vital functions has been attained, neurologic and radiologic evaluations are performed.

With control of systemic functions attention is directed toward correcting malalignment or instability of the vertebral column. In cervical fracture-dislocation, this is usually done by external skeletal traction (e.g., with Crutchfield tongs, Gardner-Wells tongs, or halo fixation). Thoracolumbar injuries do not lend themselves to external traction and accordingly, surgical attempts at stabilization using devices (such as Harrington rods or Weiss springs) can be made.

Formerly, it was customary to operate on most patients with acute spinal cord injury to decompress the damaged cord. It has become apparent that surgery has little effect on the neurologic outcome. When cord compression is certain or the neurologic disorder progresses, benefit may be seen following immediate decompression (1 to 2 hours). Comprehensive reviews of this controversial topic are given in the references.

Patients with spinal cord injury need the facilities of a special spinal care unit. After the acute treatment phase specialized and continuing therapy is required. Mechanical devices for turning patients are unnecessary; when skilled nursing is available, regular hospital beds may be used. Frequent turning of patients and the use of pillows or pads prevent pressure sores. Antiembolic stockings reduce the incidence of venous thrombosis, and administration of low-dose heparin reduces the risk of pulmonary embolus. Intermittent catheterization of the bladder has replaced use of the indwelling catheter and suprapubic cystostomy. Rehabilitation therapy should be started as soon as possible.

Complications

Bladder. Restoration of a balanced bladder implies a balance between storage and evacuation of urine. A balanced bladder shows no outlet obstruction, a sterile urine, low residual volume (less than 100 ml), and low voiding pressures. Failure to attain this requires further urodynamic studies to determine whether the problem is an obstruction (i.e., bladder neck hypertrophy, prostatism, sphincter-detrusor dyssynergia) or a disturbance of storage (i.e., uninhibited bladder contractions, outflow incontinence, decreased outlet resistance). The use of intermittent catheterization (no-touch technique) is superior to the use of indwelling catheters in reducing complications and developing bladder training.

Urinary tract complications are the result of high residual urine volume and infection. Cystitis and pyelitis respond to antibiotics. Complications occurring months or years after injury include renal and bladder stones, hydronephrosis, pyonephrosis, bladder diverticula, and ureteral reflux. The incidence of these complications has been markedly reduced in the past few decades.

Bowel Training. For several weeks after acute spinal injury, laxatives and digital removal of feces are necessary. Glycerin suppositories are useful at this time. Stretching of the anus must be avoided. Subsequent training for regular defecation includes the use of laxatives on alternate days and the judicious use of glycerin suppositories, which are inserted approximately 20 minutes before the desired time of evacuation. The goal is a consistent schedule of bowel evacuation.

Pressure Sores. Decubitus ulcers develop in almost all patients with complete transection unless preventive measures are pursued vigorously. These ulcers develop wherever bony prominences are covered by skin; the sacrum, trochanters, heels, ischium, knees, and anterior-superior iliac spine are the most common sites. Preventive measures include eliminating pressure points by padding, frequent changing of position of the patient; and keeping the bed scrupulously clean. Sheepskin, alternating pressure mattresses, Gel-Pads, and waterbeds are also commonly used for prevention. Mechanical aids (e.g., Foster or Stryker frame or Circolectric beds) are rarely necessary in well-organized and well-staffed nursing units.

Once pressure sores have developed, repeated changes of dressings, topical agents, and systemic antibiotics may be used, but these are not always successful. The most effective treatment is repositioning the patient so that pressure is continuously removed. Conservative therapy may be beneficial, but surgical debridement and early closure are usually required.

Nutritional Deficiency. Attention to general nutrition is paramount in the treatment of patients with spinal cord injuries. Early loss of weight occurs in many patients because of anorexia. In addition, protein may be lost through bedsores. A diet high in protein, calories, and vitamins is advised. If the patient cannot eat sufficient quantities by mouth, parenteral hyperalimentation may be recommended. Anemia may be treated with iron and, when severe, by blood transfusion.

Muscle Spasms. Flexor or extensor spasms require treatment when they are painful, interfere with rehabilitation, or delay healing of bedsores. The aims are reduction in the number of painful and disabling flexor spasms and a decrease in muscle tone when it interferes with function, nursing care, or rehabilitation. The most useful drugs are dantrolene, diazepam, and baclofen. Physical therapy for leg spasticity includes longitudinal myelotomy and percutaneous radiofrequency rhizotomies of the lower lumbar and upper sacral roots. Obturator neurectomy in the pelvis, myotomy of the iliopsoas at the hip, lengthening of the hamstring at the knee, and percutaneous heel cord lengthening are peripheral methods that are safe but have not been carefully evaluated. Intrathecal injections of phenol or absolute alcohol should be used only by those experienced in the treatment of spinal cord injuries.

Pain. Pain may affect anesthetic areas after complete transverse lesions. There may be sharp shooting pains in the distribution of one or more roots, burning pain may be poorly localized, or deep pain may be localized in the viscera. Treatment includes placebos, spinal anesthesia, posterior rhizotomy, sympathectomy, cordotomy, and posterior column tractotomy. None has been uniformly successful. Narcotic analgesic medication should be avoided and analgesics generally should not be prescribed routinely. Transcutaneous electrical neurostimulation has been reported to be effective.

Sexual Function. Because spinal cord injuries frequently affect sexual function and because many patients retain a normal interest in sex, counselling in sexual rehabilitation is necessary.

Rehabilitation. The ultimate aim for all patients with spinal cord injury is ambulation and economic independence. This can be accomplished in many patients with injuries below the cervical area, and is best done in a rehabilitation center with trained personnel and adequate equipment. Diligent cooperation of the patient with the physiatrist and the application of supportive braces are of major importance. When the arms are paralyzed the therapeutic goal is more limited, but devices controlled by intact muscles and appropriate surgery may permit useful motion of paralyzed arms. Implantation of diaphragmatic stimulators has permitted survival of high-level cervical cord-injured patients.

The development of spinal cord units specializing in the care of tetraplegia and paraplegia is important. An increase in life expectancy, reduction in the frequency of complications, elevation of patient morale, and development of new techniques are some of the benefits.

Finally, the best mode of treatment must be prevention. Nationwide educational programs should be concerned with motor vehicle and water safety, speed limits should be lowered; and the use of seatbelts should be mandatory to reduce the incidence of these dreadful injuries.

References

Bedbrook EM. The Care and Management of Spinal Cord Injuries. New York: Springer-Verlag, 1981.

Bennett CJ, Seager SW, Vasher EA, McGuire EJ. Sexual dysfunction and electroejaculation in men with spinal cord injury. J Urol 1988; 139:453–457.

Black P, Shepard RH Jr, Markowitz RS. Spinal cord injury in the monkey: rate of cord cooling and temperature gradient during local hypothermia. Neurosurgery 1979; 5:583–587.

Blight AR. Motor evoked potentials in CNS trauma. Cent Nerv System Trauma. 1986; 3:207–214.

Botterell EH, Jousse AT, Kraus AS, Thompson MG, Wynne-Jones M, Geisler WO. A model for the future care of acute spinal cord injuries. Can J Neurol Sci 1975; 2:361–380.

Collins WF, Chehvazi B. Concepts of the acute management of spinal cord injury. In: Mathews WB, Glaser GH, eds. Recent Advances in Clinical Neurology, No. 3. Edinburgh: Churchill Livingstone, 1982:67–82.

DeVivo MJ, et al. Seven-year survival after spinal cord injury. Arch Neurol 1987; 44:872–875.

DeVivo MJ, Fine PR, Maetz HM, Stover SL. Prevalence of spinal cord injury: a re-estimation employing life table techniques. Arch Neurol 1980; 37:707–708.

Dolan EJ, Tator CH, Endrenyi L. The value of decompression for acute experimental spinal cord compression injury. J Neurosurg 1980; 53:749–755.

Ducker TB, Salcman M, Daniell HB. Experimental spinal cord trauma. III. Therapeutic effect of immobilization and pharmacologic agents. Surg Neurol 1978; 10:71–76.

Ducker TB, Salcman M, Lucas JT, Garrison WB, Perot PL Jr. Experimental spinal cord trauma. II. Blood flow, tissue oxygen, evoked potentials in both paretic and paraplegic monkeys. Surg Neurol 1978; 10:64–70.

Epstein N, Epstein JA, Benjamin V, Ransohoff J. Traumatic myelopathy in patients with cervical spinal stenosis without fracture or dislocation. Methods of diagnosis, management and prognosis. Spine 1980; 5:489–496.

Geisler WO, Jousse AT, Wynne-Jones M. Survival in traumatic transverse myelitis. Paraplegia 1977; 14:262–275.

Geisler WO, Jousse AT, Wynne-Jones M, Breithaupt D. Survival in spinal cord injury. Paraplegia 1983; 21:364–373.

Gibson CJ. Spinal cord injury rehabilitation. Editorial. Arch Neurol 1985; 42:113.

Glaser RM. Physiologic aspects of spinal cord injury and functional neuromuscular stimulation. Cent Nerv Syst Trauma. 1986; 3:49–62.

Guthkelch AN, Fleischer AS. Patterns of cervical spine injury and their associated lesions. West J Med 1987; 147:428–431.

Hughes JT, Pathology of the Spinal Cord, 2nd ed. Philadelphia: WB Saunders, 1978.

Illis LS, Sedgwick EM, Glanville HJ. Rehabilitation of the Neurological Patient. Oxford: Blackwell Scientific Publications, 1982.

Kraus JF. Epidemiologic features of head and spinal cord injury. Adv Neurol 1978; 19:261–279.

Laitinen LV, Nilsson J, Fuglmeyer AR. Selective posterior rhizotomy for treatment of spasticity. J Neurosurg 1983; 58:895–899.

Marar BC. The pattern of neurological damage as an aid to the diagnosis of the mechanism in cervical spine injuries. J Bone Joint Surg [Am] 1974; 56:1648–1654.

McComas CF, Frost JL, Schochet SS. Post-traumatic syringomyelia with paroxysmal episodes of unconsciousness. Arch Neurol 1983; 40:322–324.

Murpy M, Ogden JA, Southwick WO. Spinal stabilization in acute spinal injuries. Surg Clin North Am 1980; 60:1035–1047.

Osterholm JL. The pathophysiological response to spinal cord injury. J Neurosurg 1974; 40:5–33.

Schneider RC, Cherry G, Pantek H. The syndrome of
  acute central cervical spinal cord injury. J Neurosurg
  1954; 11:546–577.

Sneed RC, Stover SL. Undiagnosed spinal cord injuries
  in brain-injured children. Am J Dis Child 1988;
  142:965–967.

Tator CH. Early Management of Acute Spinal Cord Injury. New York: Raven Press, 1982.

Tator CH, Rowed DW. Current concepts in the immediate
  management of acute spinal cord injuries. Can Med
  Assoc J 1979; 121:1453–1464.

The National Institute of Neurological and Communicative Disorders and Stroke. The national head and
  spinal cord injury survey. J Neurosurg 1980;
  53:S1–S43.

White RJ. Advances in the treatment of cervical cord
  injuries. In: Carmel PW, ed. Clinical Neurosurgery,
  Vol. 26. Baltimore: Williams & Wilkins,
  1979:556–569.

Wilkins RH, Rengachary SS. Neurosurgery, Vol. II, Pt
  VIII. Sect B. New York: McGraw-Hill, 1985.

Woolsey RM. Rehabilitation outcome following spinal
  cord injury. Arch Neurol 1985; 42:116–119.

Yarkony GM, et al. Benefits of rehabilitation for traumatic
  spinal cord injury. Arch Neurol 1987; 44:93–96.

56. INTERVERTEBRAL DISKS
Edward B. Schlesinger

Rupture of the intervertebral disk into the body of a vertebra was first described by Schmorl in 1927. Earlier, in a 1909 text on neurologic surgery, Krause described operating on an iceman who had been diagnosed by Oppenheimer as suffering from a lesion localized to L4. Krause found an extradural mass that was described pathologically as a chondroma; the operation apparently effected a cure. There were other reports of similar "chondromas" removed at explorations of the intervertebral area. It remained for Mixter and Barr, in 1934, to point out that these lesions were actually fragments of intervertebral disk material and that they were responsible for sciatica.

Pathogenesis. The displaced disk material may create signs and symptoms by bulging or protruding beneath an attenuated annulus fibrosis or the material may extrude through a tear in the annulus and project directly into the spinal canal itself. In either case, the encroaching disk material may irritate or compress nerve roots that are coursing to foramina of exit. In the cervical or thoracic region the problem is more complex neurologically because the spinal cord itself as well as the adjacent nerve roots may be involved. Neurologic signs and symptoms are caused either by cord compression or a combination of cord and root compression. In the lumbar region the signs and symptoms relate to an individual root lesion (compressed laterally) or to compression of the cauda equina if the disk is large enough to crowd the entire spinal canal.

In the cervical region the levels most commonly affected are in the C5 to C7 segments (Table 56–1). In the lumbar area most disk protrusions occur at the last two movable spaces (L4–L5, L5–S1). This pattern suggests that the dynamics of pathologic change are partly related to the trauma of motion and wear and tear. Thoracic disk protrusion, except at the lower thoracic levels, differs from the cervical and lumbar disorders in genesis and histopathology. Motion plays no role there because the thoracic vertebrae are designed for stability rather than motion, and the heavy rib cage contributes to the rigidity of this structure. One must therefore look elsewhere for the cause of thoracic disk rupture. On gross and microscopic examination the lesion is unique, markedly degenerated, characterized by gritty calcified deposits, and almost never of the consistency of the cervical and lumbar ruptured disk; thoracic disk protrusion is more granular and yellowish.

Although trauma has been accepted as the prime cause of disk herniation, it is by no means the only cause. There seems to be a genetic predisposition in many cases. Trauma can aggravate this propensity and cause the ultimate rupture. In the most florid preordained presentation there may be multiple levels of severe disk degeneration throughout the spine, with progressive clinical involvement in different areas. Understanding the implications of this syndrome is imperative in surgical decision making and may explain why surgical stabilization of the spine (fusion) often fails to prevent recurrent symptoms.

Spinal stenosis, which is an abnormally narrow spinal canal, is an excellent example of an inherited anomaly, as are the spinal abnormalities of the achondroplastic dwarf. These abnormal spinal configurations, along with spondylosis, are major contributors to compression syndromes of the cord and cauda equina. When disk protrusion occurs in a patient with spinal stenosis it further compromises a canal capacity that is already limited, as do changes caused by arthritic proliferation or ligamentous degeneration.

The signs and symptoms of invasion of the spinal canal by disk material relate not only to the size and strategic location of the disk fragments, but also to the size and configu-

Table 56–1. Common Root Syndromes of Intervertebral Disk Disease

Disk space	L3–L4	L4–L5	L5–S1	C4–C5	C5–C6	C6–C7	C7–T1
Root affected	L4	L5	S1	C5	C6	C7	C8
Muscles affected	Quadriceps	Peroneals; anterior tibial; extensor hallucis longus	Gluteus maximus; gastrocnemius; plantar flexors of toes	Deltoid; biceps		Triceps; wrist extensors	Intrinsic hand muscles
Area of pain and sensory loss	Anterior thigh, medial shin	Great toe, dorsum of foot	Lateral foot, small toe	Shoulder, anterior arm, radial forearm		Thumb, middle fingers	Index, fourth, fifth fingers
Reflex affected	Knee jerk	Posterior tibial	Ankle jerk	Biceps		Triceps	Triceps
Straight leg raising	May not increase pain	Aggravates root pain	Aggravates root pain				

ration of the canal. The anteroposterior and lateral dimensions of the canal, particularly the foramina, play a key role because they determine the design of the canal. Abnormalities of architecture as seen in spinal stenosis and subsequent osteoarthritic changes may compress roots as they course to the exit foramina, even with small disk protrusions. In a canal of normal dimensions the severity of compression depends more on the site of rupture and the volume of the extruded material. Symptoms and signs range from single root compression to cauda equina compression. A laterally placed lesion in the cervical region may involve a single root but, if it is large enough, it may compromise the total intraspinal space and compress the adjacent cord. This is also true in the thoracic region, where a small lesion can be significant because the canal is normally narrower here than in cervical or lumbar segments. Although single root syndromes in the lumbar region are usual, truly ventral or unusually large lesions can cause less easily recognized pictures. For instance, scoliosis may be the major feature, with severe back pain and muscle splinting, but without signs of mechanical root compression in the straight leg-raising test. With a paucity of neurologic deficit and seemingly atypical signs the diagnosis may be obscure.

Incidence. Rupture of an intervertebral disk is common in the general population, especially in the fourth to sixth decades of life. It is rare before the age of 25 and uncommon after the age of 60. About 80% of patients are men. Many patients have a history of earlier trauma.

Lumbar Intervertebral Disk Rupture

Root syndomes of intervertebral disk disease are often episodic, so that periods of remission are characteristic of disk disease affecting the nerve roots. When pain is present it may be aggravated by Valsalva maneuvers (coughing, sneezing, or straining at defecation). The pain may be restricted to the back or follow a radicular distribution in one or both legs. The pain of lumbar disk disease may increase after heavy lifting or twisting of the spine. No matter how severe it is when the patient is erect the pain is characteristically relieved promptly when the patient lies down. Some patients, however, are more comfortable sitting and some can find no comfortable position. Relief of pain on bed rest is considered a useful feature in delineating disk disease from intraspinal tumor, in which pain is often not relieved or may be worsened.

On examination, the patient with a herniated lumbar disk usually shows loss of lumbar lordosis, or flattening of the lumbar spine, with splinting and asymmetric prominence of the long erector muscles. A list or tilt may be present, with one iliac crest elevated. This asymmetry is responsible for the commonly diagnosed "longer leg on one side" and the erroneous assignment of the back pain to asymmetry of leg length. (This asymmetry often causes a patient to raise the heel on the shoe of the "short" leg to level the pelvis.) Range of motion of the lumbar spine is reduced by the protective splinting of paraspinal muscles and attempted movement in some planes induces severe back pain. There may be tenderness of the adjacent vertebrae. When the patient is erect, one gluteal fold may hang down and show added skin creases because the gluteus is wasted, evidence of involvement of the S1 root. Passive straight leg raising is reduced in range and increases back and leg pain. Muscle atrophy and weakness occur in intractable cases, along with sciatic tenderness and discomfort on direct pressure at some point along the nerve from the sciatic notch to the calf. This is particularly true in older patients or in diabetics of any age. Paresthesias in the realm of the involved root are common. Reproduction of the discrete radicular pain by jugular compression is an unequivocal sign of a severe compressive lesion. Muscle weakness or atrophy is detected in a minority of cases; fasciculation is rare.

There are typical patterns of symptoms and signs for each level of root involvement; variations depend chiefly on structural anomalies, canal capacity, and osteoarthritic reaction. All share basic features related to the musculoskeletal responses—splinting of the erector muscles, dynamic list, and acute lumbosacral discomfort. The eventual superimposition of focal radicular pain on these musculoskeletal responses and evidence of neurologic deficit mark the transition from degenerative changes in the intervertebral disk and structural responses to actual impingement on an exiting root.

The typical syndromes of root compression at lumbar levels are given in Table 56–2, although the signs may not be as distinct in actual practice as the table implies. More than 80% affect L5 or S1 (Figs. 56–1 and 56–2). When the lesion affects L4 or higher roots,

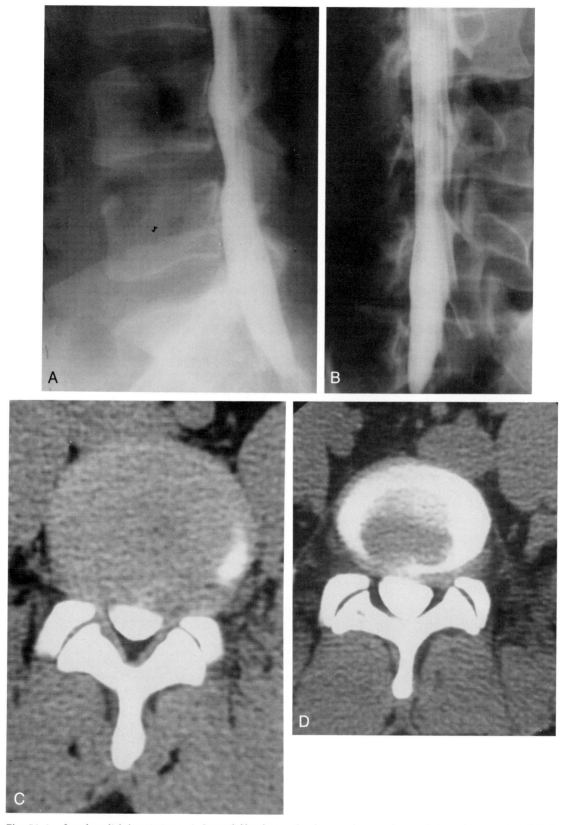

Fig. 56–1. Lumbar disk herniations. *A,* Lateral film from a lumbar myelogram demonstrates a large ventral defect at L4–L5. The L5–S1 level is unremarkable. *B,* Left posterior oblique projection demonstrates swelling and amputation of the left L5 root and possible compression of the left S1 root, with subtle thinning of the contrast. *C,* Postmyelogram axial CT scanning at the L4–L5 level confirms a large HNP obliterating the neural foramina bilaterally, with eccentric deformity of the sac on the left. *D,* At the L5–S1 level, CT is more sensitive than myelography in diagnosing lateral disk herniation into the left foramen. Compare its appearance with that of the preserved lucent fat in the right foramen. Minimal deformity of the sac ventrally accounts for the unimpressive myelogram at this level. (Courtesy of Drs. J.A. Bello, T.L Chi, and S.K. Hilal.)

Table 56–2.   Signs of Lumbar Disk Herniation in 97 Patients

Disk Space	L2–L3	L3–L4	L4–L5	L5–S1
Number of patients	1	9	45	42
Weak muscles				
Anterior tibial, extensor hallucis	0	3	13	3
Gastrocnemius, plantar responses of foot	0	0	2	3
Quadriceps	0	3	0	0
Reflex affected				
Knee jerk	1	6	4	0
Ankle jerk	0	1	12	23

(Data from Hardy RW Jr, Plank NM. Clinical diagnosis of herniated lumbar disc. In: Hardy RW, ed. Lumbar Disc Disease. New York: Raven Press, 1982:17–27.)

straight leg raising does not stretch the roots above L5. The affected roots may be tensed, however, by extending the limb with the knee flexed when the patient is prone, thus reproducing the typical radicular spread of pain.

Thoracic Disk Rupture

Because the thoracic spine is designed for rigidity rather than excursion, wear and tear from motion and stress cannot cause thoracic disk protrusion and clinical disorders are therefore rare. The substratum of thoracic disk disease may be the chronic vertebral changes incident to Scheuermann disease or juvenile osteochondritis, possibly with some late trauma. The radiographic changes of Scheuermann disease, when seen with thoracic cord compression, should raise the possibility of disk protrusion (Figs. 56–3 and 56–4). Calcific changes in the intervertebral disk and the typical vertebral changes of that disease are diagnostic markers.

The small capacity of the thoracic canal makes clinical syndromes of cord compression more critical than at other levels. By the same token, decompressive operations are more precarious and require meticulous care and planning to avoid damaging the compromised spinal cord. The lower thoracic levels, however, are more capacious and, although the conus or cauda equina may be damaged by disk protrusions, surgical approaches are less hazardous than at higher levels.

Cervical Disk Disease

Cervical disk herniation may involve both the existing root and the spinal cord, depending on two factors—the volume of the canal and the size of the lesion. Cord compression is uncommon, except in patients with spinal stenosis or massive rupture of a disk. The sites of the most frequent disk herniations are C5 to C6 and C6 to C7; C4 to C5 and C7 to T1 are less frequently affected, and other levels are rarely involved (Table 56–3). Because movement of the cervical spine is normally incremental, any process contributing to focal stress at individual levels adds

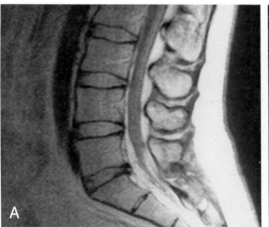 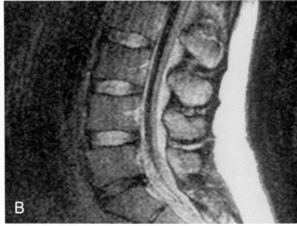

Fig. 56–2. L5–S1 herniated nucleus pulposus. *A,* Sagittal T1-weighted MRI demonstrates disk herniation at L5–S1 and bulge at L4–L5. *B,* Sagittal T2-weighted image shows decreased intensity of the degenerated disk relative to the normal disks. (Courtesy of Drs. T.L. Chi, J.A. Bello, and S.K. Hilal.)

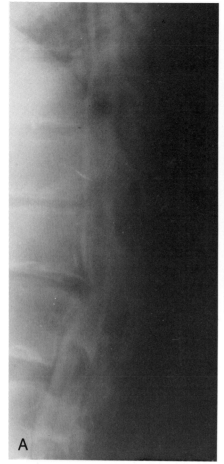

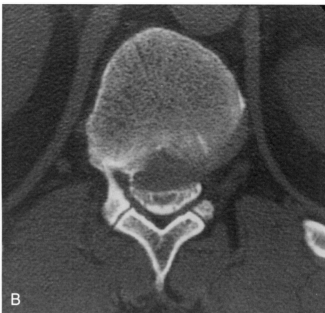

Fig. 56–3. Lower thoracic disk herniation. *A*, Lateral view from a water-soluble contrast myelogram demonstrates a ventral defect at T11–T12. *B*, Postmyelography axial CT scan at this level demonstrates deformity of the sac and cord impingement by ventral soft tissue at the intervertebral disk space consistent with disk herniation. (Courtesy of Drs. J.A. Bello and S.K. Hilal.)

to local wear and tear and to progressive pathologic changes in the disk and in joint mechanics. The development of a new fulcrum of motion above a fusion or congenital block vertebrae increases susceptibility to these changes.

Signs and Symptoms. Cervical disk disease usually begins with symptoms and signs of stiff neck and reactive splinting of the erector capital muscles, along with discomfort at the medial order of the scapula. Radicular paresthesias and pain supervene when the root is more severely compromised. These symptoms are worsened on particular movements on the head and neck, and often by stretching the dependent arm. For relief the patient often adopts a position with the arm elevated and flexed behind the head, unlike the patient with shoulder disease who maintains the arm in a dependent position, avoiding elevation or abduction or excursion at the shoulder joint.

As compression proceeds, discrete root syndromes appear (see Tables 56–1 and 56–2).

Dominant features of C5 lesions include pain in the shoulder cap with dermatomic sensory diminution with weakness and atrophy of the deltoid. The clinical picture of C6 lesions includes paresthesias of the thumb and depression of the biceps reflex with weakness and atrophy of that muscle. The pattern of C7 lesions includes paresthesias that may involve the index and middle finger and even the thumb, with atrophy and weakness in triceps, wrist extensors, and pectoral muscles, and a parallel reflex depression. C8 subserves important intrinsic muscle functions in the hand and sensation in the fourth and fifth fingers. Because these are important in discriminatory and fine finger maneuvers, C8 damage can be disabling. Large disk protrusions, particularly with spinal stenosis, can cause dramatic clinical pictures of cord compression that are indistinguishable from tumors.

Lesions such as supraspinatus tendonitis, arthritic changes in the acromioclavicular joint, and cuff tears may be difficult to dif-

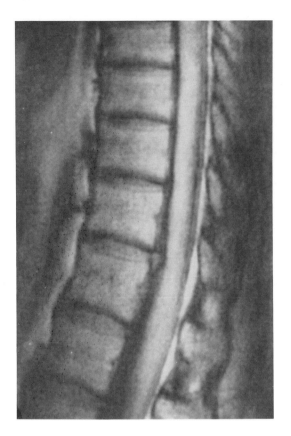

Fig. 56–4. Lower thoracic disk herniation. Sagittal T1-weighted MR scan demonstrates a soft tissue intensity signal impinging on the cord at a disk level consistent with disk herniation. (Courtesy of Drs. J.A. Bello and S.K. Hilal.)

ferentiate from cervical root compression, especially because prolonged pain and lack of range of motion lead to atrophy and frozen shoulder in all of these syndromes. C8 and T1 lesions commonly cause a partial Horner syndrome. A diagnostic workup for syndromes of these levels must include apical lordotic views of the chest and special care must be taken to rule out sulcus neoplasms or abnormal cervical ribs.

Other Diagnostic Features. Because many disk syndromes are basically genetic, significant abnormal skeletal features throughout the spine should be sought on radiographs. These include spinal stenosis, spondylolis-

Table 56–3. Frequency of Compression of the Cervical Roots by Ruptured Intervertebral Disk

Root	%
C5	2
C6	19
C7	69
C8	10
	100

(Modified from Yoss RE, Corbin KB, MacCarty CS, Love JG. Neurology 1957; 7:63.)

thesis, widespread disk disease, or Marfan disease. Acquired disorders such as osteochondritis juvenilis and metabolic states such as osteoporosis may contribute to pathologic changes in the disk and adjacent joints, as do several forms of arthritis. Recognition of the spectrum of progressive abnormalities of structure is critical in determining choice of treatment.

The myelogram affords important information about gross deformities of the intraspinal contents, and allows easy scrutiny of extended areas of the canal. CT in combination with myelography has the virtue of positive contrast and allows more accurate evaluation of abnormalities of the nerve roots or dural sac (Figs. 56–5 and 56–6). MRI is irreplaceable in revealing volume lesions of the spinal canal, particularly tumors and cysts, and extradural compression is shown well at cord levels (Fig. 56–7). Because the midline sagittal cuts are of primary importance, the lateral extradural lesions and their relationship to the lateral recess and foramen are not seen as well as on CT. MRI depiction of disk pathology at individual levels, however, can be valuable in differentiating confusing syndromes. Advances in technology continue to

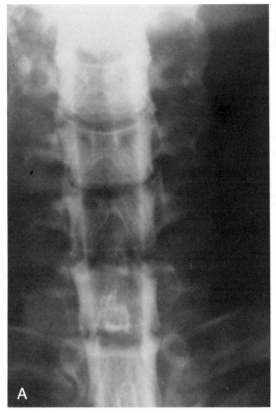

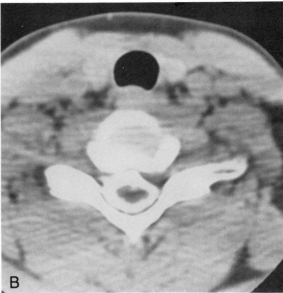

Fig. 56–5. Lower cervical disk herniation. *A,* Antero-posterior projection from a cervical myelogram demonstrates deformity of the left C7 root pouch and, to a lesser degree, of the left C6 root pouch. *B,* Postmyelography axial CT scan at the C6–C7 interspace shows soft tissue density deforming the left corner of the thecal sac, indicating herniated disk. (Courtesy of Drs. J.A. Bello and S.K. Hilal.)

enhance the diagnostic usefulness of MRI and include improved resolution and cross sectional cuts.

EMG and evoked potential studies can be helpful in localizing root involvement but are not essential. The CSF protein level varies widely and is probably a function of the degree of subarachnoid block; it is only rarely higher than 100 mg/dl or the higher values seen with tumors.

Mechanically induced disk syndromes can be duplicated by tumors (primary or metastatic), infections (e.g., epidural abscess), and arachnoiditis. When features are atypical an exhaustive workup is essential, ranging from psychiatric evaluation to sophisticated studies to rule out rheumatoid arthritis, ankylosing spondylitis, and even gout or parathyroid disease.

Treatment. Conservative treatment should continue as long as the patient improves. Most acute attacks subside spontaneously, with analgesics and bed rest for lumbar disk disorders and immobilization of the neck by a collar for cervical disk disorders. Surgery for a lumbar disk disorder is indicated when there is no improvement over a reasonable

period of strict bed rest, or when a severe neurologic disorder is found on examination. Excessively prolonged physiotherapeutic measures, bed rest, and other nonspecific measures that may cause emotional exhaustion, muscle loss, or drug dependence should, however, be avoided. The use of chymopapain or collagenase to digest the disk material is controversial.

Cord compression requires consideration of decompressive measures as soon as it is recognized. Root syndromes of the cervical spine can be separated into those that require careful supervision and early operation and those that tolerate and may respond to further conservative care. The muscles served by C5 may atrophy rapidly, leaving abduction paresis, poor prognosis for restoration of function, and a painful frozen shoulder. C8 is also vulnerable, and unrelieved compression may lead to irreversible atrophy with complex shoulder-arm-hand disorders that include circulatory and sweating abnormalities.

C6 and C7 subserve large muscles and tolerate pressure more benignly, even for long periods, and with good functional return. Cervical root syndomes are less likely to recur

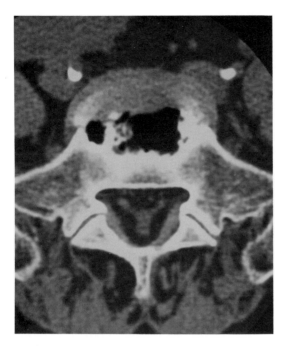

Fig. 56–6. Epidural lipomatosis. Noncontrast axial CT scan at the L5–S1 level demonstrates deformity of the thecal sac by extensive intracanalicular epidural fat. Despite obvious disk degeneration (note vacuum phenomenon) there was no evidence of disk herniation to account for symptoms. (Courtesy of Drs. J.A. Bello and S.K. Hilal.)

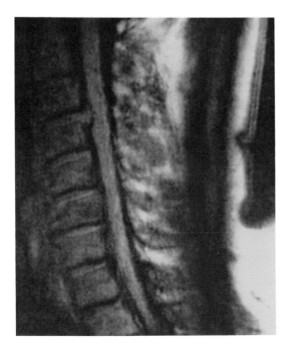

Fig. 56–7. Traumatic cervical disk herniation. Sagittal T1-weighted MR scan shows soft tissue density disk herniated posteriorly at C3–C4, with obvious cord impingement. (Courtesy of Drs. J.A. Bello and S.K. Hilal.)

than lumbar disorders and conservative therapy is worthwhile within the outlines described.

Spinal fusion is generally unnecessary for the single-level cervical disk and may create an abnormal fulcrum of motion with increased stress at adjacent joints. In the lumbar region, except when skeletal anomalies overtly contribute to the pathology, the L5 to S1 level does not require fusion. At L4 to L5 lesions that require bilateral removal create abnormal stress on joints; fusion in young adults is useful. When there is widespread involvement, as with spinal stenosis or diffuse disk disease, fusion is theoretically ideal but not practical, and may lead to increased wear and tear with later disk herniation rostral to the fusion.

Success in disk surgery depends on adequate evaluation of psychologic patterns and motivation, the thoroughness of investigation and, finally, the meticulousness of the procedure in eliminating the pathologic variables involved in the syndrome.

References

Coin CG, Coin JT. Computed tomography of cervical disk disease; technical considerations with representative case reports. J Comput Assist Tomogr 1981; 51:275–280.

Deyo RA. Conservative therapy for low back pain. Distinguishing useful from useless therapy. JAMA 1983; 250:1057–1062.

Esses SI, Morley TP. Spinal arachnoiditis. Can J Neurol Sci 1983; 10:2–10.

Francavilla TL, Powers A, Dina T, Rizzoli HV. Case report: MR imaging of thoracic disk herniations. J Comput Assist Tomogr 1987; 2:1062–1065.

Frymoyer JW. Back pain and sciatica. N Engl J Med 1988; 318:291–300.

Hardy RW Jr, ed. Lumbar Disc Disease. New York: Raven Press, 1982.

Haughton VM, Eldevik OP, Magnaes B, Amundsen P. A prospective comparison of computed tomography and myelography in the diagnosis of herniated lumbar disks. Radiology 1982; 143:103–110.

Junck L, Marshall WH. Neurotoxicity of radiological contrast agents. Ann Neurol 1983; 13:469–484.

Kirwan EOG, Parry CBW. Electric studies in the diagnosis of compression of the lumbar roots. J Bone Joint Surg [Br] 1981; 63B:71–75.

Kurihara A, Kataoka O. Lumbar disc herniation in children and adolescents. Spine 1980; 5:443–451.

Long DM, Filtzer DL, Bendebba M, Hendler NH. Clinical features of the failed-back syndrome. J Neurosurg 1988; 69:61–71.

Lufkin RB, Votruba J, Reicher M, Bassett LW, Smith S, Hanafee W. Solenoid surface coils in magnetic resonance. AJR 1986; 146:409–412.

Mixter WJ, Barr JS. Rupture of the intervertebral disc with involvement of the spinal canal. N Engl J Med 1934; 211:210.

O'Connell JEA. The indications for and results of the excision of lumbar intervertebral disc protrusions. A review of 500 cases. Ann R Coll Surg Engl 1950; 6:403.

Patterson RH Jr, Arbit E. Surgical approach through the pedicle to protruded thoracic discs. J Neurosurg 1978; 48:768–772.

Post MJD, ed. Radiographic Evaluation of the Spine. New York: Masson Publishing, 1979.

Powers SK, Bolger CA, Edwards MSB. Spinal cord pathways mediating somatosensory evoked potentials. J Neurosurg 1982; 57:472–482.

Pyeritz RE, Sack GH, Jr, Udvarhelyi GB. Thoracolumbosacral laminectomy in achondroplasia: long-term results in 22 patients. Am J Med Genet 1987; 28:433–444.

Raskin SP, Keating JW. Recognition of lumbar disk disease: comparison of myelography and computed tomography. AJR 1982; 139:349–355.

Schlesinger EB. Injuries to the low back mechanism: injuries of the intervertebral discs. In: McLaughlin HL, ed. Trauma. Philadelphia: WB Saunders, 1959:639–647.

Schlesinger EB, Taveras J. Factors in the production of "cauda equina" syndromes in lumbar discs. Trans Am Neurol Assoc 1953; 78:263–265.

Semmes RE. Ruptures of the Lumbar Intervertebral Disc: Their Mechanism, Diagnosis and Treatment. Springfield IL: Charles C Thomas, 1964.

Shaw MDM, Russell JA, Grossart KW. Changing pattern of spinal arachnoiditis. J Neurol Neurosurg Psychiatry 1978; 41:97–107.

Yoss RE, Corbin KB, MacCarty CS, Love JG. Significance of symptoms and signs in localization of involved root in cervical disc protrusion. Neurology 1957; 7:673–683.

Young A, Dixon A, Getty J, Renton P, Vacher H. Cauda equina syndrome complicating ankylosing spondylitis: use of EMG and CT in diagnosis. Ann Rheum Dis 1981; 40:317–322.

57. MYELOPATHY CAUSED BY CERVICAL SPONDYLOSIS

Lewis P. Rowland

Cervical spondylosis has been defined as a condition in which there is progressive degeneration of the intervertebral disks, leading to proliferative changes of surrounding structures, especially the bones and meninges. Damage to the spinal cord can be demonstrated at autopsy. The myelopathy is attributed to one or more of three possible mechanisms: direct compression of the spinal cord by bony or fibrocalcific tissues; ischemia caused by compromise of the vascular supply to the cord; and repeated trauma in the course of normal flexion and extension of the neck. It is difficult, however, to be precise in identifying this type of myelopathy in living patients. The very concept may be one of the persistent myths of clinical neurology and the situation begs for critical review.

Incidence. Radiographic evidence of cervical spondylosis increases in each decade of life. It is seen in from 5 to 10% of those between the ages of 20 and 30 and increases to more than 50% by the age of 45 and to more than 90% after the age of 60. Signs of cervical myelopathy of unknown cause appear in only a few patients. Victims of myelopathy do not usually have a history of repeated single root syndromes; that is, radiculopathy caused by cervical disk herniation and myelopathy seem to be distinct syndromes that affect different populations.

Pathology. The water content of the intervertebral disk and annulus fibrosis declines progressively with advancing age. Concomitantly, there are degenerative changes in the disk. The intervertebral space narrows and may be obliterated and the annulus fibrosis protrudes into the spinal canal. Osteophytes form at the margins of the vertebral body, converge on the protruded annulus and may convert it into a bony ridge or bar. The bar may extend laterally into the intervertebral foramen; there is also fibrosis of the dural sleeves of the nerve roots. All these changes narrow the canal, a process that may be aggravated by fibrosis of the ligamentum favum. The likelihood of cord compression or vascular compromise increases in direct relation to the decrease in the original diameter of the spinal canal.

The spondylotic bars may leave deep indentations (visible at autopsy) on the ventral surface of the spinal cord. At the level of the lesion (there may be several levels) there is degeneration of the gray matter, sometimes with necrosis and cavitation. Above the compression there is degeneration of the posterior columns; below the compression corticospinal tracts are demyelinated.

Symptoms and Signs. Neck pain may be prominent. Root pain is uncommon, but paresthesias may indicate the most affected root. The most common symptom is spastic gait disorder (Table 57–1). Weakness and wasting of the hands may be seen. (Fasciculations have been reported in the legs as well as the arms; how this arises is uncertain, but it has been attributed to interference with descending blood supply to the lumbar segments because the fasciculations in the legs may disappear after cervical laminectomy.) Urinary sphincter symptoms occur in a minority of patients. Overt sensory loss is uncommon, but the diagnosis is facilitated if there is a sensory level or if there is sensory loss in the distribution of a cervical dermatome. The course of the disorder is slowly progressive,

Table 57–1. Clinical Manifestations of Cervical Spondylotic Myelopathy

Symptom or Sign	%
Reflexes	
Hyperreflexia	87
Babinski sign	51
Hoffmann sign	13
Spastic gait disorder	49
Bladder symptoms	49
Sensation	
Vague sensory level	41
Proprioceptive sensory loss	39
Cervical dermatome sensory loss	33
Motor functions	
Arm weakness	31
Paraparesis	21
Hemiparesis	18
Quadriparesis	10
Brown-Sequard	18
Hand atrophy	13
Fasciculation	13
Pain	
Radicular arm	41
Radicular leg	13
Neck	8

(Data from Lunsford LD, Bissonette DJ, Zarub DS. J Neurosurg 1980; 53:87–100.)

but the natural history is not well delineated. Study of patients who were not treated surgically indicates that the condition may become arrested or even improve spontaneously. In one report, 39 of 45 patients were unchanged or better many years after the original diagnosis, without surgery.

Laboratory Data. Formerly, the most important diagnostic tests were plain radiographs of the cervical spine and myelography. Plain radiographs show narrowing of the disk spaces and the presence of osteophytes, especially at C5 to C6 and C6 to C7. Posterior osteophytes tend to be smaller than anterior projections and may not be seen without tomography. The disk bodies may be normal or show sclerosis. Changes in the zygapophyseal joints account for the designation "osteoarthritis" and may encroach on the intervertebral foramen; the changes may cause subluxation of the articular surfaces, or may compress the vertebral arteries.

In the past few years CT has largely supplanted plain radiographic examination because it can show evidence of disk degeneration and protrusion of bars into the spinal canal. The next step was to combine CT with intrathecal injection of water-soluble contrast agents to show where and how severely the spinal cord itself was compressed or dis-

torted, and spinal cord "atrophy" became a new diagnosis. Now, MRI has begun to replace both CT and CT-iohexol myelography because MRI can reveal osteophyte or disk protrusion and, more importantly, can show the spinal cord directly. In one noninvasive study it is possible to evaluate the diagnosis of spondylosis and alternative possibilities (e.g., Chiari malformation, arteriovenous malformation, extramedullary tumor, or syringomyelia). It seems merely a matter of time before the technical advances of MRI will make the use of myelography obsolete.

Somatosensory evoked responses have been used to aid in diagnosis but are not crucial. The CSF is usually normal or has a protein concentration of between 50 and 100 mg/dl. Higher protein levels or CSF pleocytosis should raise the question of multiple sclerosis or tumor, including carcinomatosis of the meninges.

Differential Diagnosis. There are two types of problems of differential diagnosis. In one group, there is compression of the cervical spinal cord, but not by spondylosis (or at least not by spondylosis alone). Cervical spinal tumors are the best example of this category. Such lesions are revealed by myelography. In other compressive lesions the primary bony changes are congenital (anomalies of the craniocervical junction) or acquired (rheumatoid arthritis or basilar impression), and may be further complicated by spondylosis. These disorders are recognized by radiography. Arteriovenous malformation may also be found.

Another group of myelopathies presents more of a diagnostic problem; cervical spondylosis is so common in the general population that it may be present by chance and harmless in a person with another disease of the spinal cord. The ultimate test of the pathogenic significance of spondylosis would be complete relief of symptoms after decompressive surgery, but this is rarely seen. Among the other diseases that can cause clinical syndromes similar to those attributed to spondylosis are multiple sclerosis, ALS, neurosyphilis, and possibly subacute combined system disease. In 12% of cases diagnosed as spondylotic myelopathy some other diagnosis was ultimately made.

Multiple sclerosis is probably the most common cause of spastic paraplegia in middle life and is probably the actual cause of the disorder in some people who have had cervical laminectomies. Therefore, before laminectomy, it is imperative to test for multiple sclerosis by use of the following: visual, somatosensory, and brain stem evoked responses; CSF gamma globulin and oligoclonal bands; and MRI examinations of the cerebral white matter, foramen magnum, brain stem, and cervical spinal cord. Proper use and interpretation of the test results will often remove diagnostic uncertainty.

ALS must be considered whenever wasting and fasciculations are seen in arm and hand muscles, as well as whenever there are fasciculations in the legs. The presence of overt fasciculation makes it unlikely that spondylotic myelopathy is the cause of symptoms; in such cases caution is warranted when considering laminectomy. There is no diagnostic test for ALS, however, and the distinction may be difficult.

Treatment. Decompressive laminectomy is the conventional treatment for the myelopathy ascribed to cervical spondylosis and many clinicians report improvement in more than 50% of patients (Table 57–2), but there have been no controlled trials or even attempts to refer patients to a regional research unit for analysis of cases. Operations are done throughout the United States. It is therefore not surprising that there is no convincing evidence that the surgery is actually helpful, that either anterior or posterior decompression is preferable, or that spinal fusion operations are good or bad. In one United States university hospital the surgical mortality rate was 3% in the years 1971 to 1977; the complication rate, including both transient and permanent effects, was 23%. Only 41% of patients could return to their normal daily activities. Decisions about surgery must therefore depend on local practices and findings in individual cases.

Without surgery, conservative therapy includes use of a soft collar to reduce cervical motion and pain and a rehabilitation program to preserve gait and ameliorate problems in activities of daily living.

References

Adams CBT, Logue V. Movement and contour of spine in relation to neural complications of cervical spondylosis. Brain 1971; 94:569–586.

Adams CBT, Logue V. Some functional effects of operations for cervical spondylotic myelopathy. Brain 1971; 94:587–594.

Barnes MP, Saunders M. The effect of cervical mobility on the natural history of cervical spondylotic myelopathy. J Neurol Neurosurg Psychiatry 1984; 47:17–20.

Dunsker SB, ed. Cervical Spondylosis. New York: Raven Press, 1981.

Hirose G, Kadoya S. Cervical spondylotic radiculo-myelopathy in patients with athetoid-dystonic cerebral palsy; clinical evaluation and surgical treatment. J Neurol Neurosurg Psychiatry 1984; 47:775–780.

Irvine DH, Foster JB, Newell DJ, Klutkvin BN. Prevalence of cervical spondylosis in a general practice. Lancet 1965; 2:1089–1092.

Jinkins JR, Bashir R, Al-Mefty O, Al-Kawi MZ, Fox JL. Cystic necrosis of the spinal cord in compressive myelopathy. AJR 1986; 147:767–775.

Kardon D. Cervical spondylotic myelopathy with reversible fasciculations in the lower extremities. Arch Neurol 1977; 34:774–776.

Lees F, Turner JWA. Natural history and prognosis of cervical spondylosis. Brit Med J 1963; 2:1607–1610.

Lunsford LD, Bissonette DJ, Zorub DS. Anterior surgery for cervical disc disease. II. Treatment of cervical spondylotic myelopathy in 32 cases. J Neurosurg 1980; 53:12–19.

MacFadyen DJ. Posterior column dysfunction in cervical spondylotic myelopathy. Can J Neurol Sci 1984: 11:365–370.

Masaryk TJ, Modic MT, Geisinger MA, et al. Cervical myelopathy: a comparison of magnetic resonance

Table 57–2. Effects of Surgical or Conservative Therapy of Cervical Spondylosis Myelopathy

Source	Treatment	Number of Patients	Results (%)		
			Improved	Unchanged	Worse
Surgical therapy:					
Symon (1971)	Posterior approach	330	61	23	16
	Anterior approach	42	60	31	9
Nurick (1972) (literature)		474	56	25	19
Nurick (1972) (personal)	Posterior approach	43	33	47	18
Scoville (1976)	Posterior approach	36	65	35	0
Lunsford, et al. (1980)	Both	32	22		71*
					45*
Nonsurgical therapy:					
Nurick (1972) (literature)		104	40	36	24
Lees & Turner		44	20	77	3

*Data in this report are given in different terms; 71% of patients noted a progressive postoperative gait disorder and 45% had a second myelogram after surgery because of persistent or progressive symptoms.

and myelography. J Comput Assist Tomogr 1986;
10:184–194.

Nurick S. The pathogenesis of the spinal cord disorder
associated with cervical spondylosis. Brain 1972;
95:87–100.

Nurick S. The natural history and results of surgical treatment of the spinal cord disorder associated with cervical spondylosis. Brain 1972; 95:101–108.

Scoville WB, Dohrmann GJ, Corkhill G. Late results of
cervical disc surgery. J Neurosurg 1976; 45:203–210.

Symon L. Surgical treatment. In: Wilkinson H, ed. Cervical Spondylosis; Its Early Diagnosis and Treatment. Philadelphia: Saunders, 1977: 154–171.

Wilkinson H, ed. Cervical Spondylosis. Philadelphia: WB
Saunders, 1971.

Yu YL, DuBoulay GH, Stevens JM, Kendall BE. Computed tomography in cervical spondylotic myelopathy and radiculopathy. Neuroradiology 1986;
28:221–236.

Yu YL, Moseley IF. Syringomyelia and cervical spondylosis: a clinicoradiological investigation. Neuroradiology 1987; 29:143–151.

Yu YL, Woo E, Huang CY. Cervical spondylotic myelopathy and radiculopathy. Acta Neurol Scand 1987;
75:367–373.

58. LUMBAR SPONDYLOSIS

Lewis P. Rowland

The same pathologic changes that define cervical spondylosis may affect the lower spine. Here, however, the roots of the cauda equina are affected rather than the spinal cord. Congenital narrowing of the canal (i.e., spinal stenosis) makes a person more vulnerable to these changes, a fact documented by Schlesinger and Taveras as well as by Verbiest in the early 1950s.

The resulting syndrome differs from acute herniation in many respects. Most patients are older than 40; many are older than 60. The progression of symptoms is likely to be gradual rather than acute; twisting the back, lifting, or falling are precipitating factors in less than a third of cases, and back pain is not the dominant symptom but may be reported in more than half. Leg pain, when present, is as often bilateral as unilateral. Weakness of the legs and urinary incontinence are symptoms in a minority of patients, but many show weakness of isolated muscles and loss of reflexes on examination. Straight leg raising is limited in only a minority of cases.

The characteristic symptom is *pseudoclaudication*, which is seen in almost all patients and is defined as unilateral or bilateral discomfort in buttock, thigh, or leg on standing or walking that is relieved by rest. Patients use the words "pain," "numbness," or "weakness" to describe the discomfort, but there is often no objective sensory loss or focal muscle weakness. The discomfort is relieved by lying down, sitting, or flexing at the waist. Sometimes pain persists in recumbency until the spine is flexed. Unlike vascular claudication the pain persists if the patient stops walking without flexing the spine, and sometimes the discomfort is brought on by prolonged standing without walking.

The pathogenesis of pseudoclaudication is uncertain. Sometimes myelography shows that hyperextension of the spine increases the protrusion of intervertebral discs, with relief of nerve root compression in flexed postures. Also, blood flow to the lumbar spinal cord may increase when leg muscles are exercised. As a result, vessels on nerve roots dilate but are then confined by the bony changes and thus compress the nerve roots. This is relieved by cessation of activity.

The diagnosis is made from the characteristic history, clinical findings, and radiography. Formerly the syndrome was defined by changes in plain spine radiographs and by evidence of partial or complete subarachnoid block found by contrast myelography. Diagnosis was facilitated by the advent of CT, alone or with intrathecal contrast agents. Now, however, it seems that MRI alone may suffice to show the specific patterns and extent of compression. Electromyography (EMG) can reveal that denervation is restricted to muscles innervated by lumbosacral roots. The CSF protein level may be normal if the tap is performed above the level of the block but values over 100 mg/dl may be found if there are multiple blocks.

The differential diagnosis includes intermittent claudication caused by peripheral arterial occlusive disease, which is recognized by the loss of pulses and characteristic trophic changes in the skin of the feet. Aortoiliac occlusive disease may spare peripheral pulses but the femoral pulse is usually affected; it may cause claudication and wasting of leg muscles but does not cause postural claudication. The pain of aortoiliac disease is localized to exercising muscles. The radicular pattern of spinal claudication is not seen. The pain of aortoiliac disease persists as long as exercise is continued, regardless of body position.

Patients older than 60 usually tolerate the prescribed decompressive laminectomy, often at several levels. In one series more than two-thirds of patients reported considerable and sustained improvement 3 or more years after surgery.

References

DeVilliers JC. Combined neurogenic and vascular claudicaton. S Afr Med J 1980; 57:650–654.

Epstein NE, Epstein JA. Lumbar spinal stenosis. In: Camins M, O'Leary P. The Lumbar Spine. New York: Raven Press, 1987:149–162.

Hall S, Bartelson JD, Onofrio BM, Baker HL, Okazaki H, O'Duffy JD. Lumbar spinal stenosis. Clinical features, diagnostic procedures, and results of surgical treatment in 68 patients. Ann Intern Med 1985; 103:271–275.

Hood SA, Weigl K. Lumbar spinal stenosis: Surgical intervention for the older person. Israel J Med Sci 1983; 19:169–172.

Modic MT, Masaryk T, Boumphrey F, Goormastic M, Bell G. Lumbar herniated disk disease and canal stenosis. Prospective evaluation by surface coil MR, CT, and myelography. Am J Roentgenol 1986; 147:757–765.

Schlesinger EB, Taveras J. Factors in the production of "cauda equina" syndromes in lumbar discs. Trans Am Neurol Assoc 1953; 78:263–265.

Verbiest H. A radicular syndrome from developmental narrowing of the lumbar vertebral canal. J Bone Joint Surg [Br] 1954; 36:230—237.

Verbiest H. Further experiences on the pathological influence of a developmental narrowness of the bony lumbar vertebral canal. J Bone Joint Surg [Br] 1955; 37:576–583.

Weinstein PR. Lumbar stenosis. In: Hardy RW Jr, ed. Lumbar Disc Disease. New York: Raven Press, 1982:257–276.

Weinstein PR, Enni G, Wilson CB, eds. Lumbar Spondylosis. Chicago: Year Book Medical Publishers, 1977.

59. INJURY TO CRANIAL AND PERIPHERAL NERVES

Lewis P. Rowland

Neuritis, Neuropathy, and Nerve Injury

The term "neuritis" has been used to denote damage to nerves from any cause. In most instances, dysfunction of the nerve is not caused by an infection and the term "neuropathy" is therefore preferred.

Etiology. The peripheral and cranial nerves are subject to many different types of injury, including trauma, infections, tumors, toxic agents, and vascular or metabolic disorders. Trauma is the most common cause of localized injury to a single nerve (mononeuritis). Toxic and metabolic disorders usually affect many nerves (polyneuritis or multiple symmetric polyneuropathy).

Pathology. The pathologic changes that develop in a damaged nerve depend on the severity of the injury. Rapidly reversible *physiologic block* is recognized as the condition in which an arm or leg "goes to sleep" momentarily; it is attributed to ischemia of a nerve and is promptly relieved by changing the position of the limb to relieve pressure on the artery and restore blood flow to the nerve. Temporary interruption of function may occur when the nerve is subjected to moderate pressure or when it is slightly damaged by some other process. Paresis and sensory loss outlast the compression and local block of conduction can be demonstrated by stimulating points proximal and distal to the site of injury. Muscle action potentials can be evoked by distal but not proximal stimulation. In these cases there is local demyelination without physical interruption of the axons; this condition is called *acute demyelinating block*. The time for recovery depends on the length of the affected segment but is usually complete in a month. Temporary interruption of function may occur when the nerve is subjected to a moderate pressure or when it is only slightly damaged by some other process.

When the injury is severe enough to damage the axis cylinder and myelin sheath, the nerve undergoes degeneration and subsequent regeneration *(wallerian degeneration)*. When there is a severe injury to a peripheral nerve at any one point the sheath at the point of injury is destroyed. Subsequently there is a degeneration of the axon and myelin sheaths along the entire length of the nerves distal to the point of injury and a similar degeneration proximal to the next node of Ranvier. This process starts within 24 hours but takes many days for completion. The axons become enlarged and fragmented and then disappear. The myelin sheaths swell and break up into globules of fatty material. If continuity of the nerve has not been interrupted the subsequent regeneration usually proceeds in an orderly fashion. In the degenerated portion of the nerve the Schwann cells in the sheath undergo changes in form and increase in number. There is also an increase in the endoneural cells. These, together with other phagocytic cells, clear away the debris resulting from the breakdown of the myelin and axon. This process is well advanced within 2 weeks of the injury and usually complete at the end of 1 to 2 months. At this stage, in contrast to demyelinating block, the nerve distal to the injury is not excitable. After all the debris has been removed the nuclei of the Schwann cells are arranged in orderly rows, which apparently serve to guide the course of the axon from its point of regeneration to its end-organ in the muscle, skin, blood vessels, or glands. The rate of regrowth of the axon is variable, but it is roughly 1 mm/day. Deposition of myelin around the axon follows its regeneration. Therefore, the time between injury and restoration of function is usually measured in months when a nerve is injured.

If the nerve has been completely severed the orderly process described above is interfered with in proportion to the width of the separation of continuity of the proximal and distal ends. If this distance is great, regeneration is not possible unless the ends are apposed at operation. When the distance is small, the fibrillary process of the axon penetrates the fibrin and connective tissue in the scar and enters the distal end of the nerve. Some of these may be deflected from the proper path by the scar and become entangled to form *a neuroma.*

There is usually no significant change in the spinal cord after injury to the peripheral nerves. The ventral horn cells that are the origin of the damaged peripheral nerve fibers undergo changes described by the terms *axonal reaction* or *chromatolysis.* The cell loses its pyramidal shape, the Nissl granules are displaced to the periphery, and the nucleus is eccentric. This is a reversible reaction and the cell soon returns to normal except when the damage to the axon is close to the spinal cord or brain stem. When there is a long-standing severe degeneration of sensory or mixed nerves, there may be degeneration of the axons and myelin sheaths in the posterior funiculi.

Symptoms. The symptoms and signs that appear after injury to a nerve are related to the type of nerve affected. If the nerve subserves mainly a motor function there is flaccid paralysis with wasting and loss of the reflexes of the muscles innervated by the nerve. If the affected nerve contains sensory fibers there is loss of sensation in an area that is usually slightly smaller than that of the anatomic distribution of the nerve. Vasomotor disorders and so-called "trophic disturbances" are more common when a sensory or mixed type of nerve is injured than when a motor nerve is damaged.

Partial injury or incomplete division of a nerve may be accompanied by pain that may be stabbing in character, by dysesthesias in the form of pins-and-needles sensation, or, rarely, by severe burning pains described by the term *causalgia.*

Complete or incomplete interruption of the nerve may be followed by changes in the skin, mucous membranes, bones, and nails classified as *vasomotor* or *trophic disturbances.*

Diagnosis. The diagnosis of injury to one or more peripheral nerves can usually be made by the distribution of the motor and sensory abnormalities. These patterns are considered in connection with the description of isolated peripheral nerve lesions. The differentiation between lesions of the spinal roots and one or more peripheral nerves can usually be made by determining whether the muscular weakness and sensory loss are of a segmental nature rather than in the pattern of a nerve distribution. EMG can be used to study the patterns of denervation and later reinnervation; nerve conduction studies can ascertain the site of injury and determine the nature of the injury.

The differential diagnosis between polyneuropathy and other causes of generalized weakness is discussed in Article 103, Acquired Neuropathies.

Prognosis. The prognosis after injury of peripheral nerves is related to the severity of the injury and, to some extent, the site of the injury.

As a rule, the nearer the site of the injury is to the CNS, the lower the probability of regeneration of a completely severed nerve. This is particularly true of the cranial nerves. Regeneration does not occur in the first or second cranial nerves, which are really part of the CNS.

When the injury to a peripheral nerve is minor and there is no degeneration, complete recovery may take place in a few days or weeks. Recovery, however, is slow and not complete if the nerve is severely injured; loss of function is usually permanent when the nerve is severed and the gap between the two ends or the severity of the scar formation is such that the regenerating axon cannot reach the distal end of the nerve.

Treatment. When a peripheral nerve is severed by trauma the ends should be anastomosed during surgery. There is no agreement about the best time to explore and treat lesions of the peripheral nerves by surgical methods if it cannot be determined whether there has been anatomic or physiologic interruption of the nerve. It is widely believed that surgery should be performed as soon as possible whenever there is any doubt about the state of the nerve.

After surgical therapy, or in patients who do not need operative therapy, there should be immediate cooperation with the rehabilitation service. Paralyzed muscles should be given passive movements and weak muscles should be given re-educative exercises. It is doubtful whether electrical stimulation is worthwhile but some clinicians claim that there is less muscular wasting when electrotherapy is used.

Splints, braces, and other corrective appliances should be used when the lesion produces a deformity. These should be removable for the regular application of physiotherapy.

Cranial Nerves

OLFACTORY NERVE AND TRACT

Disturbances of the sense of smell may occur as a result of injury to the nasal mucosa, the olfactory bulb, its filaments, or its CNS connections. Lesions of the nerve cause diminution or loss of the sense of smell. Injury to the CNS connections is not usually accompanied by any detectable loss of olfactory sense. Occasionally, however, olfactory hallucinations of a transient and paroxysmal nature occur in patients with lesions in the temporal lobe. Loss of the sense of smell is often accompanied by an impairment of taste because taste depends to a great extent on volatile substances in foods and beverages.

Temporary impairment of the sense of smell is seen frequently in connection with the common cold. Inflammatory or neuritic lesions of the bulb or tract are uncommon, although these structures may be involved in meningitis or in multiple peripheral neuritis. The olfactory bulb or tract may be compressed by meningiomas, metastatic tumors, or aneurysms in the anterior fossa or by infiltrating tumors of the frontal lobe. The filaments of the olfactory nerve may be torn from the cribriform plate, or the olfactory bulb may be contused or lacerated in injuries to the head. Leigh reported disturbances of olfactory sense in 7.2% of 1000 cases of head injury observed at a military hospital. The loss was complete in 4.1% and partial in 3.1%. Recovery of the sense of smell occurred in only 6 of the 72 patients. Parosmia (perversion of sense of smell) was present in 12 cases. In a study of head injuries in civilians, Friedman and Merritt found that the olfactory nerve was damaged in 11 of 430 cases, or 2.6%. In all cases the anosmia was bilateral. In three cases the loss was transient and disappeared within 2 weeks of injury.

Parosmia is not accompanied by impairment of olfactory acuity, and is most commonly caused by lesions of the temporal lobe, but it has been reported when the injury was probably in the olfactory bulb or tract. Hallucinations of smell may occur in psychotics, or may be an aura of seizures in patients with convulsive seizures (hippocampal or uncinate gyrus fits). The aura in such cases is usually an unpleasant odor that is described with difficulty.

Increased sensitivity to olfactory stimuli is rare, but cases have been reported in which the sense of smell is so acute that it is a source of discomfort. That symptom is usually psychogenic.

OPTIC NERVE AND TRACT

The retina, optic nerve, and optic tract are subject to injury from many causes with resulting loss of vision, impairment of the pupillary light reflexes, and abnormalities in the size of the pupil (Table 59–1).

Changes in the retina or optic nerve occur as the result of direct trauma, damage by toxins, systemic diseases (e.g., chronic nephritis, diabetes mellitus, leukemia, anemia, polycythemia, nutritional deficiencies, syphilis, tuberculosis, the lipodystrophies, giant cell arteritis, generalized arteriosclerosis), demyelinating hereditable diseases, local conditions (e.g., chorioretinitis, glaucoma, tumors, congenital anomalies, thrombosis or embolism of the veins or arteries of the retina), infiltration or compression of the nerve (e.g., by gliomas, meningiomas, pituitary tumors, craniopharyngiomas, metastatic tumors, or aneurysms), and increased intracranial pressure of whatever cause. Most of the conditions enumerated above are considered elsewhere, and discussion here is limited to optic neuritis and atrophy.

Optic Neuritis and Atrophy

Optic neuritis is a term that is loosely used to describe lesions of the optic nerves accompanied by diminution in visual acuity, with or without changes in the peripheral fields of vision caused by inflammatory, degenerative, or demyelinating disorders or toxic agents. On ophthalmoscopic examination in the early stage of optic neuritis the disc may appear normal or there may be swelling and congestion of the nerve. In the later stage, the disc is pale and smaller than normal.

The optic nerve or retina may be injured by a great variety of toxic substances, including

Table 59–1. Effects of Lesions of the Optic, Oculomotor, and Sympathetic Pathways on the Pupils

Site of Lesion on Right Side	Size of Pupil		Reaction of Homolateral Pupil to Stimulation by Light Directed Into		Consensual Reaction of Contralateral Pupil to Stimulation by Light Directed Into		Accommodation-Convergence Reaction
	Right	Left	Right	Left	Right	Left	
Retina	Dilated	Normal	Impaired	Normal	Impaired	Normal	Normal
Optic nerve	Dilated	Normal	Lost	Normal	Lost	Normal	Normal
Optic chiasm	Normal	Normal	Normal*	Normal*	Normal*	Normal*	Normal
Optic tract	Normal	Normal	Normal*	Normal*	Normal*	Normal*	Normal
Optic radiation	Normal	Normal	Normal	Normal	Normal	Normal	Normal
Periaqueductal region†	Contracted	Normal	Lost	Normal	Lost	Normal	Normal
Oculomotor nuclear complex or nerve	Dilated	Normal	Lost	Normal	Normal	Lost	Lost on right
Sympathetic pathways	Contracted	Normal	Normal	Normal	Normal	Normal	Normal

*No reaction of the pupils if the beam of light is focused sharply on the amblyopic portions of the retina.
†Argyll Robertson pupil.

methyl alcohol, ethyl alcohol and tobacco, quinine, pentavalent arsenicals, thallium, lead, mercury, and other metals.

Alcohol-Tobacco Amblyopia

This term is used to describe the optic neuritis that is attributed to long-continued use of both tobacco and ethyl alcohol. It has been postulated that the lesion is primarily an interstitial neuritis with destruction of the papillomacular bundle. A more reasonable hypothesis, however, is that the ganglion cells in the macular region of the retina are damaged. The neuritis, most commonly seen in middle-aged or elderly men who smoke a pipe and drink alcohol in large quantities, affects both eyes. At the onset there is a central or paracentral scotoma for colors that progresses to a complete central scotoma. The peripheral fields of vision are normal. The occurrence of alcohol-tobacco amblyopia in association with pernicious anemia has been noted; malabsorption of vitamin B_{12} may be a factor in the cause of alcohol-tobacco amblyopia. Some authorities believe that the condition is primarily a nutritional disorder in alcoholics who are not eating properly. Absolute withdrawal of all forms of alcohol and tobacco may improve vision unless the disease has progressed to the point of complete atrophy of the retinal cells or of the optic nerve.

Optic or Retrobulbar Neuritis

Optic neuritis is an acute infection of the optic nerve accompanied by loss of visual acuity, with or without objective changes in the fundus. In most cases optic neuritis is an episode in the course of multiple sclerosis, and is readily diagnosed as such. Spontaneous improvement, the rule in optic neuritis, is often attributed to whatever treatment is given.

The symptoms of optic neuritis consist of a rapid loss of vision in one (Fig. 59–1) or both eyes, often accompanied by slight pain, especially on movement of the eyeball. The pupillary reactions are usually preserved. Presence or absence of changes in the optic disc is presumably related to the distance of the lesions from the nerve head. If the lesion is near the chiasm the fundus appears normal or there is only slight congestion. When the lesion is in the distal portion of the nerve the optic disc is swollen, with hemorrhages in the nerve head or adjacent retina. Visual acuity is usually reduced because of the presence of a central scotoma. Various types of visual field

defects are found, depending on whether the lesion is in the proximal portion of the nerve, the chiasm, or the optic tract.

In most cases of retrobulbar neuritis the course is one of gradual improvement, with return of vision to or near to normal. Steroid therapy may relieve the local pain but has no demonstrable effect on outcome. With recurrent attacks the degree of permanent visual loss is greater and atrophy of the nerve is apparent, especially in the temporal half of the disc *(temporal pallor)*. Total loss of vision, however, is rare.

Optic neuritis is the first manifestation in about 15% of patients with multiple sclerosis, and occurs at some time in 50% of all patients with multiple sclerosis. When optic neuritis occurs without prior attacks it is difficult to predict whether other signs of multiple sclerosis will follow because figures in different reports vary (from 17% in Minnesota to 87% in Australia). The differences have been attributed to length of follow-up after optic neuritis, criteria for both diagnoses, HLA types of the local population, and geographic variables. The risk of later development of multiple sclerosis is probably greater for women than for men and if the patient is older than 20 at the time of the first attack of optic neuritis. Recurrent attacks of optic neuritis probably increase the risk of later multiple sclerosis but some patients have been followed for many years without any evidence of multiple sclerosis. Some patients with optic neuritis have no other symptoms but nevertheless show lesions of MS on MRI. It remains to be seen whether those patients develop other clinical manifestations of MS.

In older individuals, especially after the age of 60, *ischemic optic neuropathy* may cause unilateral visual loss and swelling of the disc. The onset is abrupt, with altitudinal or other visual field defects. Age of the patient, lack of local pain, and lack of improvement differentiate this condition from optic neuritis. The ESR is normal in contrast to that of temporal arteritis, and there are no clinical or laboratory signs of brain tumor.

Recognition of multiple sclerosis as the cause of optic neuritis is not difficult when other signs of the disease are present. In the absence of these signs optic neuritis must be differentiated from papilledema or optic neuritis from other causes. The severe degree of visual loss and the tenderness of the eyeballs to pressure serve to distinguish the swelling of the optic disc that occurs in optic neuritis

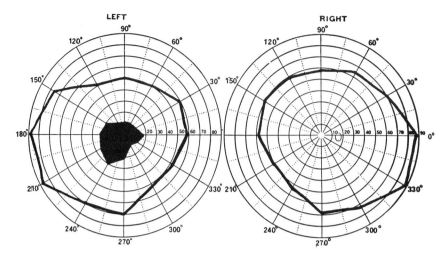

Fig. 59–1. Chart of visual fields in a patient with retrobulbar neuritis, indicating large central scotoma in left eye. Visual acuity, OD 15/15, OS 1/400. (Courtesy of Dr. M. Chamlin.)

from the papilledema resulting from increased intracranial pressure. The improvement in the degree of visual loss as well as the results of orbital and brain CT or MRI scans differentiate the optic atrophy secondary to optic neuritis from that which occurs with aneurysms, pituitary adenomas, and other tumors in the anterior fossa, or as the result of sustained increased intracranial pressure.

Optic Chiasm and Tract Lesions

Lesions of the optic chiasm are usually caused by aneurysms or pituitary and other tumors. These lesions are discussed in Chapter V, Tumors. Diminution of visual acuity and visual field defects have been reported as the result of damage of the optic nerve, chiasm, or tracts by thickening of the meninges surrounding them. This *chiasmal arachnoiditis* has been found at surgery in patients who have suffered minor or severe cerebral trauma or who have had a previous meningeal infection, particularly syphilitic meningitis. Improvement in vision sometimes occurs when the thickened adherent meninges are separated from the optic chiasm. Necropsy examinations of such cases are rare and at present there is not sufficient evidence to delineate the syndrome.

OCULOMOTOR, TROCHLEAR, AND ABDUCENS NERVES

Injury to the nerves or nuclei that innervate the ocular muscles causes diplopia, deviation of the eyeball, and impairment of ocular movements.

Complete lesions of the third nerve, or its nucleus, produce paralysis of the extrinsic muscles of the eye supplied by this nerve (medial rectus, superior rectus, inferior rectus, inferior oblique, and levator palpebrae superior) as well as the constrictor of the ciliary muscles. There is ptosis of the lid, with loss of the ability to open the eye; the eyeball is deviated outward and slightly downward; the pupil is dilated, does not react to light, and loses the power of accommodation. Partial lesions of the third nerve or its nucleus produce fragments of the above picture according to the extent of involvement of the nerve fibers or neurons.

Lesions of the fourth nerve or nucleus cause paralysis of the superior oblique muscle with impairment of the ability to turn the eye downward and inward. Deviation of the eyeball is slight and diplopia is prevented by inclining the head forward and to the side of the normal eye.

Injury to the sixth nerve causes paralysis of the lateral rectus muscle. The eyeball is deviated inward and diplopia is present in almost all ranges of movement of the eye, except on gazing to the side opposite the lesion. Lesions in the brain stem that involve the sixth nerve nucleus are accompanied by a paralysis of lateral gaze. On attempting to look toward the affected side neither eyeball moves beyond the midline. The intactness of the third nerve on the opposite side can be demonstrated by the ability of the patient to innervate the internal rectus muscle of that eye in accommodation-convergence movements.

Paralysis of the ocular muscles may result from injury to the corresponding motor nerves or cells of origin by many conditions, including trauma, neurosyphilis, multiple sclerosis and other demyelinating diseases, tumors or aneurysms at the base of the skull, acute or subacute meningitis, thrombosis of intracranial venous sinuses, encephalitis, acute anterior poliomyelitis, diphtheria, diabetes mellitus, syringobulbia, vascular accidents in the brain stem, lead poisoning, botulism, alcoholic polioencephalitis (Wernicke encephalitis), osteomyelitis of the skull, and following spinal anesthesia or simple lumbar puncture. Intraorbital lesions may cause ophthalmoplegia, proptosis, and local pain; retro-orbital lesions may cause similar symptoms. Intracavernous inflammation is held to be responsible for a form of painful ophthalmoplegia known as the *Tolosa-Hunt syndrome* but the pathology has been documented in few cases; most would also be considered examples of *orbital myositis* or *orbital pseudotumor,* in which swelling of the muscles within the orbit can be demonstrated by CT. Ocular palsies are frequently seen in myasthenia gravis, ocular myopathy, and rarely in polyneuropathy. Discussion in this section is restricted to the disturbance of eye movements in patients with increased intracranial pressure.

Paralysis of Eye Muscles Associated with Increased Intracranial Pressure

The sixth nerve has a long course from its point of emergence from the brain stem to the lateral rectus muscle in the orbit. Although it lies in a fluid-cushioned channel for a portion of this course, the nerve is peculiarly subject to injury by compression against the floor of the skull when intracranial pressure is increased from any cause. Thus, unilateral or bilateral paralysis of the lateral rectus muscle may develop in patients with increased intracranial pressure. In these cases the paralysis is of no value in localizing the site of the lesion (Table 59–2).

The third nerve is rarely injured by increased intracranial pressure. The nerve may be damaged when the increase in pressure develops slowly, as with tumors of the brain, but is more likely to be injured when the increased pressure is of sudden onset, with herniation of the uncinate gyrus through the tentorial notch and compression of the nerve. It is most commonly seen in patients with massive intracerebral hemorrhage or in those with extradural or subdural hematomas. These patients are usually comatose, making it impossible to test movements of the eyes, except by doll's eye or caloric tests that may not suffice to show paresis of muscles innervated by the third neck cranial nerve. However, compression of the third nerve may be manifest by a dilated pupil that does not respond to light, ipsilateral to the herniation.

FIFTH (TRIGEMINAL) NERVE

Injury to the fifth cranial nerve causes paralysis of the muscles of mastication with deviation of the jaw toward the side of the lesion, loss of ability to appreciate soft tactile, thermal, or painful sensations in the face, and loss of the corneal and sneezing (sternutatory) reflexes.

Lesions in the pons usually involve the motor and main sensory nuclei, causing paralysis of the muscles of mastication and loss of sensation of light touch in the face. Lesions in the medulla affect only the descending root and cause loss of the sensations of pain and temperature together with loss of the corneal reflex.

The fifth nerve may be injured by trauma, neoplasms, aneurysms, or meningeal infections. Occasionally it may be involved in poliomyelitis and generalized polyneuropathy. The sensory and motor nuclei in the pons and medulla may be destroyed by intramedullary tumors or vascular lesions. In addition, the descending root is frequently damaged in syringobulbia and multiple sclerosis. The fifth nerve is the site of trigeminal neuralgia (tic douloureux).

Trigeminal Neuralgia (Tic Douloureux)

This is a disorder of the sensory division of the trigeminal nerve characterized by recurrent paroxysms of sharp stabbing pains in the distribution of one or more branches of the nerve. Its cause is unknown. In most cases there is no organic disease of the fifth nerve or CNS. Degenerative or fibrotic changes in the gasserian ganglion have been reported, but are too inconstant to be considered as having any causal relationship to the symptoms. In some cases the trigeminal nerve has been found to be compressed by tumors or anomalous blood vessels. Pains typical of trigeminal neuralgia have occasionally occurred in patients with lesions in the brain stem as a result of multiple sclerosis or vascular lesions that involve the descending root of the fifth nerve. It has been suggested that the attacks of facial pain in trigeminal neuralgia are

Table 59–2.　Causes of Third and Sixth Cranial Nerve Palsies

	Third Nerve		Sixth Nerve	
	No. of Cases	*% of Cases*	*No. of Cases*	*% of Cases*
Total	290	100	419	100
Undetermined	67	23.1	124	29.6
Head trauma	47	16.2	70	16.7
Neoplasm	34	11.7	61	14.6
Vascular	60*	20.7	74†	17.7
Aneurysm	40‡	13.8	15§	3.6
Other	42	14.5	75	17.9

*25 had diabetes mellitus
†24 had diabetes mellitus
‡8 had subarachnoid hemorrhage
§11 had subarachnoid hemorrhage
(From Rush JA, Younge BR. Paralysis of cranial nerves III, IV, and VI. Cause and prognosis in 1000 cases. Arch Ophthalmol 1981; 99:76–79.)

caused by a paroxysmal discharge in the descending nucleus of the nerve. The discharge is presumed to be related to an excessive inflow of impulses to the nucleus. This hypothesis is supported by evidence that typical attacks of trigeminal neuralgia have been relieved occasionally by section of the greater auricular of occipital nerves and that an episode of trigeminal neuralgia can be interrupted by the intravenous injection of phenytoin.

Trigeminal neuralgia is the most frequent of all neuralgias. The onset is usually in middle or late life, but may occur at any age. Typical trigeminal neuralgia has occasionally been reported in children under the age of 10 years, although it is distinctly uncommon before the age of 35. The incidence is slightly greater in women than in men.

The pains of trigeminal neuralgia occur in paroxysms. In the interval between attacks the patient is free of symptoms except for fear of an impending attack. The pains are described by the patients as searing or burning in nature, coming in lightning-like jabs in the distribution of one or more branches of the nerve. A paroxysm may last only 1 or 2 minutes or it may be prolonged for 15 minutes or longer. The frequency of attacks varies from many times daily to a few times a month. The patient ceases to talk when the pains strike. The affected individual may occasionally rub or pinch the face or make violent convulsive movements of the face and jaw (i.e., *tic convulsif*). Watering of the eye on the involved side may occur. There is no objective loss of cutaneous sensation during or following the paroxysms, but the patient may complain of hyperesthesia of the face. A characteristic feature of many cases is the presence of a trigger

zone, stimulation of which sets off one of the typical paroxysms. This is often a small area on the cheek, lip, or nose. The trigger zone may be stimulated by facial movements or by chewing. The patient may avoid making facial expressions during conversation or go without nourishment for days to prevent an attack of pain.

The pain is strictly limited to one or more branches of the fifth nerve and does not spread beyond the distribution of this nerve. The second or third division is more frequently involved, although the third branch is involved less frequently than the second. The first division is primarily affected in less than 5% of patients. Pain originally confined to one division may spread to one or both of the other divisions. In cases of long duration, all three divisions are affected in approximately 15%. The pain is occasionally bilateral (5%), but paroxysms on both sides at one time are rare.

The physical findings in patients with trigeminal neuralgia are normal. The patients may be undernourished or emaciated because of the fear of provoking an attack by eating. There is no objective sensory loss and motor function of the nerve is normal. The results of laboratory examinations are normal.

The diagnosis of trigeminal neuralgia can usually be made without difficulty from the description of the pain. Also characteristic is the method used by many patients to demonstrate the site of origin and mode of spread of the pain. They will not touch the area but with the tip of the index finger held a short distance fom the face they indicate the site of origin and spread of the painful spasm.

Trigeminal neuralgia must be differentiated from other types of pain that occur in the face or head, particularly infections of the teeth and nasal sinus. Although the pains of dental and nasal sinus disease differ from those of trigeminal neuralgia in that they are usually steady and throbbing and persist for many hours, many patients with trigeminal neuralgia have numerous operations on the sinuses and most of the teeth are removed before the diagnosis is established. Conversely, many patients with diseased teeth are referred to neurologists with the diagnosis of trigeminal neuralgia. In these cases, the role of the diseased tooth in the production of pain can be demonstrated by syringing it and the surrounding gum tissue with ice water.

The pain of herpes zoster may simulate that of trigeminal neuralgia, but the appearance of the vesicles establishes the correct diagnosis. Postherpetic neuralgia in the face is practically always in the distribution of the first division and differs from trigeminal neuralgia in its continuous nature.

Glossopharyngeal neuralgia may be confused with neuralgia of the third division of the trigeminal nerve. The diagnosis of glossopharyngeal neuralgia can be established by spraying the tonsillar region with local anesthetics.

Tumors of the gasserian ganglion, as well as tumors and other lesions in the cerebellopontine angle, may produce pain in the face. The facial pain that results from lesions of the nerve differs from that of trigeminal neuralgia in that it is steady and lasts for many hours or days, although it is occasionally paroxysmal. Areas of anesthesia in the face, loss of the corneal reflex, atrophy and weakness of the masticatory muscles, and evidence of involvement of other cranial nerves exclude the diagnosis of trigeminal neuralgia.

Persistent or remitting neuralgic pains in the head, face, and neck that differ from trigeminal neuralgia in that they are not confined to the distribution of the trigeminal nerve have been classified under the term of *atypical facial pain*. It is thought by some that they are caused by a disturbance of the sympathetic nervous system or that they are a variant of migraine. Relief of symptoms has been reported following surgery on the cervical and dorsal sympathetic ganglia and after sectioning of the greater petrosal nerve or of the periarterial sympathetic nerves. The area adjacent to the temporal artery is most frequently the site of this type of pain. In some cases these pains are a manifestation of conversion hysteria or depression.

Pains in the face may occur in patients who have degenerative changes in the temporomandibular joint as a result of malocclusion of the teeth. Radiographic evidence of changes in the joint helps to establish this diagnosis. The symptoms are relieved by the correction of malocclusion.

The course of trigeminal neuralgia is characterized by remissions. In most patients the paroxysms of pain are present for several weeks or months and then cease spontaneously. The remission may be of short duration or the pains may be entirely absent for months or even years. There is a tendency for the attack-free intervals to become shorter as the patient grows older, but a permanent disappearance of the symptoms is rare. Trigeminal neuralgia is never fatal in itself but frequent paroxysms may incapacitate the patient; even the fear of an impending attack may prevent activity. Most of the patients bear their pains stoically and suicide or morphine addiction is rare.

Many unsuccessful forms of medical therapy have been recommended in the past for the treatment of trigeminal neuralgia. The pains are so severe that they are not relieved by analgesic drugs except opiates, the use of which is contraindicated. Phenytoin injected intravenously aborts an acute attack and daily administration of the drug prevents recurrence of the pain in many of the patients. The dosage needed, 0.4 to 0.7 g daily, is greater than that tolerated by most patients. Another anticonvulsant has been found to be more effective with less toxic side effects; this drug, carbamazepine, produces a complete remission of symptoms in a high percentage of cases when used alone or in combination with phenytoin. The dose is 200 mg, 2 to 5 times daily.

Operative procedures have included alcohol injection of the nerve or ganglion, partial section of the nerve in the middle or posterior fossa, decompression of the root, and medullary tractotomy. The number of operations indicates that none of them has been entirely satisfactory because of complications of the procedure, failure to obtain relief, or numbness and paresthesias in the anesthetic areas. At present, percutaneous thermal destruction of the affected branch extracranially is the preferred treatment when medical therapy is ineffective. Decompression by separating anomalous vessels from the nerve root is increasingly popular.

SEVENTH (FACIAL) NERVE

As it leaves the brain stem, the facial nerve has two divisions, the motor root and the nervous intermedius. These two divisions have little in common from a physiologic point of view. The functions of the intermedius are much like those of the glossopharyngeal. It conducts taste sensation from the anterior two-thirds of the tongue and supplies autonomic fibers to the submaxillary and sphenopalatine ganglia that innervate the salivary and lacrimal glands. There is disagreement whether the seventh nerve has any somatic sensory function. It is thought to carry proprioceptive impulses from the facial muscles and cutaneous sensation from a small strip of skin on the posteromedial surface of the pinna and around the external auditory canal. In fact, however, sensory loss can rarely be detected in patients with lesions of the seventh nerve. Similarly, impairment of hearing is seldom found, although the ear may become more sensitive to low tones when the stapedius is paralyzed.

Injuries to the facial nerve cause paralysis of the facial muscles with or without loss of taste on the anterior two-thirds of the tongue and a disturbance in the secretion of the lacrimal and salivary glands depending on the portion of the nerve that is involved. Lesions of the nerve near its point of origin or in the region of the geniculate ganglion are accompanied by a paralysis of the motor, gustatory, and autonomic functions of the nerve. Lesions of the nerve between the geniculate ganglion and the point of separation of the chorda tympani produce the same dysfunction as that of injury in the region of the geniculate ganglion except that lacrimal secretion is not affected. Involvement of the nerve at the region of the stylomastoid foramen results only in paralysis of the facial muscles.

Lesions of the facial nucleus in the brain stem cause paralysis of all facial muscles. Lesions of the motor cortex or the connections between the cortex and the facial nucleus are accompanied by a partial paralysis, which is usually most severe in the muscles of the lower half of the face (supranuclear palsy). There may also be an inequality of the movement of the facial muscles to voluntary and emotional stimuli.

Because of their superficial site the peripheral branches of the seventh nerve are subject to injury by stab wounds, cuts, gunshot wounds, and the pressure of forceps at birth.

The nerve may occasionally be injured by pressure against a hard object in sleep. It may be injured in operations on the mastoid, in the operative treatment of acoustic neuromas or trigeminal neuralgia, and in operations on the parotid gland. Foerster reported facial nerve injury in 120 of 3907 cases (3%) of head injury in World War I. Comparable figures were reported by Russell in World War II. In a series of civilian head injuries, Friedman and Merritt found that the seventh nerve was injured in 7 of 430 patients (1.6%). Damage to the seventh nerve that accompanies head injury is commonly associated with fracture of the temporal bone and is usually present immediately after the injury. Occasionally, however, facial paralysis may not be manifested for several days after the accident. The mechanism of this delayed paralysis is not clear. Improvement is the rule when damage to the nerve is associated with head trauma, but recovery may not be complete.

Within the skull the nerve may be damaged by tumors, aneurysms, infections of the meninges, leukemia, osteomyelitis, herpes zoster, Paget disease, and sarcomas or other tumors of the bone. The nerve is occasionally affected in the course of generalized polyneuritis. It is involved in a large percentage of patients with Guillain-Barré syndrome and in diphtheritic polyneuropathy, but seldom in the diabetic or alcoholic forms. Involvement of the facial nerve is common in leprosy. The peripheral portion of the nerve may be compressed by tumors of the parotid gland. A few cases with recurrent facial palsy in association with facial edema, cheilitis, lingua plicata, and migraine (Melkersson syndrome) have been reported. Facial palsy is rare in mumps but is common in uveoparotid fever or meningeal forms of sarcoidosis.

Bilateral facial palsy may be caused by many of the conditions that produce unilateral paralysis. It is most frequently seen in polyneuritis, leprosy, leukemia, and meningococcal meningitis.

The facial nucleus may be damaged by tumors, inflammatory lesions, vascular lesions, acute poliomyelitis, and multiple, sclerosis.

Bell Palsy

Paralysis of the seventh nerve may occur without any known cause. Bell palsy often follows exposure to cold as in riding in an open car, and is thought to be caused by swelling of the nerve within the fallopian canal. Bell palsy occurs at all ages, but is slightly more common in the third to fifth decades. The frequency of involvement on the two sides is approximately equal. The paralysis may recur occasionally, either on the same or the opposite side. There may be a tendency for familial occurrence of Bell palsy.

The onset of facial paralysis may be accompanied by a feeling of stiffness of the muscles, but facial pain is rarely present, except when the paralysis is the result of herpes zoster. There may be pain in the ipsilateral ear.

The signs of complete paralysis of the seventh nerve can be divided into motor, secretory, and sensory. When the damage is severe the facial paralysis is obvious, even when the face is at rest. There is sagging of the muscles of the lower half of the face and occasionally of the lower lid. The normal folds and lines around the lips, nose, and forehead are ironed out and the palpebral fissure is wider than normal. There is complete absence of all voluntary and associated movements of the facial and platysmal muscles. When the patient attempts to smile the lower facial muscles are pulled to the opposite side. This distortion of the facial muscles may give the false appearance of deviation of the protruded tongue or the open jaw. Saliva and food are likely to collect on the paralyzed side. The patient is unable to close the eye and, on attempting to do so, the eyeball can be seen to be diverted upward and slightly inward *(Bell phenomenon)*. When the lesion is peripheral to the ganglion the lacrimal fibers are spared and there is excessive collection of tears in the conjunctival sac because of failure of the tears to be expressed into the lacrimal duct by movements of the lids. The corneal reflex is absent as a result of paralysis of the upper lid; preservation of corneal sensation is manifested by blinking of the other lid. Secretion of tears is diminished only when the lesion is proximal to the geniculate ganglion. Decrease in salivary secretion and loss of the sense of taste in the anterior two-thirds of the tongue are present when the chorda tympani is affected.

Although the seventh nerve presumably transmits proprioceptive sense from the facial muscles and cutaneous sensation from a small area of the pinna and the external auditory canal, loss of these sensations is rarely detected.

Partial injury to the facial nerve causes weakness of the upper and lower halves of the face. Occasionally, however, the lower half may be more affected than the upper half. More rarely, the opposite occurs.

Recovery from facial paralysis depends on the severity of the lesion. If the nerve is anatomically sectioned the chances of complete or even partial recovery are remote. In the vast majority of patients, especially those with Bell palsy, partial or complete recovery occurs. With complete recovery there is no apparent difference between the two sides of the face, either at rest or on motion. When recovery is partial there is a tendency for contractures to develop on the paralyzed side so that on superficial inspection it appears that there is weakness of the muscles on the normal side. The inaccuracy of this impression becomes obvious as soon as the patient smiles or attempts to move the facial muscles. Abnormal movements of the facial muscles and disturbance in the secretion of the lacrimal gland are not infrequent sequelae of a facial palsy. There may be a slight twitch of the labial muscles whenever the patient blinks or an excess secretion of tears when the salivary glands are activated in eating. In addition to the twitching movements of the labial muscles synchronous with blinking there may be paroxysmal clonic contractions of all facial muscles, simulating focal jacksonian seizures. These spasms are occasionally seen in patients who have never had any obvious lesion of the facial nerve. The cause of these sequelae is not known. They are attributed by some researchers to misdirection of the regenerated fibers and by others to the result of spread of impulses in the fibers of the nerve.

The differential diagnosis between facial paralysis caused by a cortical lesion and that resulting from a lesion of the nucleus or nerve can be made without difficulty except when weakness is barely evident. Other signs of cortical involvement, sparing of the muscles of the forehead and upper lid, and the preservation of electrical reactions all indicate a supranuclear lesion. In addition, the weakness of a peripheral lesion is equal for all movements, whereas in supranuclear lesions there may be a discrepancy between the extent of volitional and emotional movements. Volitional contractions may be greater or less than those that occur when the patient smiles or laughs.

The differentiation between lesions of the nucleus and the nerve is made by associated findings. Lesions in the tegmentum of the brain stem are accompanied by paralysis of lateral gaze caused by concomitant injury to the sixth nucleus. Lesions in the basal part of the brain stem are accompanied by signs of involvement of the corticospinal tract. Lesions of the nerve at the point of emergence from the brain stem by tumors, meningitis, or other infections are manifested by the association of paralysis of the facial nerve with paralysis of the eighth, sixth, and possibly, the fifth nerves.

It is obvious that attempts should be made to remove the lesion that is causing the facial paralysis when a lesion is found. Local treatment of the facial muscles is considered desirable by some clinicians. The purpose of this treatment is to relieve the strain on the relaxed muscles and to preserve tone by splinting and massaging the paralyzed muscles. Others advise electrical stimulation but these treatments are of unproven value.

Surgical procedures are often helpful when spontaneous recovery does not occur. Neurolysis or end-to-end suture may be indicated in extra-cranial lesions of the nerve or its branches. When the nerve damage is proximal to the stylomastoid foramen end-to-end suture is not possible, and restoration of innervation of the facial muscle can only be obtained by suturing the distal portion of the seventh nerve with the central portion of one of the other cranial nerves. Either the eleventh or twelfth cranial nerve can be used. When the eleventh nerve is used there is permanent paralysis of the sternomastoid and upper fibers of the trapezius. This results in slight deformity, but contractions of the facial muscles occur whenever the patient attempts to turn the head or elevate the shoulder. Sooner or later a new motor pattern is developed in the cerebral cortex and the movements of the facial muscles are dissociated from those of the shoulder. Anastomosis of the twelfth nerve with the seventh nerve is followed by atrophy and paralysis of half of the tongue. This causes little discomfort and control of the facial muscles is developed without any apparent adventitious movement of other muscles.

Anastomosis of the facial nerve with either the eleventh or twelfth nerve should be performed as soon as possible when the nerve is cut in mastoid surgery or in the removal of acoustic neuromas. In other types of peripheral facial paralysis it should be delayed for 6 months or more to determine whether spontaneous regeneration is likely to occur.

Steroids have been recommended for Bell palsy on the basis of relieving edema. Reports of this form of therapy have not been convincing because therapeutic trials have not been adequately controlled and because some improvement is seen spontaneously in almost all cases.

Decompression of the nerve in the canal is recommended by some otologists to expedite and enhance return of function in patients with Bell palsy. The operation is usually performed 6 weeks after the onset of the paralysis but the value of this approach is debated.

Surgery may be necessary to alleviate the facial spasm that occurs spontaneously or after partial regeneration of the injured nerve. The nerve or one of its branches can be injected with alcohol or partially sectioned when the spasms are localized. These operations occasionally give permanent relief from the spasms but the spasms usually recur when the nerve regenerates. Permanent relief can be obtained by anastomosing the seventh nerve with the eleventh or twelfth cranial nerve.

Blepharospasm, Myokymia, and Hemifacial Spasm

Blepharospasm is a state of forceful closure of the eye. Unilateral and repeated brief blepharospasm is now regarded as a form of focal dystonia, and may be part of hemifacial spasm. Bilateral blepharospasm may be seen in basal ganglia disorders, especially parkinsonism. The combination of blepharospasm and oromandibular movement is called *Meige syndrome.* Injections of small amounts of botulinum toxin have been shown to be effective and safe in treating blepharospasm.

The term *facial myokymia* refers to a condition of fine rippling movements of facial muscles. Persistent facial myokymia is sometimes a manifestation of multiple sclerosis, brain stem glioma, or other pathology in the brain stem. These CNS lesions presumably interrupt descending inhibitory impulses that act on motor neurons in the facial nucleus, releasing the involuntary activity. Myokymia can also arise peripherally, however, and is frequently seen in the acute phase of the Guillain-Barré syndrome.

Hemifacial spasm is characterized by clonic spasms of facial muscles, usually starting around the eye and then spreading to other muscles of one side of the face. It does not have the same ominous implications of myokymia but the cosmetic effects are often distressing and interfere with the patient's daily life. The cause is often obscure, but Jannetta has reported relief of the involuntary movements by exploring the facial nerve in the posterior fossa and then removing aberrant blood vessels that may compress the nerve.

EIGHTH (ACOUSTIC) NERVE

Symptoms of involvement of the cochlear branch of the eighth nerve are tinnitus and loss of hearing; those of involvement of the vestibular portion are vertigo, disturbance of equilibrium, and impairment of ocular movements.

The loss of hearing that follows infections in the middle ear or changes in the ossicles without injury to the nerve is only for air conduction. Bone conduction is normal, although it may appear to be more acute than normal in the Weber test. Loss of hearing is total and permanent when the cochlear branch is anatomically severed. Partial lesions of the nerve or the nuclei in the brain stem produce a diminution of auditory acuity that is greatest for high tones and is frequently accompanied by tinnitus; bone conduction and air conduction are equally diminished. Unilateral lesions of the secondary connections in the brain stem or thalamus are not accompanied by loss of hearing because of the bilateral nature of these connections. Bilateral loss of hearing is possible with destructive lesions of the trapezoid body in the pons. There is no unilateral degradation in auditory acuity or differential tonal discrimination when one insulotemporal region of the cortex is destroyed because each cochlea has a physiologic representation of equal value in both medial geniculate bodies and in both cerebral hemispheres. There is, however, slight reduction in acuity of bilateral audition without any loss in differential tonal discrimination. Bilateral destruction of the primary auditory receptive cortex causes serious loss of auditory acuity. The threshold rises about 60 dB, which means that all but the loudest sounds of daily life become inaudible. In addition there is complete loss of ability to distinguish between tones and configurations of sound.

Lesions in the secondary auditory centers in the superior temporal convolution of the dominant cortex impair the understanding of spoken words (auditory agnosia). This is often accompanied by loss of ability to understand writing because of the association of the printed image with the sound of the word.

Acquired (unbalanced) disturbance of the function of the vestibular nerves or nuclei produces vertigo, disturbance of equilibrium, and nystagmus. These symptoms are most prominent in acute unilateral lesions that do not completely destroy the nerve or the nucleus and are minimal when the nerve is sectioned or completely destroyed. Lesions of the vestibular connections with the cerebellum produce a less severe disturbance of equilibrium. Injury to the medial longitudinal fasciculus, which is one of the main connections of the vestibular nuclei with other nuclei in the brain stem, causes nystagmus when the lesion is in the medulla or the upper part of the cervical cord. If the medial longitudinal fasciculus is damaged in the pons there is a peculiar dissociation of eye movements (*internuclear ophthalmoplegia*). The main feature of this condition, when it is unilateral, is failure of the medial rectus on that side to function on attempted lateral gaze. There is also likely to be impairment of movement of the opposite lateral rectus (so that there is a gaze palsy) and nystagmus in the abducting eye. In young adults internuclear ophthalmoplegia is usually caused by multiple sclerosis. In older people the syndrome is usually caused by brain-stem infarction. Tumors may also cause the disorder.

The nuclei of the eighth nerve may be involved in infections, tumors, vascular lesions, and demyelinating diseases. The peripheral portion of the nerve may be damaged by inflammatory processes in the meninges (especially acute purulent tuberculous or mumps meningitis), tumors in the cerebellopontine angle, infections in the ear and mastoid process, or degenerative or toxic disorders in the middle or inner ear. The auditory portion of the nerve is often involved in spinocerebellar degenerations and other hereditary diseases.

The eighth nerve can be damaged by many toxic substances, including drugs. The most common of the toxic drugs are acetylsalicylic acid, quinine, and streptomycin. The site of the damage caused by these substances is not known but it is presumed to be labyrinthine or retrolabyrinthine. A high incidence of vestibular disturbance and a sizable number of cases of deafness, either transient or permanent, occur with the use of streptomycin if large doses of the drug are given over prolonged periods. Generally, the otitic symptoms appear between the seventeenth and twentieth day if a dosage as high as 3 g daily is given.

Impairment of hearing in one or both ears occurs in about 8% of those with craniocerebral injuries. Fracture of the middle fossa of the skull is the usual cause. The fracture generally involves the middle ear and the resulting loss of hearing is partial and of the middle ear type. When the inner ear or the nerve is damaged the hearing loss is likely to be total and there is a loss of vestibular reactions. Traumatic lesions of the eighth nerve are often associated with injury to the facial nerve. Tinnitus usually follows damage to the inner or middle ear. True vertigo in patients with head injury is usually caused by concussion of or hemorrhage into the labyrinth. Some clinicians attribute the dizziness on change of posture, which is a prominent feature of the post-traumatic syndrome, to minor damage to the labyrinth.

Impairment of hearing is a common accompaniment of aging, occurring in more than 60% of patients older than 80. Dizziness and vertigo are also present in many elderly patients.

Damage to the eighth nerve from whatever cause is likely to have permanent effects. Improvement in hearing occurs in a fair percentage of patients with traumatic injury to the nerve. Loss of hearing as a result of damage to the nerve by infections in the meninges or by toxic substances is usually permanent, probably as a result of destruction of the inner ear.

Complete destruction of one labyrinth or the vestibular portion of the eighth nerve is not usually accompanied by any disturbance of equilibrium. Ataxia of a moderate or severe degree occurs when both labyrinths or vestibular nerves are affected. The degree of ataxia decreases when the patient learns to compensate for this defect, but difficulty will always be present on attempts to walk in the dark. Functional disturbance of the labyrinth may occur as an isolated event (acute labyrinthitis) or there may be recurrent attacks (Meniere syndrome; see Section 147).

The acute onset of symptoms of dysfunction of the labyrinth—vertigo, disturbance of equilibrium, nausea, and vomiting—is known as *acute labyrinthitis*. These symptoms are the same as those of Meniere syndrome, although in acute labyrinthitis the symptoms are not recurrent and the duration is much longer than that of Meniere syndrome.

The cause of acute labyrinthitis is unknown. It often follows a head cold. It is presumed that the infection spreads to the inner ear. Against this hypothesis, however, is the fact that the symptoms may occur without any antecedent infection of the nasopharynx.

Acute labyrinthitis may occur in patients at any age and affects both sexes equally. The signs and symptoms (i.e., severe vertigo, nausea, disturbance of equilibrium, nystagmus) are of sudden onset and may last for several days or weeks. Tinnitus and loss of hearing are usually absent or inconspicuous. During the attack there is photophobia and headache and the gait is ataxic. The patient prefers a darkened room and lies quietly in bed without turning the head. Food may be refused because of the nausea and vomiting. After several days or weeks the vertigo diminishes and the nystagmus disappears. There is no specific treatment. Antihistamines or small doses of tranquilizer may be of value.

Acute labyrinthitis must be distinguished from stroke and multiple sclerosis. Stroke can usually be diagnosed by the signs and symptoms of involvement of other structures in the brain stem. Multiple sclerosis is recognized by the history of previous attacks of the disease or evidence of injury to other parts of the nervous system. Involvement of the vestibular nuclei may occasionally be the first manifestation of multiple sclerosis. A definite diagnosis cannot be made until further evidence of the disease develops. Persistence of nystagmus after complete subsidence of the vertigo favors the diagnosis of multiple sclerosis.

NINTH (GLOSSOPHARYNGEAL) NERVE

The ninth nerve contains both motor and sensory fibers. The motor fibers supply the stylopharyngeus muscle and the constrictors of the pharynx. The sensory fibers carry general sensation from the upper part of the pharynx and the special sensation of taste from the posterior third of the tongue.

Isolated lesions of the peripheral nerve or its nuclei are rare and are not accompanied by any significant disability. Taste is lost on the posterior third of the tongue and the gag reflex is absent on the side of the lesion. Injuries of the ninth nerve by infections or tumors are usually accompanied by signs of involvement of the neighboring nerves. The tractus solitarius receives taste fibers from both the seventh and ninth nerves and may be destroyed by vascular or neoplastic lesions in the brain stem. The ninth nerve is occasionally the seat of glossopharyngeal neuralgia.

Glossopharyngeal neuralgia (tic douloureux of the ninth nerve) is characterized by paroxysms of excruciating pain in the region of the tonsils, posterior pharynx, back of the tongue, and middle ear. The cause of glossopharyngeal neuralgia is unknown and there are no significant pathologic changes in most cases. Pains in the distribution of the nerve may occasionally be associated with injury to the nerve in the neck by tumors.

Glossopharyngeal neuralgia is rare, occurring about 5% as often as trigeminal neuralgia. Men are more frequently affected than women. The symptoms may develop in patients at any age, but the onset is most frequently in the fourth and fifth decades.

The pain of glossopharyngeal neuralgia, except for its distribution, is exactly like that of trigeminal neuralgia. The pains occur in paroxysms, are burning or stabbing in nature, and are localized to the region of the tonsils, posterior pharynx, back of the tongue, and the middle ear. They may occur spontaneously but are often precipitated by swallowing, talking, or touching the tonsils or posterior pharynx. The attacks usually last only a few seconds but are occasionally prolonged for several minutes. The frequency of attacks varies from many times daily to once in several weeks. Long remissions are common.

The diagnosis of glossopharyngeal neuralgia can be made from the description of the pain. The only differential diagnosis of any importance is neuralgia of the mandibular branch of the fifth nerve. The diagnosis of glossopharyngeal neuralgia is established when an attack of pain can be precipitated by stimulation of the tonsils, posterior pharynx, or base of the tongue, or when the pains are relieved by spraying the affected area with local anesthetic. When the membrane becomes anesthetic the pains disappear and they cannot be precipitated by stimulation with an applicator. During this period the patient can swallow food and talk without discomfort.

The paroxysms of pain occur at irregular intervals and there may be long remissions. During a remission the trigger zone disappears. The pains almost always recur unless they are prevented by medical therapy or the nerve is sectioned surgically. The disease does not shorten life but affected patients may become emaciated because of the fear that each morsel of food will precipitate a pain paroxysm.

Carbamazepine, alone or in combination with phenytoin, is effective in producing a remission of symptoms in many patients. If medical therapy is not effective the nerve can

be sectioned intracranially. The results of the operation are satisfactory. The patient is relieved of the pains and there are no serious sequelae. The mucous membrane supplied by the ninth nerve is permanently anesthetized with loss of the gag reflex of this side. Taste is lost on the posterior third of the tongue. There are no motor difficulties, such as dysphagia or dysarthria, unless the tenth nerve is injured during surgery.

TENTH (VAGUS) NERVE

The fibers of the tenth nerve from the nucleus ambiguus innervate the muscles of the pharynx and larynx; the fibers from the dorsal motor nucleus supply the autonomic innervation of the heart, lungs, esophagus, and stomach.

Unilateral lesions of the nucleus ambiguus in the medulla cause dysarthria and dysphagia. Because the nucleus has a considerable longitudinal extent in the medulla lesions in the brain stem may produce dysarthria without dysphagia, or vice versa, according to the site of the lesion. Lesions confined to the lower portion of the nucleus cause dysphagia, whereas lesions of the upper portion produce dysarthria.

The dysphagia or dysarthria that follows unilateral lesions of the nucleus ambiguus is rarely severe. The voice may be hoarse but speech is intelligible. There is usually only slight difficulty in swallowing solid food but occasionally there is a transient aphagia that necessitates the administration of food by tube for a few days or weeks. On examination the palate on the affected side is lax and the uvula deviates to the opposite side on phonation. The palatal reflex is absent on the affected side. Lesions of the nucleus ambiguus on both sides cause complete aphonia and aphagia. Bilateral destruction of this nucleus is rare except in the terminal stages of ALS.

Selective destruction of cells in the nucleus ambiguus may occur in syringobulbia or intramedullary tumors, causing paralysis of the vocal cords in adduction. The patient can talk and swallow without difficulty but inspiratory stridor and dyspnea may be severe enough to require tracheotomy.

Unilateral lesions of the dorsal motor nucleus are not accompanied by any symptoms of autonomic dysfunction. Bilateral lesions are life-threatening.

The nuclei of the tenth nerve may be damaged by infections (especially acute polio-

myelitis), intramedullary tumors, syringobulbia, vascular lesions, and ALS.

The nerve or its branches may be involved
in polyneuropathy, especially in the diphtheritic and Guillain-Barré forms, or may be compressed by tumors or aneurysms.

Injury to the pharyngeal branches of the
nerve results in difficulty swallowing. Lesions
of the superior laryngeal nerve produce anesthesia of the upper part of the larynx and
paralysis of the cricothyroid muscle. The
voice is weak and soon tires. Involvement of
the recurrent laryngeal nerve, which is frequent with aneurysms of the aorta and which
occasionally occurs after operations in the
neck, causes hoarseness and dysphonia as a
result of paralysis of the vocal cords. Complete paralysis of both recurrent laryngeal
nerves produces aphonia and inspiratory stridor. Partial bilateral paralysis may produce a
paralysis of both abductors with severe dyspnea and inspiratory stridor; it does not, however, cause any alteration in the voice.

Unilateral lesions of the vagus nerve do not
produce any constant disturbance of the autonomic functions of the nerve. The heart rate
may be unchanged, slowed, or accelerated.
The respiratory rhythm is not affected and
there is no significant disturbance in the action of the gastrointestinal tract.

ELEVENTH (SPINAL ACCESSORY) NERVE

The spinal portion of the eleventh nerve
innervates the sternomastoid and part or all
of the trapezius muscles. The fibers from the
accessory portion of the nerve have their origin in the nucleus ambiguus and join with
the tenth nerve to innervate the larynx. Paralysis of the spinal portion causes weakness
and atrophy of the sternomastoid muscle and
partial atrophy of the trapezius muscles.
There is weakness of rotary movements of the
head to the opposite side and weakness of
shrugging movements of the shoulder.

The nucleus of the eleventh nerve may be
destroyed by infections and degenerative disorders in the medulla (e.g., syringobulbia,
ALS). The peripheral portion of the nerve
may be involved in polyneuropathy, infections of the meninges, extra-medullary tumors, or necrotic processes in the occipital
bone. The muscles supplied by this nerve are
frequently involved in myotonic muscular
dystrophy, polymyositis, and myasthenia
gravis.

TWELFTH (HYPOGLOSSAL) NERVE

The hypoglossal nerve is the motor nerve
to the tongue. The nucleus in the medulla or
the peripheral nerve may be injured by all the
processes mentioned in connection with the
tenth and eleventh nuclei. Occlusion of the
short branches of the basilar artery that nour-
ish the paramedian area of the medulla causes
paralysis of the tongue on one side and of the
arm and leg on the opposite side (alternating
hemiplegia).

Unilateral injury to the nucleus or nerve
results in atrophy and paralysis of the muscles of half of the tongue. When the tongue
is protruded it deviates toward the paralyzed
side and, while protruded, movement toward
the normal side is absent or weakly performed. When the tongue lies on the floor of
the mouth it deviates slightly toward the
healthy side and movement of the tongue toward the back of the mouth on this side is
impaired. Fibrillation of the muscles is seen
in chronic processes involving the hypoglossal nucleus (e.g., syringobulbia, ALS).

Bilateral paralysis of the nucleus or nerve
produces atrophy of both sides of the tongue
and paralysis of all movements, with severe
dysarthria and resultant difficulty in manipulating food in the process of eating.

The tongue is only rarely affected by lesions
in the cerebral hemispheres or corticobulbar
connections. Homolateral weakness of the
tongue may occasionally accompany severe
hemiplegia. This is manifested by a slight deviation of the tongue to the paralyzed side
when it is protruded. Moderate weakness of
the tongue may accompany pseudobulbar
palsy, but this is never as severe as that which
occurs with destruction of both medullary nuclei.

Tremors of the tongue are seen in chronic
alcoholism. Apraxia of the tongue (i.e., inability to protrude the tongue on command,
but preservation of the associated movements
in eating or licking the lips) is a frequent accompaniment of motor aphasia.

Peripheral Nerves

The peripheral nerves are subject to injury
by pressure, constriction by fascial bands, and
trauma associated with injection of drugs,
perforating wounds, fractures of the bones,
or stretching of the nerves. Isolated or multiple nerve paralysis may also be associated
with a reaction to the injection of serum or to
certain toxic or metabolic disturbances.

The radial, common peroneal, ulnar, and long thoracic nerves are subject to damage by external pressure. The median nerve is most frequently affected by constriction by fascial bands at the wrist. The axillary nerve is commonly affected in an allergic reaction to injections of serum. The sciatic nerve is affected by direct injection of drugs. Any of the peripheral nerves may be damaged by perforating wounds or fractures of the bones. The frequency of the involvement of the peripheral nerves by trauma is shown in Table 59–3.

NERVES OF THE ARM

Radial Nerve

The radial nerve arises from the posterior secondary trunk of the brachial plexus (C5–C8). It is predominantly a motor nerve and innervates the chief extensors of the forearm, wrist, and fingers (Table 59–4).

The radial nerve may be injured by cuts, gunshot wounds, callus formation after fracture of the humerus, pressure of crutches, or

Table 59–3.   The Incidence of Peripheral Nerve Lesions by Trauma

Nerve	No. of Cases	% of Cases
Medial	707	19.3
Radial	516	14.1
Ulnar	1000	27.4
Musculocutaneous	44	1.2
Axillary	9	.2
Sciatic-peroneal	404	11.1
Sciatic-tibial	394	10.8
Peroneal	341	9.3
Tibial	235	6.4
Femoral	6	0.2
	3656	100.0

(Modified from Woodhall B, Beebe GW. Peripheral Nerve Regeneration. A Follow-Up Study of 3656 World War II Injuries. Washington DC: Veterans Administration Monographs, 1956.)

Table 59–4.   Muscles Innervated by the Radial Nerve

In the Arm	In the Forearm
Triceps	Extensor digitorum
Anconeus	Extensor digiti minimi
Extensor carpi radialis longus	Extensor carpi ulnaris
Extensor carpi radialis brevis	Abductor pollicis longus
Brachioradialis	Extensor pollicis brevis
	Extensor indicis

pressure against some hard surface, especially in sleep ("Saturday night palsy").

A complete lesion of the nerve in the axilla is characterized by paralysis of the triceps and abolition of the triceps reflex in addition to the other signs of radial nerve palsy discussed below. Lesions of the radial nerve in the axilla are usually accompanied by evidence of injury to other nerves in this region. When the nerve is injured in the posteromedial surface of the arm one or more of the branches to the triceps may be spared so that weakness of extension of the forearm is minimal.

The most common site of injury to the radial nerve is in the middle third of the arm proximal to the branch to the brachioradialis muscle. Lesions of the nerve at this level result in weakness of flexion of the forearm caused by the paralysis of the brachioradialis muscle, which is a stronger flexor of the forearm than the biceps, and paralysis of extension of the wrist, thumb, and fingers at the proximal joints. Extension at the distal phalanges is performed by the interossei. There is weakness of adduction of the hand as a result of loss of action of the extensor carpi ulnaris and loss of supination when the forearm is extended because the supinating action of the biceps is evident only when the forearm is flexed. In addition there is an apparent weakness of flexion of the fingers. This weakness is not real and is a result of the faulty posture of the hand. If the wrist is passively extended it will be seen that the fingers have normal power of flexion.

Sensory loss associated with lesions of the radial nerve is slight and is confined in most cases to a small area on the posterior radial surface of the hand and of the first and second metacarpals of the thumb and of the index and middle fingers.

Lesions of the nerve or its branches in the forearm or wrist are accompanied by fragments of the syndrome described above, according to the site of the lesion.

Complete lesions of the radial nerve are followed by atrophy of the paralyzed muscles. Vasomotor or trophic disturbances are rare unless there is an associated vascular lesion. Causalgia rarely follows partial injury to the nerve.

Median Nerve

The median nerve is composed of fibers from the sixth, seventh, and eighth cervical and first thoracic roots. It arises in two heads (outer and inner), which are derived from the upper and lower secondary trunks of the brachial plexus. It has important motor and sensory functions. The following movements are controlled by this nerve: pronation of the forearm by the pronator quadratus and pronator radii teres; flexion of the hand by the flexor carpi radialis and palmaris longus; flexion of the thumb and index and middle fingers by the superficial and deep flexors; and opposition of the thumb (Table 59–5).

The sensory region of the median nerve comprises the radial side of the palm of the hand, the palmar surface of the thumb, and index, middle, and neighboring half of the ring finger, the dorsal surface of the middle and terminal phalanges of the index finger, and the radial half of the ring finger.

The median nerve may be injured by dislocation of the shoulder, perforating wounds of the arm, or the pressure of a tourniquet. It may be cut at the wrist by glass or other sharp-edged instruments in attempts at suicide and by constriction in the carpal tunnel.

Injury to the median nerve in the arm is characterized by loss of ability to pronate the forearm, weakness of flexion of the wrist, paralysis of flexion of the thumb and index finger, weakness of flexion of the middle finger, paralysis of opposition of the thumb, atrophy of the muscles of the thenar eminence, and loss of sensation in an area somewhat smaller than that of the anatomic distribution of the nerve.

Lesions of the median nerve at the wrist cause paralysis and atrophy of the thenar muscles and sensory loss in the characteristic distribution.

There is absolute paralysis of few movements of the wrist or fingers in isolated lesions of the median nerve because of the compensatory action of unparalyzed muscles. Pronation can be accomplished by the action of the deltoid in holding the arm outward

when the forearm is flexed and by rotation of the arm inward by the subscapularis when the arm is extended. Flexion of the wrist can be performed by the action of the flexor carpi ulnaris, with deviation of the hand toward the ulnar side of the arm. There is absence of flexion in the index and middle fingers, although the middle finger is usually influenced by movements of the ring finger and its deep flexor may be supplied by the ulnar nerve. In addition, flexion of the proximal phalanx of the fingers, including the index finger in association with extension of the distal phalanges, is possible through the action of the interossei. Although the opponens pollicis is paralyzed, feeble movements of opposition can be made by energetic contraction of the adductors that cause the thumb to move to the ulnar edge of the hand by pressing against the base of the fingers.

Partial lesions of the median nerve are more frequent than complete interruption, with dissociation in the degree of involvement of the various muscles supplied by the nerve and with little or no sensory loss. Flexion of the index finger and opposition of the thumb are the movements that are usually most affected in partial lesions.

Vasomotor disturbances are common with median nerve lesions, probably because of associated lesions of blood vessels. The syndrome of causalgia is most commonly associated with lesions of the median nerve.

A slowly developing atrophy limited to the muscles of the outer radial side of the thenar eminence has been described by the term *partial thenar atrophy.* The atrophy is often bilateral and exceeds the motor weakness. Pain, paresthesias, and a mild degree of impairment of sensation in the distribution of the nerves, with or without motor weakness, are fairly common as result of compression of the nerve by the transverse carpal segment *(carpal tunnel syndrome).* The pain is quite severe, often waking patients from sleep. The pain is usually in the thumb and index finger but may spread to other fingers or up the arm to the axilla. These symptoms occur most commonly in middle-aged patients and are often associated with arthritis or other changes in the tendons and connective tissues of wrists in amyloid disease, myxedema, gout, or acromegaly. Surgical division of the transverse ligament results in relief of the pains and paresthesias and gradual decrease of the weakness.

Table 59–5.   Muscles Innervated by the Median Nerve

In the Forearm	In the Hand
Pronator teres	Abductor pollicis
Flexor carpi radialis	Flexor pollicis brevis
Palmaris longus	Opponens pollicis
Flexor digitorum sublimis	First and second lumbricals
Flexor digitorum profundus (radial half)	
Flexor pollicis longus	
Pronatus quadratus	

Table 59–6. Muscles Innervated by the Ulnar Nerve

In the Forearm	In the Hand
Flexor carpi ulnaris	Adductor pollicis
Flexor digitorum profundus (ulnar half)	Flexor pollicis brevis
	Interossei
	Third and fourth lumbricals
	Palmaris brevis
	Abductor digiti minimi
	Opponens digiti minimi
	Flexor digiti minimi
	Lumbricalis (ulnar half)

Ulnar Nerve

The ulnar nerve is the main branch of the lower secondary trunk of the brachial plexus. The fibers arise from the eighth cervical and first thoracic segments. The motor fibers innervate the muscles shown in Table 59–6. The sensory portion of the nerve supplies the skin on the palmar and dorsal surfaces of the little finger, the inner half of the ring finger, and the ulnar side of the hand.

The ulnar nerve is frequently injured by gunshot wounds, stab wounds, and fractures of the lower end of the humerus, olecranon, or head of the radius. The nerve may be compressed in the axilla by a cervical rib. More frequently, it is compressed at the elbow in sleep or as an occupational neuritis in workers who rest their elbows on hard surfaces for prolonged periods.

Complete lesions of the ulnar nerve are characterized by weakness of flexion and adduction of the wrist and of flexion of the ring and little fingers, paralysis of abduction and opposition of the little finger, paralysis of adduction of the thumb, and paralysis of adduction and abduction of the fingers. There is atrophy of the hypothenar muscles and the interossei. Atrophy of the interossei is especially obvious between the thumb and index finger on the dorsal surface of the hand. Sensory loss is greatest in the little finger and is present to a lesser extent on the inner side of the ring finger. There is clawing of the hand.

Dissociated paralysis of the muscles supplied by the ulnar nerve may occur with partial lesions of the nerve in the arm or forearm.

Trophic and vasomotor symptoms are not a prominent feature of complete lesions of the nerve. There may be some hyperkeratosis or changes in the palmar fascia. Irritative lesions may be accompanied by pain, but injuries to the ulnar nerve are only rarely accompanied by causalgia.

The diagnosis of ulnar palsy can usually be made without difficulty by the posture of the hand, which is always clawed, by the atrophy of the hypothenar eminence and the first dorsal interosseous space, and by the characteristic muscular paralysis. One of the diagnostic signs of ulnar palsy, the *Froment sign,* is flexion of the terminal phalanx of the thumb when the patient attempts to hold a sheet of paper between the thumb and index finger.

Musculocutaneous Nerve

The musculocutaneous nerve is the main branch of the upper secondary trunk of the brachial plexus. Its fibers arise in the fifth, sixth, and seventh cervical segments. The musculocutaneous nerve is a mixed nerve, innervating the coracobrachialis, biceps brachii, and brachialis anticus muscles and transmitting cutaneous sensation from the anterior outer part and a small area on the posterior outer surface of the forearm. Isolated injuries of the nerve are rare. It may be involved in traumatic lesions of the brachial plexus.

Lesions of the musculocutaneous nerve produce weakness of flexion and supination of the forearm, a small area of hypesthesia or anesthesia on the anterior outer surface of the forearm, atrophy of the muscles on the anterior surface of the arm, and loss of the biceps reflex.

Flexor movements of the forearm can still be vigorously performed by the brachioradialis muscle, which is innervated by the radial nerve. If flexion is performed against resistance it can be noted by palpation that the biceps muscle is inactive. If the forearm is kept in supination forearm flexion is impossible. Because the biceps is the chief supinator of the forearm, this movement is paralyzed. Loss of function of the coracobrachialis muscle is compensated for by the action of other adductor muscles of the arm.

Axillary Nerve

The axillary nerve, which is a branch of the posterior secondary cord of the plexus with fibers from the fifth and sixth cervical segments, innervates the deltoid muscle and transmits cutaneous sensation from a small area on the lateral surface of the shoulder.

Lesions of the axillary nerve by trauma or by fractures or dislocation of the head of the humerus are usually associated with injury to the brachial plexus. The axillary nerve may be involved alone or in combination with other nerves in the neuritis that follows serum (especially antitetanus) therapy.

Lesions of the axillary nerve are characterized by loss of power in outward, backward, and forward movements of the arm because of paralysis of the deltoid muscle. The area of hypesthesia or anesthesia is inconstant and is much smaller than the anatomic distribution of the nerve.

Long Thoracic Nerve

The long thoracic nerve arises from the fifth, sixth, and seventh cervical roots. It is the motor nerve to the serratus magnus muscle.

Lesions of the long thoracic nerve are most common in men who do heavy labor. It may be injured by continued muscular effort with the arm extended or by carrying heavy sharp-cornered objects on the shoulder ("hod carrier's palsy").

Injury of the nerve following acute or chronic trauma is characterized by weakness in elevation of the arm above the horizontal plane. Winging of the scapula is a constant sign when the arm is fully abducted or elevated anteriorly (Fig. 59–2). Winging is usually absent when the arm is held at the side.

Brachial Cutaneous and Antebrachial Cutaneous Nerves

The brachial and antebrachial cutaneous nerves, branches of the lower secondary trunk of the plexus (C8–T1), are purely sensory in function. They transmit cutaneous sensation from the inner surface of the arm and upper two-thirds of the forearm.

These nerves are rarely affected except in injuries of the lower secondary trunk of the brachial plexus. Lesions of these nerves produce hypesthesia on the inner surface of the arm and forearm.

Suprascapular Nerve

The suprascapular nerve arises from the posterior surface of the outer trunk of the brachial plexus; most of its fibers come from the fifth and sixth cervical roots. It is primarily motor and innervates the supraspinatus and infraspinatus muscles.

Isolated lesions of the nerve are rare. It may be wounded directly, injured in falls, or stretched by muscular overaction. It may be involved in association with the axillary nerve in serum reactions or it may be injured in traumatic lesions of the brachial plexus.

Lesions of the nerve produce an atrophic paralysis of the supraspinatus and infraspinatus muscles. Weakness of movements performed by these muscles (i.e., abduction of

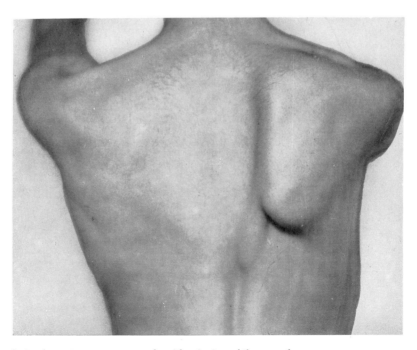

Fig. 59–2. Paralysis of serratus magnus muscle with winging of the scapula.

the shoulder and external rotation of the shoulder) is masked by the action of the deltoid and teres minor muscles.

THE BRACHIAL PLEXUS

The fourth, fifth, sixth, seventh, and eighth cervical roots and the first thoracic root contribute to the formation of the brachial plexus (Fig. 59–3). These roots intermingle to form three primary trunks (upper, middle, and lower). The upper primary trunk is composed of fibers from the fourth, fifth, and sixth cervical roots; the middle primary trunk is made of fibers from the seventh cervical roots; and the lower primary trunk is composed of fibers from the eighth cervical and first thoracic roots. From the primary trunks there is further redistribution of the fibers, which results in the formation of secondary trunks or cords (upper, posterior, and lower). The secondary trunks contribute to the formation of the peripheral nerves of the upper extremity as follows: upper secondary trunk, the musculocutaneous nerve and the outer head of the median; posterior trunk, the axillary and radial nerves; lower secondary trunk, the brachial and antebrachial cutaneous nerves, the ulnar nerve, and the inner head of the median nerve.

In addition to these major nerves, which are formed by fibers in the secondary trunks, collateral branches from the roots and trunks form nerves that innervate the shoulder and scapular muscles and supply fibers to the interior cervical ganglion.

From the arrangement of the plexus it is obvious that trauma affects different groups of nerve fibers according to the site of the lesion. Lesions in the axilla, where all the fibers converge, affect several trunks. Isolated trunk lesions are more likely to occur when the injury is in the supraclavicular fossa.

The roots or trunks of the brachial plexus may be damaged by cuts, gunshot wounds, or direct trauma. They may be compressed by tumors or aneurysms or stretched and torn by violent movements of the shoulder in falls, dislocations of the shoulder, the carrying of heavy packs on the shoulder ("rucksack paralysis"), and by traction in delivery at birth.

Unilateral or bilateral disorders of the brachial plexus may follow respiratory infections. The combination of local pain, weakness, and wasting of muscle had led to the popular terms "neuralgic amyotrophy" and "brachial plexus neuritis." Weakness is maximal within a few days. The CSF is normal. A similar disorder may affect the lumbosacral plexus. Myelography excludes intraspinal lesions. Nerve conduction studies may localize lesions of the brachial plexus. The condition remains stable for days or weeks and then improves. Some patients recover completely; others are left with moderate or severe disability.

Various complex syndromes result from injuries to the plexus. The number of combinations of motor paralysis and sensory loss are great but several root and trunk syndromes are relatively frequent. Only the trunk syndromes are discussed here. A minute examination of muscular and sensory disability must be made and studied in connection with anatomic charts of the plexus to determine the site of the lesion and whether the fibers have been injured at their point of

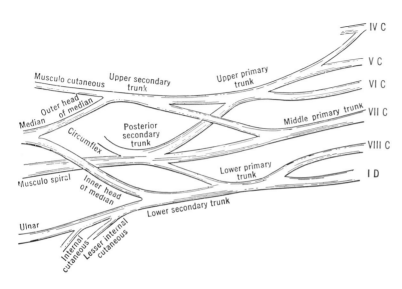

Fig. 59–3. Brachial plexus. Tinel J. Nerve Wounds. London: Balliere, Tindall & Cox, 1917.

emergence from the spinal cord or after the formation of the primary or secondary trunks (Tables 59–7, 59–8, and 59–9).

Radicular Syndromes (Roots and Primary Trunks)

The syndromes of the roots and primary trunks are essentially those of the roots involved but partial paralysis and incomplete sensory loss are common because many muscles of the arm receive innervation from two or more roots and there are extensive substitutions among the various roots.

Upper Radicular (Erb-Duchenne) Syndrome. Lesions of the upper roots (fourth, fifth, and sixth cervical roots or upper primary trunk) are characterized by paralysis of the deltoid, biceps, brachialis anticus, brachioradialis, pectoralis major, supraspinatus, intraspinatus, subscapularis, and teres major muscles. If the lesion is near the roots the serratus magnus, rhomboids, and levator anguli scapulae are also paralyzed. In addition, there is partial paralysis of the muscles supplied by the radial nerve because the upper primary trunk contributes to the formation of this nerve.

The motor disability resulting from lesions of the upper radicular group is essentially a paralysis of flexion of the forearm and of abduction and internal and external rotation of the arm. There is also weakness or paralysis of apposition of the shoulder blade and backward-inward movements of the arm. Sensory loss is incomplete and consists of hypesthesia on the outer surface of the arm and forearm. The biceps reflex is absent and percussion of the styloid process of the radius produces flexion of the fingers instead of the normal flexion of the forearm.

Middle Radicular Syndrome. Injury to the seventh cervical root or the middle primary trunk causes paralysis of the muscles supplied by the radial nerve with the exception of the brachioradialis, which is spared entirely, and the triceps, which is only partially paralyzed because it receives partial innervation from the upper primary trunk.

Weakness is essentially similar to that seen in paralysis of the radial nerve below the origin of the fibers to the brachioradialis or in lead palsy. Sensory loss is inconstant and, when present, is limited to hypesthesia over the dorsal surface of the forearm and the external part of the dorsal surface of the hand.

Lower Radicular (Klumpke) Syndrome. Injury to the lower primary trunk or eighth cervical and first thoracic root is characterized by paralysis of the flexor carpi ulnaris, the flexor digitorum, the interossei, and the thenar and hypothenar muscles. The motor disability is similar to that of a combined lesion of the median and ulnar nerves with a flattened or simian hand.

The sensory disturbance is hypesthesia on the inner side of the arm and forearm and on the ulnar side of the hand. The triceps reflex is abolished. If the communicating branch to the inferior cervical ganglion is injured there is paralysis of the sympathetic nerves, with resulting Horner syndrome.

Secondary Trunk Syndromes

Lesions of the secondary trunks of the brachial plexus produce motor and sensory dis-

Table 59–7.   Innervation of the Important Muscles of the Shoulder Girdle

Muscle	Nerve	Roots
Sternocleidomastoid	Spinal accessory	XI, C2, C3
Trapezius	Spinal accessory	C3, C4
Deltoid	Axillary	C5, C6
Pectoralis major	Exterior and interior anterior thoracic	C5–T2
Pectoralis minor	Exterior and interior anterior thoracic	C7–T2
Serratus magnus	Long thoracic	C5–C7
Levator anguli scapulae	Dorsal scapular	C5
Rhomboideus major	Dorsal scapular	C5
Rhomboideus minor	Dorsal scapular	C5
Latissimus dorsi	Long subscapular	C7, C8
Coracobrachialis	Musculocutaneous	C7
Supraspinatus	Suprascapular	C5, C6
Infraspinatus	Suprascapular	C5, C6
Teres major	Lower subscapular	C5, C6
Teres minor	Axillary	C5, C6
Subscapularis	Upper and lower subscapular	C5, C6

Table 59–8.   Innervation of the Important Muscles of the Arm and Forearm

Muscle	Nerve	Root
Biceps	Musculocutaneous	C5, C6
Brachialis {	Musculocutaneous	C5, C6
	Radial	C5, C6
Triceps	Radial	C6–C8
Anconeus	Radial	C7, C8
Pronator radii teres	Median	C6
Flexor carpi radialis	Median	C6
Palmaris longus	Median	C6
Flexor carpi ulnaris	Ulnar	C8
Flexor sublimis digitorum	Median	C7–T1
Flexor profundus digitorum	Median, ulnar	C7–T1
Pronator quadratus	Median	C8, T1
Brachioradialis	Radial	C5, C6
Extensor carpi radialis	Radial	C6, C7
Extensor communis digitorum	Radial	C6–C8
Extensor digiti minimi	Radial	C6–C8
Extensor carpi ulnaris	Radial	C6–C8
Extensor longus pollicis	Radial	C6–C8
Extensor brevis pollicis	Radial	C6–C8
Extensor indicis	Radial	C7, C8

turbances that resemble those seen after injuries to two or more peripheral nerves.

The syndrome of the upper secondary trunk is a combination of the signs and symptoms caused by injury to the musculocutaneous nerve and the outer head of the median nerve. These injuries are accompanied by a paralysis of the pronator radii teres, almost complete paralysis of the flexor carpi radialis, and weakness of the flexor pollicis and opponens.

Injury to the *posterior secondary trunk* produces paralysis similar to that which results from injury to the radial and axillary nerves.

The syndrome of the lower secondary trunk is the same as that of the ulnar nerve combined with a paralysis of flexion of the fingers as a result of injury to the inner head of the median nerve.

Ischemic Paralysis of the Arm

Paralysis of arm muscles may follow injury to large arteries. Ischemic paralysis may follow ligation of the major vessels when the collateral circulation is inadequate or it may follow prolonged constriction of the arm by plaster casts.

In the initial stages of ischemic paralysis the distal part of the extremity is cyanotic and edematous. Active movements of the finger and wrist muscles are possible but are of a limited range. There is diminution of cutaneous sensibility; all stimuli are poorly localized and have a painful quality. With the passage of time the cyanosis and edema disappear, the skin becomes smooth and shiny, and the muscles undergo fibrotic changes; anesthesia extends in a glove-like

Table 59–9.   Innervation of the Muscles of the Hand

Muscle	Nerve	Root
Palmaris brevis	Ulnar	T1
Abductor pollicis	Median	C6, C7
Opponens pollicis	Median	C6, C7
Flexor brevis pollicis	Median	C6, C7
Abductor digiti minimi	Ulnar	C8, T1
Opponens digiti minimi	Ulnar	C8, T1
Flexor brevis digiti minimi	Ulnar	C8, T1
Lumbricales	Medial, ulnar	C6–T1
Abductor pollicis	Ulnar	C8, T1
Interossei palmaris	Ulnar	C8, T1
Interossei dorsales	Ulnar	C8, T1

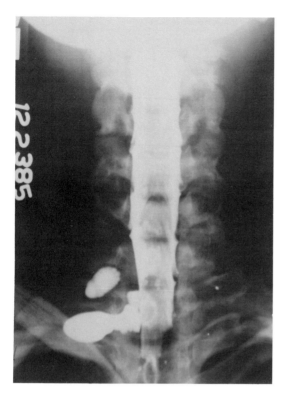

Fig. 59–4. Traumatic avulsion of lower cervical nerve roots. Pantopaque cervical myelogram (anteroposterior view) demonstrates contrast in avulsed right C8 an T1 root pouches. (Courtesy of Drs. S.K. Hilal and J.A. Bello.)

distribution to the wrist or middle of the forearm. The hand is held extended and the fingers are slightly flexed except when there are associated nerve lesions.

Ischemic paralysis can be differentiated from paralysis caused by lesions of the nerves by the absence of pulsations in the radial artery, the glove-like distribution of sensory loss, which does not correspond to that of any peripheral nerve, the fibrous consistency of the tissues and, in some cases, by the persistence of feeble imperfect movements of some of the muscles.

Ischemic paralysis is frequently permanent. Improvement in some cases can be obtained by hot baths, massage, passive movements, and electrical stimulation.

NERVES OF THE LEG

Obturator Nerve

The obturator nerve is a mixed nerve that originates in the lumbar plexus from the second, third, and fourth lumbar roots. It transmits cutaneous sensation from a small area on the inner surface of the middle side of the hip, thigh, and knee joint. It innervates the obturator externus muscle, the adductor longus, adductor brevis, gracilis, and adductor magnus muscles.

Lesions of the obturator nerve are uncommon. It may be injured by pressure within the pelvis by tumors, obturator hernias, or the fetal head in difficult labor.

Injuries to the obturator nerve result in severe weakness of adduction and, to a lesser extent, of internal and external rotation of the thigh. Pain in the knee joint is sometimes caused by pelvic involvement of the geniculate branch of the obturator.

Iliohypogastric Nerve

The iliohypogastric nerve is a mixed nerve that originates from the uppermost part of the lumbar plexus and is derived from the twelfth thoracic and first lumbar roots. It transmits cutaneous sensation from the outer and upper part of the buttocks and the lower part of the abdomen and supplies partial innervation to the internal oblique and transversalis muscles. Lesions of the iliohypogastric nerve are rare. It may be divided by incisions in kidney operations or together with the iliolingual nerve in operations in the inguinal region. Lesions of these nerves do not produce any significant motor loss and there is only a small area of cutaneous anesthesia.

Ilioinguinal Nerve

The ilioinguinal nerve, a branch of the lumbar plexus, arises from the twelfth thoracic and first lumbar roots. It transmits cutaneous sensation from the upper inner portion of the thigh, the pubic region, and the external genitalia. Motor filaments are given off to the transversalis, internal oblique, and external oblique muscles. The ilioinguinal nerve is usually injured in connection with the iliohypogastric nerve.

Genitofemoral Nerve

This nerve originates from the second lumbar root and is primarily a sensory nerve. It transmits cutaneous sensation from an oval area on the thigh in the region of Scarpa's triangle and from the scrotum and the contiguous area of the inner surface of the thigh. Lesions of the genitofemoral nerve are rare. Irritative lesions of the nerve in the abdominal wall are accompanied by painful hyperesthesia at the root of the thigh and the scrotum.

Lateral Cutaneous Nerve of Thigh

This nerve is formed by fibers from the second and third lumbar roots. It crosses beneath the fascia iliaca to emerge at the anterior superior iliac spine, descends in the thigh beneath the fascia lata, and divides into two branches. The posterior branch passes obliquely backward through the fascia lata and transmits cutaneous sensation from the superior external part of the buttocks. The anterior branch, which is more important clinically, pierces the fascia lata through a small fibrous canal about 10 cm below the ligament and transmits cutaneous fibrous sensation from the outer surface of the thigh.

The anterior portion of the nerve is occasionally the site of *meralgia paresthetica*, which is a sensory neuritis with dysesthesias in the nature of tingling, burning, prickling, or pins-and-needles sensations, with or without sensory loss, in the cutaneous distribution of the nerve. The long superficial course exposes it to various forms of trauma, but in most cases there is no history of trauma to explain the onset of symptoms. Various factors that are said to play a contributing role include pressure of tight belts or corsets and intermittent stretching by extensor movements of the thigh in walking. The involvement is unilateral in the vast majority of cases. Men are affected about three times as frequently as women.

The diagnosis is not difficult when the dysesthesias are limited to the distribution of the anterior division of the nerve. Pains in the lateral surface of the thigh caused by spinal lesions or pelvic tumors must be excluded by appropriate diagnostic studies.

The course of meralgia paresthetica is variable. The symptoms occasionally disappear spontaneously after a few weeks. In the vast majority of cases, they clear up by the removal of tight belts and avoidance of excessive walking. It is rarely necessary to split the fascia lata at the point of emergence of the nerve or correct the angulation of the nerve at the iliac spine.

Femoral Nerve

The femoral nerve arises from the second, third, and fourth lumbar nerves. It innervates the iliacus, psoas magnus, pectineus, sartorius, and quadriceps femoris muscles. It also transmits cutaneous sensation from the anterior surface of the thigh and, by its internal saphenous branch, from the entire inner surface of the leg and the anterior internal surface of the knee.

Traumatic lesions of the femoral nerve are uncommon. It may be compressed by tumors and other lesions in the pelvis or it may be injured by fractures of the pubic ramus or femur. Often there is no adequate explanation for the occurrence of an isolated femoral nerve palsy. In such cases it is presumed that the lesion of the nerve is a result of some toxic factor such as diabetes, typhoid, or gout.

Injury to the femoral nerve produces paralysis of extension of the leg and weakness of flexion of the thigh. When the patient stands erect the leg is held stiffly extended by contraction of the tensor fasciae femoris and the gracilis. Walking on level ground is possible as long as the leg can be kept extended but, if the slightest flexion occurs, the patient sinks down on the suddenly flexed knee. Climbing stairs or walking uphill is difficult or impossible. The quadriceps reflex is lost on the affected side and cutaneous sensation is impaired in an area somewhat smaller than the anatomic distribution of the nerve.

Paralysis of the femoral nerve must be distinguished from hysterical paralysis and reflex muscular atrophies that follow fractures of the femur or lesions of the knee joint. Hysterical paralysis can be diagnosed by the presence of the knee jerk and by special tests. In hysterical paralysis, when the patient is in the recumbent position and attempts to elevate the "paralyzed" limb, there is an absence of the normal fixing movements (downward pressure of the heel) of the opposite leg (*Hoover sign*).

Orthopedic appliances that fix the knee joint in extension are of value in the treatment of femoral nerve paralysis. Transplantation of tendons should be considered when the paralysis persists.

Sciatic Nerve

The sciatic nerve is the largest nerve in the body. Its terminal branches consist of two distinct nerves, which are antagonists of each other: the common peroneal (external popliteal) and the tibial (internal popliteal) nerves. The common peroneal arises from the posterior and the tibial nerve arises from the anterior portion of the sacral plexus (i.e., L4–S3). The main trunk of the sciatic nerve innervates the semitendinosus, the long and short heads of the biceps, the adductor magnus, and the semimembranosus muscles. The terminal branches of the nerve are considered separately below.

Total paralysis of the sciatic nerve is rare; even with a lesion in the thigh the common peroneal nerve is often more severely damaged than the tibial nerve. The sciatic nerve is frequently injured by gunshot, shrapnel, or stab wounds, although it is rarely injured in civilian life. Partial rupture may result from violent muscular contractions or the nerve may be injured by fractures of the pelvis or femur, dislocations of the hip, pressure of the fetal head on the plexus in the mother's pelvis, or pelvic tumor. The nerve is sometimes inadvertently injured by intramuscular injection of drugs, especially in infants.

Total involvement of the sciatic nerve produces complete paralysis of all movements of the ankle and toes, as well as weakness or paralysis of flexion of the leg. The patient can stand but the leg must be raised unduly high to correct for the foot drop when the patient walks. The ankle jerk is lost and cutaneous sensation is lost on the outer surface of the leg, on the instep and sole of the foot, and over the toes. Vasomotor and trophic disturbances may also be present.

The sciatic nerve is the seat of *sciatica*. This term is loosely used to describe pains that occur in the low back and in the leg along the course of the nerve. The term merely describes a set of symptoms that may be caused by involvement of any portion of the nerve, including its intraspinal roots. The concept of the etiology of sciatica has changed with the elucidation of the syndrome of the ruptured intervertebral disk. In the older literature the list of causes of sciatica was long and included so-called toxic or infectious processes, such as alcohol, arsenic, lead, diabetes, gout, syphilis, gonorrhea, phlebitis, and tuberculosis; arthritis of sacroiliac joint; arthritis of the hip; fibrositis; gluteal bursitis; osteitis deformans; sacralization of the fifth lumbar vertebra; pelvic tumors; and an inflammatory neuritis of the nerve. Although pain in the low back that extends down the posterior surface of the leg may be associated with pathologic processes in the pelvis and lower portion of the spine, in most patients the pains are caused by a ruptured intervertebral disk. In some patients the symptoms are produced by arthritis in the sacroiliac joint or spine. The distinctive features of ruptured intervertebral disks are considered more fully in Article 51, Intervertebral Disks.

Sciatica is most common in the third to sixth decade of life and occurs about three times more frequently in men than in women. The pain of sciatica varies in severity. In some patients there is a feeling of discomfort in the low back and down the posterior surface of the leg. In others the pain may be so intense as to incapacitate the afflicted individual totally. The pain may be limited to the buttocks and sacroiliac region, it may extend only to the knee, or it may involve the calf and outer surface of the foot. There is usually no weakness, but the patient may keep the knee slightly flexed in walking to prevent stretching of the nerve. On examination, the nerve may be sensitive to pressure at any point along its course. Any movement of the leg that stretches the nerve is accompanied by pain and involuntary resistance to the movement. There is limitation of straight leg raising on the affected side and complete extension of the leg is not possible when the hip is flexed. Similar movements of the unaffected limb can be more fully performed, but may produce slight pain on the opposite side. Sensory loss and diminution or loss of the Achilles reflex are rarely found in the sciatica associated with osteoarthritis of the spine or sacroiliac joint and suggest involvement of the nerve roots in the spinal canal.

The clinical course of sciatica depends on the nature of the underlying pathology. In most patients the symptoms last for several weeks or months and disappear, only to recur after a remission of months or years.

The diagnosis of the cause of pain in the low back and along the course of the sciatic nerve presents one of the most difficult problems in neurology. Thorough study is usually necessary. This must include radiographic examination of the hips, pelvis, sacroiliac joint, and lumbosacral spine, examination of the CSF and, in selected cases, CT or myelography. Only by the results of these studies can it be determined whether the symptoms are caused by a ruptured intervertebral disk, primary or metastatic tumor of the spine, osteoarthritic changes, or other factors.

The treatment of sciatica is essentially that of the underlying cause. The criteria for the operative removal of ruptured intervertebral disks are discussed elsewhere. Sciatica associated with osteoarthritis of the spine or sacroiliac joint is treated by complete rest in bed for several weeks. Traction on the affected leg often lessens the pain and speeds recovery but occasionally this cannot be tolerated. Heat may be applied. Analgesic drugs such as aspirin or codeine may be used. With subsidence of pain the patient should be allowed out of bed and to gradually assume usual activities. A back brace may be worn during waking hours and the patient's bed should have a firm mattress. Injection of the nerve or the epidural space with anesthetic solutions was quite widely used in the past but is rarely necessary. The treatment of causalgic pains following trauma to the sciatic nerve is discussed later in this section.

Common Peroneal (External Popliteal) Nerve

The common peroneal is a mixed nerve that innervates the extensor muscles of the ankle and toes, and the evertor (abductor) muscles of the foot. It transmits cutaneous sensation from the outer side of the leg, the front of its lower third, the instep, and the dorsal surface of the four inner toes over their proximal phalanges.

The common peroneal nerve is more frequently subjected to trauma than any other nerve of the body. It may be damaged by wounds in the region of the knee or in the trunk of the sciatic nerve in the thigh. Because of its superficial position in close relation to the head and neck of the fibula it is injured readily by pressure against hard objects while the patient is asleep, intoxicated, or under an anesthetic. It may be stretched by prolonged squatting or compressed by crossing the knees while sitting or by lying on a hard or uneven mattress during sleep, especially in acutely or chronically ill patients. Many cases of simple pressure neuritis of the common peroneal nerve are falsely recorded as being caused by such conditions as malarial, typhoid or tuberculous neuritis. The nerve may be injured by ganglion cysts. The cysts, which can usually be palpated at the head of the fibula, compress the nerve and produce footdrop accompanied by burning pains on the lateral aspect of the leg and in the ankle or foot. Relief of symptoms can be obtained by excision of the cyst.

Paralysis of the common peroneal nerve results in footdrop and inversion of the foot. The patient cannot dorsiflex the ankle, straighten or extend the toes, or evert the foot. The gait is characterized by overflexion of the knee and slapping of the foot on the floor (steppage gait). Sensory loss is present in an area less extensive than the anatomic distribution of the nerve or it may be entirely absent when the injury is caused by pressure. Vasomotor and trophic disturbances consist-

ing of swelling, local cyanosis, and anhidrosis may also be present.

Complete or partial recovery is the rule when the paralysis is caused by transient pressure. Treatment consists of physiotherapy and the use of a foot brace to overcome the footdrop.

Tibial (Internal Popliteal) Nerve

The tibial branch of the sciatic nerve innervates the muscles on the posterior surface of the leg and the plantar muscles. It transmits sensation from the entire sole of the foot, the back and lower part to the middle third of the leg, to the outer dorsal surface of the foot, and to the terminal phalanges of the toes.

Lesions of the tibial nerve are uncommon. It may be injured by gunshot wounds or fractures of the legs. A complete lesion of the nerve is characterized by paralysis of plantar flexion and adduction of the foot, flexion and separation of the toes, and a sensory loss in an area less extensive than the anatomic distribution of the nerve. The ankle jerk and plantar reflex are lost. Causalgia is occasionally seen.

Compression of the posterior tibial branch at the medial malleolus produces pain and paresthesias in the soles of the feet in a manner similar to compression of the medial nerve at the wrist. Decompression results in relief of the symptoms.

CAUSALGIA

Neuralgic pains in the limbs after injury of the nerves were first described by Weir Mitch-

Table 59–10. Lesions Producing Causalgia in 100 Cases

Type of Lesion	Arm	Leg
Median nerve	17	
Multiple nerve injuries	28	
Brachial plexus	10	
Ulnar nerve	9	
Radial	6	
Cutaneous nerves of forearm	2	
Digital nerve	2	
Sciatic nerve		8
Tibial nerve		2
Injuries to soft tissues	4	1
Fracture of bone or injury to joint	4	6
	82	17

(Modified from Rasmussen TB, Freedman H. Treatment of causalgia. J Neurosurg 1946; 3:165–173.)

Table 59–11.   Results of Treatment of Causalgia of the Arms and Legs

Treatment	No. of Cases	Relief of Pain			Adequate but Incomplete	Inadequate
		Immediate	Within 1 Month	Within a Few Months		
Paraverterbral block with Novocain	91	6	7		32	46
Sympathectomy						
Postganglionic	21	5	5	4		7
Preganglionic	14	13	1	0		0

(Modified from Rasmussen TB, Freedman H. Treatment of causalgia. J Neurosurg 1946; 3:165–173.)

ell. It was formerly considered that this type of neuralgia was found only after injury to the median nerve, but it may develop after an injury to any of the sensory or mixed nerves or damage to the plexuses, with or without damage to the major arteries of the limbs.

The pain is usually described as burning in nature (hence the name causalgia) and is constantly present. There is considerable variation in the severity of the pain. In some cases it is so extreme that the patient is completely incapacitated. The affected limb is constantly protected from movement or external stimuli. Examination of the affected limb is strenuously resisted by the patient. In other patients the pain is severe but the affected limb can be used (minor causalgia).

Causalgia is usually associated with an incomplete lesion of a nerve. Partial or complete continuity of the nerve may be preserved even though functional loss is complete. The pain is usually limited to the skin distribution of the affected nerve but it may spread to involve the distal part of the limb or the entire limb. When more than one nerve is injured the pain is often in the distribution of only one of the affected nerves. In injuries to the plexus the pain is present in the palm, fingertips, and entire hand or arm, rather than in a nerve or root distribution.

Causalgia is an uncommon complication of nerve injury. It is most frequently seen in those in the military. The onset of pain varies from immediately to several weeks after injury. It usually appears within a few days of the injury. In most patients the injury affects the median or sciatic nerves, either alone or in combination with other nerves (Table 59–10).

The pathogenesis of the pain is not known but it is attributed to injury to the sympathetic fibers in the nerve trunks. This concept is supported by the fact that relief of symptoms follows interruption of sympathetic pathways,

whereas such operations as neurolysis, removal of neuromas, sectioning, and resuturing of the nerve are usually of no value.

Examination of motor and sensory function in the affected limb is made with difficulty in severe cases because any stimulation causes an exacerbation of the pain. In most patients there is extreme vasodilatation and the limb is pink, warm, and velvety to the touch. Perspiration may be increased or decreased. When the pain is severe enough to prevent use of the limb there is rapid development of trophic changes in the skin and nails and periarticular fibrosis; these changes are also called *reflex sympathetic dystrophy.*

The course of the condition is variable. In mild cases the pain may disappear spontaneously after a few weeks or months without the development of any trophic changes in the affected limb. Spontaneous remission is less common in severe cases and permanent contractures may result unless the condition is relieved by therapy.

Operative procedures on the nerve are rarely followed by relief of the symptoms. The most successful form of therapy is sympathectomy or sympathetic block (Table 59–11). Preganglionic denervation of the limb is more effective than postganglionic denervation or paravertebral sympathetic block. In a few patients, a remission is induced by hyperpyrexia produced by the intravenous injection of typhoid vaccine or by means of the fever cabinet.

References

Neuritis, Neuropathy, and Nerve Injury

Aminoff MJ. Electromyography in Clinical Practice: Electrodiagnostic aspects of neuromuscular disease. 2nd ed. New York: Churchill Livingstone, 1987.

Dyck PJ, Thomas PK, Lambert EH, eds. Peripheral Neuropathy, 2nd ed. Philadelphia: WB Saunders, 1983.

Harris W. Neuritis and Neuralgia. London: Oxford University Press, 1926.

Haymaker W, Woodhall B. Peripheral Nerve Injuries, 2nd ed. Philadelphia: WB Saunders, 1953.

Kimura J. Electrodiagnosis in Diseases of Nerve and Muscle: Principles and Practice. 2nd ed. Philadelphia: FA Davis, 1989.

Liveson JA, Spielholz NI. Peripheral Neurology: Case Studies in Electrodiagnosis. Philadelphia: FA Davis, 1979.

Omer GE Jr, Spinner M, eds. Management of Peripheral Nerve Problems. Philadelphia: WB Saunders, 1980.

Seddon HJ. Peripheral nerve injuries. Medical Research Council Special Report Series No. 282. London: Her Majesty's Stationary Office, 1954.

Stewart JD, Siminovitch M. Focal Peripheral Neuropathies. Amsterdam: Elsevier, 1987.

Stookey B. Surgical and Mechanical Treatment of Peripheral Nerves. Philadelphia: WB Saunders, 1922.

Sumner AJ, ed. The Physiology of Peripheral Nerve Disease. Philadelphia: WB Saunders, 1980.

Sunderland S. Nerves and Nerve Injuries, 2nd ed. Edinburgh: Churchill, 1979.

Tinel J. Nerve Wounds. Symptomatology of Peripheral Nerve Lesions Caused by War Wounds. London: Balliere, Tindall and Cox, 1917.

Cranial Nerves

Auger RG, Pipegras DG, Laws ER Jr. Hemifacial spasm: results of microvascular decompression of the facial nerve in 54 patients. Mayo Clin Proc 1986; 61:640–644.

Battista AF. Hemifacial spasm and blepharospasm. Percutaneous fractional thermolysis of branches of facial nerve. NY State J Med 1977; 77:2234–2237.

Birkhead R, Friedman JH. Hiccups and vomiting as initial manifestations of multiple sclerosis. J Neurol Neurosurg Psychiatry 1987; 50:232–234.

Brisman R. Trigeminal neuralgia and multiple sclerosis. Arch Neurol 1987; 44:379–381.

Boghen DR, Glaser JS. Ischemic optic neuropathy; the clinical profile and natural history. Brain 1975; 98:689–708.

Chavis RM, Garner A, Wright JE. Inflammatory orbital pseudotumor. A clinicopathologic study. Arch Ophthalmol 1978; 96:1817–1822.

Choudury AG. Pathogenesis of unilateral proptosis. Acta Ophthalmol 1977; 55:237–251.

Cohn DF, Carasso R, Steifler M. Painful ophthalmoplegia: the Tolosa Hunt syndrome. Eur Neurol 1979; 18:373–381.

Croft CB, McKelvie P, Fairley JW, Hol-Allen RTJ, Shaheen O. Treatment of paralysis of the vocal cords: a review. J Roy Soc Med 1986; 79:473–475.

Dunphy EB. Alcohol-tobacco amblyopia; a historical survey. Am J Ophthalmol 1969; 68:569–578.

Ehni G, Woltman HWW. Hemifacial spasm; review of 106 cases. Arch Neurol Psychiatry 1945; 53:205–211.

Ferguson GG, Brett DC, Peerless SJ, Barr HWK, Girvin JP. Trigeminal neuralgia: comparison of percutaneous rhizotomy and microvascular decompression. Can J Neurol Sci 1981; 8:207–214.

Ford FR, Woodhall B. Phenomena due to misdirection of regenerating fibers of cranial, spinal and autonomic nerves. Clinical observations. Arch Surg 1938; 36:480–496.

Friedman AP, Merritt HH. Damage to cranial nerves resulting from head injury. Bull Los Angeles Neurol Soc 1944; 9:135–139.

Fromm GH, Terrence CF, Maroon JC. Trigeminal neuralgia. Current concepts regarding etiology and pathogenesis. Arch Neurol 1984; 41:1204–1207.

Gary-Babo A, Fuentes JM, Guerrier B. Cross-facial nerve anastomosis in treatment of facial paralysis. Br J Plast Surg 1980; 33:195–201.

Graham MD, House WF, eds. Disorders of the Facial Nerve: Anatomy, Diagnosis, and Management. New York: Raven Press, 1982.

Hassler R, Walker AE. Trigeminal Neuralgia. Philadelphia: WB Saunders, 1970.

Holinger LD, Holinger PC, Holinger PH. Etiology of bilateral abductor vocal cord paralysis. A review of 389 cases. Ann Otol 1976; 85:428–436.

Huizing EH, Mechelse K, Staal A. Treatment of Bell's palsy: analysis of the available studies. Acta Otolaryngol (Stockh) 1981; 92:115–121.

Isamat F, Ferran E, Acebes JJ. Selective percutaneous thermocoagulation rhizotomy in essential glossopharyngeal neuralgia. J Neurosurg 1981; 55:575–580.

Jankovic J, Ford J. Blepharospasm and orofacial-cervical dystonia: clinical and pharmacological findings in 100 patients. Ann Neurol 1983; 13:402–411.

Jannetta P. Observations on the etiology of trigeminal neuralgia, hemifacial spasm, acoustic nerve dysfunction and glossopharyngeal neuralgia. Definitive microsurgical treatment and results in 11 patients. Neurochirurgia 1977; 20:145–154.

Juncos JL, Beal MF. Idiopathic cranial polyneuropathy. A 15-year experience. Brain 1987; 110:197–212.

Kalovidouris A, Mancuso AA, Dillon W. A CT-clinical approach to patients with symptoms related to the V, VII, IX–XII cranial nerves and cervical sympathetics. Radiology 1984; 151:671–6.

Konigsmark BW. Hereditary deafness. N Engl J Med 1969; 281:713–720, 827–832.

Lecky BRF, Hughes RAC, Murray NMF. Trigeminal sensory neuropathy. Brain 1987; 110:1463–1486.

Leigh RJ, Zee DS. The Neurology of Eye Movements. Philadelphia: FA Davis, 1983.

Lisney SJW. Current topics of interest in the physiology of trigeminal pain: a review. J Roy Soc Med 1983; 76:292–296.

Loeser JD, Chen J. Hemifacial spasm: treatment by microsurgical facial nerve decompression. Neurosurgery 1983; 13:141–146.

Massey EW, Moore J, Schold SC Jr. Mental neuropathy from systemic cancer. Neurology 1981; 31:1277–1281.

May M, Klein SR, Taylor FH. Idiopathic Bell's facial palsy: natural history defies steroid and surgical treatment. Laryngoscope 1985; 95:406–409.

Menon V, Singh J, Prakash P. Aetiological patterns of ocular motor nerve palsies. Ind J Ophthalmol 1984; 32:447–453.

Mills R. Meniere's syndrome: pathogenesis and treatment. Br Med J 1986; 293:463–464.

Moffie D, Ongeboer de Visser BW, Stefanko SZ. Parinaud's syndrome. J Neurol Sci 1983; 58:175–183.

Moller AR, Jannetta PJ. Hemifacial spasm. Electrophysiologic recording during microvascular decompression operations. Neurology 1985; 35:969–974.

Moller AR, Jannetta PJ. Monitoring facial EMG responses during microvascular decompression operations for hemifacial spasm. J Neurosurg 1987; 66:681–685.

Nadeau SE, Trobe JD. Pupil sparing in oculomotor palsy: a brief review. Ann Neurol 1983; 13:143–148.

Nielsen VK. Electrophysiology of the facial nerve in hemifacial spasm: ectopic/ephaptic excitation. Muscle Nerve 1985; 8:545–555.

Pulsinelli WA, Rottenberg DA. Painful tic convulsif. J. Neurol Neurosurg Psychiatry 1977; 40:192–195.

Portenoy RK, Duma C, Foley KM. Acute herpetic and postherpetic neuralgia. Clinical review and current management. Ann Neurol 1986; 20:651–664.

Rudge P. Clinical Neuro-Otology. New York: Churchill Livingstone, 1983.

Rush JA, Younge BR. Paralysis of cranial nerves III, IV and VI. Cause and prognosis in 1000 cases. Arch Ophthalmol 1981; 99:76–79.

Rushton JG, Stevens JC, Miller RH. Glossopharyngeal (vagoglossopharyngeal) neuralgia. Arch Neurol 1981; 38:201–205.

Schwartz JF, Chutorian AM, Evans RA, Carter S. Optic atrophy in childhood. Pediatrics 1964; 34:670–679.

Searles RP, Mladinich K, Messner RP. Isolated trigeminal sensory neuropathy: early manifestations of mixed connective tissue disease. Neurology 1978; 28:1286–1289.

Spillane JD, Wells CEC. Isolated trigeminal neuropathy. Brain 1959; 82:391–416.

Stevens H. Melkersson's syndrome. Neurology 1965; 15:263–266.

Tenser RB. Myokymia and facial contraction in multiple sclerosis. Arch Intern Med 1976; 136:81–83.

Troost BT, Daroff RB. The ocular motor defects in progressive supranuclear palsy. Ann Neurol 1977; 2:397–403.

Van Zandyke M, Martin JJ, VanderGaer L, Van den Heyning P. Facial myokymia in the Guillain-Barre syndrome: a clinicopathologic study. Neurology 1982; 32:744–748.

Victor M, Dreyfus PM. Tobacco-alcohol ambylopia. Further comments on its pathology. Arch Ophthalmol 1965; 74:649–657.

Wartenberg R. Hemifacial Spasm: A Clinical and Pathological Study. London: Oxford University Press, 1952.

Westmoreland, BF, Sharborough FW, Stockard JJ, Dale AJD. Brain stem auditory evoked potentials in 20 patients with palatal myoclonus. Arch Neurol 1983; 40:155–158.

Willoughby EW, Anderson NE. Lower cranial nerve motor function in unilateral vascular lesions of the cerebral hemisphere. Br Med J 1984; 289:791–794.

Peripheral Nerves

Aguayo AJ. Neuropathy due to compression and entrapment. In: Dyck PJ, Thomas PK, Lambert EH, eds. Peripheral Neuropathy, 2nd ed. Philadelphia: WB Saunders, 1983.

Asbury AK, Fields HL. Pain due to peripheral nerve damage: an hypothesis. Neurology 1984; 34:1587–1594.

Buchthal F, Rosenfalck A, Trojaborg W. Electrophysiological findings in entrapment of the median nerve at the wrist and elbow. J Neurol Neurosurg Psychiatry 1974; 37:340–360.

Castellanos AM, Glass JP, Yung WKA. Regional nerve injury after intra-arterial chemotherapy. Neurology 1987; 37:834–837.

D'Amour ML, Lebrun LH, Rabbat A, Trudel J, Daneault N. Peripheral neurological complications of aorto-iliac vascular disease. Can J Neurol Sci 1987; 14:127–130.

Downie A. Peripheral nerve compression syndromes. In: Matthews WB, Glaser GH, eds. Recent Advances in Clinical Neurology, No. 3. Edinburgh: Churchill Livingstone, 1982.

Eisen A, Schomer D, Melmed C. The application of F-wave measurements in the differentiation of proximal and distal upper limb entrapments. Neurology 1977; 27:662–668.

England JD, Sumner AJ. Neuralgic amyotrophy: an increasingly diverse entity. Muscle Nerve 1987; 10:60–68.

Evans BA, Stevens JC, Dyck PJ. Lumbosacral plexus neuropathy. Neurology 1981; 31:1327–1331.

Fernandez E, Pallini R, Talamonti G. Sleep palsy (Saturday-night palsy) of the deep radial nerve. J Neurosurg 1987; 66:460–462.

Friedman AH, Nashold BS Jr, Ovelmen-Levitt J. Dorsal root entry zone lesions for the treatment of post-herpetic neuralgia. J Neurosurg 1984; 60:1258–1262.

Gilliatt RW. Acute compression block. In: Sumner AJ, ed. The Physiology of Peripheral Nerve Disease. Philadelphia: WB Saunders, 1980: 287–315.

Gilliatt RW, Willison RG, Dietz V, et al. Peripheral nerve conduction in patients with a cervical rib and band. Ann Neurol 1978; 4:124–129.

Goodgold J, Eberstein A. Electrodiagnosis of Neuromuscular Diseases. Baltimore: Williams & Wilkins, 1977.

Haymaker, W, Woodhall B. Peripheral Nerve Injuries. Principles of Diagnosis, 2nd ed. Philadelphia: WB Saunders, 1953.

Kline DG, Judice DJ. Operative management of selected brachial plexus lesions. J Neurosurg 1983; 58:631–649.

Kopell HP, Thompson WA. Peripheral Entrapment Neuropathies. Baltimore: Williams & Wilkins, 1963.

Kori SH, Foley KM, Posner JB. Brachial plexus lesions in patients with cancer: 100 cases. Neurology 1981; 31:45–50.

Mastroianni PP, Roberts MP. Femoral neuropathy and retroperitoneal hemorrhage. Neurosurgery 1983; 13:44–47.

Miller RG. Injury to peripheral nerves. Muscle Nerve 1987; 10:698–710.

Morris HH, Peters PH. Pronator syndrome: clinical and electrophysiological features in seven cases. J Neurol Neurosurg Psychiatry 1976; 39:461–464.

Nakano KK, Lundergan C, Okharo MM. Anterior interosseous syndromes: diagnosic methods and alternative treatments. Arch Neurol 1977; 34:477–480.

Omer GE, Spinner M, eds. Management of Peripheral Nerve Problems. Philadelphia: WB Saunders, 1980.

Schott GD. Mechanisms of causalgia and related clinical conditions. The role of the central and of the sympathetic nervous systems. Brain 1986; 109:717–738.

Schwartzman RJ, McLellan TL. Reflex sympathetic dystrophy; a review. Arch Neurol 1987; 44:555–561.

Seddon HJ. Peripheral nerve injuries. Medical Research Council Special Report, Series No. 282. London: Her Majesty's Stationery Office, 1954.

Stewart JD. The variable clinical manifestations of ulnar neuropathies at the elbow. J Neurol Neurosurg Psychiatry 1987; 50:252–258.

Subramony SH. Neuralgic amyotrophy (acute brachial neuropathy). Muscle Nerve 1988; 11:39–44.

Swash M. Diagnosis of brachial root and plexus lesions. J Neurol 1986; 233:131–135.

Synek VM. Cowan JC. Somatosensory evoked potentials in supraclavicular brachial plexus injuries. Neurology 1982; 32:1347–1352.

Thomas JE, Pipegras DG, Scheithauer B, Onofrio BM, Shives TC. Neurogenic tumors of the sciatic nerve. A clinicopathologic study of 35 cases. Mayo Clin Proc 1983; 58:640–647.

Trojaborg W. Early electrophysiological changes in conduction block. Muscle Nerve 1978; 1:400–403.

Trojaborg W. Electrophysiological finding in pressure palsy of the brachial plexus. J Neurol Neurosurg Psychiatry 1977; 40:1160–1167.

Trojaborg W. Rate of recovey in motor and sensory fibres

of the radial nerve. J Neurol Neurosurg Psychiatry 1970; 33:625–638.

Tsairis P, Dyck P, Mulder D. Natural history of brachial plexus neuropathy. Arch Neurol 1972; 27:109–117.

Wiles CM, Whitehead S, Ward AB, Fletcher CDM. Not tarsal tunnel syndrome: a malignant "triton" tumour of the tibial nerve. J Neurol Neurosurg Psychiatry 1987; 50:479–482.

Wulff CH, Hansen K, Strange P, Trojaborg W. Multiple mononeuritis and radiculitis with erythema, pain, elevated CSF protein and pleocytosis (Bannwarth's syndrome). J Neurol Neurosurg Psychiatry 1983; 46:485–490.

60. THORACIC OUTLET SYNDROME

Lewis P. Rowland

The term "thoracic outlet syndrome," singular though it may be, encompasses different syndromes that arise from compression of the nerves in the brachial plexus or blood vessels (subclavian or axillary arteries, or veins in the same area). The compressing lesions are also diverse.

How often these lesions are actually responsible for symptoms, and how the symptoms should be treated, are matters of intense debate. Studies done mainly by orthopedists, vascular surgeons, and neurosurgeons have included reports on several hundred patients who were treated surgically for this syndrome. When neurologists write about this neurologic disorder, however, the tone is always skeptical and the syndrome is described as exceedingly rare, with an annual incidence of about 1/1,000,000. The debate warrants separate consideration although this is actually another disorder of the peripheral nervous system.

Pathology. The T1 and C8 nerve roots and the lower trunk of the brachial plexus are exposed to compression and angulation by anatomic anomalies that include cervical ribs and fibrous bands of uncertain origin. Among the more imaginative lesions are those ascribed to hypertrophy of the scalenus muscles. Cervical ribs are commonly found in asymptomatic people and it is difficult to assume that the mere presence of a cervical rib automatically explains local symptoms. In addition to the neural syndromes the same anomalies may compress local blood vessels and cause vascular syndromes.

Symptoms and Signs. The patients have pain in the shoulder, arm, and hand or in all three locations. The hand pain is often most severe in the fourth and fifth fingers. The pain is aggravated by use of the arm, and "fatigue"

of the arm is often prominent. There may or may not be hypesthesia in the affected area.

Critics have divided the cases into two groups, those with the "true" neurogenic thoracic outlet syndrome and those with the "disputed" syndrome. In the *true* syndrome there are definite clinical and electrical abnormalities. This syndrome is rare but is almost always caused by a cervical band that extends from a cervical rib and compresses the C8 and T1 roots or lower brachial plexus. There is unequivocal wasting and weakness of muscles in the hand that are innervated by these segments, and results of electrodiagnostic studies are compatible with the site of the nerve lesion.

In the *disputed* form there are no objective signs and there are no consistent laboratory abnormalities. Attempts to reproduce the syndrome by abducting the arm (the Adson test) or other maneuvers have been cited repeatedly, but the same "abnormalities" can be demonstrated in normal people and have no diagnostic value.

Similarly, application of electrodiagnostic techniques has not been blinded or controlled, so different abnormalities have been reported, then refuted. The list includes low amplitude of the sensory evoked potential in the ulnar nerve, slowing of proximal conduction after stimulation at Erb's point, ulnar F-wave determination, and abnormality of somatosensory evoked potentials from the ulnar nerve.

Diagnosis and Management. In cases of true thoracic outlet syndrome diagnosis must exclude entrapment syndromes in the arm and compressive lesions in the cervical spine. Arteriography may be indicated if there is any suggestion of aneurysm of the subclavian artery. Surgery is indicated when the diagnosis is unequivocal.

In the disputed form when no objective findings are noted on neurologic examination, there is a problem. Each case must be evaluated separately but, in the absence of objective changes, it would seem reasonable to be cautious. Psychogenic factors should be considered. Conservative therapy should be given a trial; postural adjustments, manual therapy to increase mobility of the shoulder girdle, and an exercise program have all been advocated. The results of surgery are difficult to evaluate when there are no objective signs or diagnostic laboratory abnormalities; placebo effects are rarely considered in the evaluation of surgery. Success rates of 90% for a particular operation may be followed by equally enthusiastic reports for reoperation after the "failed operation." Surgery is not without hazard; complications include causalgia, injury of the long thoracic nerve, infection, and laceration of the subclavian artery.

References

Carroll RE, Hurst LC. The relationship of thoracic outlet syndrome and carpal tunnel syndrome. Clin Orthop 1982; 164:149–153.

Cherington M, Harper I, Machanic B, Parry L. Surgery for thoracic outlet syndrome may be hazardous to your health. Muscle Nerve 1986; 9:632–4.

Gilliatt RW. Thoracic outlet syndrome. In: Dyck RJ, Thomas PK, Lambert EH, Bunge R, eds. Peripheral Neuropathy. Philadelphia: WB Saunders, 1984; 1409–1424.

Gregoudis R, Barnes RW. Thoracic outlet arterial compression: prevalence in normal persons. Angiology 1980; 31:538–541.

Huffman JD. Electrodiagnostic techniques for and conservative treatment of thoracic outlet syndrome. Clin Orthop 1986; 207:21–23.

Jerrett SA, Cuzzone LJ, Pasternak BM. Thoracic outlet syndrome. Electrophysiologic reappraisal. Arch Neurol 1984; 41:960–963.

Roos DB. Congenital anomalies associated with thoracic outlet syndrome. Am J Surg 1976; 132:771–778.

Smith T, Trojaborg W. Diagnosis of thoracic outlet syndrome. Arch Neurol 1987; 44:1161–1166.

Swift TR, Nicholas FT. The droopy shoulder syndrome. Neurology 1984; 34:212–215.

Veilleux M, Stevens JC, Campbell JK. Somatosensory evoked potentials: lack of value for diagnosis of thoracic outlet syndrome. Muscle Nerve 1988; 11:571–575.

Wilbourn AJ, Lederman RJ. Evidence for conduction delay in thoracic outlet syndrome is challenged. N Engl J Med 1984; 310:1052–1053.

61. IONIZING RADIATION
Bertram E. Sprofkin

The adult nervous system is relatively resistant to ionizing radiation but the fetal nervous system may be damaged by comparatively small doses.

Experimental work in mammals has shown that the embryonic nervous system is readily injured by radiation; it is now commonly accepted that microcephaly, hydrocephalus, and other development anomalies may occur in the human fetus as result of pelvic irradiation of the pregnant mother. This is particularly true if the radiation is given during the early stages of development of the fetus.

Little is known about acute damage to the adult nervous system as a result of excessively large doses of ionizing radiation. Fatalities after explosion of an atom bomb were usually related to blast injury and the systemic effects of radiation. The adult nervous system may be damaged occasionally by accidental application of an overdose of radium or other forms of radiation energy or by apparently safe doses of these agents for the treatment of tumors of the skin or other structures overlying the brain or spinal cord.

Unless the dose is excessively high, damage to the nervous tissue usually does not become evident until 6 months or more after the course of therapy. There are thickening and proliferation of the blood vessels and necrosis of the parenchyma in the affected areas. Radiation injury of the brain may cause slowly progressive symptoms suggesting the presence of an intracranial tumor. Injury to the cord is followed by subacute development of the syndrome of transverse myelitis. Roots, plexuses, and nerves may be damaged by radiation, with resultant motor and sensory defects that tend to progress. Because of the progressive nature of these radiation-induced lesions an erroneous diagnosis of tumor regrowth might lead to further radiation and additional tissue damage. Occasionally evidence of damage to the nervous system may appear within 3 months as a result of demyelinating lesions similar to those of multiple sclerosis without evidence of damage to the blood vessels.

Although MRI can depict radiation necrosis with greater sensitivity than CT, neither technique can reliably discriminate between recurrent or residual brain tumor and radiation necrosis. The use of contrast-enhancing paramagnetic substances, however, such as gadolinium, may extend the diagnostic capabilities of MRI.

References

Abbatucci JS, Delozier T, Quint R, Roussel A, Brune D. Radiation myelopathy of the cervical spinal cord: time, dose and volume factors. Int J Radiat Oncol Biol Phys 1978; 4:239–248.

Ashenhurst EM, Quartey GRC, Starreveld A. Lumbrosacral radiculopathy induced by radiation. Can J Neurol Sci 1977; 4:259–263.

Bleyer WA. Neurologic sequelae of methotrexate and ionizing radiation: a new classification. Cancer Treat Rep 1981; 65(suppl 1): 89–98.

Brasch RC, Nitecki DE, Brant-Zawadzki M, et al. Brain nuclear magnetic resonance imaging enhanced by a paramagnetic nitroxide contrast agent. Am J Radiol 1983; 141:1019–1023.

Dooms GC, Hecht S, Brant-Zawadzki M, et al. Brain radiation lesions: MR imaging. Radiology 1986; 158:149–155.

Dorfman LJ, Donaldson SS, Gupta PR, Bosley TM. Electrophysiologic evidence of subclinical injury to the posterior columns of the human spinal cord after therapeutic radiation. Cancer 1982; 50:2815–2819.

Ducatman BS, Scheithauer BW. Postirradiation neurofibrosarcoma. Cancer 1983; 51:1028–1033.

Felix R, Schörner W, Laniado M, et al. Brain tumors: MR imaging with gadolinium-DPTA. Radiology 1985; 156:681–688.

Fitzgerald RHJ, Marks RD Jr, Wallace KM. Chronic radiation myelitis. Radiology 1982; 144:609–612.

Foley KM, Woodruff JM, Ellis FT, Posner JB. Radiation-induced malignant and atypical schwannomas. Ann Neurol 1979; 7:311–318.

Gilbert HA, Kagan AR, eds. Radiation Damage to the Nervous System—A Delayed Therapeutic Hazard. New York: Raven Press, 1980.

Haymaker W, Shiraki H, Natsuoka S, et al. Effects of atomic radiation of the brain in man. A study of forty-nine Hiroshima and Nagasaki casualties. J Neuropathol Exp Neurol 1958; 17:79–137.

Holdorff B. Radiation damage of the brain. In: Vinken PJ, Bruyn GW, eds. Handbook of Clinical Neurology (vol 23). New York: Elsevier-North Holland, 1976:639–663.

Horowitz SL, Stewart JD. Lower motor neuron syndrome following radiotherapy. Can J Neurol Sci 1983; 10:56–58.

Kim YH, Fayos JV. Radiation tolerance of the cervical spinal cord. Radiology 1981; 139:473–478.

Marks JE, Baglan RJ, Prassad SC, Blank WF. Cerebral radionecrosis: incidence and risk in relation to dose, time, fractionation, and volume. Int J Radiat Oncol Biol Phys 1981; 7:243–252.

Regan TJ, Thomas JE, Colby MY Jr. Chronic progressive radiation myelopathy. JAMA 1968; 203:106–110.

62. ELECTRICAL INJURIES
Bertram E. Sprofkin

Injury to the CNS or the peripheral nerves may result from the passage of electricity through the body. As a rule, the passage of a current sufficient to damage the nervous system is fatal. The patient may survive, however, and show evidence of damage to the brain, spinal cord, or cranial or spinal nerves.

Accidental contact with high-tension current in the home or industry is the most common cause of electrical injury. Less common causes of serious electrical injury to the nervous system are lightning strokes, and electric shock therapy.

Pathology. Respiratory arrest or ventricular fibrillation is the cause of death in fatal cases. Peripheral nerves may be injured by direct effects of the current, but lesions in the CNS are more probably caused by damage to blood vessels or by cerebral anoxemia secondary to the temporary cardiac and respiratory failure. These include edema, perivascular hemorrhages, and areas of cellular loss or demyelination secondary to vascular damage.

Signs and Symptoms. The symptoms of severe electrical injury are divided into two groups, acute symptoms and late manifestations. In the acute state there is loss of consciousness, often accompanied by convulsive seizures. Death results if ventricular fibrillation occurs or if there is a prolonged arrest of respiration.

Late manifestations of electrical injury are rare. Atrophic paralysis as a result of injury to the peripheral nerves or spinal cord is the most common sign. Hemiplegia and other focal cerebral symptoms, chorea, dystonia, and other signs of injury to the basal ganglia, and mental disturbances have been reported as a result of injury to the brain. In some of these cases there was no doubt about the relationship of the shock to the symptoms. In others cerebral arteriosclerosis was probably a contributing factor.

Treatment. Cardiopulmonary resuscitation should be instituted immediately to save the patient's life and to prevent further damage to the nervous system by anoxia. The treatment of neurologic residuals is the same as for similar defects from other causes.

References

Kotagal S, Rawlings CA, Chen SC, Burris G, Nouri S. Neurologic, psychiatric, and cardiovascular complications in children struck by lightning. Pediatrics 1982; 7:190–192.

Panse F. Electrical trauma. In: Vinken PJ, Bruyn GW, eds. Handbook of Clinical Neurology (vol 23). New York: Elsevier-North-Holland, 1976:683–729.

Petty PG, Parkin G. Electrical injury to the central nervous system. Neurosurgery 1986; 19:282–284.

Sances A, Larson SJ. Myklebust J, Cusick JF. Electrical injuries. Surg Gynecol Obstet 1979; 49:97–108.

Solem L, Fischer RP, Strate RG. The natural history of electrical injury. J Trauma 1977; 17:487–492.

63. DECOMPRESSION SICKNESS
Leon D. Prockop

In scuba diving, caisson work, flying, and simulated altitude ascents, rapid reduction in ambient pressure may cause the formation and growth of gas bubbles within supersaturated blood and tissues. Resultant lesions involve the limbs, cardiorespiratory system, and CNS. In divers most neurologic lesions affect spinal cord segments. In fliers cerebral damage is most common.

Pathology. Those involved in diving accidents have the greatest incidence of decompression sickness; thoracic, upper lumbar, and lower cervical cord segments are affected, in that order of frequency. Ischemic perivascular lesions are usually confined to the white matter but subsequent petechial hemorrhage may occur and extend into the gray matter. Pathologic mechanisms include tissue disruption with intra- and extracellular bubbles as well as vascular occlusion by bubbles. Although it is a distinct entity, coincident intra-arterial embolism may cause cerebral damage.

Signs and Symptoms. With cord damage back pain is followed by leg paresthesias, paresis, and urinary retention. Unless recompression is achieved promptly the signs, including paralysis, may be permanent. When the brain is affected focal or generalized neurologic signs and symptoms include visual impairment, loss of consciousness, hemiparesis, seizures, and vertigo.

Treatment. Serious manifestations of decompression sickness, including any neurologic signs, are a medical emergency. They require recompression therapy, which is directed at maintaining proper pressure long enough for residual gas bubbles to be recompressed and absorbed; oxygen must be supplied at increased partial pressure to the damaged tissues. Results of treatment vary, but the sooner recompression is begun, the better the results. Rapid transport to a hyperbaric chamber while the patient is breathing 100% oxygen is essential. For chamber locations, physicians should contact the local United States Coast Guard marine and air rescue centers, listed in telephone directories in coastal areas.

References

Crockett ATK, Pauley SM, Zehl DN, Pimanis AA, Crockett WF. Pathophysiology of bends and decompression sickness; an overview with emphasis on treatment. Arch Surg 1979; 114:296–301.

Department of the Navy. U.S. Navy Diving Manual. Washington, DC: Department of the Navy, June 1984 (NAVSEA 0994-LP-001-9101).

Dick APK, Massey EW. Neurological presentation of decompression sickness and an embolism in sports divers. Neurology 1985; 35:667–671.

Green RD, Leitch DR. Twenty years of treating decompression sickness. Aviat Space Environ Med 1987; 58:362–6.

Hallenbeck JM, Andersen J. Pathogenesis of decompression disorders. In: Bennett PB, Elliot DH, eds. The Physiology and Medicine of Diving. Carson, CA: Best Bookbinders, 1983:L435–L460.

Haymaker W. Decompression sickness. In: Lubarsch O, Henke F, Rossle R, eds. Handbuch der Speziellen Pathologischen Anatomie und Histologie (vol 13). Berlin: Springer-Verlag, 1957:1600–1672.

Haymaker W, Johnston AD. Pathology of decompression sickness; comparison of lesions in airmen with those in caisson workers and divers. Milit Med 1955; 117:285–306.

Lambertsen CJ. Concepts for advances in the therapy of bends in undersea and aerospace activity. Aerosp Med 1968; 39:1086–93.

Leitch DR, Hallenbeck JM. Oxygen and pressure in the treatment of spinal cord decompression sickness. Undersea Biomed Res 1985; 12:269–289.

Neuman TS, Spragg RG, Wagner PD, Moser KM. Cardiopulmonary consequences of decompression stress. Respir Physiol 1980; 41:143–53.

Strauss RH, Prokop LD. Decompression sickness among scuba divers. JAMA 1973; 223:637–40.

Chapter VII

Birth Injuries and Developmental Abnormalities

64. NEONATAL NEUROLOGY
M. Richard Koenigsberger

Intracranial Hemorrhage

Intracranial hemorrhage is becoming more common than asphyxia in neonates. Gestational age is the best statistical indicator of the probable site of hemorrhage. *Supratentorial subdural hemorrhage* is becoming rare, and occurs almost exclusively in full-term or large babies after difficult deliveries. *Parenchymal cerebral hemorrhage* that originates in the periventricular area, with or without secondary subarachnoid bleeding, is common in infants of 35-weeks gestation or less; it is unusual after 36 weeks. *Primary subarachnoid supratentorial hemorrhage* of venous origin occurs in full-term newborns who have focal seizures and a benign clinical course. Subarachnoid hemorrhage may be found at autopsy in premature babies, but there is no recognized clinical syndrome. Posterior fossa hemorrhages are usually fatal in preterm infants, but may be amenable to surgical or medical treatment in full-term infants.

PERIVENTRICULAR-INTRAVENTRICULAR HEMORRHAGE

Periventricular-intraventricular hemorrhage occurs in nearly half of infants who weigh less than 1500 g; most of these infants are less than 35 weeks of gestational age.

Pathology and Pathophysiology. In most cases, the hemorrhage arises in the vascular germinal plate between the thalamus and caudate, near the foramina of Monro. Periventricular hemorrhage may be confined to this friable matrix area (Type I); 75% to 80% extend into the lateral ventricles (Type II), sometimes enlarging them (Type III) or extending into the brain substance (Type IV). It is not known whether the source is arterial (recurrent artery of Heubner from the anterior cerebral artery)

or venous (thalamostriate veins as they enter the internal cerebral vein). Proponents of the arterial theory cite hypotension followed by hypertension in an asphyxiated, softened brain that has lost autoregulation. The venous hypothesis suggests that increased venous pressure leads to stasis, thrombosis, rupture, and bleeding from the thin-walled venules. Whatever the mechanism, periventricular bleeding is often associated with hyaline membrane disease or pneumothorax. Hypercarbia, hypo- or hypertension, or increased venous pressure are encountered in severe respiratory distress. It is not clear which factors are the main cause of hemorrhage. Bleeding usually occurs in the first 48 hours after birth, but has been reported in utero as well as several days after birth.

Signs and Symptoms. Type I hemorrhage is usually asymptomatic. In Type II, there is nonspecific irritability or lethargy but no ventricular dilatation. In Types III and IV, deterioration may ensue soon after onset with at least 50% chance of mortality; signs include severe apnea and bradycardia, extensor posturing and opisthotonos, deviated eyes converged or diverged, and pupils fixed, usually in midposition. Many neonates become flaccid and unresponsive, and die within minutes or hours. Clonic limb movements may occur concurrently. The posturing and movements have been called "seizures," but there is no EEG seizure activity. Less dramatic deterioration may occur in a few days and ventricular dilatation may be severe with few symptoms or little increase in head size.

Diagnosis. In preterm infants, gestation of less than 35 weeks places an infant at risk for periventricular-intraventricular hemorrhage. The laboratory features of the more severe kinds include: fall of hematocrit of 10% or more, hypercarbia, acidosis, hypocalcemia, and hypo- or hyperglycemia. The CSF contains many red blood cells and has a protein content of 250 to 1200 mg/dl. Lumbar puncture is not always diagnostic because traumatic taps are common. Conversely, CSF may be normal, possibly because blood has not descended to the lumbar level or because blood occludes the aqueduct. A few days later, the CSF is xanthochromic with white and red blood cells and low sugar content; meningitis is ruled out by cultures.

Sonography has replaced CT as the cornerstone of diagnosis. This portable cribside technique delineates the site of blood in the parenchyma and ventricles, ventricular size, and shifts of major structures (Fig. 64–1). White matter infarctions and cystic periventricular leukomalacia can also be identified. Subarachnoid blood and subdural collections that are nearer the transducer applied at the fontanelle are harder to identify; when necessary they may be confirmed by CT. The role of MRI remains to be defined, but it may prove useful in demonstrating anatomic changes created by various lesions plus their effects on myelinization.

Prognosis and Therapy. In Types I and II hemorrhage, prognosis is good, with an 80%

to 90% survival rate without neurologic abnormality. Morbidity is attributed to coexisting ischemic damage after respiratory distress. In Types III and IV hemorrhage, early mortality is as high as 50% and survivors often show clinical evidence of brain damage. Ventricular dilatation after intraventricular hemorrhage may resolve spontaneously or may progress. Death may be due to parenchymal extension of hemorrhagic complications of cardiopulmonary disease.

No treatment is necessary for Types I and II hemorrhages. In Types III and IV, serial lumbar punctures have been used. They are most effective when large volumes can be drained, e.g. 10 ml, or when sonography after lumbar puncture shows diminished ventricular size. If sonographic evidence of ventricular enlargement and signs of intracranial pressure persist, external ventriculostomy is used for periods not exceeding 5 days (because of the danger of infection). Lastly, ventriculoperitoneal shunt may be installed, but this procedure has a high complication rate in small infants. Every attempt should be made to delay shunting until the infant has shown as much somatic growth as possible.

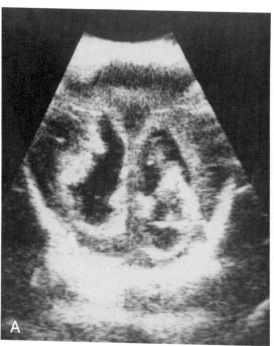 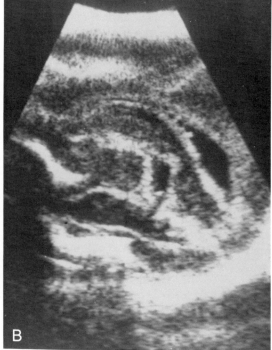

Fig. 64–1. Real-time sonography of intraventricular hemorrhage. *A,* Coronal plane shows hypoechoic CSF within lateral ventricles. Echogenic clots are present bilaterally, larger on left. *B,* Left lateral ventricle in sagittal plane. Hypoechoic CSF in temporal horn and clot of mixed echogenicity in frontal and occipital horns. (Courtesy of Dr. J. Amodio.)

Although medical therapy to decrease production of CSF and osmodiuresis with acetazolamide or glycerol remain of questionable efficacy, they may postpone shunt placement.

Prevention. Many treatments for the prevention and spread of germinal hemorrhage have been attempted. Pharmacologic agents administered to small preterm infants include phenobarbital, ethamsylate, vitamin E, and indomethacin. None has been proven clearly beneficial; also, all side-effects have yet to be documented. Steroids and phenobarbital have been given to the mother antepartum. Again, their effect in reducing germinal plate hemorrhage is not well established. Bedside pharmacologic treatments and nursing therapies aimed at reducing the infant's systemic blood pressure with subsequent effects on cerebral blood flow may diminish the incidence of hemorrhage and its spread. Among these, the technique of pancuronium paralysis, while the infant is ventilated during the highest risk first 48 hours of life, has drawn much attention and controversy. The best prevention of intracranial hemorrhage remains avoidance of premature birth, if possible.

Asphyxia

Incidence. Largely because of improved obstetric techniques, asphyxia neonatorum has become less frequent; however, it remains a leading cause of static encephalopathy. Anoxic or asphyxial brain injury probably occurs with equal frequency in preterm and full-term infants, but the overt clinical patterns are seen mainly after 35 weeks gestational age and especially in the postmature infant.

Pathology and Pathophysiology. The anoxic-ischemic insult occurs before or during labor in 90% of cases. Concomitant cardiopulmonary or renal dysfunction may add to postnatal anoxic injury. The resulting brain pathology depends on the maturity of the brain at the time of insult and the duration of the ischemia. Preterm infants develop periventricular leukomalacia with puncta or islands of ischemia in the centrum semiovale often affecting the frontal periventricular myelinated fibers that project to the legs. The periventricular area is a vascular watershed region in premature infants and is especially vulnerable. After 36 weeks of gestation, lesions involve the cerebral gray matter, basal ganglia, brain stem, or cerebellar Purkinje cells. Acute neuronal necrosis is sometimes accompanied by hemorrhage, edema, or infarction. The chronic picture reveals neuronal loss and astrocytosis, and there may be ulegyria of the cortex, status marmoratus of the basal ganglia, or cerebellar atrophy. (See Article 66, Cerebral Palsy and Mental Retardation.)

Severe, brief, total asphyxia results in diffuse lesions that are rarely compatible with life. Experimentally, similar lesions can be induced in monkeys by complete intrauterine asphyxia for less than 13 minutes. Human cases could be caused by abruptio placentae or by the umbilical cord being wrapped tightly around the neck.

Partial asphyxia for minutes or hours results in predominantly supratentorial lesions, with generalized cerebral edema and hemorrhage or laminar neuronal necrosis in the depths of the sulci. Some lesions have a parasagittal or watershed distribution, especially after fetal hypotension. These are the subacute variants most often recognized in the neonatal period. They are attributed to impaired placental exchange and result in fetal heart tone abnormalities in the first or second stages of labor. Less severe intrauterine anoxic episodes of undetermined duration or timing may involve neurons diffusely or may preferentially affect the hippocampal areas.

Signs and Symptoms. Infants who sustain hypoxic or ischemic insults weeks or months before birth may seem normal at birth, but later show signs of static encephalopathy or seizures. Others, however, already exhibit signs of chronic cerebral disease at birth, with overt microcephaly and spasticity. In the perinatal period, asphyxia results in Apgar scores or less than 6 at 1 and 5 minutes after delivery. The infant may have poor color and a reduced heart rate; respiration, muscle tone, and reflexes are depressed or absent; and there is respiratory acidosis.

The clinical pattern in infants of less than 34-weeks gestation differs from that of full-term infants because the findings are nonspecific. Unless there is concurrent intraventricular hemorrhage (Type III or IV), preterm infants may show only poor response to stimulation, frequent apnea, and bradycardia. After resuscitative efforts, full-term infants may exhibit brain-stem involvement with respiratory problems, stupor, and severe hypotonia. There are oculomotor and pupillary abnormalities, ptosis, disturbed sucking, tongue fasciculations, and palatal myoclonus. There is also pooling of secretions and dysphagia.

The more common clinical patterns of sub-acute asphyxia involving the cerebral cortex of infants of more than 36-weeks gestation include three patterns: minimal lethargy and hypotonia; hyperalertness, often with hypertonia; or depression and severe hypotonia. Seizures are common in this last clinical pattern. In any of these patterns, there may have been evidence of intrauterine distress by fetal monitoring or meconium staining, and low Apgar scores at 1, 5, and even 10 or more minutes after delivery.

Some children gradually improve in alertness and tone from the beginning. Others have a few seizures before they improve. Infants with severe encephalopathy become more stuporous in the first 24 hours and have seizures, respiratory depression, brain-stem abnormalities, and intermittent decerebration. They lose Moro and sucking reflexes and become unresponsive. Even with vigorous anticonvulsant and supportive therapy, 20 to 30% die. If the infants survive the first 48 to 72 hours, seizures usually stop. The patients remain hypotonic and stuporous for a variable period, depending on the severity of brain damage and the amount of drugs given to control the seizures.

Laboratory Data. The most useful laboratory test in perinatal asphyxia is performed before birth during the first and second stages of labor. Fetal heart tone records that indicate late and variable deceleration of heart rate relative to uterine contractions, or fixed intrauterine heart rate, are evidence of placental insufficiency and fetal distress, which lead to postnatal anoxic encephalopathy.

After birth, arterial blood gases shows low pO_2, high pCO_2, and low pH. Serum glucose may be below 40 μg/100 ml. Serum sodium may be decreased. Serum CK-BB isoenzyme activity may be elevated. CSF is usually normal but the CSF lactic acid level may be increased. An EEG may reveal seizure activity that is clinically inapparent. In the interictal period, relatively inactive and burst-suppression patterns have been consistently correlated with poor outcome in infants of 36-weeks gestational age or older. Impaired visual evoked responses (VER) and brain-stem auditory evoked responses (BAER) may imply poor prognosis. Areas of decreased uptake of isotope may correlate with CT evidence of extensive areas of hypodensity of both gray and white matter; these findings imply poor prognosis.

Treatment and Prognosis. Because the hypoxic insult involves several body systems, attention must be directed to the respiratory, cardiovascular, and renal systems plus the brain. Measures include respiratory support and maintenance of normal blood pressure and renal output while specific treatment of seizures and brain edema are undertaken. The treatment of seizures is discussed below. Steroids and osmotic agents have been used to treat brain edema in this setting with equivocal results.

The prognosis is always guarded. The more rapid the recovery from initial depression, the better the outlook. Of infants with a benign neonatal course 20 to 30% may still have neurologic sequelae ranging from intellectual impairment to spastic diplegia and seizures. At least 50% of those with seizures have serious morbidity. Some early predictive statements can be made by judicious interpretation of the laboratory studies and clinical course. Prevention, by rapid delivery (caesarean section) when there is evidence of intrauterine distress, is the best method of avoiding sequelae.

Neonatal Infections

Bacterial infections commonly are acquired perinatally. Viral or protozoan infections may be acquired in utero from the first trimester to delivery; the TORCH quadrad (TO for toxoplasmosis, R for rubella, C for cytomegalic virus, and H for herpes simplex) is discussed in Chapter II, Infections of the Nervous System.

Bacterial meningitis is usually seen in association with sepsis. The incidence of sepsis neonatorum is about 0.51/1000 live births. In cases of neonatal sepsis, about 30% have spread to the meninges. The predominating organism in neonatal septicemia and meningitis varies with the year and locale. Gram-negative organisms (Escherichia coli, Pseudomonas vulgaris or aeruginosa) account for about 30%; however, in North America in the last decade, group B Streptococcus has replaced Staphylococcus as the most common cause of neonatal meningitis and now accounts for about 40%. Listeria and other rare organisms cause the others. Susceptibility to these organisms is attributed to immaturity of immune responses or of the blood-brain barrier. Pathologic changes in the newborn brain are like those in older children or adults.

The clinical presentation of meningitis in the newborn is more subtle than in older individuals. Meningeal signs are rarely elicited; lassitude and poor feeding may be the only abnormalities. Hypothermia, rather than fever, is a suggestive sign. Seizures may be the first sign. Only when the course is advanced does the fontanelle bulge and the infant assume a position of opisthotonos. Diagnosis is by lumbar puncture; the CSF changes are like those in older children, but hypoglycorrhachia is difficult to evaluate because newborns may have blood glucose levels of 30 to 40 mg/dl and CSF blood–glucose ratios are less valid. Culture of the CSF is often positive even when antibiotics have been administered; cultures may also remain positive for 3 or 4 days after initiation of proper therapy.

Because the disease may be advanced when it is clinically manifest, both mortality and morbidity remain high. Appropriate intravenous antibiotic therapy should be given for 3 weeks because both gram-negative and streptococcal infections may recur without an obvious focus being found. Intrathecal and intraventricular therapy have not been effective. Parenchymal invasion and clinically significant subdural effusions are rare at this age. Gram-negative organisms are implicated most frequently in neonatal abscess, which is rare.

Neonatal Seizures

Seizures in the neonatal period should always be considered symptomatic of serious underlying neurologic or systemic disease. Neonatal convulsions imply at least 17% mortality and 30% serious morbidity. The prognosis depends mainly on the cause of the seizures and on rapid establishment of diagnosis and treatment; however, it is difficult to recognize the clinical expressions of abnormal cortical discharges, particularly in infants of less than 35 weeks gestation; conventional clinical and EEG seizure patterns are rarely seen.

Classification. Neonatal seizures occur in several forms. Focal and multifocal clonic varieties are the most frequent that have clear electrical concomitants. They constitute 50% of neonatal convulsions and may begin as unifocal jerking of a single limb, one side of the face, or rhythmic horizontal deviation of the eyes. More often than not, the convulsions become multifocal; clonus or "jitteriness" may be misinterpreted as a seizure. The rhythm of a seizure is slow, three to four jerks/second; clonus or nonspecific tremor is about six to 12 jerks/second. Moreover, clonus or tremulousness can be started or stopped by altering the position of a limb.

Tonic postures are the next most common kind of neonatal seizure. An arm may be extended with or without horizontal eye deviation or head-turning. Abnormal EEG activity may originate from the frontal or temporal lobe. These seizures may not be recognized by nursery personnel and may look like yawning or stretching. On the other hand, total body extension with arm flexion or opisthotonic postures and vertical eye movements may be overinterpreted as seizures. These decerebrate or decorticate postures have no electrical correlation and are likely to occur in infants of less than 34 weeks gestational age with intraventricular hemorrhage.

Classic grand mal seizures or infantile myoclonic seizures are rare in the newborn. Myoclonus is often stimulus-sensitive and suggests severe brain damage or drug withdrawal. Adventitious movements are frequently described in mature infants with severe anoxic encephalopathy; these include mouthing movements, tongue thrusting, pedaling movements, writhing, and chaotic eye movements. These movements of uncertain pathogenesis are often witnessed in the late stages of an encephalopathy with no epileptiform discharges in the EEG.

Apneic spells may be manifestations of seizure in the full-term infant. On the other hand, in infants of less than 35-weeks gestation, apnea is rarely a convulsion. Apnea, accompanied by bradycardia in the preterm infant, is a frequent but poorly understood event. In infants of 36-weeks gestation or older, apnea without bradycardia is usually accompanied by other types of seizures, and is an important type of convulsion to recognize. It responds to anticonvulsants, whereas depressant agents are contraindicated in the apnea of the premature.

Diagnosis. Once a seizure is identified, diagnostic evaluation should proceed as rapidly as possible. Family, pregnancy, and delivery history and physical examination may provide the essential clues to etiology. The first laboratory tests evaluate the common metabolic and infectious disorders that require specific treatment. A dipstick test for hypoglycemia and lumbar puncture to exclude meningitis or hemorrhage are essential. Then blood glucose, calcium, magnesium, sodium, and acid-base values should be obtained plus a blood culture. EEG studies must be undertaken promptly if abnormal movements are not clearly identified as seizures. CT may confirm subarachnoid or parenchymal blood collections, major congenital anomalies, or ischemic damage, but is usually not immediately essential. If necessary, sonography can provide early information about large hemorrhages. If a congenital infection is suspected, TORCH titers should be drawn. If seizures do not respond to the usual treatment, pyridoxine (50 mg) should be given intravenously to rule out rare pyridoxine dependency. Blood, urine, and CSF should then be analyzed for errors of inborn metabolism that may present in the neonatal period: phenylketonuria, maple sugar urine disease, organic acidemias, ammonia cycle abnormalities, and ketotic and nonketotic hyperglycinemia.

Etiology and Prognosis. The outcome of neonatal seizures is linked to etiology (Table 64–1). In some metabolic disorders, prognosis is better the sooner treatment starts. Surveys of prognosis have given different estimates; some institutions see more neonatal seizures of benign etiology (e.g., late hypocalcemia), and adventitious movements of some other genesis may be thought to be seizures.

The EEG, judiciously interpreted, may help in determining prognosis. The proper time for an EEG is 24 to 48 hours after the last seizure. In older children, a longer interval is recommended, but in newborns, the EEG often becomes normal in a few days and may lose prognostic significance.

Five types of interictal EEG patterns are ob-served in infants of 36 to 42 weeks gestation: normal, unifocal spike with normal background, multifocal spike, burst-suppression, and inactive or flat. The first two types suggest a 70% chance of good outcome. However, a poor prognostic etiology is more important than any EEG pattern. Multifocal spikes, especially with abnormal backgrounds, imply only a 20% chance of a good prognosis. The burst-suppression pattern, not to be confused with the normal deep-sleep pattern, almost invariably implies severe static encephalopathy. The inactive or flat EEG has the same poor prognosis, although it may be hard to interpret when anticonvulsant drug levels are high; it is not synonymous with brain death.

Treatment. Treatment of neonatal seizures is either specific or symptomatic. The metabolic encephalopathies require specific therapy. Documented neonatal hypoglycemia (defined as a blood glucose of less than 40 mg/dl in a full-term infant and less than 30 mg/dl in a premature infant) is usually treated with an intravenous bolus of 25 to 50% glucose followed by a maintenance infusion of 10% dextrose. If there is difficulty in maintaining blood glucose, 1 mg dexamethasone is given every 6 hours for 1 or 2 days to promote gluconeogenesis.

Hypocalcemia (defined as a blood calcium level of less than 7 mg/dl) is of two varieties.

Table 64–1.   Relationship of Neurologic Disease to Prognosis in Neonatal Seizures

Disease	Percentage of Children Who Survive and Become Normal	Comment
Perinatal asphyxia	50	
Subarachnoid hemorrhage	90	
Intraventricular hemorrhage	10	Seizures rare in prematures
Hypoglycemia	50	Outcome may be related to early-onset therapy
Late hypocalcemia	90	Presents day 5–10
Early hypocalcemia	50	Presents day 1–3 in conjunction with other encephalopathies
Inborn metabolic errors	10	A few with phenylketonuria or pyridoxine dependency may do well
Bacterial meningitis	30	
Congenital anomalies	0	Defects include lissencephaly, polymycrogyria, pachygyria
Drug withdrawal	?	Good follow-up series unavailable; drugs include heroin, methadone
Cause unknown	67	10–20% of neonatal seizures, including benign familial seizure

(Modified from Volpe JJ, Koenigsberger MR. Neonatology: Pathophysiology and Management of the Newborn. Philadelphia: JB Lippincott, 1981.)

The late-onset (after day 5) benign type is usually seen in full-term infants who are given high-phosphate formulas and who have multifocal seizures. When hypocalcemia is suspected, blood should be drawn for calcium level tests. Treatment begins with intravenous doses of calium gluconate with EKG monitoring. When the blood calcium level does not rise in response to this therapy, hypomagnesemia is a possibility. Recalcitrant hypocalcemia may respond to intramuscular therapy with magnesium sulfate. The seizures of infants with hypocalcemia in the first 2 or 3 days of life may not respond to therapy because early hypocalcemia often accompanies severe intracranial hemorrhage or asphyxia. Severe encephalopathy with inappropriate antidiuretic hormone secretion causes hyponatremia, which may also result from iatrogenic overhydration. It is controlled by fluid restriction. Other metabolic encephalopathies are difficult to treat and have a poor prognosis.

Symptomatic treatment of neonatal seizures can be divided into management of a single seizure (or a few widely separated seizures) and the management of continuous seizures. General supportive care should not be forgotten; when possible, therapy should be carried out in a neonatal intensive care unit. An adequate airway should be assured and means for mechanical respiration should be available. Intravenous administration of glucose and electrolytes provides energy and osmotic balance, but fluid intake should be restricted to avoid brain edema.

A single seizure is treated with a loading intravenous dose of 15 to 20 mg/kg body weight of phenobarbital, followed by a maintenance dosage of 5 mg/kg/day in two 12-hour doses. Blood phenobarbital levels of 20 to 40 µg/dl should be established and maintained. In status epilepticus, a loading dose of 20 mg/kg of body weight of phenobarbital is given intravenously over 2 minutes. If the seizures continue or recur, two more 10 mg/kg doses can be administered slowly within 1 or 2 hours. If this is not adequate, phenytoin can be given intravenously (20 mg/kg) over 15 minutes with cardiac monitoring. Maintenance dosage of phenobarbital, administered orally, intramuscularly, or intravenously, should be 3 to 7 mg/kg/day. A blood level of 20 to 40 µg/dl is suggested, but a blood level of 40 to 60 µg/dl for 1 or 2 days is not harmful (if respiration is maintained) is attempts to suppress potentially harmful continuous epileptic activity. Phenytoin maintenance doses of 7 to 10 mg/kg of body weight/day can also be given intravenously; neither intramuscular nor oral routes are effective for this drug. If status epilepticus continues, a 4% paraldehyde intravenous drip is adjusted against seizure activity. Diazepam is not given to the neonate because its anticonvulsant action is too brief and, in combination with barbiturates, may be harmful.

In infants with single or easily controlled seizures, anticonvulsants may be tapered on discharge. Others remain on phenobarbital maintenance (5 µg/kg/day).

References

Intracranial Hemorrhage

Allan WC, Volpe JJ. Periventricular-intraventricular hemorrhage. Pediatr Clin North Am 1986; 36:47–63.

Ahman PA, Lazarra A, Dykes FD, et al. Intraventricular hemorrhage in the high risk preterm infant: Incidence and outcome. Ann Neurol 1980; 7:118–124.

Bergman I, Bauer RE, Barmada MH. Intracerebral hemorrhage in the full-term neonatal infant. Pediatrics 1985; 75:488–496.

Connell J, et al. Predictive value of early continuous EEG monitoring in ventilated preterm infants with intraventricular hemorrhage. Pediatrics 1988; 82:337–343.

Dubowitz IMS, Bydder GM. Nuclear magnetic resonance imaging in the diagnosis and follow-up of neonatal cerebral injury. Clinics in Perinatology 1985; 12:245–260.

Goddard-Finegold J. Periventricular intraventricular hemorrhage in the premature newborn. Update on pathologic features, pathogenesis and possible means of prevention. Arch Neurol 1984; 41:766–771.

Goddard-Finegold J, Mizrani EM. Understanding and preventing perinatal peri- and intraventricular hemorrhage. Jour Child Neurol 1987; 2:170–185.

Hill A, Volpe JJ. Normal pressure hydrocephalus in the newborn. Pediatrics 1981; 68:623–629.

Kauffman RE. Therapeutic interventions to prevent intracerebral hemorrhage in preterm infants: J Pediatr 1986; 108:323–26.

Kreusser KL, Tarby T, Taylor D, et al. Rapidly progressive post hemorrhagic hydrocephalus; treatment with external ventricular drainage. Am J Dis Child 1984; 138:633–637.

Levine M, Williams J, Fawer C. Ultrasound of the Infant Brain. Philadelphia: JB Lippincott, 1985.

Ment LR, Duncan CC, Ehrenkranz RA, et al. Intraventricular hemorrhage in the preterm neonate: Timing and cerebral blood flow changes. J Pediatr 1984; 104:419–425.

Pape KE, Wigglesworth JS. Hemorrhage, Ischemia and the Perinatal Brain. Philadelphia: JB Lippincott, 1979.

Papile LA, Burstein J, Burstein R, et al. Incidence and evolution of subependymal and intraventricular hemorrhage: A study of infants with birth weight less than 1500 g. J Pediatr 1978; 92:529–534.

Pearlman JM, Goodman S, Kreuser KL, et al. Reduction in intraventricular hemorrhage by elimination of fluctuating cerebral blood flow velocity in preterm infants with respiratory distress syndrome. N Engl J Med 1985; 312:1353–56.

Volpe JJ. Neurology of the Newborn. Philadelphia: WB Saunders, 1987.

Welch K, Strand R. Traumatic parturitional intracranial hemorrhage. Dev Med Child Neurol 1986; 28:156–164.

Asphyxia

Adsett DB, Fitz CR, Hill A. Hypoxic-ischemic injury in the term newborn; correlation of CT findings with neurological outcome. Dev Med Child Neurol 1985; 27:155–160.

Amiel-Tison C, Ellison P. Birth asphyxia in the fullterm newborn; early assessment and outcome. Dev Med Child Neurol 1986; 28:671–682.

Banker BA, Larroche JC. Periventricular leukomalacia of infancy. Arch Neurol 1962; 7:386–410.

Fenichel GM. Hypoxic-ischemic encephalopathy in the newborn. Neurology 1983; 40:261–266.

Freeman J, Nelson KB. Intrapartum asphyxia and cerebral palsy. Pediatrics 1988; 82:240–249.

Hill A, Volpe JJ. Pathogenesis and management of hypoxic-ischemic encephalopathy in the term newborn. Neurol Clin North Am 1986; 3:3–46.

Lupton BA, et al. Brain swelling in the asphyxiated term newborn: pathogenesis and outcome. Pediatrics 1988; 82:139–146.

Majnemmer A, Rosenblatt B, Riley P. Prognostic significance of auditory brain stem evoked response in high risk neonates. Dev Med Child Neurol 1988; 30:36–42.

Myers RE. Experimental models of periventricular brain damage: Relevance to human pathology. In: Gluck L, ed. Intrauterine Asphyxia and the Developing Brain. Chicago: Year Book Medical, 1977:337–397.

Nelson KB, Ellenberg, JH. Antecedents of cerebral palsy. N Engl J Med 1986; 315:81–86.

Skow B, Lou H, Pederson H. Perinatal brain ischemia: Impact at 4 years of age. Dev Med Child Neurol 1984; 26:353–356.

Volpe JJ, Hirscovitch P, Perlman JM, et al. Positron emission tomography in the asphyxiated term newborn: Parasagittal impairment of cerebral blood flow. Ann Neurol 1985; 17:287–296.

Wilson DA, Steiner RA. Periventricular leukomalacia: evaluation with MR imaging. Radiology 1987; 160:507–512.

Infections

Bell WE, McCormick WF. Neurologic Infections in Children, 2nd ed. Philadelphia: WB Saunders, 1981.

Edwards MS, Rench MA, Haffer AA, et al. Long-term sequelae of group B streptoccocal meningitis in infants. J Pediatr 1985; 106:717–722.

Harriss MC, Polin RA. Neonatal septicemia. Pediatr Clin North Am 1983; 30:243–258.

Klein JO, Feigin RD, McCracken GH. Report of the task force on diagnosis and management of meningitis. Pediatrics [Suppl]1986; 78:959–982.

Mises J, Daviet F, Mousalli-Salefranque F, et al. Brain abscesses in neonates (27 cases): electroclinical evolution. Revue d'Electroencephalographie et de Neurophysiologie Clinique 1987; 17:301–308.

Seizures

Brown JK. Convulsions in the newborn period. Dev Med Child Neurol 1973; 15:823–846.

Cockburn F, Brown JK, Belton NR, et al. Neonatal convulsions associated with primary disturbance of calcium, phosphorus and magnesium metabolism. Arch Dis Child 1973; 48:99–108.

Holden KR, Mellitis ED, Freeman JM. Neonatal seizures I. Correlation of prenatal and perinatal events with outcome. Pediatrics 1982; 70:165–176.

Koenigsberger MR. Abnormal neonatal movements, intracranial hemorrhage, asphyxia. Pediatr Annals 1983; 12:798–804.

Koivisto M, Blanco-Sequieros M, Krause U. Neonatal symptomatic hypoglycemia: A follow-up study of 151 children. Dev Med Child Neurol 1972; 14:603–609.

Legido A, Clancy RR, Berman PH. Recent advances in the diagnosis, treatment, and prognosis of neonatal seizures. Pediatric Neurology 1988; 4:79–86.

Mizrani EM, Kellaway P. Characterization and classification of neonatal seizures. Neurology 1987; 37:1837–1844.

Painter MJ, Bergmann I, Crumrine P. Neonatal seizures. Pediatr Clin North Am 1986; 33:91–109.

Perlman JM, Volpe JJ. Seizures in the preterm infant: Effects on cerebral blood flow velocity, intracranial pressure, and arterial pressure. J Pediatr 1983; 102:228–293.

Petit RE, Fenichel GM. Benign familial neonatal seizures. Arch Neurol 1980; 37:47–48.

Rose AL, Lombroso CT. Neonatal seizures states. A study of clinical features in 137 full term babies with long term follow-up. Pediatrics 1970; 45:404–425.

Volpe JJ. Neonatal seizures. Clin Perinatol 1977; 4:43–53.

65. THE FLOPPY INFANT SYNDROME
Darryl C. DeVivo

When a normal infant is suspended in the prone position, the arms and legs move out and the head is held in line with the body. In many different disorders, the child does not respond in this fashion. Rather, the limbs and head all hang limply—"like a rag doll." That is why *the floppy infant syndrome* has caught on as a popular term. In addition to these abnormal postures, some clinicians have extended the use of the term to include children with diminished resistance of limbs to passive movement and to children with abnormal extensibility of joints.

The number of conditions that sometimes cause these manifestations seems endless, including disorders of the brain, spinal cord, peripheral nerves, neuromuscular junction, muscles, ligaments, and some disorders of unknown origin. The number of possible causes of floppy infant syndrome makes diagnosis of the primary disorder seem impossible. However, there are almost always clues of some kind that narrow the list of possible causes to a few choices. An essential division separates conditions found in the newborn infant from those that occur later (Table 65–1).

Table 65–1. Floppy Infant Syndromes

	Neuromuscular Disorders (weakness prominent)	Central Disorders with Abnormal Neurologic Signs or Peripheral Disorders (little or no weakness)
Neonatal	Infantile spinal muscular atrophy[1] Congenital myotonic dystrophy Neonatal myasthenia gravis Congenital myopathies[1,2] Infantile acid-maltase deficiency (Pompe disease) Congenital muscular dystrophy (Fukuyama and Zellweger types)	Perinatal asphyxia or cerebral hemorrhage Sepsis Intoxication Spinal-cord injury or malformation Failure-to-thrive syndromes Congenital hypothyroidism Dysgenetic syndromes (e.g., Down disease) Prader-Willi syndrome
Age 1–6 months (or later)	Infantile spinal muscular atrophy Infantile Guillain-Barré or other peripheral neuropathy Congenital myasthenia gravis[3] Botulism	Metabolic cerebral degenerations[4] Hypotonic cerebral palsy Connective tissue disorders[5] Metabolic and endocrine diseases[6] Essential hypotonia
Failure to reach developmental stages but not really floppy	Congenital myopathies[2] Some Duchenne muscular dystrophy	

1. Spinal muscular atrophy and congenital myopathies are more likely to cause symptoms *after* the neonatal period.
2. Congenital myopathies include those characterized by specific histochemical abnormality (nemaline, central core, myotubular, and other structures).
3. Congenital myasthenia does not usually cause infantile symptoms other than ophthalmoplegia.
4. Leucodystrophies, lipid storage diseases, mucopolysaccharidoses, aminoacidurias, Leigh syndrome.
5. Congenital laxity of ligaments, Ehlers-Danlos syndrome, Marfan syndrome.
6. Organic acidemia, hypo- or hypercalcemia; hypothyroidism; renal tubular acidosis.

A second division separates conditions that are characterized by true limb weakness (often with no tendon reflexes) from those with clear neurologic signs or cerebral injury without true limb weakness. Among the latter, there are likely to be signs of mental retardation, dysmorphic physical evidence of chromosomal abnormality, or evidence of metabolic abnormality.

A third diagnostic consideration concerns illness in the mother and the perinatal history. If the mother is known to have myotonic muscular dystrophy or myasthenia gravis, depressed movement in the infant is immediately recognized. On the other hand, the correct diagnosis in the child may be the first clue to explain previously unrecognized manifestations of illness in the mother. Similarly, maternal narcotic drug abuse, alcoholism, or use of anticonvulsant medications may affect the infant. Perinatal events may lead to suspicion of asphyxia or cerebral hemorrhage.

A fourth consideration is the distribution of abnormality. Are all four limbs affected? Only the legs? One arm? Are sucking and swallowing impaired? The answers have different diagnostic implications.

The most common causes of hypotonia are perinatal insult to the brain or spinal cord, spinal muscular atrophy, and dysgenetic syndromes. About 75% of cases fall into these categories. However, spinal muscular atrophy is only rarely evident immediately after birth. The neonatologist considers common perinatal insults such as birth asphyxia, hypoxic-ischemic insults, intracranial hemorrhage, bacterial or viral infections, metabolic disturbances, and extreme prematurity as principal causes of hypotonia in the newborn nursery. Congenital hypoglycemia or hypothyroidism may be suggested by hypothermia. Spinal cord injuries usually follow intrauterine malpositioning or traumatic birth. In these conditions, the perinatal history is informative and the hypotonic infant has associated behavioral alterations including decreased responsiveness or seizures. Dysmorphic features are absent and tendon reflexes are present.

Focal Neonatal Hypotonia

This disorder may be caused by trauma or developmental abnormality. A flaccid arm usually implies brachial plexus injury. Signs of injury to the upper brachial plexus may be associated with ipsilateral paralysis of the diaphragm; lower brachial plexus lesions may be accompanied by an ipsilateral Horner syndrome. EMG and spinal evoked potentials help to define the severity of the nerve root injury. Metrizamide myelography may document nerve root avulsion.

Hypotonia and weakness of the legs indicate spinal cord pathology. Spinal dysraphism and the caudal regression syndrome are obvious on inspection of the back. An arthrogrypotic leg deformity or gross maldevelopment of the legs is associated with sacral agenesis. Fifteen percent of patients with sacral agenesis are infants of diabetic mothers.

Dysgenetic Syndromes

These syndromes are often associated with distinctive dysmorphic physical features. The neurologic disorder may not be recognized until the infant fails to reach certain developmental stages. Common syndromes associated with hypotonia are Down syndrome, Prader-Willi syndrome, Lowe syndrome, Zellweger syndrome, Smith-Lemli-Opitz syndrome, and the Riley-Day (familial dysautonomia) syndrome. Environmental toxins also may produce hypotonia and dysmorphism. Common examples include fetal exposure to heroin, phenytoin, trimethadione, or alcohol. Strength is normal in these syndromes, but the tendon reflexes may vary from nondetectable to brisk.

Neuromuscular Disorders

Neuromuscular disorders that cause infantile hypotonia do not impair mental alertness but are characterized by decreased limb movement (because of muscle weakness) and decreased tendon reflexes. Dysmorphic features accompany many congenital myopathies. After the immediate neonatal period, spinal muscular atrophy is the most common cause of infantile hypotonia. This autosomal recessive disorder (Werdnig-Hoffmann disease) may sometimes be evident at birth. The characteristic findings include limb weakness, areflexia, and fasciculations of the tongue. Although most affected infants die before age 2, some survive for decades.

Poliomyelitis is now uncommon as a cause of limb weakness. The neurologic findings are asymmetric and are accompanied by signs of meningeal irritation with (CSF) pleocytosis and elevated protein content.

Infantile neuropathies are uncommon causes of weakness, areflexia, and hypotonia. Examples include metachromatic leukodystrophy, globoid cell leukodystrophy, infantile neuroaxonal dystrophy, giant axonal neuropathy, neonatal adrenoleukodystrophy, hypertrophic interstitial polyneuropathy, and peroneal muscular atrophy. Important clues may include a family history, palpably enlarged peripheral nerves, upper motor neuron signs, elevated CSF protein concentration, and slowed nerve conduction velocities. Guillain-Barré syndrome rarely presents in infancy.

Disturbances at the myoneural junction may cause limb weakness. Fluctuating signs intensified by vigorous crying or limb activity are important observations. *Congenital myasthenia gravis* often affects siblings and is thought to be inherited as an autosomal recessive disorder. This condition is considered nonimmunologic. Clinically, the infant may display external ophthalmoplegia and generalized weakness; sudden respiratory failure rarely occurs. Autoimmune forms of myasthenia gravis in infancy include the transient *neonatal form* in infants of myasthenic mothers. The *juvenile form* does not ordinarily cause symptoms before age 2 years. Acetylcholine receptor antibodies, sensitivity to curare, and responsiveness to plasmapheresis distinguish these myasthenic syndromes from the inherited nonimmunologic forms.

Another condition that affects neuromuscular transmission is *infantile botulism,* which results from the ingestion of Clostridium botulinus spores that germinate in the intestinal tract. Manifestations include ileus, constipation, hypotonia, weakness, pupillary dilatation, and apneic spells. The clinical picture is distinctive and diagnosis can be confirmed by the recovery of the bacterium and the exotoxin in the feces. A facilitating response to repetitive stimulation (like that of the Eaton-Lambert syndrome) can usually be demonstrated and may be an important diagnostic clue. Complete recovery follows appropriate supportive care.

Myopathies that cause infantile limb weakness include the *congenital myopathies* with specific structural abnormalities, myotonic muscular dystrophy, and metabolic myopathies. Although the term "muscular dystrophy" usually implies progressive disease, the term has been applied to apparently static congenital disorders in which the changes in muscle biopsy are myopathic but have no specific features. In Japan, the Fukuyama type of *congenital muscular dystrophy* is characterized by severe mental retardation in all cases and seizures in about 50%. Symptoms may start soon after birth, with difficulty nursing and impoverished movement. The children never walk but may live for decades. The cerebral pathology is distinctive, with polymicrogyria of the occipital lobes in a pattern that can be recognized by CT. Similar cases have been seen in the United States and Europe.

The *histochemically-defined myopathies* may be inherited as autosomal dominant or recessive traits or as a sex-linked recessive trait. These disorders share many phenotypic features that overlap other syndromes. Examples include central core disease, multicore disease, nemaline myopathy, myotubular (centronuclear) myopathy, congenital-fiber-type disproportion, sarcotubular myopathy, fingerprint-body myopathy, and reducing-body myopathy. Muscular weakness, decreased tendon reflexes, dysmorphic physical features, a predisposition to congenital hip dislocation, and later, development of scoliosis characterize most of the histochemically defined myopathies. The similarities often outweigh the differences.

Infantile acid maltase deficiency (Pompe disease) is the classic example of a metabolic myopathy and motor neuron disease that causes infantile hypotonia. The affected infant is mentally alert, but weak and areflexic. Enlargement of the tongue and heart are associated findings; congestive heart faiure is the cause of death before age 6 months. Other *metabolic myopathies* that may cause infantile hypotonia and weakness include cytochrome-C oxidase deficiency, glycogenosis type IV (debrancher enzyme deficiency), and glycogenosis Type V (myophosphorylase deficiency). Cytochrome-C oxidase deficiency is associated with lactic acidosis.

A few hypotonic infants eventually develop normally after several years. The term *essential hypotonia* should be reserved to describe an otherwise healthy infant with unexplained hypotonia with normal strength, tendon reflexes, and general physical features.

References

Brooke MH, Carroll JE, Ringel SP. Congenital hypotonia revisited. Muscle Nerve 1979; 2:84–100.

DiMauro S, Hartlage PL. Fatal infantile form of muscle phosphorylase deficiency. Neurology 1978; 28:1124–1129.

DiMauro S, Mendell JR, Sahenk Z, et al. Fatal infantile mitochondrial myopathy and renal dysfunction due to cytochrome c-oxidase deficiency. Neurology 1980; 30:795–804.

DiMauro S, Nicholson JF, Hays AP, et al. Mitochondrial myopathy due to reversible cytochrome-c oxidase deficiency. Ann Neurol 1983; 14:226–234.

Dubowitz V. The floppy infant. London: Spastics International Medical Publications, 1969.

Dubowitz V. Muscle Disorders in Childhood. Philadelphia: WB Saunders, 1978.

Egger J, Kendall BE, Erdohazi M, et al. Involvement of the central nervous system in congenital muscular dystrophies. Dev Med Child Neurol 1983; 25:32–42.

Fukuyama Y, Osawa M, Suzuki H. Congenital progressive muscular dystrophy of the Fukuyama type. Clinical, genetic and pathological considerations. Brain Dev 1981; 3:1–29.

Hagberg B, Sanner G, Steen M. The dysequilibrium syndrome in cerebral palsy: Clinical aspects and treatment. Acta Paediatr Scand 1972; 61 (suppl 266):1–63.

Pickett J, Berg B, Chaplin E, Brunstetter-Shaffer MA. Syndrome of botulism in infancy: Clinical and electrophysiological study. N Engl J Med 1976; 295:770–772.

Rabe EF. The hypotonic infant (a review). J Pediatr 64:422–440.

Sarnat HB. Neuromuscular disorders in the neonatal period. In: Korobkin R, Guilleminault C, eds. Advances in Perinatal Neurology (vol 1). New York: SP Medical & Scientific Books, 1979:153–203.

66. CEREBRAL PALSY AND MENTAL RETARDATION

Sidney Carter
Niels L. Low

The brain of a child can be adversely affected at any time from the fertilization of the ovum through infancy. Severe insults lead to death or major degrees of brain injury, whereas mild degrees of the same kind of insult may produce only minor deviations. The clinical results are functional handicaps that are static, or nonprogressive.

If the functional handicap primarily affects motor performance, it is assumed that the motor areas of the brain are predominantly involved and the child is said to have *cerebral palsy* (CP). If learning and reasoning are significantly impaired, the term *mental retardation* is applied and is attributed to diffuse cerebral involvement of small lesions that occurred early in gestation and may have interfered with normal cerebral maturation. Some children are not retarded, although their powers of concentration and attention are diminished; they are hyperactive, easily distracted, and impulsive. Many of these children have circumscribed learning disorders or coordination difficulties. The terms *minimal brain dysfunction* (MBD) and *attention deficit disorder* are applied to this group to indicate attention deficit hyperactivity, and learning disabilities. Impairment of the senses of sight and hearing follows lesions of appropriate areas of the brain. Convulsions are attributed to cortical lesions. Speech disturbances may result from diffuse cerebral involvement or a focal lesion involving the speech area. These syndromes may occur as isolated clinical phenomena or in any combination.

Cerebral Palsy

The term "cerebral palsy" encompasses many different conditions that include some specific criteria. The pathology is in the brain; there is a motor disorder; the disorder is not progressive; and the etiologic insult occurred before birth, in the perinatal period, or during the first few years of life.

Etiology. We have only limited knowledge of the causes of cerebral structural anomalies that arise during gestation, but it is believed that CP can be caused by anomalies resulting from abnormal implantation of the ovum or fetus, maternal diseases, threatened miscarriage, external toxins, or metabolic disorders. The single, most frequent factor associated with CP is a birth weight below 2500 g, which may occur in premature delivery, small-for-gestational-age infants, or multiple births. All complications of childbirth, including abruptio placentae, prolapsed umbilical cord, and complicated breech deliveries, predispose to hypoxia or intracranial bleeding in the neonate. The location of intracranial bleeding may be subependymal or intraventricular. Sonography and CT have enabled the diagnosis and location of these hemorrhages and provide information about the incidence and consequences. Infections and trauma are the chief causes of CP in the postnatal period.

Pathology. Because CP is not a single clinical entry and many etiologic factors may cause these syndromes or contribute to them, there is no single pathology; the findings depend primarily on the cause. The most common causes are primarily germinal layer and intraventricular hemorrhage or periventricular leukomalacia in the preterm infant, and ischemic brain damage in the birth-asphyxiated child.

Classification. There are three major types of CP: spastic, dyskinetic, an ataxic. Combinations of two (or, rarely, all three) types may occur. The following list shows the clinical classification of CP:

Spastic
  hemiparesis
  tetraparesis
  diplegia (diparesis)
    hypertonic
    hypotonic ("atonic")

paraparesis
mono- and triparesis
Dyskinetic
athetosis
other dyskinesias
Ataxic
Mixed

Course. By definition, CP is not progressive, although the clinical manifestations may change. The untreated spastic child may develop fixed deformities due to nonusage of muscles and joints. Some walking patients become nonambulatory if they gain too much weight because the energy then required for walking becomes prohibitive. The possibility of glutaric aciduria, Type I, should be considered in children whose CP seems progressive. The child with uncontrolled seizures may lose mental ability; therefore, the child may become functionally worse although the disorder is static. On the other hand, some children seem to become more intelligent. The apparent improvement follows underestimates at an age when psychometric testing depends too much on motor performance.

Age at Diagnosis. Hemiparesis is the easiest syndrome to diagnose early in life because there is a built-in control, the opposite side. Asymmetry of arm or fist posture is often first noticed by the parent, or asymmetric kicking of the legs is seen during the first few months of life, even by an untrained observer.

A physician or therapist who is experienced with both normal children and those with CP can often detect abnormal postures (opisthotonos, backward head thrust, abnormal turning) that lead to diagnosis of CP in infancy. Dyskinesia is difficult to diagnose during the first year of life because athetosis is so similar to the normal random movements of infancy. But even then, abnormal postures may be apparent by age 6 months.

Treatment. CP cannot be cured; however, function can be improved in almost all cases, especially when treatment starts early. Although this is not the text for detailed description of treatment, a few points can be made. There is no standard therapy; the physician must recommend what is best for each individual patient at a particular time and age. The goals of therapy are to improve function, control seizures, select the most suitable type and place of education, and help the patient to establish an emotional life that approaches normal.

Treatment includes physical and occupa-

tional therapy, speech therapy, and judicious use of orthoses. Surgery may be indicated when specific goals cannot be obtained by other means and when a particular surgical procedure can be expected to improve function. In all forms of therapy, the family or other caretakers should be intimately involved.

School placement should depend primarily on learning ability, rather than the physical handicap. The normally intelligent child, with or without CP, learns best in a regular class. The retarded child should be in school with other retarded children, regardless of any physical problem.

Emotional Life. The emotions experienced by a child with CP differ from those of normal children; their families also have special emotional experiences. Unless the parents can adjust early to the presence of a handicapped child, the child has no chance to adapt to the handicap. The physician who first recognizes CP in a child, and the professionals who treat the patient, must begin to help the family early and continue helping them to adjust thereafter. The child's adjustment follows. In certain periods, especially during puberty and sexual awakening, individual psychotherapy and guidance are helpful.

SPASTIC CEREBRAL PALSY

Hemiparesis. This term implies that limbs are affected on one side of the body while the other side is normal. In most instances, the arm is more affected than the leg. The spastic limbs are usually thinner and smaller than the other extremities. These changes in part are attributed to parietal lobe lesions, which may also lead to impairment of sensory-cortical function such as diminished or absent discrimination of size, shape, and texture of objects (astereognosis). Children with spastic hemiparesis tend to have increased tone predominantly in the flexors of the arms, hip adductors and flexors, knee flexors, and plantar extensors; the combination causes a characteristic gait and posture. The disorder may be minimal or severe. Walking may seem normal, but the abnormality becomes apparent when the child runs. Tendon reflexes are increased on the affected side, and clonus may be present; the Babinski sign is often absent in congenital CP, but is usually present in postneonatal cases.

Tetraparesis. This term is applied when the trunk and all four limbs are equally affected with only minor asymmetry. Because both cerebral hemispheres are involved, supra-nuclear (pseudobulbar) palsy is often found, with dysarthric speech, dysphagia, and drooling.

Spastic Diplegia (Diparesis). This term was coined by Sigmund Freud to describe cases in which all four limbs are involved, but with the legs and feet more severely affected than the arms and hands. The borderline between tetra- and diparesis is not sharp; in fact, it is a continuum. In children with little impairment of arm and hand function, only an experienced examiner can demonstrate the impairment. Fine finger skills, rapid hand movements, and asymmetric forearm function have to be evaluated. This is the most common form of CP that complicates prematurity, and has been attributed to parasagittal ischemia and can be corroborated by positron emission tomography (PET).

Hypotonic (atonic) diplegia is only seen in young children and the physiologic basis for the decreased tone is not understood. Tone always increases as these children mature. Monoparesis and triparesis are uncommon. Paraparesis attributable to a cerebral lesion is rare.

DYSKINETIC CEREBRAL PALSY

This major category is characterized by abnormal involuntary movements, especially athetosis, which is seen in young children. In infants, athetosis is difficult to recognize and, with increasing age, dystonic movements or chorea may be superimposed. Ultimately, there is hypertrophy of the continually moving muscles, especially those of the neck and shoulders. Dyskinesia subsides in sleep. Many children with dyskinetic CP also have some spasticity.

The seat of pathology is presumably in the basal ganglia, especially the globus pallidus. Kernicterus (especially due to Rh-type incompatibility) was once the major cause of athetosis, but with modern methods of prevention and treatment it is now uncommon.

ATAXIC CEREBRAL PALSY

In less than 5% of children with CP, ataxia is the main manifestation. The pathology is not well understood. In young children, other causes of ataxia should be excluded before assuming that the ataxia is static and nonprogressive. Children with this syndrome tend to improve functionally as they learn to compensate for the ataxia.

ASSOCIATED CONDITIONS

Any disease that involves the brain and impairs motor function can also impair intellectual development, attention, activity and impulse control, vision and hearing, and can cause seizures. Thus, mental retardation, MBD, and epilepsy are often associated with CP. Published incidence figures of these associated conditions vary enormously, but more than half the children with CP have one or more of these associated disturbances.

The Minimal Brain Dysfunction Syndrome

The terms *minimal brain dysfunction* (MBD) and *attention deficit disorder* are applied to children with normal or nearly normal intelligence who demonstrate abnormal behavior patterns or specific learning disabilities. The deviant behavior is manifested by hyperactivity, short attention span, distractibility, and poor impulse control. About 5 to 10% of all school-age children are thought to have this syndrome in whole or in part. Boys outnumber girls at least four to one.

Etiology. Two kinds of parallel evidence imply that brain damage or neurologic dysfunction causes this syndrome. First, similar patterns of behavior are seen in survivors of encephalitis and in those who have suffered severe head trauma. Second, similar behavior and learning characteristics have been observed in children born after difficult or complicated pregnancies and in those who experienced overt trauma at time of delivery, circumstances that might be expected to increase the likelihood of cerebral injury.

Follow-up studies of children born prematurely or who suffered anoxia at birth indicated that these children were at increased risk of developing hyperkinetic syndromes, often with perceptual deficits or other cognitive deficiencies. Pasamanick and Knobloch demonstrated the relationship between prematurity, prenatal difficulties, and perinatal medical complications to numerous psychological, neurologic, and behavioral disorders. They evolved the concept of "a continuum of reproductive casualty." Severe insults (e.g., extreme prematurity, prolonged anoxia) lead to death or major degrees of brain injury manifested by marked retardation and spasticity; they postulated that mild, often unnoticed, injury of the same kind might cause minor deviations of intelligence, behavior, and coordination.

Other possible causes of the syndrome include chronic lead intoxication or excessive alcohol intake by pregnant women. Genetic factors were suggested because parents of hyperactive children also had histories of similar behavior and learning problems. The paradoxic effect of the amphetamines on hyperactivity, inattentiveness, and distractibility has led to consideration of a neurochemical cause. Human and animal studies have implicated dopamine depletion.

Studies have not supported claims that hyperactivity is caused, aggravated, or worsened by a diet containing artificial food colors or other additives.

Pathology. It has not yet been possible to perform pathologic studies of the brains of children diagnosed as having the MBD syndrome. Those who favor the explanation of a structural disturbance of the brain would expect similar, but less severe, lesions than those found in children who have suffered profound brain injury.

Clinical Manifestations. The clinical syndrome of MBD is variable and the manifestations may change with age. Deviant behavior, learning disabilities, speech disorders, and poor coordination are most common. The behavioral patterns most frequently encountered relate to hyperactivity (i.e., short attention span, distractibility, and impulsivity). The hyperactive behavior may be noted in infancy as restlessness, irritability, or poor sleep patterns. In older children, hyperactivity is manifested by excessive running, difficulty sitting still or staying seated, or fidgeting. The hyperkinesis fluctuates. It is most marked when the child is confronted with new or stressful situations, and tends to be less in familiar or one-on-one personal encounters. Hyperactivity tends to diminish spontaneously at about age 12 years and is significantly modified by age 15.

Not all affected children are hyperactive; some are hypoactive. In almost all affected children, however, distractibility and short attention span are significant features. They cannot focus and maintain attention on a task because they cannot disregard the distractions of minimal or trivial auditory, visual, or tactile stimuli. Perseverance may alternate with shortened attention. There may be rigidity of behavior, abnormal preoccupation with a single object or detail, resistance to change, and failure to respond appropriately to changing stimuli. Emotional lability may be prominent. Some behavioral disorders are reminiscent of those seen after brain injury:

frequent temper outbursts, inappropriate aggressiveness, and low frustration threshold, so that seemingly insignificant conditions provoke uncontrolled rage. Many affected children are emotionally immature and prefer to play with younger children.

Failure in school in one or more areas is a frequent sign of MBD. Specific learning problems unrelated to intellectual potential or deviant behavior are additional features. Impaired perceptual performance results in academic difficulties, especially for reading and mathematical concepts. Specific reading disability or dyslexia implies that the inability to read is not related to mental retardation, sensory impairment, inadequate schooling, or proper motivation; it is the single most commonly encountered isolated cognitive dysfunction. Either the child cannot read or reads below age level. Some children also cannot write or spell properly, and some are poor performers in calculations. Difficulties with abstract concepts are common and are more evident with increasing age. Many of these children are ambidextrous, which has been taken to imply failure in developing cerebral dominance.

Language difficulties are common and are frequently manifested by a delay in the development of speech. There may be a tendency to preserve immature modes of expression. Speech may be characterized by a paucity or misuse of words and by poor articulation.

Impaired coordination is another feature of MBD. Affected children tend to be awkward and clumsy. Fine motor coordination is poor and they have difficulty learning to manipulate a button, close a zipper, or tie a knot. This may become evident later in manipulating scissors, coloring within a figure, and handwriting. Impaired gross coordination delays learning how to hop, skip, catch a ball, or ride a bicycle.

Secondary emotional symptoms are common; these result from the poor self-image that follows school failures, deviant behavior, and peer rejection. The emotional symptoms sometimes include aggression, destruction, withdrawal, or fantasy life. In others, there is significant depression.

Physical and Neurologic Examination. General examination should include inspection of the skin after the child has undressed completely. Cafe-au-lait spots should be sought carefully because children with neurofibromatosis may present with the MBD syndrome. The usual neurologic examination is frequently normal, but it may be possible to demonstrate soft signs. The gait may be lumbering and awkward. There may be impaired ability to hop after age 5. The most frequent finding is clumsiness in executing rapid alternating movements with the arms; there may be choreic movements of the extended fingers. Increased tone may be manifested by tightness of the hamstrings, posterior tibials, or pronators of the forearm. There may be right-left confusion and handedness may not be established. Eye-muscle imbalance of the convergent or divergent type is common.

Ancillary Tests. There are no specific laboratory studies to confirm the clinical diagnosis. The EEG is frequently normal but may show abnormalities of organization with voltage and frequency changes or even multispike and spike-and-wave activity. Plain radiographs of the skull, CT of the brain, and auditory and visual evoked response studies are normal.

Psychological testing is the most helpful ancillary study, providing further evidence of impaired cerebral function and an estimate of intellectual potential. Discrepancy between high verbal scores and low performance scores and scatter on the subtests on the Wechsler Intelligence Scale for Children-Revised (WISC-R) and perceptual difficulties on the Bender Visual Motor Gestalt Test are signs of organic brain impairment.

Diagnosis. It is relatively easy to identify children who present with all the features of MBD; difficulties arise when only a few of the manifestations are evident. No single clinical or laboratory test can confirm the diagnosis of the MBD syndrome. The history is of paramount importance. Documenting minor signs of neurologic dysfunction on formal examination is an aid to diagnosis, but not the major determinant. Examination helps to exclude more serious neurologic disorders. The EEG is of limited benefit, but psychological testing by an experienced psychologist can aid immeasurably in reaching a final diagnosis.

Mental retardation, variants of the norm, and psychiatric disorders must be considered in the differential diagnosis. Many mentally retarded children are hyperactive and have a short attention span; it may be difficult to evaluate the initial response to psychological testing. The hyperactivity of many normal children is more readily controlled and is not associated with short attention span, distractibility, or low frustration tolerance. Psychiatric disorders that may require differentiation include anxiety states, character disorders, and some psychoses. However, the child with MBD may present with prominent emotional manifestations.

Treatment. The therapeutic program for MBD includes family counseling, proper school placement, and medication to improve behavior when indicated. Family counseling is critically important; parental anxiety and guilt are often relieved when the physical nature of the disability is explained.

Ideally, educational planning is made after a detailed diagnostic educational evaluation. The school is responsible for establishing the program, which is done with the cooperation of the physician. Some children can be maintained in a regular class supplemented by a resource program, but others require placement in special classes.

Medication may be indicated in addition to the educational therapy when the child is hyperactive, has a short attention span, and is excessively distractible. Inattentiveness alone may be responsible for most of the social and academic dysfunction. Psychostimulants are used most frequently in treatment, although the paradoxic effect of the stimulants is unexplained. Dextroamphetamine is the most effective amphetamine and is given in doses of 2.5 to 30 mg/day; half the daily dose is given after breakfast and half after lunch. It is best to begin with a small dose, gradually increasing the amount each day until the desired clinical effect is observed or until toxic reactions become apparent. Parents should be informed that there may be difficulty with sleep for the first 3 or 4 nights and that anorexia generally improves after a few weeks.

Methylphenidate is also effective in children with MBD syndrome. The response is similar to that observed with amphetamines. Some investigators believe that therapeutic doses of methylphenidate are less likely to result in sedation, lethargy, anorexia, and insomnia. It is best to begin with a small dose, 2.5 to 5 mg daily. This is gradually increased to 5 mg given 3 times a day, after which it can be further increased up to 60 mg/day. The side-effects are similar to those of the amphetamines.

Pemoline, another stimulant, has the advantage that a single daily dose can produce sustained improvement of behavior and performance. It is best to begin with smallest dose available, 18.75 mg, given each morning. The dosage is increased by 18.75-mg increments at 4- to 7-day intervals up to a daily dose of 75 mg. Side-effects include facial grimacing and myoclonic or choreic movements of the limbs.

Medications that are used to treat the behavioral disturbances include the diphenylmethane derivatives, phenothiazines, chlordiazepoxides, tricyclic antidepressants, and the anticonvulsants.

Psychotherapy is indicated in some, but not all, children. The superimposed emotional problems can compound and add to the child's inability to learn. Psychotherapy, combined with proper school placement, may help the child cope and to become more available for learning. Psychotherapy for one or both parents is indicated when there is a seriously disturbed parent-child relationship.

Prognosis. MBD is not always a benign disorder and may presage serious adjustment difficulties in later life. Children identified in elementary school after second grade as being hyperactive are more likely than a control population to have academic and disciplinary problems in early adolescence. Many children with MBD have more social problems, educational deficits, vocational failure, psychopathology, and neuropsychological abnormalities than other children. Some symptoms and adjustments can persist into adulthood.

Mental Retardation

Normal infancy, childhood, and adolescence are characterized by the gradual acquisition of higher cortical functions, of cognitive skills, of adaptation to the environment (especially to other people), and by attainment of independence.

Mental retardation is the absence or incomplete development of these accomplishments. The World Health Organization defines it as "an incomplete or insufficient general development of mental capacities." A manual of the American Association on Mental Deficiency defines it as a "significantly subaverage general intellectual functioning existing concurrently with deficits in adaptive behavior, and manifested during the developmental period."

The borderline between so-called normal and retarded children is ill-defined, depending somewhat on the subjective opinion of the observer and on the criteria used. The incidence of retardation is highest during school years; before and after that period there often is less societal pressure on performance. IQs vary with the examiner, the test used, and the expectations of the caretakers (families, teachers).

Classifications of retardation are useful as long as one is not too rigid about the borders between the categories. Children with an IQ between 50 and 75 are classified as mildly retarded or educable; those with an IQ between 30 and 50 are called moderately retarded or trainable; and those with an IQ below 30 cannot be trained for adequate self-care and are severely retarded.

It is said that 3% of the general population is retarded, but 75% of these people are only mildly retarded and are therefore educable. Only about 5% of the entire group are severely affected. The distribution of these subgroups depends partly on location. Urban societies with higher expectations, more sophisticated technical requirements for social survival, better transportation, and emphasis on personal interactions discover more retardation and tend to put the retardates into lower classifications. Rural communities are often less competitive, tend to be more tolerant, and require less IQ-testing in school; the result is lower figures on the incidence of retardation.

Causes. The causes of mental retardation can be classified into major groups, but in some conditions, retardation is not obligatory. For instance, in neurofibromatosis and Duchenne muscular dystrophy, the IQ is statistically lower than in controls, but retardation may be absent and, if present, is usually mild. The following list is not an attempt to give a complete listing of all causes of mental retardation.

Chromosomal: trisomies (e.g., Down syndrome is usually trisomy 21), translocations, deletions, fragile X-syndrome, mosaicism

Gene Disorders: These conditions may present either as static mental retardation or progressive mental deterioration

Dominant: tuberous sclerosis, neurofibromatosis, congenital myotonic muscular dystrophy

Recessive: lipidoses, most leukodystrophies, ceroid storage diseases, amino acidurias (e.g., phenylketonuria, maple syrup urine disease, histidinemia), congenital muscular dystrophy

X-linked: adrenoleukodystrophy, incontinentia pigmenti, Lesch-Nyhan syndrome, Duchenne muscular dystrophy

Maternal Diseases and Complications

Infections acquired in utero: rubella, cytomegalic inclusion disease, toxoplasmosis, syphilis

Maternal infections: extreme maternal starvation, intrauterine radiation, other teratogens (e.g., alcohol, drugs)

Complications of labor and delivery

Malnutrition

Caloric deficiency

Protein deficiencies

Postnatal Infections

Meningitis

Encephalitis

Toxins

Trauma

Vascular Conditions: thromboses, emboli, hemorrhages

Environmental Causes: isolation, understimulation, neglect, abuse

Most mentally retarded persons do not fit into any of the above named groups because the cause of retardation remains unknown.

Diagnosis. The diagnosis of mental retardation may be difficult in preschool children. However, certain physical features, such as those of Down syndrome, may enable the diagnosis of retardation immediately after birth. In some severe congenital anomalies (e.g., anencephaly, microcephaly, holoprosencephaly), the diagnosis is also easy. In the milder cases, only the gradual recognition of delayed motor development, delayed interpersonal relationships, or poor achievement of speech alerts parents or professionals to the probability of mental retardation. Head circumference below the third percentile should also alert the examiner. Mild mental retardation is usually first suspected in school because of poor performance and standardized IQ tests.

Evaluators other than teachers and school psychologists should be employed to make the definite diagnosis because "pseudoretardation" must be excluded; some children appear to be retarded but are not. For instance, children with impaired vision or hearing may be misdiagnosed as retarded; tests to rule out these handicaps are therefore necessary.

Laboratory tests, while not always helpful, should be done because defining the cause of retardation can be important for therapy and genetic implications. Routine screening of

urine usually can detect all common disorders of amino acid and carbohydrate metabolism. These urinary screening tests include ferric chloride, dinitrophenylhydrazine, sodium nitroprusside, cetyltrimethyl ammonium bromide, and Benedict's. Thin layer chromatography or paper electrophoresis of urine should be done to detect abnormal amino acids. Routine screening for organic acids (e.g., lactic and pyruvic acids) should be performed. Additional tests may include chromosomal analysis and determination of thyroid function. Radiologic studies such as plain skull films, computed tomography and magnetic resonance imaging may reveal underlying congenital anomalies, calcifications or abnormal blood vessels.

Mental retardation may be the first or dominant feature of a degenerative disease of the brain. Children who are suspected of such disorder (familial occurrence or progression of symptoms) require a more sophisticated investigation.

Management. The management plan can be divided into: (1) medical management, (2) education and training, and (3) location of management (home or institution).

Few children with mental retardation can be intellectually improved by medical management. There are some important exceptions; for example, if phenylketonuria or hypothyroidism is diagnosed soon after birth a low phenylalanine diet or thyroid administration can prevent or minimize retardation.

Because restlessness, explosive reactions, and inappropriate behavior are often present in mentally retarded children and adults, treatment with drugs may be beneficial; medications include sedatives, tranquilizers, amphetamines, and methylphenidate. Psychotherapy (especially for the family), therapeutic behavior-modification techniques, and general psychological guidance often help patients and relatives.

Medical management also includes the treatment of associated conditions. The incidence of seizures is higher in retardates than in the general population. When seizures occur, appropriate therapy is mandatory.

The education and training of the mentally retarded patient depend on the degree of retardation, on the patient's behavior, and on community resources. The mildly retarded child should be exposed to other children and to a stimulating environment to foster development near the true potential. Nursery school programs for these children are highly desirable, and guidance for home management should also be supplied through these centers.

Educable children (i.e., IQ 50–75) should attend school at the appropriate age. Larger communities (because of larger numbers of retarded children) find it financially more feasible to supply special schools or classes for retarded children. These classes require an adequate number of trained teachers. Small towns or villages may find the cost of special classes prohibitive, but they may be able to combine with neighboring communities to supply services jointly.

Whether a mentally retarded child should live at home or in an institution is an old problem. The pendulum of public opinion has recently swung toward home care. The young child normally receives the best care from the family; however, if the family is unable or unwilling to keep the child at home, they must consider foster care, adoption, or placement in an institution. Family members should not be pressured to give up a retarded child, nor should they be forced to maintain the child at home against their wishes. The very best of parents reach their limitations when the retarded children become older and are not self-supporting. In these cases, the appropriate plan for a home-substitute (group homes or institutions) must be made. Guidance to that end must be individualized; no undue burden should be placed on normal siblings.

References

Cerebral Palsy

Bard G. Energy expenditure of hemiplegic subjects during walking. Arch Phys Med Rehabil 1963; 44:368–370.

Courville CB. Birth and brain damage. Pasadena: MF Courville, 1971.

Crothers B, Paine RS. The natural history of cerebral palsy. Cambridge: Harvard University Press, 1959.

Diamond LJ, Jaudes PK. Child abuse in a cerebral-palsied population. Dev Med Child Neurol 1983; 25:169–174.

Freud S. Infantile cerebral paralysis. Coral Gables: University of Miami Press, 1968.

Goodman SI, Moe PG, Miles BS, Ting CC. Glutaric aciduria: A "new" disorder of amino acid metabolism. Biochem Med 1975; 12:12–21.

Ingram TTS. Paediatric aspects of cerebral palsy. Edinburgh: E & S Livingstone, 1964.

Lademann A. Postneonatally acquired cerebral palsy. Copenhagen: Munksgaard, 1978.

Little WJ. On the influence of abnormal parturition, difficult labor, premature birth, and asphyxia neonatorum on the mental and physical conditions of the child, especially in relation to deformities. Trans Obstet Soc Lond 1862; 3:293–344.

Low NL, Downey JA. Cerebral palsy. In: Downey JA, Low NL, eds. The Child with Disabling Illness, 2nd ed. New York: Raven Press, 1982:93–104.

Palmer FB, et al. The effects of physical therapy in cerebral palsy: a controlled trial. N Engl J Med 1988; 318:803–808.

Rose J, Medeiros JM, Parker R. Energy cost index as an estimate of energy expenditure of cerebral palsied children during assisted ambulation. Dev Med Child Neurol 1985; 27:485–490.

Stutchfield P, Edwards MA, Gray RGF, Crawley P, Green A. Glutaric aciduria Type I misdiagnosed as Leigh's encephalopathy and cerebral palsy. Dev Med Child Neurol 1985; 27:514–517.

Volpe JJ, Herscovitch P, Perlman JM, Kreusser KP, Raichle ME. Positron emission tomography in the asphyxiated term newborn: Parasagittal impairment of cerebral blood flow. Ann Neurol 1985; 17:287–296.

Volpe JJ, Pasternak J. Parasagittal cerebral injury in neonatal hypoxic-ischemic encephalopathy: Clinical and neuroradiologic features. J Pediatr 1977; 91:472–476.

Mental Retardation

Crome L, Stern J. Pathology of mental retardation. Edinburgh: Churchill Livingstone, 1972.

Eichenwald HF. Prevention of mental retardation. In: Proceedings of a conference of Prevention of Mental Retardation through Control of Infectious Diseases. Bethesda: USDHEW, 1968; Public Health Service Publication No. 1692.

Fuller PW, Guthrie RD, Alvord EC Jr. Proposed neuropathologic basis for learning disabilities in children born prematurely. Dev Med Child Neurol 1983; 25:214–231.

Kinsbourne M. Disorders of mental development. In: Menkes J, ed. Textbook of Child Neurology, 3rd ed. Philadelphia: Lea & Febiger, 1985:764–801.

Koch R. The child with mental retardation. In: Kelley VC, ed. Practice of Pediatrics. Hagerstown: Harper & Row, 1980.

Menkes JH. Textbook of Child Neurology, 3rd ed. Philadelphia: Lea & Febiger, 1985.

Penrose LS. The biology of mental deficit. London: Sedgwick & Jackson, 1972.

Swaiman KJ, Wright FS. The Practice of Pediatric Neurology, 2nd ed. St. Louis: CV Mosby, 1982.

Minimal Brain Dysfunction or Attention Deficit Disorder

Berry CA, Shaywitz SE, Shaywitz BA. Girls with attention deficit disorders—a silent minority. A report on behavioral and cognitive characteristics. Pediatrics 1985; 16:801–809.

Cantwell DP. Genetics of hyperactivity. J Child Psychol Psychiatry 1975; 16:261–264.

Clements SD. Minimal brain dysfunction in children. NINDB Monograph No. 3. DC: USDHEW, 1966.

Committee on Children with Disabilities. Medication for children with attention deficit disorder. Pediatrics 1988; 80:758–760.

Harper PA, Fischer LK, Ryder RV. Neurological and intellectual status of prematures at three to five years of age. J Pediatr 1959; 55:679–690.

Hart EJ, Carter S. Attention deficit disorder, hyperactivity and learning disabilities: The minimal brain dysfunction syndrome. In: Downey JA, Low NL, eds. The Child with Disabling Illness. New York: Raven Press, 1982:145–174.

Huessy HR, Cohen AH. Hyperkinetic behaviors and learning disabilities followed over seven years. Pediatrics 1976; 57:4–10.

Huessy HR, Metoyer M, Townsend M. Eight to ten year follow-up of 84 children treated for behavioral disorder in rural Vermont. Acta Paedopsychiatr (Basel) 1974; 40:230–231.

Kinsbourne M. Disorders of mental development. In: Menkes J, ed. Textbook of Child Neurology, 3rd ed. Philadelphia: Lea & Febiger, 1985: 764–801.

Ottenbacher KJ, Cooper HM. Drug treatment of hyperactivity. Dev Med Child Neurol 1983; 25:358–366.

Pasamanick B, Knobloch H. Syndrome of minimal cerebral damage. JAMA 1959; 170:1384–1387.

Rapoport J, Ferguson HB. Biological validation of the hyperkinetic syndrome. Dev Med Child Neurol 1981; 23:669–682.

Shaywitz BA, Yager RD, Klopper JH. Selective brain dopamine depletion in developing rats: an experimental model of minimal brain dysfunction. Science 1976; 191:305–309.

Shaywitz SE, Cohen DJ, Shaywitz BA. The biochemical basis of minimal brain dysfunction. J Pediatr 1978; 92:179–187.

Shaywitz SE, Cohen DJ, Shaywitz BA. Behavioral and learning difficulties in children of normal intelligence born to alcoholic mothers. J Pediatr 1980; 96:978–982.

Silver LB. Acceptable and controversial approaches to treating the child with learning disabilities. Pediatrics 1975; 55:406–415.

Strauss AA, Lehtinen LE. Psychopathology and Education of the Brain Injured Child (vol 1). New York: Grune & Stratton, 1947.

Strauss AA, Kephart NC. Psychopathology and Education of the Brain Injured Child. (vol 2). New York: Grune & Stratton, 1955.

Strecker EA. Behavior problems in encephalitis; clinical study of relationship between behavior and acute and chronic phenomena of encephalitis. Arch Neurol Psychiatry 1929; 21:137–144.

Swanson JM, Sandman CA, Deutsch C, Baren M. Methylphenidate hydrochloride given with or before breakfast: Behavioral, cognitive, and electrophysiologic effects. Pediatrics 1983; 72:49–55.

Shaywitz SE, Shaywitz BA. Attention deficit disorder: Current perspectives. Ped Neurol 1987; 3:129–135.

Taylor EA. The overactive child. London: Spastics International Medical Publications, 1986.

Towbin A. Organic causes of minimal brain dysfunction: perinatal origin of minimal cerebral lesions. JAMA 1971; 217:1207–1214.

Towen BCL, Prechtl HFR. The neurological examination of the child with minor nervous dysfunction. Philadelphia: JB Lippincott, 1970.

U.S. Department of Health, Education and Welfare. Minimal brain dysfunction in children. DC: USDHEW, 1969; Public Health Service Publication No. 2015.

Weiss G, Trokenberg Hechtman L. Hyperactive children grownup. New York: Guilford Press, 1986.

Wender PH. Minimal Brain Dysfunction in Children. New York: John Wiley & Sons, 1971.

67. AUTISM

Alan M. Aron

This syndrome of unknown cause was described by Kanner in 1943. He called attention to a situation in which a child, from the beginning of life, could not relate to others in the usual way. Speech failed to develop. There was an obsessive desire to maintain sameness in the environment. This desire for constancy ranged from such trivia as furniture arrangement to activities of the day. Today we recognize a range in the degree of severity of autism. Lack of specific physical diagnostic signs makes diagnosis difficult. Most patients with autism are first evaluated between the ages of 2 and 3 years because of delayed speech development. Earlier symptoms of impaired affective contact are frequently overlooked or minimized by parents.

Clincal Symptoms. Two courses in autism have been described. In the first, deviant behavior is evident shortly after birth. These autistic infants cry infrequently; they do not seek to be held. They are "unusually good." In the second, autistic infants seem to develop normally until age 18 to 24 months when regressive changes appear. The subsequent clinical course is similar despite the age of onset. Autism has been reported to occur with a frequency of 0.7 to 4.5/10,000 children.

The behavioral symptoms of autism involve disturbances of perception, cognitive development, social interaction, speech and language, and motility. Both hypo- and hyperresponsivity may occur in the same child. Examples include inattention to auditory stimuli and decreased responsiveness to tactile and painful stimuli. The diminished response to sound may falsely suggest a primary auditory deficit. Whirling, rocking and head rolling, repetitive hand-clapping, and teeth-grinding have all been interpreted as behavior that actively induces vestibular and proprioceptive stimulation.

Delayed development of speech and language may range from total failure (muteness) to echolalia. When speech does develop, it is frequently rudimentary, atonal and arrhythmic without inflection or emotion. Use of pronouns is typically confused; the self is referred to in the third person. Nonsense rhyming is common.

Motility disturbances are characterized by frequent stereotyped movements of the hands and arms. Hand-flapping, posturing, and twirling are frequent. Autistic children tend to rub surfaces and to put objects in their mouths more often than do normal children.

Disturbances of social interaction are characterized by poor eye contact, delayed social smiling, and preferring objects to human contact, which is avoided. The child's activities and utterances are designed to maintain a sense of sameness and solitude. A small percentage of autistic children make some social adjustment. They frequently appear odd, humorless, or socially immature. Autistic adolescents and adults lack social skills. They rarely make personal friendships. They lack empathy. They rarely marry.

There is an increased incidence of prenatal and perinatal morbidity in patients with autism. Some 7.7% of autistic males show the fragile X-syndrome. Appropriate karyotype study should be performed to screen for this condition. Genetic counseling and prenatal diagnosis should be available to the family. A 4:1 male to female ratio in autism, a 2% incidence of autism in siblings of affected individuals, and a 36% concordance rate in monozygotic twins are factors that suggest genetic influences. Of autistic children 7 to 28% develop seizures by age 18 years. Seventy-five percent of all autistic patients are classified as mentally retarded throughout life.

The neurologic examination can be unremarkable or there may be soft neurologic signs such as decreased tone and impaired fine- or gross-motor coordination. Evidence of ventricular enlargement of mild to moderate degree has been reported in a subgroup of young autistic children. The neocerebellar vermal lobules VI and VII were demonstrated on magnetic resonance imaging to be significantly smaller in autistic patients then in controls. This appeared to be a result of developmental hypoplasia. EEGs show variable findings. No specific biochemical abnormality has been defined.

Differential Diagnosis. The diagnosis of autism can be made if the patient shows the characteristic abnormalities before age 36 months. Childhood schizophrenia is a diagnostic categorization that should be reserved for children who first have symptoms after 4 to 5 years of age; they often show regression from a previously normal developmental baseline.

Some specific disorders may present with autistic features. Deafness and blindness should be apparent but must be carefully ruled out. Autistic syndromes have been described in metabolic diseases such as phenylketonuria, congenital hyperthyroidism or Hurler disease, abnormalities of cerebral development (e.g., arrested hydrocephalus Dandy-Walker syndrome), perinatal injuries, specific organic brain syndrome, Rett syndrome, fragile X-syndrome, mental retarda-

tion, and seizure disorders such as infantile spasms. Mental retardation and autism can coexist. Clinical evidence suggests 65 to 75% of all autistic patients later perform at retarded levels. Emotional deprivation may cause developmental disturbances, but it does not cause the syndrome of autism. Studies have shown that parents of autistic children are not psychopathic and do not induce the disorder in their children.

Treatment and Prognosis. Behavior modification techniques, including operant conditioning, special education, speech therapy, use of sign language, psychotherapy, and counseling for parents have all been used. However, an intensive behavioral educational approach seems to offer the greatest promise for treatment. This includes a full-time individual therapeutic program in school and incorporates the parents in maintaining behavioral modification techniques at home. Tranquilizing medication can be useful if uncontrolled aggressiveness occurs. Treatment in a residential setting can be helpful when parents feel unable to cope. The best approach to therapy should be flexible, concentrating on long-term management and guidance for the individual. A multidisciplinary approach including physiologic, genetic, psychological, biochemical, and neurologic studies is required for future study.

The prognosis is guarded. Failure to develop appropriate play with toys is associated with a poor prognosis. Failure to develop communicative language by age 5 has a poor prognosis for future development. Some patients, especially those who do develop speech, may become marginally self-sufficient. Patients with higher IQ scores, communicative speech, and appropriate play have responded best to intensive therapeutic treatment techniques. Most patients are ultimately placed in an institution for chronic care. Whether there is a relationship between autism and adult schizophrenia is unknown.

References

Brown TW, Jenkins EC, Cohen IL, et al. Fragile X and autism: A multi-center survey. Am J Med Genet 1986; 23:341–352.

Campbell M, Rosenblum S, Perry R, et al. Computerized axial tomography in young autistic children. Am J Psychiatry 1982; 139:510–512.

Cox A, Rutter M, Newman S. A comparative study of infantile autism and specific developmental receptive language disorder. Br J Psychiatry 1975; 126:146–159.

Courchesne E, Yeung-Courchesne R, Press, GA, et al.

Hypoplasia of cerebellar vermal lobules VI and VII in autism. N Eng J Med 1988; 318:1349–1354.

DeMeyer MK, Hingtgen JN, Jackson RK. Infantile autism revisited: A decade of research. Schizophr Bull 1981; 7:388–451.

Folstein S, Rutter M. Infantile autism: a genetic study of 21 twin pairs. J Child Psychol Psychiat 1977; 18:297–321.

Hauser SL, DeLong GR, Rosman NP. Pneumographic findings in the infant autism syndrome: A correlation with temporal lobe disease. Brain 1975; 98:667–688.

Kanner L. Autistic disturbances of affective contact. Nerv Child 1943; 2:217–250.

Kanner L. Early infantile autism. J Pediatr 1944; 25:211–217.

Kanner L. Childhood Psychosis: Initial Studies and New Insights. DC: H Winston & Sons, 1973.

Lovaas OI. Behavioral treatment and normal educational and intellectual functioning in young autistic children. J Consult Clin Psychol 1987; 55:3–9.

McGillivray BC, Herbst DS, Dill FJ, Sandercock HJ, Tischler B. Infantile autism: An occasional manifestation of fragile (X) mental retardation. Am J Med Genet 1986; 23:353–358.

Olsson I, Steffenburg S, Gillberg C. Epilepsy in autism and autistic like conditions. Arch Neurol 1988; 45:666–668.

Omitz EM, Ritvo ER. Autism: Diagnosis, current research and management. In: Ritvo ER, ed. Autism: Diagnosis, Current Research and Management. New York: Halstead Press, 1976.

Opitz JM, Reynolds JF, Ed. The Rett syndrome. Amer J Med Gen 1986; Supp 1 23:1–402.

Rett Syndrome Diagnostic Criteria Work Group. Diagnostic criteria for Rett syndrome. Ann Neurol 1988; 23:425–428.

Turner G, Jacobs P. Marker (X)-linked mental retardation. Adv Hum Genet 1983; 13:83–112.

Young JG, Leven LI, Newcorn JH, Knott PJ. Genetic and neurobiological approaches to the pathophysiology of autism and the pervasive developmental disorders. In Meltzer H.Y. Ed. Psychopharmacology: The third generation of progress. New York: Raven Press, 1987; 825–836.

68. CHROMOSOMAL DISORDERS
William G. Johnson

Chromosomal disorders have become increasingly important in neurology because improved methods permit detection of previously unrecognized clinical disorders and because chromosome abnormalities have assumed a major role in neurologic disease research.

Types of Abnormalities. Chromosome abnormalities may involve the number or the structure of either the autosomes or the sex chromosomes. Humans have 46 chromosomes; 44 are autosomes, two are sex chromosomes. Human cells are normally *diploid,* that is they contain twice the *haploid* number of chromosomes, which is 23. Triploid or tet-

raploid cells contain three or four times the haploid number of chromosomes, respectively. Cells not containing an exact multiple of the haploid number of normal chromosomes are *aneuploid.* A trisomic cell has 47 normal chromosomes and three copies of a chromosome; a *monosomic* cell has 45 normal chromosomes and only a single copy of an autosome.

Structural abnormalities include deletions, insertions, duplications, inversions (pericentric or paracentric), translocations (reciprocal or Robertsonian), and ring chromosomes. Improved banding techniques and the use of prometaphase spreads have enabled recognition of increasingly smaller structural abnormalities. However, with minor or inconsistent abnormalities, it is not always possible to be sure the chromosomal finding is the cause of the patient's clinical disease.

Mosaicism occurs when some of a patient's cells show an abnormality and others do not. Because of this, a normal study does not exclude a chromosomal disorder. Finding mosaicism, for example, in a culture of amniotic fluid cells does not mean the fetus is abnormal because mosaicism may arise independently in culture. A patient with mosaicism is usually more mildly affected clinically that a patient with a consistent abnormality in every cell.

Incidence of Disorders. Different populations have been extensively surveyed for chromosomal abnormalities.[*] Chromosomal abnormalities are far from rare; unbalanced chromosome abnormalities are found in 10 to 30% of the institutionalized mentally retarded, the largest number have Down syndrome. About 2.5% of psychiatric hospital and prison residents are 47 XXY men. Chromosomal abnormalities are also associated with a large proportion of spontaneous abortions; only a small percentage of aneuploid fetuses come to term. Trisomy 16 is the most common trisomy; affected fetuses never survive to term. *Trisomy 21 (Down syndrome)* is the most common postnatal trisomy, because a relatively high proportion survive to term. Chromosome abnormalities are found in about 75% of spontaneous abortuses at 9 weeks gestation, in 33% at 19 to 30 weeks gestation, and in 1% of unselected newborns.

Clinical Features. Autosomal chromosomal abnormalities produce a large variety of clin-

---

[*]There are problems and controversies regarding ascertainment, methodology, and interpretation, but some general conclusions are possible.

ical features but some are seen frequently and relatively consistently. Mental deficiency, often severe and disproportionately involving language, is probably the most consistent feature; it is especially important for neurologists to consider chromosomal disorders in the differential diagnosis of mental retardation. Of equal importance is growth retardation, both intrauterine and postnatal. A third type of finding is the congenital malformation, which is usually multiple. Finally, the possibility of autosomal chromosomal disorder is suggested by a pattern of dysmorphic signs, especially that which involves the face, distal limbs, and genitalia.

Brain malformations are relatively common in autosomal chromosome disorders, for example agenesis of the corpus callosum and holoprosencephaly. Common abnormalities include lumbar or occipital spina bifida; microphthalmia; ocular coloboma; kidney and urinary tract malformations; heart and great vessel malformations; and cleft lip, cleft palate, or both.

Dysmorphic features are more subtle than outright malformations and may be considered normal variants or even within the range of normal. Examples are variations in the shape of the face, the size or shape of the palpebral fissures; interocular distance; epicanthic folds; ocular ptosis; strabismus; size, shape, or position of the ears; size or shape of the nose or nasal bridge; and palatal configuration. Similar dysmorphic variants are found for the distal limbs or genitalia. Minor, often rather nonspecific radiographic skeletal abnormalities are frequent. In most autosomal chromosomal disorders, there are multiple dysmorphic features, and the pattern of dysmorphism is more important than any individual feature.

Reduced fertility, genital hypoplasia, and delayed or defective puberty are commonly seen in autosomal chromosomal disorders, especially in males. Likewise, the family history may show higher than expected fetal wastage, prematurity, neonatal deaths, reduced fertility, and difficulties in pregnancy.

Disorders of the sex chromosomes differ clinically from disorders of the autosomes. Mental deficiency is seldom a feature and is usually not severe. Likewise, growth retardation is rarely a feature; height may even be increased. Major malformations are much less frequent and dysmorphic features are usually rare and nonspecific. Infertility is the most prominent feature of most sex chromosome disorders.

Diagnosis. A banded chromosome study on blood leukocytes should be obtained when the presence of mental defect, growth retardation, congenital malformations, or dysmorphic features suggests a chromosomal disorder. Sometimes comparison of the patient's appearance and clinical features with those in standard illustrated texts and catalogues will suggest a specific disorder. However, the number of chromosomal syndromes is huge and growing; moreover, many disorders lack features of sufficient specificity to be diagnostic. It is important to establish a specific diagnosis for at least three reasons: (1) to enable an accurate prognosis; (2) to assure accurate genetic counseling if other family members are at risk; and (3) to enable prenatal diagnosis of chromosomal disorders.

If the chromosomal study is normal but clinical suspicion of a chromosomal disorder remains, the possibility of a mosaic should be considered. Other tissues can be sampled; cultured bone marrow cells or cultured skin fibroblasts may reveal the chromosomal disorder. Fragile sites such as the fragile-X syndrome, which is a common cause of mental retardation in males, may remain undetected unless the cells are cultured in folate-deficient medium. If the laboratory is not told the fragile X-syndrome is suspected, the diagnosis may be missed. Also, an increasing number of neurologic disorders are associated with tiny deletions that previously were undetected. Prometaphase banding may reveal these; even so, a detectable deletion may be missed unless attention is drawn to a particular chromosome or region. For instance, the *Prader-Willi syndrome* (see Section 70), has been associated with small deletions and other abnormalities of the proximal long arm of chromosome 15. That syndrome may be the most common autosomal structural abnormality, more common than the *cri du chat* (cat cry) syndrome, which results from deletion of part of the short arm of chromosome 5. Nonetheless, unless the Prader-Willi phenotype is recognized clinically and attention is drawn to chromosome 15, a small deletion may go unrecognized. In a less frequent disorder, the *Miller-Dieker syndrome,* microcephaly and lissencephaly may be associated with deletion or other abnormality of the short arm of chromosome 17.

Research Implications. Documenting the chromosomal cause of a clinical syndrome is important for patients, families, and research, because identifying a damaged chromosome in only a few patients with a clinical disorder can lead to chromosomal localization of the gene for that disorder. Identifying a suitable chromosomal defect in even a single case of a genetic disorder can lead to cloning of the gene, as already illustrated by Duchenne muscular dystrophy and perhaps soon for Prader-Willi syndrome.

Patients with genetic disorders have one or more damaged copies of a particular gene. The damage can occur several ways. In one, a DNA point mutation in the coding region of a gene may lead to an amino acid substitution in the protein gene product. Also, a small deletion may remove part or all of the DNA sequence of a gene. A larger deletion may remove the entire DNA sequence of one gene plus that of one or more neighboring genes. The deletion may be large enough to be visible on a banded chromosome preparation.* Another possibility is that the gene is damaged when one breakpoint of a chromosome translocation cuts through its DNA sequence. Such a translocation will likely be visible on a banded chromosome preparation.

It is probable that a subgroup of patients for nearly every genetic disease has sufficiently significant chromosome damage to be visible in banded chromosome preparations. Although this group is not large, it is important because the site of chromosome damage gives the chromosomal location of the disease gene directly. Moreover, the abnormal chromosomes can be used to clone the gene for the disease even though the gene product is unknown. Thus, it is essential to study patients with genetic diseases for chromosome morphology, especially if there is something atypical about the disease in an individual patient.

It is useful to obtain banded chromosome studies to seek deletions, translocation, or other chromosome damage in patients with typical and atypical cases of genetic disorders and from selected apparently nongenetic disorders. Finding a consistent location for chromosome damage in even a few patients will enable rapid localization and cloning of the responsible gene and will document the origin of disorders not previously known to be genetic.

---

*Or the same patient may have clinical features of two distinct genetic disorders because the corresponding genes are next to one another.

References

Borgaonkar DS, Shaffer R, Reisor N. Repository of Human Chromosomal Variants and Anomalies, 12 listings, December 1987, Medical Center of Delaware & University of Delaware, Newark, Delaware.

Dobyns WB. Developmental aspects of lissencephaly and the lissencephaly syndromes. Birth Defects 1987; 23:225–241.

Franke U, Ochs HD, de Martinville B, et al. Minor Xp21 deletion chromosome deletion in a male associated with expression of Duchenne muscular dystrophy, chronic granulomatous disease, retinitis pigmentosa and McLeod syndrome. Am J Hum Genet 1985; 37:250–267.

Human Gene Mapping 9. Cytogenetics & Cell Genetics 1987; 46:1–762.

Labidi F, Cassidy SB. A blind prometaphase study of Prader-Willi syndrome: Frequency and consistency in interpretation of del 15q. Am J Hum Genet 1986; 39:452–460.

Ledbetter DH, Mascarello JT, Riccardi VM, Harper VD, Airhart SD, Strobel RJ. Chromosome 15 abnormalities and the Prader-Willi syndrome: A follow-up report of 40 cases. Am J Hum Genet 1982; 34:278–285.

McKusick VA. The Morbid Anatomy of the Human Genome. Bethesda, Maryland; Howard Hughes Medical Institute, 1988.

Schinzel A. Catalogue of Unbalanced Chromosome Aberrations in Man. New York: Walter de Gruyter, 1984.

Therman E. Human Chromosomes—Structure, Behavior, Effects, 2nd ed. New York: Springer-Verlag, 1986.

Worton RG, Duff C, Sylvester JE, et al. Duchenne muscular dystrophy involving translocation of the dmd gene next to ribosomal RNA genes. Science 1984; 224:1447–1449.

---

69. LAURENCE-MOON-BIEDL SYNDROME
Melvin Greer

Among the rare syndromes characterized by obesity and hypogonadism, that described by Laurence and Moon in 1866 is the prototype. Also called Laurence-Moon-Biedl-Bardet syndrome, it consists of obesity, hypogonadism, hypogenitalism, polydactyly, retinitis pigmentosa, and mental retardation. The mode of inheritance is autosomal recessive. Males are more likely to be affected by hypogenitalism. Testicular atrophy, decrease in germinal cells, and spermatogenic arrest have been described. Debate continues about the fundamental cause of the hypogonadism. Measurement of hormone levels and hormone stimulation studies provide evidence of target organ unresponsiveness in some patients; in others there seems to be a fundamental disturbance in the hypothalamic-pituitary axis. Testosterone is ineffective in treating hypogonadism or hypogenitalism. Diabetes insipidus has been reported occasionally, but other endocrine abnormalities are absent. Signs and symptoms are stationary except for the visual loss, which is usually progressive. Although the condition is compatible with a normal life span, early death often occurs due to coincidental kidney abnormalities or congenital heart disease. No specific neuropathologic changes have been described (Fig. 69–1).

The *Alström-Hallgren syndrome* is transmitted as an autosomal recessive disorder. Obesity, hypogonadism, retinitis pigmentosa, nerve deafness, and diabetes mellitus are major features. Neither polydactyly nor significant mental retardation is observed.

The *Biemond syndrome* is characterized by hypogonadotrophic hypogonadism, obesity, postaxial polydactyly, mental retardation, and coloboma of the iris rather than retinitis pigmentosa.

The *Prader-Willi syndrome* has an autosomal recessive mode of inheritance and includes obesity, hypogonadism, and mental retardation. Micromelia, shortness of stature, and

hypotonia are distinguishing features along with the absence of visual problems.

The occurrence of retinitis pigmentosa, adiposity, and impotence in association with spinocerebellar degeneration suggests a relationship between these syndromes and the cerebellar ataxias.

References

Biedl A. Über das Laurence-Biedlsche Syndrom. Med Klin 1933; 29:839–840.

Churchill DN, McManamon P, Hurley RM. Renal disease—a sixth cardinal feature of the Laurence-Moon-Biedl syndrome. Clin Nephrol 1981; 16:151–154.

Goldstein JL, Fialkow, PJ. The Alström syndrome. Medicine 1973; 52:53–71.

Klein D, Ammann, F. The syndrome of Laurence-Moon-Bardet-Biedl and allied diseases in Switzerland. J Neurol Sci 1969; 9:479–513.

Koepp P. Laurence-Moon-Biedl syndrome associated with diabetes insipidus neurohormonalis. Eur J Pediatr 1975; 121:59.

Leroith D, Farkash Y, Bar-Ziev J, Spitz IM. Hypothalamic-pituitary function in the Bardet-Biedl syndrome. Isr J Med Sci 1980; 16:514–518.

Linné T, Wikstad I, Zetterstrom R. Renal involvement in the Laurence-Moon-Biedl syndrome. Acta Paediatr Scand 1986; 75:240–244.

McLoughlin TG, Shanklin DR. Pathology of Laurence-Moon-Bardet-Biedl syndrome. J Pathol Bacteriol 1967; 93:65.

Mosaffarian G, Nakhjavani MK, Farrahi A. The Laurence-Moon-Bardet-Biedl syndrome: Unresponsiveness to the action of testosterone, a possible mechanism. Fertil Steril 1979; 31:417–422.

Pagon RA, Haas JE, Bunt AH, Rodaway KA. Hepatic involvement in the Bardet-Biedl syndrome. Am J Med Genet 1982; 13:373–381.

Price D, Gartner JG, Kaplan BS. Ultrastructural changes in the glomerular basement membrane of patients with Laurence-Moon-Biedl-Bardet syndrome. Clin Nephrol 1981; 16:283–288.

Tieder M, Levy M, Gubier MC, Gaguadoux MF, Broyer M. Renal abnormalities in the Bardet-Biedl syndrome. Int J Pediatr Nephrol 1982; 3:199–203.

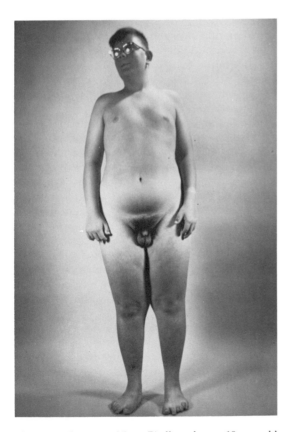

Fig. 69–1. Laurence-Moon-Biedl syndrome. 19-year-old with obesity, hypogenitalism, polydactyly (toes), retinitis pigmentosa, and mental retardation.

70. PRADER-WILLI SYNDROME
Melvin Greer

The Prader-Willi syndrome consists of hypotonia (often noted in the neonatal period), short stature, obesity, hypogonadism, micromelia, and mental retardation. An autosomal-recessive inheritance is probable. There is a high frequency of chromosome-15 abnormalities; a small deletion with breakpoints in bands 15q11 and 15q13 has been described.

Serious postnatal feeding problems are replaced by hyperphagia toward the end of the first year. Alimentary hyperglycemia in early life may be mistaken for diabetes mellitus, although an inadequate insulin response may be identified to establish a true diabetic state later in life. Other endocrine abnormalities are often present. Both hypothalamic-pituitary dysfunction and primary target-organ unresponsiveness have been considered the underlying cause of hypogonadism. In boys, the small penis and biopsy of the testes reveal signs of immaturity. Inadequate breast and pubic-hair development and lack of menstruation are noted in girls. Growth-hormone deficiency is detected in some. No pathologic changes in the hypothalamus have been described, although, in one patient, the pituitary stalk was thin and there were minor pituitary gland abnormalities.

Additional variable findings include acromicria, abnormalities of the central visual pathways, straight ulnar border of the hand, keratosis pilaris, stringy saliva, and diminished sensitivity to pain; scoliosis is attributed to both obesity and associated congenital anomaly. A pleasant and ingratiating personality has been described, although later in life there may be temper outbursts. Psychometric tests reveal levels of functioning from merely educable to nearly normal learning capability.

In 30 to 50% of patients, a retarded bone age is noted after age 5 years. The hypotonia becomes less prominent in adolescence. Muscle biopsies have been unrevealing. Dietary restriction is attempted to control obesity, but is effective in only a few patients.

Some patients have had bypass bowel surgery without controlling the overeating-obesity component of the syndrome. Death is attributable to cardiorespiratory failure when obesity is not controlled.

References

Bray GA, Dahms WT, Swerdloff RS, Fiser RH, Atkinson RL, Carrel RE. The Prader-Willi syndrome: 40 cases. Medicine 1983; 62:59–80.

Burke CM, Kousseff BG, Gleeson M, O'Connell BM, Devlin JG. Familial Prader-Willi Syndrome. Arch Int Med 1987; 147:673–675.

Creel DJ, Bendel CM, Wiesner GL, Wirtschafter JD, Arthur DC, King RA. Abnormalities of the central visual pathways in Prader-Willi syndrome associated with hypopigmentation. N Engl J Med 1986; 314:1606–1609.

Donlon TA, Lalande M, Wyman A, Bruns G, Latt SA. Isolation of molecular probes associated with chromosome 15 in Prader-Willi syndrome. Proc Natl Acad Sci 1986; 83:4408–4412.

Jeffcoate WJ, Laurance BM, Edwards CR, Besser GM. Endocrine function in the Prader-Willi syndrome. Clin Endocrinol 1980; 12:81–89.

Laurance BM, Brito A, Wilkinson J. Prader-Willi syndrome after age 15 years. Arch Dis Child 1981; 56:181–186.

Ledbetter DH, Riccardi VM, Airhart SD, Strobel RJ,

Keenan BS, Crawford JD. Deletions of chromosome 15 as a cause of the Prader-Willi syndrome. N Engl J Med 1981; 304:325–328.

Prader A, Labhart A, Willi H. Ein Syndrom von Adipositas, Kleinwuchs, Kryptorchismus und Oligophrenie nach myatonieartigem Zustand in Neugeborenenalter. Schweiz Med Wochenschr 1956; 86:1260–1261.

Second Annual Prader-Willi Syndrome Scientific Conference. Houston, June 17, 1987. Proceedings and Abstracts. Am J Med Genet 1987; 28:779–924.

71. AGENESIS OF THE CORPUS CALLOSUM
Abe M. Chutorian

Defective embryogenesis of the midline telencephalic structures may cause total or partial absence of the corpus callosum. The hippocampal and anterior commissures are also absent in many cases. This anomaly may be present without signs or symptoms of neurologic dysfunction, although it is most commonly associated with seizures and varying degrees of mental retardation. Seizures are frequently focal, probably owing to failure of propagation of unilaterally derived seizures to the opposite hemisphere. In addition to frank mental deficiency attributed to associated cerebral defects, disorders of perceptual and cognitive function have been described. These vary from little or no apparent defect to variants of the *"disconnection"* syndromes in which each cerebral hemisphere functions independently of the other. It is generally believed that the disconnection syndromes occur only in patients with acquired callosal defects (following commissurotomy), but patients with agenesis of the corpus callosum may show impaired integrative capacities for fine motor, kinesthetically mediated, and visual capacities. The occurrence of clinical symptoms is usually related to other cranial or spinal abnormalities that are present in most patients (i.e., hydrocephalus, microgyri, heterotopias, arachnoid cysts, cerebellar dysgenesis, spina bifida, meningomyelocele). Partial or complete agenesis is frequently present with lipomas or cysts in the region of the corpus callosum. Clinically, agenesis of the corpus callosum may occur as a severe syndrome in infancy or childhood, as a milder syndrome in young adults, or as an asymptomatic incidental finding. When callosal agenesis is found in infancy or early childhood, hydrocephalus is usual; seizures and signs of diffuse or focal brain dysfunction are seen in a minority. In one study of a large

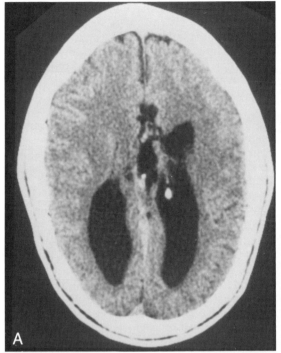

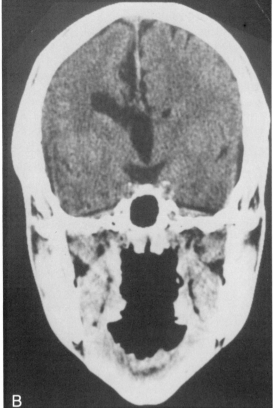

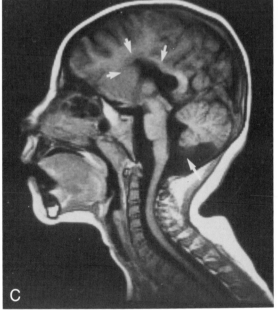

Fig. 71–1. Agenesis of corpus callosum. Noncontrast CT scans. *A*, axial, and *B*, coronal, planes show high-riding third ventricle. *C*, Sagittal MRI showing agenesis of the anterior portion of the corpus callosum (multiple arrows). An associated anomaly, aplasia of the inferior portion of the cerebellar vermis, is indicated by the single arrow. (Courtesy of Dr. S.K. Hilal.)

developmentally disabled population, 2.3% had agenesis of the corpus callosum.

Specific clinical syndromes or chromosome abnormalities may be associated with dysgenesis of the corpus callosum. These include extra-ring chromosome with mosaicism; trisomy; pituitary endocrine dysfunction with septo-optic dysplasia, holoprosencephaly, familial occurrence; Andermann syndrome (with progressive neuropathy) and Aicardi syndrome (i.e., agenesis of corpus callosum with retardation, seizures, and characteristic retinal patches of pigment, epithelial and choroidal atrophy).

The diagnosis of agenesis of the corpus callosum is made by computed tomography (Fig. 71–1) and magnetic resonance imaging (MRI). The anomaly produces marked separation of the lateral ventricles, a concave configuration of the medial walls and dilatation of the caudal portions of the lateral ventricles and a dorsal extension and dilatation of the third ventricle. The ability of MRI to project a detailed sagittal section of the brain makes it the study of choice.

References

Bernardi F, Zamboni G, del Majno UM, Zoppi G. Small supernumerary ring chromosome in a subject with agenesis of the corpus callosum. Pathologica 1979; 71:406–407.

Bertoni JM, von Loh S, Allen RJ. The Aicardi syndrome: Report of 4 cases and review of the literature. Ann Neurol 1979; 5:475–482.

Curnes JT, Laster DW, Koubek TD, Moody DM, Ball MR. MRI of corpus callosal syndromes. AJNR 1986; 7:617–622.

de Johg JGY, Delleman JW, Houben M, et al. Agenesis of the corpus callosum, infantile spasm, ocular anomalies (Aicardi's syndrome). Neurology 1976; 26:1152–1158.

Field M, Ashton R, White K. Agenesis of the corpus callosum: Report of two preschool children and review of the literature. Dev Med Child Neurol 1978; 20:47–61.

Gotts PS, Saul RE. Agenesis of the corpus callosum: Limits of functional compensation. Neurology 1978; 28:1272–1279.

Harner RN. Agenesis of the corpus callosum and associated defects. In: Appel S, Goldensohn ES, eds. Scientific Approaches to Clinical Neurology. Philadelphia: Lea & Febiger 1977:616–621.

Jeret JS, Serur D, Wisniewski KE, Lubin RA. Clinicopathological findings associated with agenesis of the corpus callosum. Brain Dev 1987; 9:255–264.

McLeod NA, Williams JP, Machen B, Lum, GB. Normal and abnormal morphology of the corpus callosum. Neurology 1987; 37:1240–1242.

Kazner E, Lanksch W, Steinhoff H. Cranial computerized tomography in the diagnosis of brain disorders in infants and children. Neuropädiatrie 1976; 7:136–174.

Loeser JD, Alvord EC. Agenesis of the corpus callosum. Brain 1968; 91:553–570.

Loeser JD, Alvord EC. Clinicopathological correlations in agenesis of the corpus callosum. Neurology 1968; 18:745–756.

Lynn RB, Buchanan DC, Fenichel GM, Freeman FR. Agenesis of the corpus callosum. Arch Neurol 1980; 37:444–445.

Sadowsky C, Reeves AG. Agenesis of the corpus callosum with hypothermia. Arch Neurol 1975; 32:774–776.

Wollschlaeger G, Wollschlaeger PB, Brannan DD, Segal AJ. Lipoma of the corpus callosum. AJR 1961; 86:142–147.

72. MEGALENCEPHALY

Abe M. Chutorian

Megalencephaly is a condition in which the brain is abnormally large and heavy. Factors such as hydrocephalus, severe brain edema, or hematoma, which may produce increased weight of the cranial contents, are generally absent. Megalencephaly owing to increased brain water content, with or without mild ventricular enlargement, appears to occur in some conditions that are not viewed traditionally as associated with either hydrocephalus or brain edema. These will be described presently. Structural abnormalities and a variety of malformations may or may not be found in megalencephalic brains. The clinical signs and symptoms are variable and depend on the extent and severity of such malformations and on multiple other factors associated with specific syndromes.

Familial megalencephaly, which may be entirely benign, is seen when otherwise normal individuals with megalencephaly transmit megalencephaly as an autosomal dominant trait to their otherwise normal children. Dominant inheritance also occurs in symptomatic megalencephaly, however, in the absence of otherwise identifiable metabolic, neurocutaneous, or other syndromic features. In this form of familial megalencephaly there is a 4:1 ratio of males to females, virtually uniform increase in birth weight and occipital frontal circumference, and a high frequency of intellectual deficit and seizure disorder. There is also a tendency to abnormal stature, equally divided between excessively tall and excessively short individuals. Recent studies have indicated that megalencephaly occurs 4 times more frequently in the learning disabled than in otherwise normal children.

Other children with megalencephaly may harbor metabolic disorders, such as leukodystrophies or lysosomal enzyme disorders, or may have gigantism-associated megalencephaly (as in achondroplastic dwarfism), a variety of other cranioskeletal dysplasias, and neurocutaneous disorders such as neurofibromatosis. Specific examples of these disorders include craniometaphyseal dysplasia, marble bone disease, lipidoses such as Tay-Sachs disease, mucopolysaccharidoses such as Hurler disease, and leukodystrophies such as Canavan and Alexander diseases. In some of these disorders, the abnormal storage of cerebral metabolites may involve the leptomeninges, causing frank communicating hydrocephalus, which compounds abnormal head growth (e.g., Hurler disease).

Some of these disorders are associated with increased brain fluid content, and while not ordinarily or traditionally perceived as being associated with cerebral edema or hydrocephalus, one or the other of these conditions may actually be incipient and aggravate the megalencephaly. This is particularly apt to occur in certain conditions in which impedance of cranial venous outflow occurs on a chronic basis, especially during infancy and early childhood, when the cranial sutures easily accommodate expansion of brain volume. Thus, in Sotos syndrome, CT and MRI have shown mild ventriculomegaly in this disorder, and sometimes distension of the sulci and subarachnoid cisterns, due to impaired cerebrospinal fluid egress from the brain, as shown by intrathecal isotope studies. Similar studies, as well as venous angiography, have shown that cerebral venous outflow may also be compromised in achondroplastic dwarfism, with either ventriculomegaly or increase in brain volume. Similarly, arterial venous malformations, or anomalous venous cranial outflow without arterial venous malformation, at times associated with a variety of cutaneous angiomatous syndromes, may be associated with impedance of cranial venous outflow. Vigilance is required in all of these conditions for either progressive ventriculomegaly or unduly rapid expansion of brain size, because either ventricular shunting or dural venous sinus shunting may be warranted in some of these cases. More often, however, the rate of increase in head and brain size is modest.

Megalencephaly with dwarfism includes achondroplasia, thanatophoric dwarfism, small stature with endocrinopathy, and certain unusual forms of muscular dystrophy. Megalencephaly with gigantism includes Sotos syndrome, pituitary gigantism, arachnodactyly, and Weaver-Smith syndrome.

Other syndromes associated with megalencephaly include "external hydrocephalus" (combined modest ventriculomegaly with distension of sulci cisterns and fissures, at times associated with "benign subdural effusions"), agenesis of the corpus callosum, Bannayan-Zonana syndrome (familial, with mesodermal hematomas), macrocephaly with osteopathic striata and cranial sclerosis, hypomelanosis of Ito, and sundry others.

References

Chutorian, AM, Carmel, PW. Cerebral fluid malabsorption in cerebral gigantism (Sotos syndrome). Neurology 1988; 38:283.

Crome L, Stern J. The Pathology of Mental Retardation, 2nd ed. Edinburgh: Churchill Livingstone, 1972.

DeMeyer W. Megalencephaly in Children. Neurology 1972; 22:634.

DeMeyer W. Megalencephaly: Types, clinical syndromes, and management. Pediatr Neurol 1986; 2:321–328.

Miles JH, Zovana J, McFarlane J. Macrocephaly with

hamartomas: Bannayan-Zovana syndrome. Am J Med Genet 1984; 19:225–234.

Modic MT, Kaufman B, Bonstelle CT, Tomsick TA, Weinstein MA. Megaloencephaly and hypodense extracerebral fluid collections. Radiology 1981; 141:93–100.

Portnoy, HD, Crossant, PD. Megalencephaly in infants and children: The possible role of increased dural sinus pressure. Arch Neurol 1978; 35:306–316.

Robinow M, Unger F. Syndrome of osteopathia striata, macrocephaly and cranial sclerosis. Am J Dis Child 1984; 138:821–823.

Ross DL, Liwnicz BH, Chun RW, Gilbert E. Hypomelanosis of Ito—a clinicopathologic study: Macrocephaly and gray matter heterotopias. Neurology 1982; 32:1013–1016.

Shapiro K, Shulman K. Facial nevi associated with anomalous venous return. J Neurosurg 1976; 45:20–25.

Stephan MJ, Bryan DH, Smith DW, Cohen MM. Macrocephaly in association with unusual cutaneous angiomatosis. J Pediatr 1975; 87:353–359.

Williams JP, Blalock CP, Dunaway CL, Chalhub EG. Schizencephaly. J Comp Tomogr 1983; 7:135–139.

Yamanda H, Shigetoshi N, Tajima M, Kageyama N. Neurological manifestations of pediatric achondroplasia. J Neurosurg 1981; 54:49–57.

Zonana, J, Rimoin DL, Davis DC. Macrocephaly with multiple lipomas and hemangiomas. J Pediatr 1976; 89:600.

73. SPINA BIFIDA AND CRANIUM BIFIDUM
Abe M. Chutorian

Failure of closure of the bony spine or cranium is known as spina bifida or cranium bifidum. This failure of closure may occur at any level but it is most common in the lumbosacral region of the spine (Table 73–1).

Spina Bifida

Spina bifida is defined as a failure in the closure of the spinal column due to a defect in the development of vertebrae. It may be associated with defects in the development of the spinal cord, brain stem, cerebellum or cerebrum, meningoceles, meningomyeloceles, congenital tumors, hydrocephalus, or developmental defects in other areas of the body.

Pathology and Pathogenesis. The spinal canal closes by the fourth week and the bony canal by the twelfth week of intrauterine life. The combination of genetic and environmental factors (multifactorial inheritance) is postulated to be the underlying mechanism in the cause of neural tube defects. Patients with spina bifida can be classified into two large groups: (1) spina bifida occulta, in which there is a simple defect in the closure of the vertebrae, and (2) spina bifida with meningocele or meningomyelocele, where the defect in the spinal column is associated with a

Table 73–1. Site of Lesions in Spina Bifida and Cranium Bifidum

Site of Lesion	No. of Cases
Cranial	84
Nasal	5
Nasopharyngeal	1
Frontal	6
Parietal	9
Occipital	63
Cervical	23
Thoracic	39
Thoracolumbar	43
Lumbar	205
Lumbosacral	87
Sacral	46
Thoracolumbosacral	10
Pelvic	1
Undesignated	8
Total	546

(From Ingraham FD et al. Spina Bifida and Cranium Bifidum. Cambridge: Harvard University Press, 1944)

Table 73–2. Incidence of Various Lesions in Patients with Spina Bifida and Cranium Bifidum

Type of Lesion	No. of Cases
Spina bifida occulta (13 with lipomas)	65
Meningocele	98
Lipomeningocele	14
Meningomyelocele	279
Lipomyelomeningocele	18
Encephalocele	84
Total	558

(From Ingraham FD et al. Spina Bifida and Cranium Bifidum. Cambridge: Harvard University Press, 1944)

sac-like protrusion of the skin and meninges overlying the vertebral defect. The sac may contain meninges or portions of the spinal cord.

Incidence. The incidence of meningomyelocele varies with geographic location: 0.3/1000 live births in Japan; 4.2/1000 live births in Dublin; and 12.5/1000 live births in Monmouthshire, Wales. There is a slight female preponderance (1.25:1.0). Simple failure of closure of one or more vertebral arches in the lumbar or sacral region without other anomaly in the nervous system is a relatively common finding (estimated at 25% by Ingraham and Lowrey) in routine examination of the spine at autopsy or by radiograph. Spinal defects of clinical importance are much more

rare, occurring in about 1 in 4000 cases admitted to the Children's Hospital in Boston (Ingraham). The incidence is slightly greater among girls. There was a history of similar defects in the spinal column in other members of the family in 6% of Ingraham's 546 cases. This figure is consistent with subsequent reports that indicate a recurrence risk of 5% after one affected offspring. Rarely, inheritance is autosomal recessive as in the syndrome of sacral and conotruncal heart defects with minor head and neck anomalies (Kouseff syndrome). X-linked inheritance is postulated in a few instances. Fortunately, recent studies cite a progressive decline in the incidence of myelomeningocele.

The coincidence of spina bifida and other developmental defects is common. Ingraham and his associates found 570 developmental anomalies in 232 of their 546 patients (Table 73–3). Hydrocephalus was present in 208 cases, clubfoot in 102, and other defects in the vertebrae in 49 cases, including seven cases of the Klippel-Feil anomaly. Defects in the nervous system were noted in 58 cases, with the Arnold-Chiari malformation occurring in 20.

Although the defect is present before birth, there may be a delay of several or many years

Table 73–3. Developmental Anomalies Associated with Spina Bifida and Cranium Bifidum in 546 Cases

Anomaly	No. of Cases
Hydrocephalus	208
Clubfoot	102
Bone defects	94
Vertebrae (including 7 cases of Klippel-Feil's syndrome)	49
Skull	16
Other bones	29
Central nervous system defects	58
Cerebrum	20
Cerebellum and brainstem (including 20 cases of Arnold-Chiari malformation)	26
Other portions	12
Hernia	27
Dislocated hip	23
Genitourinary anomaly	11
Congenital heart disease	4
Other	43
Total	570

(From Ingraham FD et al. Spina Bifida and Cranium Bifidum. Cambridge: Harvard University Press, 1944)

before sufficient symptoms develop for the patient to seek medical aid. This is important, because all patients with this developmental defect are not seen in pediatric clinics.

Symptoms and Signs. Spina bifida occulta may be present without any neurologic symptoms. Symptoms and signs, when they occur, are related to a concomitant defect in the development of the spinal cord (diastematomyelia, tethered cord, ectopic nerve roots) or the presence of lipomas, dermoids, or other tumors. The symptoms and signs in these cases include weakness and atrophy of the muscles of the legs, disturbances of the gait, urinary incontinence, impairment of cutaneous and proprioceptive sensations in the lumbar and sacral segments, and loss of tendon reflexes in the legs. Maldevelopment of the feet with valgus, varus or cavus deformities, usually unilateral, and scoliosis are the most common associated structural deformities. Progressive spasticity or scoliosis may occur due to associated hydromyelia or brain stem compression, requiring surgical treatment for these lesions.

Not infrequently, the defect in the spine can be detected by palpation or is evident by the presence of a localized overgrowth of hair, a hard lump, a shallow pit or sinus, or a capillary angioma *(naevus flammeus)* in the skin near the site of the defect. The most common dermal anomaly of the lumbosacral region without underlying neurologic or bony defect of the spine is a small naevus flammeus. A lipoma was present at the site of the defect in 13 of the 65 cases of Ingraham and Lowrey. These lipomas consist of lobules of gritty firm fat bound together by fibrous septa, and may extend from any tissue level of the back of the spinal cord binding the various tissues together and preventing the normal rostral movements of the lower end of the cord with growth. The lipomatous masses may extend into the epidural and subdural spaces and compress the roots of the cauda equina or the lower end of the cord. The lipoma may also extend widely over the subcutaneous region of the lumbosacral region causing obvious visible and palpable deformation of these areas. There is evidence from a large experience at Toronto's Hospital for Sick Children that early surgical treatment of these lesions prevents permanent neurologic deficit.

Simple meningoceles may occur without any symptoms, but when elements of the spinal cord are present in the sac (meningomyelocele) (Fig. 73–1), some disability is almost invariably present. The nature of the symptoms is related to the level of the lesion. In the lumbar region (Fig. 73–2), they are similar to those that may occur in association with spina bifida occulta. At higher levels, there may be symptoms and signs of complete or incomplete transection of the cord, or combined root and cord symptoms of a syringomyelic character.

Diagnosis. The diagnosis of spina bifida is obvious when the defect is associated with a mass protruding from the spine. In other cases it can be readily diagnosed by radiographic examination. The finding of a spinal defect on the radiograph does not always indicate the symptoms are due to this defect. However, it should lead to the consideration of the possibility of the presence of a congenital tumor or some other developmental defect. Fawcitt described an 82% incidence of unfused vertebral arches at one or more levels in the radiologic examination of 500 asymptomatic children; the incidence in adults is an estimated 25% of patients, indicating progressive closure of these defects until maturation. The lesion that generates the greatest controversy about diagnosis and management is the tethered cord (i.e., anchoring of the cones of the spinal cord at the lower end of the bony spinal canal by a tight filum terminale, with or without spina bifida). The diagnosis depends on myelographic (CT or MRI) evidence of abnormally low placement (below L2) of the conus medullaris, together with progressive neurologic deficit. Some patients improve clinically, and the prolonged latency of somatosensory-evoked responses may be reversed after resection of the filum terminale, providing objective evidence of benefit. For occult spinal dysraphism, MRI is considered by some to be superior to CT or myelography. Cerebral sonography is useful for the detection or confirmation of hydrocephalus in infants with myelomeningocele.

Approaches to antenatal diagnosis of neural tube defects include determination of serum and amniotic fluid alpha-fetoprotein (AFP), amniotic fluid acetylcholinesterase (AChE), amniotic-fluid culture for glial cells, fetal ultrasonography, and contrast-enhanced amniography. Maternal serum-AFP screening is relatively invalid, with a 20% false-negative rate, but it lends itself to mass screening, and has a proven cost-benefit advantage. Ultrasound techniques miss 5 to 10% of spina bifidas, comparing favorably both as a screening and diagnostic test with serum-AFP de-

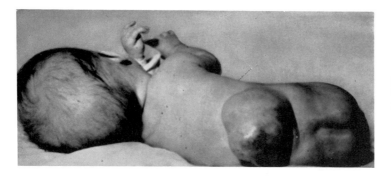

Fig. 73–1. Spina bifida in lumbosacral region with meningomyelocele and hydrocephalus.

termination. Amniotic-fluid AChE determination, in a large population of women with positive amniotic-fluid AFP, substantially reduced the number of false-positive results of the AFP test. Among women with positive AFP, the risk of having a fetus with an open neural-tube defect compared to having one without serious malformation or miscarriage is raised about 16-fold if the AChE test is also positive. Amniotic-fluid culture yields glial cells arising from the open neural tube, and this method may further reduce the incidence of false-positive AFP or AChE results.

Course. The course of patients with defects in the closure of the spine depends on the extent of the lesion and the nature of other congenital defects. Death may occur in infancy after infection of the nervous system secondary to rupture of the sac or because of the associated hydrocephalus. Spina bifida occulta with minor defects in the development of the nervous system is compatible with a relatively normal span of life. Neurologic signs may increase, however, in severity or redevelop at any time. Lorber has shown that 33% of meningomyelocele survivors are totally dependent, 50% are of normal intelligence but severely handicapped, and about 20% are completely independent.

Treatment. Increases in the numbers of surviving children with dysraphic disorders is chiefly due to advances in antibiotic therapy of neonatal meningitis and to the widespread practice of surgical intervention in the first day of life.

Hydrocephalus is the most significant complicating factor in the course of meningomyelocele, occurring in 50 to 80% of infants studied in the early weeks of life. Closure of the meningomyelocele may precipitate hydrocephalus from latent to active and progressive disease. Ventricular shunting can be avoided in as many as one third of infants owing to spontaneous arrest. The favorable signs in

this regard include slow head growth and normal psychomotor development.

The treatment of spina bifida an its complications is by surgery. Lipomatous or other types of intraspinal tumors should be removed. Simple meningoceles can be excised when hydrocephalus is not present, after hydrocephalus has been stabilized spontaneously, or after surgical treatment. The excision of spinal sacs that contain neural elements usually shows poor results due in part to the frequency of coincidental spinal or cerebral defects. The management of infants and children with meningomyelocele often requires the protracted and dedicated involvement of the pediatric neurosurgeon, neurologist, orthopedic surgeon, urologist, and physiatrist. The goals of rehabilitation include bladder asepsis, prevention of hydronephrosis and of joint contractures, maintenance of stability of the spine and legs, and management of associated cerebral deficits.

Reduction in the incidence of severe defects may be effected by antenatal diagnosis and termination of pregnancy.

Cranium Bifidum

Defects in the fusion of the cranial bone are known as cranium bifidum. These defects occur in the midline and are most common in the occipital region. The skull defects are usually accompanied by sac-like protrusions of the overlying skin. This sac contains meninges (*meningocele*) or meninges and cerebral tissue (*encephalocele*). Other congenital malformations of the nervous system may be present. Hydrocephalus is common when the defect in the skull is in the occipital region.

Occasionally, nasal or sphenoethmoid encephalocele is encountered. Meckel syndrome refers to the association of occipital encephalocele with cystic kidneys and hepatic fibrosis. The disorder is recessively inherited. Other syndromes include encephalocele with amniotic band, cryptophthalmos, frontonasal

The occurrence of clinical symptoms and signs in patients with cranial meningoceles or encephaloceles is usually related to the presence or absence of hydrocephalus or other congenital malformations of the nervous system. The actual size of the sac is important only because rupture of the skin and infection of the meninges are more likely when the sac is large.

The treatment of cranial meningoceles or encephaloceles is excision of the sac with its contents and firm closure of the dura. The prognosis is good when only meninges and CSF are contained in the sac. It is poor if large amounts of cerebral tissue are present, if the ventricular system extends into the mass, if hydrocephalus is present, or if there are other serious defects in the nervous system. It is estimated that less than 5% of infants with encephalocele are normal at follow-up.

References

Anderson FM. Occult spinal dysraphism. Pediatrics 1975; 55:826–835.

Aula P, von Koskull H, Teramo K, et al. Glial origin of rapidly adhering amniotic fluid cells. Br Med J 1980; 281:1456–1457.

Bell WD, Charney EB, Bruce DA, Sutton LN, Schut L. Symptomatic Arnold-Chiari malformation: Review of experience with 22 cases. J Neurosurg 1987; 66:812–816.

Bell WD, Sumner TE, Volberg FM. The significance of ventriculomegaly in the newborn with myelodysplasia. Childs Nerv Syst 1987; 3:234–241.

Bennett MJ, Blaw K, Johnson RD, Chamberlain GVP. Some problems of alpha-fetoprotein screening. Lancet 1978; 2:1296–1297.

Brunberg JA, Latchow RE, Kanal E, Burk DL Jr, Albright L. Magnetic resonance imaging of spinal dysrhaphism. Radiol Clin North Am 1988; 26:181–205.

Burton BK. Alpha-fetoprotein screening. Adv Pediatr 1986; 33:181–196.

Cohen MM Jr, Lemire RJ. Syndromes with cephaloceles. Teratology 1982; 25:161–172.

Crandell PF, ed. The Prevention of Neural Tube Defects: The Role of Alpha-Fetoprotein. New York: Academic Press, 1978.

Donnenfeld AE, Hughes H, Weiner S. Prenatal diagnosis and perinatal management of frontoethmoidal meningoencephalocele. Am J Perinatol 1988; 5:51–53.

Fawcitt J. Some aspects of congenital anomalies of the spine in childhood and infancy. Proc Roy Soc Med 1959; 52:331–333.

Fisher NL, Smith DW. Occipital encephalocele and early gestational hyperthermia. Pediatrics 1981; 68:480–483.

Fishman MA. Recent advances in the treatment of dysraphic states. Pediatr Clin North Am 1976; 23:517–526.

Gilbert JN, Jones KL, Rorke LB, Chernoff GF, James HE. Central nervous system anomalies associated with meningomyelocoele, hydrocephalus and the Arnold-Chiari malformation. Neurology 1986; 18:559–564.

Griscomb NT, Frigoletto FD, Harris GBC. Amniography in the early prenatal detection of thoracic, lumbar

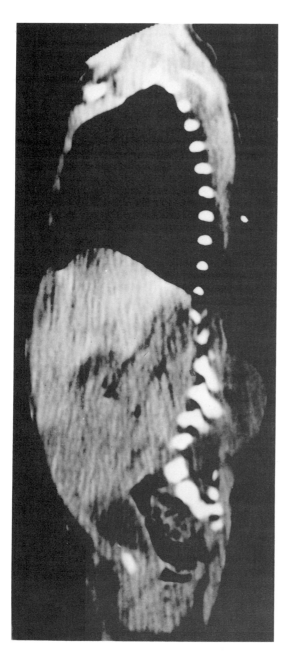

Fig. 73–2. Lumbosacral meningocele. Direct sagittal CT scan shows spinal dysraphism with distal lumbar meningocele; this is contiguous with thecal sac at lumbosacral junction. (Courtesy of Drs. J.A. Bello and S.K. Hilal.)

dysraphism, and maternal Warfarin ingestion. First-trimester hyperthermia has been associated with isolated occipital encephalocele; experimental encephalocele has been produced by hyperthermia in the rat.

The antenatal diagnostic techniques described for meningomyelocele apply equally to the diagnosis of bifid cranial abnormalities.

and sacral myelomeningocoeles. Am J Roentgen 1979; 133:438–439.

Hagberg B, Nagle AS. The conservative management of infantile hydrocephalus. Acta Paediatr Scand 1972; 61:165–177.

Harris R, Read AP. New uncertainties in preventive screening for neural tube defects. Br Med J 1981; 282:1416.

Heins ER, Rosenbaum AE, Scarff TB, Reigel DH, Drayer BP. Tethered spinal cord following meningomyelocoele repair. Radiology 1979; 131:153–160.

Hilal SK, Marton D, Pollack E. Diastematomyelia in children. Radiology 1974; 112:609–622.

Hoffman HJ, Hendrick EB, Humphreys RP. The tethered spinal cord. Child Brain 1976; 2:145–155.

Hoffman HJ, Taecholarn C, Hendrick EB, Humphreys RP. Management of lipomyelomeningocoeles. Experience at the Hospital for Sick Children, Toronto. J Neurosurg 1985; 62:1–8.

Holmes LB, Driscoll SG, Atkins L. Etiologic heterogeneity of neural-tube defects. N Engl J Med 1976; 294:365–369.

Hormann D, Grafe G. Results of cerebral sonography in children with myelomeningocoeles. Monatsschr Kinderheilkd 1986; 134:263–268.

Hunt GM, Whitaker RH. The pattern of congenital anomalies associated with neural tube defects. Dev Med Child Neurol 1987; 29:91–95.

Ingraham FD, Swan H, Hamlin H, Lowrey JJ, et al. Spina Bifida and Cranium Bifidum. Cambridge, Mass: Harvard University Press, 1944.

Laurence KM. The natural history of spina bifida cystica. Arch Dis Child 1964; 39:41–57.

Laurence KM, Carter CO, David PA. The major central nervous system malformations in South Wales. I. Incidence, local variations and geographical factors. Br J Prev Soc Med 1968; 22:146–158.

Layde PM, von Allmen SD, Oakley GP Jr. Maternal serum alpha-fetoprotein screening: a cost-benefit analysis. Am J Pub Health 1979; 69:566–573.

Liptak GS, Bloss JW, Briskin H, Campbell JE, Hebert EB, Revell GM. The management of children with spinal dysrhaphism. J Child Neurol 1988; 3:3–20.

Lorber J. The family history of spina bifida cystica. Pediatrics 1968; 35:589–595.

Lorber J. Results of treatment of myelomeningocoele. Dev Med Child Neurol 1971; 13:279–303.

Lorber J. Spina bifida cystica. Results of treatment of 270 consecutive cases with criteria for selection for the future. Arch Dis Child 1972; 47:854–873.

Lorber J, Schofield JK. The prognosis of occipital encephalocele. Kinderchir Grenzgeb 1979; 28:347–351.

Lorber J, Ward AM. Spina bifida—a vanishing nightmare? Arch Dis Child 1985; 60:1086–1091.

McLaughlin JF, Shurtleff DB. Management of the newborn with myelodysplasia. Clin Pediatr (Phila) 1979; 18:463–480.

Park TS, Cail WS, Maggio Wm, Mitchell DC. Progressive spasticity and scoliosis in children with myelomeningocele: Radiological investigation and surgical treatment. J Neurosurg 1985; 62:367–375.

Report of the Collaborative Acetylcholinesterase Study. Amniotic fluid acetylcholinesterase electrophoresis as a secondary test in the diagnosis of anencephaly and open spina bifida in early pregnancy. Lancet 1981; 2:321–324.

Roos RA, Vielvoye GJ, Voormolen JH, Peters AC. Magnetic resonance imaging in occult spinal dysrhaphism. Pediatr Radiol 1986; 16:412–416.

Rubin JM, DiPietro MA, Chandler WF, Venes JL. Spinal ultrasonography: Intraoperative and pediatric applications. Radiol Clin North Am 1988; 26:1–27.

Salonen R. The Meckel syndrome: Clinicopathologic findings in 67 patients. Am J Genet 1984; 18:671–689.

Sargent LA, Seyfer AE, Gruby EN. Nasal encephaloceles: Definitive one stage reconstruction. J Neurosurg 1988; 68:571–575.

Second Report of the U.K. Collaborative Study on Alpha-Fetoprotein in Relation to Neural-Tube Defects. Amniotic-fluid alpha-fetoprotein measurement in antenatal diagnosis of anencephaly and open spina bifida in early pregnancy. Lancet 1979; 2:651–661.

Shurtleff DB, Hayden PW, Loeser JD, Kronmal RA. Myelodysplasia: decision for death or disability. N Engl J Med 1974; 291:1105–1111.

Simpson DA, David DJ, White J. Cephaloceles: Treatment, outcome and antenatal diagnosis. Neurology 1984; 15:14–21.

Third Report of the U.K. Collaborative Study on Alpha-Fetoprotein in Relation to Neural-Tube Defects. Survival of infants with open spina bifida in relation to maternal serum alpha-fetoprotein level. Br J Obstet Gynaecol 1982; 89:3–7.

Thompson MW, Rudd NL. The genetics of spinal dysraphism. In: Morley TP, ed. Current Controversies in Neurosurgery. Philadelphia: WB Saunders, 1976; 126.

Toriello HV, Sharda K, Beaumont EJ. Autosomal recessive syndrome of sacral and conotrunkal developmental field defects (Kouseff syndrome). Am J Med Genet 1985; 22:357–360.

Vogl D, Ring-Mrozik E, Baierl P, Vogl T, Zimmerman K. Magnetic resonance imaging in children suffering from spina bifida. Z-Kinderchir 1987; 42(Suppl):60–64.

Wippold FJ, Citrin C, Barkovich AJ, Sherman JS. Evaluation of MR in spinal dysrhaphism with lipoma: comparison with metrizamide computed tomography. Pediatr Radiol 1987; 17:184–188.

---

74. ARNOLD-CHIARI MALFORMATION
Melvin Greer

A congenital anomaly of the hindbrain characterized by a downward elongation of the brain stem and cerebellum into the cervical portion of the spinal cord was originally described by Arnold in 1894 and Chiari in 1895.

Pathology. The cause of this defect is not entirely clear. Because of its common association with spina bifida occulta or the presence of a meningocele or meningomyelocele in the lumbosacral region, it is thought that the downward displacement of the brain stem and cerebellum is due to the fixation of the cord at the site of the spinal defect early in fetal life. With the growth of the spine in the later months of intrauterine life, the adhesions in the lumbar or sacral region prevent the cord from ascending in a normal manner and pull the brain stem and cerebellum downward into the cervical canal. This hypothesis is not applicable to the cases in which there is no defect in the lower spine and fails to account for the other anomalies commonly associated with the hindbrain malformation (e.g., absence of the septum pellucidum, fusion of the thalami, hypoplasia of the falx cerebri, fusion of the corporea quadrigemina and microgyri). Some type of developmental arrest and overgrowth of the neural tube in embryonic life is a more plausible explanation of the anomaly.

The gross description of the abnormality has been remarkably similar in all the reported cases. The inferior poles of the cerebellar hemispheres extend downward through the foramen magnum in two tongue-like processes and are often adherent to the adjacent medulla, more than half is usually below the level of the foramen magnum (Fig. 74–1). The medulla is elongated and flattened anteroposteriorly and the lower cranial nerves are stretched.

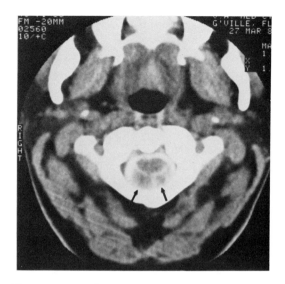

Fig. 74–2. Arnold-Chiari malformation. Post myelography CT. At level of odontoid in high cervical region spinal cord is flattened by cerebellar tonsils (arrows). (Courtesy of Drs. S.K. Hilal and M. Mawad.)

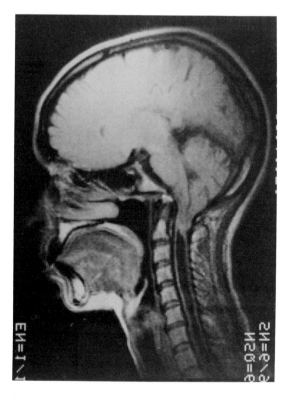

Fig. 74–1. Arnold-Chiari malformation. Magnetic resonance T1-weighted image of midsagittal section of brain and cervical cord. Note small and elongated fourth ventricle, low position of obex of fourth ventricle below plane of foramen magnum, cerebellar tonsillar ectopia, short clivus, wide foramen magnum, kinked cervical medullary junction and prominent superior vermis. Large hydromyelia in cervical cord.

Incidence. The Arnold-Chiari malformation is not as rare as would be expected from the small number of cases reported in the literature. Ingraham and Swan found 20 instances of this abnormality in 290 cases with myelomeningoceles (see Table 73–3). The defect is almost always, but not invariably, associated with a meningomyelocele or spina bifida occulta in the lumbosacral region. Hydrocephalus is present in most cases. Other associated defects of development include rounded defect in the bones of the skull (craniolacunia, Lückenschädel), defects in the spinal cord (hydromyelia, syringomyelia, double cord), and defects in the spinal column (basilar impression).

Symptoms and Signs. The neurologic signs and symptoms of the Arnold-Chiari malformation that appear in the first few months of life are usually due to hydrocephalus and other developmental defects in the nervous system. The prognosis is poor in these cases. The onset of symptoms is rarely delayed until adult life. There may be signs and symptoms of injury to the cerebellum, medulla, and the lower cranial nerves, with or without evidence of increased intracranial pressure. Progressive ataxia, leg weakness, and visual complaints are characteristic. Oscillopsia at rest and visual blurring of fixated targets are described. Downbeat nystagmus and see-saw nystagmus may be noted in lesions of the cervicomedullary region.

Diagnosis. The presence of the Arnold-

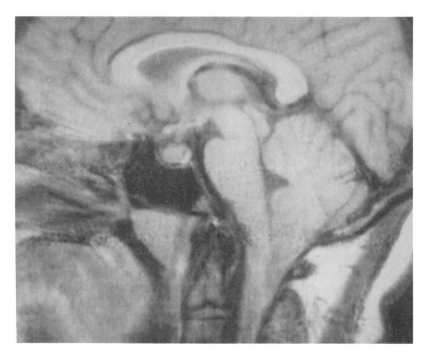

Fig. 74–3.   Type I Arnold-Chiari malformation. Sagittal T1-weighted scan shows tonsillar herniation through foramen magnum. Fourth ventricle is of normal size and position as are aqueduct and brainstem. There is no hydrocephalus. (Courtesy of Drs. J.A. Bello and S.K. Hilal.)

Chiari malformation is probable when there is the coincidence of a meningomyelocele, hydrocephalus, and craniolacunia in infancy. The diagnosis in adults should be considered whenever signs and symptoms of damage to the cerebellum, medulla, and the lower cranial nerves appear. The clinical signs and symptoms of the Arnold-Chiari malformation in adults may simulate the syndromes produced by tumors of the posterior fossa, multiple sclerosis, syringomyelia, or basilar impression. The diagnosis can be established by myelography, computed tomography (Fig. 74–2), and magnetic resonance imaging (Fig. 74–3).

Treatment. The treatment of the condition in infants includes excision of the sac in the spinal region and a ventriculoperitoneal shunt to relieve the hydrocephalus. In adults the posterior fossa should be decompressed. The best results are obtained when there are few neurologic symptoms caused by the spinal defect or other congenital anomalies.

References

Arnold J. Myelocyste. Transposition von Gewebskeimen und Sympodie. Beitr Pathol Anat 1894; 16:1–28.

Balagura S, Kuo DC. Spontaneous retraction of cerebellar tonsils after surgery for Arnold-Chiari malformation and posterior fossa cyst. Surg Neurol 1988; 29:137–140.

Banerji NK, Millar JHD. Chiari malformation presenting in adult life. Its relationship to syringomelia. Brain 1974; 97:157–168.

Caviness VS Jr. The Chiari malformations of the posterior fossa and their relation to hydrocephalus. Dev Med Child Neurol 1976; 18:103–116.

Chiari H. Über Veranderungen des Kleinhirns, des Pons und der Medulla oblongata in Folge von congenitaler Hydrocephalie des Grosshirns. Denkschr Akad Wiss Wien 1896; 63:71–116.

DeBarros MC, Farias W, Ataide L, Lins S. Basilar impression and Arnold-Chiari malformation. J Neurol Neurosurg Psychiatry 1968; 31:596–605.

Dehaene I, Pattyn G, Calliauw L. Megadolicho-basilar anomaly, basilar impression and occipito-vertebral anastomosis. Clin Neurol Neurosurg 1975; 78:131–138.

Dunsker SB, Brown O, Thomson N. Cranioverterbral anomalies. Clin Neurosurg 1980; 27:430–439.

el Gammal T, Mark EK, Brooks BS. MR imaging of Chiari II malformation. Am J Radiol 1988; 150:163–170.

Gilbert JN, Jones KL, Rorke LB, Chernoff GF, James HE. Central nervous system anomalies associated with meningomyelocele hydrocephalus and the Arnold-Chiari malformation. Neurosurgery 1986; 18:559–564.

Levy WJ, Mason L, Hahn JF. Chiari malformation presenting in adults: A surgical experience in 127 cases. Neurosurgery 1983; 12:377–390.

Naidich TP. Cranial CT signs of the Chiari II malformation. J Neuroradiol 1981; 8:207–227.

Paul KS, Lye RH, Strang A, Dutton J. Arnold-Chiari malformation. Review of 71 cases. J Neurosurg 1983; 58:183–187.

Salam MZ, Adams RD. The Arnold-Chiari malformation. In: Vinken P, Bruyn G, eds. Handbook of Clinical

Neurology (vol 32). New York: American Elsevier-North Holland, 1978:99–110.

Spooner JW, Baloh RW. Arnold-Chiari malformation: Improvement in eye movements after surgical treatment. Brain 1981; 104:51–60.

Venes JL. Multiple cranial nerve palsies in an infant with Arnold-Chiari malformation. Dev Med Child Neurol 1974; 16:817–820.

Weisberg L. Computed tomographic findings in the Arnold-Chiari type malformation. Comput Tomogr 1981; 5:1–9.

Welch K, Shillito J, Strand R, Fischer EG, Winston KR. Chiari I "malformations"—an acquired disorder? J Neurosurg 1981; 55:604–608.

Woolsley RE, Whaley RA. Use of metrizamide in computerized tomography to diagnose the Chiari I malformation. J Neurosurg 1982; 56:373–376.

Zimmerman CF, Roach ES, Troost BT. See-saw nystagmus associated with Chiari malformation. Arch Neurol 1986; 43:299–300.

75. MALFORMATIONS OF OCCIPITAL BONE AND CERVICAL SPINE

Melvin Greer

The defects in the development of the cervical spine and base of the skull may be divided into the following groups:

1. Basilar impression
2. Malformation of the atlas and axis
3. Malformation or fusion of other cervical vertebrae (Klippel-Feil anomaly)

Any of these malformations may occur singly or together; they also may be associated with developmental defects in the skull, spine, CNS, or other organs. These deformities can be present without clinical symptoms, but symptoms may appear because of mechanical compression of the neuraxis or due to an associated malformation of the nervous system.

Basilar Impression

Platybasia, basilar impression, and basilar invagination are names frequently used interchangeably for the skeletal malformation in which the base of the skull is flattened on the cervical spine. *Platybasia* (flat base skull) is present if the angle formed by a line connecting the nasion, tuberculum sella, and anterior margin of the foramen magnum is greater than 143° (Fig. 75–1). *Basilar invagination* refers to an upward indentation of the base of the skull, which may be present in Paget disease, osteomalacia, or other forms of bone disease associated with softening of the bones of the skull. An upward displacement of the occipital bone and cervical spine with protrusion of the odontoid process into the foramen magnum constitutes *basilar impression*. Compression of the pons, medulla, cerebellum, and cervical cord and stretching of the cranial nerves may result from the upward ascent of the occipital bone and cervical spine and from narrowing of the foramen magnum.

Pathology and Pathogenesis. Minor degrees of platybasia and basilar invagination may produce no symptoms. In most symptomatic cases the deformity is due to a congenital maldevelopment or hypoplasia of the basiocciput which causes basilar impression, platybasia, partial or complete atlanto-occipital fusion, atlantoaxial dislocation, and a narrowed foramen magnum (see Fig. 75–1). An autosomal dominant mode of inheritance has been suggested, with male preponderance. The pons, medulla, and cerebellum may be distorted and the cranial nerves stretched. Vertebral artery obstruction may be significant in the production of brain-stem symptoms (e.g., vertigo and drop attacks with head-turning) in basilar impression.

Symptoms and Signs. Basilar impression is rare. Neurologic symptoms, when present, usually develop in childhood or early adult life. The head may appear to be elongated and its vertical diameter reduced. The neck appears shortened and its movements may be limited by anomalies of the upper cervical vertebrae. Neurologic symptoms include spastic weakness of the limbs, unsteadiness of gait, cerebellar ataxia, nystagmus, and paralyses of the lower cranial nerves. Papilledema and signs of increased pressure may occur when the deformity interferes with the circulation of the CSF. Partial or complete subarachnoid block is present at lumbar puncture in most cases. CSF protein levels are increased in 50% of patients.

Diagnosis. The diagnosis of basilar impression is usually obvious from the general appearance of the patient. It can be established with certainty by the characteristic radiographic appearance of the base of the skull. The clinical syndromes produced by the anomaly can simulate those caused by multiple sclerosis, syringomyelia, the Arnold-Chiari malformation, and posterior fossa tumors. These diagnoses are readily excluded radiographically.

Treatment. The treatment is surgical decompression of the posterior fossa and the upper cervical cord.

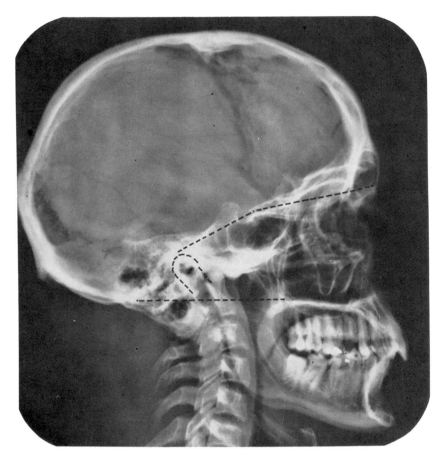

Fig. 75–1.   Basilar impression with platybasia. The odontoid process is entirely above Chamberlain's line (hard palate to base of skull). Basal angle is flat. (Courtesy of Dr. Juan Taveras.)

Malformations of the Atlas and Axis

Maldevelopments of the atlas and axis may be found with basilar impression or may occur independently. Congenital defects resulting in weakness or absence of the structures maintaining stability of the atlantoaxial joints predispose to subluxation and dislocation. These include dens aplasia, a condition in which part of the odontoid process remains on the body of the second cervical vertebra, thereby reducing the stability of the joint. Neurologic symptoms may be produced by anterior dislocation of the atlas and compression of the cord between the protruding odontoid process and the posterior rim of the foramen magnum. There may be mild or severe spastic quadriplegia, with or without evidence of damage to the lower cranial nerves. Head movement causes pain. Sensory loss may be absent or of only mild degree. Transitory signs or symptoms of a progressive myelopathy may occur, often following exaggerated movements of the neck or mild

trauma. Respiratory embarrassment is prominent when the thoracic muscles are affected. The diagnosis is by the finding of anterior dislocation of the atlas in the radiographs. When the bony changes are slight, and especially when there is little or no posterior dislocation of the odontoid process, the symptoms may be due to other congenital defects, such as syringomyelia or Arnold-Chiari malformation.

Fusion of the Cervical Vertebrae

Fusion of the upper thoracic vertebrae and the entire cervical spine into a single bony mass was reported by Klippel and Feil in 1912. Since that time, numerous cases have been reported with variations of this deformity. In most, the abnormality consists of the fusion of the cervical vertebrae into one or more separate masses (Fig. 75–2). This vertebral fusion is the result of maldevelopment in utero and there is evidence of both autosomal dominant and recessive transmission. This anomaly is

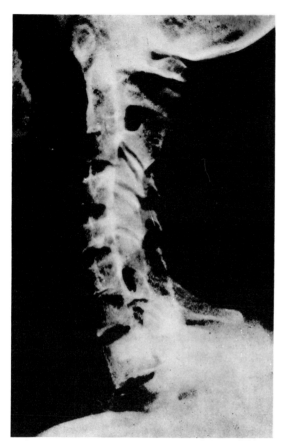

Fig. 75–2. Fusion of cervical vertebrae (Klippel-Feil syndrome).

associated with a short neck, low hairline, and limitation of neck movement, especially in the lateral direction. The fusion of the vertebrae is not in itself of any great clinical importance except for the resulting deformity in the appearance of the neck. Clinical symptoms are usually due to the presence of syringomyelia or other developmental defects of the spinal cord, brain stem, or cerebellum. Congenital cardiovascular defects have been reported in 4% and genitourinary anomalies in 2% of patients. Congenital deafness due to faulty development of the osseous inner ear was estimated by Palant and Carter to occur in up to 30% of patients.

Gunderson and Greenspan emphasized the much more frequent occurrence of fusion of only two adjacent cervical vertebrae. These patients have a normal morphologic appearance, the limited anomaly causing only accentuation of symptoms in the presence of cervical osteoarthritis.

A curious neurologic symptom (i.e., the presence of mirror movements in the arms and hands) has been reported to occur in conjunction with the anomaly of the cervical spine. Voluntary movements of one arm are involuntarily imitated to a more or less degree by the other. The pathophysiology of these mirror movements is not known. In the reported cases, they were present from birth, but became less evident as the child grew older.

References

DeBarros MC, Farias W, Ataide L, Luis S, et al. Basilar impression and Arnold-Chiari malformation. J Neurol Neurosurg Psychiatry 1968; 31:596–605.

Dehaene I, Pattyn G, Calliauw L. Megadolicho-basilar anomaly, basilar impression and occipitovertebral anastomosis. Clin Neurol Neurosurg 1975; 78:131–138.

Dunsker SB, Brown O, Thomson N. Craniovertebral anomalies. Clin Neurosurg 1980; 27:430–439.

Greenberg AD. Atlanto-axial dislocations. Brain 1968; 91:655–684.

Gunderson CH, Greenspan RH, Glaser GH. The Klippel-Feil syndrome: Genetic and clinical reevaluation of cervical fusion. Medicine 1967; 46:491–512.

Janeway R, Toole JF, Leinbach LB, Miller HS. Vertebral artery obstruction with basilar impression. Arch Neurol 1966; 15:211–214.

Kaplan JG, Rosenberg RS, DeSouza T, et al. Atlantoaxial subluxation in psoriatic arthropathy. Ann Neurol 1988; 23:522–524.

Lee CK, Weiss AB. Isolated congenital cervical block vertebrae below the axis with neurological symptoms. Spine 1981; 6:118–124.

Murtagh FR. Visualization of basilar invagination by computerized tomography. Arch Neurol 1979; 36:659–660.

Norot JC, Stauffer ES. Sequelae of atlanto-axial stabilization in two patients with Down's syndrome. Spine 1981; 6:437–440.

Sakai M, Shinkawa A, Miyake H, Komatsu N. Klippel-Feil syndrome with conductive deafness: Histological findings of removed stapes. Ann Otol Rhinol Laryngol 1983; 92:202–206.

Vangilder JC, Menezes AH, Dlan KD. The Craniovertebral Junction and its Abnormalities. Mt. Kisco, NY: Futura Publishing Co., 1987.

Wilkinson M. The Klippel-Feil syndrome. In: Vinken P, Bruyn G, eds. Handbook of Clinical Neurology (vol 32). New York: Elsevier-North Holland, 1978:111–122.

76. PREMATURE CLOSURE OF THE CRANIAL SUTURES

Charles Kennedy

The bones of the cranium are normally separated by fibrous tissue in fetal life. During the first postnatal year, the borders meet and interdigitations develop to form the sutures that partially unite the individual bones into a functionally continuous calvarium. These sutures normally yield to the forces of the growth of the underlying brain and allow symmetric expansion. With the completion of brain growth, the sutures become increasingly resistant to separation; eventually fusion takes place. When fusion occurs prematurely (before completion of brain growth), the term *craniosynostosis* is applied. This is usually a selective pathologic process that involves one or a pair of sutures, but all sutures may be affected or different combinations may be seen (Table 76–1). Fusion prevents expansion of the cranium in a direction perpendicular to the line of the suture, and the normal cranial configuration is therefore distorted.

Craniosynostosis may result from metabolic disorders (e.g., hypercalcemia, hypophosphatasia, hyperthyroidism, rickets). It is also a secondary consequence of a failure of brain development (microcephaly) and may be seen after decompression in the treatment of hydrocephalus. Normal patency of the sutures seems to depend on sustained expansile forces of the growing brain.

Most often, however, the cause of premature suture closure is unknown and no distinctive histopathlogy has been observed. The defective growth process is usually confined to one or more of the cranial sutures and marks a largely sporadic disorder with an incidence of 0.6/1000 live births. Occasionally craniosynostosis is but one manifestation of a more generalized dysmorphic state in which there are other skeletal defects or malformations in other tissues. Mental retardation is often present. More than 50 syndromes with craniosynostosis in common have been described. Some are accompanied by chromosomal defects; a few are hereditary.

A clinical distinction is made according to the abnormal configuration of the skull, which is determined by which sutures are fused. When the sagittal suture is affected, growth is in the anteroposterior axis and the skull becomes elongated and narrow or dolicocephalic *(scaphocephaly)*. If the fusion is at the coronal sutures, anteroposterior growth is restricted and compensatory expansion is lateral; the skull becomes broad and short *(brachycephaly)* and the forehead is flattened. If only one coronal suture is closed, the flattening is unilateral *(plagiocephaly)*. Involvement of the lambdoidal suture results in flattening of the occiput and prominence of the parietal regions. In the case of metopic suture, the forehead becomes pointed with flattening in the supraorbital areas *(trigonencephaly)*. If all sutures are symmetrically fused, the cranial configuration may be normal, but the brain may be displaced upward to produce a tower-like shape *(oxycephaly)*. The circumference is often below the norm, and the signs are those of increased intracranial pressure, including papilledema. Proptosis, impaired ocular movement, and corneal drying have also been attributed to elevated intracranial pressure; however, it is likely that shallow orbits due to abnormal growth of facial bones are more important contributing factors. Oxycephaly accompanied by maxillary hypoplasia with shortness of the upper lip, prognathism, and a small pointed nose with a depressed bridge is characteristic of *craniofacial dysostosis (Crouzon syndrome)*, which is an autosomal dominant disorder. Similar to this, but also accompanied by syndactyly of the hands and feet, is *acrocephalosyndactyly (Apert syndrome)*—Fig. 76–1.

The diagnosis of premature suture fusion can be established by radiographic examination, but the full extent of involvement is best established by high-resolution computed tomography. This not only confirms the altered cranial contour but may demonstrate an increased relative density of bone along the line of the suture. An important early sign is local bony thickening, either internally or externally, which is seen in a plane perpendicular to the suture. A corresponding ridge may be palpable. Prominence of digital marks, generalized thinning of the cranial vault, and erosion of the posterior clinoids are evidence of long-standing elevation of intracranial pressure. Radiographs may also reveal premature

Table 76–1.   The Frequency of Involvement of Various Sutures in 370 Patients with Craniosynostosis

Sutures Involved	No. of Patients	%
Sagittal alone	205	55
Coronal	72	20
Bilateral, 23		
Unilateral, 49		
Metopic	13	4
Any three sutures	19	5
Four or more sutures	15	4
Any two unpaired sutures	12	3
Lambdoid	16	4
Acrocephalosyndactyly	18	5
Total	370	100

Modified from Hunter AGW, Rudd NL. Teratology 1976; 14:185–194.

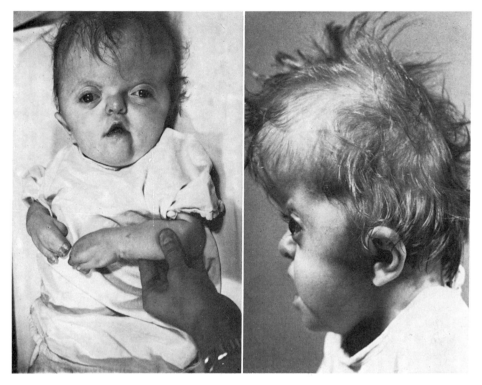

Fig. 76–1. Acrocephalosyndactyly (Apert syndrome). Head is shortened in anterioposterior dimension, forehead is prominent, and occiput flat. Typical facies showing shallow orbits and proptosis of eyes, downward slanting palpebral fissures, small nose, and low-set ears. Osseous and cutaneous syndactyly of hands and feet.

suture closure and associated malformation of the orbital, nasal, sphenoid, and maxillary bones (Fig. 76–2). In radionuclide scans, local accumulations of ^{99m}Tc-polyphosphate mark regions of osteoblastic activity so that the timing of fusion can be established.

The course of untreated craniosynostosis is variable and dependent both upon which sutures are involved and the timing of their early closure. Except for the distortion of the cranial vault, most patients with one suture prematurely closed (typically the sagittal or metopic suture) have no symptoms or signs referable to brain function. With multiple suture involvement, however, intracranial pressure may be elevated due to confinement of the growing brain and a concomitant impairment in the resorption of cerebrospinal fluid over the cortical surface. Headache-related behavior, altered patterns of sleep, and developmental delay may be present in infancy. Later, seizures may occur followed by blindness and irreversible mental retardation.

Surgical treatment is directed to restoring a normal contour of the head, enlarging the cranial cavity, and assuring its capacity to accommodate brain growth. Generally, results are better when the operative procedure is performed early in life. Often there are indications for surgery before 6 months of age. Linear craniectomy suffices when a single or a pair of sutures are involved, but in dysmorphic syndromes in which bones of the face and base of the skull are also fused, complex, multistage procedures may be necessary. In some cases the rate of progression of suture closure is slow, albeit premature, so that signs do not develop until the late preschool or early school years. In these children, signs are nonspecific, e.g., impaired mental function, behavioral changes, and restlessness. Because the brain has attained all but about 5% of its mature size by the age of 6 years, the value of surgical intervention at this age is questionable, especially when lumbar puncture fails to reveal elevated cerebrospinal pressure. Further deterring any consideration of surgical intervention is the often reported coexistence of mental impairment unrelated to the sutural disorder. However, there have been sufficiently frequent anecdotes of remarkable postoperative improvement in behavior and learning to sustain a controversy. This may well be resolved by continuous

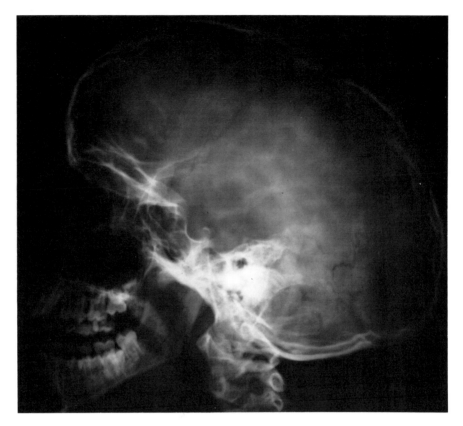

Fig. 76–2.   Head radiograph of 12-year-old with craniosynostosis of sagittal suture. There is elongation of anterio-posterior diameter (dolichocephaly). Digital markings are prominent. (Courtesy of Dr. Clifton A. Leftridge.)

monitoring of intracranial pressure. Centers in which monitoring is done as part of the evaluation of craniosynostosis have found that those with episodic, if not sustained, intracranial hypertension, especially as it occurs in rapid-eye-movement sleep, are among those likely to benefit from surgical treatment.

References

Anderson FM. Treatment of coronal and metopic synostosis: 107 cases. Neurosurgery 1981; 8:143–149.

Andersson H, Gomes SP. Craniosynostosis: Review of the literature and indications for surgery. Acta Paediatr Scand 1968; 57:47–54.

Apert E. De l'acrocéphalosyndactylie. Bull Soc Med Hop Paris 1906; 23:1310–1330.

Barrett J, Brooksbank M, Simpson D. Scaphocephaly: Aesthetic and psychosocial considerations. Dev Med Child Neurol 1981; 23:183–191.

Carmel PW, Luken MG III, Ascherl GF. Craniosynostosis: computed tomographic evaluation of skull base and calvarial deformities and associated intracranial changes. Neurosurgery 1981; 9:366–372.

Cohen MM. Craniosynostosis and syndromes with craniosynostosis: Incidence, genetics, penetrance, variability, and new syndrome updating. Birth Defects 1979; 15:13–63.

Cohen MM ed. Craniosynostosis: Diagnosis, Evaluation and Management. New York: Raven Press, 1986.

Crouzon Q. Dysostose cranio-faciale hereditaire. Bull Mem Soc Med Hop Paris 1912; 33:545.

Furuya Y, Edwards MSB, Alpers CE, Tress BM, Norman D, Ousterhout DK. Computerized tomography of cranial sutures. J Neurosurg 1984; 61:59–70.

Hemple DJ, Harris LE, Svien HJ, Holman CB. Craniosynostosis involving the sagittal suture only: Guilt by association? J Pediatr 1961; 58:342–355.

Hunter AGW, Rudd NL. Craniosynostosis: I. Sagittal synostosis; its genetics and associated clinical findings in 214 patients who lacked involvement of the coronal suture(s). Teratology 1976; 14:185–194.

Hunter AGW, Rudd NL. Craniosynostosis: II. Coronal synostosis; its familial characteristics and associated clinical findings in 109 patients lacking bilateral polysyndactyly or syndactyly. Teratology 1977; 15:301–310.

Matson DD. Neurosurgery of Infancy and Childhood, 2nd ed. Springfield, Ill: Charles C Thomas, 1969.

Mohr G, Hoffman HJ, Munro IR, Hendrick EB, Humphreys RP. Surgical management of unilateral and bilateral coronal craniosynostosis: 21 years of experience. Neurosurgery 1978; 2:83–92.

Renier D, Sainte-Rose C, Marchac D, Hirsch J-F. Intracranial pressure in craniostenosis. J Neurosurg 1982; 57:370–377.

Shillito J, Matson DD. Craniosynostosis. A review of 519 surgical patients. Pediatrics 1968; 41:829–853.

Shuper A, Merlob P, Grunebaum M, Reisner SH. The

incidence of isolated craniosynostosis in the newborn infant. Am J Dis Child 1985; 139:85–86.

Tessier P. Relationship of craniostenosis to craniofacial depostosis and to faciostenosis. Plast Reconstr Surg 1971; 48:224–237.

Whittle IR, Johnston IH, Besser M. Intracranial pressure changes in craniostenosis. Surg Neurol 1984; 21:367–372.

77. THE MARCUS GUNN AND MÖBIUS SYNDROMES

Abe M. Chutorian

Marcus Gunn Syndrome

Reflex elevation of the eyelid in association with movements of the jaw was described by Marcus Gunn. The cause and the anatomic pathway of this reflex are unknown. The reflex is unilateral and occurs in patients who have partial ptosis of one lid. Movements of the jaw, particularly those that involve lateral deviation of the jaw, are accompanied by elevation of the affected lid and widening of the palpebral fissure. The reflex movement causes no disability except for the embarrassment it may cause the patient while eating in public places. Familial occurrence of the syndrome has been described by Falls and associates. Amblyopia and strabismus are common. Unilateral levator excision, bilateral facial suspension, and other surgical procedures may be helpful. Abnormal auditory brain stem reflexes in some patients suggest developmental pathology in the pons. Neurogenic changes in the levator palpebrae superioris muscle are described. Association with other syndromes (e.g. Waardenberg) suggests a common origin of neurocrestopathy.

Möbius Syndrome

Congenital facial diplegia (Möbius syndrome) is rare. In 1939, Henderson found only 60 cases in the literature since the first description by von Graefe in 1868. The paralysis of the facial muscles may be complete or partial, and is frequently associated with paresis of other cranial muscles, particularly the ocular and oropharyngeal muscles. Other congenital defects are also common; these include skeletal abnormalities, such as joint contractures, clubfoot, and limb hypoplasia, mental deficiency of variable degree, dextrocardia and ventricular septal deficit, and pituitary dysfunction. The symptoms are usually static, but there have been three reported cases of progressive peripheral neuropathy with hypogonadotrophic hypogonadism. In a fourth case with these characteristics, the disorder seemed to be a slowly progressing neuropathy. Sometimes congenital facial diplegia proves to be part of facioscapulohumeral or myotonic muscular dystrophy.

There are probably multiple causes of this congenital defect. Hereditary factors are clearly involved; some families include two or more patients with this rare disorder. Most such cases appear to involve dominant inheritance, but recessive (and possibly sporadic) cases do occur. In one three-generation pedigree of a Möbius-syndrome variant, all affected members had reciprocal translocation between chromosomes 1 and 13. Poland-Möbius syndrome represents the association of two rare congenital disorders, Möbius syndrome with skeletal bone and muscle aplasia, and in some cases, dextracardia. Computed tomography and magnetic resonance imaging are helpful in evaluating the brain, pons, orbits, and facial nerves in Möbius syndrome.

The association of Möbius syndrome with Poland and Klippel-Feil syndromes is hypothesized to result from a vascular lesion termed "subclavian artery supply description sequence."

Pathologic studies may show a hypoplasia of the nuclei in the brain stem and of the nerves and muscles connected with them. Evidence of in utero necrosis of brain-stem nuclei has been reported in several cases. This necrosis may have resulted from an episode of anoxia in utero; the brain stem is known to be susceptible at this age. In other cases, the primary defects appear to have involved facial muscles indirectly. In the case reported by Pitner and his associates, there was dysplasia of the facial muscles. Although hypoplastic changes were found in the cerebellum and medulla, the facial nucleus and the facial nerves were normal. In a literature review of the available pathology, together with a case report of Möbius syndrome associated with pontine tegmental necrosis, Towfighi points out that pontine nuclear atrophy, peripheral nerve lesions, and muscle atrophy have all been reported as isolated and presumably primary lesions, which suggests the heterogeneous character of the disorder. Embryonic experimental failure of myeogenesis and of neurogenesis have been shown to cause atrophy and regression of the reciprocal tissue. Thus, Möbius syndrome may originate in either abnormality.

When the paralysis is complete, it is usually evident immediately after birth owing to the difficulty in nursing or failure of the eyes to close during sleep. Partial paralysis may not be detected until it is noted that the child's face does not move normally in crying or laughing. The paralysis is complete in about 35% of the cases. In the rest, the muscles of the upper half of the face are more severely affected than those of the lower half, a condition that is different from that usually seen in either supranuclear or peripheral palsies. Facial diplegia occurred as an isolated phenomenon in only about 15% of the reported cases. In the original description of Möbius syndrome, patients also had abducens paralysis (70%). Other congenital abnormalities include ophthalmoplegia externa (25%), ptosis (10%), either unilateral or bilateral lingual palsy (18%), clubfoot (30%), brachial malformations (22%), pectoral-muscle defects (13%), and mental deficiency (10%).

References

Marcus Gunn Syndrome

Creel DJ, Kivlin JD, Wolfley DE. Auditory brain stem responses in Marcus-Gunn ptosis. Electroencephalogr Clin Neurophysiol 1984; 59:341–344.

Doucet TW, Crawford JS. The quantification, natural course, and surgical results in 57 eyes with Marcus Gunn (jaw winking) syndrome. Am J Ophthalmol 1981; 92:702–707.

Falls HF, Kruse WT, Cotterman CW. Three cases of Marcus Gunn phenomenon in two generations. Am J Ophthalmol 1949; 32:53–59.

Grant FC. The Marcus Gunn phenomenon. Arch Neurol Psychiatry 1936; 35:487–500.

Lewy FH, Groff RA, Grant FC. Autonomic innervation of the eyelids and the Marcus Gunn phenomenon. Arch Neurol Psychiatry 1937; 37:1289–1297.

Lyness RW, Collin JR, Alexander RA, Garner A. Histologic Appearances of the Levator Palpebral Superioris Muscle in the Marcus Gunn Phenomenon. Br J Ophthalmol 1988; 72:104–9.

Meirez F, Standaert L, Delaey JJ, Zeng LH. Waardenberg Syndrome, Hirschprung Megacolon, and Marcus Gunn Ptosis. Am J Med Genet 1987; 27:683–6.

Pratt SG, Beyer CK, Johnson CC. The Marcus Gunn phenomenon. A review of 71 cases.

Möbius Syndrome

Abid F, Hall R, Hudgson P, Weiser R. Möbius syndrome, peripheral neuropathy and hypogonadotrophic hypogonadism. J Neurol Sci 1978; 35:309–315.

Baraitser M. Genetics of Möbius syndrome. J Med Genet 1977; 14:415–417.

Bavinck JN, Weaver DD. Subclavian artery supply description sequence: hypothesis of a vascular etiology for Poland, Klippel-Feil, and Möbius anomalies. Am J Med Genet 1986; 23:903–18.

Brill CB, Peyster RG, Keller MS, Galtman L. Isolation of the right subclavian artery with subclavian steal in a child with Klippel-Feil anomaly: An example of the subclavian artery supply description sequence. Am J Med Genet 1987; 26:933–40.

Carlson BM. The development of facial muscles and nerves in relation to the Moebius syndrome. Otolaryngol Head Neck Surg 1981; 89:903–906.

Hanson PA, Rowland LP. Möbius syndrome and facioscapulohumeral muscular dystrophy. Arch Neurol 1971; 24:31–39.

Henderson JL. The congenital facial diplegia syndrome. Brain 1939; 62:381–403.

Hopper KK, Haas DK, Rice MM, Freeley DA, Taubner RW, Ghaed N. Poland-Moebius syndrome: Evaluation by computerized tomography. South Med J 1985; 78:523–527.

Olson WH, Bardin CW, Walsh GO, Engel WK. Möbius syndrome, lower motor neuron involvement and hypogonadotropic hypogonadism. Neurology 1970; 20:1002–1008.

Pitner SE, Edwards JE, McCormick WF. Observations on the pathology of the Moebius syndrome. J Neurol Neurosurg Psychiatry 1965; 28:362–374.

Rubenstein AE, Lovelace RE, Behrens MM, Weisberg LA. Moebius syndrome in Kallmann syndrome. Arch Neurol 1975: 32:480–482.

Sprofkin BE, Hillman JW. Moebius's syndrome—Congenital oculofacial paralysis. Neurology 1956; 6:50–54.

Thakkar N, O'Neil W, Duvally J, Liu C, Ambler M. Möbius syndrome due to brain stem tegmental necrosis. Arch Neurol 1977; 34:124–126.

Towfighi J, Marks K, Palmer E, Vanucci R. Möbius syndrome. Neuropathologic observations. Acta Neuropathol (Berl) 1979; 48:11–17.

Ziter FA, Wiser WC, Robinson A. Three generation pedigree of a Möbius syndrome variant with chromosome translocation. Arch Neurol 1977; 34:437–442.

Chapter VIII

Genetic Diseases of Recognized Biochemical Abnormality

78. DISORDERS OF AMINO ACID METABOLISM
John H. Menkes

Mass screening for disorders of amino-acid metabolism has resulted in early biochemical diagnosis of phenylketonuria and other aminoacidopathies. In one screening program, the incidence of phenylketonuria was 1:10,000 in New South Wales, Australia; the incidence of defects of amino-acid transport was about 2:10,000, and the combined incidence of all other aminoacidopathies was less than 8:100,000. Although these conditions are rare, they are important because they provide information about the development and functions of the brain.

Phenylketonuria

Phenylketonuria is an inborn error of metabolism transmitted as an autosomal recessive disorder and manifested by an impairment in the hepatic hydroxylation of phenylalanine to tyrosine. Untreated, the disorder causes a clinical picture that is highlighted by mental retardation, seizures, and imperfect hair pigmentation. Inasmuch as phenylketonuria is the prototype for demonstrating the interrelation between genetic alterations and neurologic dysfunction, it deserves more space than its frequency in the panoply of neurologic disorders would otherwise warrant.

The disease has been found in all parts of the world. The frequency in the general population of the United States, as determined by screening programs, is about 1:11,700.

Pathogenesis and Pathology. The hydroxylation of phenylalanine to tyrosine is an irreversible and complex reaction that requires at least three enzymes and several nonprotein components. Phenylalanine hydroxylase is normally found in liver, kidney, and pancreas, but not in brain or skin fibroblasts. In phenylketonuria, as a result of multiple and distinct mutations in the gene for phenylalanine hydroxylase, enzyme activity is completely or nearly completely abolished. Cloning of a full-length complementary DNA (cDNA) has enabled characterization of the normal and mutant genes. The most prevalent of the seven mutations identified to date has been a single base substitution, which interferes with RNA splicing and results in a shortened and unstable phenylanine hydroxylase.

Dihydropteridine reductase, the second enzyme required for phenylalanine hydroxylation, is present in normal amounts in classic phenylketonuria, but is absent or defective in a rare variant of the disease, which manifests itself by elevated serum phenylalanine levels and progressive neurologic dysfunction.

The hydroxylation of phenylalanine also requires oxygen and dihydrobiopterin. The latter is converted to tetrahydrobiopterin, the active cofactor. Defects in the synthetic pathway account for 1 to 3% of infants with phenylalanine elevation. The condition leads to a syndrome of progressive neurologic deterioration, accompanied by a variety of involuntary movements.

Phenylketonuric children are born with only slightly elevated phenylalanine blood levels, but because of the absence of phenylalanine-hydroxylase activity, the amino acid derived from food proteins accumulates in serum and CSF and is excreted in large quantities. In lieu of the normal degradative pathway, phenylalanine is converted to phenylpyruvic acid, phenylacetic acid, and phenylacetylglutamine.

The transamination of phenylalanine to phenylpyruvic acid is sometimes deficient for the first few days of life, and the age when phenylpyruvic acid may be first detected ranges from 2 to 34 days.

Alterations within the brain are nonspecific and diffuse, involving both gray and white matter. There are three types of alterations within the brain:

1. *Interference with normal maturation of the brain.* Brain growth is reduced; there is microscopic evidence of impaired cortical layering, delayed outward migration of neuroblasts, and heterotopic gray matter. These changes suggest there is a period of abnormal brain development during the last trimester of gestation.

2. *Defective myelination.* This may be generalized or limited to areas in which postnatal deposition of myelin is normal. Except in some older patients, products of myelin degeneration are not seen. Generally, there is relative pallor of myelin, sometimes with mild gliosis and irregular areas of vacuolation (i.e., status spongiosus). The vacuoles are usually seen in central white matter of the cerebral hemispheres and in the cerebellum.

3. *Diminished or absent pigmentation* of the substantia nigra and locus ceruleus.

Symptoms and Signs. Phenylketonuric infants appear normal at birth. During the first 2 months, there is vomiting (sometimes projectile) and irritability. Delayed intellectual development is apparent within 4 to 9 months; mental retardation may be severe, precluding speech or toilet training. Seizures, common in more severely retarded infants, usually start before age 18 months and may cease spontaneously. In infants, seizures may appear as infantile spasms, later changing to grand mal attacks.

The typical affected child is blond and blue-eyed with normal and often pleasant features. The skin is rough and dry, sometimes with eczema. A peculiar musty odor, attributable to phenylacetic acid, may suggest the diagnosis. Significant focal neurologic abnormalities are rare. Microcephaly may be present and there may be a mild increase in muscle tone, particularly in the legs. A fine, irregular tremor of the hands is seen in about 35% of subjects. The plantar response is often variable or extensor. EEG abnormalities include hypsarrhythmic patterns, recorded even in the absence of seizures, and single or multiple foci of spike and polyspike discharges.

Diagnosis. The diagnosis of phenylketonuria may be suspected from the clinical features and by ferric chloride testing of the patient's urine. Because there may be a delay in the urinary excretion of phenylpyruvic acid, the ferric chloride and 2,4-dinitrophenylhydrazine tests are inadequate during the neonatal period. Thus, screening programs have been designed to measure blood phenylalanine in infants just before they are discharged from the nursery.

If a case of classic phenylketonuria is missed, the most likely reason is laboratory error rather than insufficient protein intake or too early testing of the infant.

The high frequency of restriction fragment length polymorphism (RFLP) sites at or near the gene for phenylalanine hydroxylase has facilitated carrier detection and the prenatal diagnosis of phenylketonuria in families with at least one previously affected child.

The widespread screening programs that detect newborns with blood phenylalanine concentrations higher than normal have also uncovered other conditions in which blood phenylalanine levels are increased in the neonatal period. Patients with the hyperphenylalaninemias, as these entities are termed collectively, have phenylalanine levels that tend to be lower than those seen in classic phenylketonuria. Hepatic phenylalanine hydroxylase activity ranges from 1.5 to 34.5% of normal. As a rule, the greater the phenylalanine hydroxylase activity, the less the likelihood for mental retardation. The hyperphenylalaninemias either represent compound heterozygotes of one phenylketonuria gene and one of several hyperphenylalaninemia genes or homozygotes for two hyperphenylalaninemia genes.

Treatment. Upon referral of an infant with a positive screening test, the first step is quantitative determination of serum phenylalanine and tyrosine levels. If serum phenylalanine is higher than 20 mg/dl and tyrosine concentration is normal (1–4 mg/dl), the infant may have classic phenylketonuria and should be hospitalized; the infant suspected of having phenylketonuria should be given an evaporated-milk formula for 3 days. At the end of this period, an affected child shows a rise in serum phenylalanine and consistently normal tyrosine levels; the affected child usually excretes urine that contains considerable amounts of phenylpyruvic acid and o-hydroxyphenylacetic acid. When these biochemical abnormalities are found, the infant is started on a low-phenylanine diet.

The distinction between phenylketonuria and the other phenylalaninemias is more than academic. Children with phenylalaninemia do not fare well on dietary therapy. Phenylalanine levels tend to fall precipitously, and side-effects such as hypoglycemia or symptoms of protein deficiency are likely; intellectual retardation and other neurologic symptoms may ensue.

The generally accepted therapy for treatment of phenylketonuria is restriction of the dietary intake of phenylalanine by placing the infant on a low-phenylalanine formula such as Lofendac. To avoid symptoms of phenylalanine deficiency, milk is added to the diet in amounts sufficient to maintain serum levels of the amino acid between 4 and 15 mg/dl. Generally, patients tolerate this diet quite well, and within 1 to 2 weeks the serum concentration of phenylalanine becomes normal.

Serum phenylalanine determinations are essential to assure adequate regulation of diet. Preliminary results suggest that infants with phenylalaninemia do not require dietary therapy if blood levels stay below 20 mg/dl on a full protein intake. Most professionals, however, treat infants during the early period of life, when the diagnosis is still in doubt, and some insist that dietary restriction is necessary for all infants with serum phenylalanine levels higher than 8 mg/dl.

Some physicians briefly reinstate a normal protein intake at about age 6 months in all patients on a restricted phenylalanine diet. In some infants who initially had blood phenylalanine concentrations of 20 mg/dl or higher, amino acid levels did not rise when a normal diet was given for 72 hours 3 months after diagnosis.

At present there is no consensus when if ever the special diet should be ended. It is clear, however, that termination before 8 years of age has a deleterious effect on IQ and school performance.

Treatment of phenylalaninemia due to biopterin deficiency involves administration of tetrahydrobiopterin or a synthetic pterin, and replenishment of the neurotransmitters (levodopa, 5-hydroxy-tryptophan) because synthesis of these substances is also impaired.

Early detection and dietary control of phenylketonuria has increased the number of homozygous phenylketonuric women who are of child-bearing potential. The harmful effects of maternal hyperphenylalaninemia on the heterozygous offspring include mental retardation, microcephaly, seizures, and congenital heart defects. There is no convincing evidence that maintenance of the prospective mother on a low-phenylalanine diet during pregnancy, or even before conception, can prevent these defects.

Prognosis. When the patient with classic phenylketonuria is maintained on a low-phenylalanine diet, seizures disappear and the EEG tends to revert to normal. Abnormally blond hair regains natural color.

The effects on mental ability are less clear-cut. In most studies, some deficit in intellectual development has been found, even in infants who had been diagnosed and treated as neonates. When the measured IQ is normal, children may exhibit significantly impaired perceptual functions, and their progress in school is poorer than expected from the IQ score.

This failure to prevent mild mental retardation or cognitive deficits, even with optimal control, may be a consequence of prenatal brain damage induced by high phenylalanine levels in the fetus.

Maple Syrup Urine Disease

Maple syrup urine disease is a familial cerebral degenerative disease caused by a defect in branched-chain amino-acid metabolism and marked by the passage of urine with a sweet, maple-syrup-like odor. Its incidence is

Table 78–1. Aminoacidurias Detected by Newborn-Infant Urine Screening

Condition	Cases/ 100,000 6-week-old infants
Disorders of amino-acid metabolism	
Phenylketonuria	10
Histidinemia	5.2
Hyperprolinemia	1.0
Cystathioninuria	0.33
Tyrosinemia	0.33
Argininosuccinic aciduria	0.25
Hyperlysinemia	0.1
Nonketotic hyperglycinemia	0.1
Homocystinuria	0.1
α-ketoadipic aciduria	0.1
Others	0
Disorders of amino-acid transport	
Iminoglycinuria	10
Cystinuria	5.8
Hartnup disease	4.0
Cystinosis	0.33

Table 78–2.   Some Uncommon Errors of Amino Acid Metabolism

Disease	Enzymatic Defect	Clinical Features	Diagnosis
Argininosuccinic aciduria	Argininosuccinase	Recurrent generalized convulsions, poorly pigmented hair, ataxia, hepatomegaly, mental retardation	CSF shows large amounts of argininosuccinic acid, elevated blood ammonia
Citrullinemia	Argininosuccinic acid synthetase	Mental retardation, vomiting, irritability, seizures	Serum and urine citrulline elevated, elevated blood ammonia
Hyperammonemia	a) Ornithine transcarbamylase	Recurrent changes in consciousness, hepatomegaly, males succumb early	Elevated blood ammonia, assay of liver enzymes
	b) Carbamyl phosphate synthetase	Episodic vomiting, lethargy	Elevated blood ammonia, assay of liver enzymes
Hyperlysinemia	Lysine-α-ketoglutarate reductase	Severe retardation, hypotonia (some normal)	Elevated plasma lysine, elevated urine lysine, also seen in heterozygotes for cystinuria
Saccharopinuria	Aminoadipic semialdehyde-glutamate reductase	Mental retardation, progressive spastic diplegia	Elevated urine, serum lysine, saccharopine in urine and serum
Aspartylglucosaminuria	Aspartylglucosaminidase	Mental retardation, hepatosplenomegaly, vacuolated lymphocytes in 75%, coarse facial features	Elevated urine aspartylglucosamine
Carnosinemia	Carnosinase	Mental retardation, mixed major and minor motor seizures	Elevated serum, urine carnosine, elevated CSF homocarnosine
Hyperargininemia	Arginase	Spastic diplegia, seizures	Elevated plasma and CSF arginine, elevated blood ammonia

Disorder	Enzyme defect	Clinical features	Biochemical findings
Hypervalinemia	Valine transaminase	Vomiting, failure to thrive, nystagmus, mental retardation	Increased blood and urine valine; no increase in keto-acid excretion
Sarcosinemia (folic acid dependent)	Impaired sarcosine-glycine conversion	Emotional disturbance in some; normal intelligence in most others	Increased blood and urine sarcosine, ethanolamine
Hyperbeta-alaninemia	β-Alanine-α-ketoglutarate transaminase	Seizures commencing at birth, somnolence	Plasma, urine-β-alanine and β-aminoisobutyric acid elevated, urinary γ-amino-butyric acid elevated
β-Methylcrotonic aciduria	a) β-Methylcrotonyl-CoA carboxylase b) Biotin metabolism	Similar to infantile spinal muscular atrophy, persistent vomiting, mental retardation, urine smells like that of cat	Increased urine β-hydroxyisovaleric acid, β-methylcrotonylglycine; some patients are biotin-responsive
α-Methyl-β-hydroxy-butyric aciduria	Defective conversion of α-methylaceto-acetate to propionate	Recurrent severe acidosis	α-Methyl acetoacetate and α-methyl-β-hydroxy-butyric acid in urine
Cytosol tyrosine aminotransferase deficiency	Soluble tyrosine amino transferase	Multiple congenital anomalies	p-Hydroxyphenylpyruvic and p-hydroxyphenyl lactic acid excretion increased
Hypertryptophanemia	Tryptophan pyrrolase	Ataxia, spasticity, mental retardation, pellagra-like skin rash	Elevated serum tryptophan, diminished kynurenine
Glutamyl cysteine synthetase deficiency	γ-Glutamylcysteine synthetase	Hemolytic anemia, spinocerebellar degeneration, peripheral neuropathy	Reduced erythrocyte glutathione, generalized aminoaciduria
5-Oxoprolinuria	Glutathione synthetase	Mental retardation, metabolic acidosis	Elevated urinary 5-oxoproline

1:220,000 newborns. The disorder is characterized by accumulation of three branched-chain keto acids: α-keto-isocaproic acid, α-keto-isovaleric acid, and α-keto-β-methylvaleric acid, which are the respective derivatives of leucine, valine, and isoleucine. Accumulation of these substances results from a defect in oxidative decarboxylation of branched-chain keto acids.

Plasma levels of the corresponding amino acids are also elevated because the keto acids are transaminated. In some cases, the branched-chain hydroxyacids, most prominently α-hydroxyisovaleric acid, are also excreted, and a derivative of α-hydroxybutyric acid, the decarboxylation of which is impaired by accumulation of α-keto-β-methylvaleric acid, is responsible for the characteristic odor of the urine and sweat.

Structural alterations in the brain are similar to, but more severe than, those in phenylketonuria. Also, the cytoarchitecture of the cortex is generally immature with fewer cortical layers and persistence of ectopic foci of neuroblasts.

Manifestations of the untreated condition include opisthotonos, intermittent increase of muscle tone, seizures, and rapid deterioration of all cerebral functions. Some patients have presented with pseudotumor cerebri or with fluctuating ophthalmoplegia. About half the infants develop hypoglycemia.

The condition is diagnosed by the characteristic odor of the patient, and by a positive 2,4-dinitrophenylhydrazine test on the urine. It is confirmed by chromatography of urine for keto acids or of serum for amino acids.

Treatment is based on a commercially available diet that contains restricted amounts of leucine, isoleucine, and valine. For optimal results, dietary management should be initiated during the first few days of life. It is complex and requires frequent quantitative measurement of serum amino acids. A few children maintained on this regimen have achieved some intellectual development, with IQ scores ranging from 55 to 100. As a consequence of dietary therapy, the reduced white matter density demonstrable on CT scan reverts to normal.

Some patients have residual amounts of branched-chain keto-acid-decarboxylase activity in skin fibroblasts and peripheral leukocytes. The clinical picture includes intermittent periods of ataxia, drowsiness, behavior disturbances, and seizures that appear between 6 and 9 months of age. In other

children, there is only mild or moderate mental retardation.

Defects in the Metabolism of Sulfur Amino Acids

Of the several defects in the metabolism of sulfur-containing amino acids, the most common is homocystinuria. This inborn error of methionine metabolism is manifested by multiple thromboembolic episodes, ectopia lentis, and mental retardation. It is transmitted by an autosomal recessive gene. The condition occurs in 1:45,000 newborns; it is second in frequency only to phenylketonuria among metabolic errors responsible for brain damage, and accounts for about 0.02% of inmates of institutions for the retarded in the United States.

In the most common form of homocystinuria, the metabolic defect affects cystathionine synthase, the enzyme that catalyzes the formation of cystathionine from homocysteine and serine. In most homocystinuric subjects, activity of this enzyme is completely absent, but there is some residual activity in some affected families. In the latter group, addition of pyridoxine may stimulate enzyme activity and partially or completely abolish the excretion of homocystine. As a result of the enzymatic block, increased amounts of homocystine, the oxidized derivative of homocysteine, and its precursor, methionine, are found in urine and plasma.

Primary structural alterations are noted in blood vessels of all calibers. In most vessels, there is intimal thickening and fibrosis; in the aorta and its major branches, fraying of elastic fibers may be found. Both arterial and venous thromboses are common in different organs. In the brain, there are usually multiple infarcts of varying age. Dural sinus thrombosis has been recorded. The relationship between the metabolic defect and the predisposition to vascular thrombosis is unclear. Increased platelet turnover, abnormal platelet aggregation, activation of factor XII, and activation of endogenous factor V by homocysteine have all been implicated.

Homocystinuric infants appear normal at birth, and early development is unremarkable until seizures, developmental slowing, or strokes occur between 5 and 9 months of age. Ectopia lentis has been recognized by age 18 months and is invariable in older children. The typical older homocystinuric child's hair is sparse, blond, and brittle. There are multiple erythematous blotches over the skin, particularly across the maxillary areas and cheeks. The gait is shuffling, the limbs and digits are long, and genu valgum is usually present.

In about half, major thromboembolic episodes occur once or more. These include fatal thromboses of the pulmonary artery and vein. Multiple major strokes may result in hemiplegia and, ultimately, in pseudobulbar palsy. Minor and unrecognized cerebral thrombi may be the direct cause of the mental retardation that occurs in more than 50% of homocystinuric patients.

The diagnosis of homocystinuria is suggested by the appearance of the patient and can be confirmed by a positive urinary cyanide-nitroprusside reaction, by the increased urinary excretion of homocystine, and by an elevated plasma methionine level.

Administration of a commercially available low-methionine diet lowers plasma methionine content and eliminates the abnormally high homocystine excretion. Large doses of pyridoxine reduce the homocystine excretion of pyridoxine-responsive patients. Although the biochemical picture can be improved by these means, the variable clinical picture, particularly the thromboembolic episodes and mental retardation, has up to now rendered useless any evidence for clinical benefit.

Heterozygotes for homocystinuria have an increased propensity to peripheral vascular disease and premature cerebrovascular accidents. However, the incidence of myocardial infarcts in this population is no higher than normal.

Four other genetic entities are known to manifest themselves by homocystinuria due to an impaired conversion of homocysteine to methionine, the result of various defects in the conversion of cobalamine to methyl cobalamine, the active cofactor in the methylation of homocysteine to methionine. In three of these, homocystinuria is accompanied by methylmalonic aciduria.

OTHER DEFECTS OF AMINO ACID METABOLISM

There have been numerous reports of a neurologic disorder apparently associated with some abnormality in the amino-acid pattern of serum or urine. The frequency in the general population can be gauged by routine, mass newborn screening, such as the one conducted by Wilcken and associates (Table 78–1). Other screening programs have found similar incidences.

Aside from phenylketonuria, neurologic

complications in some of the more common conditions (such as histidinemia, hyperprolinemia, and cystathioninuria) are considered unrelated to the metabolic defect, and the result of screening mentally retarded individuals. Some of the less uncommon disorders are summarized in Table 78–2.

Disorders of Amino Acid Transport

Renal amino-acid transport is handled by five specific systems that have nonoverlapping substrate preferences. The disorders that result from genetic defects in each of these systems are listed in Table 78–3.

LOWE SYNDROME

Lowe syndrome (oculocerebrorenal syndrome) is a sex-linked recessive disorder characterized clinically by severe mental retardation, delayed physical development, myopathy, and congenital glaucoma or cataract. Biochemically, there is generalized aminoaciduria of the Fanconi type, with renal tubular acidosis and rickets. Neuropathologic examination has disclosed rarefaction of the molecular layer of the cerebral cortex and parenchymal vacuolation. The fundamental biochemical defect is unknown, but is believed to be a defect in membrane transport. The urinary levels of lysine are more elevated than those of the other amino acids, and defective uptake of lysine and arginine by the intestinal mucosa has been demonstrated in two patients.

HARTNUP DISEASE

This rare familial condition is characterized by photosensitive dermatitis, intermittent cerebellar ataxia, mental disturbances, and renal aminoaciduria. The name is that of the family in which the disorder was first detected.

Symptoms are caused by an extensive disturbance in the transport of neutral amino acids. There are four main biochemical abnormalities: renal aminoaciduria, increased excretion of indican, increased excretion of nonhydroxylated indole metabolites, and increased fecal amino acids.

Symptoms usually occur in mildly malnourished children. When present, they are intermittent and variable, tending to improve with age. They include a red, scaly rash on the exposed areas of the body (resembling the dermatitis of pellagra), intermittent personality disorders, migraine-like headaches, photophobia, and bouts of cerebellar ataxia.

Table 78–3. Defects in Amino Acid Transport

Transport System	Condition	Biochemical Features	Clinical Features
Basic amino acids	Cystinuria (three types)	Impaired renal clearance, defective intestinal transport of lysine, arginine, ornithine, and cystine	Renal stones, no neurologic disease. Increased prevalence in subjects with mental disease
	Lowe syndrome	Impaired intestinal transport of lysine and arginine, impaired tubular transport of lysine	Severe mental retardation, glaucoma, cataracts, myopathy, sex-linked transmission
Acidic amino acids	Dicarboxylic aminoaciduria	Increased excretion of glutamic, aspartic acids	Harmless variant
Neutral amino acids	Hartnup disease	Defective intestinal and renal tubular transport of tryptophan and other neutral amino acids	Intermittent cerebellar ataxia, photosensitive rash
Proline, hydroxyproline, glycine	Iminoglycinuria	Impaired tubular transport of proline, hydroxyproline, and glycine	Harmless variant
β-amino acids	None known	Excretion of β-aminoisobutyric acid and taurine in β-alaninemia is increased due to competition at the tubular level	

The similarity of Hartnup disease to pellagra has prompted treatment with nicotinic acid. However, the tendency for symptoms to remit spontaneously and for general improvement to occur with improved dietary intake and advancing age makes such therapy difficult to evaluate.

References

Phenylketonuria

DiLella AG, Huang WM, Woo SLC: Screening for phenylketonuria mutations by DNA amplification with the polymerase chain reaction. Lancet 1988; 1:497–499.

Güttler F, Ledley FD, Lidsky AS: Correlation between polymorphic DNA haplotypes at phenylalanine hydroxylase locus and clinical phenotypes of phenylketonuria. J Pediatr 1987; 110:68–71.

Holtzman NA, Kronmal RA, van Doorninck W, Azen C, Koch R. Effect of age at loss of dietary control of intellectual performance and behavior of children with phenylketonuria. N Engl J Med 1986; 314:593–598.

Kaufman S, Kaufman S, Kapatos G, Rizzo WB, et al. Tetrahydropterin therapy for hyperphenylalaninemia caused by defective synthesis of tetrahydrobiopterin. Ann Neurol 1983; 14:308–315.

Koch R, Friedman EG. Accuracy of newborn screening programs for phenylketonuria. J Pediatr 1981; 98:267–268.

Ledley FD, Levy HL, and Woo SLC. Molecular analysis of the inheritance of phenylketonuria and mild hyperphenylalaninemia in families with both disorders. N Engl J Med 1986; 314:276–280.

Lenke RR, Levy HL. Maternal phenylketonuria and hyperphenylalaninemia. N Engl J Med 1980; 302:1202–1208.

Lidsky AS, Ledley FD, DiLella AG, et al. Extensive restriction site polymorphisms at the human phenylalanine hydroxylase locus and application in prenatal diagnosis of phenylketonuria. Am J Hum Genet 1985; 37:19–34.

Malamud N. Neuropathology of phenylketonuria. J Neuropathol Exp Neurol 1966; 25:254–268.

Partington MW. The early symptoms of phenylketonuria. Pediatrics 1961; 27:465–473.

Schneider AJ. Newborn phenylalanine tyrosine metabolism. Implications for screening for phenylketonuria. Am J Dis Child 1983; 137:427–432.

Smith I, Leeming RJ, Cavanagh NPC, Hyland K. Neurologic aspects of biopterin metabolism. Arch Dis Child 1986; 61:130–137.

Waisbren SE, Mahon BE, Schnell RR, et al.: Predictors of intelligence quotient and intelligence quotient change in persons treated for phenylketonuria early in life. Pediatrics 1987; 79:351–355.

Wilcken B, Smith A, Brown DA. Urine screening for amino-acidopathies: Is it beneficial? J Pediatr 1980; 97:492–497.

Maple Syrup Urine Disease

Dancis J, Hutzler J, Cox RP. Enzyme defect in skin fibroblasts in intermittent branched-chain ketonuria and in maple syrup urine disease. Biochem Med 1969; 2:407–411.

Haymond MW, Karl IE, Feigin RD. Hypoglycemia and maple syrup urine disease: Defective gluconeogenesis. Pediatr Res 1973; 7:500–508.

Mantovani JF, Naidich TP, Prensky AL, Dodson WE, Williams JC. MSUD: Presentation with pseudotumor cerebri and CT abnormalities. J Pediatr 1980; 96:279–281.

Menkes JH. Maple syrup disease: Isolation and identification of organic acids in the urine. Pediatrics 1959; 23:348–353.

Menkes JH, Hurst PL, Craig JM. A new syndrome: Progressive familial infantile cerebral dysfunction associated with unusual urinary substance. Pediatrics 1954; 14:462–466.

Yoshida II, Sweetman L, Nyhan WL. Metabolism of branched-chain amino acids in fibroblasts from patients with maple syrup urine disease and other abnormalities of branched-chain ketoacid dehydrogenase activity. Pediatr Res 1986; 20:169–174.

Defects in the Metabolism of Sulfur Amino Acids

Boers GHJ. Heterozygosity for homocystinuria in premature peripheral and cerebral occlusive arterial disease. N Engl J Med 1985; 313:709–715.

Mitchell GA, Watkins D, Melancon SB, et al. Clinical heterogeneity in cobalamin C variant of combined homocystinuria and methylmalonic aciduria. J Pediatr 1986; 108:410–415.

Mudd SH, Levy HC. Disorders of transsulfuration. In: Stanbury JB, Wyngaarden JB, Fredrickson DS, Goldstein JL, Brown MS, eds. The Metabolic Basis of Inherited Disease, 5th ed. New York: McGraw-Hill, 1983:522–559.

Rodgers GM, Kane WH. Activation of endogenous factor V by a homocysteine-induced vascular endothelial cell activator. J Clin Invest 1986; 77:1909–1916.

Schimke RN, McKusick VA, Huang T. Homocystinuria: Studies of 20 families with 38 affected members. JAMA 1965; 193:711–719.

Disorders of Amino Acid Transport

Lowe Syndrome

Charnas L, Bernar J, Pezeshkpour GH, et al. MRI findings and peripheral neuropathy in Lowe's Syndrome. Neuropediatrics 1988; 19:7–9.

Chutorian A, Rowland LP. Lowe's syndrome. Neurology 1966; 16:115–122.

Hodgson SV, Heckmatt JZ, Hughes E, et al. A balanced de novo X/autosome translocation in a girl with manifestations of Lowe syndrome. Am J Med Genet 1986; 23:837–847.

Kornfeld M, Synder RD, MacGee J, Appenzeller O. The oculo-cerebral-renal syndrome of Lowe. Arch Neurol 1975; 32:103–107.

Lowe CU, Terrey M, MacLachlan EA. Organic aciduria, decreased renal ammonia production, hydrophthalmos, and mental retardation. Am J Dis Child 1952; 83:164–184.

Martin MA, Sylvester PE. Clinico-pathological studies of oculo-cerebral-renal syndrome of Lowe, Terrey and MacLachlan. J Ment Defic Res 1980; 24:1–16.

Menkes JH. Textbook of Child Neurology, 3rd ed. Philadelphia: Lea & Febiger, 1985: 1–122.

Tripathi RC, Cibis GW, Harris DJ, Tripathi B. Lowe's syndrome. Birth Defects 1982; 18:629–644.

Hartnup Disease

Baron DN. Hereditary pellagra-like skin rash with temporary cerebellar ataxia, constant renal amino-aciduria, and other bizarre chemical features. Lancet 1956; 2:421–428.

Jepson JB. Hartnup disease. In: Stanbury JB, Wyngaarden JB, Fredrickson DS, eds. The Metabolic Basis of Inherited Disease, 4th ed. New York: McGraw-Hill, 1978:1563–1577.

Tahmousch AJ, Alpers DH, Feigen RD, Armbrustmacher V, Prensky AL. Hartnup disease. Arch Neurol 1976; 33:797–807.

Wilcken B, Yu JS, Brown DA. Natural history of Hartnup disease. Arch Dis Child 1977; 52:38–40.

79. DISORDERS OF PURINE METABOLISM

Harry H. White
Lewis P. Rowland

Lesch-Nyhan Syndrome

In 1964, Lesch and Nyhan described two brothers with hyperuricemia, mental retardation, choreoathetosis, and self-destructive biting of the lips and fingers. All known cases have affected boys; the trait is inherited as an X-linked recessive trait and the gene has been localized to the long arm of the X-chromosome. The basic defect is lack of hypoxanthine-guanine phosphoribosyltransferase (HPRT) in all body fluids. The gene was one of the first human genes to be cloned. Because of the enzyme deficiency, the rate of purine biosynthesis is increased and the content of the end product of purine metabolism, uric acid, reaches high values in blood, urine, and CSF. Deposits of urate are found in the kidneys and joints and may result in debilitating nephropathy and gout.

The neurologic manifestations include severe mental retardation, spasticity, and choreoathetosis that start in the first year of life. The characteristic self-mutilating behavior appears in the second year. Death is usually due to renal failure and may occur in the second or third decade of life. The pathogenesis of the cerebral symptoms is not known. Although low levels of dopamine metabolites have been found in postmortem samples of tissue from the basal ganglia, it is not known how these abnormalities lead to the symptoms or how they relate to the enzyme disorder.

Diagnosis depends on recognition of the clinical manifestations and can be made precisely by biochemical assay of the enzyme in erythrocyte hemolysates or cultured fibroblasts. Hair root analysis of HPRT has become a convenient way to analyze activity. Prenatal enzymatic diagnosis is possible in the first trimester with chorionic villus sampling. DNA haplotype analysis can be used for prenatal diagnosis and carrier detection but not to determine individual cases because only some 20% show deletions with available DNA probes.

Treatment is not satisfactory. Gout can be treated with allopurinol but the neurologic disorder is daunting. Restraints may be needed to prevent the child from damaging himself or others; sometimes teeth must be removed. Enzyme replacement therapy with long-term erythrocyte transfusions in three patients gave only modest improvement of the neurologic symptoms, and drug therapy to modify dopamine metabolism has not yet been effective. Gene therapy is being evaluated in animals, because the human gene has been introduced into transgenic mice and enzyme activity is expressed in the brain of the recipient animals.

There is evidence of both clinical and biochemical heterogeneity. Hyperuricemia and cerebellar ataxia have been noted in individuals with normal HPRT activity. Patients with partial enzyme deficiency may have gout without neurologic symptoms, or there may be varying severity of mental retardation, movement disorders, spastic tetraplegia, or seizures. The self-mutilating behavior may be restricted to the classic form, which lacks all enzyme activity.

Neurologic abnormalities are also seen in patients without other enzymes of purine nucleoside metabolism. Adenosine deaminase (ADA) deficiency causes severe combined immunodeficiency in infants; some patients have extrapyramidal or pyramidal signs and psychomotor development and may be retarded. Partial exchange transfusion may be clinically beneficial. Also, a few patients lacking purine nucleoside phosphorylase (PNP), with impaired cellular immunity, may show neurologic abnormality.

References

Baumeister AA, Frye GD. The biochemical basis of the behavioral disorder in Lesch-Nyhan syndrome. Neurosci Biobehav Rev 1985; 9:169–178.

Coleman MS, Danton MJ, Philips A. Adenosine deaminase and immune dysfunction. Ann NY Acad Sci 1985; 451:54–65.

Edwards NL. Immunodeficiencies associated with errors in purine metabolism. Med Clin North Am 1985; 69:505–518.

Edwards NL, Fox IH. Disorders associated with purine and pyrimidine metabolism. Spec Top Endocrinol Metab 1984; 6:95–140.

Edwards NL, Jeryc W, Fox IH. Enzyme replacement in the Lesch-Nyhan syndrome with long-term erythrocyte transfusions. Adv Exp Med Biol 1984; 165:23–26.

Gibbs DA, McFadyen IR, Crawford MDA, DeMuinck Keizer EE, et al. First-trimester diagnosis of Lesch-Nyhan syndrome. Lancet 1984; 2:1180–1183.

Gibbs RA, Caskey CT. Identification and localization of mutations at the Lesch-Nyhan locus by ribonuclease A cleavage. Science 1987; 236:303–305.

Hirschhorn R. Complete and partial adenosine deaminase deficiency. Ann NY Acad Sci 1985; 451:20–25.

Hirschhorn R, Ellenbogen A. Genetic heterogeneity in adenosine deaminase (ADA) deficiency: Five different mutations in five new patients with partial ADA deficiency. Am J Hum Genet 1986; 38:13–25.

Jankovic J, Caskey TC, Stout JT, Butler IJ. Lesch-Nyhan syndrome: motor behavior and CSF neurotransmitters. Ann Neurol 1988; 23:466–468.

Kelley WM, Wyngaarden JB. Clinical syndromes associated with hypoxanthineguanine deficiency. In: Stanbury JB, Wyngaarden JB, Fredrickson DS, Goldstein JL, Brown MS, eds. The Metabolic Basis of Inherited Disease, 5th ed. New York; McGraw-Hill, 1983:1115–1143.

Kuehn MR, Bradley A, Robertson EJ, Evans MJ. A potential animal model for Lesch-Nyhan syndrome through introduction of HPRT mutations into mice. Nature 1987; 326:295–298.

Monk M, Handyside A, Hardy K, Whittingham D. Preimplantation diagnosis of deficiency of hypoxanthine phosphoribosyl transferase in a mouse model for Lesch-Nyhan syndrome. Lancet 1987; 2:423–425.

Nelson DL, Chang SM, Henkel-Tigges J, et al. Gene replacement therapy for inborn errors of purine metabolism. Cold Spring Harbor Symp Quant Biol 1986; 51:1065–1071.

Nyhan WL, Parkman R, Page T, et al. Bone marrow transplantation in Lesch-Nyhan disease. Adv Exp Med Biol 1986; 195:167–170.

Shapira J, Ziberman Y, Becker A. Lesch-Nyhan syndrome: A nonextracting approach to prevent mutilation. Spec Care Dentist 1985; 5:210–212.

Silverstein FS, Johnson MV, Hutchinson RJ, Edwards NL. Lesch-Nyhan syndrome: CSF neurotransmitter abnormalities. Neurology 1985; 35:907–911.

Stout JT, Caskey CT. HPRT: Gene structure, expression and mutation. Ann Rev Genet 1985; 19:127–148.

Stout JT, Chen HY, Brennand J, Caskey CT, Brinster RL. Expression of human HPRT in the central nervous system of transgenic mice. Nature 1985; 317:250–251.

Stout JT, Jackson LG, Caskey CT. First trimester diagnosis of Lesch-Nyhan syndrome: Applications to other disorders of purine metabolism. Prenat Diagn 1985; 5:183–189.

Watson AR, Simmonds HA, Webster DR, Layward L, Evans DIK. Purine nucleoside phosphorylase (PNP) deficiency: A therapeutic challenge. Adv Exp Med Biol 1984; 165:53–59.

Watts RWE, Spellacy E, Gibbs DA, Allsop J, et al. Clinical, postmortem, biochemical and therapeutic observations on the Lesch-Nyhan syndrome with particular reference to the neurologic manifestations. Q J Med 1982; 201:43–78.

Wilson JM, Kelley WN. Molecular genetics of hypoxanthine-guanine phosphoribosyltransferase deficiency in man. Arch Intern Med 1985; 145:1895–1900.

Wilson JM, Stout JT, Palella TD, Davidson BL, et al. A molecular survey of hypoxanthine-guanine phosphoribosyltransferase deficiency in man. J Clin Invest 1986; 77:188–195.

80. LYSOSOMAL DISEASES AND OTHER STORAGE DISEASES
William G. Johnson

In some diseases, storage material accumulates inside cells because of a genetically determined deficiency of a catabolic enzyme. Although these diseases are individually rare, they are not uncommon in the aggregate. They often appear in the differential diagnosis of patients seen by the neurologist. In most of these conditions, a lysosomal enzyme is deficient and the storage occurs in lysosomes. The stored material is usually of a complex lipid or saccharide nature; the nervous system is usually affected. The inheritance pattern is recessive, usually autosomal but occasionally X-linked. Carrier detection and prenatal diagnosis have been accomplished in most of these disorders, but there is as yet no specific treatment for any of the lysosomal storage diseases. Dietary therapy is effective for Refsum disease. Kidney transplant corrects the renal dysfunction in Fabry disease. Bile acid therapy decreases cholestanol production in cerebrotendinous xanthomatosis and may prove to be effective for therapy. Enzyme-infusion therapy is being tried experimentally for adult Gaucher disease and Fabry disease in which the nervous system is unaffected. Osmotic opening of the blood-brain barrier is being explored to deliver infused enzyme to the nervous system. Bone marrow transplantation is being tried experimentally for the mucopolysaccharidoses.

The Lipidoses

Storage disorders involve all three major lipid classes: neutral lipids (i.e., cholesterol ester, fatty acid, and triglycerides), polar lipids (glycolipids and phospholipids), and very polar lipids (gangliosides). The largest group of stored lipids is the sphingolipids, based on sphingosine (Fig. 80–1A). When a long chain fatty acid is attached to the 2-amino group of sphingosine, the resulting compounds are called ceramides. Further hydrophilic residues are attached at the 1-hydroxyl group to give the sphingolipids (Fig. 80–1B–E).

GM$_2$-GANGLIOSIDOSES

Hexosaminidase-deficiency diseases result from a genetically determined deficiency of the enzyme hexosaminidase (reaction 3, Figs. 80–1B and C, 80–2, and 80–3), which causes accumulation in cells (especially in neurons) of GM$_2$-ganglioside, certain other glycosphingolipids, and other compounds containing a terminal β-linked, N-acetylgalactosaminide or N-acetylglucosaminide moiety.

For full activity, hexosaminidase requires at least two different subunits, α and β, which are specified by gene loci on chromosomes 15

and 5, respectively. At least three isozymes of hexosaminidase have a defined subunit structure: hexosaminidase A (α β)$_n$; hexosaminidase B (β β)$_n$; and hexosaminidase S (α α)$_n$. Hexosaminidase A is required for cleavage of GM$_2$-ganglioside, but the true substrate may be the ganglioside bound to a heat-stable protein activator. Deficiency of the protein activator also causes a GM$_2$-gangliosidosis (the so-called AB variant). The GM$_2$-gangliosidoses are classified according to the phenotype, the genetic locus, and the allele involved.

Progressive infantile encephalopathy was the most common clinical presentation in the past. The success of carrier screening among couples of Ashkenazi Jewish background dramatically reduced the incidence of this condition, and later-onset variants are now seen more commonly. Hexosaminidase deficiencies present with a variety of phenotypes (Table 80–1) from infancy to adulthood. This diagnosis can reasonably be suspected with nearly any degenerative neurologic disorder except demyelinating neuropathy or myopathy. Sensory dysfunction, ocular palsies, neurogenic bladder, or extraneural involvement are not prominent features.

The diagnosis is made by measuring the amount of hexosaminidase in blood serum and leukocytes. Hexosaminidase determination in cultured skin fibroblasts of the patient and of the patient's family members is advised both to detect additional carriers and to document a genetic compound. Rectal biopsy for electron microscopy of neurons is useful to confirm the diagnosis in variant phenotypes.

Infantile Encephalopathy with Cherry-Red Spots. Three biochemical disorders in this group are well known: classic infantile *Tay-Sachs* disease (homozygous for the HEXα^2- allele), infantile *Sandhoff disease* (homozygous for the HEXβ^2 allele), and the so-called AB variant (deficiency of the HEX A activator protein). The HEXα^2 allele occurs with high frequency among persons of Ashkenazi background (1 in 30 compared with 1 in 300 for the general population), accounting for the ethnic concentration of classic Tay-Sachs disease and genetic compounds containing the HEXα^2 allele.

In all three conditions, the infants appear normal until 4 to 6 months of age. They learn to smile and reach for objects, but do not sit or crawl. A myoclonic jerk reaction to sound (so-called hyperacusis) and the macular

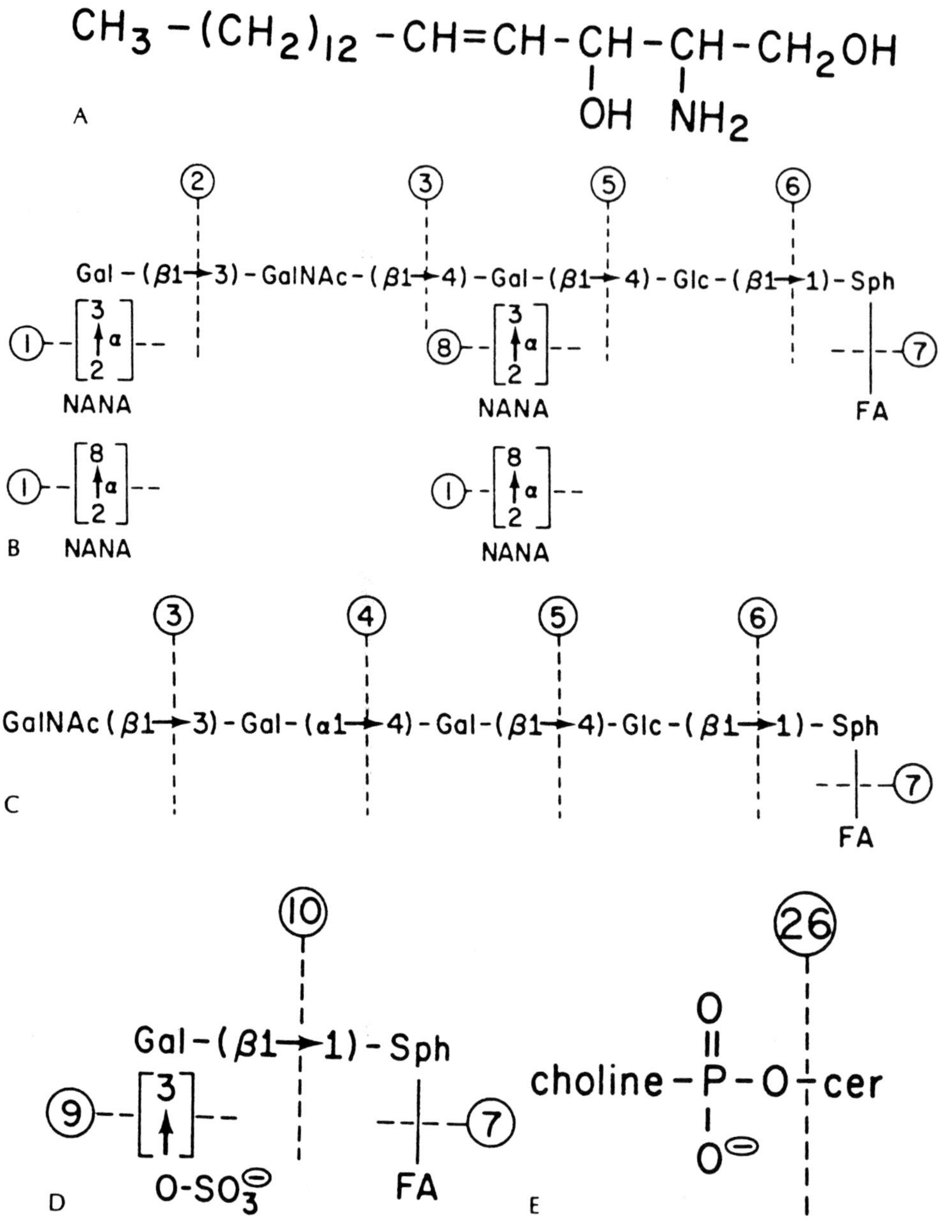

$$CH_3-(CH_2)_{12}-CH=CH-CH-CH-CH_2OH$$

with OH and NH_2 substituents

A

B

C

D

E

Fig. 80–1. *A.* Sphingosine. Addition of fatty acid in amide linkage gives ceramide (Cer). *B.* Structure of a ganglioside (here, a tetrasialoganglioside, GQ_{1a}) containing sphingosine (Sph), fatty acid (FA), neutral hexoses (glucose = Glc, galactose = Gal), hexosamine (GalNAc = N-acetylgalactosamine, and sialic acid (NANA = N-acetylneuraminic acid). *C.* Structure of a glycolipid, globoside (GL-4), containing sphingosine, fatty acid, neutral hexoses and hexosamine. *D.* Structure of sulfatide (a major glycolipid of myelin) containing sphingosine, fatty acid, and galactose, which is sulfated on the 3-hydroxyl group. *E.* Structure of sphingomyelin or ceramide phosphorylcholine.
1. Sialidase (sialidoses). 2. Beta-galactosidase (GM_1-gangliosidoses, Morquio syndrome type B, secondarily deficient in galactosialidosis). 3. Hexosaminidase (GM_2-gangliosidoses). 4. Alpha-galactosidase (Fabry disease). 5. Ceramide lactosidase. 6. Beta-glucosidase (Gaucher disease). 7. Ceramidase (Farber disease). 8. Ganglioside sialidase (?mucolipidosis IV). 9. Sulfatase A (Metachromatic leukodystrophy, mucosulfatidosis, MSD). 10. Galactocerebrosidase (Krabbe disease). 11. Alpha-L-iduronidase (Hurler syndrome, Scheie syndrome, Hurler-Scheie compound). 12. Iduronate-2-sulfate sulfatase (Hunter syndrome, MSD). 13. Sulfamidase (Sanfilippo A, MSD). 14. Alpha-N-acetylglucosaminidase (Sanfilippo B). 15. N-acetyl transferase (Sanfilippo C). 16. Galactose-6-sulfate sulfatase or N-acetylgalactosamine-6-sulfate sulfatase (Morquio syndrome type A, MSD). 17. N-acetylgalactosamine-4-sulfate sulfatase or sulfatase B (Maroteaux-Lamy syndrome, MSD). 18. Beta-glucuronidase (Sly syndrome). 19. N-acetylglucosamine-6-sulfate sulfatase (DiFerrante syndrome, MSD). 20. Dermatan sulfate N-acetylgalactosamine-6-sulfate sulfatase. 21. Alpha-L-fucosidase (fucosidosis). 22. Alpha-mannosidase (mannosidosis). 23. Beta-mannosidase (caprine and human beta-mannosidosis). 24. Endoglucosaminidase. 25. Aspartylglucosaminidase (aspartylglucosaminuria). 26. Sphingomyelinase (Niemann-Pick disease, types A, B, and F).

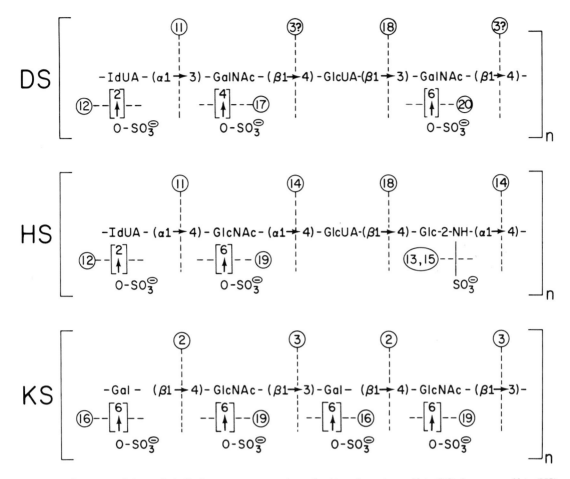

Fig. 80–2. Structure of three clinically important mucopolysaccharides: dermatan sulfate (DS), heparan sulfate (HS), and keratan sulfate (KS). Each consists of repeating dimers of uronic acid (IdUA = iduronic acid, GlcUA = glucuronic acid), hexosamine (GlcNAc = N-acetylglucosamine, GalNAc = N-acetylgalactosamine), and sulfate (O-SO$_3$). In DS, the hexosamine is GalNAc. In HS, the hexosamine is α-linked glucosamine, sometimes N-acetylated, sometimes N-sulfated. In KS, uronic acid is replaced by galactose (Gal). The glycan portion is bound to protein (not shown).

cherry-red spot (Fig. 80–4) are constant findings. The infants become floppy and weak but have hyperactive reflexes, clonus, and extensor plantar responses. Visual deterioration, apathy, and loss of developmental milestones lead to a vegetative state by the second year. Seizures and myoclonus are prominent for the first 2 years. The infants eventually become decorticate. They need tube feeding, have difficulty with secretions, and are blind. Head circumference enlarges progressively to about the 90th percentile from 1 to 3 years, and then stabilizes. Death is due to intercurrent infection, usually pneumonia. The disease is confined to the nervous system.

By light microscopy, grossly ballooned neurons (Fig. 80–5) are found throughout the brain, cerebellum, and spinal cord. The cytoplasm is filled with pale homogeneous-appearing material that pushes the nucleus and

Nissl substrate to a corner of the cell. By electron microscopy, membranous cytoplasmic bodies (MCBs—distended lysosomes) are seen with regularly spaced concentric dark and pale lamellae.

GM$_2$-ganglioside (see Fig. 80–1B) content is markedly increased in the brain and, to a much lesser degree, in the viscera. Other glycosphingolipids with a terminal β-linked N-acetylgalactosamine moiety, such as asialo-GM$_2$ (see Fig. 80–1B) and globoside (see Fig. 80–1C) accumulate to a lesser degree. The storage results from deficiency of hexosaminidase (reaction 3).

In classic Tay-Sachs disease, hexosaminidase A (α β)$_n$ and hexosaminidase S (α α)$_n$ are absent. Hexosaminidase B (β β)$_n$ is present in normal or increased amounts. These findings implicate the α subunit of hexosaminidase as the site of the abnormality. It is likely that the

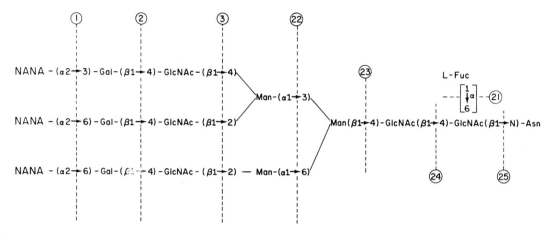

Fig. 80–3. Structure of an asparagine-linked glycoprotein consisting of asparagine (Asn), neutral sugars (Man = mannose, Gal = galactose, L-Fuc = L-fucose), hexosamine (GlcNAc = N-acetylglucosamine), and sialic acid (NANA = N-acetylneuraminic acid). The mannose-6-phosphate recognition marker is formed by transfer of GlcNAc-1-P to the 6-hydroxyl groups of the alpha-linked mannose residues and subsequent removal of the phosphate-linked GlcNAc residues.

primary abnormality is a mutation at the hexosaminidase α locus on chromosome 15. Heterozygous carriers have a partial decrease of hexosaminidase A.

In infantile Sandhoff disease, hexosaminidase A and B are deficient. Hexosaminidase S, normally barely detectable, is increased to about 5% of the normal total hexosaminidase level. This implicates the hexosaminidase β subunit and the β locus on chromosome 5. Cross-reacting material has been found. Carriers have partially decreased hexosaminidase, the B isoenzyme being decreased more than the A isoenzyme.

In one form of the AB variant, a hexosaminidase A activating protein is missing. Although levels of hexosaminidase A and B are decreased, GM₂-ganglioside cannot be cleaved. Diagnosis requires use of the radiolabelled natural substrate, GM₂-ganglioside or direct testing for the activator. In a second form of the AB variant, the residual hexosaminidase A cleaves artificial but not sulfated artificial or natural substrate. Although this is detected as an AB variant, it in fact results from an α-locus disorder rather than an activator-locus disorder.

In a case clinically similar to infantile Tay-Sachs disease, there was subtotal hexosaminidase A deficiency when the assay was done with an artificial substrate, but with radiolabelled GM₂-ganglioside natural substrate, hexosaminidase was totally absent. The patient appeared to have a genetic compound of two abnormal alpha-locus alleles, HEXα², and HEXα⁴. It is important to identify such

cases because conventional methods of prenatal diagnosis using artificial substrates may fail in such families. Alternate methods such a natural substrate assay or assay with sulfated artificial substrate may be used.

Late Infantile, Juvenile, and Adult GM₂-Gangliosidoses. These are present with dementia and ataxia with or without macular cherry-red spot. Spasticity, muscle wasting due to anterior horn cell disease, and seizures are frequently seen. Hexosaminidase A deficiency or hexosaminidase A and B deficiency are found on biochemical study of serum, leukocytes, and cultured skin fibroblasts.

Other late-onset forms of GM₂-gangliosidosis present as cerebellar ataxia or spinocerebellar ataxia, resembling Ramsay-Hunt dyssynergia cerebellaris progressiva, Menzel ataxia, Friedreich ataxia, Holmes ataxia, or atypical spinocerebellar ataxias. Hexosaminidase A or hexosaminidase A and B deficiency are found on biochemical study.

Motor neuron disease may be the presenting feature of late-onset GM₂-gangliosidoses. Lower motor neuron disease may resemble Kugelberg-Welander or Aran-Duchenne syndrome. Upper motor neuron disease may be present, giving an amyotrophic lateral sclerosis-like phenotype. Thus far, only hexosaminidase A deficiency has been found with this clinical presentation.

Many, perhaps most, of these late-onset cases are genetic compounds. Rectal biopsy for electron microscopy of autonomic neurons and natural substrate hexosaminidase assays are recommended for diagnosis of these late-

Table 80–1. Clinical Presentation of Hexosaminidase Deficiencies

Clinical Presentation	Disorder	Abnormal HEX allele number*	Clinical Features
Infantile Encephalopathy			
α-Locus	Classic infantile Tay-Sachs disease	(α^2,α^2)	Onset of dementia at about 6 months, visual loss, myoclonic seizures, and macular cherry-red spot; progressive loss of milestones to vegetative state; death by 6th year.
	Tay-Sachs disease (genetic compound) with residual HEX A	(α^2,α^4)	
β-Locus	Sandhoff disease	(β^2,β^2)	
	Sandhoff disease (genetic compound)	—	
Activator-locus	AB-variant		
Late-infantile or Juvenile Encephalopathy			
α-Locus	Juvenile Tay-Sachs disease	(α^3,α^3)	Onset at 1–4 years of dementia, seizures and ataxia with or without macular cherry-red spot; progressive deterioration may be slow or rapid.
	Juvenile Tay-Sachs disease (genetic compound)	(α^2,α^7)	Similar to above
β-Locus	Juvenile Sandhoff disease	—	Static or progressive mental defect with spasticity, ataxia, and seizures.
Activator-locus	—	—	—
Cerebellar Ataxia			
α-Locus	Atypical spinocerebellar ataxia	—	Onset at 4–12 years of slowly progressive limb and gait ataxia, with or without mental defect, spasticity, or muscle wasting; dystonic postures and psychosis may occur.
β-Locus	Juvenile cerebellar ataxia	—	Onset at 3–5 years of slowly progressive cerebellar-outflow tremor; resembles dyssynergia cerebellaris progressiva of Ramsey Hunt.
	Adult-onset cerebellar ataxia	—	Onset in late adolescence or young adulthood of progressive cerebellar syndrome.
Activator-locus	—	—	—
Motor-Neuron Disease			
α-Locus	Juvenile spinal muscular atrophy (genetic compound)	(α^2,α^7)	Resembles adolescent-onset Kugelberg-Welander phenotype.
	Adult spinal muscular atrophy	—	Resembles adult-onset Aran-Duchenne phenotype.
	ALS phenocopy	—	Early adult onset upper and lower motor neuron disease.
β-Locus	Juvenile spinal muscular atrophy	—	Resembles childhood onset Kugelberg-Welander phenotype.
Activator-locus	—	—	—
Adult-Onset Encephalopathy			
α-Locus	—	—	—
β-Locus	—	—	—
Activator-locus	Adult GM$_2$-gangliosidosis	—	Early adult dementia, seizures, and normal pressure hydrocephalus (incompletely studied).
Asymptomatic or Presymptomatic Adults			
α-Locus	"Total" HEX A deficiency	(α^2,α^5)	Asymptomatic (? presymptomatic)
	"Near total" HEX A deficiency	(α^2,α^6)	Presymptomatic
β-Locus	HEX A and B deficiency		Asymptomatic
Activator-locus	—	—	—

*Allele numbering according to system proposed by JS O'Brien. suggestions for a nomenclature for the GM$_2$-gangliosidoses making certain assumptions. (From O'Brien JS. Am J Hum Genet 1978; 30:672–675.)

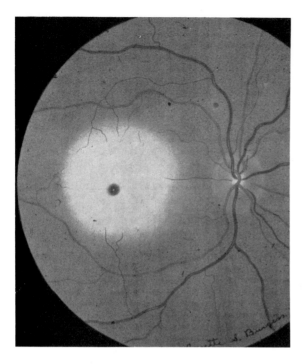

Fig. 80–4. Macular cherry-red spot in Tay-Sachs disease. (Courtesy of Dr. Arnold Gold.)

onset phenotypes because some asymptomatic (or presymptomatic) adults, usually relatives of GM_2-gangliosidosis patients, have severe hexosaminidase A or hexosaminidase A and B deficiency.

GM_1-GANGLIOSIDOSIS

This group of disorders is characterized by deficiency of GM_1-ganglioside β-galactosidase (see reaction 2, Figs. 80–1B and C, 80–2,

80–3) and storage of compounds that contain a terminal beta-linked galactose moiety. These include GM_1-ganglioside, asialo-GM_1, keratan sulfate-like oligosaccharides, and glycoproteins. Other β-galactosidases, such as those that cleave galactosylceramide (see reaction 10, Fig. 80–1D) and lactosylceramide (see reaction 5, Fig. 80–1B and C) are not deficient and those compounds do not accumulate. The enzyme GM_1-ganglioside β-galactosidase is believed to consist of only one kind of subunit and therefore is coded by a single gene locus. There are at least three forms of deficiency of this enzyme: (1) primary deficiency of β-galactosidase, causing infantile and late-infantile GM_1-gangliosidosis and an adult form; (2) combined neuraminidase and β-galactosidase deficiency, galactopialidosis; and (3) combined deficiency of β-galactosidase and several other lysosomal enzymes in I-cell disease, mucolipidosis II. The latter two types are discussed under mucolipidosis.

Infantile GM_1-Gangliosidosis. Infantile GM_1-gangliosidosis is earlier in onset, more severe, and more rapidly progressive than infantile Tay-Sachs disease. Soon after birth, these infants become hypotonic, with poor sucking ability and slow weight gain. Their faces have frontal bossing, coarsened features, large low-set ears, and elongated philtrum. Gum hypertrophy, macroglossia, peripheral edema, and often faint corneal haze are noted. Strabismus and nystagmus may be seen. About half the patients develop macular cherry-red spot (see Fig. 80–4). Development is slow and they do not sit or crawl. By age 6 months, liver and spleen are enlarged; joint

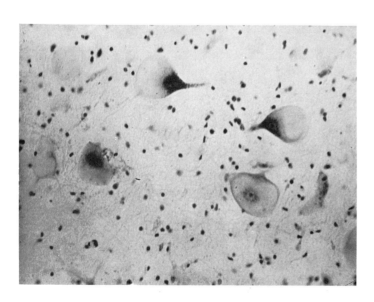

Fig. 80–5. Ballooned spinal cord ventral horn cells in Tay-Sachs disease. (Courtesy of Dr. Abner Wolf.)

stiffness and claw-hand deformities may be seen, and the skin is coarse and thickened. Seizures may develop. The infants enter a vegetative state and die before age 2 of pneumonia or cardiac arrhythmias.

Bone radiographs after 6 to 12 months show changes similar to those of Hurler syndrome, with anterior beaking of vertebral bodies and J-shaped sella turcica. Lymphocytes from peripheral smear are vacuolated and histiocytes in the bone marrow are foamy.

Diagnosis is made by the characteristic oligosaccharide pattern in urine, assay of GM_1-ganglioside β-galactosidase (see reaction 2, Fig. 80–2) in blood leukocytes or cultured skin fibroblasts, and demonstration of partially decreased enzyme levels in the obligate carrier parents. It is important to exclude sialidosis and to be prepared for prenatal diagnosis.

Late Infantile GM_1-Gangliosidosis. This is probably an allelic variant of the infantile disorder because genetic complementation between them does not occur in fibroblast culture. Onset is usually between 1 and 3 years with gait ataxia, hypotonia, hyperreflexia, dysarthria, and speech regression. Seizures, dementia, and spastic quadriplegia lead to death, usually by pneumonia. Optic atrophy and evidence of anterior horn cell disease may be found. Corneas are clear, organomegaly is absent, and bony changes are scanty. Diagnosis is made in the same manner as for the infantile form.

FABRY DISEASE

Angiokeratoma corporis diffusum is an X-linked disorder affecting the skin, kidney, peripheral and autonomic nervous systems, and blood vessels with storage of trihexosyl-ceramide, galactosyl-galactosyl-glucosyl-ceramide, a break-down product of globoside (see Fig. 80–1C). Trihexosylceramide accumulates because of a deficency of trihexosylceramide α-galactosidase (see reaction 4, Fig. 80–1C), also known as *alpha-galactosidase A.* Fabry disease is the only sphingolipidosis that is X-linked. It is incompletely recessive; that is, some female heterozygotes are clinically affected.

Symptoms usually begin in childhood or adolescence, with lancinating pains in the limbs, especially the feet and hands, often brought on by temperature changes, and accompanied by paresthesia or abdominal crises. Anhydrosis and unexplained fever are common.

The characteristic skin lesions, which become more numerous with age, are purple, macular and maculopapular hyperkeratotic and are 1 to 3 mm in size with a predilection for the groin, buttocks, scrotum, and umbilicus. Glycolipid storage in the renal glomeruli and tubules begins with asymptomatic proteinuria in children; it progresses to renal failure and hypertension in the third or fourth decade. Glycolipid storage in blood-vessel walls may cause stroke. Edema of the limbs, faint haziness of the cornea visible by slit lamp, and myocardial involvement may occur. There is no specific treatment. Renal transplant is lifesaving when renal failure supervenes. The lancinating pains may respond to phenytoin.

Heterozygous females may also be affected, but manifestations are less marked. Skin lesions are few or absent. Corneal opacity is more common. If renal or cardiac involvement occurs, they are later in onset and less severe.

GAUCHER DISEASE

This entity embraces several autosomal recessive sphingolipidoses in which glucocerebroside (see Fig. 80–1B and C) is stored as a result of deficiency of glucocerebroside beta-glucosidase (or glucocerebrosidase, see reaction 6, Fig. 80–1B and C). At least four forms are known (Table 80–2): the infantile neuronopathic form, the juvenile neuronopathic form, the adult neuronopathic form, and the adult non-neuronopathic form. The juvenile form is probably heterogeneous and some cases may be genetic compounds. The severity of the enzyme deficiency correlates well with clinical severity. Patients with infantile neuronopathic Gaucher disease have almost no residual glucocerebrosidase activity; patients with the adult non-neuronopathic form may have one fourth to one third of the control enzyme activity. Carrier detection and prenatal diagnosis are possible. The adult (non-neuropathic) form is more common in persons of Ashkenazi background. Diagnosis of all forms is made by the characteristic clinical picture, finding of Gaucher cells in bone marrow, and by finding reduced glucocerebroside β-glucosidase in cultured skin fibroblasts or blood leukocytes.

Infantile Neuronopathic Gaucher Disease. This disease occurs in the first year of life, often in the first 3 months. The course is rapid with developmental regression and death before age 2 years. Although the spleen and liver enlarge, the infants lose weight. They have stridor, difficulty in sucking and swallowing, strabismus, opisthotonic head retraction, spasticity, and hyperreflexia. Later they enter a vegetative state, becoming flaccid and weak. Seizures may occur. Macular cherry-red spot and optic atrophy do not occur.

Juvenile Neuronopathic Gaucher Disease. This form is characterized by splenomegaly, Gaucher's cells in bone marrow, mental deficiency (retardation or dementia), seizures, incoordination, and tics. Neurologic signs develop in childhood or adolescence. This group is probably heterogeneous.

Adult Gaucher Disease. Characteristics are splenomegaly and bony lesions but not neurologic disorders. It is most common in individuals of Ashkenazi background. Despite the name, the disease may be found even in young children. Although thrombocytopenia may be a problem, splenectomy should be avoided if possible; however, severe and prolonged thrombocytopenia is an indication for splenectomy. Lesions of long bones, pelvis, or vertebral bodies may be painful. Live, skin, lymph nodes and lungs may be involved. Multiple myeloma may be a late complication.

Adult Neuronopathic Gaucher Disease. Although resembling adult-onset Gaucher's disease, symptoms also include seizures and dementia.

NIEMANN-PICK DISEASE

This group of disorders is characterized by lysosomal storage of the glycosphingolipid sphingomyelin (ceramide phosphorylcholine (see Fig. 80–1E). Cholesterol storage is thought to be a secondary phenomenon except in Type C. Several clinical types have been described. Deficiency of a sphingomyelin-cleaving enzyme, sphingomyelinase (see reaction 26, Fig. 80–1E), has been found in Types A, B, and F; deficiency of one sphingomyelinase subfraction has been reported in Type C. Diagnosis is made by the clinical evidence of hepatosplenomegaly, with or without cerebral symptoms, by finding characteristic "mulberry" storage cells (which appear different from Gaucher cells) in bone marrow, and by demonstrating decreased sphingomyelinase activity in cultured skin fibroblasts, leukocytes, or tissue (for Types A, B, and F), or increased sphingomyelin in tissue (for Types C and D).

Infantile Niemann-Pick Disease. This is the most common and most severe form (infantile neuronopathic form, type A) of Niemann-Pick disease and occurs more commonly in individuals of Ashkenazi background. Transient neonatal jaundice is followed by progressive hepatosplenomegaly; developmental regression and weight loss lead to death by age 2. Dementia and hypotonia are noted. About one third of patients develop macular cherry-red spots (see Fig. 80–4). Seizures are uncommon. Bony involvement is mild. Skin often has a brownish-yellow tinge. Most patients have diffuse haziness or patchy infiltrates in the lungs.

Diagnosis is by the characteristic clinical picture, the finding of foam cells in the bone marrow, and by demonstration of nearly total sphingomyelinase (see reaction 26, Fig. 80–1E) deficiency in leukocytes and cultured skin fibroblasts.

Juvenile Non-Neuronopathic, Type B. This form presents with asymptomatic splenomegaly or hepatosplenomegaly without neurologic disorder in infants, children, or adults. Foam cells appear in the bone marrow, and sphingomyelinase (see reaction 26, Fig. 80–1E) is reduced in cultured skin fibroblasts and leukocytes. These patients have more residual sphingomyelinase (15–20% of normal) than those with type A (up to 10%).

Niemann-Pick Disease Type C. Patients are normal in infancy but after 1 to 2 years develop progressive dementia, seizures, spasticity, vertical gaze paresis, and ataxia. Hepatosplenomegaly is less prominent than in other types. Diagnosis is by demonstration of foam cells (sea-blue histiocytes) in bone marrow and the elevation of cholesterol and sphingomyelin (see Fig. 80–1E) in involved tissue (liver, spleen, or lymph node). It is not clear whether sphingomyelinase (see reaction 26, Fig. 80–1E) is deficient in Type-C disease. However, the primary defect may be an abnormality of cholesterol metabolism; cholesterol may be stored in lysosomes because of tardy translocation of cholesterol from lysosomes to endoplasmic reticulum and Golgi. At present, this metabolic abnormality is the most specific method of diagnosis, although its molecular basis remains unknown.

Other types of Niemann-Pick disease have been designated Types D, E, and F. In Type D, found in Yarmouth County Acadians of Nova Scotia, other phospholipids are stored with sphingomyelin, and sphingomyelinase is not deficient. Type-E patients may simply be adult Type-B patients. Type F resembles Type B except that sphingomyelinase is heat-labile in Type F.

FARBER LIPOGRANULOMATOSIS

In the first few months of life, as early as 2 weeks of age, infants with this disease have painful, swollen joints, hoarseness, vomiting, respiratory difficulty, or limb edema. Subcutaneous nodules are found near joints and tendon sheaths, especially on the hands, arms, and at pressure points such as the occiput or lumbosacral spine. Other findings include cardiac enlargement and murmurs, lymphadenopathy, hepatomegaly, splenomegaly, enlarged tongue, difficulty in swallowing, and pulmonary granulomata. Tendon reflexes may be hyper- or hypoactive. Mental development may be normal or impaired. Seizures do not occur. CSF protein may be elevated.

Ceramide (see Fig. 80–1B, C, D, and E) and some related compounds accumulate in foam cells in affected tissues, because of severe diminution of acid ceramidase (see reaction 7, Fig. 80–1B, C, D, and E), an enzyme that catabolizes ceramide to sphingosine and fatty acid. Neutral ceramidase is not decreased. Diagnosis is made by the clinical picture, finding foam cells and elevated ceramide in tissue (for example, a biopsied skin nodule), and deficiency of acid ceramidase in cultured skin fibroblasts or leukocytes. Prenatal diagnosis and carrier testing are possible. Most patients die of pulmonary disease before age 2 years, but some survive into adolescence.

WOLMAN DISEASE

Infants affected by Wolman disease are normal at birth, but in the first few weeks of life have severe vomiting, abdominal distention, diarrhea, poor weight gain, jaundice, and unexplained fever. Hepatosplenomegaly may be massive and there may be a papulovesiculopustular rash on face, neck, shoulders, and chest. The extent of neurologic disorder is not clear, because the infants are so sick and die so early. Initially, they are active and alert, but activity decreases. Corticospinal signs have been found in some. Laboratory findings include anemia and foam cells in bone marrow. A distinctive finding is calcification of the adrenals on radiographic examination. The course is usually rapidly progressive. Death usually occurs within 3 to 6 months, but some survive into the second year. The lipid storage consists primarily of cholesterol ester and smaller amounts of triglyceride because there is severe deficiency of a lysosomal fatty acid ester acid hydrolase (acid lipase, acid esterase, or acid cholesteryl ester hydrolase), which cleaves cholesterol ester, triglycerides, and artificial substrates. Nearly total deficiency of this acid lipase is found in tissues, leukocytes, and cultured fibroblasts from patients; carriers have been detected and prenatal diagnosis is possible.

A milder, probably allelic, form of Wolman disease with deficiency of the same enzyme is called *cholesterol ester storage disease.* These patients have hepatomegaly (with or without splenomegaly), hypercholesterolemia, and foam cells in the bone marrow.

REFSUM DISEASE

This recessive disease (also known as heredopathia atactica polyneuritiformis) is unique among the lipidoses because the stored lipid is not synthesized in the body, but is exclusively dietary in origin. This has enabled successful therapy by dietary management. Refsum disease belongs in the newly defined group of *peroxisomal disorders* in which lipids normally oxidized in peroxisomes accumulate because of abnormality or absence of these subcellular organelles. Others in this group include: adrenoleukodystrophy, adrenomyeloneuropathy, cerebrotendinous xanthomatosis, hyperpipecolic acidemia, neonatal adrenoleukodystrophy, and Zellweger disease.

Onset is in early childhood in some patients, but delayed until the fifth decade in others. Progressive night blindness usually appears in the first or second decade, followed by limb weakness and gait ataxia. Symptoms are progressive, but abrupt exacerbations and gradual remissions may occur with intercurrent illness or pregnancy. There are no seizures, but some patients have psychiatric symptoms. Peripheral neuropathy is manifest by loss of tendon reflexes, weakness and wasting, and distal sensory loss. Ataxia of gait and limbs is prominent and nystagmus may be seen. Retinitis pigmentosa is usually found, but is less constantly present than night blindness. Other findings include ichthyosis, nerve deafness (often severe), cataracts, miosis and pupillary asymmetry, pes cavus, and bony deformities with shortening of the metatarsal bones, epiphyseal dysplasia, and in some, kyphoscoliosis. CSF protein is elevated. Nerve conduction velocities are slowed. EKG changes may be seen, including conduction abnormalities. Peripheral nerves may feel thickened, and on histologic study, may have hypertrophic interstitial changes

Table 80-2. Lipidoses

Disorder	Defective Enzyme (reaction number)	Stored Material	Clinical Features
A. GM$_2$-Gangliosidoses	Hexosaminidase (#3)	GM$_2$, GA$_2$, GL-4 globoside, OLS, ?GP, ?MPS	See Table 80-1
B. GM$_1$-Gangliosidoses	β-galactosidase (#2)	GM$_1$, GA$_1$, OLS, KS-like material	
1. Infantile form			Infantile encephalopathy, organomegaly, skeletal involvement, macular cherry-red spot (50%), corneal haze (occasionally)
2. Late-infantile form			Onset at age 1–3 years of dementia, seizures, ataxia, dysarthria, spastic quadriplegia
C. Fabry disease	α-galactosidase (#4)	Ceramide trihexoside, ? blood group substance type B	Purple skin lesions, painful hands and feet, renal disease, leg edema, stroke
D. Gaucher disease	β-glucosidase (#6)	Glucocerebroside	
1. Infantile neuronopathic form			Onset at age 3 months of dementia, organomegaly, poor suck and swallowing, opisthotonus, spasticity, seizures
2. Juvenile neuronopathic form			Variable onset of mental defect, splenomegaly, incoordination, seizures
3. Adult non-neuronopathic form			Splenomegaly (sometimes in infancy) and bony involvement; Ashkenazi Jewish predilection
4. Adult neuronopathic form			Splenomegaly, bony involvement, seizures, dementia
E. Nieman-Pick Disease			
1. Infantile neuronopathic form, Type A	Sphingomyelinase (#26)	Sphingomyelin, cholesterol	Infantile encephalopathy, organomegaly, macular cherry-red spot (30%), lung infiltrates; Ashkenazi Jewish predilection
2. Juvenile non-neuronopathic form, Type B	Sphingomyelinase (#26)	Sphingomyelin, cholesterol	Hepatosplenomegaly
3. Juvenile neuronopathic form, Type C	?Sphingomyelinase (#26)	Sphingomyelin, cholesterol	Onset at age 1–3 years of dementia, seizures, spasticity, ataxia; hepatosplenomegaly less prominent

Disease	Enzyme defect	Storage material	Clinical features
4. Nova Scotia variant, Type D	?	Cholesterol, cholesterol ester, sphingomyelin, bis(monoacylglyceryl) phosphate	Infantile hepatosplenomegaly, onset age 2–5 years of dementia, seizures, ataxia, spasticity
5. Adult non-neuronopathic form, Type E	?	Sphingomyelin	Adult hepatosplenomegaly
6. Juvenile non-neuronopathic form, Type F	Sphingomyelinase (#26)	Sphingomyelin	Resembles type B, juvenile hepatosplenomegaly, sea-blue histiocytes, heat-labile sphingomyelinase
F. Farber disease	Acid ceramidase (#7)	Ceramide	Early infantile painful swollen joints, subcutaneous nodules, organomegaly, enlarged heart, dysphagia, vomiting, normal or impaired mentation
G. Wolman disease	Acid lipase	Cholesterol ester, triglyceride	Early infantile organomegaly, vomiting, diarrhea, jaundice, variable nervous system involvement
H. Refsum disease	Phytanic acid α-hydroxylase	Phytanic acid	Night blindness, retinitis pigmentosa, ataxia, demyelinating neuropathy, ichthyosis
I. Cerebrotendinous Xanthomatosis	?	Cholestanol, cholesterol	Static encephalopathy in 1st decade, adolescent or adult-onset cataracts, tendon xanthomas, ataxia, spasticity
J. Neuronal lipofuscinoses (Batten disease)	?	Retinoic acid derivatives, dolichol derivatives (whether this storage is primary or secondary is unclear)	
1. Infantile (Finnish) form (Santavuori disease)			Infantile onset of progressive visual loss, retinal degeneration, myoclonic jerks, microcephaly
2. Late-infantile form (Jansky-Bielschowsky)			Onset at age 1–4 years of seizures, ataxia, dementia, then visual deterioration and retinal degeneration
3. Juvenile form (Spielmeyer-Sjögren)			Onset at age 5–10 years of progressive visual loss and pigmentary retinal degeneration then seizures and dementia
4. Adult form (Kufs)			Adult onset of dementia, ataxia, seizures, and myoclonus

GM_2 = GM_2-ganglioside, GA_2 = asialo-GM_2-ganglioside, GP = glycoprotein, MPS = mucopolysaccharide, GM_1 = GM_1-ganglioside, GA_1 = asialo-GM_1-ganglioside, KS = keratan sulfate, DS = dermatan sulfate, HS = heparan sulfate, GM_3 = GM_3-ganglioside, GD_3 = GD_3-ganglioside.

and onion-bulb formation. The course is generally progressive with exacerbations and remissions. Peripheral visual fields may ultimately be lost with resulting telescopic vision. Sudden death may result from cardiac arrhythmia.

There is accumulation in the liver and kidneys of phytanic acid due to lack of phytanic acid alpha-hydroxylase, which converts phytanic acid to alpha-hydroxyphytanic acid. The enzyme deficiency has been demonstrated in cultured skin fibroblasts. Diagnosis is made by the characteristic clinical picture and biochemical patterns.

Therapy limits dietary phytanic acid and its precursor, phytol. When dairy products, ruminant fat, and chlorophyll-containing foods are eliminated, plasma phytanic acid levels are reduced and tissue stores are mobilized, with improvement of symptoms. Paradoxically, symptoms may worsen and plasma phytanic acid levels may rise shortly after institution of dietary therapy, especially if patients reduce caloric intake and lose weight. Increased plasma phytanic acid causes anorexia, increased weight loss, and still more severe symptoms. Adequate caloric intake helps prevent weight loss and abrupt fat mobilization. Plasmapheresis has also been helpful in preventing or treating such exacerbations.

CEREBROTENDINOUS XANTHOMATOSIS (CHOLESTANOL STORAGE DISEASE)

Although patients with cholestanol storage disease often have mental defect of early onset, the diagnosis is difficult in the first decade because cataracts, tendon xanthomas, and progressive spasticity, usually associated with ataxia, commonly do not begin before adolescence or young adulthood. The spasticity and ataxia are severe and progressive. Speech is affected. Neuropathy may appear with distal muscle wasting. Sensory deficits and Babinski signs are seen. Pseudobulbar palsy develops terminally. Death usually occurs in the fourth to sixth decade, caused by neurologic disease or myocardial infarction. Some patients have apparently normal mental function.

Tendon xanthomas are almost always seen on the Achilles tendon and may occur elsewhere. The cerebellar hemispheres contain large (up to 1.5 cm), yellowish, granulomatous, xanthomatous lesions with extensive demyelination of white matter. Microscopically, cystic areas of necrosis and clear, nee-

dle-shaped clefts contain birefringent material surrounded by macrophages with foamy vacuolated cytoplasm and multinucleated giant cells. The brain stem and spinal cord may be involved.

Cholestanol is increased in plasma, brain, and tendon xanthomas. Cholesterol is increased in tendon xanthomas but is usually normal in plasma. Cholestanol is increased in bile, but chenodeoxycholic acid (a major component of normal bile) is virtually absent. The basic defect is unknown.

Diagnosis is by the characteristic clinical picture and biochemical findings. Neither carrier testing, prenatal diagnosis, nor treatment are yet possible, but genetic counseling is of value.

THE NEURONAL CEROID LIPOFUSCINOSES

The neuronal ceroid lipofuscinoses are defined by histologic and ultrastructural features. By light microscopy, neurons are engorged with PAS-positive material, a finding that placed these disorders in the older classification of "amaurotic family idiocy." However, the storage material in the neuronal ceroid lipofuscinoses is autofluorescent; ultrastructurally, abnormal lipopigments resembling ceroid and lipofuscin are found in distinctive, abnormal cytosomes such as curvilinear and finger-print bodies. Although the signs and symptoms are confined to the nervous system, the abnormal cytosomes are widely distributed in skin, muscle, peripheral nerves, and viscera. The basic defect and the precise composition of the stored material are unknown. The abnormal lipopigment might be formed by peroxidation of fatty acids, but deficiency of peroxidase in leukocytes seems to be a secondary and variable finding. The autofluorescent material in neurons contains a retinoic acid-like compound. Dolichol is elevated in tissue and urine sediment.

Diagnosis is made by the characteristic clinical picture, abnormal electroretinogram (in the infantile, late-infantile, and juvenile forms), and by electron microscopic examination of tissue (skin, nerve, muscle, or rectal biopsy for autonomic neurons). Abnormal autofluorescence is seen on examination of frozen section of biopsied muscle, enabling rapid diagnosis. The abnormal storage material has been seen by electron microscopy of leukocytes and urine sediment.

Carrier testing and prenatal diagnosis are not yet available. Genetic counseling is important. The neuronal ceroid lipofuscinoses are autosomal recessive.

Infantile (Finnish) Variant (Santavuori Disease). This variant of neuronal ceroid lipofuscinosis begins at about 8 months with progressive visual loss, loss of developmental milestones, myoclonic jerks, and microcephaly. There is optic atrophy, macular and retinal degeneration, and no response in the electroretinogram. Progression is rapid but infants may survive for several years.

Late-Infantile Variant (Jansky-Bielschowsky Disease). This begins between 1½ and 4 years with seizures and ataxia. Seizures respond poorly to anticonvulsants. There is progressive visual deterioration with abolished electroretinogram and retinal deterioration. Progression is usually rapid to a vegetative state, but some affected children may survive several years.

Juvenile Variant (Spielmeyer-Sjögren Disease). This variant of neuronal ceroid lipofuscinosis begins with progressive visual loss, between the ages of 5 and 10 years, with pigmentary degeneration of the retina. Seizures, dementia, and motor abnormalities occur later and progress to death by the end of the second decade.

Adult Variant (Kuf Disease). This begins in the third or fourth decade with progressive dementia, seizures, myoclonus, and ataxia. Blindness and retinal degeneration are *not* features of the adult form.

Leukodystrophies

Historically, the concept of leukodystrophies began when "diffuse sclerosis" was described by Heubner in 1887 and "encephalitis periaxialis diffusa" was reported by Schilder in 1912. What became known as "Schilder's disease" was a heterogeneous group of disorders that included demyelinating diseases related to multiple sclerosis, inflammatory disorders with secondary demyelination, and progressive genetic metabolic disorders affecting myelin metabolism. The last group now comprises the leukodystrophies (Table 80–3).

The leukodystrophies were further subdivided by specific outstanding features, leaving a heterogeneous residual group of "nonspecific leukodystrophies," which will no doubt be further subdivided in the future. Krabbe leukodystrophy (globoid cell leukodystrophy, GLD) was initially defined by the presence of globoid cells in demyelinated portions of the brain. Metachromatic leukodys-

trophy (MLD) was set apart by abnormal tissue metachromasia. Adrenoleukodystrophy (ALD) was set apart by involvement of adrenal glands and by X-linked inheritance (see Article 84, Adrenoleukodystrophy). Classic Pelizaeus-Merzbacher disease was set apart by X-linked inheritance, very early onset, a long course, and islands of preserved myelin in the demyelinated areas. This leaves a heterogeneous group of unclassified leukodystrophies. These are sometimes called orthochromatic or sudanophilic leukodystrophies, but the term *unclassified leukodystrophies* seems preferable.

Three leukodystrophies have been associated with enzyme deficiencies (GLD, ALD, and MLD). In all three, the findings suggest that the leukodystrophies arise from abnormal metabolism of myelin constituents.

KRABBE LEUKODYSTROPHY (GLOBOID CELL)

Patients are normal at birth. Symptoms begin at age 3 to 6 months with irritability, inexplicable crying, fevers, limb stiffness, seizures, feeding difficulty, inexplicable vomiting, and slowing of mental and motor development. Later mental and motor deterioration occur with marked hypertonia and extensor postures. Early, tendon reflexes may be increased or already decreasing. Optic atrophy may be seen. Later, tendon reflexes decrease or disappear. Patients may develop flaccidity or flexor postures before death occurs at about age 2 years.

Important diagnostic features are increased CSF protein and decreased nerve conduction velocities. On electron microscopy, sural nerve biopsies show needle-like inclusions in histiocytes and Schwann cells, also seen in globoid cells in demyelinated brain regions (Fig. 80–6).

Galactocerebrosidase is deficient in serum, leukocytes, and cultured skin fibroblasts. Both galactosylcerebroside and galactosylsphingosine (psychosine) are substrates for that enzyme. Galactosylcerebroside is markedly decreased in the brains of patients with Krabbe disease (to a lesser extent than other myelin lipids), but galactosylsphingosine is increased at least 200-fold over levels in the normal brain, where it is barely detectable. Psychosine storage is probably the cause of the disease because, injected into brain, it causes cessation of myelination and severe demyelination.

A few patients with juvenile onset and slower progression of dementia, optic atro-

Table 80-3. Leukodystrophies

Clinical Disorder	Defective Enzyme (reaction number)	Stored Material	Clinical Features
A. Krabbe leukodystrophy (GLD)			
1. Infantile form	Galactocerebrosidase (#10)	Psychosine Galactocerebroside	Onset at age 3–6 months of irritability, spasticity, seizures, fevers. Progressive mental and motor loss to blind decerebrate vegetative state, with optic atrophy, decreased tendon reflexes, decreased nerve conduction velocities, increased CSF protein
2. Juvenile form	Galactocerebrosidase (#10)	Galactocerebroside ? Psychosine	Juvenile onset of dementia, optic atrophy, pyramidal tract disorder
3. Adult form	? Galactocerebrosidase (#10)	? Galactocerebroside ? Psychosine	Adult onset of slowly progressive dementia, optic atrophy, and pyramidal signs
B. Metachromatic leukodystrophy (MLD)			
1. Late-infantile form	Sulfatase A (#9)	Sulfatide	Onset at age 1–2½ years of walking difficulty with weakness, ataxia or spasticity; progressive dementia, optic atrophy, loss of deep tendon reflexes; slow nerve conduction velocities, increased CSF protein
2. Juvenile form	Sulfatase A (#9)	Sulfatide	Onset at age 3–10 years of dementia, gait difficulty, neuropathy, elevated CSF protein; more slowly progressive
3. Adult form	Sulfatase A (#9)	Sulfatide	Adult onset dementia, often with ataxia and pyramidal findings; slowly progressive
4. MLD without sulfatase A deficiency	? Sulfatase A (#9) activator	Sulfatide	Same as late-infantile or juvenile form
5. Asymptomatic or presymptomatic adults with sulfatase A deficiency	Sulfatase A (#9)	Sulfatide	Normal

6. Multiple sulfatase deficiency (mucosulfatidosis, MSD)	Sulfatase A (#9) Sulfatase B (#17) Sulfatase C cholesterol sulfate sulfatase dehydroepiandrosterone sulfate sulfatase iduronate-2-sulfate sulfatase (#12) sulfamidase (#13) N-acetylgalactosamine-6-sulfate sulfatase (#16) N-acetylglucosamine-6-sulfate sulfatase (#19) basic defect unknown	Sulfatide MPS	Slowed early development. Onset at age 1–2 years of mental and motor deterioration and seizures; mildly coarsened facial features, ichthyosis, organomegaly, skeletal changes
C. X-linked leukodystrophies 1. With adrenal involvement a. Adrenoleukodystrophy	Peroxisomal fatty acid oxidation system (?bifunctional enzyme or fatty acyl Co-A synthetase)	Very long chain fatty acids	X-linked recessive; onset at age 8 years (3–12) of behavioral change followed by dementia, visual loss (often cortical), gait disturbance, pyramidal signs, optic atrophy, and variable adrenal insufficiency
b. Adrenomyeloneuropathy	Peroxisomal fatty acid oxidation system (?bifunctional enzyme or fatty acyl Co-A synthetase)	Very long chain fatty acids	X-linked (incompletely) recessive; adrenal insufficiency in childhood; onset in third decade of progressive spastic paraparesis and neuropathy often with hypogonadism, dementia, and cerebellar dysfunction
2. Without adrenal involvement a. Classic Pelizaeus-Merzbacher disease	?	Proteolipid protein	X-linked (incompletely) recessive, severely delayed motor milestones, infantile trembling eye movements; juvenile mental defect and slowly progressive spasticity, ataxia, and optic atrophy; long survival (4th decade or longer)
b. Seitelberger variant	?	?	More severe than classic Pelizaeus-Merzbacher disease with death early in first decade

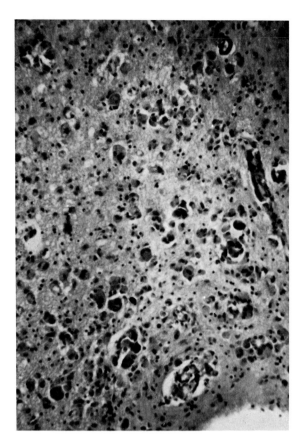

Fig. 80–6. Globoid cells in white matter, Krabbe leukodystrophy (H&E stain).

phy, and pyramidal-tract signs without neuropathy have had galactocerebrosidase deficiency. An adult-onset disorder with similar, but more slowly progressive course, has been described based on the pathologic findings of globoid cell leukodystrophy, however, the biochemical basis has not been established.

The Mucopolysaccharidoses

The mucopolysaccharidoses are recognizable by a characteristic phenotype, and by the tissue storage and urinary excretion of acid mucopolysaccharide (Table 80–4). They were originally regarded as a single disease, but eight clinical types and numerous subtypes are now known. Each is caused by deficiency of a lysosomal hydrolase enzyme required for degradation of one or more of three sulfate mucopolysaccharides: dermatan sulfate, heparan sulfate, and keratan sulfate (see Fig. 80–2).

Diagnosis is based on the clinical picture, excessive amounts of one or more acid mucopolysaccharides in urine, and the presence

of the enzyme defect. Urine screening tests for excess mucopolysaccharide are useful but show both false-positive and false-negative results. Positive screening tests require confirmation by quantitative and qualitative determination of urinary mucopolysaccharides, radiographic and histologic evidence of tissue storage, and demonstration of the enzyme defect. Screening tests may be falsely negative, especially in Sanfilippo and Morquio syndromes. If clinical suspicion of mucopolysaccharidosis is strong, diagnostic evaluation should be pursued even with a negative urine screening test. Prenatal diagnosis of these disorders is possible.

HURLER SYNDROME (MPS IH)

This is the most severe of the mucopolysaccharidoses, characterized by onset in infancy, progressive disability, and death usually occurring before 10 years of age. Nearly all the features found in other types are present in Hurler syndrome. Corneal clouding and lumbar gibbus are noted in the first year of life. Patients develop stiff joints with periarticular swelling, short stubby hands and feet, claw hands, lumbar lordosis, chest deformity, and dwarfing, which are usually apparent by 2 or 3 years of age. The facial features become coarsened and grotesque, with thickened eyelids and lips, frontal bossing, bushy eyebrows, depressed nasal bridge, hypertelorism, enlarged tongue, noisy breathing, rhinorrhea, and widely spaced peglike teeth. Mental retardation and deterioration, but not seizures, are noted. Deafness is frequent. Few patients develop speech. Leptomeningeal thickening, arachnoid cysts, and hydrocephalus may occur. Cardiac murmurs due to valvular heart disease, coronary occlusion, and cardiac enlargement may occur and cause death. Abdominal distension is commonly noted, with inguinal and umbilical hernias and hepatomegaly. Corneal clouding becomes progressively more severe and, with retinal degeneration, impairs vision. Cervical-cord compression with quadriplegia may occur.

Radiographic changes are often helpful for the diagnosis of mucopolysaccharidosis, but do not reliably distinguish the various types. These changes include ovoid or beaked lumbar vertebrae, peg-shaped metacarpals, a J-shaped sella turcica, and spatulate ribs. Peripheral leukocytes and bone marrow cells contain metachromatic granules. Clear vacuoles are seen in liver cells and cells of other

Table 80-4. Mucopolysaccharidoses

Syndrome Number	Syndrome Name	Stored Material	Deficient Enzyme	Reaction Number*	Mental defect	Cloudy corneas	Hearing loss	Coarse facial features	Dwarfing	Dysostosis multiplex	Heart disease	Organomegaly	Other Features
MPS IH	Hurler	DS,HS	α-L-iduronidase	11	3+	3+	2+	3+	3+	3+	3+	3+	Cord compression Pigmentary retinopathy
MPS IH/S	Hurler-Scheie compound	DS,HS	α-L-iduronidase	11	±	3+		2+	1+	2+	1+	2+	Severe arachnoid cysts
MPS IS	Scheie	DS	α-L-iduronidase	11	0	3+	±	±	0	1+	1+	±	Pigmentary retinopathy Carpal tunnel syndrome
MPS II A	Hunter (severe)	DS,HS	Iduronate-2-sulfate sulfatase	12	+	0	3+	2+	2+	2+	±	1+	Nodular skin lesions
MPS II B	Hunter (mild)	DS,HS	Iduronate-2-sulfate sulfatase	12	0	0	2+	1+	1+	1+	±	±	Pigmentary retinopathy Carpal tunnel syndrome Nodular skin lesions
MPS III A	Sanfilippo A	HS	Sulfamidase	13	3+	0	2+	1+	0	1+	1+	1+	Retinal degeneration May have seizures
MPS III B	Sanfilippo B	HS	α-N-acetylglucosaminidase	14	3+	0	2+	1+	0	1+	1+	1+	Retinal degeneration
MPS III C	Sanfilippo C	HS	N-acetyltransferase	15	3+	0	2+	1+	0	1+	1+	1+	
MPS IV A	Morquio A	KS	Galactose-6-sulfate sulfatase	16	0	2+	2+	1+	3+	3+	2+	±	Cord compression Odontoid hypoplasia
MPS IV B	Morquio B	KS,OLS	β-galactosidase	2	0	1+	0	0	0	2+	0	0	
MPS V	Category vacant	—	—										
MPS VI A	Maroteaux-Lamy (severe)	DS	Sulfatase B	17	0	2+	2+	2+	2+	2+	2+	±	Cord compression Carpal tunnel syndrome Hydrocephalus
MPS VI B	Maroteaux-Lamy (intermediate)	DS	Sulfatase B	17	0	2+		±	1+	2+	2+	0	Carpal tunnel syndrome
MPS VI C	Maroteaux-Lamy (mild)	DS	Sulfatase B	17	0	1+		±	1+	1+	1+	0	Cord compression Carpal tunnel syndrome
MPS VII	Sly	DS,HS	β-glucuronidase	18	2+	±	1+	1+	2+	2+	1+	1+	Hydrocephalus Odontoid hypoplasia
MPS VIII	DiFerrante	HS,KS	N-acetylglucosamine-6-sulfate sulfatase	19	2+	0	1+	0	1+	1+	0	1+	

*See Figs. 80–1 through 80–3.

GM_2 = GM_2-ganglioside, GA_2 = asialo GM_2-ganglioside, OLS = oligosaccharide, GP = glycoprotein, MPS = mucopolysaccharide, GM_1 = GM_1-ganglioside, GA_1 = asialo-GM_1-ganglioside, KS = keratan sulfate, DS = dermatan sulfate, HS = heparan sulfate, GM_3 = GM_3-ganglioside, GD_3 = GD_3-ganglioside.

tissues. Zebra bodies containing lipids occur in the brain. Both dermatan sulfate and heparan sulfate (see Fig. 80–2) are stored. Alpha-L-iduronidase (see reaction 11, Fig. 80–2), required for degradation of both, is deficient. The diagnosis is made by demonstrating severe deficiency of alpha-L-iduronidase in cultured skin fibroblasts and leukocytes.

Hurler-Scheie Compound (MPS IH/S) patients lack alpha-L-iduronidase (see reaction 11, Fig. 80–2). This disorder is milder than the Hurler syndrome, but more severe than Scheie-syndrome. Distinction from Hurler and Scheie syndromes is solely by the clinical features.

Scheie Syndrome (MPS IS) is characterized by juvenile onset of stiff joints with the development of claw hands and deformed feet. Corneal clouding causes visual impairment; corneal grafts may become opacified. Other features are pigmentary degeneration of the retina, glaucoma, coarse facial features, genu valgus, carpal tunnel syndrome, and involvement of the aortic valve. Deafness may occur. Stature and intelligence are normal. Psychological disturbances have been noted. Life span may be normal unless cardiac involvement becomes severe. Distinction from other alpha-L-iduronidase deficiency disorders is solely on clinical grounds.

HUNTER SYNDROME (MPS II)

This mucopolysaccharidosis includes at least two forms, mild and severe. Both forms (presumably allelic) in boys are X-linked recessive and show iduronate-2-sulfatase deficiency (see reaction 12, Fig. 80–2). A Hunter phenotype in girls with iduronate-2-sulfatase deficiency is due to total sulfatase deficiency (MLD, Austin type).

Boys with the severe form have juvenile onset of joint stiffness, coarse facial features, dysostosis multiplex, hepatosplenomegaly, diarrhea, dwarfing, and mental deterioration. Progressive deafness is prominent. Pigmentary retinal deterioration, papilledema, and hydrocephalus may be seen. Nodular or pebbled skin change over the scapulae and absence of corneal clouding are important features distinguishing Hunter from Hurler syndrome. Patients usually die by age 15 years.

Patients with the mild form of Hunter syndrome may be asymptomatic. They have short stature, joint stiffness and limitation of motion, coarse feature, and hepatosplenomegaly. They may have hernias and carpal tunnel syndrome. Intelligence is normal but they may develop papilledema and neurologic deterioration late in the course. Life span may be normal. Diagnosis is by finding excess urinary dermatan sulfate and heparan sulfate (Fig. 80–2), and demonstration of iduronate-2-sulfatase deficiency (see reaction 12, Fig. 80–2) in serum or cultured skin fibroblasts.

SANFILIPPO SYNDROME (MP III)

Patients with this syndrome have prominent mental involvement, mild somatic involvement, and urinary excretion of heparan sulfate alone. Three biochemically distinct forms reflect three metabolic steps required for the degradation of heparan sulfate, but not that of dermatan sulfate or keratan sulfate.

These patients have the juvenile onset of mental deterioration with delay or deterioration of speech or school performance. On evaluation for psychiatric disorder, mental retardation, or dementia, the examiner notes mild coarsening of facial features, hepatosplenomegaly, hirsutism, joint stiffness, and radiographic changes of dysostosis multiplex. These patients deteriorate neurologically with progressive dementia, spastic quadriparesis, tetraballism, athetosis, incontinence, and seizures. Cardiac involvement may occur. Corneal clouding is absent. Bone changes, dwarfing, and organ enlargement are slight. Patients may die in adolescence or survive into the third decade.

The diagnosis is made by the characteristic clinical picture, excess heparan sulfaturia, and demonstration of the enzyme defect. Urinary screening tests for mucopolysacchariduria may be negative in Sanfilippo syndrome. In Sanfilippo syndrome Type A, the enzyme heparan sulfate N-sulfatase (sulfamidase, see reaction 13, Fig. 80–2) is deficient. In Type B, alpha-N-acetylglucosaminidase (see reaction 14, Fig. 80–2) is lacking. In Type C, an N-acetyl transferase is deficient (see reaction 15, Fig. 80–2); this enzyme acetylates the amino group from which sulfamidase removes the sulfate (reaction 13, Fig. 80–2) thus allowing the alpha-N-acetylglucosaminidase (see reaction 14, Fig. 80–2) to act. Type A is by far the most common.

MORQUIO SYNDROME (MPS IV)

This mucopolysaccharidosis is characterized by a severe skeletal disorder, little neurologic abnormality, and the urinary excretion of keratan sulfate (see Fig. 80–2). Two biochemically distinct forms are known, reflecting the two metabolic steps specifically required to degrade keratan sulfate.

Skeletal manifestations appear in the first year, as in Hurler syndrome, but corneal clouding is not prominent (corneas usually become mildly cloudy). Patients develop severe dwarfing, pectus carinatum joint laxity, knock-knees, short neck, sensorineural deafness, abnormal facies, and hepatosplenomegaly. Intelligence is normal. Because of odontoid process hypoplasia and joint laxity, atlantoaxial subluxation may cause cervical cord compression even in young children; this may be prevented by posterior spinal fusion. Cardiac or respiratory disease may cause death in the third or fourth decade.

The diagnosis of Type A is made by finding excess urinary keratan sulfate; that of Type B, by finding excess urinary oligosaccharides as well. Patients with Type A Morquio syndrome lack an enzyme that cleaves 6-0-sulfate groups from galactose-6-sulfate (see reaction 16, Fig. 80–2) and N-acetylgalactosamine-6-sulfate, causing the storage of keratan sulfate (which contains galactose-6-sulfate) and chondroitin-6-sulfate (which contains N-acetylgalactosamine-6-sulfate). The milder Type B form of Morquio syndrome is caused by deficiency of beta-galactosidase (see reaction 2, Fig. 80–2), apparently the same enzyme that is deficient in GM$_1$-gangliosidosis. Presumably, the Morquio mutation severely affects the enzyme's ability to cleave the beta-galactoside linkage in keratan sulfate, but leaves sufficient activity against that linkage in GM$_1$-ganglioside to prevent brain disease.

MAROTEAUX-LAMY SYNDROME (MPS VI)

This syndrome resembles MPS Type I syndrome because of the prominent skeletal disease, but intelligence is normal and the predominant urinary mucopolysaccharide is dermatan sulfate. It is distinguished from Scheie syndrome by the affected patient's short stature.

At least three forms of Maroteaux-Lamy syndrome are known, all with deficiency of N-acetylgalactosamine-4-sulfate sulfatase or arylsulfatase B (see reaction 17, Fig. 80–2). In the severe form, growth retardation is noted by 2 or 3 years of age. Coarse facial features, marked corneal clouding, and severe skeletal disease develop. Valvular heart disease and heart failure develop. Intelligence is normal, but neurologic complications include hydrocephalus and cervical-cord compression resulting from hypoplasia of the odontoid process. Patients may survive into the second or third decade. In milder forms, cervical-cord compression and carpal tunnel syndrome may occur.

The Mucolipidoses

The mucolipidoses (Table 80–5) resemble the Hurler phenotype but lack excess urinary mucopolysaccharide, having instead excess urinary oligosaccharides or glycopeptides, most of which are fragments of more complex structures (see Fig. 80–3). Urinary thin-layer chromatography for oligosaccharides is a useful screening test.

SIALIDOSIS

Patients with sialidoses have deficiency of alpha-L-neuraminidase, also known as sialidase (see reaction 1, Figs. 80–1B and 80–3). In most forms, sialic acid-containing glycoproteins, oligosaccharides, and glycolipids accumulate in tissue, and sialo-oligosaccharides are excreted in urine.

The diagnosis is based on clinical findings, the presence of abnormal sialo-oligosaccharides in the urine, and deficiency of the appropriate sialidase in cultured skin fibroblasts, tissue, or leukocytes. There are at least two distinct lysosomal sialidases, one that cleaves the (alpha 2,3)-linked sialic acid in monosialoganglioside (see reaction 8, Fig. 80–1B) and the other that cleaves (alpha 2,3)-linked and (alpha 2,6)-linked sialic acid in polysialogangliosides, oligosaccharides, and glycoproteins (see reaction 1, Figs. 80–1B and 80–3). The former sialidase is reportedly deficient in mucolipidosis IV, as discussed later. The latter enzyme is deficient in the other sialidoses. In addition to the isolated sialidase deficiencies, two other groups of mucolipidoses have sialidase deficiency. In one, galactosialidosis, both sialidase and beta-galactosidase are deficient because a stabilizing protein they share is defective. In the second group, mucolipidosis II and III, sialidase and several other lysosomal hydrolases are deficient.

Sialidoses with isolated sialidase deficiency have a highly variable clinical picture. Neonates with congenital sialidoses have hydrops fetalis, hepatosplenomegaly, and short survival times. They resemble infants with congenital lipidosis of Norman and Wood. Infants with nephrosialidosis resemble the Hurler phenotype and develop macular cherry-red spot and renal disease. Children with mucolipidosis I (lipomucopolysaccharidosis), a milder

Table 80–5. Mucolipidoses

Clinical Disorder	Defective Enzyme (reaction number)*	Stored Material	Clinical Features
A. Sialidoses			
1. Sialidoses with isolated sialidase deficiency		GP, OLS, ? ganglioside	
a. Congenital sialidosis	Oligosaccharide sialidase (#1)		Premature birth, congenital hydrops fetalis, organomegaly, severe mental and motor defect, death 0–5 months
b. Severe infantile sialidosis	Oligosaccharide sialidase (#1)		Similar to congenital sialidosis, but with renal disease and survival until age 2
c. Nephrosialidosis	Oligosaccharide sialidase (#1)		Onset age 4–6 months of organomegaly, facial dysmorphism and psychomotor retardation; progressive renal disease, macular cherry-red spot and fine corneal opacities develop
d. Mucolipidosis I	Oligosaccharide sialidase (#1)		Onset at age 6 months of mild Hurler-like facial and skeletal changes, corneal clouding, macular cherry-red spot, mental defect, myoclonic jerks, cerebellar syndrome, seizures, neuropathy
e. Macular cherry-red spot myoclonus syndrome	Oligosaccharide sialidase (#1)		Onset around age 10 years of myoclonus, decreasing visual activity, and macular cherry-red spot; predilection for Italians
2. Sialidoses with additional beta-galactosidase deficiency (galactosialidosis)			
a. Infantile sialidosis (GM$_1$-gangliosidosis phenotype)	Stabilizing protein for: Oligosaccharide sialidase (#1) β-galactosidase (#2)		Same as GM$_1$ gangliosidosis
b. Goldberg syndrome	Stabilizing protein for: Oligosaccharide sialidase (#1), and β-galactosidase (#2)		Similar to mucolipidosis I but juvenile or adolescent onset and slow progression, most common among Japanese

B. Salla disease	Sialic acid egress from lysosomes	Free sialic acid	Infantile onset of hypotonia, developmental delay; juvenile ataxia, mental and motor retardation, spasticity, athetosis, dysarthria, and sometimes convulsions; short stature
C. Fucosidosis	α-L-fucosidase (#21)	GP, OLS, fucolipids	Some resemble Hurler phenotype; some have coarse features and neurologic disorder resembling leukodystrophy
D. α-Mannosidosis	α-mannosidase (#22)	GP, OLS	Mild or severe disorder with mental defect, mild organomegaly, coarse features, and skeletal involvement; may have gingival hyperplasia, lenticular opacities, and survival into third decade
E. β-Mannosidosis	β-mannosidase (#23)	GP, OLS	Juvenile onset of mental retardation, speech delay, ± coarsened facial features, ± mild bony changes, ± angiokeratoma
F. Aspartylglycosaminuria	Aspartylglucosaminidase (#25)	Aspartylglucosamine, OLS	Predilection for those of Finnish descent; characteristic facies, thickened skull, scoliosis, diarrhea, frequent respiratory infections, dementia, psychosis, and seizures
G. Mucolipidosis II (I-cell disease)	UDP-N-acetylgalactosamine-1-phosphate: glycoprotein N-acetylgalactosaminylphosphotransferase.	GP, OLS, MPS, Ganglioside	Infantile onset of Hurler-like disorder, but corneas are usually clear
H. Mucolipidosis III (Pseudopolydystrophy)	Same as Mucolipidosis II	GP, OLS, MPS, Ganglioside	Onset at age 2–4 of coarse facies, dwarfism, short neck, claw hands, shoulder stiffness; clear corneas, carpal tunnel syndrome, mental defect, and long survival
I. Mucolipidosis IV	? Soluble ganglioside sialidase (#8)	GM_3, GD_3	Early infantile corneal clouding; juvenile mental and motor defect; Ashkenazi Jewish predilection

*See Figs. 80–1 through 80–3.
GM_2 = GM_2-ganglioside, GA_2 = asialo-GM_2-ganglioside, OLS = oligosaccharide, GP = glycoprotein, MPS = mucopolysaccharide, GM_1 = GM_1-ganglioside, GA_1 = asialo-GM_1-ganglioside, KS = keratan sulfate, DS = dermatan sulfate, HS = heparan sulfate, GM_3 = GM_3-ganglioside, GD_3 = GD_3-ganglioside.

disorder, are similarly affected but develop ataxia, myoclonic jerks, and seizures. The mildest form is the cherry-red spot myoclonus disorder in which adolescents, who are usually mentally normal, develop macular cherry-red spot, myoclonus, and myoclonic seizures. There is a predilection for individuals of Italian descent.

Sialidosis with combined sialidase and beta-galactosidase deficiency (galactosialidosis) includes two forms: an infantile sialidosis with the clinical phenotype of GM$_1$-gangliosidosis, and the Goldberg syndrome. The first disorder should be considered in any patient who is suspected of having GM$_1$-gangliosidosis or is found to have beta-galactosidase deficiency. Goldberg syndrome resembles mucolipidosis I, but is milder with a predilection for those of Japanese origin; there is an adult form as well.

SALLA DISEASE

Onset of this disorder is between ages 4 and 12 months with hypotonia, developmental delay, or both. Ataxia of trunk and limbs follow and, by age 2 years, there is mental and motor retardation. Patients are invariably severely mentally retarded and may never speak or walk. Usually they develop spasticity, athetosis, dysarthria, and sometimes convulsions. They are short, often with strabismus and with thickened calvaria. Ultrastructural analysis of blood lymphocytes, skin, and liver reveals abnormal lysosomal morphology. Free sialic acid is markedly increased in urine; defective sialic acid egress has been noted from isolated fibroblast lysosomes. There is a predilection for those of Finnish descent.

Some patients with *fucosidosis* have severe neurologic disease that resembles a leukodystrophy. Others with fucosidosis resemble the Hurler phenotype. Some have survived into the second or third decade. Fucose residues form part of the structure of oligosaccharides, glycoproteins, and glycolipids, including "fucogangliosides."

The diagnostic findings are excessive urinary abnormal oligosaccharides (see Fig. 80–3) and by demonstrating severely decreased levels of alpha-L-fucosidase (reaction 21, Fig. 80–3) in serum, leukocytes, and cultured skin fibroblasts.

α-*Mannosidosis* may be mild or severe. In severely affected patients, the diagnosis has been confused with mucolipidosis I. Other patients have slower progression of the disorder with greater dysmorphism, cataracts, and longer survival. Others have presented primarily with marked mental defect, striking gingival hyperplasia, and survival into the third decade or longer. Facial dysmorphism, skeletal involvement, and organ enlargement have been slight in these patients.

Diagnosis requires a high index of suspicion and findings of excessive abnormal urinary oligosaccharides, and decreased α-mannosidase (reaction 22, Fig. 80–3) in leukocytes and cultured skin fibroblasts.

HUMAN β-MANNOSIDOSIS

This disorder, originally described in goats, has been found in at least three patients. One patient presented at 16 months with slowing of speech development and at 46 months had coarsened facial features, mild bony changes, speech delay, and mental retardation. Two brothers, aged 44 and 19 years, had angiokeratoma on the penis and scrotum, mental retardation from age 5 years or earlier, and no coarse features, organomegaly, or bony changes. Diagnosis was by lack of β-mannosidase in plasma, leukocytes, and fibroblasts and by presence of a mannose-containing disaccharide in urine. Interestingly, the first patient had absent sulfamidase, low sulfamidase in one parent, and urinary mucopolysaccharide excretion identical to that in Sanfilippo syndrome, Type A, a clinically similar disorder.

Aspartylglycosaminuria occurs almost solely in Finland. Patients have juvenile onset of somatic and mental changes. Somatic changes include coarse facial features anteverted nostrils, short neck, and scoliosis. Intellectual deterioration leads to severe mental defect in the adult. Episodic hyperactivity, psychotic behavior, and seizures may occur.

Patients excrete large amounts of aspartylglucosamine in their urine because of deficiency of N-aspartyl-beta-glucosaminidase (reaction 25, Fig. 80–3). Diagnostic findings are aspartylglucosamine in the urine and deficiency of N-aspartyl-beta-glucosaminidase (reaction 25, Fig. 80–3) in cultured skin fibroblasts.

Mucolipidosis II (I-cell disease) is a severe disorder that resembles Hurler syndrome, but the patient's corneas are clear. Cultured fibroblasts have coarse inclusions (I-cells). Diagnosis is made by finding excess sialo-oligosaccharides in the urine and deficiencies of multiple lysosomal enzymes in cultured skin fibroblasts with elevated levels of these enzymes in plasma. In brain and viscera, only β-galactosidase is consistently deficient. The basic defect is deficiency of the enzyme, UDP-N-acetylglucosamine: glycoprotein N-acetylglucosaminylphosphotransferase. This enzyme attaches the N-acetylglucosamine-1-phosphate of UDP-GlcNAc-1-P to the 6-position of alpha-linked mannose residues of glycoproteins. The N-acetylglucosamine is subsequently removed to leave a mannose-6-phosphate residue, an important recognition marker for uptake of certain glycoproteins (including many lysosomal hydrolase enzymes) into the cell.

Mucolipidosis III (pseudo-Hurler polydystrophy) is a milder clinical disorder than mucolipidosis II but is caused by a deficiency of the same enzyme. Diagnosis is made as for mucolipidosis II.

Patients with *mucolipidosis IV* present with corneal clouding as early as 6 weeks of age. Mild retardation progresses to severe mental and motor defect. There is a predilection for those of Ashkenazi Jewish descent. Diagnosis is by the clinical picture, light microscopic findings (lipid-laden marrow histiocytes), and electron microscopic findings (vacuoles and membranous bodies in skin, conjunctiva, and cultured fibroblasts).

Gangliosides GM_3 and GD_3 (Fig. 80–1B) accumulate in fibroblasts. Soluble ganglioside sialidase (reaction 8, Fig. 80–1B) is reportedly deficient.

References

General

Barringer JA, Brady RO, eds. Molecular Basis of Lysosomal Storage Disorders. New York: Academic Press, 1984.

Callahan JW, Lowden JA, eds. Lysosomes and Lysosomal Storage Diseases. New York: Raven Press, 1981.

Johnson WG. Sphingolipid storage diseases. In: Conn RB, ed. Current Diagnosis, 7th ed. Philadelphia: WB Saunders, 1985:770–777.

Johnson WG. Mendelian and non-Mendelian inheritance. In: Rowland LP, ed. Molecular Genetic of Neuromuscular Diseases. New York: Oxford University Press, 1988.

Kolodny EH, Cable WJL. Inborn errors of metabolism. Ann Neurol 1982; 11:221–232.

McKusick VA. Mendelian Inheritance in Man, 8th ed. Baltimore: Johns Hopkins University Press, 1988.

Myrianthropoulos NC. Neurogenetic Directory Part I. In: Vinken PJ, Bruyn GW, eds. Handbook of Clinical Neurology (vol 42). New York: Elsevier-North Holland, 1981.

Lipidoses

GM₂-Gangliosidoses

Brett EM, Ellis RB, Haas L, et al. Late onset GM₂-gangliosidosis: clinical, pathological and biochemical studies on 8 patients. Arch Dis Child 1973; 48:775–785.

Hardie RJ, Young EP, Morganhughes JA. Hexosaminidase a deficiency presenting as juvenile progressive dystonia. J Neurol Neurosurg Psychiat 1988; 52:446–447.

Johnson WG. The clinical spectrum of hexosaminidase deficiency disorders. Neurology 1981; 31:1453–1456.

Johnson WG. Genetic heterogeneity of hexosaminidase deficiency diseases. Res Publ Assoc Res Nerv Ment Dis 1983; 60:215–238.

Johnson WG. Neurological disorders with hexosaminidase deficiency. In: Moss AJ. ed. Pediatrics Update. New York: Elsevier Science, 1987:91–104.

Johnson WG, Wigger HJ, Karp HR, Glaubiger LM, Rowland LP. Juvenile spinal muscular atrophy: a new hexosaminidase deficiency phenotype. Ann Neurol 1982; 11:11–16.

Korneluk RG, Mahuran DJ, Neote K, et al. Isolation of cDNA clones coding for the α-subunit of human β-hexosaminidase: Extensive homology between the α and β subunits and studies on Tay-Sachs disease. J Biol Chem 1986; 261:8407–8413.

Little LE, Lau MMH, Quon DVK, Fowler AV, Neufeld EF. Proteolytic processing of the α-chain of the lysosomal enzyme β-hexosaminidase, in normal human fibroblasts. J Biol Chem 1988; 263:4288–4292.

Myerowitz R, Piekarz R, Neufeld EF, Shows TB, Suzuki K. Human β-hexosaminidase α chain: Coding sequence and homology with the β chain. Proc Natl Acad Sci USA 1986; 82:7830–7834.

Navon R, Argov Z, Frisch A. Hexosaminidase A deficiency in adults. Am J Med Genet 1986; 24:179–196.

O'Dowd BF, Klavins MH, Willard HF, Gravel R, Lowden JA, Mahuran DJ. Molecular heterogeneity in the infantile and juvenile forms of Sandhoff disease (O-variant G_{M2}-gangliosidosis). J Biol Chem 1986; 261:12,680–12,685.

Proia RL. Gene encoding the human β-hexosaminidase β chain: Extensive homology of intron placement in the α- and β-chain genes. Proc Nat Acad Sci USA 1988; 85:1883–1887.

Willner JP, Grabowsky GA, Gordon RE, et al. Chronic G_{M2}-gangliosidosis masquerading as atypical Friedreich ataxia: chemical, morphologic, and biochemical studies of nine cases. Neurology 1981; 31:787–798.

GM₁-Gangliosidoses

Goldman JE, Katz D, Rapin I, Purpura DP, Suzuki K. Chronic G_{M1}-gangliosidosis presenting as dystonia. I. Clinical and pathological features. Ann Neurol 1981; 9:465–475.

Kobayashi T, Suzuki K. Chronic G_{M1}-gangliosidosis presenting as dystonia. II. Biochemical studies. Ann Neurol 1981; 9:476–483.

Landing BH, Silverman FN, Craig JM, Jacoby MD, Lahey ME, Chadwick DL. Familial neurovisceral lipidosis. Am J Dis Child 1964: 108:503–522.

Lowden JA, Callahan JW, Gravel RA, Skomorowski MA, Becker L, Groves J. Type 2 G_{M1}-gangliosidosis with long survival and neuronal ceroid lipofuscinosis. Neurology 1981; 31:719–724.

O'Brien JS, Gugler E, Giedion A, et al. Spondyloepiphyseal dysplasia, corneal clouding, normal intelligence, and acid beta-galactosidase deficiency. Clin Genet 1976; 9:495–504.

O'Brien JS, Ho HW, Veath ML, et al. Juvenile G_{M1}-gangliosidosis. Clinical, pathological, chemical, and enzymatic studies. Clin Genet 1972; 3:411–434.

Okada S, O'Brien JS. Generalized gangliosidosis: Beta-galactosidase deficiency. Science 1968; 160:1002–1004.

Wenger DA, Sattler M, Mueller OT, Myers GG, Schneiman RS, Nixon GW. Adult G_{M1}-gangliosidosis: clinical and biochemical studies on two patients and comparison to other patients called variant or adult G_{M1}-gangliosidosis. Clin Genet 1980; 17:323–334.

Fabry Disease

Bishop DF, Calhoun DH, Bernstein HS, Hantzopoulos P, Quinn M, Desnick RJ. Human α-galactosidase A: Nucleotide sequence of a cDNA clone encoding the mature enzyme. Proc Natl Acad Sci USA 1986; 83:4859–4863.

Brady RO, Gal AE, Bradley RM, Martensson E, Warshaw AL, Laster L. Enzymatic defect in Fabry's disease: ceramide trihexosidase deficiency. N Engl J Med 1967; 276:1163–1167.

Brady RO, Tallman JF, Johnson WG, et al. Replacement therapy for inherited enzyme deficiency in Fabry's disease. N Engl J Med 1973; 289:9–14.

Kaye EM, Kolodny EH, Logigian EL, Ullman MD. Nervous system in Fabry's disease. Ann Neurol 1988; 23:505–509.

Wise D, Wallace HJ, Jellinek EH. Angiokeratoma corporis diffusum: A clinical study of eight affected families. Q J Med 1962; 31:177–206.

Gaucher Disease

Brady RO, Kanfer JN, Shapiro D. Metabolism of glucocerebrosides. II. Evidence of an enzymatic deficiency in Gaucher's disease. Biochem Biophys Res Commun 1965; 18:221–225.

Dreborg S, Erikson A, Hayberg B. Gaucher Disease—Norbottnian type. Eur J Pediatr 1980; 133:107–118.

Gonzalez-Sastre F, Pampols T, Sabater J. Infantile Gaucher's disease: A biochemical study. Neurology 1974; 24:162.

Ginns EI, Choudary PV, Martin BM, et al. Isolation of cDNA clones for human β-glucocerebrosidase using the lambda-gt11 expression system. Biochem Biophys Res Commun 1984; 123:574–580.

Herrlin KM, Hillborg PO. Neurological signs in a juvenile form of Gaucher's disease. Acta Paediatr 1962; 51:137–154.

King JO. Progressive myoclonic epilepsy due to Gaucher's disease in an adult. J Neurol Neurosurg Psychiatry 1975; 38:849–854.

Melamed E, Cohen C, Soffer D, Lavy S. Central nervous system complication in a patient with chronic Gaucher's disease. Eur Neurol 1975; 13:167–175.

Miller JD, McCluer R, Kanfer JN. Gaucher's disease: neurologic disorder in adult siblings. Ann Intern Med 1973; 78:883–887.

Neil JF, Glew RH, Peters SP. Familial psychosis and diverse neurologic abnormalities in adult-onset Gaucher's disease. Arch Neurol 1979; 36:95–99.

Schneider EL, Ellis WG, Brady RO, McCulloch JR, Epstein CJ. Infantile (type II) Gaucher's disease: in utero diagnosis and fetal pathology. J Pediatr 1972; 81:1134–1139.

Winkelman MD, Banker BQ, Victor M, Moser HW. Noninfantile Gaucher's disease. A clinicopathologic study. Neurology 1983; 33:994–1008.

Niemann-Pick Disease

Brady RO, Kanfer JN, Mock MB, Fredrickson DS. The metabolism of sphingomyelin. II. Evidence of an enzymatic defect in Niemann-Pick disease. Proc Natl Acad Sci USA 1966; 55:366.

Crocker AC, Farber S. Niemann-Pick disease: A review of eighteen patients. Medicine 1958; 37:1.

Gal AE, Brady RO, Barranger JA, Pentchev PG. The diagnosis of type A and type B Niemann-Pick disease and detection of carriers using leukocytes and a chromogenic analogue of sphingomyelin. Clin Chim Acta 1980; 104:129–132.

Huterer S, Wherrett SR, Poulos A, Callahan JW. Deficiency of phospholipase C acting on phosphatidylglycerol in Niemann-Pick disease. Neurology 1983; 33:67–73.

Neville BGR, Lake BD, Stephens R, Sanders MD. A neurovisceral storage disease with vertical supranuclear ophthalmoplegia, and its relation to Niemann-Pick disease: A report of nine patients. Brain 1973; 96–97.

Pentchev PG, Comely ME, Kruth HS, et al. A defect in cholesterol esterification in Niemann-Pick disease (Type C) patients. Proc Nat Acad Sci USA 1985; 82:8247–8251.

Pentchev PG, Comely ME, Kruth HS, et al. Group C Niemann-Pick disease; faulty regulation of low density lipoprotein uptake and cholesterol storage in cultured fibroblasts. FASEB J 1987; 1:40–45.

Rao BG, Spence MW. Niemann-Pick disease type D: Lipid analyses and studies on sphingomyelinases. Ann Neurol 1977; 1:385–392.

Savitzky A, Rosner F, Chodsky S. The sea-blue histiocyte syndrome, a review: Genetic and biochemical studies. Semin Hematol 1972; 9:285.

Schneider EL, Pentchev PG, Hibbert SR, Sawitsky A, Brady RO. A new form of Niemann-Pick disease characterized by temperature-labile sphingomyelinase. J Med Genet 1978; 15:370–374.

Farber Disease

Farber S, Cohen J, Uzman LL. Lipogranulomatosis: A new lipoglycoprotein "storage" disease. Mt Sinai J Med 1957; 24:816–837.

Sugita M, Dulaney JT, Moser HW. Ceramidase deficiency in Farber's disease (lipogranulomatosis). Science 1972; 178:1100–1102.

Wolman Disease

Patrick AD, Lake BD. Deficiency of an acid lipase in Wolman's disease. Nature 1969; 222:1067–1068.

Wolman M, Sterk VV, Gatt S, Frenkel M. Primary family xanthomatosis with involvement and calcification of the adrenals. Report of two more cases in siblings of a previously described infant. Pediatrics 1961; 28:742–757.

Young ER, Patrick AD. Deficiency of acid esterase activity in Wolman's disease. Arch Dis Child 1970; 45:664–668.

Refsum Disease

Djupesland G, Flottorp G, Refsum S. Phytanic acid storage disease; hearing maintained after 15 years of dietary treatment. Neurology 1983; 33:237–239.

Nevin NC, Cumings JN, McKeown F. Refsum's syndrome: Heredopathia atactica polyneuritiformis. Brain 1967; 90:419.

Refsum S. Heredopathia atactica polyneuritiformis. Acta Psychiatr Scand 1946; (suppl 38):1.

Refsum S. Heredopathia atactica polyneuritiformis. J Nerv Ment Dis 1952; 116:1046–1050.

Steinberg D, Herndon JH Jr, Uhlendorf BW, Mize CE, Avigan J, Milne GWA. Refsum's disease; nature of the enzyme defect. Science 1967; 156:1740–1742.

Steinberg D, Mize CE, Herndon JH Jr, Fales HM, Engel WK, Vroom FQ. Phytanic acid in patients with Refsum's syndrome and response to dietary treatment. Arch Intern Med 1970; 125:75–87.

Cerebrotendinous Xanthomatosis

Berginer VM, Salen G, Shefer S. Long-term treatment of cerebrotendinous xanthomatosis with chenodeoxycholic acid. N Engl J Med 1984; 311:1649–1652.

Bjorkhem I, Fausa O, Hopen G, Oftebro H, Pedersen JI, Skrede S. Role of the 26-hydroxylase in the biosynthesis of bile acids in the normal state and in cerebrotendinous xanthomatosis: An in vivo study. J Clin Invest 1983; 71:142–148.

Menkes JH, Schimshock JR, Swanson PD. Cerebrotendinous xanthomatosis. The storage of cholestanol within the nervous system. Arch Neurol 1968; 19:47.

Oftebro H, Bjorkhem I, Stormer FC, Pederson JI. Cerebrotendinous xanthomatosis: Defective liver mitochondrial hydroxylation of chenodeoxycholic acid precursors. J Lipid Res 1981; 22:632–640.

Salen G, Shefer S, Cheng FW, Dayal B, Batta AK. Tint GS. Cholic acid biosynthesis: the enzymatic defect in cerebrotendinous xanthomatosis. J Clin Invest 1979; 63:38–44.

Neuronal Ceroid-Lipofuscinoses

Boehme DH, Cottrell JC, Leonberg SC, Zeman W. A dominant form of neuronal ceroid-lipofuscinosis. Brain 1971; 94:745.

Carpenter S, Karpani G, Andermann F. Specific involvement of muscle, nerve, and skin in late-infantile and juvenile amaurotic idiocy. Neurology 1972; 22:170.

Hagberg B, Haltia M, Sourander P, et al. Polyunsaturated fatty acid lipidosis—infantile form of so-called ceroid lipofuscinosis. I. Clinical and morphological aspects. Acta Paediatr Scand 1974; 57:495.

Santavuori P, Haltia M, Rapola J. Infantile type of so-called neuronal ceroid-lipofuscinosis. Dev Med Child Neurol 1974; 16:644.

Wolfe LS, Kin NY, Palo J, Haltta M. Dolichols in brain and urinary sediment in neuronal ceroid lipofuscinosis. Neurology 1983; 33:103–106.

Wolfe LS, Kin NY, Baker RR, Carpenter S, Andermann F. Identification of retinoyl complexes as the autofluorescent component of the neuronal storage material in Batten disease. Science 1977; 195:1360–1362.

Leukodystrophies

Krabbe Disease

Crome L, Hanefeld F, Patrick D, Wilson J. Late onset globoid cell leucodystrophy. Brain 1973; 96:841.

Dunn HG, Lake BD, Dolman CL, Wilson J. The neuropathology of Krabbe's infantile cerebral sclerosis (globoid cell leucodystrophy). Brain 1969; 92:329.

Hagberg B, Kollberg H, Sourander P, Akesson HO. Infantile globoid cell leukodystrophy (Krabbe's disease). A clinical and genetic study of 32 Swedish cases (1953–1967). Neuropediatrics 1969; 1:74.

Suzuki Y, Suzuki K. Krabbe's globoid cell leukodystrophy: deficiency of galactocerebrosidase in serum, leukocytes, and fibroblasts. Science 1971; 171:73.

Svennerholm L, Vanier MT, Mansson JE. Krabbe disease: A galactosylsphingosine (psychosine) lipidosis. J Lipid Res 1980; 21:53–64.

Mucopolysaccharidoses

General

Dorfman A, Matalon R. The mucopolysaccharidoses (a review). Proc Natl Acad Sci USA 1976; 73:630–637.

Neufeld EF. The biochemical basis of mucopolysaccharidase and mucolipidoses. Prog Med Genet 1974; 10:81–101.

Spranger J. The systemic mucopolysaccharidoses. Ergeb Inn Med Kinderheilkd 1971; 32:166–265.

The Alpha-Iduronidase Deficiency Diseases

Bach G, Friedman R, Weisman B, et al. The defect in Hurler and Scheie syndromes deficiency of alpha-L-iduronidase. Proc Natl Acad Sci USA 1972; 60:2048.

Matalon R, Dorfman A. Hurler's syndrome, an alpha-L-iduronidase deficiency. Biochem Biophys Res Commun 1972; 47:959.

Stevenson RE. The iduronidase-deficient mucopolysaccharidoses: clinical and roentgenographic features. Pediatrics 1976; 57:111.

Hunter Syndrome (MPS II)

Ballenger CE, Swift TR, Leshner RT, Gammal TAE, McDonald TF. Myelopathy in mucopolysaccharidosis type II (Hunter syndrome). Ann Neurol 1980; 7:382–385.

DiFerrante N, Nichols BL. A case of the Hunter syndrome with progeny. Johns Hopkins Med J 1972; 130:325–328.

Migeon BR, Sprenkle JA, Liebaers I, Scott JF, Neufeld EF. X-linked Hunter syndrome: The heterogeneous phenotype in cell culture. Am J Hum Genet 1977; 29:448–454.

Sanfilippo Syndrome (MPS III)

Danks DM, Campbell PE, Cartwright E, et al. The Sanfilippo syndrome, clinical biochemical, radiological, haematological and pathological features of nine cases. Aust Paediatr J 1972; 8:174.

Klein U, Kress H, von Figura K. Sanfilippo syndrome type C; deficiency of acetyl-CoA: Alpha-glucoside N-acetyltransferase in skin fibroblasts. Proc Natl Acad Sci USA 1978; 75:5185–5189.

Kress H. Mucopolysaccharidosis III A (Sanfilippo A disease): deficiency of a heparan sulfamidase in skin fibroblasts and leucocytes. Biochem Biophys Res Commun 1973; 54:1111.

Kress H, Von Figura K, Klein U. A new biochemical subtype of the Sanfilippo syndrome: Characterization of the storage material in cultured fibroblasts of a Sanfilippo C Patient. Eur J Biochem 1978; 92:333–339.

O'Brien JS. Sanfilippo syndrome: Profound deficiency of alpha-acetylglucosaminidase activity in organs and skin fibroblasts from type-B patients. Proc Natl Acad Sci USA 1972; 69:1720–1722.

van de Kamp JJP. The Sanfilippo syndrome. A clinical and genetic study of 75 patients in the Netherlands. 'S-Gravenhagen: JH Pasman, 1979.

Morquio Syndrome (MPS IV)

Arbisser AI, Donnelly KA, Scott Jr CI, et al. Morquio-like syndrome with beta-galactosidase deficiency and normal hexosamine sulfatase activity: Mucopolysaccharidosis IV B. Am J Med Genet 1977; 1:195–205.

Groebe H, Krins M, Schmidberger H, et al. Morquio syndrome (mucopolysaccharidosis IV B) associated with beta-galactosidase deficiency. Report of two cases. Am J Hum Genet 1980; 32:258–272.

Matalon R, Arbogast B, Justile P, et al. Morquio's syndrome: deficiency of a chondroitin sulfate N-acetyl-hexosamine sulfate sulfatase. Biochem Biophys Res Commun 1974; 61:759.

O'Brien JS, Gugler E, Giedion A, et al. Spondyloepiphyseal dysplasia, corneal clouding, normal intelligence, and acid beta-galactosidase deficiency. Clin Genet 1976; 9:495–504.

Trojak JE, Ho CK, Roesel RA. Morquio-like syndrome (MPS IV B) associated with deficiency of a beta-galactosidase. Johns Hopkins Med J 1980; 146:75–79.

Maroteaux-Lamy Syndrome (MPS VI)

Peterson DI, Bacchus H, Seaich L, Kelly TE. Myelopathy associated with Maroteaux-Lamy syndrome. Arch Neurol 1975; 32:127.

Pilz H, von Figura K, Goebel HH. Deficiency of aryl sulfatase B in two brothers aged 40 and 38 years (Maroteaux-Lamy syndrome, type B). Ann Neurol 1979; 6:315–325.

Wilson CS, Mankin HT, Pluth JR. Aortic stenosis and mucopolysaccharidoses. Ann Int Med 1980; 92:496–498.

Sly Syndrome (MPS VII)

Benson PF, Dean MF, Muir H. A form of mucopolysaccharidosis with visceral storage and excessive urinary excretion of chondroitin sulphate. Dev Med Child Neurol 1972; 14:69.

Guise NS, Korneluk RG, Waye J, et al. Isolation and expression in Escherichia coli of a cDNA clone encoding human β-glucuronidase. Gene 1985; 34:105–110.

Sly WS, Quinton BA, McAlister WH, Rimoin DL. Beta-glucuronidase deficiency: report of clinical, neurological and biochemical features of a new mucopolysaccharidosis. J Pediatr 1973; 82:249.

DiFerrante Syndrome (MPS VIII)

Ginsberg LC, Donnelly PV, DiFerrante DT, DiFerrante NM, Caskey CT. N-acetylglucosamine-6-sulfate sulfatase in man: Deficiency of the enzyme in a new mucopolysaccharidosis. Pediatr Res 1978; 12:805–809.

Mucolipidoses

General

Durand P, O'Brien JS. Genetic Errors of Glycoprotein Metabolism. New York: Springer-Verlag, 1982.

Neufeld EF. The biochemical basis of mucopolysaccharidoses and mucolipidoses. Prog Med Genet 1974; 10:81–101.

Spranger JW, Widemann HR. The genetic mucolipidoses. Diagnosis and differential diagnosis. Hum Genet 1970; 9:113–139.

Sialidoses

Aylsworth AS, Thomas GH, Hood JL, Malouf N, Libert J. A severe infantile sialidosis: Clinical, biochemical, and microscopic features. J Pediatr 1980; 96:662–668.

Gravel RA, Lowden JA, Callahan JW, Wolfe LS, Kin NY. Infantile sialidosis: A phenocopy of type I G$_{M1}$-gangliosidosis distinguished by genetic complementation and urinary oligosaccharides. Am J Hum Genet 1979; 31:669–679.

Johnson WG, Thomas GH, Miranda AF, Driscoll JM. Congenital sialidosis, a new form of alpha-L-neuraminidase deficiency—its possible relation to hydrops fetalis. Neurology 1980; 30:377.

Lowden JA, O'Brien JS. Sialidosis: A review of human neuraminidase deficiency. Am J Hum Genet 1979; 31:1–18.

Maroteaux P, Humbel R, Strecker G, Michalski JC, Maude R. Un nouveau type de sialidose avec atteinte renele: la nephrosialidose. I. Etude clinique, radiologique, et nosologique. Arch Fr Pediatr 1978; 35:819–829.

Rapin I, Goldfischer S, Katzman R, Engel J, O'Brien JS. The cherry-red spot-myoclonus syndrome. Ann Neurol 1978; 3:234–242.

Renlund M, Aula P, Kari OR, et al. Salla disease. A new lysosomal storage disorder with disturbed sialic acid metabolism. Neurology 1983; 33:57–66.

Renlund M, Tietze F, Gahl WA. Defective sialic acid egress from isolated fibroblast lysosomes of patients with Salla disease. Science 1986; 232:759–762.

Ylitalo V, Hagberg B, Rapola J, et al. Salla disease variants. Sialoylaciduric encephalopathy with increased sialidase activity in two non-Finnish children. Neuropediatrics 1986; 17:44–47.

Fucosidosis

Fukushima H, de Wet JR, O'Brien JS. Molecular cloning of cDNA for human α-L-fucosidase. Proc Natl Acad Sci USA 1985; 82:1262–1265.

Patel V, Watanabe I, Zeman W. Deficiency of alpha-L-fucosidase. Science 1972; 176:426.

Wiederschain GYA, Kolibaba LG, Rosenfeld EL. Human alpha-L-fucosidosis. Clin Chim Acta 1973; 46:305.

α- and β-Mannosidosis

Autio S, Norden N, Ockerman PA, Reikkinen P, Rapola J, Louhimo T. Mannosidosis: Clinical, fine structural and biochemical findings in three cases. Acta Paediatr Scand 1973; 62:555–565.

Carroll M, Dance N, Masson PK, Robinson D, Winchester BG. Human mannosidosis—the enzymic defect. Biochem Biophys Res Commun 1972; 49:579–583.

Cooper A, Sardharwalla IB, Roberts MM. Human β-mannosidase deficiency. N Engl J Med 1986; 315:1231.

Jones MZ, Dawson G. Caprine beta-mannosidosis. J Biol Chem 1981; 256:5185–5188.

Kister JP, Lott IT, Kolodny EH. Mannosidosis. New clinical presentation, enzyme studies, and carbohydrate analysis. Arch Neurol 1977; 34:45–51.

Vidgoff J, Lovrien EW, Beals RK, Buist NRM. Mannosidosis in three brothers—A review of the literature. Medicine 1977; 56:335–348.

Wenger DA, Sujansky E, Fennessey PV, Thompson JN. Human β-mannosidase deficiency. N Engl J Med 1986; 315:1201–1205.

Yamashita K, Tachibana Y, Mihara K, Okada S, Yabuuchi H, Kobata A. Urinary oligosaccharides of mannosidosis. J Biol Chem 1980; 255:5126–5133.

Yamashita K, Tachibana Y, Takada S, Matsuda I, Arashima S, Kobata A. Urinary glycopeptides of fucosidosis. J Biol Chem 1979; 254:4820–4827.

Aspartylglucosaminuria

Arstila AU, Palo J, Haltia M, et al. Aspartylglucosaminuria. I. Fine structure studies on brain, liver and kidney. Acta Neuropathol (Berl) 1972; 20:207.

Aula P, Nanto V, Laipio ML, et al. Aspartylglucosaminuria: Deficiency of aspartylglucosaminidase in cultured fibroblasts of patients and their heterozygous parents. Clin Genet 1973; 4:297.

Autio S, Visakarpi JK, Jarvinen H. Aspartylglucosaminuria (AGU). Further aspects of its clinical picture, mode of inheritance and epidemiology based on a study of 57 patients. Ann Clin Res 1973; 5:149.

Mucolipidoses II and III

Haselik A, Neufeld EF. Biosynthesis of lysosomal enzymes in fibroblasts: phosphorylation of mannose residues. J Biol Chem 1980; 255:4946–4950.

Haselik A, Waheed A, von Figura K. Enzymatic phosphorylation of lysosomal enzymes in the presence of UDP-N-acetylglucosamine. Absence of activity in I-cell fibroblasts. Biochem Biophys Res Commun 1981; 98:761–767.

Leroy LG, Spranger JW, Feingold M, et al. I-cell disease: A clinical picture. J Pediatr 1971: 79:360.

Melham R, Dorst JP, Scott CI, McKusick VA. Roentgen findings in mucolipidosis III (pseudo-Hurler polydystrophy). Radiology 1973; 106:153.

Reitman ML, Kornfeld S. UDP-N-acetylglucosamine: Glycoprotein N-acetylglucosamine-I-phosphotransferase. J Biol Chem 1981; 256:4275–4281.

Reitman ML, Varki A, Kornfeld S. Fibroblasts from patients with I-cell disease and pseudo-Hurler polydystrophy are deficient in uridine 5'-diphosphate-N-acetylglucosamine: Glycoprotein N-acetylglucosaminylphosphotransferase activity. J Clin Invest 1981; 67:1574–1579.

Taber P, Gyepes MT, Philippart M, Ling S. Roentgenographic manifestations of Leroy's I-cell disease. AJR 1973; 118:213.

Tanaka T, Kobayashi M, Fukuda T, Tsugi Y, Usui T. I-cell disease: nine lysosomal enzyme levels in lymphocytes and granulocytes. Hiroshima J Med Sci 1979; 28:189–193.

Mucolipidosis IV

Bach G, Zeigler M, Schaap T, Kohn G. Mucolipidosis IV: Ganglioside sialidase deficiency. Biochem Biophys Res Commun 1979; 90:1341–1347.

Berman ER, Livni N, Shapira E, et al. Congenital corneal clouding with abnormal systemic storage bodies: A new variant of mucolipidosis. J Pediatr 1974; 84:519.

Kohn G, Livni M, Beyth Y. Prenatal diagnosis of mucolipidoses IV by electronmicroscopy. Pediatr Res 1975; 9:314.

Merin S, Livni N, Berman ER, Yatziv S. Mucolipidosis IV: Ocular, systemic, and ultrastructural findings. Investig Ophthal 1975; 14:437.

81. METACHROMATIC LEUKODYSTROPHY
James H. Austin

Metachromatic leukodystrophy (MLD) was the first lipidosis to be linked to a specific enzyme deficiency. The normal function of this catabolic enzyme—sulfatase A or cerebroside sulfatase—is to hydrolyze sulfate groups from cerebroside sulfate (sulfatide). In MLD, the enzyme is not "missing"; an imperfect protein still remains. What is missing is its normal hydrolase activity. As a result, sulfated lipids increase and the membranes of the myelin sheath break down in both the central and the peripheral nervous systems.

Sulfate groups are a strong locus of net negative charge. Therefore, high concentrations of sulfatides can form a complex with dye molecules that carry an opposing positive charge. In doing so, dye molecules such as cresyl violet or toluidine blue are reoriented and turn a different color. For example, acid

solutions of cresyl violet stain sulfatides a *brown* color, not a violet color. This phenomenon, termed metachromasia, gives the disease its name.

A profound leukodystrophy that tends to spare the arcuate fibers predominates in the CNS. Despite myelin dissolution, there are few sudanophilic neutral lipids so typical of other forms of myelin breakdown. Relatively few oligodendroglia are seen, even in the least affected areas of white matter. A sulfatide lipidosis is also evident, especially in the dentate and brain-stem nuclei. Intracellular sulfatide deposits also occur in some systemic organs, notably in kidney tubules and gallbladder epithelium, but also in endocrine tissues.

Normally, at the cellular level, sulfatides are synthesized in microsomes. Their sulfate group is later split off in the acid pH inside lysosomes, where sulfatase A is concentrated. A complementary activator protein, acting in concert with the enzyme, normally enhances sulfatase activity. In MLD, the cause of the defective structure and function of the enzyme is still not clear; in rare instances, MLD is caused by a defect of the activator protein. Whatever the mechanism of the sulfatase deficiency, the resulting lipidosis concentrates sulfatides in the plasma membranes of many cells, including the myelin-forming membranes of Schwann cells and oligodendroglia. One cause of the leukodystrophy may lie in some intrinsic instability of a high-sulfatide low-cerebroside ratio in MLD myelin. Other possibilities, such as a metabolic derangement in mitochondria or a toxic sulfated compound like psychosine sulfate, remain to be critically tested.

Incidence. MLD cases have occurred worldwide with equal frequency in both sexes. The disorder appears to be inherited as an autosomal recessive trait. Genetic heterogeneity introduces clinical variability and complications in biochemical diagnosis. Presumably, most of this heterogeneity reflects three or more alleles for the structural sulfatase gene. Valid prenatal screening methods, combined with genetic counseling, should help decrease the incidence of late infantile and juvenile MLD. Using radio-labelled substrates to "load" cultured cells, prenatal tests and detection of carriers have become increasingly sophisticated. For example, if leukocyte sulfatidase activity, measured against ^{35}S-labelled sulfatide, is completely absent, this finding helps separate clinically atypical cases of MLD from other causes of low arylsulfatase A activity. The in vitro laboratory finding that sulfatase levels are very low in tests of leukocytes or fibroblasts does not mean a person has MLD. Indeed, the term, "pseudoarylsulfatase A deficiency," has been introduced to describe situations in which arylsulfatase A activity is low, ranging from 10 to 50% of normal when tested against nitrocatechol sulfate. Such persons do not have clinical MLD; they excrete normal amounts of sulfatide in urine; sulfatase activity is normal when tested against the lipid substrate cerebroside sulfate. Diagnostic difficulties are compounded when those tested have another neurologic disorder that may resemble MLD. In prenatal testing, moreover, even if sulfatase A activity is absent in cultured amniotic-fluid cells, the enzyme activity must be known in both parents to exclude the possibility that the fetus has inherited only the low normal carrier state of a parent rather than the disease.

Signs and Symptoms. Four forms of MLD are commonly recognized: late infantile, juvenile, adult, and multiple sulfatase deficiency. The late infantile form is the most common, having an incidence in Sweden of about 1:40,000. The child is normal at birth, but becomes unsteady between 12 and 18 months of age, losing previously gained abilities in the use of the legs both for locomotion and for support. Neurologic examination shows weakness and hypotonia with decreased to absent reflexes, especially in the legs. These findings frequently coexist with genu recurvatum and bilateral extensor plantar responses. Thereafter, incoordination involves the arms; speech becomes indistinct, swallowing is impaired, and a dementia emerges with superimposed optic atrophy. Occasionally, the macula appears grayish, but this subtle, ocular finding is far less evident than in Tay-Sachs disease.

The juvenile form of MLD includes, by convention, those patients whose symptoms present between the ages of 4 and 21 years. Most are affected before the age of 10. Impaired school performance and emotional lability (including euphoria) may be heralding complaints. Early findings include cerebellar incoordination, pyramidal-tract findings with extensor plantar responses, and diminished reflexes in the legs.

The adult form of MLD was described by Alzheimer and Nissl in 1910, well before the childhood and other forms. Patients present with mental disturbances and subtle symptoms of an organic mental syndrome. These include: impaired concentration, failing memory, schizophrenic-like symptoms, and emotonal lability with euphoria and depression. A few patients have unusual spasmodic movements. Seizures are infrequent and occur less commonly than in the other forms. In one series, the average age of onset was 29; the oldest age of onset was 46. The average duration of the illness was 14 years, though the range of duration was from 3 to 36 years. Chemically, the sulfatide lipidosis is minimal in adult MLD.

The fourth form of MLD is more appropriately described as multiple sulfatase deficiency, rather than as mucosulfatidosis. After a slow development that may be apparent during the first year, the neurologic signs develop in a manner similar to late infantile MLD. In addition, the skin may be scaly, thickened, loose, and dry, and the children seem deaf. The sternum may be convex or show pectus excavatum; ribs may be flared. Hepatosplenomegaly is sometimes present, but the corneas are not cloudy.

Laboratory Data. Demyelination in peripheral nerves causes an early and sometimes profound slowing of nerve conduction, a point especially helpful in childhood onset forms of MLD. CSF protein content is frequently elevated near or above 100 mg/dl in the late infantile form, is usually elevated in multiple sulfatase deficiency, but may be normal in juvenile or adult forms.

CT scans show a symmetrically reduced volume of cerebral white matter with corresponding ventricular enlargement. Distinctive focal areas of accentuated white matter loss are superimposed bifrontally and biparietally, especially in juvenile and adult MLD. T2-weighted magnetic resonance scans show a confluent hyperintense signal in shrunken white matter (Fig. 81–1).

Involvement of the gallbladder wall causes inability to concentrate contrast material in a cholecystogram; thus, a nonfilling gallbladder is frequently found, however, cholecystography is difficult to carry out in younger children. EEG changes are nonspecific. Frozen tissue sections, stained with acetic cresyl violet and examined microscopically, show distinctive brownish metachromasia. The biopsy sites include peripheral nerves (usually sural), the conjunctiva, and the skin (for its small superficial nerves). The nerves in the pulp of an extracted tooth can be stained.

The excess sulfatides in the urine can be

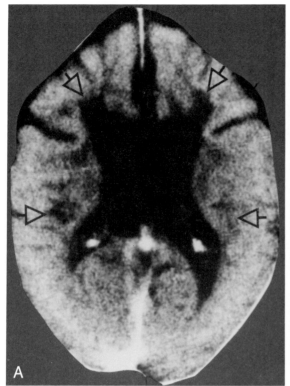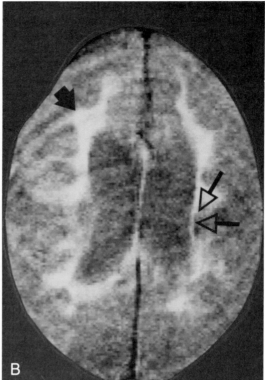

Fig. 81–1. A, standard CT projection through the central cerebrum. Open arrows indicate symmetrical lesions of markedly decreased absorption in white matter. Adult MLD, age 36. B, A more T_2 weighted MRI scan of same patient. Black arrow shows the confluent hyperintense signal in diseased white matter. So shrunken is this ribbon of white matter that gyri now extend down next to the ventricle (open arrows).

extracted, concentrated on filter paper, and stained with toluidine blue in a rapid spot test. The requisite color for diagnosis is red-pink against a blue background. Controls are necessary. The sulfatase deficiency is demonstrated in leukocytes obtained at venipuncture, in urine supernatant, or in cultured skin fibroblasts using nitrocatechol sulfate or ^{35}S-labelled sulfatide. The heterozygote state can also be shown in cultured skin fibroblasts. In multiple sulfatase deficiency, Wright- or Giemsa-stained blood smears show a hypergranulation abnormality in the polymorphonuclear cells; urine supernatant shows an excess of sulfated glycosaminoglycans (mucopolysaccharides) attributable to the sulfatase deficiency. Also, the sulfatase C deficiency causes increased steroid sulfates in the tissues. The quantity of an apparently normal enzyme protein may be reduced by increased degradation in this form. BAER tests show hearing is impaired both peripherally and centrally.

Diagnosis and Differential Diagnosis. Clinically, MLD resembles many other diseases.

In a child, the diagnosis can be suspected when a progressive difficulty in walking is coupled with hypoactive tendon reflexes and extensor plantar responses. The diagnosis is facilitated if there is a positive family history in siblings or first cousins. Given these, plus prolonged peripheral nerve conductions and increased CSF protein, the diagnostic workup proceeds to the appropriate tests for the sulfatase deficiency or for the sulfatide excess. The infantile form needs to be distinguished from other leukodystrophies (e.g., the later onset form of globoid leukodystrophy), Tay-Sachs disease, the Jansky-Bielschowski form of ceroidosis, the Type A form of Niemann-Pick disease, subacute necrotizing encephalopathy, various types of GM_1 and GM_2 gangliosidosis, and the amino-acidopathies. Cerebellar tumors, polyneuritis, and myopathies may also be included in the differential diagnosis. Multiple sulfatase deficiency needs to be further distinguished from the Type-1 form of GM_1 gangliosidosis and from the mucopolysaccharidoses.

Later juvenile forms of MLD require differentiation from adreno- and other sudano-philic leukodystrophies, from Pelizaeus-Merzbacher disease, subacute sclerosing panencephalitis, the hereditary ataxias, and childhood forms of multiple or diffuse sclerosis. It is difficult to diagnosis adult MLD on clinical grounds alone because it can be confused with schizophrenia and with the many other slowly progressive dementias and with Binswanger disease (due to similar CT findings).

Course and Prognosis. In general, the earlier the onset, the sooner death occurs. However, some cases of late infantile onset last 7 to 8 years. Juvenile cases may have an apparent temporary plateau, whereas an occasonal adult case may pursue a more rapid course.

Treatment. Allogenic bone marrow transplantation from a normal histocompatible sibling has been associated with a delay in progression of some aspects of the disease. Some recent evidence suggest that the mutant sulfatase A is more susceptible to cysteine proteinases in MLD patients whose disease begins clinically after the late infantile stage. Inhibiting such proteinases has yet to be shown to be clinically effective.

References

Austin J. Metachromatic leukodystrophy (sulfatide lipidosis). In: Hers H, Van Hoof F, eds. Lysosomes and Storage Diseases. New York: Academic Press, 1973:411–437.

Austin J. Some mechanisms of disease in metachromatic leukodystrophy (MLD). In: Goldensohn E, Appel S, eds. Scientific Approaches to Clinical Neurology. Philadelphia: Lea & Febiger, 1977:342–362.

Austin J, Armstrong D, Fouch S, et al. Metachromatic leukodystrophy (MLD). VIII. Metachromatic leukodystrophy in adults; diagnosis and pathogenesis. Arch Neurol 1968; 18:225–240.

Farrell K, Applegarth D, Toone J, McLeod P, Savage A. Pseudoarylsulfatase-A deficiency in the neurologically impaired patient. Can J Neurol Sci 1985; 12:274–277.

Inui K, Emmett G, Wenger D. Immunological evidence for deficiency in an activator protein for sulfatide sulfatase in a variant form of metachromatic leukodystrophy. Proc Natl Acad Sci USA 1983; 80:3074–3077.

Kolodny E, Moser H. Sulfatide lipidosis: Metachromatic leukodystrophy. In: Stanbury J, Wyngaarden J, Fredrickson D, Goldstein J, Brown M, eds. The Metabolic Basis of Inherited Disease, 5th ed. New York: McGraw-Hill, 1983:881–905.

Krivit W, Lipton ME, Lockman LA, Tsai M, et al. Prevention of deterioration in metachromatic leukodystrophy by bone marrow transplantation. Am J Med Sci 1987; 30:80–85.

McKhann G. Metachromatic leukodystrophy—clinical and enzymic parameters. Neuropediatrics 1984; 15(suppl):4–10.

Skomer C, Stears J, Austin J. Metachromatic leukodystrophy (MLD). XV. Adult MLD with focal lesions by computed tomography. Arch Neurol 1983; 40:354–355.

von Figura K, Steckel F, Conary J, Hasilik A, Shaw E. Heterogeneity in late-onset metachromatic leukodystrophy. Effect of inhibitors of cysteine proteinases. Am J Hum Genet 1986; 39:371–382.

82. DISORDERS OF CARBOHYDRATE METABOLISM
Salvatore DiMauro

Glycogen Storage Diseases

Abnormal metabolism of glycogen and glucose may occur in a series of genetically determined disorders, each representing a specific enzyme deficiency (Table 82–1). The signs and symptoms of each disease are largely determined by the tissues in which the enzyme defect is expressed. Those that affect the neuromuscular system primarily are discussed in Chapter XVII, Myopathy.

Severe fasting hypoglycemia may result in periodic episodes of lethargy, coma, convulsions, and anoxic brain damage in glucose-6-phosphatase deficiency or glycogen synthetase deficiency. The liver is enlarged in both diseases. Clinical manifestations tend to become milder in patients who survive the first few years of life.

The nervous system is directly affected by the enzyme defect in generalized glycogen storage diseases, even though neurologic symptoms are lacking in some disorders and, in others, may be ascribed to liver rather than to brain dysfunction. The following enzyme defects seem to be generalized: acid maltase (Type II), debrancher (Type III), brancher (Type IV), and phosphoglycerate kinase (PGK, Type IX).

In the infantile form of acid maltase deficiency (Pompe disease), pathologic involvement of the CNS has been documented, with accumulation of both free and intralysosomal glycogen in all cells, especially spinal motor neurons and neurons of the brain-stem nuclei. Peripheral nerve biopsies showed accumulation of glycogen in Schwann cells. The profound generalized weakness of infants with Pompe disease is probably due to combined effects of glycogen storage in muscle, anterior horn cells, and peripheral nerves. In the childhood form of acid maltase deficiency, increased glycogen deposition in the CNS was found in two children (one of whom was mentally retarded), but not in two other patients. No morphologic changes were seen in the CNS of a patient with adult-onset acid maltase deficiency despite marked decrease of enzyme activity.

Patients with debrancher deficiency (glycogenosis Type III) have hepatomegaly, fasting hypoglycemia, and seizures in infancy and childhood, which usually remit around puberty. Clinical manifestations are similar to those of glucose-6-phosphatase deficiency, but tend to be less severe. In branching enzyme deficiency (glycogenosis Type IV), the clinical picture is dominated by liver disease, with progressive cirrhosis and chronic hepatic failure causing death in childhood. Deposits of a basophilic, intensely PAS-positive material that is partially resistant to β-amylase digestion, have been found in all tissues; in the CNS, spheroids composed of branched filaments were present in astrocytic processes, particularly in the spinal cord and medulla. Ultrastructurally, the storage material was composed of aggregates of branched osmiophilic filaments, 6 nm in diameter often surrounded by normal glycogen particles.

In phosphoglycerate kinase (PGK) deficiency (glycogenosis Type IX), type and severity of clinical manifestations vary in different genetic variants of the disease, and are probably related to the severity of the enzyme defect in different tissues. In several families, the clinical picture was characterized by the association of severe hemolytic anemia with mental retardation and seizures.

Lafora Disease and Other Polyglucosan Storage Diseases

Myoclonus epilepsy with Lafora bodies (Lafora disease) is a hereditary neurologic disease that is transmitted as an autosomal recessive trait and affects both sexes equally. Clinically, the disease is characterized by the triad of epilepsy, myoclonus, and dementia. Inconstant other neurologic manifestations include ataxia, dysarthria, spasticity, and rigidity. Onset is in adolescence and the course rapidly progresses to death in 90% of patients between 17 and 24 years of age. Negative criteria or manifestations that imply some other disease include onset before age 6 or after age 20, optic atrophy, macular degeneration, prolonged course, and normal intelligence. Epilepsy, with generalized seizures, is the first manifestation in most patients; status epilepticus is common in terminal stages. Myoclonus usually appears 2 or 3 years after the onset of epilepsy, may affect any area of the body, is sensitive to startle, and is absent during sleep. Intellectual deterioration generally follows the appearance of seizures by 2 or 3 years and progresses rapidly to severe dementia. Therapy is symptomatic and is designed to suppress seizures and reduce the number and severity of myoclonic jerks; some control of myoclonus is achieved by benzodiazepines.

Laboratory findings are normal, except for EEG changes; bilaterally synchronous discharges of wave-and-spike formations are commonly seen in association with myoclonic jerks. EEG abnormalities may be found in asymptomatic relatives. The pathologic hallmark of the disease is the presence in the CNS of the bodies first described by Lafora in 1911: round, basophilic, strongly PAS-positive intracellular inclusions that vary in size from small "dust-like" bodies less than 3 μm in diameter to large bodies up to 30 μm in diameter. The medium and large bodies often show a dense core and a lighter periphery. Lafora bodies are seen only in neuronal perikarya and processes and are most numerous in cerebral cortex, substantia nigra, thalamus, globus pallidus, and dentate nucleus.

Ultrastructurally, Lafora bodies are not limited by a membrane. They consist of two components in various proportions: amorphous electron-dense granules and irregular filaments. The filaments, which are about 6 nm in diameter, are often branched and frequently continuous with the granular material.

Irregular accumulations of a material similar to that of the Lafora bodies are found in liver, heart, skeletal muscle, skin, and retina, suggesting that Lafora disease is a generalized storage disease. Both histochemical and biochemical criteria indicate that the storage material is a branched polysaccharide composed of glucose (polyglucosan) similar to the amylopectin-like polysaccharide that accumulates in branching enzyme deficiency. However, the activity of branching enzyme was normal in several tissues, including brain, of patients with Lafora disease. The biochemical defect remains unknown.

A clinically distinct form of polyglucosan body disease was described in 10 patients with a complex but stereotyped chronic neurologic disorder characterized by progressive upper and lower motor neuron involvement, sensory loss, sphincter problems, neurogenic bladder, and in four patients, dementia; there

Table 82–1. Classification of Glycogen Storage Disease

Type	Affected Tissues	Clinical Presentation	Glycogen Structure	Enzyme Defect	Mode of Transmission*
I	Liver and kidney	Severe hypoglycemia; hepatomegaly	Normal	Glucose-6-phosphatase	AR
II Infancy	Generalized	Cardiomegaly; weakness; hypotonia; death < age 1 year	Normal	Acid maltase	AR
Childhood	Generalized	Myopathy simulating Duchenne dystrophy; respiratory insufficiency	Normal		
Adult	Generalized	Myopathy simulating limb-girdle dystrophy or polymyositis; respiratory insufficiency	Normal		
III	Generalized	Hepatomegaly; fasting hypoglycemia; progressive weakness	PLD†	Debrancher	AR
IV	Generalized	Hepatosplenomegaly; cirrhosis of liver; hepatic failure	Longer peripheral chains; fewer branching points	Brancher	AR
V	Skeletal muscle	Intolerance to intense exercise; cramps; myoglobinuria	Normal	Muscle phosphorylase	AR

Type	Tissue	Clinical Features	Glycogen Structure	Deficient Enzyme	Inheritance*
Vi	Liver; RBC	Mild hypoglycemia; hepatomegaly	Normal	Liver phosphorylase	AR
VII	Skeletal muscle; RBC	Intolerance to intense exercise; cramps; myoglobinuria	Normal (± longer peripheral chains)	Muscle phosphofructokinase (PFK-M)	AR
VIII	Liver	Asymptomatic hepatomegaly	Normal	Phosphorylase kinase	XR
	Liver and skeletal muscle	Hepatomegaly, growth retardation, hypotonia	Normal	Phosphorylase kinase	AR
	Skeletal muscle	Exercise intolerance, myoglobinuria	Normal	Phosphorylase kinase	AR
	Heart	Fatal infantile cardiomyopathy	Normal	Phosphorylase kinase	AR
IX	Generalized	Hemolytic anemia; seizures; mental retardation / Intolerance to intense exercise; myoglobinuria	Normal (?)	Phosphoglycerate kinase (PGK)	XR
X	Skeletal muscle	Intolerance to intense exercise; myoglobinuria	Normal (?)	Muscle phosphoglycerate mutase (PGAM-M)	AR
XI	Skeletal muscle	Intolerance to intense exercise; myoglobinuria	Normal (?)	Muscle lactate dehydrogenase (LDH-M)	AR
	Liver	Severe hypoglycemia; hepatomegaly		Glycogen synthetase	AR (?)

*AR = Autosomal recessive; XR = X-linked recessive
†PLD = Phosphorylase-limit dextrin

was no myoclonus or epilepsy. Onset was in the fifth or sixth decade of life; the course ranged from 3 to 20 years. Electrophysiologic studies showed axonal neuropathy. Throughout the CNS, polyglucosan bodies were present in processes of neurons and astrocytes, but not in perikarya. Polyglucosan accumulations were also seen in peripheral nerve and in several other tissues (i.e., liver, heart, and skeletal and smooth muscle). As in debranching enzyme deficiency and Lafora disease, the abnormal polysaccharide in these cases seems to have longer peripheral chains than normal glycogen, but the metabolic error is not known. Branching enzyme activity was normal in muscle biopsies from two patients.

Another form of polyglucosan is represented by corpora amylacea, which accumulate progressively and nonspecifically with age. They are more commonly seen within astrocytic processes in the hippocampus, and in the subpial and subependymal regions; however, they also occur in intramuscular nerves in patients older than 40.

References

Carpenter S, Karpati G, Andermann, F, Jacob JC, Andermann E. Lafora's disease: Peroxisomal storage in skeletal muscle. Neurology 1974; 24:531–538.

Coleman DL, Gambetti PL, DiMauro S. Muscle in Lafora disease. Arch Neurol 1974; 31:396–406.

DiMauro S. Metabolic myopathies. In: Vinken PJ, Bruyn GW, Ringel SP, eds. Handbook of Clinical Neurology (vol 41). New York: Elsevier-North Holland, 1979:175–234.

DiMauro S, DeVivo DC. Disorders of glycogen metabolism. In: Lajtha A, ed. Handbook of Neurochemistry (vol 10). New York: Plenum Press, 1984.

DiMauro S, Stern LZ, Mehler M, Nagle RG, Payne C. Adult-onset acid maltase deficiency: A postmortem study. Muscle Nerve 1978; 1:27–36.

Gambetti PL, DiMauro S, Baker L. Nervous system in Pompe's disease. J Neuropathol Exp Neurol 1971; 30:412–430.

Gambetti PL, DiMauro S, Hirt L, Blume RP. Myoclonic epilepsy with Lafora bodies. Arch Neurol 1971; 25:483–493.

Huijing F. Glycogen metabolism and glycogen storage diseases. Physiol Rev 1975; 609–658.

Lafora GR. Über das Vorkommen amyloider Körperchen in Innern der Ganglienzellen. Virchows Arch Pathol Anat 1911; 205:295–303.

McMaster KR, Powers JM, Hennigar GR, Wohltmann HJ, Farr GH. Nervous system involvement in type IV glycogenosis. Arch Pathol Lab Med 1979; 103:105–111.

Okamoto K, Llena JF, Hirano A. A type of adult polyglucosan body disease. Acta Neuropathol 1982; 58:73–77.

Peress NS, DiMauro S, Roxburgh VA. Adult polysaccharidosis. Arch Neurol 1979; 36:840–845.

Robitaille Y, Carpenter S, Karpati G, DiMauro S. A distinct form of adult polyglucosan body disease with massive involvement of central and peripheral neu-

ronal processes and astrocytes. Brain 1980; 103:315–336.

Sakai M, Austin J, Witmer F, Trueb L. Studies in myoclonus epilepsy (Lafora body form). II. Polyglucosans in the systemic deposits of myoclonus epilepsy and in corpora amylacea. Neurology 1970; 20:160–176.

Sakai M, Austin J, Witmer F, Trueb L. Studies of corpora amylacea. Arch Neurol 1969; 21:526–544.

Spencer-Peet J, Norman ME, Lake BD, McNamara J, Patrick AD. Hepatic glycogen storage disease. Q J Med 1971; 40:95–114.

83. HYPERAMMONEMIA

John M Freeman
Mark L. Batshaw

The urea cycle is the mammalian system for the detoxification of ammonia. The cycle converts NH_3 produced by the catabolism of protein and amino acids to nontoxic urea that can be excreted; enzymatic defects have been described at each step (Fig. 83–1). Untreated infants with these diseases usually die or are left with brain damage. Early recognition may enable specific therapy to avoid toxic accumulation of ammonia.

Diagnosis. The newborn with hyperammonemia presents with lethargy, apneic episodes, vomiting, coma, and seizures. At this age, enzyme deficiencies are usually relatively complete and ammonia intoxication is severe and often lethal. Because symptoms are caused by the accumulation of ammonia, the infant appears normal at birth and then shows progressive deterioration after the first 12 to 24 hours of life. A high index of suspicion and prompt determination of plasma ammonia level are essential for diagnosis and management. Any newborn with unexplained lethargy should have a plasma analysis for NH_3; elevated levels deserve further evaluation.

In older children, a urea cycle abnormality is usually caused by an incomplete block. Clinical manifestations differ from those in the newborn. Intermittent lethargy, vomiting, or coma may be preceded by irritability or hyperactivity. Developmental delay is common and there may be a history of protein intolerance.

Major causes of increased blood ammonia levels are shown in Table 83–1. In the newborn, hyperammonemia associated with asphyxia and liver damage can usually be distinguished by birth history. Organic acidurias such as methylmalonic and propionic acidemia are usually distinguished by ketosis, ac-

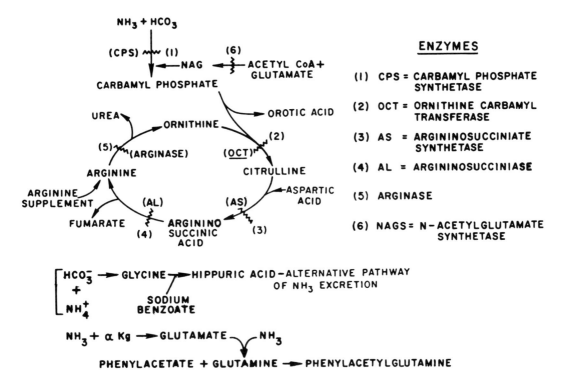

Fig. 83–1. The urea cycle.

idosis, and an increased anionic gap in serum; specific identification requires gas-liquid chromatography of urine. Lack of ketosis does not completely exclude the diagnosis. Congenital lactic acidosis caused by pyruvate dehydrogenase or pyruvate carboxylase deficiency also leads to hyperammonemia. If the anionic gap is normal, a specific urea cycle defect can be differentiated from transient hyperammonemia of the newborn by plasma amino acid chromatography (Table 83–2).

In older children, acute or chronic liver disease can usually be diagnosed by history and liver function tests. Elevated plasma content of alanine, glutamine, and glutamic acid may suggest congenital hyperammonemia; the specific urea cycle defect can be discriminated by the plasma amino acid pattern (see Table 83–2). N-acetyl glutamate synthetase and carbamyl phosphate synthetase deficiencies are clinically identical, but distinguishable by enzymatic assay. In the other disorders, it is usually not necessary to measure enzymatic activity directly to make a diagnosis.

Ornithine carbamyl transferase (OCT) and carbamyl phosphate synthetase (CPS) activities can only be measured in liver tissue; other defects are expressed in fibroblasts in other tissues.

OCT deficiency is inherited as a sex-linked

Table 83–1. Major Causes of Hyperammonemia

Newborn
  Transient hyperammonemia of the newborn
  Asphyxia
  Urea cycle defects
  Organic acidurias
    Methylmalonic acidemia
    Propionic acidemia
    Isovaleric acidemia
    Multiple carboxylase deficiency
  Congenital lactic acidosis
    Pyruvate dehydrogenase
    Pyruvate carboxylase
Older children
  Urea cycle defects
  Severe liver disease
    Chronic hepatitis
    Acute hepatitis
    Reye syndrome
  Dibasic amino acidurias
    Lysinuric protein intolerance
    Hyperammonemia-hyperornithinemia-homocitrullinemia (HHH syndrome)
    Systemic carnitine deficiency
  Drugs
    Valproic acid
    Salicylic acid

Table 83–2. Plasma Amino Acid and Urinary Orotic Acid Findings in Urea Cycle Defects

Enzymatic Deficiency	Citrulline	Arginino-succinic Acid	Orotic Acid	Arginine
Carbamyl phosphate synthetase (CPS deficiency)	0 to Trace	0	↓	↓
Ornithine carbamyl transferase (OTC deficiencies)	0 to Trace	0	↑ ↑	↓
Argininosuccinate synthetase (citrullinuria)	↑ ↑	0	↑	↓
Argininosuccinase (argininosuccinic aciduria)	↑	↑ ↑	nl	↓
Arginase	nl	0	↑	↑ ↑
Transient hyperammonemia of newborn	nl or sl ↑	0	nl	nl

Note: nl = normal in plasma and urine; ↑ = increased in plasma and urine; ↓ = decreased. (Modified from Batshaw ML, Brusilow SW, Waber L, et al. N Engl J Med 1982; 306: 1387–1392.)

disorder; the others are all autosomal recessive traits. Heterozygote detection may be possible in OCT deficiency by giving a protein load (1 g/kg body weight), followed by plasma ammonia determinations at 2 and 4 hours. Urinary orotate excretion also increases in the OCT heterozygote. Recently, recombinant DNA techniques have been used successfully for both heterozygote detection and prenatal diagnoses in OCT and CPS deficiencies. Heterozygote and prenatal diagnoses of the other urea cycle disorders are possible by enzyme determinations in fibroblasts or leukocytes.

Management of Coma. Acute hyperammonemic coma in the newborn is a medical emergency; rapid reduction of the ammonia level is necessary. Peritoneal dialysis is more effective than exchange transfusion; hemodialysis may also be effective. Useful adjuncts include intravenous administration of sodium benzoate (250 mg/kg body weight), followed by a constant infusion of 250 to 500 mg/kg body weight every 24 hours and a loading dose of arginine hydrochloride 0.8 g per kg body weight followed by 0.2 g kg body weight/day as a constant infusion for deficiency of N-acetyl glutamic acid synthetase (NAGS), CPS, and OCT. Patients with citrullinemia and argininosuccinic aciduria require 0.8 g per kg body weight. Protein deletion and caloric supplementation are also used.

Long-Term Treatment. The therapy of the urea cycle enzymopathies depends on the specific enzyme abnormality, as discussed by Batshaw (see references). Several basic principles have improved therapy:

1. Nitrogen intake must be decreased by restriction of protein intake. Further nitrogen restriction can take place by the use of essential amino acids or by their ketoanalogues.
2. The use of arginine supplementation for argininosuccinic aciduria increases waste nitrogen excretion.
3. Excretion can also be increased by using sodium benzoate supplementation, which increases nitrogen excretion by conjugation with glycine to form hippurate and sodium phenylacetate, which acetylates glutamine to form phenylacetyl glutamine. This is also readily excreted in the urine.

References

Batshaw ML. Hyperammonemia. Curr Probl Pediatr 1984; 14:1–69.
Batshaw ML, Brusilow SW, Waber L, et al. Long-term survival in neonatal onset urea cycle enzymopathies. N Engl J Med 1982; 306:1387–1392.
Brusilow SW, Batshaw ML, Waber L. Neonatal hyperammonemic coma. Adv Pediatr 1982; 29:69–103.
Brusilow SW, Danney M, Waber LT, et al. Treatment of episodic hyperammonemia in children with inborn errors of urea synthesis. N Engl J Med 1984; 310:1630–1634.

84. ADRENOLEUKODYSTROPHY
William G. Johnson

Adrenoleukodystrophy (ALD) is a distinct entity that is well defined clinically, genetically, and pathologically. There are both biochemical and genetic markers available for ALD. The basic defect involves the fatty acid β-oxidation system in subcellular organelles, called peroxisomes, which break down very long chain fatty acids (VLCFAs). Consequently, these acids accumulate in tissue and plasma.

The defective enzyme in the peroxisomal

fatty acid β-oxidation pathway has not been conclusively identified, although two candidates have been suggested: (1) fatty acyl Co-A synthetase and (2) the bifunctional enzyme, enoyl-CoA hydratase/3-hydroxyacyl-CoA dehydrogenase. The latter has been mapped to the Xq26-Xqter segment of the X chromosome.

Adrenoleukodystrophy is inherited as an X-linked, incompletely recessive disorder that maps to the distal end of the long arm of the X chromosome (Xq27-28) near the loci for hemophilia A and red-green color blindness. Although the gene for red-green color vision has been cloned, the ALD gene has yet to be. Interestingly, defects in red-green color discrimination seem to be frequent in ALD patients. At least one ALD patient lacked the red-green color vision gene, suggesting that ALD arose in that patient because of a small deletion affecting both the genes for ALD and red-green color vision.

Adrenoleukodystrophy appears in boys who had normal early development. Onset is most common about 8 years of age, although it may occur as early as 3 years or as late as 12 years. Neurologic manifestations usually precede symptoms of adrenal involvement and are relentlessly progressive. Behavioral change is the most common presenting feature and may consist of abnormal withdrawal or aggression, poor memory or school performance, and leading ultimately to progressive dementia. Visual loss, often a form of cortical blindness, may be a presenting factor and occurs sooner or later in most patients. Optic atrophy is eventually seen in all patients. Progressive gait disturbance with pyramidal tract signs is an important feature and may occur early. Dysarthria, dysphagia, and deafness may occur. Seizures are common later in the course, but may be the presenting manifestation. Some patients have overt signs of adrenal failure including fatigue, intermittent vomiting, and melanoderma that is most prominent in skin folds. In other patients, mild symptoms may be overlooked. The course is relentlessly progressive. Patients enter a vegetative state and die from adrenal crisis or other cause from 1 year to a decade after onset of symptoms. Spinal fluid protein is often elevated. CT scans show characteristic findings of hyperdense and hypodense band-like regions in posterior areas of the hemispheres; if found, these are virtually diagnostic of ALD. Adrenal function tests, especially the ACTH stimulation test, usually show adrenal insufficiency even in the absence of clinical signs. In the zona fasciculata and reticularis the finding of adrenal biopsy material with abundant ballooned cortical cells and striated cytoplasm and microvacuoles is specific for ALD. Characteristic inclusions, accumulations of lamellar lipid profiles, may also be seen in the brain, sural nerve biopsy, or testis. The primary finding in the brain is extensive diffuse demyelination with sparing of U-fibers in the centrum semiovale and elsewhere.

Biochemical studies of lipids in brain, adrenal, plasma, and cultured skin fibroblasts reveal an unusual but highly specific change. Cholesterol esters have an unusually high proportion of VLCFAs, fatty acids larger than C_{22} with the peak being C_{25} or C_{26}. These changes are also seen in white matter gangliosides.

Diagnosis is by the characteristic clinical findings of neurologic deterioration, the demonstration of adrenal hypofunction, and by CT scan. Definitive diagnosis is by the presence of elevated VLCFAs in plasma and cultured skin fibroblasts. To date, elevated VLCFAs have been found only in adrenoleukodystrophy, adrenomyeloneuropathy (see below), and in patients with generalized peroxisomal disorders. Patients on a ketogenic diet may show elevated VLCFAs in plasma but not cultured skin fibroblasts.

The diagnosis has important genetic counseling implications. Prenatal diagnosis is by amniotic fluid cells or chorionic villus sampling. About 85% of female carriers of ALD are detected by determination of VLCFAs in plasma and cultured skin fibroblasts. The polymorphic DNA marker St14 may enable improved carrier detection.

Patients should receive steroid replacement therapy during stressful periods, such as intercurrent illness, or if there is evidence of adrenal insufficiency. Although there is as yet no specific therapy, two approaches seem promising. First, because much VLCFA is of dietary origin, dietary restriction has been tried; however, this did not reduce plasma VLCFA or cause clinical improvement in ALD. Second, addition of oleic acid as synthetic glycerol trioleate to the diet reduces endogenous VLCFA in ALD. Combined therapy with dietary restriction and glycerol trioleate lowered plasma VLCFA in ALD by nearly half. Current trials are assessing clinical benefit in patients and possible prevention of disease in presymptomatic individuals.

Adrenomyeloneuropathy and Related Phenotypes

A related X-linked leukodystrophy, adrenomyeloneuropathy (AMN), has been defined with later onset and slower course. These patients have adrenal insufficiency beginning in childhood and usually in the third decade develop neurologic disease with progressive spastic paraparesis and peripheral neuropathy. Hypogonadism, impotence, and sphincter disturbance are also features. Cerebellar dysfunction and dementia have been reported. The patients are mostly males in pedigrees suggesting X-linked inheritance. A few females have been involved in pedigrees compatible with X-linked dominant inheritance.

Pathologic findings in AMN include demyelination and dying-back changes in the cord and lamellar cytoplasmic inclusions in brain, adrenal, and testis similar to those found in ALD. The fatty acid profile is altered with an increased percentage of VLCFA in cholesterol esters. The occasional finding of ALD and AMN in the same family suggests they may be variable manifestations of the same abnormal gene. Diagnosis and treatment are as for adrenoleukodystrophy.

Neonatal ALD is an autosomal recessive disorder with more generalized peroxisomal dysfunction, which closely resembles Zellweger cerebrohepato-renal syndrome. Seizures in the first few days of life, psychomotor retardation in infancy, pigmentary retinal disturbance, and death before age 4 years are common. However, there is a range of phenotypes and survival sometimes is into the midteens or longer.

X-linked ALD similar to the childhood form, but with adolescent onset, is occasionally seen. In adults, X-linked ALD may present with symptoms chiefly of cerebral origin such as dementia, schizophrenia or focal cerebral syndromes such as aphasia, Klüver-Bucy syndrome, or hemoanopsia; usually evidence of adrenal insufficiency can be found. Adult ALD may also present as spastic paraparesis, cerebellar syndrome, or olivopontocerebellar atrophy. Female heterozygotes may become symptomatic with adult ALD. Finally, adults with the biochemical defect may be asymptomatic or presymptomatic for ALD.

References

Aubourg PR, Sack GH Jr, Meyers DA, Lease JJ, Moser HW. Linkage of adrenoleukodystrophy to a polymorphic DNA probe. Ann Neurol 1987; 21:349–352.

Aubourg PR, Sack GH Jr, Moser HW. Frequent alterations of visual pigment genes in adrenoleukodystrophy. Am J Hum Genet 1988; 42:408–414.

Kolodny EH. The adrenoleukodystrophy—adrenomyeloneuropathy complex: Is it treatable? Ann Neurol 1987; 21:230–231.

Moser HW. Adrenoleukodystrophy: From bedside to molecular biology. J Child Neurol 1987; 2:140–150.

Moser AB, Borel J, Odone A, et al. A new dietary therapy for adrenoleukodystrophy: Biochemical and preliminary clinical results in 36 patients. Ann Neurol 1987; 21:240–249.

Moser HW, Naidu S, Kuma AJ, Rosenbaum AE. The adrenoleukodystrophies. CRC Crit Rev Neurobiol 1987; 3:29–88.

Poll-The BT, Roels F, Opier H, Scotto J, et al. A new peroxisomal disorder with enlarged peroxisomes and a specific deficiency of acyl-CoA oxidase (Pseudo-neonatal adrenoleukodystrophy). Am J Hum Genet 1988; 42:422–435.

Rizzo WB, Phillips MW, Dammann AL, et al. Adrenoleukodystrophy: Dietary oleic acid lowers hexacosanoate levels. Ann Neurol 1987; 21:232–239.

Schaumberg H, Powers J, Raine C, Suzuki K, Richardson E. Adrenoleukodystrophy—a clinical and pathological study of 17 cases. Arch Neurol 1975; 32:577–591.

Tanaka K, Shimada M, Naruto T, et al. Very long-chain fatty acids in erythrocyte membrane sphingomyelin: Detection in ALD hemizygotes and heterozygotes. Neurology 1986; 36:791–795.

85. DISORDERS OF METAL METABOLISM
John H. Menkes

Hepatolenticular Degeneration (Wilson Disease)

Wilson disease is an inborn error of copper metabolism that is associated with cirrhosis of the liver and degenerative changes in the basal ganglia.

During the second half of the 19th century, a condition termed pseudosclerosis was distinguished from multiple sclerosis by the lack of nystagmus and visual loss. In 1902, Kayser observed green corneal pigmentation in one such patient; Fleischer commented on the association of the corneal rings with pseudosclerosis in 1903. In 1912, Wilson gave the classic description of the disease and its pathologic anatomy.

Pathogenesis and Pathology. Wilson disease is an autosomal recessive disorder; the gene is located on the long arm of chromosome 13 near the esterase D locus. The worldwide prevalence of the disease is about 30/million, with a gene frequency of 1:180. Although most patients show markedly diminished serum ceruloplasmin concentrations, the localization of the gene for ceruloplasmin to chromosome 3 indicates that failure to form the copper protein is not the primary defect. Studies with radioisotopes indicate that the dynamic turnover of copper is disturbed. After intravenous administration of ^{64}Cu to a normal person, there is a rapid rise of serum copper content followed by an equally rapid fall and, commencing at about 6 hours post-infusion, a secondary slow rise as ceruloplasmin enters the serum. In Wilson disease, the initial rise is more extensive, the secondary rise is not observed, and no radioactivity enters the globulin fraction where ceruloplasmin is normally found. This phenomenon is also noted in patients who have nearly normal ceruloplasmin concentrations and in asymptomatic children who lack the protein, which is an indication that the rate of copper transfer from the albumin into the globulin fraction is reduced.

In addition to these abnormalities, plasma levels of nonceruloplasmin copper are increased, and the biliary excretion of copper is reduced. Equally unexplained are the low to low-normal levels of plasma iron-binding globulin. These abnormalities also occur in asymptomatic carriers and suggest that Wilson disease may also involve a disorder of iron metabolism; ceruloplasmin directly affects the transfer of iron from tissue cells to plasma transferrin.

Another metabolic feature is a persistent aminoaciduria. This is most marked during the later stages, but may be noted in some asymptomatic patients. The presence of other tubular defects (e.g., impaired phosphate resorption in patients without aminoaciduria) suggests that a toxic action of the metal on renal tubules causes the aminoaciduria.

The most plausible explanation of the copper accumulation and other features of Wilson disease is that there is a defect of an energy-mediated secretory mechanism for the metal in hepatocytes, possibly in hepatic lysosomes, and that a similar defect prevents copper from entering the ceruloplasmin compartment.

The abnormalities in copper metabolism result in a deposition of the metal in several tissues. Anatomically, the liver shows focal necrosis that leads to a coarsely nodular, post-necrotic cirrhosis; the nodules vary in size and are separated by bands of fibrous tissue of different width. Some hepatic cells are enlarged and contain fat droplets, intranuclear glycogen, and clumped pigment granules; other cells are necrotic and there are regenerative changes in the surrounding parenchyma.

Electron microscopic studies have shown that copper is sequestered by lysosomes that become more than normally sensitive to rupture and therefore lack normal alkaline phosphatase activity. Copper probably initiates and catalyzes oxidation of the lysosomal membrane lipids, resulting in lipofuscin accumulation. Within the kidneys the tubular epithelial cells may degenerate and the cytoplasm may contain copper deposits.

In brain, the basal ganglia show the most striking alterations (Fig. 85–1). They have a brick-red pigmentation; spongy degeneration of the putamen frequently leads to the formation of small cavities. Microscopic studies reveal a loss of neurons, axonal degeneration, and large numbers of protoplasmic astrocytes, including giant forms known as *Alzheimer cells*. The cortex of the frontal lobe may also show spongy degeneration and astrocytosis. Copper is deposited in the pericapillary area and within astrocytes, where it is located in the subcellular soluble fraction and bound not only to cerebrocuprein but also to other cerebral proteins. Copper is uniformly absent from neurons and ground substance.

Lesser degenerative changes are seen in the brain stem, the dentate nucleus, the substantia nigra, and the convolutional white matter. Copper is also found throughout the cornea, particularly the substantia propria. In the periphery of the cornea, the metal appears in granular clumps close to the endothelial surface of the Descemet membrane. The deposits in this area are responsible for the appearance of the Kayser-Fleischer ring. The color of this ring varies from yellow to green to brown. Copper is deposited in two or more layers, with particle size and distance between layers influencing the ultimate appearance of the ring.

Symptoms and Signs. Wilson disease is a progressive condition with a tendency toward temporary clinical improvement and arrest. It is transmitted in an autosomal recessive manner with a high rate of consanguinity in parents of affected children. The condition occurs in all races, with a particularly high incidence among Eastern European Jews, Italians from Southern Italy and Sicily, and people from some of the smaller islands of Japan—groups in which there is a high rate of inbreeding.

In most patients, symptoms begin between the ages of 11 and 25 years. Onset as early as age 4 and as late as the fifth decade have been

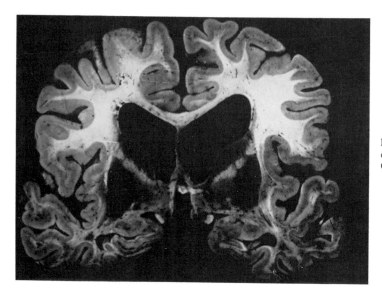

Fig. 85–1. Wilson disease. Ventricular dilation, atrophy of caudate nucleus. Cyst in lower half of putamen.

recorded. In reported cases, there is a slight preponderance of men.

The signs and symptoms of hepatolenticular degeneration are those of damage to the liver and brain. Although it was formerly thought that the cirrhosis of the liver was always asymptomatic, signs of liver damage, ascites, or jaundice may occur at any stage of the disease. They have been observed in some cases several or many years before the onset of neurologic symptoms.

The neurologic manifestations are so varied that it is impossible to describe a clinical picture that is characteristic. In the past, texts have distinguished between pseudosclerotic and dystonic forms of the disease: the former dominated by tremor, the latter by rigidity and contractures. In actuality, most patients, if untreated, ultimately develop both types of symptoms. In essence, Wilson disease is a disorder of motor function; despite often widespread cerebral atrophy, there are no

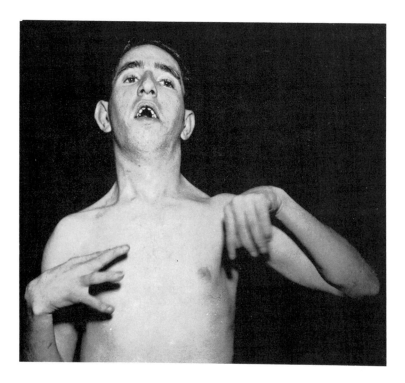

Fig. 85–2. Wilson disease. Open mouth, athetoid posture of arms, and wing-beating movements of left hand.

sensory symptoms or reflex alterations. Symptoms at onset are shown in Table 85–1. Symptoms of basal ganglia damage usually predominate, but cerebellar symptoms may occasionally be in the foreground. Tremors and rigidity are the most common early signs. The tremor may be of the intention type, or it may be the alternating tremor of Parkinson disease. More commonly, however, it is a bizarre tremor, localized to the arms and best described by the term "wing-beating" (Fig. 85–2). This tremor is usually absent when the arms are at rest; it develops after a short latent period when the arms are extended. The beating movements may be confined to the muscles of the wrist, but it is more common for the arm to be thrown up and down in a wide arc. The movements increase in severity and may become so violent that the patient is thrown off balance. Changing the posture of the outstretched arms may alter the severity of the tremor. The tremor may affect both arms, but is usually more severe in one. The tremor may occasionally be present even when the arm is at rest. Many patients have a fixed, open-mouth smile.

Rigidity and spasms of the muscles are often present. In some cases, a typical parkinsonian rigidity may involve all muscles. Torticollis, tortipelvis, and other dystonic movements are not uncommon. Spasticity of the laryngeal and pharyngeal muscles may lead to dysarthria and dysphagia. Drooping of the lower jaw and excess salivation are common. Other symptoms include convulsions, transient periods of coma, and mental changes. Mental symptoms may dominate the clinical course for varying periods and simulate an affective disorder of functional psychosis.

Tendon reflexes are increased, but extensor plantar responses are exceptional. Somatosensory evoked potentials are abnormal in most patients with neurologic symptoms.

The intracorneal, ring-shaped pigmentation first noted by Kayser and Fleischer may be evdent to the naked eye or may be seen only by slit-lamp examination. The ring may be complete or incomplete and is present in 75% of patients who present with hepatic symptoms and in all patients with cerebral symptoms alone or both cerebral and hepatic symptoms. The Kayser-Fleischer ring may antedate overt symptoms and has been detected even with normal liver functions. In the larger clinical series of Arima, it was never present in patients younger than 7.

CT usually reveals ventricular dilatation and diffuse atrophy of the cortex, cerebellum, and brain stem. In about half the patients, there are hypodense areas in the thalamus and basal ganglia. Increased density due to copper deposition is not observed. As a rule, magnetic resonance (MR) scans correlate better with the clinical symptoms than CT, demonstrating abnormal signals in the lenticular, caudate, and dentate nuclei and thalamus and, in a few subjects, focal white matter lesions (Fig. 85–3).

Diagnosis. The clinical picture of Wilson

Table 85–1. Clinical Manifestations at Onset of Wilson Disease

Symptoms	Percentage
Hepatic or hematologic abnormalities	35
Behavior abnormalities	25
Neurologic symptoms	40
Pseudosclerotic form—one or more of the following:	40
Tremor at rest or purposive	
Dysarthria or scanning speech	
Diminished dexterity or mild clumsiness	
Unsteady gait	
Tremor, alone	33
Dysarthria, alone	5
Dystonic form—one or more of the following:	60
Hypophonic speech or mutism	
Drooling	
Rigid mouth, arms, or legs	
Seizures	1
Chorea or small-amplitude twitches	<1

Table prepared with Drs. I.H. Scheinberg and I. Sternlieb, Department of Medicine, Albert Einstein College of Medicine, Bronx, New York.

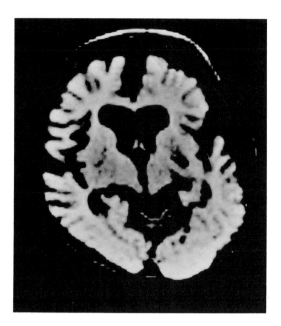

Fig. 85–3. Axial T_1 weighted MRI in patient with kinky hair disease. Patient was a 2-year-old girl with psychomotor retardation, seizures, and characteristic hair. No family history of neurologic disease. Chromosomal analysis revealed X/2 translocation. There is considerable periventricular and cortical atrophy. Fluid collection over left cortical margin represents old subdural hematoma.

disease is fairly clear-cut when the disease is advanced. The important features are the family history of hepatic or neurologic disease, progressive extra-pyramidal symptoms commencing during the first or second decade of life, abnormal liver function, aminoaciduria, cupriuria, and absent or decreased ceruloplasmin. The Kayser-Fleischer ring is the most important diagnostic feature; absence of corneal pigmentation in untreated patients with neurologic symptoms rules out the diagnosis. The ring is not seen in most presymptomatic patients or in some children with hepatic symptoms. Although 96% of patients with Wilson disease have low or absent serum ceruloplasmin, some cases have been reported with normal ceruloplasmin levels. In affected families, the differential diagnosis between heterozygotes ad presymptomatic homozygotes is of utmost importance because homozygotes should be treated preventively.

Low ceruloplasmin levels in an asymptomatic patient are indicative of the presymptomatic stage of the disease. However, because 6% of heterozygotes also have low ceruloplasmin levels, which is a phenomenon that tends to be familial, the ceruloplasmin levels of the affected patient's parents should

be determined. Whenever the diagnosis remains unresolved, a liver biopsy must be performed to measure hepatic copper content. The relatively close linkage to esterase D should facilitate diagnosis in families with a previously affected member.

A variant of Wilson disease begins in adolescence and is marked by progressive tremor, dysarthria, disturbed eye movements, and dementia. Biochemically, it is characterized by low serum levels of copper and ceruloplasmin. Kayser-Fleischer rings are absent and liver copper concentrations are low. Metabolic studies using labelled copper suggest a failure in copper absorption from the lower gut. Another recently discovered variant, in which there is a familial apoceruloplasm deficiency but no neurologic symptoms other than blepharospasm, confirms that ceruloplasm plays only a secondary role in the pathogenesis of Wilson disease.

Treatment. The aim of treatment is to prevent tissue accumulation of copper by restricting the intake of the metal, and by removing excessive amounts already deposited. A copper-poor diet and potassium sulfide, 20 mg with each meal, are recommended to minimize copper absorption. Penicillamine, 1 to 3 g daily in divided doses, on an empty stomach, is given to promote urinary excretion of copper. Improvement of neurologic symptoms and signs and fading of the Kayser-Fleischer rings result from this therapy. As a rule, patients with the predominantly pseudosclerotic form of the disease fare better than those with dystonia as the main manifestation. In some dystonic patients, addition of L-dopa to the penicillamine regimen has been beneficial. Serial CT demonstrates progressive reduction of the hypodense areas in the basal ganglia. Survival for many years with complete or almost complete remission of symptoms has been reported.

Kinky Hair Disease (Menkes Syndrome)

Trichopoliodystrophy (kinky hair disease) is a focal degenerative disorder of gray matter that is transmitted by a sex-linked gene, due to an undefined defect in copper metabolism.

The characteristic feature is maldistribution of body copper; the metal accumulates to abnormal levels in a form or location that makes it inaccessible for the synthesis of copper enzymes. Copper levels are low in liver and all areas of the brain but are elevated in some other tissues, notably intestinal mucosa and kidney. Patients absorb little or no orally administered copper, but when the metal is given intravenously there is a prompt rise in serum copper and ceruloplasmin. In fibroblasts the copper content is markedly elevated as is metallothionein; synthesis of metallothionein is increased as a consequence of abnormally high intracellular copper levels.

As a consequence of tissue copper deficiency, several pathologic changes are set into motion. Cerebral and systemic arteries are tortuous with irregular lumens and frayed and split intimal linings. In the brain, there is extensive focal degeneration of cortical gray matter with neuronal loss and gliosis. Cellular loss is prominent in the cerebellum where many Purkinje cells are lost; others show grotesque proliferation of the dendritic network. In the thalamus, there is primary cellular degeneration that spares the smaller inhibitory neurons.

The incidence is thought to be about 2/100,000 male live births. Symptoms appear in the neonatal period. Most commonly, hypothermia, poor feeding, and impaired weight gain are observed. Seizures soon become apparent with progressive deterioration of all neurologic functions. The most striking finding is the appearance of the hair, which is colorless and friable. On microscopic examination, a variety of abnormalities are evident, most often *pili torti* (twisted hair) and *trichorrhexis nodosa* (fractures of the hair shaft at regular intervals).

Radiographs of long bones reveal metaphyseal spurring and a diaphyseal periosteal reaction. On arteriography, the cerebral vessels are markedly elongated and tortuous. Similar changes are seen in systemic blood vessels. CT or MR may reveal areas of cortical atrophy or tortuous and enlarged intracranial vessels. Subdural effusions are not unusual (Fig. 85–4).

The clinical history and appearance of the infant suggest the diagnosis. Serum ceruloplasmin and copper levels are normally low in the neonatal period and do not reach adult levels until age 1 month. Thus, these determinations must be performed serially to demonstrate that the expected rise does not occur. The increased copper content of fibroblasts permits intrauterine diagnosis. Even though copper infusions raise serum copper and ceruloplasmin, neurologic symptoms are neither alleviated nor prevented. Several variants of Menkes syndrome have been recognized on the basis of low serum copper concentrations. Symptoms include ataxia, mild mental retardation, and extrapyramidal movement disorders.

References

Aisen AM, Martel W, Gabrielsen TO, et al. Wilson disease of the brain. MR imaging. Radiology 1985; 157:137–141.

Arima M, Takeshita K, Yoshino K, Kitahara T, Suzuki Y. Prognosis of Wilson's disease in childhood. Eur J Pediatr 1977; 126:147–154.

Brewer GJ, Hill GM, Prasad AS, Cossack ZT, Rabbani P. Oral zinc for Wilson's disease. Ann Intern Med 1983; 99:314–320.

Chu NS. Sensory evoked potentials in Wilson's disease. Brain 1986; 109:491–507.

Danks DM. Hereditary disorders of copper metabolism in Wilson's disease and Menkes' disease. In: Stanbury JB, Wyngaarden JB, Fredrickson DS, eds. The Metabolic Basis of Inherited Diseases, 5th ed. New York: McGraw-Hill, 1982: 1251–1268.

Danks DM, Campbell PE, Stevens BJ, Mayne V, Cartwright E. Menkes' kinky hair syndrome: An inherited defect in copper absorption with widespread effects. Pediatrics 1972; 50:188–201.

Gibbs K, Walshe JM. Biliary excretion of copper in Wilson's disease. Lancet 1980; 2:538–539.

Grover WD, Johnson WC, Henkin RI. Clinical and biochemical aspects of trichopoliodystrophy. Ann Neurol 1979; 5:65–71.

Heckmann J, Saffer D. Abnormal copper metabolism: another "non-Wilson's" case. Neurology 1988; 38:1493–1496.

Horn N, Morton NE. Genetic epidemiology of Menkes disease. Genetic Epidemiol 1986; 3:225–230.

Labadie GU, Hirschhorn K, Katz S, Beratis NG. Increased copper metallothionein in Menkes cultured fibroblasts. Pediatr Res 1981; 15:257–261.

Leone A, Pavlakis GN, and Hamer DH. Menkes' disease: Abnormal metallothionein gene regulation in response to copper. Cell 1985; 40:301–309.

Menkes JH, Alter M, Steigleder GK, Weakley DR, Sung JH. A sex-linked recessve disorder with growth retardation, peculiar hair, and focal cerebral and cerebellar degeneration. Pediatrics 1962; 29:764–779.

Miyajima H, Nishimura Y, Mizoguchi K, et al: Familial apoceruloplasmin deficiency associated with blepharospasm and retinal degeneration. Neurology 1987; 37:761–767.

Owen CA. Copper and hepatic function: Biological roles of copper. Ciba Found Symp 1980; 79:267–282.

Packman S, Palmiter RD, Karin M, et al.: Metallothionein messenger RNA regulation in the mottled mouse and Menkes kinky hair syndrome. J Clin Invest 1987; 79:1338–1342.

Polson RJ, Rolles K, Calne RY, Williams R, Marsden D. Reversal of severe neurological manifestations of Wilson's disease following orthoptic liver transplantation. Q J Med 1987: 64:685–692.

Royce PM, Camakaris J, Danks DM. Reduced lysyl oxidase activity in skin fibroblasts from patients with Menkes' syndrome. Biochem J 1980; 192:579–586.

Scheinberg IH, Jaffe ME, Sternlieb I. The use of trientine in preventing the effects of interrupting penicillamine therapy in Wilson's disease. N Engl J Med 1987; 317:209–213.

Scheinberg IH, Sternieb I. Wilson's Disease. Philadelphia: WB Saunders, 1984.

Starosta-Rubenstein S, Young AB, Kluin K, et al. Clinical

assessment of 31 patients with Wilson's disease. Arch Neurol 1987; 44:365–370.

Takano K, Kuroiwa Y, Shimada Y, Mannen T, Toyokura Y. CT of cerebral white matter in Wilson disease. Ann Neurol 1983; 13:108–109.

Varki A, Muchmore E, Diaz S. A sialic acid-specific O-acetylesterase in human erythrocytes: Possible identity with esterase D, the genetic marker of retinoblastomas and Wilson disease. Proc Nat Acad Sci USA 1986; 83:882–886.

Whiting DA. Structural abnormalities of the hair shaft. J Am Acad Dermatol 1987; 16:1–25.

Wilson SAK. Progressive lenticular degeneration: A familial nervous disease associated with cirrhosis of the liver. Brain 1912; 34:295–509.

86. ACUTE INTERMITTENT PORPHYRIA

Lewis P. Rowland

Excessive excretion of porphyrins makes the urine appear bright red, a change so dramatic that one form of genetic porphyria was among the first inborn metabolic errors discovered when that class of disease was identified by Garrod. We now recognize both acquired and heritable forms; the genetic categories are further divided into hepatic and erythropoietic types, depending on the site of the enzymatic disorder. Neurologic manifestations are encountered in two classes of porphyria. *Acute intermittent porphyria* (AIP) occurs worldwide; *variegate porphyria* occurs only in Sweden and South Africa. These two forms differ primarily in that a rash occurs in the variegate form but not in AIP. Both are inherited as autosomal dominant traits.

Pathogenesis. There are eight steps in the biosynthesis of heme. The crucial steps in understanding porphyria are: (1) delta *aminolevulinic acid* (ALA) is formed from succinyl CoA and glycine under the influence of ALA synthetase; (2) two molecules of ALA are joined by ALA-dehydratase to form a monopyrrole, *porphobilinogen* (PBG); (3) four molecules of porphobilinogen are linked to form a *porphyrin* by *uroporphyrinogen-1 synthase*—rearrangements of the side-chains of this tetrapyrrole follow under the action of a series of other enzymes, including *protoporphyrinogen oxidase;* and (4) the process culminates in the formation of heme by the addition of an iron molecule.

In AIP, there is excessive urinary excretion of ALA, PBG, and several porphyrins. Suggestions that there might be a block in an alternate pathway of ALA metabolism have not been confirmed. It is still not certain how this pattern of metabolite excretion arises. The

popular theory is that there is a block in the activity of PBG deaminase in AIP and of protoporphyrinogen oxidase in the variegate form; this causes decreased amounts of heme to be formed downstream and the lack of normal inhibitory feedback from heme on ALA synthetase releases that enzyme to account for overproduction of ALA and PBG. However, there is no evidence of deficiency of heme compounds in blood or tissues, and activity of PBG deaminase is about 50% of normal (the expected level of asymptomatic carriers of autosomal recessive diseases). The decreased activity of PBG deaminase has been demonstrated in liver biopsies, cultured skin fibroblasts, amniotic cells, and erythrocytes, but some unequivocally affected individuals have normal activity of the enzyme. Neurologic symptoms do not appear in other genetic disorders of porphyrin synthesis. It has not been possible to attribute the characteristic neuropathy of AIP to the increased amounts of circulating ALA or PBG. Clinical symptoms of porphyria are similar to those of lead poisoning, in which ALA excretion also increases, but PBG excretion is normal in lead intoxication.

Whatever the abnormality, clinical symptoms seem to be caused by the interaction of genetic and environmental factors. Porphyric crises seem to result most often from ingestion or administration of drugs that adversely affect porphyrin metabolism, especially barbiturates taken for sedation or for general anesthesia. Attacks are also attributed to menses, starvation, emotional stress, intercurrent infections, or other drugs.

Pathology. It seems clear that the functional disorder is not due to structural change. Even in fatal cases it may be difficult to demonstrate any histologic lesions. Demyelinating lesions of central and peripheral nerves have been observed, but modern electrophysiologic studies show normal or nearly normal conduction velocities with signs of denervation in muscle, a pattern that suggests primarily axonal neuropathy. This view has been supported by morphometric studies of peripheral nerves and nerve roots, with evidence also of a dying-back process. Large and small fibers are affected in peripheral nerves and autonomic fibers are also affected.

Incidence. In South Africa, Dean and Barnes traced most current cases to a single colonist who arrived there in 1688. In Sweden the prevalence varies from 1:1000 in the north to 1:100,000 population in other parts. Prevalence figures for other countries are also about 1:100,000. In one psychiatric hospital the prevalence was 2:1000. Acute symptoms are rare, however, and in major academic medical centers in New York, new cases are seen less often than once a year. All races seem to be affected. In most series, women are more often affected than men. Symptoms are rare in childhood and are most likely to affect adolescents or young adults.

Symptoms and Signs. Asymptomatic individuals with acute porphyria or variegate porphyria are identified by biochemical tests. Symptoms of either disease occur in attacks that may be induced by commonly used drugs; these will be described below. The symptoms of an attack are most commonly gastrointestinal (attributed to autonomic neuropathy), psychiatric, and neurologic (Table 86–1). Abdominal pain is most common, and may occur alone or with a neurologic or psychiatric disorder. There is usually no abdominal rigidity, but fever, leukocytosis, and diarrhea or constipation often lead to laparotomy. Patients with acute porphyria may actually have appendicitis or some other visceral emergency. The psychiatric disorder may suggest conversion reaction, acute delirium, mood change, or an acute or chronic psychosis. Symptoms of the neuropathy are like those of any peripheral neuropathy except that the signs may be purely motor and are almost always associated with abdominal

pain. In one series, 18% of the cases with neuropathy were fatal, 25% recovered completely, and the others were left with some neurologic disability. Survivors may have recurrent attacks. Cerebral manifestations are unusual except for the syndrome of inappropriate secretion of antidiuretic hormone. Unexplained transient amblyopia has been reported. Autonomic abnormalities include hypertension and tachycardia.

Laboratory Data. Routine laboratory tests usually give normal results, including CSF. EMG shows signs of denervation, but motor and sensory nerve velocities are normal or only slightly slow.

Even between attacks, affected individuals can be identified by a qualitative test for PBG in the urine. The Watson-Schwartz test depends on the action of the monopyrrole with diaminobenzaldehyde to form a reddish compound that is soluble in chloroform. The test can be performed in a few minutes and there are few false-positive or false-negative results. Quantitative measurement of urinary PBG and ALA can be achieved by column chromatography, available in many centers. The most reliable test now seems to be the assay of PBG-deaminase activity in red blood cell membranes, which is about 50% of control values in affected individuals with AIP. Variegate porphyria is rare in the United States and is identified in specialized laboratories by a different pattern of porphyrin excretion.

Diagnosis. Clinical diagnosis is not difficult if there is a family history of the disease, but the condition is so rare in the United States that physicians often do not recognize the source of unexplained abdominal pain and personality disorder. If peripheral neuropathy is added to the syndrome, however, and the appropriate biochemical tests are made, the diagnosis is ascertained. These tests are more important than looking for red urine or measurement of porphyrins in urine. Neurologically, the major disorder to be considered is the Guillain-Barré syndrome but the characteristic rise in CSF protein content of that disease is not found in AIP; the CSF protein rises so rarely in AIP that, when the protein does rise, it may be a sign of Guillain-Barré syndrome in a person with porphyria.

Treatment. The fundamental biochemical abnormality cannot be corrected, but the autonomic manifestations of an acute attack may be reversed by propanolol. Doses up to 100

Table 86–1. Clinical Manifestations of Acute Intermittent Porphyria*

	% of Patients
Abdominal pain	85–95
Vomiting	52–75
Constipation	46–70
Diarrhea	9–11
Abdominal surgery	22–46
Paresis	42–72
Myalgia	53
Convulsions	10–16
Sensory loss	9–38
Transient amaurosis	4–6
Diplopia	3
Delirium	18–52
Mood change	28
Psychosis	12
Hypertension	40–55
Tachycardia	28–60
Fever	12–37
Azotemia	6–27

*(Data from 352 reported cases in 3 series cited by Rowland LP. Dis Nerv Sys 1961; 22 (suppl): 1–12.)

Table 86–2.   Porphyrogenic Drugs in Acute Porphyria*

Drugs	Number of Exposures	Only Precipitant
Barbiturate	81	31
Analgesics	16	5
Sulfonamides	16	5
Nonbarbiturate hypnotics	15	4
Unidentified sedatives	14	10
Miscellaneous drugs	12	3
Anticonvulsants	10	5
Hormonal	6	5

*153 acute episodes in 138 patients.
(From Eales L. S Afr Med J 1979; 2:914–917.)

mg every 4 hours may reverse tachycardia, abdominal pain, and anxiety.

The neuropathy and abdominal symptoms may respond dramatically to hematin given intravenously in amounts from 200 mg to 1000 mg in attempts to suppress the activity of ALA dehydratase The optimal dosage is uncertain; one recommendation is to use 4 mg hematin/kg body weight twice daily for 3 days.

Treatment of seizures is a problem because most of the commonly used anticonvulsants have been held responsible for porphyric attacks in human patients, or they are porphyrogenic in experimental animals or cultured hepatic cells. In acute attacks of porphyria, seizures may be treated with diazepam or paraldehyde while hematin and propanolol are used to abort the attacks. Between attacks, conventional anticonvulsants may be evaluated cautiously, monitoring urinary excretion of ALA and porphobilinogen.

Other drugs that are suitable for symptomatic relief include codeine and meperidine for pain, chlorpromazine and other psychoactive drugs, and almost all antibiotics. The major drugs to avoid are barbiturates in any form, including pentobarbital for general anesthesia (Table 86–2). Barbiturates may be especially hazardous when given for sedation or anesthesia in the early stages of an attack. It is otherwise difficult to prevent attacks, but some women have symptoms only and regularly in relation to menses; both suppression of ovulation and prophylactic use of hematin have been reported to be effective.

In case of accident, patients should wear warning bracelets to identify the drug problem.

References

Anonymous. Treatment of acute hepatic porphyria (Editorial). Lancet 1978; 1:1024–1025.

Becker DM, Kramer S. The neurological manifestations of porphyria: a review. Medicine 1977; 56:411–423.

Bottomley SS, Bonkowsky HL, Birnbaum MK. The diagnosis of acute intermittent porphyria. Usefulness and limitations of the erythrocyte uroporphyrinogen-1 synthase assay. Am J Clin Pathol 1981; 76:133–139.

Brenner DA, Bloomer SR. The enzymatic defect in variegate porphyria. Studies with human cultured skin fibroblasts. N Engl J Med 1980; 302:765–769.

Brezis M, Ghanem J, Weiler-Ravell O, Epstein O, Morris D. Hematin and propanolol in acute intermittent porphyria. Full recovery from quadriplegic coma and respiratory failure. Eur Neurol 1979; 18:289–294.

Campbell BC, Brodie MJ, Thompson GG, Meredith PA, Moore MR, Goldberg A. Alterations in the activity of enzymes of haem biosynthesis in lead poisoning and acute hepatic porphyria. Clin Sci 1977; 53:335–340.

Dean G. The porphyrias. A Story of Inheritance and the Environment, 2nd ed. London: Pitman, 1971.

Desnick RJ, Ostasiewica LT, Tishler PA, Mustajoki P. Acute intermittent porphyria: Characterization of a novel mutation in the structural gene for porphobilinogen deaminase. J Clin Invest 1985; 76:1473–1478.

Eales L. Porphyria and the dangerous life-threatening drugs. S Afr Med J 1979; 2:914–917.

Flugel KA, Druschky KF. EMG and nerve conduction in patients with acute intermittent porphyria. J Neurol 1977; 214:267–279.

Goldberg A. Molecular genetics of acute intermittent porphyria. Br Med J 1985; 291:499–500.

Gorchein A, Webber R. Delata aminolaevulinic acid in normal, uraemic and porphyric subjects. Clin Sci 1987; 72:103–112.

Hindmarsh JT. The porphyrias: Recent advances. Clin Chem 1986; 32:1255–1263.

Kappas A, Sassa S, Anderson KE. The porphyrias. In: Stanbury JB, Wyngaarden JB, Fredrickson DS, Goldstein JL, Brown MS, eds. The Metabolic Basis of Inherited Disease, 5th ed. New York: McGraw-Hill, 1983:939–1007.

Lee J-S, Anvret M, Lindsten J, et al. DNA polymorphisms within the porphobilinogen deaminase gene in acute intermittent porphyria. Human Genet 1988; 79:379–381.

Llewellyn DH, Elder GH, Kalshekar NA, et al. DNA polymorphism of human porphobilinogen deaminase gene in acute intermittent porphyria. Lancet 1987; 2:706–708.

Moore MR, Disler PB. Drug induction of the acute porphyrias. Adverse Drug React Acute Poisoning Rev 1983; 2:149–189.

Mustajoki P, Desnick RJ. Genetic heterogeneity in acute intermittent porphyria: Characterisation and frequency of porphobilinogen deaminase mutations in Finland. Br Med J 1985; 291:505–509.

Pierach CA, Weimer MK, Cardinal RA, Bossenmaier IC, Blommer JR. Red blood cell porphobilinogen deaminase in the evaluation of acute intermittent porphyria. JAMA 1987; 257:60–61.

Qadri M, Church SE, McColl KEL, Moore MR, Youngs GR. Chester porphyria: A clinical study of a new form of acute porphyria. Br Med J 1986; 292:455–459.

Reynolds NC, Miska RM. Safety of anticonvulsants in hepatic porphyrias. Neurology 1981; 31:480–484.

Ridley A. The neuropathy of acute intermittent porphyria. Q J Med 1969; 1969; 38:307–333.

Rowland LP. Acute intermittent porphyria: search for an enzymatic defect with implications for neurology and psychiatry. Dis Nerv Sys 1961:22 (suppl):1–12.

Thorner PA, Bilbao JM, Sima AAF, Briggs S. Porphyric neuropathy: an ultrastructural and quantitative study. Can J Neurol Sci 1981: 8:261–287.

Tishler PV, Woodward B, O'Connor J, et al. High prevalence of intermittent acute porphyria in a psychiatric patient population. Am J Psychiatry 1985; 142:1430–1436.

Yamada M, Kondo M, Tanaka M, et al. An autopsy case of acute porphyria with a decrease of both uroporphyrinogen I synthetase and ferrochetalase activities. Acta Neuropathol (Berl) 1984; 64:6–11.

Yeung AC, Moore MR, Goldberg A. Pathogenesis of acute porphyria. Q J Med 1987; 163:377–392.

87. ABETALIPOPROTEINEMIA

James F. Schwartz

Abetalipoproteinemia is an inherited disorder of lipid metabolism manifested clinically by a progressive neurologic syndrome of ataxia, dysarthria, areflexia, muscle weakness, impaired proprioception, retinitis pigmentosa, and ophthalmoparesis. Other cardinal manifestations include acanthocytosis (a term that describes the unusual appearance of erythrocytes that have spiny or thorn-like projections), fat malabsorption with steatorrhea, and impaired physical growth. The disease is also called *Bassen-Kornzweig syndrome* after two physicians who described the first patient in 1950. Although the condition is rare it is important because it was one of the first hereditary ataxias in which a basic metabolic abnormality was identified. The primary metabolic defect is inability to synthesize the apoprotein of β-lipoprotein, the major protein of chylomicrons and very-low-density lipoproteins; β-lipoprotein is absent from both plasma and intestinal mucosa. As a consequence, the serum content of lipids is much reduced—including cholesterol, triglycerides and the three major phospholipids, lecithin, cephalin, and sphingomyelin. Other markedly decreased plasma concentrations include low-density and very-low-density lipoproteins and chylomicrons. The concentration of high-density lipoproteins is reduced by about 50% and there are alterations of the protein and lipid compositions of these lipoproteins, too. Another consequence of the markedly decreased chylomicrons and low-density lipoproteins is a severe deficiency of the fat soluble vitamins, A and E.

Signs and Symptoms. The earliest clinical symptom is fatty diarrhea with abdominal distention and impaired physical growth, which is evident in infancy, years before any neurologic symptoms become apparent. Loss of tendon reflexes is the earliest neurologic sign, which is noted by the age of 5. Gait unsteadiness and weakness are evident by the end of the first decade. Subsequently, there is progressive limb ataxia with impaired vibratory and position sensation and mild cutaneous sensory loss in stocking-glove distribution. Both distal and proximal muscle weakness occur, and scoliosis and foot deformities (including pes cavus) are evident by the age of 20. Extensor plantar reflexes have been noted in a few patients.

Abnormal ocular movements with progressive esotropia, paresis of the medial recti, dissociated nystagmus on lateral gaze, and mild ptosis develop insidiously. It is not clear whether the ocular motor abnormalities are primarily myopathic or neuropathic. Retinitis pigmentosa with progressive constriction of visual fields, central scotoma, and gradual reduction of visual acuity occur late in the second decade; electroretinographic studies have shown both rod and cone abnormalities, with rod responses more severely limited and these have been documented before the patients are aware of any visual loss. Signs of cardiomyopathy have been prominent in some patients with EKG abnormalities, cardiac enlargement, and murmurs. Neurophysiologic studies have shown consistently low-sensory nerve action potentials and denervation on needle EMG compatible primarily with axonal peripheral neuropathy. Brain stem auditory evoked potentials are normal. Abnormal somatosensory evoked potentials are consistent with the clinical signs of posterior column damage.

Pathology. Pathologic studies of abetalipoproteinemia have been limited. The neurologic findings of ataxia, dysarthria, impaired proprioception, muscle weakness and wasting, areflexia, and cutaneous sensory loss suggest involvement of cerebellum, posterior columns, and peripheral nerves. Extensor plantar reflexes, which are an inconstant finding, imply lateral column disease. Pathologic findings include marked demyelination of posterior columns and spinocerebellar tracts and, to a lesser extent, the corticospinal tracts. There is also loss of nuclei in the molecular layer of the cerebellum and in Purkinje cells and, to a lesser degree, in anterior horn cells.

Peripheral nerves show focal areas of segmental demyelination; in one patient morphometric analysis revealed a reduction of large myelinated fibers in the sural nerve. No lesions of ocular motor nuclei, pontine reticular formation, or medial longitudinal fasciculus have been described to account for the abnormal eye movement. Interstitial myocardial fibrosis was described in one autopsy.

The erythrocyte malformation, acanthocytosis, affects 50 to 90% of the red cells. The basic defect in the acanthocyte is in the cell membrane that contains increased amounts of sphingomyelin, decreased lecithin, and a profound deficiency of linoleic acid, despite normal total lipids, cholesterol, and phospholipids. Even the normal-appearing erythrocytes in patients with abetalipoproteinemia have the chemical abnormality of red-cell membranes that may be shared by membranes of neural tissues, including the retina.

Acanthocytes are also found in several other neurologic syndromes that differ in clinical and biochemical manifestations. In one form, adult-onset ataxic neuropathy is associated with steatorrhea, reduced but not absent low-density lipoproteins, and acanthocytosis. A less distinct hereditary neurologic syndrome with choreic movements, ataxia, areflexia, muscle weakness, and seizures was described by Levine and associates in a family whose blood contained acanthocytes but had normal plasma lipids and low-density lipoproteins. A third hereditary syndrome with acanthocytosis was described by Critchley and co-workers with manifestations of areflexia, chorea, involuntary tongue and lip-biting, and mental deficiency, but without any disorder of lipid metabolism or plasma lipid concentrations.

Treatment. Treatment of abetalipoproteinemic patients has included dietary manipulation. Restricted intake of long-chain fats by substitution of polyunsaturated fats or medium-chain triglycerides controls the fatty diarrhea and improves nutritional status but not the neurologic disease, even after prolonged diet therapy. Parenteral infusions of lipid emulsions or plasma rich in β-lipoproteins have not produced any clinical improvement. Because there are severe deficiencies of fat-soluble vitamins A, E, and K, it was thought that marked vitamin E deficiency might cause enhanced peroxidation of unsaturated fatty acids with secondary changes in the phospholipids of myelin and other membranes. Similar neurologic abnormalities appear in other forms of vitamin E deficiency and can be reversed by vitamin E therapy.

There is strong evidence that vitamin E deficiency may be the primary cause of the neurologic disorder in abetalipoproteinemia. Patients with abetalipoproteinemia and vitamin E–defcient mammals have identical neuropathologic findings. The clinical and neuropathologic features of abetalipoproteinemia are similar to other chronic fat malabsorption disorders associated with vitamin E deficiency. Also, the arrest of progression of both the retinal and neurologic disease in abetalipoproteinemia patients treated with large doses of oral vitamin E supplements lends credence to the vitamin E deficiency association.

References

Brin MF, Pedley TA, Lovelace RE, et al. Electrophysiologic features of abetalipoproteinemia: Functional consequences of vitamin E deficiency. Neurology 1986; 36:669–673.

Critchley EMR, Clark DB, Wikler A. Acanthocytosis and neurological disorder without abetalipoproteinemia. Arch Neurol 1968; 18:134–140.

Fagan ER, Taylor MJ. Longitudinal multimodal evoked potential studies in abetalipoproteinemia. Can J Neurol Sci 1987; 14:617–621.

Guggenheim MA, Ringel SP, Silverman A, Grabert BE. Progressive neuromuscular disease in children with chronic cholestasis and vitamin E deficiency: Diagnosis and treatment with alpha tocopherol. J Pediatr 1982; 100:51–58.

Herbert PN, Gotto AM, Fredrickson DS. Familial lipoprotein deficiency. In: Stanbury JB, Wyngaarden JB, Fredrickson DS, eds. The Metabolic Basis of Inherited Disease. 5th ed. New York: McGraw-Hill, 1983:589–622.

Levine IM, Estes JW, Looney JM. Hereditary neurological disease with acanthocytosis. Arch Neurol 1968; 19:403–409.

Miller RG, Davis CJ, Illingworth DR, Bradley W. The neuropathology of abetalipoproteinemia. Neurology 1980; 30:86–91.

Muller DPR, Lloyd JK, Wolff OH. The role of vitamin E in the treatment of the neurological features of abetalipoproteinemia and other disorders of fat absorption. J Inherited Metab Dis 1985; (8 Suppl)1:88–92.

Rowland LP. Molecular genetics, pseudogenetics and clinical neurology. Neurology 1983; 33:1179–1195.

Runge P, Muller DP, McAllister J, et al. Oral vitamin E supplements can prevent the retinopathy of abetalipoproteinemia. Br J Ophthalmol 1986; 70:166–173.

Satya-Murti S, Howard L, Krohel G, Wolf B. The spectrum of neurologic disorder from vitamin E deficiency. Neurology 1986; 36:917–921.

Scanu AM. Abetalipoproteinemia: What is the primary defect? Adv Neurol 1978; 21:125–130.

Schwartz JF, Rowland LP, Eder H, et al. Bassen-Kornzweig syndrome: Deficiency of serum B-lipoprotein. Arch Neurol 1963; 8:438–454.

Werlin SL, Harb JM, Swick H, Blank E. Neuromuscular dysfunction and ultrastructural pathology in children with chronic cholestasis and vitamin E deficiency. Ann Neurol 1983; 13:291–296.

88. XERODERMA PIGMENTOSUM

Lewis P. Rowland

This rare condition is not a metabolic disorder in the conventional sense. Rather, cultured cells from affected patients are hypersensitive to being killed or to mutagenesis by ultraviolet light and chemical carcinogens. The disorder is attributed to autosomal recessive inheritance that results in lack of a gene product that is responsible for the excision of damaged DNA or for replication past the damaged site of DNA.

The syndrome was first described by Kaposi in 1874. Affected individuals show marked cutaneous hypersensitivity to sunlight beginning in early childhood. Erythema and blisters are followed by freckling, keratosis, and skin cancers. Neurologic disorders include microcephaly, mental retardation, chorea, ataxia, corticospinal signs, and either motor neuron disorders or segmental demyelination of peripheral nerves. Hearing loss and supranuclear ophthalmoplegia have been prominent in some cases. In others, the neurologic disorder is more disabling than the cutaneous problems (see Section 109, Hereditary Ataxias).

In the only autopsy case, the outstanding change was selective neuronal loss in the cerebral cortex, basal ganglia, olivary nuclei, and cerebellum.

Management includes avoidance of sunlight. Antenatal diagnosis is possible because cultured amniotic cells show the abnormal patterns of excision repair of DNA. There is no effective treatment for the neurologic disorders.

References

Cleaver JE. Xeroderma pigmentosum. In: Stanbury JB, Wyngaarden JB, Fredrickson DS, Goldstein JL, Brown MS, eds. The Metabolic Basis of Inherited Disease, 5th ed. New York: McGraw-Hill, 1982. 1227–1248.

Hakamada S, Watanbe K, Sobue G, Hara K, Miyazaki S. Xeroderma pigmentosum: neurological, neurophysiological and morphological studies. Eur Neurol 1982; 21:69–76.

Kenyon GS, Booth JB, Prasher DK, Rudge P. Neurootological abnormalities in xeroderma pigmentosum with particular reference to deafness. Brain 1985; 108:771–784.

Kraemer KH, Lee MM, Scotto J. Xeroderma pigmentosum. Cutaneous, ocular, and neurologic abnormalities in 830 published cases. Arch Dermatol 1987; 123:241–250.

Neurologic Disorders of Uncertain Etiology or Pathogenesis

Chapter IX

Cerebral Degenerations of Childhood

89. PROGRESSIVE SCLEROSING POLIODYSTROPHY (ALPERS DISEASE)
Isabelle Rapin

It is doubtful that progressive sclerosing poliodystrophy, also known as spongy glioneuronal dystrophy, is a nosologic entity. The term *Alpers disease* is best reserved for children who have intractable seizures, myoclonic jerks, progressive spasticity, and optic atrophy in early infancy and who fail to reach any meaningful developmental milestones. In some cases, the onset is subacute rather than insidious. Affected infants may linger for several years in a vegetable state.

The brain becomes severely shrunken; affected children are microcephalic. CT shows the basal ganglia, thalamus, and cerebellum as hyperdense in contrast to the decreased density of the cerebral hemispheres. Both external and internal hydrocephalus are severe. CSF protein and cell count may be normal or elevated.

Pathologic examination shows severe atrophy of the cortex due to diffuse neuronal loss. Changes are less severe in the basal ganglia, cerebellum, and brain stem. The white matter is demyelinated and gliotic, with severe loss of axons. The long tracts are thin and pale. The neuropil appears spongy because of perivascular and astroglial vacuolation. This predominates in the superficial layers of the cortex and may be severe enough to obliterate cortical lamination. In typical cases, the atrophy is diffuse and does not follow the distribution of the cerebral blood vessels. The end result is a "walnut brain" that may weigh as little as 500 g at autopsy.

Some infants with progressive glioneuronal dystrophy have increased levels of lactic acid in the CSF and, in some cases, in the blood. Several different mitochondrial enzyme deficiencies affecting pyruvate metabolism have been reported in brain, liver, muscle, or fibroblasts in some, but not all, children with the phenotype of Alpers poliodystrophy. A variant associated with liver failure and selective involvement of the visual cortex may be a specific syndrome. Giant mitochondria in the cortex of some infants with the Alpers phenotype and a lipid myopathy in others suggest that this disorder, like Leigh syndrome, Kearns-Sayre syndrome, Friedreich ataxia, and other mitochondrial cytopathies, involves a defect of energy metabolism.

Unfortunately, none of the therapeutic attempts to correct deficiency of pyruvate metabolism have been successful, including high-dose thiamine, lipoic acid, and the ketogenic diet. Because several different diseases probably produce the Alpers phenotype as an end-result, detailed studies of living children are essential if rational therapies are to be devised.

References

Alpers B. Progressive cerebral degeneration in infancy. J Nerv Ment Dis 1960; 130:442–448.

Gabreels PJ, Prick MJ, Trijbels JM, et al. Defects in citric acid cycle and electrontransport chain in progressive poliodystrophy. Acta Neurol Scand 1984; 70:145–154.

Harding BN, Egger J, Portmann B, Erdohazi M. Progressve neuronal degeneration of childhood with liver disease. Brain 1986; 109:181–206.

Janota I. Spongy degeneration of gray matter in three children: Neuropathological report. Arch Dis Child 1974; 49:571–575.

Jellinger K, Seitelberger F. Spongy glio-neuronal dystrophy in infancy and childhood. Acta Neuropathol (Berl) 1970; 16:125–140.

90. SPONGY DEGENERATION OF THE NERVOUS SYSTEM
Isabelle Rapin

This autosomal recessive illness is one of the more common cerebral degenerative diseases of infancy. Although van Bogaert and

Bertrand should be credited with the nosologic identification, it is often called *Canavan disease* in this country. It affects all ethnic groups, but is especially prevalent among Ashkenazi Jews from eastern Poland, Lithuania, and western Russia. One of the most characteristic clinical features, which it shares with Alexander disease and classic Tay-Sachs disease, is megalencephaly. The clinical picture is often sufficiently distinctive to suggest the diagnosis. It is occasionally manifested at birth by severe floppiness; more often, symptoms begin later in the first year. Extremely poor control of the enlarged head, spasticity, optic atrophy, and lack of psychomotor development are the main features. The children may achieve smiling, but they are characteristically quiet and apathetic. Few progress far enough to reach for objects or sit, and none ever walk independently. Seizures or massive myoclonic jerks occur infrequently. By age 2, head growth reaches a plateau as progressive parenchymal destruction leads to hydrocephalus ex vacuo. The children eventually become decerebrate and die of intercurrent illness after a few years in a vegetative state.

CT shows increased lucency of the white matter, poor demarcation of gray and white matter (Fig. 90–1), and later, severe brain atrophy with ventricular enlargement and gaping sulci. CSF and nerve conduction velocities are usually normal. Up to now, cortical biopsy has been needed to verify the diagnosis. The biopsy shows two characteristic abnormalities: intramyelinic vacuolation of the deep layers of the cortex and superficial layers of the white matter, and gigantic abnormal mitochondria that contain a dense filamentous granular matrix and distorted cristae in the watery cytoplasm of hypertrophied astrocytes. Fibrous astrocytes lack the normal histochemical reaction for ATPase. Sponginess eventually becomes diffuse and involves the centrum semiovale, brain stem, cerebellum, and spinal cord. As the disease progresses, the vacuoles enlarge and split the myelin sheath to form cysts that communicate with the extracellular space. This leads to extensive demyelination and tissue destruction with loss of neurons, axons, and oligodendroglia; extensive gliosis follows. Chemical analysis of the brain reveals markedly increased water content, nonspecific loss of myelin and other tissue constituents.

A very recent report indicates that children with spongy degeneration have greatly elevated amounts of N-acetylaspartate in their plasma and excrete it in their urine. Three children with the disease had profound deficiency of aspartocylase in their skin fibroblasts, and it was deficient in the brain of one of them. The enzyme is active in chorionic villi and amniocytes, which suggests that prenatal diagnosis may be possible.

Spongy degeneration of the brain also occurs in other conditions, notably intoxication by triethyl tin or hexachlorophene, some neonatal aminoacidurias and organic acidurias, disorders of pyruvate metabolism, and the Kearns-Sayre syndrome. In fact, cases labelled *juvenile* spongy degeneration that

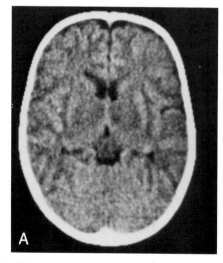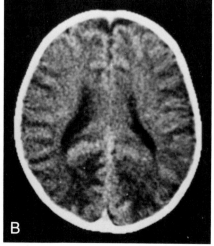

Fig. 90–1. Axial noncontrast CT scans of 11-month-old boy with spongy degeneration. Note diffuse low density of white matter with occipital preponderance and poor demarcation between gray and white matter. Sulci are mildly widened.

started in childhood with external ophthal-moplegia and pigmentary degeneration of the retina, with or without other neurologic or systemic abnormalities may be Kearns-Sayre syndrome or some other mitochondrial dis-order. Giant mitochondria have also been seen in children with the phenotype of Alpers disease. Nosologic classification based on morphology is clearly inadequate and will re-main so until the biochemical pathology of all these conditions is clarified.

References

Adachi M, Schneck L, Cara J, Volk BW. Spongy degen-eration of the central nervous system (von Bogaert and Bertrand type; Canavan's disease): a review. Hum Pathol 1973; 4:331–347.

Banker BQ, Robertson JT, Victor M. Spongy degeneration of the central nervous system in infancy. Neurology 1964; 14:981–1001.

van Bogaert L., Bertrand I. Spongy Degeneration of the Brain in Infancy. Springfield: CC Thomas, 1967.

Jellinger K, Seitelberger F. Juvenile form of spongy de-generation of the CNS. Acta Neuropathol (Berl) 1969; 13:276–281.

Johnson AB. Deficiency of ATPase-positive astrocytic processes in spongy degeneration of the nervous system (Canavan's disease). J Neuropathol Exp Neu-rol 1970; 29:136.

Kamoshita S, Rapin I, Suzuki K, Suzuki K. Spongy de-generation of the brain: A chemical study of two cases including isolation and characterization of my-elin. Neurology 1968; 18:975–985.

Matalon R, Michals K, Sebesta D, Deanching M, Gash-koff P, Casanova J. Aspartoacylase deficiency and N-acetylaspartic aciduria in patients with Canavan dis-ease. Am J Med Genet 1988; 29:463–471.

Ungar M, Goodman, RM. Spongy degeneration of the brain in Israel: A retrospective study. Clin Genet 1983; 23:23–29.

91. INFANTILE NEURAXONAL DYSTROPHY
Isabelle Rapin

Infantile neuraxonal dystrophy *(Seitelberger disease)* is an autosomal recessive disease that typically become manifest between the ages of 6 and 18 months and leads to death before the end of the first decade, usually after a variable period of purely vegetative existence. The first symptom is arrest of motor devel-opment, which is followed by loss of skills. The children may be floppy or spastic or show a combination of both. Most never achieve independent walking or speaking. In some, the motor disorder progresses from the legs to the arms and finally to the cranial muscles, causing severe dysphagia. There may be loss of sensation in the legs and urinary retention. Ataxia, nystagmus, and optic atrophy are

common, but seizures are relatively rare. The degree of dementia is difficult to ascertain be-cause of anarthria; at first, affected children appear alert and seem to understand some language, but intellectual deterioration even-tually becomes severe.

Atypical variants occur. A few infants are symptomatic from birth, whereas others ex-perience a later onset and more protracted course, some with prominent myoclonus, others with dystonic features. The relation-ship of these more chronic cases to Haller-vorden-Spatz disease is controversial. Some researchers consider neuraxonal dystrophy and Hallervorden-Spatz disease to be the same nosologic entity because spheroid for-mation is seen in both and because there are clinical similarities. However, spheroids are not pathognomonic of either disease and the distribution of these lesions differs in the two disorders; brown discoloration of the globus pallidus occurs only in Hallervorden-Spatz disease. The typical forms of the two diseases are clinically distinct. The disease tends to run a similar course in siblings, whereas affected individuals in families with atypical variants differ, which argues for genetic heterogene-ity. The absence of a biochemical marker makes it impossible to resolve the question of the disease's relation to Hallervorden-Spatz disease.

The characteristic pathologic picture of neuraxonal dystrophy is the profusion of ax-onal spheroids in the brain, spinal cord, and peripheral nerves. Spheroids are eosino-philic, argyrophilic, ovoid inclusions that dis-tend axons and myelin sheaths. They may be found anywhere along axons, but are espe-cially numerous in axon terminals, including at the neuromuscular junction. Electron-mi-croscopy shows that they contain tubular structures, vesicles, and masses of smooth membranes that are arranged in stacks or, less often, in circular concentric arrays. The rela-tion of these structures to synaptic vesicles or smooth endoplasmic reticulum is speculative. Spheroids also contain membrane-bound clefts and accumulations of mitochondria. Spheroids are particularly prevalent in the cerebellum, basal ganglia, thalamus, cuneate, gracile, and the brain-stem nuclei. The cere-bellum is strikingly atrophic because of loss of Purkinje and granular cells. The basal gan-glia show neuronal loss and may appear spongy, with demyelinated axons and sphe-roid deposition. Although lipopigment gran-ules are found in basal ganglia, there is no discoloration visible to the naked eye. The long tracts of the visual system, corticospinal system, spinocerebellar pathways, and posterior columns are degenerated, and there is pallor of the myelin. No characteristic lesions have been described in the viscera. Biochemical changes found in the brain are viewed as nonspecific.

Laboratory tests are not very helpful. The CSF is usually normal; EEG changes are absent or nonspecific. Nerve conduction velocities may be normal or slow. EMGs usually suggest denervation. Definite diagnosis requires autopsy. Nerve, muscle, rectal, or conjunctival biopsy is confirmatory when spheroids are found in nerves or at the neuromuscular junction but, because of sampling problems, normal peripheral nerve or even cortical biopsy does not exclude the diagnosis. Because nothing is known of the pathogenesis of this illness, there is no chemical or enzymatic test available; intrauterine diagnosis is not feasible. Treatment is limited to symptomatic measures and to the providing of support and genetic counseling to the child's family.

References

Arsénio-Nunes ML, Goutières F. Diagnosis of infantile neuroaxonal dystrophy by conjunctival biopsy. J Neurol Neurosurg Psychiatry 1978; 41:511–515.

Dorfman LJ, Pedley TA, Tharp BR, Scheithauer BW. Juvenile neuroaxonal dystrophy: Clinical, electrophysiological, and neuropathological features. Ann Neurol 1978; 3:419–428.

Gilman S, Barrett RE. Hallervorden-Spatz disease and infantile neuroaxonal dystrophy. J Neurol Sci 1973; 19:189–205.

Herman MH, Huttenlocher PR, Bensh KG. Electronmicrosopic observations in infantile neuroaxonal dystrophy: Report of a cortical biopsy and review of the recent literature. Arch Neurol 1969; 20:19–34.

Martin JJ, Martin L. Infantile neuroaxonal dystrophy: Ultrastructural study of the peripheral nerves and of the motor end plates. Eur Neurol 1972; 8:239–250.

Scheithauer BW, Forno LS, Dorfman LJ, Lane CA. Neuroaxonal dystrophy (Seitelberger's disease) with late onset, protracted course and myoclonic epilepsy. J Neurol Sci 1978; 36:247–258.

92. HALLERVORDEN-SPATZ DISEASE
Isabelle Rapin

Hallervorden-Spatz disease is an insidiously progressive, autosomal recessive disease of childhood and adolescence in which motor symptoms predominate. It usually presents with stiffness of gait and is eventually associated with distal wasting, pes cavus or equinovarus, and toe-walking. The arms are held stiffly with hyperextended fingers; the hands may become useless when the child is still ambulatory. The children often have a characteristically frozen, pained expression with risus sardonicus and contracted platysma muscles. They speak through clenched teeth and have difficulty eating. Eventually, they become anarthric, although they continue to understand language. Muscle tone is both spastic and rigid, often with painful spasms, yet passive movement with the patient supine reveals an underlying hypotonia. Reflexes are hyperactive, including facial reflexes, and the toes are usually, but not always, upgoing. Some children become dystonic and assume bizarre postures that suggest dystonia musculorum deformans. Ataxia, tremor, nystagmus, and facial grimacing are seen in some patients, usually early in the illness. Pigmentary degeneration of the retina occurs in some families; in others the eyegrounds are normal or show primary optic atrophy. Assessing intellectual function is difficult; affected children remain alert and, if it occurs, dementia may not be severe. Death is usually due to an intercurrent illness that is poorly tolerated by the emaciated and immobilized patient.

The course of the illness typically spans a dozen years. Death occasionally supervenes after only 6 to 8 years; survival may extend over several decades. Variants with mid- or late-adult onset and symptoms reminiscent of Parkinson disease also occur. The several clinical variants, with relatively stereotyped course within families, suggest genetic heterogeneity.

Once the illness is full-blown, the clinical picture is sufficiently characteristic to suggest the diagnosis. Demonstration of increased uptake of the iron isotope ^{59}Fe by scanning the basal ganglia is said to be confirmatory. Definite diagnosis requires autopsy because the biochemical basis of the illness is unknown. CT shows mild atrophy with flattening of the caudate nucleus. Magnetic resonance (MR) demonstrates nonspecific changes in the globus pallidus. Prenatal diagnosis is not available and therapy is limited to symptomatic measures.

The pathology is so restricted in distribution that biopsy diagnosis is not practical. Olive or golden-brown discoloration of the medial segment of the globus pallidus is the macroscopic hallmark of Hallervorden-Spatz disease. Less striking discoloration occurs in the red nucleus and zona reticulata of the substantia nigra. This appearance is due to granules of an iron-containing lipopigment (similar to neuromelanin) that are located inside and outside the neurons and hyperplastic astrocytes. Irregular mulberry concretions, some calcified, lie free in the tissue. Increased amounts of iron and other metals (e.g., zinc, copper) and calcium are found in the affected tissue, which contains axonal spheroids identical to those seen in neuraxonal dystrophy. Neuronal loss and thinning of myelin sheaths are prominent in the globus pallidus, less severe in the rest of the basal ganglia, and uncommon elsewhere, although mild cerebellar atrophy does occur. Spheroids are found in small numbers of the cerebral cortex.

References

Elejalde BR, Elejalde MMJ, Lopez F. Hallervorden-Spatz disease. Clin Genet 1979; 16:1–18.

Jankovic J, Kirkpatrick JB, Blomqvist KA, Langlais PJ, Bird ED. Late-onset Hallervorden-Spatz disease presenting as familial parkinsonism. Neurology 1985; 35:227–234.

Littrup PJ, Gebarski SS. MR imaging of Hallervorden-Spatz disease. J Comput Assist Tomogr 1985; 9:491–493.

Newell FW, Johnson RO II, Huttenlocher PR. Pigmentary degeneration of the retina in Hallervorden-Spatz syndrome. Am J Ophthalmol 1979; 88:467–471.

Swaiman KF, Smith SA, Trock GL, Siddiqui AR. Hallervorden-Spatz disease or ceroid storage disease with abnormal isotope scan? Neurology 1983; 33:301–306.

Szanto J, Gallyas F. A study of iron metabolism in neuropsychiatric patients. Hallervorden-Spatz disease. Arch Neurol 1966; 14:438–442.

Tennison MB, Bouldin TW, Whaley RA. Mineralization of the basal ganglia detected by CT in Hallervorden-Spatz syndrome. Neurology 1988; 38:154–155.

Wigboldus JM and Bruyn GW. Hallervorden-Spatz disease. In: Vinken PJ, Bruyn GW, eds. Handbook of Clinical Neurology (vol 6). New York: Elsevier-North Holland, 1968: 604–631.

93. PELIZAEUS-MERZBACHER DISEASE

Isabelle Rapin

Two clinical forms of Pelizaeus-Merzbacher disease, both X-linked recessive, are recognized; one is present at birth, the so-called *connatal variant* of Seitelberger, and the other is an infantile variant with a more protracted course, which is the *classic form*. In addition, some cases that clinically and histologically resemble Pelizaeus-Merzbacher disease have been described in girls. These autosomal recessive phenocopies and the report of patients with late onset and protracted course strongly suggest genetic heterogeneity.

A prominent, irregular nystagmus and head-tremor or head-rolling from birth or the first few months of life are the most striking features of both forms of the illness. In the connatal form, these symptoms are associated with floppiness, headlag, grayness of the optic discs, and stridor. Meaningful development does not occur. The boys develop ataxia, severe spasticity, and optic atrophy. Seizures, microcephaly, and failure to thrive supervene, and most infants succumb in the first years of life. Others survive for 8 to 12 years but are mute with limited intellect, despite apparent alertness. In the classic form, slow motor development may enable the children to reach for objects, roll over, crawl, and say a few words. Independent ambulation is not achieved; even these few developmental milestones are lost as increasing ataxia, spasticity with hyperreflexia, and choreoathetotic movements develop. By school age the affected boy is usually mute and confined to a wheelchair.

Affected boys are likely to develop kyphoscoliosis and joint contractures; they become incontinent. Sensory loss does not occur. Dementia is difficult to assess but may not be profound. Optic atrophy is not severe. Hearing is preserved. Despite severe growth failure and small muscle mass, there is little further deterioration until the patient dies of an intercurrent illness, usually in late adolescence or early adulthood.

Normal nerve conduction velocities and usually normal CSF protein help differentiate the connatal variant from Krabbe disease and metachromatic leukodystrophy. The prominent nystagmus is the main differentiating symptom from infantile neuraxonal dystrophy and early-onset Hallervorden-Spatz disease. The EEG is normal or mildly slow. CT shows ventricular dilatation, decreased differentiation between gray and white matter, and cerebellar atrophy. The diagnosis can be made by cerebral biopsy.

At autopsy, the brain, cerebellum, brain stem, and spinal cord of children with the connatal variant are essentially devoid of myelin. In the late infantile variant, characteristic changes are limited to the white matter of the cerebral hemispheres and cerebellum; a so-called tigroid appearance is seen on myelin stains because islands of preserved myelin are found against a nonmyelinated background. The brain stem and spinal cord may show pallor of long fiber tracts, but are otherwise normal. There is no sparing of U-fibers in either type and the demarcation of gray and white matter is blurred in both. Axons are present in the demyelinated areas and are almost devoid of oligodendroglia. Sparse myelin-breakdown products are seen as sudanophilic-lipid droplets consisting of cholesterol esters. The severity of gliosis varies with the duration of the illness. The cerebral cortex is preserved, although large pyramids in layer V of the motor cortex (Betz cells) may be lacking in the connatal form. Neuronal dropout is not severe, with the possible exception of granular cell loss in the cerebellum where axon torpedoes may be seen in Purkinje cells. Areas of cerebral dysgenesis and micropolygyria have been observed too often to be coincidental. Peripheral nerves are characteristically well myelinated, which suggests that the disease may affect oligodendroglia rather than myelin. Chemical studies have shown only a decrease in myelin components, especially extra-long-chain fatty acids. There is a drastic reduction of proteolipid protein in the connatal variant (and in rodent models of the disease).

Pelizaeus-Merzbacher disease has been classified among the sudanophilic leukodystrophies. The course of the illness suggests progressive deterioration, although it has not been established whether it results from a failure of myelination or from demyelination with accelerated breakdown of an unstable myelin. Because the pathogenesis of the disease is unknown, genetic counseling is limited to an explanation of recurrence risks in families in which the patterns of inheritance and diagnosis are clear.

References

Garg BP, Markand OH, DeHyer WE. Usefulness of BAER studies in early diagnosis of Pelizaeus-Merzbacher disease. Neurology 1983; 33:955–956.

Koepper AH, Ronca NA, Greenfield EA, Hans MB. Defective biosynthesis of proteolipid protein in Pelizaeus-Merzbacher disease. Ann Neurol 1987; 21:159–170.

Renier WO, Gabreëls FJM, Hastinx TWJ, et al. Connatal Pelizaeus-Merzbacher disease with congenital stridor in two maternal cousins. Acta Neuropathol (Berl) 1981; 54:11–17.

Seitelberger F. Pelizaeus-Merzbacher disease. In: Vinken PJ, Bruyn GW, eds. Handbook of Clinical Neurology (vol 10). New York: Elsevier-North Holland, 1970: 150–202.

Witter B, Debuch H, Klein H. Lipid investigation of central and peripheral nervous system myelin in connatal Pelizaeus-Merzbacher disease. J Neurochem 1980; 34:957–962.

Yokoi S, Amano N, Oanawa H, Isoyama K, Ishikawa A, Ogino T. Postnatal sudanophilic leukodystrophy in two siblings. Acta Neuropathol 1985; 67:103–113.

94. ALEXANDER DISEASE
Isabelle Rapin

Two main variants of Alexander disease, which appears to affect astrocytes primarily, occur in children. The first is a rapidly progressive *infantile variant* that causes megalencephaly, severe motor and developmental deficits, and seizures. The large head is usually due to an enlarged brain, but some develop hydrocephalus and signs of increased intracranial pressure with lethargy and vomiting due to an obstruction of the aqueduct of Sylvius by Rosenthal fibers. The children are usually, but not invariably, spastic. Most die in a vegetative state in infancy or during the preschool years. A few children survive into the second decade. CT suggests the diagnosis when there is marked demyelination with frontal predominance, especially if there are enlarged ventricles with a zone of increased density in the subependymal region (Fig. 94–1). Occasionally, the basal ganglia appear necrotic on CT, as in the infantile variant of Leigh disease. The main differential diagnosis is spongy degeneration, which is suggested by the enlarged head, early dementia, and decreased density of the white matter, although optic atrophy is not characteristic of Alexander disease. Autosomal recessive inheritance is suggested by some pedigrees, but there is an unexplained predominance of affected boys and sporadic cases. No clear instance of an X-linked inheritance is known.

The *juvenile variant* (or variants) may resemble the infantile variant, except for a later onset and a more indolent, protracted course (usually without seizures), or it may present like some adult cases, all of which are sporadic, with signs of bulbar palsy and ataxia, with or without intellectual deterioration and spasticity. Few of these late-onset cases are familial, and both sexes are equally affected. It is not even clear that these adult cases should be classified with the infantile cases with megalencephaly because only the pathology is similar.

The pathogenesis and chemical pathology of this illness are unknown. Thus, it is defined by the principal histologic characteristic, the so-called *Rosenthal fibers*, which are hyaline, eosinophilic, and argyrophilic inclusions found exclusively in astrocytic footplates. They are characteristically distributed in subpial, subependymal, and perivascular locations. In some cases, especially in infants, the

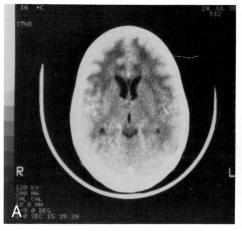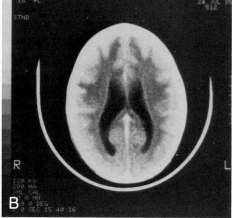

Fig. 94–1. Axial contrast CT scans of 29-month-old girl with Alexander disease. Note low density of white matter with frontal to occipital gradient and increased periventricular density.

fibers are found diffusely in the brain and spinal cord; in others, especially the juvenile and adult cases, they are restricted to the brain stem and spinal cord, especially the floor of the fourth ventricle. Demyelination, with loss of oligodendroglia and sparing of axons, occurs in regions rich in Rosenthal fibers. In infantile cases, demyelination of the centrum semiovale is so severe that it may lead to cavitation; loss of myelin is most severe frontally and has a characteristic frontal-to-occipital gradient. The myelin of peripheral nerves is spared. Neurons are also spared with the exception of brain-stem motor neurons in some juvenile and adult cases with bulbar symptoms and of basal ganglia neurons in some infantile cases. No characteristic biochemical abnormality has been reported except for the loss of myelin constituents in cases with severe demyelination. The fibers are proteinaceous, but whether they are derived from degraded glial filaments is not certain.

Rosenthal fibers are not pathognomonic of this illness; they occur in pilocytic astrocytomas, are rarely associated with multiple-sclerosis plaques, and have been reported in adolescents and adults without known neurologic symptoms. Rosenthal fiber formation has been induced in rats by the implantation of wires made of nickel but not of other metals. Diagnosis may be made on clinical grounds and by cortical biopsy. Prenatal diagnosis is not yet possible. Therapy remains purely symptomatic.

References

Borrett D, Becker LE. Alexander disease: A disease of astrocytes. Brain 1985; 108:367–385.

Escourolle R, DeBaecque C, Gray F, Baumann N, Hauw J-J. Etude en microscopie électronique et neurochimique d'un cas de maladie d'Alexander. Acta Neuropathol (Berl) 1979; 45:133–140.

Holland IM, Kendall BE. Computed tomography in Alexander's disease. Neuroradiology 1980; 20:103–106.

Kress Y, Gaskin F, Houroupian DS, Grosman C. Nickel induction of Rosenthal fibers in cat brain. Brain Res 1981; 210:419–425.

Russo LS Jr, Aron A, Anderson PJ. Alexander's disease: A report and reappraisal. Neurology 1976; 26:607–614.

95. COCKAYNE SYNDROME
Isabelle Rapin

Cockayne syndrome is a progressive multisystem disease with autosomal recessive inheritance characterized by extreme dwarfing, a peculiar cachectic appearance, and neurologic deterioration. The children are of normal size at birth. Failure to thrive and grow with progressive drop-off of health, weight, and head circumference to many standard deviations below the mean becomes apparent before the child reaches 2 years of age. Affected children have an arresting facies with large ears, long aquiline nose, deep set eyes, thin lips, and jutting chin; the appearance is often accentuated by the loss of severely carious teeth. Some children have atrophic or hyperpigmented skin changes over exposed areas, especially the face. Body proportions, although miniature, are appropriate for the child's age. Signs of maturation, such as the shedding of deciduous teeth and puberty, occur on time, although testes and breasts are usually underdeveloped. The children may suffer from carbohydrate intolerance and anomalies of renal function. Most of these children survive at least into the second decade.

Intellectual development is extremely limited, but affected children remain alert and have pleasant personalities. Most do not speak and many do not walk independently because of progressive spasticity, widespread joint contractures, and deformities of the feet. Some have signs of a peripheral neuropathy and are ataxic. Many become deaf and vision is impaired as the result of variable combinations of corneal opacity, cataract, pigmentary degeneration of the retina, and optic atrophy. The pupils are miotic and respond poorly to mydriatics. Tearing is reduced or absent. Plain radiographs of the skull and CT typically show stippled calcification in the basal ganglia. Nerve conduction velocities are slow and CSF protein may be elevated. Because not all children who are considered to have Cockayne syndrome have all of the described signs, it may not be genetically homogenous. Therapy is purely symptomatic.

The diagnosis is suggested by the clinical features. The main differential diagnosis is Seckel (bird-headed) dwarfs, who are invariably dwarfed at birth with extremely low weights for gestational age; they do not suffer from progressive physical and neurologic deterioration; they learn to walk and speak despite their extreme microcephaly; they are less retarded than children with Cockayne syndrome but share similar dysmorphic features. Children with progeria are usually normally intelligent and have much more prominent signs of premature aging than children with Cockayne syndrome, who do not lose their hair, for example, even though mild, early graying can occur.

Brains of children with Cockayne syndrome (and those of Seckel dwarfs) are tiny, weighing about 500 g. A prominent feature is extreme thinness of the white matter, which has a tigroid aspect on myelin stains because of islands of myelinated fibers amid areas without myelin, a pattern reminiscent of that seen in Pelizaeus-Merzbacher disease. Calcification of the basal ganglia and cerebellar atrophy are typical. Developmental anomalies include areas of deficient gyration of the neocortex and hippocampus, defective cell migration and cortical lamination, and evidence of diffuse neuronal and axonal loss. These findings indicate that the disease starts prenatally, despite allegedly normal head circumference and development in infancy.

Other pathology features include grotesque dendrites of Purkinje cells and multinucleated astrocytes. Although the disease is clearly progressive, it is characterized by both developmental anomalies and degenerative changes. Fibroblasts and amniocytes of children with Cockayne syndrome are hypersensitive to ultraviolet radiation. This characteristic has been exploited for prenatal diagnosis and to demonstrate genetic heterogeneity in this disease. A few children suffer from both Cockayne disease and xeroderma pigmentosum, another disease affecting DNA repair mechanisms; these children are sensitive to both ultraviolet light and ionizing radiation.

References

Cockayne EA. Dwarfism with retinal atrophy and deafness. Arch Dis Child 1946; 21:52–54.

Giannelli F. DNA maintenance and its relation to human pathology. J Cell Sci 1986; (Suppl)4:383–416.

Goldstein S. Human genetic disorders which feature accelerated aging. In: Schneider EL, ed. The Genetics of Aging. New York: Plenum Press, 1978.

Kraemer KH, Lee MM, Scotto J. Xeroderma pigmentosum. Cutaneous, ocular, and neurologic abnormalities in 830 published cases. Arch Dermatol 1987; 123:241–250.

Lehmann AR, Francis AJ, Giannelli P. Prenatal diagnosis of Cockayne's syndrome. Lancet 1985; 1:486–488.

Seckel HPG. Birdheaded Dwarfism. Basel: Karger, 1960.

Sofer D, Grotsky HW, Rapin I. Suzuki K. Cockayne syndrome: Unusual pathological findings and review of the literature. Ann Neurol 1979; 6:340–348.

96. ZELLWEGER SYNDROME AND OTHER PEROXISOMAL DISEASES
Isabelle Rapin

Peroxisomal Diseases

Peroxisomes are subcellular organelles surrounded by a single membrane that are present in virtually all cell types. They are particularly prominent in hepatocytes and renal tubular cells but are also demonstrable in fibroblasts, amniocytes, retinal pigment epithelium, astrocytes, oligodendroglia, and neurons. At least 40 enzymes are localized in peroxisomes, some in their matrix, others membrane-bound. Peroxisomes contain catalase, a variety of oxidases (in particular phytanic acid and very long chain fatty acid β-oxidases), and enzymes required for synthesis of bile acids and plasmalogens and the degradation of pipecolic acid.

Many genetic-metabolic diseases of the nervous system are known to be associated

Table 96–1. Neurologic Diseases with Peroxisomal Defects

Disease Classification

Absent or malformed peroxisomes
   Zellweger cerebrohepatorenal syndrome
   Neonatal adrenoleukodystrophy
   Infantile Refsum syndrome
   Cerebrotendinous xanthomatosis
   Leber congenital amaurosis?

Structurally normal peroxisomes
   Adrenoleukodystrophy and adrenomyelo-
     neuropathy
   Classic Refsum disease
   Pseudo-Zellweger disease

with abnormalities of peroxisomal structure or enzymatic activity (Table 96–1). A single peroxisomal enzyme is inactive in some diseases while in others, notably Zellweger and infantile adrenoleukodystrophy, peroxisomes are absent or malformed and multiple peroxisomal enzymes are deficient. Mitochondria and peroxisomes are malformed with deficient mitochondrial enzyme activities in some disorders. How abnormalities in these two distinct organelles are related is unknown. There appears to be a defect in the import of matrix proteins into the organelle in Zellweger disease.

Zellweger Syndrome

The Zellweger syndrome (cerebrohepatorenal syndrome) is an autosomal recessive disease that seems to have no racial predilection. It is manifest at birth. Affected infants are strikingly floppy and inactive and lack Moro, stepping, and placing reflexes. The facial appearance is characteristic with a high narrow forehead, round cheeks, flat root of the nose, wide-set eyes with shallow orbits, puffy eyelids, corneal opacities, pursed lips, narrow high-arched palate, and small chin. The head circumference is normal but the fontanelles and sutures are widely open. The pinnas may be abnormal and posteriorly rotated. Affected infants suck and swallow so poorly that they often require tube feeding. Some have congenital heart disease, notably patent ductus arteriosus or septal defects. The liver is cirrhotic and either enlarged or shrunken; some children are jaundiced and some develop splenomegaly and a bleeding diathesis. Cystic dysplasia. of the kidneys may be palpable and may cause mild renal failure. Genital anomalies include an enlarged clitoris, hypospadias, and cryptorchidism.

Minor skeletal anomalies such as contractures of large and small joints, polydactyly, low-set rotated thumbs, and club feet are typical, as are stippled calcifications of the patella and epiphyseal cartilage. The children are apathetic, poorly responsive to environmental stimuli, and limp. Tendon reflexes are absent or hypoactive. Many children have seizures, and fail to thrive or develop; most succumb within the first few months of life.

Typical, but nonspecific, laboratory findings include elevated bilirubin, abnormal liver function tests, elevated serum iron, saturated iron binding-capacity, and transferrin. The CSF protein may be elevated. The EEG is abnormal and CT scans show poor myelination and brain atrophy. Signs of peroxisomal dysfunction include elevated levels of several acids: C_{26} and C_{24} long chain fatty acids, trihydroxycoprostanic—a bile acid precursor, pipecolic, and, to a lesser extent, of phytanic acid. Plasmalogen levels are markedly reduced in many tissues. The mitochondrial electron transport chain is blocked at the succinate ubiquinone oxidoreductase step.

The absence of peroxisomes in hepatocytes is a pathognomonic feature of Zellweger syndrome and one that helps distinguish it from closely related peroxisomal diseases of infancy such as pseudo-Zellweger disease, neonatal adrenoleukodystrophy, and hyperpipecolic acidemia. Mitochondria have an abnormally dense matrix and distorted cristae. Lipid leaflets resembling those in adrenoleukodystrophy are found in several tissues, including the adrenal gland. The brain is dysgenetic with signs of disordered cell migration that results in areas of pachygyria or micropolygyria and neuronal ectopias. The inferior olive is grossly disorganized. Myelination is severely affected. Neutral fat accumulates in fibrous astrocytes, hepatocytes, renal tubules and glomeruli, and muscle. Intrauterine diagnosis is available, but therapy is purely symptomatic.

References

Goldfisher S, Collins J, Rapin I, et al. Pseudo-Zellweger syndrome: Deficiencies in several peroxisomal oxidative activities. J Pediatr 1986; 108:25–32.

Goldfisher S, Moore CL, Johnson AB, et al. Peroxisomal and mitochondrial defects in the cerebro-hepatorenal syndrome. Science 1973; 182:62–64.

Govaerts L, Monnens L, Tegelaers W, Trijbels F, Raay-Selten AV. Cerebro-hepato-renal syndrome of Zellweger: clinical symptoms and laboratory findings in 16 patients. Eur J Pediatr 1982; 139:125–128.

Kelley RI. Review: The cerebrohepatorenal syndrome of

Zellweger, morphologic and metabolic aspects. Am J Med Genet 1983; 16:503–517.

Moser HW, Goldfisher SL. The peroxisomal disorders. Hop Prac 1985; 20:61–70.

Moser HW. The peroxisome: nervous system role of a previously underrated organelle. Neurology 1988; 38:1617–1627.

Moser AE, Singh I, Brown FR III, et al. The cerebrohepatorenal (Zellweger) syndrome: Increased levels and impaired degradation of very-long fatty acids and their use in prenatal diagnosis. N Engl J Med 1984; 310:1141–1146.

Santos MJ, Imahaka T, Shio H, et al. Peroxisomal membrane ghosts in Zellweger syndrome—aberrant organelle assembly. Science 1988; 239:1536–1538.

Schram AW, Goldfisher S, van Roermund CWT, et al. Human peroxisomal 3-oxoacyl-coenzyme A thiolase deficiency. Proc Nat Acad Sci USA 1987; 84:2494–2496.

Shutgens RBH, Heymans HSA, Wanders RJA, et al. Prenatal diagnosis of the cerebro-hepato-renal (Zellweger) syndrome by detection of an impaired plasmalogen biosynthesis. J Inherit Metab Dis 1985; (Suppl 2)153–145.

Trijbels JMF, Berden JA, Monnens L, et al. Biochemical studies in the liver and muscle of patients with Zellweger syndrome. Pediatr Res 1983; 17:514–517.

Versmold HT, Bremer HJ, Herzog V, et al. A metabolic disorder similar to Zellweger syndrome with hepatic acatalasia and absence of peroxisomes, altered content and redox state of cytochromes, and infantile cirrhosis with hemosiderosis. Eur J Pediatr 1977; 124:261–275.

Volpe JJ, Adams RD. Cerebro-hepato-renal syndrome of Zellweger: An inherited disorder of neuronal migration. Acta Neuropathol (Berl) 1972; 20:175–198.

Wanders RJA, Schrakamp G, van den Bosch H, et al. A prenatal test for the cerebro-hepato-renal (Zellweger) syndrome by demonstration of the absence of catalase-containing particles (peroxisomes) in cultures of amniotic cells. Eur J Pediatr 1986; 145:136–138.

97. NECROTIZING ENCEPHALOMYELOPATHY AND LACTIC ACIDOSIS

Darryl C. DeVivo

Neurologic diseases associated with disturbances of pyruvate metabolism are being recognized with increasing frequency. The clinical phenotype varies from infantile lactic acidosis with severe psychomotor retardation to catastrophic neurologic deterioration in an otherwise healthy adult. The broad clinical spectrum and the complexity of the metabolic pathways have contributed to the current confusion about the pathophysiology and nosology of these disorders.

In 1951, Leigh described a 7-month-old infant with necrotizing lesions in the brain stem that resembled Wernicke encephalopathy. Many similar reports followed; the necrotic lesions are located in the periaqueductal areas of the midbrain and pons and in the substance of the medulla adjacent to the fourth ventricle (Table 97–1). The cerebrum, basal ganglia, thalamus, cerebellum, and central portion of the spinal cord may also be affected as may be peripheral nerves or muscle. The prominent histopathologic features include cell necrosis, demyelination, and vascular proliferation. The vascular changes and the characteristic topography of the lesions are distinctive. Pathologically, subacute necrotizing encephalomyelopathy differs from Wernicke disease because of the relative sparing of the hypothalamus and mamillary bodies.

Necrotizing encephalomyelopathy is uncommon. In several familial cases, especially in infants and children, the disorder appears to be inherited as an autosomal recessive trait. Adult cases are usually sporadic. The onset of symptoms is often insidious. Some infants develop normally for several months; others show evidence of neurologic damage from early infancy. Respiratory abnormality, a poor cry, and impairment of feeding may be observed early. Later, impairment of vision and hearing, ataxia, muscular weakness and hypotonia, progressive intellectual deterioration, and seizures can appear. Eye movement abnormalities (including rotatory nystagmus) are common, but external ophthalmoplegia is rare. Dystonia or ataxia may be the dominant clinical feature in older children. Affected patients usually die in the first few years, but some patients live until the third decade.

Routine laboratory examinations usually

Table 97–1. Comparison of Distribution of Brain Lesions in Subacute Necrotizing Encephalomyelopathy and Wernicke Disease

	SNE (%)	WD (%)
Brainstem	98	85
Midbrain	90	72
Tegmentum	78	
Substantia nigra	62	5
Pons	92	36
Medulla	84	58
Spinal cord	74	33
Cerebellum	58	19
Cerebrum	92	97
Cortex	10	33
Basal ganglia	65	11
Thalamus	51	68
Hypothalamus	27	97
Mamillary bodies	16	96

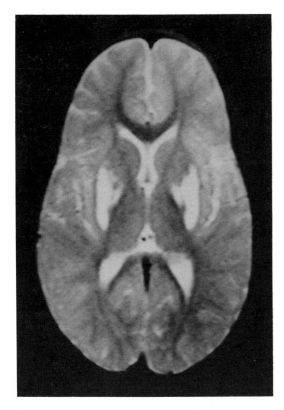

Fig. 97–1. MR scan. 2-year-old girl with cytochrome C oxidase deficiency and Leigh syndrome. Prominent signal abnormality is evident in heavily T2-weighted image with bilaterally symmetric involvement of basal ganglia. Putaminal involvement is characteristic of Leigh syndrome.

are not helpful. CSF protein content is mildly elevated in about 25% of the cases. Lactate and pyruvate are almost invariably elevated in CSF and, to a lesser degree, in blood and urine. The constancy of this finding and the resemblance of the pathology to Wernicke disease have focused attention on an inherited defect of pyruvate metabolism. The EEG may show nonspecific changes. Evoked potentials of auditory, visual, and somatosensory systems are often abnormal. CT may show symmetric lucencies in the basal ganglia and thalamus, and the ventricles may be enlarged. MRI demonstrates the distinctive topography of the brain lesions in exquisite detail (Fig. 97–1).

The biochemical defects underlying Leigh disease involve cerebral oxidative metabolism. Defective regulation of the thiamine-dependent pyruvate dehydrogenase complex has been reported and provides a central theme unifying the two clinical disorders that show similar pathology. Cytochrome C oxi-

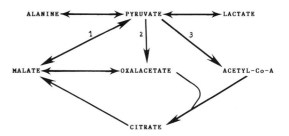

Fig. 97–2. Overlapping clinical phenotypes involving disturbances of pyruvate metabolism: mitochondrial malic enzyme (1); pyruvate carboxylase (2); and pyruvate dehydrogenase multienzyme complex (3).

dase deficiency also has been reported in cases of Leigh disease. This enzyme deficiency is partial and cross-reacting material is present in the affected tissue. Ragged-red fibers are conspicuously absent in the biopsied skeletal muscle of these patients. The association between pyruvate carboxylase deficiency and Leigh disease is more tenuous. This enzyme was linked to Leigh disease in 1968. Subsequent reports have described a different neuropathology associated with this biochemical defect. Some investigators have associated disturbances of the tricarboxylic acid cycle with progressive infantile poliodystrophies and lactic acidosis including one case of fumarase deficiency. Understanding the biochemical defects associated with Leigh disease is complicated by reports of infants with severe deficiencies of pyruvate dehydrogenase complex, cytochrome C oxidase, and pyruvate carboxylase who fail to show the distinctive neuropathology. In some, the concentration of thiamine triphosphate in the brain is decreased, especially in affected regions. An inhibitor in the urine of some patients with Leigh disease has been reported to interfere with the catalytic conversion of thiamine pyrophosphate to thiamine triphosphate. Any commonality among the several biochemical theories of the causation of Leigh disease remains to be determined.

Several investigations also have suggested abnormalities of pyruvate dehydrogenase complex and mitochondrial malic enzyme in patients with Friedreich ataxia, but other reports have failed to confirm these observations. Thus, biochemical abnormalities of oxidative metabolism, especially pyruvate metabolism, may be associated with overlapping clinical phenotypes (Fig. 97–2).

References

Atkin BM, Buist NRM, Utter MF, Leiter AB, Banker BQ. Pyruvate carboxylase deficiency and lactic acidosis in a retarded child without Leigh's disease. Pediatr Res 1979; 13:109–116.

Blass JP, Avigan J, Uhlendorf BW. A defect in pyruvate decarboxylase in a child with an intermittent movement disorder. J Clin Invest 1970. 49:423–432.

Blass JP, Schulman JD, Young DS, Hom E. An inherited defect affecting the tricarboxylic acid cycle in a patient with congenital lactic acidosis. J Clin Invest 1972; 51:1845–1851.

DeVivo DC, Haymond MW, Leckie MP, Bussmann YL, McDougal DB Jr, Pagliara AS. The clinical and biochemical implications of pyruvate carboxylase deficiency. J Clin Endocrinol Metab 1977; 45:1281–1296.

DeVivo DC, Haymond MW, Obert K, Nelson JS, Pagliara AS. Defective activation of the pyruvate dehydrogenase complex in subacute necrotizing encephalomyelopathy (Leigh Disease). Ann Neurol 1979; 6:483–494.

DeMauro S, Servidei S, Zeviani M, et al. Cytochrome C oxidase deficiency in Leigh's syndrome. Ann Neurol 1987; 22:498–506.

Farrell DF, Clark AF, Scott CR, Wennberg RP. Absence of pyruvate decarboxylase activity in man: A cause of congenital lactic acidosis. Science 1975; 187:1082.

Feigin I, Wolf A. A disease in infants resembling chronic Wernicke's encephalopathy. J Pediatr 1954; 45:243–263.

Ho L, Hu CWC, Packman S, et al. Deficiency of the pyruvate dehydrogenase component in pyruvate dehydrogenase complex-deficient human fibroblasts. J Clin Invest 1986; 78:844—847.

Hommes FA, Polman HA, Reerink JD. Leigh's encephalomyelopathy: An inborn error of gluconeogenesis. Arch Dis Child 1968; 43:423–426.

Jellinger K, Zimprich H, Muller D. Relapsing form of subacute necrotizing encephalomyelopathy. Neuropediatrics 1973; 4:314–321.

Leigh D. Subacute necrotizing encephalomyelopathy in an infant. J Neurol Neurosurg 1951; 14:216–221.

Montpetit VJA, Andermann F, Carpenter S, Fawcett JS, Zborowska-Sluis D, Giberson HR. Subacute necrotizing encephalomyelopathy: A review and a study of two families. Brain 1971; 94:1–30.

Pincus JH. Subacute necrotizing encephalomyelopathy (Leigh's disease): A consideration of clinical features and etiology. Dev Med Child Neurol 1972; 14:87–101.

Plaitakis A, Whetsell WO Jr, Cooper JR, Yahr MD. Chronic Leigh disease: A genetic and biochemical study. Ann Neurol 1980, 7:304–310.

Sheu KR, Hu CC, Utter MF. Pyruvate dehydrogenase complex activity in normal and deficient fibroblasts. J Clin Invest 1981; 67:1463–1471.

Sipe JC. Leigh's syndrome: the adult form of subacute necrotizing encephalomyelopathy with predilection for the brainstem. Neurology 1973; 23:1030–1038.

Stumpf DA, Parks JK, Eguren LA, et al. Friedreich ataxia. III. Mitochondrial malic enzyme deficiency. Neurology 1982; 32:221–227.

van Erven PMM, Ruitenbeek W, Gabreels FJM, et al. Disturbed oxidative metabolism in subacute necrotizing encephalomyelopathy (Leigh syndrome). Neuropediatrics 1986; 17:28–32.

Willems JL, Monnens LAH, Trijbels JMF, et al. Leigh's encephalomyelopathy in a patient with cytochromic c oxidase deficiency in muscle tissue. Pediatrics 1977; 60:850–857.

Worsley HE, Brookfield RW, Elwood JS, Noble RL, Taylor WH. Lactic acidosis with necrotizing encephalopathy in two sibs. Arch Dis Child 1965; 40:492–501.

Zinn AB, Kerr DS, Hoppel CL. Fumarase deficiency: A new cause of mitochondrial encephalomyopathy. N Engl J Med 1986; 315:469–475.

98. DIFFUSE AND TRANSITIONAL SCLEROSIS
Charles M. Poser

Numerous reviews have attempted to clarify the nomenclature of diffuse sclerosis, principally to better define the eponymic designation Schilder disease. Despite these efforts, nomenclatural confusion remains. The greatest confusion arises because, both clinically and by neuroimaging, it is essentially impossible to differentiate between myelinoclastic diffuse sclerosis and the somewhat more common adrenoleukodystrophy.

The basis for the confusion can be traced directly to Schilder himself, who used a single term, *encephalitis periaxialis diffusa*, to designate what later were shown to be three quite different entities. His 1912 report has become the prototype for what we now refer to as myelinoclastic diffuse sclerosis. It should be noted parenthetically that this first patient was a young girl. The second case, in 1913, was that of a leukodystrophy, almost certainly of the adrenoleukodystrophy type, and the last one, in 1936, was an early example of subacute sclerosing panencephalitis.

The problem of classification and differentiation is further complicated by the frequent difficulty in differentiating pathologically and clinically between diffuse demyelination and sclerosis resulting from so-called "primary demyelination" and the result of vascular and toxic conditions. Two examples are the *maladie de Schilder-Foix* caused by bilateral involvement of the posterior cerebral arteries and *Binswanger disease*, which is now considered a manifestation of arteriosclerosis, which mainly affects the small vessels serving the gray-white matter junction.

Diffuse Sclerosis of Schilder, 1912 Type

The disease is defined as follows: Schilder myelinoclastic diffuse sclerosis is a rare condition that affects children and adults of both genders. It is a subacute or chronic myelinoclastic disorder resulting in the formation of one or, more commonly, two roughly symmetric bilateral plaques measuring at least 3 × 2 cm in two of the three dimensions and involving the centrum semiovale of the cerebral hemispheres. These must be the only lesions that can be demonstrated on the basis of clinical, paraclinical (e.g., evoked potentials), or imaging studies. There must be no involvement of the peripheral nervous system; adrenal function must be normal; and biochemical analysis of the fatty acid components of serum cholesterol esters must yield normal carbon chain lengths. Thus, the diagnosis is essentially one of exclusion and cannot be made even on the basis of postmortem examination, but requires that adrenoleukodystrophy must be ruled out.

Pathogenesis and Pathology. The pathogenesis is considered identical with that of multiple sclerosis. Diffuse sclerosis is a variant of multiple sclerosis, the difference resulting, perhaps, from a difference in the terrain (i.e., the cerebral tissue in which the disease process occurs). The large areas of demyelination might be attributed to a child's immature nervous system, which may be more susceptible to the injurious agent. The cause of the disease remains unknown.

The close relationship to multiple sclerosis is illustrated by a closely related condition, *transitional sclerosis* or *diffuse-disseminated sclerosis.* In this condition, the areas of demyelination vary from very large, characteristic of diffuse sclerosis, to small and scattered like in multiple sclerosis. In a survey of 105 reported cases of diffuse sclerosis, only 33 had lesions that were solely bilateral, symmetric areas of demyelination involving a large area of the centrum ovale; in the other 72 there were several, or many, small isolated plaques (as seen in classic multiple sclerosis) plus the large bilateral lesions.

There are large sharply demarcated areas of demyelination in the centrum ovale of the cerebral hemispheres (Fig. 98–1). The axons are usually affected but to a lesser degree than the myelin. The subcortical U fibers are often spared. The glial reaction is similar to that of any cerebral inflammatory condition with formation of giant multinucleated or swollen astrocytes. In the acute stages there is extensive perivascular cuffing with lymphocytes and phagocytes. Areas of frank tissue necrosis may occur in severe lesions, indicating that the process may go beyond simple demyelination.

Electron-microscopic observations of diffuse sclerosis have shown that the pattern of demyelination appears to be primary and similar to that in multiple sclerosis. Evidence of Wallerian degeneration is common, and some features suggest abortive remyelination. There are many naked axons and axons partially covered with thin layers of myelin (segmental demyelination).

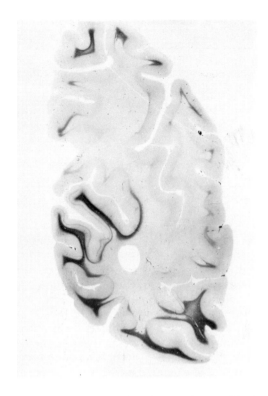

Fig. 98–1. Diffuse myelinoclastic sclerosis. Myelin sheath stain: almost complete loss of myelin in occipital white matter. U-fibers are irregularly involved. (Courtesy of Dr. H. Shiraki, Tokyo)

The differentiation between myelinoclastic diffuse scleroses and the dysmyelinating diseases is based on histopathologic characteristics (Table 98–1).

Essentially, it is assumed that in diffuse sclerosis, myelin had originally been normally constituted and was then secondarily destroyed by endogenous or exogenous factors. The disease produces periaxial demyelination that relatively spares the axons. The gliosis is a true reactive or inflammatory response and myelin breakdown proceeds in the usual fashion, similar to that in classic Wallerian degeneration, ending in cholesterol esters that are phagocytized. The lesions have the same pathologic characteristics as those seen in multiple sclerosis.

Incidence. The disease is considerably rarer than once believed because many cases previously labeled Schilder disease turned out to be something else, mostly adrenoleukodystrophy. A review of the literature of the past 15 years, revealed 32 cases. The diagnoses were based on clinical, neuropathologic, or

Table 98–1. Diseases of the Myelin Sheath Histopathologic Characteristics

	Myelinoclasia	Dysmyelination
Symmetry	Rare	Frequent
Edge of lesion	Sharply demarcated	Diffuse (to U fibers)
U fibers	Often involved	Usually spared
Gliosis	Anisomorphic	Isomorphic
Axons	Usually spared	Involved early
Peripheral nerves	Never involved	Often involved
Inflammatory reaction	Mild to moderate	Usually absent
Myelinogenesis	Normal	Abnormal
Myelin breakdown	Classical Wallerian degeneration to cholesterol esters	

neuroimaging observations. Of these, only nine can be accepted as Schilder myelinoclastic diffuse sclerosis. Ten were adrenoleukodystrophy, five were transitional or multiple sclerosis, five were acute disseminated encephalomyelitis, and three lacked sufficient information for diagnosis. Only three cases clearly could be differentiated from adrenoleukodystrophy, i.e., by analysis of the fatty acids of plasma cholesterol esters or electron-microscopic examination of brain or adrenal cortex. Although some authors have suggested that Schilder disease does not exist, these three cases, and undoubtedly many others, are proof to the contrary.

This disease is most prevalent in children, although it may be seen in adults. Conversely, the age incidence of patients with transitional sclerosis follows a distribution curve that resembles the more common multiple sclerosis.

The number of definite diagnosed cases is too small to establish any racial, ethnic, or geographic predilection, but it is probably similar to that of multiple sclerosis. The gender incidence appears to be roughly equal.

Familial Incidence. Many cases of familial Schilder disease have been reported. In most, examination of the original reports indicates that the authors were describing leukodystrophy. In others, the diagnosis was made purely on clinical grounds, which made it impossible to distinguish myelinoclastic or dysmyelinating conditions. The only documented instance of familial incidence of myelinoclastic diffuse sclerosis involved a woman with transitional sclerosis and her daughter with diffuse sclerosis.

Signs and Symptoms. It is difficult to delineate a typical clinical picture for myelinoclastic diffuse sclerosis, primarily because in 66% of the cases, the disease may be transitional sclerosis rather than true diffuse sclerosis; the ad-

ditional, scattered small lesions modify the clinical signs and symptoms.

Basically, the clinical course is that of subacute or chronic mental and neurologic deterioration after a period of normal development. As a general rule, the disease progresses slowly and relentlessly and is manifested by intellectual deterioration, increasing spasticity with signs of pyramidal-tract involvement, blindness, and deafness. In the rare adult cases, the clinical presentation may be purely psychiatric. A list of the signs and symptoms would include: headache, vertigo, convulsive seizures, optic neuritis and atrophy, true papilledema, hemianopsia, cortical blindness, extraocular muscle paralysis, internuclear ophthalmoplegia, nystagmus, facial palsy, deafness, hemiparesis, cortical sensory deficits, cerebellar and, rarely, extrapyramidal signs and symptoms, dysarthria, dysphagia, aphasic disturbances, memory impairment, dullness, irritability, change in personality, confusion, disorientation, dementia, generalized spasticity, bladder and bowel incontinence, fever of unknown origin, general malnutrition, and cachexia. Death is usually due to intercurrent pulmonary, skin, or urinary tract infection.

Increased intracranial pressure may suggest a mass lesion; the large subcortical areas of demyelination are associated with cerebral edema.

Laboratory Data. As in multiple sclerosis, the only reasonably reliable, although not definitive laboratory test, is the elevation of the CSF IgG fraction and the presence of oligoclonal bands.

CT provides accurate diagnostic information in demyelinating diffuse sclerosis, particularly when contrast enhancement provides a hyperdense border zone for the hypodense area of demyelination involving large areas of the white matter. CT and magnetic resonance imaging, in particular, considerably ease the task of differentiating between true diffuse sclerosis and transitional or multiple sclerosis. EEG may be quite helpful in showing a large slow-wave focus corresponding to the clinical localization of the myelinoclastic lesion.

Diagnosis and Differential Diagnosis. The early clinical symptoms are so nonspecific that it is difficult to differentiate from other degenerative diseases of childhood. It is almost impossible to pose this diagnosis with any degree of reliability after childhood. Absence of positive family history; early appearance of the combination of optic atrophy, pyramidal-tract signs and, in particular, deafness; nonspecific, but often large, focal EEG abnormalities and the relatively infrequent occurrence of convulsive seizures are most helpful, as is the pathognomonic CT scan.

The most important condition to be differentiated is adrenoleukodystrophy (see Article 84, Adrenoleukodystrophy). This may be difficult unless there is clear-cut involvement of the peripheral nerves, which would immediately label the case probable adrenoleukodystrophy. However, it should be noted that in some cases of adrenoleukodystrophy the white matter lesions are completely indistinguishable from those seen in the true 1912 myelinoclastic diffuse sclerosis. In such cases, there is an anisomorphic gliosis and a perivascular inflammatory reaction, which may be severe. Further confusing the issue is that CSF pleocytosis and evidence of local production of immunoglobulin G can be demonstrated. The CT image is the same as in Schilder myelinoclastic diffuse sclerosis, including the ring-like contrast enhancement. Adrenocortical function may be clinically normal in adrenoleukodystrophy and, despite the disease's sex-linked inheritance, even if the patient is a girl there is no guarantee she does not have adrenoleukodystrophy; likewise, she may be a so-called symptomatic carrier.

The differential diagnosis includes subacute sclerosing panencephalitis that can be identified by high or rising measles-antibody titers in the serum and CSF, unusually high level of CSF IgG, the invariable presence of oligoclonal bands, and the characteristic EEG changes, when present. CT may be of little diagnostic value in this instance. Progressive multifocal leukoencephalopathy is almost always associated with chronic leukemia or lymphoma.

Of the dysmyelinating diseases, metachromatic leukodystrophy (sulfatide lipidosis) frequently has a history of familial incidence; consistently elevated CSF protein with normal gamma globulin and IgG fractions; slow peripheral-nerve conduction times, nonfilling gallbladder; and some specific biochemical procedures.

There have been isolated reports of diffuse sclerosis after lead encephalopathy, ergotamine intoxication and carbon monoxide intoxication.

In the adult, the major problem in differential diagnosis is cerebral neoplasm. In the absence of elevation of CSF IgG, it may be impossible to differentiate these conditions except by CT, angiography, or cerebral biopsy. Evoked response studies may reveal the presence of additional but separate lesions.

Course and Prognosis. The number of cases of true myelinoclastic diffuse sclerosis is so small that it is difficult to generalize regarding course and prognosis. The disease usually starts during the second half of the first decade and runs a course lasting several months to 3 or 4 years. Except when modified by treatment, the disease is invariably fatal.

Of the 72 cases of transitional sclerosis, the duration of the disease was known in 70. The mean duration was 6.2 years with extremes ranging from 3 days to 45 years. It lasted 10 years in 23%. In general, transitional sclerosis leads to death much more quickly than multiple sclerosis, but not as rapidly as diffuse sclerosis.

Treatment. Few patients with this disease have been treated; however, there is one published report of arrest of the disease for several years after treatment with oral corticosteroids and intravenous ACTH. A striking reduction in the size of the lesions was demonstrated by CT. In another well documented case, similar results were obtained with cyclophosphamide treatment. Supportive treatment, in particular prevention and control of secondary infection, may prolong life without affecting nervous system deterioration.

References

Mehler M, Rabinowich L. Inflammatory myelinoclastic diffuse sclerosis. Ann Neurol 1988; 23:413–415.

Poser C. Diseases of the myelin sheath. In: Baker A, Baker L, eds. Clinical Neurology (vol 2). Philadelphia: Lea & Febiger, 1978: 1–88.

Poser C, Goutieres F, Carpentier M. Aicardi J. Schilder's myelinoclastic diffuse sclerosis. Pediatrics 1986; 77:107–112.

99. DIFFERENTIAL DIAGNOSIS

Isabelle Rapin

Although most of the degenerative diseases of infancy and childhood are not treatable today, neurologists are obligated to make as definite a diagnosis as possible. This allows the neurologist to provide the parents with a prognosis and genetic counseling. Of course physicians are on the alert for the few treatable conditions, but there is also responsibility to advance knowledge, and precise diagnosis is the first step toward unraveling the chemical pathology of the illness and devising therapy. The clinician's first concern is to determine that the illness is in fact progressive and to review the genetic evidence. Findings on physical and neurologic examination almost always narrow the diagnostic possibilities and guide the selection of laboratory tests.

Deterioration is usually obvious when a disease affects an adult or adolescent, but in infancy and early childhood the slope of the developmental curve is so steep that it can mask functional decay; the child's symptoms represent the net difference between the two opposing trends (Fig. 99–1). An early sign of insidious dementia may be slowing of development rather than loss of milestones. As long as the child continues to acquire new skills, even too slowly, the illness is likely to be misinterpreted as a static condition. When the disease is already advanced at birth, dementia can masquerade as total failure to develop, suggesting brain maldevelopment or an unrecognized perinatal catastrophe. In these situations, the correct diagnosis may not be contemplated until after the birth of an affected sibling.

A family history of similar disease or consanguinity are strong clues, but neither is frequent. Most of these diseases are recessive and the birth of the first affected child occurs as a sporadic event. It is important to detect X-linked recessive diseases (Table 99–1) because parents can be assured that they can have normal children, even in the absence of a specific method for intrauterine diagnosis, if they can accept abortion of all male fetuses. Knowing that certain diseases are particularly frequent in children of particular ethnic backgrounds is also helpful (Table 99–2).

The patient's age at onset may be a lead to the diagnosis (Table 99–3). Genetically homogeneous syndromes tend to run a predictable course and appear at about the same age, but what is considered to be genetically homogeneous today is likely to prove to be nonhomogeneous tomorrow because phenocopies are common. As a general rule, the younger the child is when the symptoms appear, the more rapid is the deterioration, but there are exceptions. For example, when Pelizaeus-Merzbacher disease is manifest before the age of 1, the patient may survive into the third decade. Two diseases of midchildhood or adolescence can progress rapidly to death from liver failure (Wilson disease) or adrenal insufficiency (adrenoleukodystrophy).

The general physical examination may provide helpful clues (Table 99–4). The neurologic symptoms and signs indicate which systems are most affected. Intractable seizures and myoclonus are more typical of diseases of gray matter than of white matter (Table 99–5), whereas severe spasticity appears early in diseases of the white matter. Because spasticity may be the result of either diffuse neuronal dropout or central demyelination, it occurs in the late stages of most diseases. Hypotonia suggests involvement of peripheral nerves, anterior horn cells, or cerebellum (Table 99–6). The combination of hypotonia and increased reflexes, which is seen in Tay-Sachs disease, suggests that both upper and lower motor neurons are affected. Ataxia and abnormal involuntary movements are particularly useful diagnostic signs. Sensory abnormalities are rarely detectable; lack of sensitivity to pain suggests dysautonomia and is reported in some cases of infantile neuraxonal dystrophy.

The eyes are so likely to provide information of diagnostic importance that detailed examination is mandatory (Table 99–7). Dilating the pupil is required to afford an adequate view of the peripheral retina, macula, and disc. The mild corneal haze of some of the mucolipidoses and mucopolysaccharidoses and the detection of early Kayser-Fleischer rings call for slit-lamp examination. Electroretinography may disclose pigmentary degeneration of the retina before it is visible with the ophthalmoscope.

Repeated neuropsychologic testing may be needed to document progressive dementia. In older children and adolescents, deterioration may be suggested by a reading age that is well above mental age. Lack of dementia, at least early, in the face of motor deterioration, suggests a disease that spares the cortex

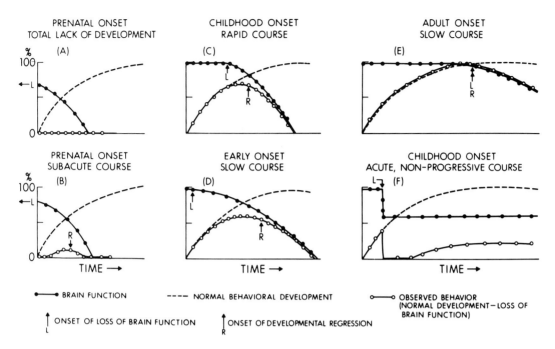

Fig. 99–1. Theoretical curves show the possible effects of progressive brain dysfunction on behavior, depending on time of onset and rapidity of course. The curve depicting observed behavior (o-o-o-o-) is the difference between the curves indicating expected development (-----) and brain function (●-●-●-●). A. Prenatal onset, with damage at birth so advanced that no development is observed, suggesting a severe static encephalopathy. B, Prenatal onset, with damage at birth somewhat less severe than in A. Development is minimal and markedly delayed, but does appear to take place initially. C and D. Onset at birth, with a less acute course. E. Onset in adulthood. Note that in B, C, and D, loss of milestones may not appear until months or years after the onset of the illness, which therefore does not appear progressive unless it is realized that deceleration of development or developmental standstill implies deteriorating function. When a progressive disease starts after adolescence (E), loss of function should be less delayed and the disease recognized as progressive virtually from its start. F. A severe static lesion acquired postnatally may produce total regression acutely, but development may be expected to resume until the time of puberty. (From Rapin I. In: Rudolph AM, ed. Pediatrics, 16th ed. New York: Appleton-Century-Crofts, 1977.)

Table 99–1. Unusual Pattern of Inheritance Other than Autosomal Recessive

X-linked Recessive	*X-linked Dominant?*
Adrenoleukodystrophy	Incontinentia pigmenti
Pelizaeus-Merzbacher disease	Pseudo- and pseudopseudohypoparathyroidism
Fabry disease	Rett syndrome
Hunter disease (MPS II)	
Ornithine transcarbamylase deficiency	*Autosomal Dominant*
Lesch-Nyhan syndrome	Neurofibromatosis
Leber optic atrophy	Tuberous sclerosis
Lowe oculocerebrorenal syndrome	Von Hippel-Lindau disease
Trichopoliodystrophy	Acute intermittent porphyria
Duchenne muscular dystrophy	Huntington disease
Norrie disease	
Fragile X-syndrome	

Table 99–2. Predominant Ethnic Background in Certain Diseases

Ashkenazi Jews
Classic Tay-Sachs disease
Infantile Niemann-Pick disease
Juvenile Gaucher disease
Recessive dystonia musculorum
   deformans
Mucolipidosis IV
Spongy degeneration
Dysautonomia

Nova Scotia
Type D Niemann-Pick disease

Japan
Sialidosis with chondrodystrophy

Scandinavia
Finnish (infantile) variant of ceroid lipofuscinosis
Juvenile ceroid lipofuscinosis
Krabbe disease
Aspartylglucosaminuria
Baltic myoclonus epilepsy (Ramsay Hunt syndrome,
   Unverricht-Lundborg syndrome)

Table 99–3. Typical Age at Onset

Neonatal or Early Infantile Onset
Aminoacidurias
Urea cycle disorders
Galactosemia
Connatal Pelizaeus-Merzbacher syndrome
Connatal Alexander disease
Alpers syndrome
Spongy degeneration (some cases)
Infantile Gaucher disease
Infantile adrenoleukodystrophy
Zellweger syndrome and variants
Infantile Refsum syndrome
GM_1 gangliosidosis (infantile variant)
I-cell disease (mucolipidosis II)
Trichopoliodystrophy
Incontinentia pigmenti
Progressive spinal muscular atrophy
   (Werdnig-Hoffmann disease)
Seckel bird-headed dwarfs

Infantile Onset
Many sphingolipidoses, mucopolysacchar-
   idoses, mucolipidoses
Infantile ceroid lipofuscinosis
Leigh syndrome (early types)
Other mitochondrial cytopathies
Lesch-Nyhan syndrome
Sjögren-Larsson syndrome
Spongy degeneration
Wolman disease
Alexander disease
Pelizaeus-Merzbacher disease
Neuraxonal dystrophy
Infantile Hallervorden-Spatz disease
Infantile fucosidosis
Nephrosialidosis
Pompe disease
Xeroderma pigmentosum
Cockayne disease
Progeria

Onset in Preschool Years
Aspartylglucosaminuria
Marinesco-Sjögren syndrome
Alexander disease
Ataxia telangiectasia
Xeroderma pigmentosum
Chédiak-Higashi disease
Metachromatic leukodystrophy
Late infantile gangliosidoses
Niemann Pick-Nova Scotia variant
Late infantile ceroid lipofuscinosis
Sanfilippo syndromes
Maroteaux-Lamy disease
Mild Hunter disease
Leigh syndrome
Kearns-Sayre syndrome

Onset School Age or Adolescence
Wilson disease
Acute intermittent porphyria
Juvenile ceroid lipofuscinosis
Adrenoleukodystrophy
Late variants of the gangliosidoses
Niemann-Pick with vertical ophthalmoplegia
Sialidosis with cherry red spot-myoclonus (var-
   iants with and without chondrodystrophy)
Fabry disease
Cerebrotendinous xanthomatosis
Leigh syndrome (some variants)
Other mitochondrial cytopathies
Refsum disease
Friedreich ataxia
Bassen-Kornzweig disease
Other spinocerebellar degenerations
Dystonia musculorum deformans
Juvenile Huntington disease
Juvenile parkinsonism
Classic Hallervorden-Spatz syndrome
Lafora disease
Baltic myoclonus
Subacute sclerosing panencephalitis (SSPE)

Table 99–4. Helpful Clues in the Physical Examination

Big Head
Tay-Sachs disease
Alexander disease
Spongy degeneration
Hurler disease
Other mucopolysaccharidoses with
  hydrocephalus

Small Head
Krabbe disease
Infantile ceroid lipofuscinosis
Alpers syndrome
Neuraxonal dystrophy
Incontinentia pigmenti
Cockayne disease
Rett syndrome
Bird-headed dwarfs

Hair Abnormalities
Stiff, wiry:
  Trichopoliodystrophy
Hirsutism:
  Infantile GM_1 gangliosidosis
  Hurler, Hunter, Sanfilippo syndromes
  I-cell disease
Gray:
  Ataxia telangiectasia
  Cockayne disease
  Chédiak-Higashi disease
  Progeria

Skin Abnormalities
Telangiectasia:
  Ataxia telangiectasia
Angiokeratoma:
  Fabry disease
  Juvenile fucosidosis
  Sialidosis with chondrodystrophy
Ichthyosis:
  Refsum disease
  Sjögren-Larsson syndrome
Hypopigmentation:
  Trichopoliodystrophy
  Chédiak-Higashi syndrome
  Tuberous sclerosis (ash leaf spots)
Hyperpigmentation:
  Niemann-Pick disease
  Adrenoleukodystrophy
  Farber disease
  Neurofibromatosis (café au lait spots)
  Xeroderma pigmentosum
Thin atrophic skin:
  Ataxia telangiectasia
  Cockayne disease
  Xeroderma pigmentosum
  Progeria

Thick skin:
  I-cell disease
  Mucopolysaccharidoses I, II, III
  Infantile fucosidosis
Subcutaneous nodules:
  Farber disease
  Neurofibromatosis
  Cerebrotendinous xanthomatosis
Xanthomas:
  Neimann-Pick disease
Blotching:
  Dysautonomia

Enlarged Nodes
Farber disease
Niemann-Pick disease
Juvenile Gaucher disease
Chédiak-Higashi disease
Ataxia telangiectasia (lymphoma)

Stridor, Hoarseness
Infantile adrenoleukodystrophy
Farber disease
Infantile Gaucher disease
Pelizaeus-Merzbacher disease

Enlarged Orange Tonsils
Tangier disease

Severe Swallowing Problems
(Present late in the course of all patients with se-
  vere bulbar, pseudo-bulbar, cerebellar, or basal
  ganglia pathology)
Infantile Gaucher disease
Dysautonomia
Hallervorden-Spatz syndrome
Dystonia musculorum deformans
Infantile adrenoleukodystrophy
Zellweger disease

Heart Abnormalities
Pompe disease
Hurler disease and other mucopolysaccharidoses
Fabry disease
Infantile fucosidosis
Refsum disease
Friedreich ataxia
Abetalipoproteinemia (Bassen-Kornzweig
  disease)
Tuberous sclerosis
Progeria
Zellweger disease

Strokes
Fabry disease
Trichopoliodystrophy
Progeria

Table 99–4. *continued*

Organomegaly
Mucopolysaccharidoses (most types)
Infantile GM$_1$ gangliosidosis
Niemann-Pick disease
Gaucher disease
Zellweger disease
Galactosemia
Pompe disease
Mannosidosis

Gastrointestinal Problems
Malabsorption:
  Wolman disease
  Bassen-Kornzweig disease
Nonfunctioning gallbladder:
  Metachromatic leukodystrophy
  Infantile fucosidosis
Jaundice:
  Infantile Niemann-Pick disease
  Zellweger disease
  Galactosemia
  Niemann-Pick disease
Vomiting
  Dysautonomia
  Urea cycle defects
Diarrhea
  Hunter syndrome

Kidney Problems
Renal failure:
  Fabry disease
  Nephrosialidosis
Cysts:
  Zellweger disease
  Von Hippel-Lindau disease
  Tuberous sclerosis
Stones:
  Lesch-Nyhan disease
Aminoaciduria:
  Aminocidurias
  Lowe syndrome
  Wilson disease

Bone and Joint Abnormalities
Stiff joints:
  Mucopolysaccharidoses (all but type
    I-S)
  Mucolipidoses (most types)

Fucosidosis
Farber disease
Sialidoses (some forms)
Zellweger disease
Cockayne disease
Scoliosis:
  Friedreich ataxia
  Ataxia telangiectasia
  Dystonia musculorum deformans
  All chronic diseases with muscle weakness,
    especially anterior horn cell involvement
Kyphosis:
  Mucopolysaccharidoses

Endocrine Dysfunction
Adrenals:
  Adrenoleukodystrophy
  Wolman disease
Hypogonadism:
  Xeroderma pigmentosum
  Ataxia telangiectasia
  Some spinocerebellar degenerations
Diabetes:
  Ataxia telangiectasia
Dwarfing:
  Morquio disease
  Other mucopolysaccharidoses
  Cockayne syndrome
  Progeria
  Diseases with severe malnutrition

Neoplasms
Ataxia telangiectasia
Xeroderma pigmentosum
Neurofibromatosis
Von Hipple-Lindau disease
Tuberous sclerosis

Hearing Loss
Hunter disease
Other mucopolysaccharidoses
Adrenoleukodystrophy
Refsum disease
Some mitochondrial cytopathies
Cockayne disease
Kearns-Sayre and Leigh syndromes
Some spinocerebellar degenerations
Usher syndrome

Table 99–5. Diseases with Prominent Seizures
            or Myoclonus

Acute intermittent porphyria
Gangliosidoses (infantile types especially)
Ceroid lipofuscinoses (late infantile variant
    especially)
Alpers syndrome
Trichopoliodystrophy
Zellweger syndrome
Adrenoleukodystrophy (infantile variant
    especially)
Infantile Alexander disease
Krabbe disease
Lafora disease
Sanfilippo disease
Juvenile Huntington disease
Tuberous sclerosis
Ramsay Hunt syndrome (Baltic myoclonus)
Some mitochondrial cytopathies
Juvenile neuropathic Gaucher disease
SSPE

Table 99–6. Motor Signs Helpful to Diagnosis*

Floppiness in Infancy
Progressive spinal muscular atrophy
Congenital myopathies
Zellweger syndrome
Pompe disease
Trichopoliodystrophy
Neuraxonal dystrophy
Gangliosidoses (early variants)
Fucosidosis (infantile variant)
Infantile ceroid lipofuscinosis
Spongy degeneration (early)
Leigh syndrome (early variant)

Peripheral Neuropathy
Acute intermittent porphyria
Metachromatic leukodystrophy
Fabry disease
Krabbe disease
Neuraxonal dystrophy
Refsum disease
Tangier disease
Bassen-Kornzweig disease
Sialidosis (some variants)
Mucolipidosis III
Cerebrotendinous xanthomatosis
Ataxia telangiectasia
Adrenomyeloneuropathy
Levy-Roussy syndrome
Mucopolysaccharidoses I, II, VI, VII
    (entrapment)
Cockayne syndrome
Some mitochondrial cytopathies

Prominent Cerebellar Signs
Wilson disease
Late infantile ceroid lipofuscinosis

Pelizaeus-Merzbacher disease
Neuraxonal dystrophy
Metachromatic leukodystrophy
Ataxia telangiectasia
Leigh syndrome
Niemann-Pick disease (Nova Scotia variant)
Some late-onset gangliosidoses
Some sialidoses
Friedreich ataxia
Bassen-Kornzweig disease
Cerebrotendinous xanthomatosis
Other spinocerebellar degenerations
Lafora disease
Ramsay Hunt syndrome (Baltic myoclonus)
Chédiak-Higashi disease
Usher syndrome

Abnormal Posture or Movements
Wilson disease
Lesch-Nyhan disease
Hallervorden-Spatz syndrome
Familial striatal necrosis
Dystonia musculorum deformans
Juvenile Niemann-Pick with ophthalmoplegia
Chronic GM_1 and GM_2 gangliosidoses
Pelizaeus-Merzbacher syndrome
Crigler-Najjar disease
Ataxia telangiectasia
Juvenile ceroid lipofuscinosis
Juvenile Huntington disease
Juvenile Parkinsonism
Gilles de la Tourette syndrome
Xeroderma pigmentosum with endocrine dys-
    function

*Spasticity is so common as to be nondiscriminating.

Table 99–7. Eye Findings

Conjunctival Telangiectasia
Ataxia telangiectasia
Fabry disease

Corneal Opacity
Wilson disease (Kayser-Fleischer ring)
Mucopolysaccharidoses I, III, IV, VI
Mucolipidoses III, IV
Fabry disease
Sialidosis with chondrodystrophy
Cockayne disease
Xeroderma pigmentosum
Zellweger disease (inconstant)

Lens Opacity
Wilson disease
Galactosemia
Marinesco-Sjögren syndrome
Lowe disease
Cerebrocutaneous xanthomatosis
Sialidosis (rarely significant clinically)
Mannosidosis
Zellweger disease

Glaucoma
Mucopolysaccharidosis I—Scheie
Zellweger disease (infrequent)

Cherry-Red Spot
Tay-Sachs disease
Sialidosis (usually)
Infantile Niemann-Pick (50% of cases)
Infantile GM_1 gangliosidosis (50% of cases)
Farber disease (inconstant)
Multiple sulfatase deficiency (metachromatic leukodystrophy variant)

Macular and Retinal Pigmentary Degeneration
Ceroid lipofuscinosis (most types)
Mucopolysaccharidoses I-H and I-S, II, III
Mucolipidosis IV
Bassen-Kornzweig syndrome (abetalipoproteinemia)
Infantile adrenoleukodystrophy
Refsum disease (all types)
Kearns-Sayre syndrome
Leber congenital amaurosis

Other mitochondrial cytopathies
Hallervorden-Spatz syndrome (some types)
Cockayne disease
Sjögren-Larsson syndrome (not always)
Usher syndrome
Some other spinocerebellar syndromes

Optic Atrophy
Krabbe disease
Metachromatic leukodystrophy
Most sphingolipidoses late in their course
Adrenoleukodystrophy
Alexander disease
Spongy degeneration
Pelizaeus-Merzbacher disease
Neuraxonal dystrophy
Alpers disease
Leber optic atrophy
Some spinocerebellar degenerations
Disease with retinal pigmentary degeneration

Nystagmus
Diseases with poor vision (searching nystagmus)
Pelizaeus-Merzbacher syndrome
Metachromatic leukodystrophy
Friedreich ataxia
Other spinocerebellar degenerations and cerebellar atrophies
Neuraxonal dystrophy
Ataxia telangiectasia
Leigh syndrome (inconstant)
Marinesco-Sjögren syndrome
Opsoclonus-myoclonus syndrome
Chédiak-Higashi syndrome

Ophthalmoplegia
Leigh syndrome
Kearns-Sayre and Leigh syndromes
Niemann-Pick variant with vertical ophthalmoplegia
Bassen-Kornzweig syndrome
Ataxia telangiectasia
Infantile Gaucher disease
Tangier disease

and selectively affects the basal ganglia, brain stem, or cerebellar pathways.

In children with an undiagnosed disease, laboratory investigations are screening devices. How many are used depends, in part, on accessibility and cost (Table 99–8). "New" diseases are often discovered serendipitously rather than after a directed diagnostic endeavor.

Electrical studies may yield clues (Table 99–9). The plain EEG rarely provides decisive information, although photomyoclonus suggests Lafora disease, somatosensory myoclonussiglidosis, and Ramsy Hunt syndrome.

Radiologic tests are crucial in some cases. Adrenal calcification is virtually pathognomonic of Wolman disease. The diagnostic yield of plain radiographs of the skull is extremely low, in contrast to the efficiency of CT. Even if CT only shows nonspecific atrophy, this is helpful if it is progressive. Spongy degeneration, Alexander disease, and adrenoleukodystrophy show a characteristic pattern of lucency of the white matter. Radionuclide scans are often positive at the margins of the area of active demyelination in adrenoleukodystrophy, but are not helpful in most other diseases. Lack of radioactive copper absorption into the liver can be shown in trich-

Table 99–8. Useful Laboratory Tests

Urine
  Aminoacids, organic acids
  Phytanic acid
  Pipecolic acid
  Galactose, other sugars
  Mucopolysaccharides, sialidated oligosac-
    charides
  Acetyl aspartic acid
  Copper excretion
  Porphyrins
  Metachromatic granules, curvilinear profiles
    in sediment
  Dolichols
 	
Blood Chemistry
  Ammonia (urea cycle disorders)
  Lactate-pyruvate ratio (Leigh syndrome,
    other mitochondrial cytopathies)
  Aminoacids, organic acids and other special
    metabolites
  C26/C22 fatty acid ratio (adrenoleukodystro-
    phy, Zellweger disease, infantile Refsum
    disease)
 	
White Blood Cells
  Lysosomal enzymes and other enzymatic
    assays
  Lipid and other inclusions (ceroid lipofusci-
    noses, gangliosidoses)
	Red Blood Cells
	  Enzymatic assays for galactosemia, porphyria
	
	Cultured Skin Fibroblasts
	  Enzymatic assays for most diseases with
	    known deficits
	  Lipid and other inclusions (in mucolipidosis
	    IV, I-cell disease, mucopolysaccharidoses,
	    Chédiak-Higashi)
	  DNA repair after ultraviolet or irradiation ex-
	    posure (ataxia telangiectasia, Cockayne syn-
	    drome, xeroderma pigmentosum)
	  Restriction length polymorphisms
	
	CSF Protein Increased
	  Metachromatic leukodystrophy, Krabbe, in-
	    fantile adrenoleukodystrophy (not always
	    in classic variant), Friedreich ataxia and
	    other spinocerebellar degenerations (incon-
	    stant), Zellweger disease (sometimes), Ref-
	    sum disease, Cockayne syndrome
	
	Amniotic Cells
	  Enzymatic assays for disease of known enzy-
	    matic defect
	  Abnormal inclusion in mucolipidosis IV
	  Karyotype in X-linked disease
	  C26/C22 fatty acid ratio
	  Restriction length polymorphisms
	
	Intradermal Histamine test
	  Dysautonomia

opoliodystrophy. Positron emission tomography (PET) and magnetic resonance (MR) hold great promise in the field of genetic diseases.

The need for a biopsy arises when noninvasive tests fail (Table 99–10). Skin biopsy is examined under the electron microscope for abnormal inclusions and is also used for tissue culture. Cultured fibroblasts may yield an enzymatic diagnosis; equally important, the cultures can be kept viable indefinitely in the frozen state and tissue will be available when

new data suggest further study, especially as molecular biologic techniques enable detection of additional mutations. Conjunctival biopsies are helpful when storage in connective tissue is suspected and enzymatic diagnosis is unavailable (e.g., in mucolipidosis IV) or when axonal spheroids are being evaluated. The main purpose of liver biopsy is to measure copper content in Wilson disease, but it is also helpful in Zellweger syndrome and Lafora disease.

Brain biopsies are reserved for cases in

Table 99–9. Electrodiagnosis

Electromyography and nerve conduction
  velocity:
	To detect neuropathy, anterior horn cell disease,
	  or muscle involvement

Electroretinography:	To detect retinitis pigmentosa.

Visual evoked responses:	Giant potentials in late infantile ceroid lipofusci-
	  nosis; delayed latency and decreased amplitude
	  in leukodystrophies or optic atrophy.

Brain-stem auditory evoked responses:	Diagnosis of hearing loss; prolonged latency in
	  leukodystrophies; delayed waves with decrease
	  of amplitude in leukodystrophies and other
	  disease of the brain stem.

Somatosensory evoked responses:	Giant potentials in sialidosis with cherry-red spot
	  myoclonus; decreased amplitude in peripheral
	  neuropathy; delayed waves with decreased am-
	  plitude in diseases of the white matter and pe-
	  ripheral nerves.

Table 99–10.   Diseases in which Biopsies are Likely to Help

Skin	*Nerve*
Ceroid lipofuscinosis	Neuraxonal dystrophy
Mucopolysaccharidoses	Metachromatic leukodystrophy
Mucolipidosis IV	Adrenoleukodystrophy
Neuraxonal dystrophy	Other diseases with neuropathies
Conjunctiva	*Liver*
Mucopolysaccharidoses	Wilson disease (copper content)
Mucolipidoses	Zellweger syndrome (absent peroxisomes,
Neuraxonal dystrophy	cirrhosis)
Bone marrow	Lafora disease
Niemann-Pick disease	Glycogenesis
Gaucher disease	*Brain*
Mucopolysaccharidoses	(rarely needed except possibly for the following)
Sea blue histiocyte syndrome	Spongy degeneration
Rectum	Alexander disease
Sphingolipidoses	Neuraxonal dystrophy
Ceroid lipofuscinoses	Undiagnosed disease with probable cortical
Sialidoses	involvement
Muscle	
Glycogenoses	
Mitochondrial myopathies	
(Kearns-Sayre, Leigh syn-	
drome)	
Other myopathies	
Neuraxonal dystrophy	
Lafora disease	

which the diagnosis remains elusive despite thorough peripheral investigation and when the CT or EEG suggest the cortex is severely affected. Brain biopsy is likely to be diagnostic in storage diseases, spongy degeneration, neuraxonal dystrophy, and Alexander disease. It is unlikely to help when the brunt of the disease is subcortical. To maximize the probability of arriving at a definite diagnosis, the biopsy is made through a small craniotomy, making certain to sample the white matter as well as the cortex. Routine histologic examination of the tissue is not sufficient because brain biopsy is reserved for disorders that are biochemical enigmas; therefore, brain biopsy should be carried out in a center that has the resources necessary for many avenues of investigation that include histochemistry, Golgi staining, electron microscopy, quantitative neurochemical analysis, and metabolic studies. In the proper hands, the informational yield of brain biopsy is sufficiently high, and its morbidity sufficiently low, to make it a rewarding procedure, both clinically and scientifically. Biopsy is not a substitute for autopsy because it may not be diagnostic

and because some studies can be done only on biopsy tissue or only on autopsy tissue.

When all diagnostic methods have failed and brain biopsy is not indicated or is not acceptable, the physician must broach the subject of an autopsy. This can be done when the parents are informed of the likelihood of a fatal outcome. Parents who understand how little is known about their child's illness are likely to want an autopsy; they will also be spared the unnecessary hurt of being pressed for an autopsy when the child actually dies and the parents are most distressed. A planned and speedy autopsy maximizes the probability of obtaining useful data. Viscera, peripheral nerves, muscle, and retina, as well as the brain, must be investigated. Tissue samples should be removed and frozen at −70°C for chemical analysis; other samples are fixed for electron microscopy before the organs are placed in formalin. If autopsy does not yield a diagnosis, the physician must explain to the parents that the child's illness may be one that is as yet unrecognized and that data of scientific importance may emerge from the study of their child, who will thus have made a unique contribution to other children and their families.

Chapter X

Neurocutaneous Disorders

Several genetic diseases involve both the skin and nervous system. These are called *neurocutaneous disorders* or *neuroectodermatoses*. In the past, they were referred to as the "phakomatoses" (*phakos* is the Greek word for lentil, flat plate, or spot). Retinal lesions are seen in tuberous sclerosis and, sometimes, in neurofibromatosis. Other distinct disorders are Sturge-Weber-Dimitri syndrome, linear nevus sebaceous, and incontinentia pigmenti.

Any portion of the central and peripheral nervous system may be affected by these heredodegenerative diseases, and different portions may be involved in various combinations. Some families breed true and show a remarkable consistency with regard to location and extent of the pathologic changes; other families demonstrate great discrepancies among individual members of the family. The clinical spectrum ranges from frequent abortive forms (*formes frustes*) to a severe, potentially lethal condition with highly protean clinical manifestations.

100. NEUROFIBROMATOSIS
Arnold P. Gold

Neurofibromatosis was first described by von Recklinghausen in 1882; it is one of the most common single genetic disorders of the CNS. The two cardinal features are multiple hyperpigmented marks on the skin (*café-au-lait spots*) and multiple neurofibromas; other symptoms may result from lesions in bone, the central and peripheral nervous system, or other organs.

Etiology. The pathogenesis of neurofibromatosis is poorly understood. Many of the clinical features, neurofibromas, and CNS lesions affect structures that originate in the neural crest. Other disorders include altered synthesis and secretion of melanin, disturbed cellular organization with hamartomatous collections, and abnormal production and distribution of nerve growth factors.

Genetics and Incidence. Neurofibromatosis is a disease of autosomal dominant inheritance with variable clinical expressivity, but penetrance is almost 100%. Mutations account for about 50% of the new cases. The disorder affects both sexes with equal frequency and involves all racial and ethnic groups with a prevalence of 1 in 3,000. This figure must be a minimal estimate because abortive or forme fruste cases are often unrecognized clinically.

Molecular genetics has altered concepts of neurofibromatosis. The gene for generalized von Recklinghausen disease, now called NF-1, has been assigned to chromosome 17. The gene for the syndrome of bilateral acoustic neuroma (NF-2) has been linked to chromosome 22. The two syndromes must therefore differ in pathogenesis as well as clinical expression.

Neuropathology. The neuropathologic changes result from changes in neural supporting tissue with resultant dysplasia, hyperplasia, and neoplasia. These pathologic changes may involve the central, peripheral, and autonomic nervous systems. Visceral manifestations result from hyperplasia of the autonomic ganglia and nerves within the organ. In addition to the neural lesions, dysplastic and neoplastic changes affect skin, bone, endocrines, and blood vessels. Developmental anomalies include thoracic meningocele and syringomyelia. People affected by neurofibromatosis seem more likely than others to have neoplastic disorders, including neuroblastoma, Wilms tumor, leukemia, pheochromocytoma, and sarcomas.

Neoplasms involving the peripheral nervous system and spinal nerve roots include schwannomas and neurofibromas. Intramedullary spinal cord tumors include ependymomas (especially of the conus medullaris and filum terminale) and, less often, astrocytomas. The most common intracranial tumors are hemisphere astrocytomas of any histologic grade from benign to highly malignant. Pilocytic astrocytic gliomas of the optic nerve and bilateral acoustic neuromas are also characteristic. Meningiomas, most commonly observed in adults, may be solitary or multicentric.

Symptoms and Signs. There are at least four genetic forms of neurofibromatosis. *Peripheral* or *classic neurofibromatosis* as described by von Recklinghausen is most commonly encountered. *Central* or *acoustic neurofibromatosis* is also of dominant inheritance. Symptoms of the bilateral acoustic neuroma appear at about age 20. Cutaneous changes are mild and there are only a few café-au-lait spots or neurofibromas. Antigenic activity of nerve growth factor is increased. *Segmental neurofibromatosis* is characterized by café-au-lait spots and neurofibromas that are limited, usually affecting an upper body segment. The lesions extend to the midline and include the ipsilateral arm but spare the head and neck. *Cutaneous neurofibromatosis* is limited to pigmentary changes; there are numerous café-au-lait spots but no other clinical manifestations of the disorder.

Peripheral neurofibromatosis often presents with protean and progressive manifestations. Not uncommonly, once the diagnosis is established, a fate like that of the grotesque Joseph Merrick (the Elephant Man) is anticipated by parents or physicians. In reality, many patients with this disease are functionally indistinguishable from normal. They often have only cutaneous lesions and are diagnosed when they see a physician because of learning disability, scoliosis, or other problem.

Cutaneous Symptoms. The café-au-lait macule is the pathognomonic lesion, being present in almost all patients (Fig. 100–1). Six or more café-au-lait spots larger than 1.5 cm in diameter are diagnostic. The spots are usually present at birth, but may not appear until age 1 or 2. Increasing in both size and number during the first decade of life, the macules tend to be less evident after the second decade because they blend into the surrounding hyperpigmented skin. These discrete, tan macules involve the trunk and limbs in a random fashion, but tend to spare the face.

Other cutaneous manifestations may include freckles over the entire body, but freckles usually involve the axilla and other intertriginous areas. Larger and darker hyperpigmented lesions (Fig. 100–2) are often associated with an underlying plexiform neu-

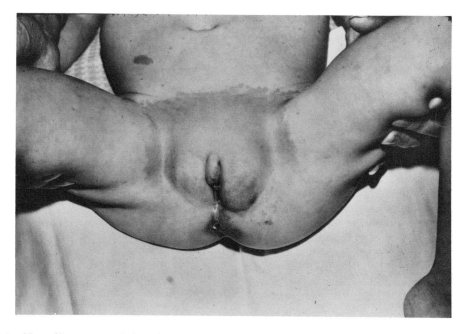

Fig. 100–1. Neurofibromatosis. Café-au-lait macule (abdomen) and larger pigmented lesion in the perineal area associated with an underlying plexiform neuroma and elephantiasis of the left labia.

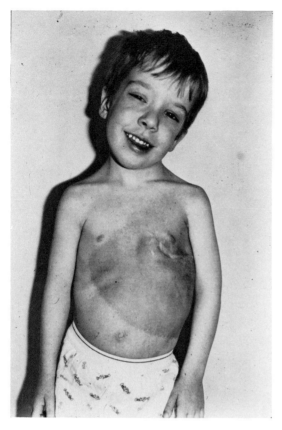

Fig. 100–2. Neurofibromatosis. Large pigmented lesion with associated progressive scoliosis.

rofibroma; if this involves the midline, it may indicate the presence of a spinal cord tumor.

Ocular Symptoms. Pigmented iris hamartomas *(Lisch nodules)*, when present, are characteristic and consist of small translucent yellow or brown elevations. The nodules increase in number with age. They are observed only in peripheral neurofibromatosis and are not seen in the normal eye.

Neurologic Symptoms. Neurofibromas, which are highly characteristic lesions, usually become clinically evident when patients are 10 to 15 years old. They always involve the skin, ultimately developing into sessile and pedunculated lesions. The nodules are found on deep peripheral nerves or nerve roots and on the autonomic nerves that innervate the viscera and blood vessels. The lesions increase in size and number during the second and third decades. There may be a few or many thousand. These benign tumors consist of neurons, Schwann cells, fibroblasts, blood vessels, and mast cells. They rarely give rise to any symptoms other than pain due to pressure on nerves or nerve roots,

but may undergo sarcomatous degeneration in the third and fourth decades of life (Fig. 100–3). Neurofibromas involving the terminal distribution of peripheral nerves form vascular plexiform neurofibromas that result in localized overgrowth of tissues or segmental hypertrophy of a limb *(elephantiasis neuromatosa).* Spinal root or cauda equina neurofibromas are often asymptomatic when they are small, but large tumors may compress the spinal cord, causing the appropriate clinical signs.

Optic gliomas, astrocytomas, acoustic neuromas, neurilemmomas, and meningiomas have a combined frequency of 5 to 10% of all patients with neurofibromatoses. Optic nerve gliomas and other intracranial neoplasms are often evident before age 10; acoustic neuromas become symptomatic at about age 20. When optic glioma is associated with neurofibromatosis, it commonly involves the optic nerve or is multicentric; less frequently, it involves the chiasm (Figs. 100–4, 100–5). Optic nerve glioma must be distinguished from the commonly observed non-neoplastic optic nerve hyperplasia. The optic glioma of neurofibromatosis is slowly progressive and has a better prognosis than similar tumors without this association. Central neurofibromatosis with bilateral acoustic neuromas is a distinct genetic disease. Clinically evident at about age 20, symptoms include hearing loss, tinnitus, imbalance, and headache. Only a

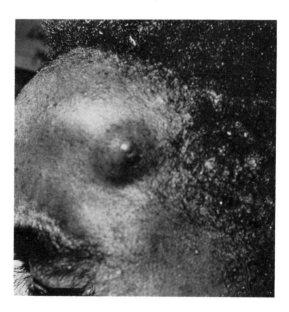

Fig. 100–3. Neurofibromatosis. Sarcomatous degeneration of a neurofibroma at 35 years.

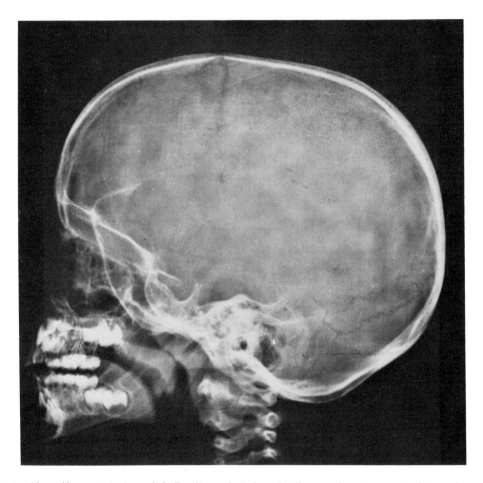

Fig. 100–4. Neurofibromatosis. Lateral skull radiograph. J-shaped sella secondary to an optic chiasm glioma.

few café-au-lait spots and neurofibromas occur.

CNS involvement in neurofibromatosis is highly variable. Macrocephaly, a common clinical manifestation of postnatal origin, is an incidental finding with no correlation with academic performance, seizures, or neurologic function. Specific learning disabilities or attention defect disorder, with or without impaired speech, is the most common neurologic complication of neurofibromatosis. Intellectual retardation or convulsive disorders each occur in about 5% of the patients.

Occlusive cerebrovascular disease is rare, but is sometimes seen in children with acute hemiplegia and convulsions. Cerebral angiography may demonstrate an occlusion of the supraclinoid portion of the internal carotid artery at the origin of the anterior and middle cerebral arteries with associated telangiectasia.

Symptoms of the Skull, Spine, and Extremities. Skeletal anomalies characteristic of neu-rofibromatosis include: (1) unilateral defects in the posterior superior wall of the orbit, with pulsating exophthalmos; (2) a defect in the lambdoid with underdevelopment of the ipsilateral mastoid; (3) dural ectasia with enlargement of the spinal canal and scalloping of the posterior portion of the vertebral bodies, which is also seen in connective tissue disorders such as the syndromes of Marfan and Ehlers-Danlos; (4) kyphoscoliosis, seen in 2 to 10% of neurofibromatosis patients, most commonly involving the cervicothoracic vertebra and, unless corrected, rapidly progressive, characterized by a short-segment angular scoliosis involving the lower thoracic vertebrae; (5) pseudoarthrosis, especially involving the tibia and radius; (6) "twisted ribbon" rib deformities; and (7) enlargement of long bones.

Miscellaneous Symptoms. Pheochromocytoma, an unusual complication of neurofibromatosis, is never seen in children. Hypertension may be due to pheochromocytoma or

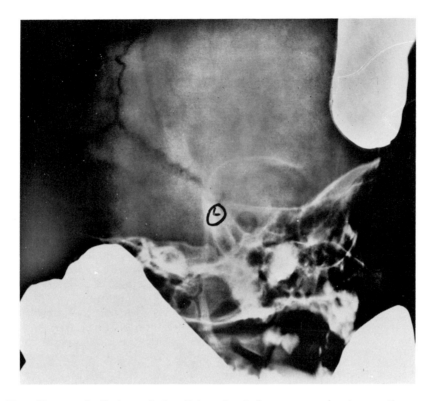

Fig. 100–5. Neurofibromatosis. Optic canal view. Enlarged optic foramen secondary to an optic nerve glioma.

neurofibromatosis of a renal artery. Malignant tumors not uncommonly complicating neurofibromatosis include sarcoma, leukemia, Wilms tumor, ganglioglioma, and neuroblastoma. Medullary thyroid carcinoma and hyperparathyroidism rarely occur. Precocious puberty and, less commonly, sexual infantilism result from involvement of the hypothalamus by glioma or hamartoma.

Diagnosis. The diagnosis of neurofibromatosis is based on clinical criteria, including one or more of the following: (1) six or more café-au-lait macules measuring more than 1.5 cm at their broadest area, or axillary freckling; (2) neurofibromas; (3) iris nodules; and (4) family history.

Laboratory Data. There is no laboratory test or prenatal procedure that is specific in making the diagnosis of neurofibromatosis. It has therefore been suggested that all patients and those at risk should receive an extensive clinical evaluation aimed at diagnosis and identification of possible complications. Ancillary laboratory studies, however, should be individualized, determined by the clinical manifestations. A complete evaluation may include psychoeducational and psychometric testing; radiographs of the skull, optic foram-

ina, internal auditory foramina, and vertebral spine; EEG; audiologic testing; cranial CT, including orbital views; CT of the spine and internal auditory foramina; MRI of brain and spine; and quantitative measurement of 24-hour urinary catecholamines. Serum nerve growth factor determinations distinguish peripheral or classic neurofibromatosis from central neurofibromatosis with bilateral acoustic neuroma.

Treatment. There is no specific treatment for neurofibromatosis, but complications may be ameliorated with early recognition and prompt therapeutic intervention. Learning disabilities should be considered in all children with neurofibromatosis and may be complicated by behavioral problems (hyperkinesis or attentional defect disorder) that warrant educational therapy or behavioral modification, psychotherapy, and pharmacotherapy. Speech problems require a language evaluation and formal speech therapy, and seizures indicate the need for anticonvulsant medication. Progressive kyphoscoliosis usually requires surgical intervention. Surgery may be necessary for removal of pheochromocytomas and intracranial or spinal neoplasms; cutaneous neurofibromas require extirpation when they compromise function or are disfiguring. Radiation therapy is reserved for some CNS neoplasms, including optic glioma. Genetic counseling and psychotherapy with family counseling are important.

References

Blatt J, Jaffe R, Deutsch M, Adkins JC. Neurofibromatosis and childhood tumors. Cancer 1986; 57:1225–1229.

Conference Statement, National Institutes of Health Consensus Development Conference: Neurofibromatosis. Arch Neurol 1988; 45:575–578.

Crowe FW, Schull WJ, Neel JV. A clinical, pathological and genetic study of multiple neurofibromatosis. Springfield: Charles C Thomas, 1956.

Holt JF. 1977 Edward BD. Neuhauser Lecture: Neurofibromatosis in children. AJR 1978; 130:615–639.

Jacoby CG, Go RT, Beren RA. Cranial CT of neurofibromatosis. AJNR 1980; 135:553–557.

Levinsohn PM, Mikhael MA. Rothman SM. Cerebrovascular changes in neurofibromatosis. Dev Med Child Neurol 1978; 20:789–792.

Martuza RL, Eldridge R. Neurofibromatosis 2 (bilateral acoustic neurofibromatosis). New Engl J Med 1988; 318:684–688.

Riccardi VM, Mulvihill JJ. Neurofibromatosis (von Recklinghausen disease). Adv Neurol 1981; 29:1–283.

Riccardi VM, Eichner JE. Neurofibromatosis. Baltimore: The Johns Hopkins Press, 1986.

Rubenstein AE, Bunge RP, Housman DE (eds). Neurofibromatosis. NY Acad Sci NY 1986; 486:1–414.

Schneider M, Obringer AC, Zackai E, Meadows AT. Childhood neurofibromatosis: risk factors for malignant disease. Cancer Genet Cytogenet 1986; 21:347–354.

Seizinger BR, Rouleau GR, Ozelius LJ, et al. Common pathogenetic mechanism for three tumor types in bilateral acoustic neurofibromatosis. Science 1987; 236:317–319.

Stern J, DiGiacinto GV, Housepian EM. Neurofibromatosis and optic glioma; clinical and morphological correlations. Neurosurgery 1979; 4:524–528.

Tibbles JAR, Cohen MM. The Proteus syndrome: the Elephant Man diagnosed. Br Med J 1986; 293:683–685.

Wanda JV, Das Gupta TK. Neurofibromatosis. Curr Probl Surg 1977; 14:1–81.

Wiedemann HR, Burgio GR, Aldenhoff P, et al. The Proteus syndrome: partial gigantism of the hands and/or feet, hemihypertrophy, subcutaneous tumors, macrocephaly or other skull anomalies and possible accelerated growth and visceral affections. Eur J Pediatr 1983; 140:5–12.

101. ENCEPHALOTRIGEMINAL ANGIOMATOSIS
Arnold P. Gold

Encephalotrigeminal angiomatosis *(Sturge-Weber-Dimitri syndrome)* classically includes the presence of a cutaneous vascular portwine nevus of the face, contralateral hemiparesis and hemiatrophy, glaucoma, seizures, and mental retardation. In 1847, Sturge

described the clinical picture and attributed the neurologic manifestations to a nevoid lesion of the brain similar to the facial lesion. In 1923, Dimitri showed the gyriform pattern of calcifications. Weber described the radiographic findings of these intracranial calcifications.

Genetics. Most cases are sporadic, but affected siblings suggest a recessive mode of inheritance. As with other neurocutaneous disorders, there is a high incidence of incomplete penetrance with marked variability of the clinical manifestations. The gene has been linked to chromosome 3.

Neuropathology. The occipital lobe is affected most often, but lesions may involve the temporal and parietal lobes or the entire cerebral hemisphere. Atrophy is characteristically unilateral and ipsilateral to the facial nevus. Leptomeningeal angiomatosis with small venules fills the subarachnoid space. Calcification of the arteries on the surface of the brain and intracerebral calcifications of small vessels are seen. The trolley-track or

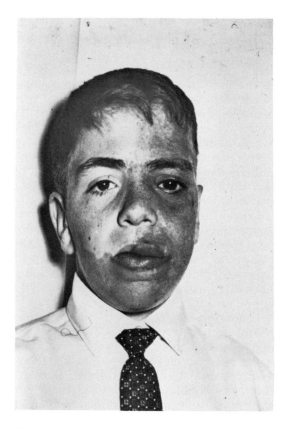

Fig. 101–1. Encephalotrigeminal angiomatosis. Facial nevus flammeus involving the cutaneous distribution of all three branches of the trigeminal nerve on one side and the mandibular branch on the contralateral side.

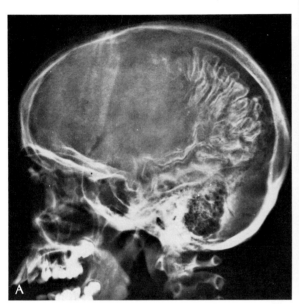
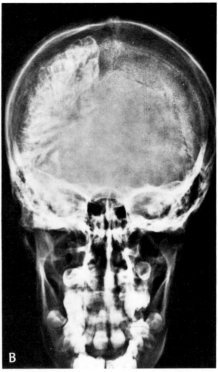

Fig. 101–2. Encephalotrigeminal angiomatosis. *A,* Skull radiography (lateral view) with characteristic calcifications consisting of paired curvilinear lines localized maximally to the occipital and parietal lobes. *B,* Encephalotrigeminal angiomatosis. Skull radiography (PA view) with calcifications outlining an atrophic right cerebral hemisphere.

curvilinear calcifications seen on skull radiographs are due to calcification of the outer cortex rather than of blood vessels.

Symptoms and Signs. Facial nevus and a neurologic syndrome of seizures, hemiplegia, retardation, and glaucoma are characteristic of encephalotrigeminal angiomatosis.

Cutaneous Symptoms. The port-wine facial nevus flammeus is related to the cutaneous distribution of the trigeminal nerve (Fig. 101–1). Most commonly involving the forehead, the nevus may involve half of the face and may extend to the neck. The nevus may cross or fall short of the midline. In rare instances, bilateral facial lesions may be seen.

Only when the entire ophthalmic sensory area (forehead and upper eyelid) is covered by the nevus flammeus (with or without involvement of the maxillary and mandibular areas) is there a high risk for glaucoma or neurologic complications. Neuro-ocular disease is rare when only part of the ophthalmic area has a port-wine stain. There is little to no risk when the nevus is localized to the maxillary or mandibular trigeminal sensory areas without involvement of the ophthalmic area.

Neurologic Symptoms. Epilepsy is the most common neurologic manifestation, usually starting in the first year of life with focal motor, generalized major motor, or partial complex convulsions. Often refractory to anticonvulsants, the focal motor seizures, hemiparesis, and hemiatrophy are contralateral to the facial nevus. Intellectual retardation often becomes more marked with age.

Ophthalmologic Symptoms. Raised intraocular pressure with glaucoma and buphthalmos occurs in approximately 30% of patients. Buphthalmos, which is more common than glaucoma, is due to antenatal intraocular hypertension. Homonymous hemianopia, a common visual field complication, is invariable when the occipital lobe is involved. Other congenital anomalies include coloboma of the iris and deformity of the lens.

Laboratory Data. The highly characteristic calcifications are rarely seen on radiographs before the patient is older than two years of age (Fig. 101–2). They appear as paired (trolley-track) curvilinear lines that follow the cerebral convolutions. Cerebral atrophy may be implied by asymmetry of the calvarium, with elevated petrous pyramid, thickening of the

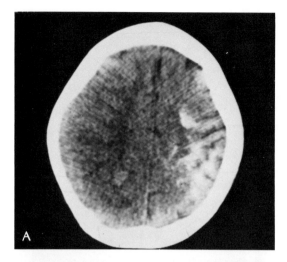

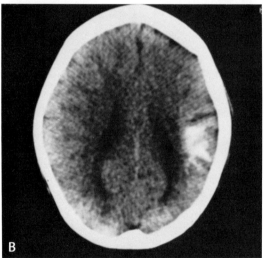

Fig. 101–3. Noncontrast CT shows subcortical calcification conforming to the gyral pattern of calcification in the Sturge-Weber syndrome. (Courtesy of Drs. S.K. Hilal and M. Mawad.)

calvarial diploë, and enlargement of the paranasal sinuses and mastoid air cells on the side of the lesion. CT documents the intracranial calcifications and unilateral cerebral atrophy (Fig. 101–3). Cerebral angiography may demonstrate capillary and venous abnormalities. The capillaries over the affected hemisphere are homogeneously increased, the superficial cortical veins are markedly decreased, and the superior sagittal sinus may be diminished or not seen.

EEG shows a wide area of low potentials over the affected areas, and this electrical silence correlates with the degree of intracranial calcification. The remainder of the hemisphere may show epileptiform activity. Visual field studies document the homonymous hemianopia.

Diagnosis. The diagnosis is based on the facial vascular port-wine nevus flammeus and one or more of the following: seizures, contralateral hemiparesis and hemiatrophy, mental retardation, and ocular findings of glaucoma or buphthalmos. The appearance of calcifications on skull radiographs or CT reinforces the diagnosis. On rare occasions, Sturge-Weber-Dimitri syndrome may occur with the neurologic syndrome and the typical intracranial calcifications, but without the facial nevus.

Treatment. The facial nevus rarely requires early cosmetic therapy. Later, this blemish can be covered with cosmetics or permanently treated with laser therapy. Seizures may be difficult to control with anticonvulsants; lobectomy or hemispherectomy may be efficacious. Physical and occupational therapy are indicated for the hemiparesis. Educational therapy and placement in a special school are important in the learning-disabled or intellectually impaired patient; vocational training is essential in affected older children and young adults. Behavioral problems are common and may include attention defect disorders or overt psychopathology that warrants psychotropic drug therapy and psychotherapy.

References

Alexander GL. Sturge-Weber syndrome. Handb Clin Neurol 1972; 14:223–240.

Alexander GL, Norman RM. The Sturge-Weber Syndrome. Baltimore: Williams & Wilkins, 1960.

Enjooras O, Riche MC, Merland JJ. Facial port-wine stains and Sturge-Weber syndrome. Pediatrics 1985; 76:48–51.

Gobbi G, Sorrenti G, Santucci M et al. Epilepsy with bilateral occipital calcifications: A benign onset with progressive severity. Neurology 1988; 38:913–920.

Poser CM, Taveras JM. Cerebral angiography in encephalotrigeminal angiomatosis. Radiology 1957; 68:327–336.

Seizinger BR, Rouleau EA, Ozelius LJ et al. Von Hippel-Lindau disease maps to chromosome 3 associated with renal cell carcinoma. Nature 1988; 332:268–269.

Sturge WA. A case of partial epilepsy, apparently due to a lesion of one of the vaso-motor centres of the brain. Trans Clin Soc London 1879; 12:162–167.

Weber FP. Right-sided hemi-hypertrophy resulting from right-sided congenital spastic hemiplegia, with a morbid condition of the left side of the brain, revealed by radiograms. J Neurol Psychopathol 1922; 3:134–139.

102. INCONTINENTIA PIGMENTI
Arnold P. Gold

Incontinentia pigmenti, described by Bloch and Sulzberger, is a genetic disorder that affects the skin in a characteristic manner and also involves the brain, eyes, nails, and hair.

Genetics. Found almost exclusively in girls, the disorder is due to an X-linked dominant gene that is prenatally lethal in males. The few cases of incontinentia pigmenti in boys are attributed to spontaneous mutation. A pregnant woman with incontinentia pigmenti runs a 25% risk of a spontaneous miscarriage (the affected male); half of her female children will be affected and will have the disease. Daughters are likely to be more severely affected than their mothers.

Neuropathology. The neuropathologic findings are nonspecific and include cerebral atrophy with microgyria, focal necrosis with formation of small cavities in the central white matter, and focal areas of neuronal loss in the cerebellar cortex.

Symptoms and Signs
Cutaneous Symptoms. Half the affected infants have the initial linear vesicobullous lesions at birth, and most of the other children show the lesions in the first two weeks of life. About 10% are delayed, appearing as late as one year of age. The skin lesions can recur and ultimately may undergo a characteristic change to linear verrucous and dyskeratotic growth, usually between the second and sixth week of life; pigmentary changes appear between the ages of 12 and 26 weeks. Some infants may show the pigmentary lesions at birth without further cutaneous progression. The pigmentation involves the trunk and extremities, is slate-gray blue or brown, and is distributed in irregular marbled or wavy lines. With age, the pigmentary lesions fade and become depigmented with atrophic skin changes.

Neurologic Symptoms. About 20% of affected children have a neurologic syndrome that may include slow motor development, pyramidal-tract dysfunction with spastic hemiparesis, quadriparesis or diplegia, mental retardation, and convulsive disorders.

Ocular Symptoms. Strabismus, cataracts, and severe visual loss occur in about 20% of affected children. Retinal vascular changes may result in blindness with ectasia, microhemorrhages, avascularity and, later, retinal pigmentation and atrophy.

Other Manifestations. Partial or total ano-dontia and peg-shaped teeth are characteristic of incontinentia pigmenti. Partial or complete diffuse alopecia with scarring and nail dystrophy may also occur.

Laboratory Data. Eosinophilia as high as 65% is often seen in infants less than 1 year old with an associated leukocytosis. Eosinophils are also found in the vesicobullous lesions and in the affected dermis.

Treatment. There is no specific treatment for incontinentia pigmenti, and management is directed at complicating problems, such as anticonvulsants for seizures. Awareness of the ocular manifestations is essential because laser coagulation in retinal ectasia prevents blindness.

Incontinentia Pigmenti Achromians

This neurocutaneous entity was originally described by Ito *(hypomelanosis of Ito)* and is distinctive in both clinical manifestations and pathologic features.

Etiology. The pathogenesis of this disease is similar to that of other neurocutaneous disorders. Migration of neural cells to the brain and melanoblasts to the skin from the neural

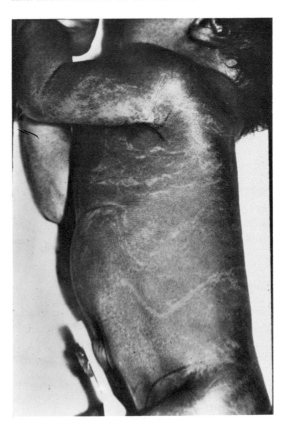

Fig. 102–1. Incontinentia pigmenti achromians. Hypopigmented skin lesions presenting as streaks or whorls.

crest occur between 3 and 6 months gestational age. A disturbance of this migration results in both brain and cutaneous pigmentary disease.

Genetics. Incontinentia pigmenti achromians is found in all races and sexes and is inherited as an autosomal dominant trait with variable penetrance. A chromosome abnormality with a balanced translocation between chromosome 2 and 8 may be significant.

Clinical Manifestations. In infancy, hypopigmented skin lesions appear as whorls or streaks on any part of the body (Fig. 102–1) and tend to progress onto uninvolved areas. This lesion is the negative image of incontinentia pigmenti. In later childhood, affected areas tend to return to normal skin color. The cutaneous lesion is often associated with developmental and neurologic abnormalities with hypotonia, pyramidal tract dysfunction and almost 80% mental retardation, and seizures. Ophthalmologic disorders, including strabismus, optic atrophy, micro-ophthalmia, tessellated fundus, eyelid ptosis, and heterochromia irides, also are present. The hair, teeth, and musculoskeletal system may be affected.

Pathology. The hypopigmented skin lesions are characterized by a decrease in the number of dopapositive melanocytes and decreased pigment production in the basal layer of the epidermis.

Diagnosis and Laboratory Data. Because there is no pathognomonic laboratory test, diagnosis must be based solely on the characteristic hypomelanosis.

Treatment. The whorly, marble-cake, hypopigmented skin lesions do not require any treatment. Therapy is directed toward the associated complications, such as anticonvulsants for seizures and specialized educational facilities for the learning-disabled or retarded child.

References

Carney RG. Incontinentia pigmenti: a world statistical analysis. Arch Dermatol 1976; 112:535–542.

Donat JF, Walsworth DM, Turk LL. Focal cerebral atrophy in incontinentia pigmenti achromians. Am J Dis Child 1980; 134:709–710.

Jelinek JE, Bart RS, Schiff GM. Hypomelanosis of Ito (incontinentia pigmenti achromians). Arch Dermatol 1973; 107:596–601.

Larsen R, Ashwal S, Peckham N. Incontinentia pigmenti: Association with anterior horn cell degeneration. Neurology 1987; 37:446–450.

Miller CA, Parker WD Jr. Hypomelanosis of Ito: association with a chromosomal abnormality. Neurology 1985; 35:607–610.

O'Brien JE, Feingold M. Incontinentia pigmenti a longitudinal study. Am J Dis Child 1985; 139:711–712.

O'Doherty NJ, Norman RM. Incontinentia pigmenti (Bloch-Sülzberger syndrome) with cerebral malformation. Dev Med Child Neurol 1968; 10:168–174.

Schwartz MF, Esterly NB, Fretzin DF, Pergament E, Rozenfeld IH. Hypomelanosis of Ito (incontinentia pigmenti achromians): a neurocutaneous syndrome. J Pediatr 1977; 90:236–240.

Sulzberger MB. Incontinentia pigmenti (Bloch-Sulzberger): report of an additional case, with comment or possible relation to a new syndrome of familial and congenital anomalies. Arch Dermatol 1938; 38:57–69.

103. TUBEROUS SCLEROSIS
Arnold P. Gold

Tuberous sclerosis was first described by von Recklinghausen in 1862. In 1880, Bourneville coined the term *sclérose tubéreuse* for the potato-like lesions in the brain. In 1890, Pringle described the facial nevi or *adenoma sebaceum*. Vogt later emphasized the classic triad of seizures, mental retardation, and adenoma sebaceum. Eponymically, tuberous sclerosis is called *Pringle disease* when there are only dermatologic findings, *Bourneville disease* when the nervous system is affected, and *West syndrome* when skin lesions are associated with infantile spasms, hypsarrhythmia, and mental retardation.

Tuberous sclerosis is a hereditable and determined progressive disorder characterized by the development in early life of hamartomas, malformations, and congenital tumors of the nervous system, skin, and viscera.

Genetics and Incidence. Tuberous sclerosis is inherited as an autosomal dominant trait with a high incidence of sporadic cases and protean clinical expressivity. These features are attributed to modifier genes, for which the homozygous condition results in a phenotypically normal individual despite the presence of the gene for tuberous sclerosis; when heterogeneous, the modifier gene results in a mildly affected patient. Evidence suggests that the gene for tuberous sclerosis is on chromosome 9. Incidence figures must be considered minimal because milder varieties are often unrecognized. Autopsy data gave an incidence of 1 in 10,000; clinical surveys gave a prevalence between 1 in 10,000 and 1 in 170,000. Although all races are affected, the disease is thought to be uncommon in blacks, and there may be a greater frequency in men.

Pathology and Pathogenesis. The pathologic changes are widespread and include lesions in the nervous system, skin, bones, retina, kidney, and other viscera.

The brain is usually normal in size, but several or many hard nodules occur on the surface of the cortex. These nodules are smooth, rounded, or polygonal, and project slightly above the surface of the neighboring cortex. They are whitish in color and firm to the touch. The nodules are of various sizes. Some involve only a small portion of one convolution. Others may encompass the convolutions of one whole lobe or a major portion of a hemisphere. In addition, there may be developmental anomalies of the cortical convolutions in the form of pachygyria or microgyria. On sectioning the hemispheres, sclerotic nodules may be found in the subcortical gray matter, the white matter, and the basal ganglia. The lining of the lateral ventricles is frequently the site of numerous small nodules that project into the ventricular cavity (*candle gutterings*—Fig. 103–1). Sclerotic nodules are less frequently found in the cerebellum, brain stem, and spinal cord.

Histologically, the nodules are characterized by the presence of a cluster of atypical glial cells in the center and giant cells in the periphery. Calcifications are relatively frequent. Other features include heterotopia, vascular hyperplasia (sometimes with actual angiomatous malformations), disturbances in the cortical architecture, and the occasional development of subependymal giant-cell astrocytomas. Intracranial aneurysm is an uncommon finding.

The lesions in the skin are multiform and include the characteristic facial nevi (*fibroma molluscum*) and patches of skin fibrosis. The facial lesions (Fig. 103–2) are not adenomas of the sebaceous glands, but are small hamartomas arising from nerve elements of the skin combined with hyperplasia of the connective tissue and blood vessels. Lesions similar in composition to those on the face are occasionally found between the nails and the digits of the hands and feet. Circumscribed areas of hypomelanosis or white nevi are common in tuberous sclerosis and are often found in infants. Although these are less specific than the *sebaceous adenoma*, they are of importance in suspecting the diagnosis in infants with seizures. Histologically, the skin appears normal except for the loss of melanin, but ultrastructural studies have shown that the melanosomes are small and have reduced content of melanin.

The retinal lesions are small congenital tumors (*phakomas*) composed of glia, ganglion cells, or fibroblasts. Glioma of the optic nerve has been reported.

Other lesions include cardiac rhabdomyomas; renal angiomyolipomas and renal cysts; cystic disease of the lungs and pulmonary lymphangiomatosis; hepatic angiomas and hamartomas; skeletal abnormalities with localized areas of osteosclerosis in the calvarium, spine, pelvis, and limbs; cystic defects involving the phalanges; and periosteal new bone formation confined to the metacarpals and metatarsals.

Symptoms and Signs. The cardinal features of tuberous sclerosis are skin lesions, con-

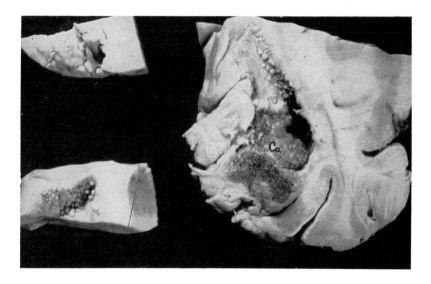

Fig. 103–1. Tuberous sclerosis. Nodules ("candle gutterings") on surface of ventricles. (Courtesy of Dr. Leon Roizin.)

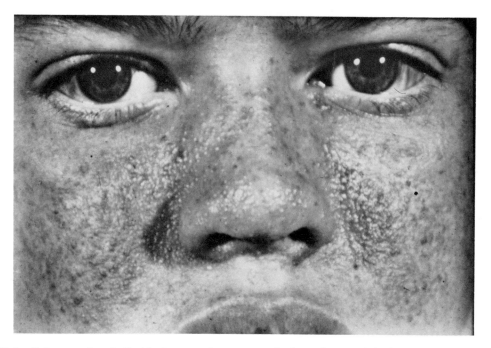

Fig. 103–2.   Tuberous sclerosis. Facial adenoma sebaceum over the butterfly area of the face sparing the upper lip.

vulsive seizures, and mental retardation. The disease is characterized by variability and expressivity of the clinical manifestations.

Cutaneous Symptoms. Depigmented or hypomelanotic macules are the earliest skin lesion (Fig. 103–3). These macules are present at birth, persist through life, and may only be found with a Wood's lamp. The diagnosis is suggested if there are three or more macules that measure 1 cm or more in length. Numerous small macules sometimes resemble confetti or depigmented freckles. Most macules are leaf-shaped, resembling the leaf of the European mountain ash tree and some-

Fig. 103–3.   Tuberous sclerosis. Hypomelanotic or ash leaf macules.

times following a dermatomal distribution. Facial adenoma sebaceum (facial angiofibroma) is never present at birth, but is clinically evident in over 90% of affected children by age 4. At first, the facial lesion is the size of a pinhead or a millet seed, and red in color because of the prominent angiomatous component. It is distributed symmetrically on the nose and cheeks in a butterfly distribution. The lesions may involve the forehead and chin, but rarely involve the upper lip. They gradually increase in size and become yellowish and glistening. *Shagreen patches*, a connective-tissue hamartoma, are also characteristic of tuberous sclerosis. Rarely present in infancy, these patches become evident after the first decade of life. Usually found in the lumbosacral region, shagreen plaques are yellowish-brown elevated plaques that have the texture of pig skin. Other skin lesions include *café-au-lait spots*, small fibromas that may be tiny and resemble coarse goose flesh, and ungual fibromas that appear after puberty.

Neurologic Symptoms. Seizures and mental retardation are indicative of diffuse encephalopathy. Infantile myoclonic spasms, with or without hypsarrhythmia, are the characteristic seizures of young infants and, when associated with hypopigmented macules, are diagnostic of tuberous sclerosis. The older child or adult has generalized tonic-clonic or

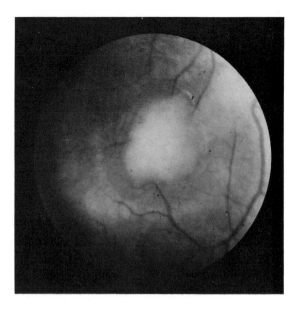

Fig. 103–5. Tuberous sclerosis. Phakoma or retinal hamartoma involving the peripheral retina.

partial complex seizures. There is a close relationship between the onset of seizures at a young age and mental retardation. Mental retardation rarely occurs without clinical seizures, but intellect may be normal, despite seizures. Other than a delayed acquisition of developmental milestones, intellectual impairment, or nonspecific language or coordinative deficiencies, a formal neurologic examination is unremarkable for tuberous sclerosis.

Ophthalmic Symptoms. Hamartomas of the retina or optic nerve are observed in about 50% of well-studied patients with tuberous sclerosis. Two types of retinal lesions are seen on funduscopic examination: (1) the easily recognized calcified hamartoma near or at the disc with an elevated multinodular lesion that resembles mulberries, grains of tapioca, or salmon eggs (Fig. 103–4); and (2) the less distinct, relatively flat, smooth-surfaced, salmon-colored, circular or oval-shaped lesion located peripherally in the retina (Fig. 103–5). Nonretinal lesions can vary from the specific depigmented lesion of the iris (Fig. 103–6) to the nonspecific nonparalytic strabismus, optic atrophy, visual-field defects, or cataracts.

Visceral Symptoms. Renal lesions include hamartomas (angiomyolipomas) and renal cysts. Typically, both are multiple, bilateral, and usually innocuous and silent. In one series, there was a 50% incidence of tuberous

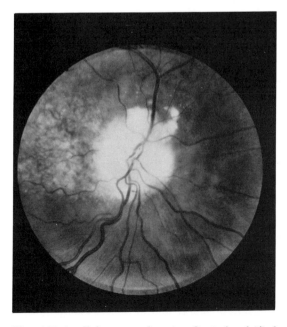

Fig. 103–4. Tuberous sclerosis. Central calcified hamartoma or so-called "mulberry phakoma" at the optic nerve.

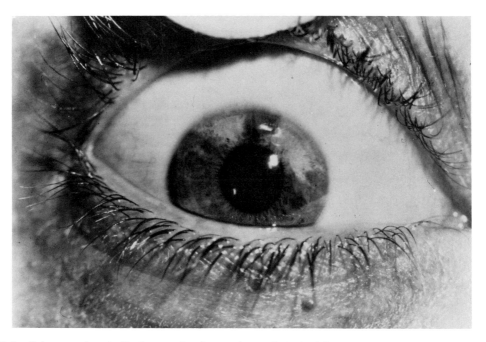

Fig. 103–6. Tuberous sclerosis. Depigmented or hypomelanotic lesions of the iris.

sclerosis in cases of cardiac rhabdomyoma. This cardiac tumor may be symptomatic at any age, even infancy, and can result in death.

Pulmonary lesions occur in fewer than 1% of patients. These become symptomatic (often with a spontaneous pneumothorax) in the third or fourth decade of life, and are progressive and often fatal. Sclerotic lesions of the calvarium and cystic lesions of the metacarpals and phalanges are asymptomatic. Hamartomatous hemangiomas of the spleen and racemose angiomas of the liver are rare and asymptomatic.

Laboratory Data. Unless renal lesions are present, routine laboratory studies are normal. Renal angiomyolipomas are usually asymptomatic and rarely cause gross hematuria, but may show albuminuria and microscopic hematuria. Sonograms, angiograms, and CT are often diagnostic (Fig. 103–7). Multiple or diffuse renal cysts may be associated with albuminuria, or azotemia and hypertension. Intravenous pyelograms are diagnostic.

Chest radiographs may reveal pulmonary lesions or rhabdomyoma with cardiomegaly. EKG findings are variable, but the echocardiogram is diagnostic.

Skull radiographs usually reveal small calcifications within the substance of the cerebrum (Fig. 103–8). CSF is normal except when a large intracerebral tumor is present. EEGs are often abnormal, especially in patients with clinical seizures. Abnormalities include slow wave activity and epileptiform discharges that include hypsarrhythmia, focal or multifocal spike or sharp-wave discharges, and generalized spike-and-wave discharges. CT is diagnostic when calcified subependymal nodules encroach on the lateral ventricle (often in the region of the foramen of Monro) and calcified cortical or cerebellar nodules (Fig. 103–9).

A few nodules appear isodense on CT and are better visualized on MRI. Calcified paraventricular and cortical lesions have been visualized shortly after birth, and the number of nodules is unrelated to intelligence.

Diagnosis. Clinical diagnosis is possible at most ages. In infancy, three or more characteristic depigmented cutaneous lesions suggest the diagnosis, and this is reinforced in the presence of infantile myoclonic spasms. In the older child or adult, the diagnosis is made by the triad of tuberous sclerosis (i.e., facial adenoma sebaceum, epilepsy, and mental retardation). Retinal or visceral lesions may be diagnostic. However, the disease is noted for protean manifestations, and a family history may be invaluable in establishing the diagnosis, which is often established by CT evidence of calcified subependymal nodules.

The differential diagnosis includes other

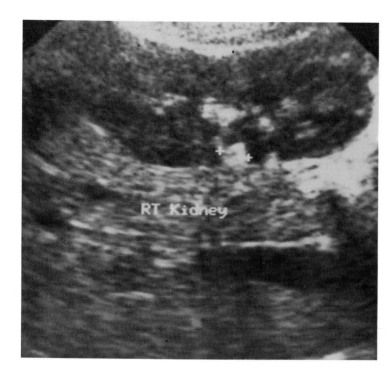

Fig. 103–7. Tuberous sclerosis. Renal sonogram demonstrating a renal angiomyolipoma.

diseases that involve skin, nervous system, and retina. Neurofibromatous and encephalotrigeminal angiomatosis are differentiated by the characteristic skin lesions of those disorders.

Multisystem involvement may result in difficulties in establishing a diagnosis of tuberous sclerosis. Gomez defined primary and secondary diagnostic criteria (Table 103–1).

There is no method for prenatal diagnosis.

Course and Prognosis. Mild or solely cutaneous involvement often follows a static course, whereas those with the full-blown syndrome have a progressive course with increasing seizures and dementia. The child with infantile myoclonic spasms is at great risk of later intellectual deficit. Brain tumor, status epilepticus, renal insufficiency, cardiac failure, or progressive pulmonary impairment can lead to death.

Treatment. There is no specific treatment. The cutaneous lesions do not compromise

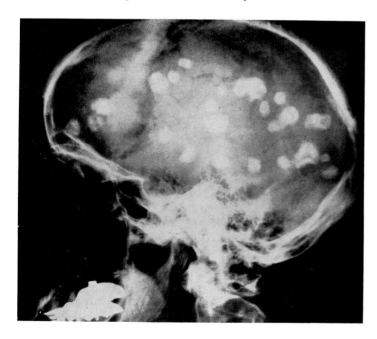

Fig. 103–8. Tuberous sclerosis. Calcified nodules in the cerebrum. (Courtesy of Dr. P.I. Yakovlev.)

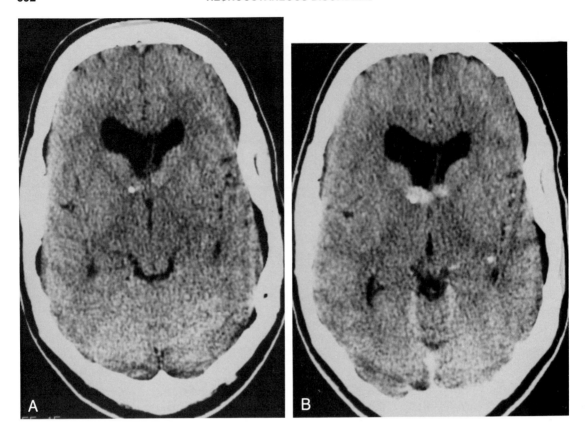

Fig. 103–9. Tuberous sclerosis. *A,* An axial noncontrast CT scan demonstrates a calcific density adjacent to the right foramen of Monro, a typical location for tubers. *B,* Post-contrast, this lesion enhances as well as additional noncalcified lesions on the contralateral side. (Courtesy of Drs. J.A. Bello and S.K. Hilal.)

function, but cosmetic surgery may be indicated for facial adenoma sebaceum or large shagreen patches. Infantile myoclonic spasms often respond to corticosteroid or corticotropin therapy; focal and generalized seizures are treated with anticonvulsants. Progressive cystic renal involvement often responds to

surgical decompression. Intramural cardiac rhabdomyoma and complicating congestive heart failure are managed medically with cardiotonics, diuretics, and salt restriction. Whole obstructive intracavity tumors and congestive heart failure require surgical extirpation of the tumor. Progressive pulmonary involvement is an indication for respiratory therapy, but response is poor and most patients die a few years after the onset of this complication.

Table 103–1. Diagnostic Criteria for Tuberous Sclerosis (Gomez 1979)

Primary Diagnosis—one of the following
Facial adenoma sebaceum
Periungual or subungual fibroma
Cortical tuber or subependymal hamartoma
Multiple retinal hamartomas

Secondary Diagnosis—two of the following
Infantile spasms
Hypomelanotic macules
Shagreen patch
Single retinal hamartoma
Intraventricular or paraventricular nodular
  calcifications
Bilateral renal angiomyolipomas
Cardiac rhabdomyoma

References

Baker RS, Ross PA, Baumann RJ. Neurologic complications of epidermal nevus syndrome. Arch Neurol 1987; 44:227–231.

Bellock GS, Shapshay SM. Management of facial angiofibromas in tuberous sclerosis: use of the carbon dioxide laser. Otolaryngol Head Neck Surg 1986; 94:37–40.

Bourneville DM. Sclérose tubéreuse des circonvolutions cérébrales: idiotie et épilepsie hémiplégique. Arch Neurol 1880; 1:81–91.

Cooper JR. Brain tumors in hereditary multiple system hamartomatosis (tuberous sclerosis). J Neurosurg 1971; 34:194–202.

Donegani G, Gratarolla FR, Wildi E. Tuberous sclerosis. In: Vinken PJ, Bruyn GW, eds. Handbook of Clinical

Neurology (vol 14). New York: Elsevier-North-Holland, 1972: 340–389.

Fryer AE, Connor JM, Povey S, Yates JRW, Chalmers A, Fraser I, Yates AD, Osborne JP. Evidence that the gene for tuberous sclerosis is on chromosome 9. Lancet 1987; 1:659–661.

Gold AP, Freeman JM. Depigmented nevi: the earliest sign of tuberous sclerosis. Pediatrics 1965; 35:1003–1005.

Gomez MR, ed. Tuberous Sclerosis. New York: Raven Press, 1979.

Gomez MR, Mellinger JF, Reese DF. The use of computerized axial tomography in the diagnosis of tuberous sclerosis. Mayo Clin Proc 1975; 50:553–556.

Kandt RS, Gebarski SS, Geotting MG. Tuberous sclerosis with cardiogenic cerebral embolism: magnetic resonance imaging. Neurology 1985; 35:1223–1225.

Lucchese NJ, Goldberg MF. Iris and fundus pigmentary changes in tuberous sclerosis. J Pediatr Ophthalmol Strabismus 1981; 18:45–46.

Martyn L: Tuberous sclerosis of Bourneville. In: Tasman W, ed. Retinal Diseases in Children. New York: Harper and Row, 1971:98–103.

Medley BS, McLeod RA, Houser OW. Tuberous sclerosis. Semin Roentgenol 1976; 11:35–54.

Palmieri A, De Vecchio E, Pirolo R, Gardeur D, Ambrosio A. The current potential of neuroradiology in the diagnosis of tuberous sclerosis. Ital J Neurol Sci 1982; 3:229–233.

Pampligione G, Moynahan EJ. The tuberous sclerosis syndome: clinical and EEG studies in 100 children. J Neurol Neurosurg Psychiatry 1976; 39:666–673.

Paulson GW, Lyle CB. Tuberous sclerosis. Dev Med Child Neurol 1966; 8:571–586.

Roach ES, Williams DP, Laster DW. Magnetic resonance imaging in tuberous sclerosis. Arch Neurol 1987; 44:301–303.

Wielderholt WC, Gomez MR, Kurland LT. Incidence and prevalence of tuberous sclerosis in Rochester, Minnesota, 1950 through 1982. Neurology 1985; 35:600–603.

Chapter XI

Cranial Nerve Disorders

104. LEBER HEREDITARY OPTIC ATROPHY
Myles M. Behrens

A hereditary disease of the optic nerve, characterized by loss of central vision with relatively normal peripheral fields, was described by von Graefe in 1858. The disease was named after Leber, who reported 15 cases in four different families in 1871. The disease usually affects young men in their late teens or early twenties. The onset is often acute, simulating optic neuritis.

The mode of inheritance of Leber disease is not fully understood. It is usually transmitted from mother to son, suggesting sex-linked inheritance, but not in strict accord with Mendelian principles: it is manifest more often than expected in female carriers; it is transmitted by symptomless women to most of their offspring; there is no transmission by men of either the carrier state or the disease. It is thought that maternal transmission is due to cytoplasmic (e.g., mitochondrial) transmission. A mutation in mitochondrial DNA has been identified.

The characteristic findings at autopsy are a primary neuronal degeneration of the retina and the central portion of the optic nerves. Occasionally there are other signs of disease of the nervous system, including nystagmus, ataxia, intention tremor, convulsive seizures, and increased reflexes; demyelination of other parts of the brain and the dorsal columns of the spinal cord may occur in such instances. CSF pleocytosis may occur, which resembles multiple sclerosis. Cardiac defects have also been reported.

The visual loss usually develops suddenly without an obvious cause. There is cloudiness of central vision that usually progresses to a larger and denser centrocecal scotoma over several weeks, only occasionally breaking out peripherally to a minor extent. There is impairment of color vision and visual acuity, usually in the 20/200 to finger-counting range. Both eyes are usually affected within days or months of each other.

At onset, the disc often appears blurred and is suggestive of edema as in papillitis. However, a characteristic disc appearance has been described: blurring of the disc margins with a glistening peripapillary opacity that is attributed to swelling of the nerve fiber layer. There is no evidence of abnormal vascular permeability on fluorescein angiography and the abnormality is not true edema but rather suggests impaired axonal transport. There is telangiectatic microangiopathy with excessive small vessels undulating in and out of the peripapillary nerve fiber layer. The vascular abnormality may long antedate visual loss and may be pathogenetic. Dilation of the vessels with increased arteriovenous shunting accompanies the thickening of the axonal layer as the acute stage approaches. This subsides after a few weeks or months, with impairment of capillary filling initially in the papillomacular bundle region and the development of optic atrophy that is primarily temporal at first, but usually becomes generalized (Fig. 104–1).

Occasionally, there is subsequent gradual decline in vision but not to blindness; more often there is some improvement, infrequently striking and occasionally sudden. The degree of visual loss generally remains relatively stationary after a certain point. Thus the patient should therefore be encouraged to adjust to the amount of vision preserved. No treatment is of proven value, including corticosteroids, hydroxycobalamin (suggested because of evidence that cyanide toxicity might be a factor), or craniotomy with lysis of optic nerve chiasm arachnoidal adhesions. Despite optimistic reports, none of these therapies has been widely confirmed and the var-

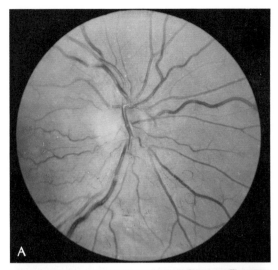

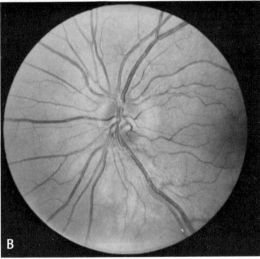

Fig. 104–1. Appearance of the fundi in a 23-year-old man wth centrocecal scotomas of 3 months duration O.D. *(A)* and 1 month O.S. *(B).* The scotoma is denser O.D. Temporal pallor has developed O.D. with some residual peripapillary nerve-fiber layer thickening as indicated by obscuration of large venous branches 1 disc diameter from the disc at 11:00 o'clock and at 6:30 o'clock with a prominent "cork screw" peripapillary vessel at 11:30 o'clock. The more acute fundus picture is seen O.S. with more hyperemic blurred disc with peripapillary excessive fine tortuous vasculature (e.g., at 5:00 o'clock).

iable natural history of untreated Leber optic atrophy makes it difficult to evaluate treatment.

The diagnosis of Leber optic atrophy is usually made when the typical course of visual loss occurs with an appropriate family history or observation of the typical acute fundus appearance in the patient or compatible fundus features in close maternal relatives. Other forms of bilateral optic neuropathy with cen-

trocecal scotomas include demyelinating, toxic-nutritional optic neuropathy (including tobacco-alcohol amblyopia), other types of hereditary optic atrophy, occasionally glaucoma, and only rarely compressive lesions. To help exclude tumors, one may use computed tomography—axial and coronal orbital views with and without contrast to include the optic nerves and chiasm—or high-quality magnetic resonance imaging of these structures.

Other forms of hereditary optic atrophy may occur as part of more extensive neurologic disorders, including the lipidoses and hereditary cerebellar ataxias. The recessive *Behr complicated optic atrophy* may be a transitional form between the ataxias and isolated hereditary optic atrophy. Other autosomal recessive forms of optic atrophy include the rare severe form of simple optic atrophy beginning in early infancy and that associated with diabetes insipidus, diabetes mellitus and hearing defect. The dominant variety of hereditary optic atrophy as initially categorized by Kjer is the most common form of hereditary optic atrophy and must be distinguished from Leber optic atrophy. It is also characterized by centrocecal scotoma, dyschromatopsia, and temporal pallor, but is generally mild, usually beginning insidiously between ages 4 and 8 years, and mildly progressive with visual acuity from 20/30 to no worse than 20/200.

A source of confusion in nomenclature is the severe congenital visual loss known as *Leber congenital amaurosis.* It is an autosomal recessive degeneration of the retina rather than of the optic nerve and is usually characterized by retinal arteriolar narrowing and retinal pigmentary degeneration. Occasionally, the fundus may appear normal at first. The electroretinogram is extinguished, whereas it is normal with optic neuropathy.

References

Adams JH, Blackwood W, Wilson J. Further clinical and pathological observations on Leber's optic atrophy. Brain 1966; 8:15–26.

Anonymous. Leber's optic neuropathy (Editorial). Br Med J 1980; 280:1097–1098.

Carroll WM, Mastaglia FL. Leber's optic neuropathy. A clinical and visual evoked potential study of affected and asymptomatic members of a six generation family. Brain 1979; 102:559–580.

Imachi J. Neuro-surgical treatment of Leber's optic atrophy and its pathogenic relationship to arachnoiditis. In: Brunette J, Barbeau A (eds). Progress in Neuro-Ophthalmology. Amsterdam: Excerpta Medica, 1969:121–127.

Kjer P. Infantile optic atrophy with dominant mode of

inheritance. In: Vinken PJ, Bruyn GW, eds. Handbook of Clinical Neurology (vol 13). New York: Elsevier-North Holland, 1972:111–123.

Kline LB, Glaser JS. Dominant optic atrophy: The clinical profile. Arch Ophthalmol 1979; 97:1680–1686.

Leber T. Über hereditäre und congenital angelegte Sehnervenleiden. Arch Ophthalmol 1871; 17:249–291.

Lundsgaard R. Leber's disease: A genealogic, genetic and clinical study of 101 cases of retrobulbar optic neuritis in 20 Danish families. Acta Ophthalmol (suppl 21) 1944, pp. 1–306.

Miller NR. Walsh and Hoyt's Clinical Neuro-Ophthalmology, 4th ed (vol 1). Baltimore: Williams & Wilkins, 1982:311–317.

Nikoskelainen E. New aspects of the genetic, etiologic, and clinical puzzle of Leber's disease. Neurology 1984; 34:1482–1484.

Nikoskelainen E, Hoyt WF, Nummelin K. Ophthalmoscopic findings in Leber's hereditary optic neuropathy. I. Fundus findings in asymptomatic family members. Arch Ophthalmol 1982; 100:1597–1602.

Nikoskelainen E, Hoyt WF, Nummelin K. Ophthalmoscopic findings in Leber's hereditary optic neuropathy. II. The fundus findings in the affected family members. Arch Ophthalmol 1983; 101:1059–1068.

Nikoskelainen E, Hoyt WF, Nummelin K, Schatz H. Fundus findings in Leber's hereditary optic neuroretinopathy. III. Fluorescein angiographic studies. Arch Ophthalmol 1984; 102:981–989.

Nikoskelainen EK, Savontaus M, Wanne OP, Katila MJ, Nummelin KU. Leber's hereditary optic neuroretinopathy, a maternally inherited disease. Arch Ophthalmol 1987; 105:665–671.

Pilley SFJ, Thompson HS. Familial syndrome of diabetes insipidus, diabetes mellitus, optic atrophy, and deafness (didmoad) in childhood. Br J Ophthalmol 1976; 60:294.

Smith JL, Hoyt WF, Susac JO. Ocular fundus in acute Leber optic neuropathy. Arch Ophthalmol 1973; 90:349–354.

'Jemura A, Osame M, Nakagawa M, Nakahara K, Sameshima M, Ohba N. Leber's hereditary optic neuropathy: Mitochondrial and biochemical studies on muscle biopsies. Br J Ophthalmol 1987; 71:531–536.

Van Senus AHC. Leber's disease in the Netherlands. Doc Ophthalmol 1963; 17:1–162.

Von Graefe. Ein ungewöhnlicher Fall von Hereditäre Amaurose. Arch Ophthalmol 1858; 4:266–268.

Wallace DC, Singh G, Lott MT, et al. Mitochondrial DNA mutation associated with Leber's hereditary optic neuropathy. Science 1988; 242:1427–1430.

105. PROGRESSIVE EXTERNAL OPHTHALMOPLEGIA

Lewis P. Rowland

Clinical Manifestations. Progressive ophthalmoplegia, a syndrome of familial or sporadic incidence, is characterized by progressive weakness of the external muscles of the eye. The syndrome is heterogeneous and comprises several different disorders. The onset is usually in early childhood, but may be delayed to middle life. The condition starts with slight ptosis of the lids and progresses

for years to complete paralysis of all external muscles of the eye. Only rarely is the pupil affected. Occasionally, paralysis of the muscles of one eye may precede that of the other eye by several or many years.

On examination, the ophthalmoplegia may be the only abnormality or there may be weakness of eye closure, oropharyngeal muscles, neck, or limbs. One special autosomal dominant form has been singled out as *oculopharyngeal muscular dystrophy.*

If the weakness is restricted to the eyes, there is a cosmetic problem and considerable inconvenience, but there is no threat to life. The ptosis can be corrected surgically (with care to avoid exposure keratitis). If limb muscles are affected, the disability may be mild or severe; in these patients there is no cardiac disorder.

Classification and Debate. The same pattern of ophthalmoplegia may occur in association with many neurologic symptoms and signs including retinitis pigmentosa, cerebellar ataxia, spastic paraplegia, dystonia, deafness, motor neuron disease, and peripheral neuropathy. There is intense controversy about the classification of these syndromes and two divergent views have emerged.

Some authorities lump the several different multisystem diseases as *ophthalmoplegia plus,* suggesting that overlapping manifestations defy isolation of specific syndromes. In general, these investigators are impressed with the almost universal appearance of mitochondrial abnormalities in biopsy of skeletal muscle. In special stains, these abnormal organelles appear bright red; hence, the term "ragged red fibers."

Moreover, they go three steps further: (1) They believe that the neurologic disorders are a consequence of the mitochondrial abnormality. Thus, the names *"mitochondrial encephalomyopathy"* or *"mitochondrial myopathy"* are given. (2) They include progressive external ophthalmoplegia with syndromes that completely lack ophthalmoplegia, as long as there are ragged red fibers in the muscle biopsy. Some of these syndromes are restricted to cerebral pathology, others include spinal cord disease, and some are manifest only by "exercise intolerance." (3) Many of these other syndromes are inherited in autosomal dominant fashion, so it is presumed that all are heritable diseases. Although there have been attempts to show mitochondrial inheritance, it has yet to be proved.

"Splitters," on the other hand, believe that

specific syndromes can be delineated on clinical grounds. They note that ragged red fibers are found with so many different clinical patterns that the histologic abnormality cannot be used as the basis of a classification. Moreover, they view as unproven the assumption that these diseases are all due to malfunction of mitochondria. The ragged red fibers, themselves, might be caused by some underlying disorder.

Kearns-Sayre Syndrome. The center of the controversy is the *Kearns-Sayre syndrome*, which the splitters regard as a specific disorder (Table 105–1). This disorder is identified by an invariant triad: onset before age 20, PEO, and pigmentary degeneration of the retina. In addition, there must be one of the following: heartblock, cerebellar syndrome, and CSF protein content of 100 mg/dl or more. Other manifestations are listed in Table 105–1.

Defined in this way, the Kearns-Sayre syndrome is almost never familial. There have been only two sets of affected siblings, and no cases in which the full condition has appeared in successive generations. For these and other reasons, it has been suggested that

Table 105–1.　Manifestations of Kearns-Sayre Syndrome

	1977[a]		1982[b]	
Number of cases (%)	35	(100)	35	(100)
Retarded	14	(40)	20	(57)
Cerebellar syndrome	24	(69)	32	(91)
Babinski signs	9	(26)	9	(26)
Limb weakness	13	(33)	29	(83)
Hearing loss	19	(54)	24	(69)
Seizures		0	3	(10)*
Short stature	22	(63)	25	(71)
Delayed puberty	11	(33)	—	—
CSF protein				
Not done		10		7
Normal		1		2
(>100 mg/dl)		20/24		26/28
Ragged red fibers in limb muscle		5/7		28/30
CT lucencies		—		4
Pontine atrophy		—		4
Calcification		—		2
Normal		—		4
Autopsies		5		8
Spongy degeneration		5		8

[a]Berenberg, Pellock, et al. (1977)
[b]Cases reported since (a).
*All three hypoparathyroidism.
(From Scarlato and Cerri, eds. Mitochondrial Pathology in Muscle Disease.)

the condition may be acquired, and the possibility of lethal dominant inheritance has been raised. If affected individuals never have children, the gene cannot be passed, and only new mutations will be seen. Which of these alternatives, or others, is correct remains to be seen.

Laboratory abnormalities include raised blood and CSF lactate and pyruvate levels (without acidosis) and low CSF folate values. Several patients have had evidence of primary hypoparathyroidism. Biochemical studies of isolated mitochondria have sometimes shown abnormalities, but none has been found consistently. At postmortem examination every typical case has had spongy degeneration of the brain. Correspondingly, computed tomography may show lucent areas in the white matter. In patients with hypoparathyroidism, there may be calcification of the basal ganglia. MRI findings have yet to be reported, partly because so many of the older patients have metal pacemakers that preclude exposure to the magnetic field.

It is important to recognize the Kearns-Sayre syndrome because sudden death due to the cardiac disorder is a threat that can be prevented. With a pacemaker, the children live longer but the natural history of the disease has not been analyzed. Patients are subject to episodic coma, perhaps because diabetic acidosis combines with the brain disease to make the individual more vulnerable. Also, the cerebellar syndrome may be severe and disabling. Treatment with coenzyme Q may retard some laboratory abnormalities, but it has not reversed the ophthalmoplegia or neurologic disorder.

Differential Diagnosis. Many other syndromes are also characterized by progressive ophthalmoplegia. Whether an ophthalmoplegic syndrome is assigned to a neurogenic or myopathic category depends on EMG and biopsy study of limb muscle, or autopsy examination. In syndromes that are characterized only by weakness, one or the other category may seem unequivocal and, usually, myopathic. Ragged red fibers are found commonly in autosomal dominant or recessive progressive external ophthalmoplegia as well as in isolated cases. In oculopharyngeal muscular dystrophy, however, there are different histologic abnormalities in muscle-rimmed vacuoles and intranuclear tubular filamentous inclusions.

When ophthalmoplegia is associated with neurologic disorders, the cause of the ocular

Table 105–2. Biochemical classification of the mitochondrial myopathies

Defects of transport
  CPT deficiency
  Carnitine deficiency
  Defect of FAD uptake (?)
Defects of substrate utilization
  Pyruvate carboxylase deficiency
  Pyruvate dehydrogenase complex deficiency
  Defects of B-oxidation
Defects of the Krebs cycle
  Fumarase deficiency
  α-Ketoglutarate dehydrogenase (dihydrolipoyl dehydrogenase) deficiency
Defects of oxidation-phosphorylation coupling
  Complex I deficiency
  Complex II deficiency (?)
  Complex III deficiency
  Complex IV deficiency
  Complex V deficiency
  Combined defects of respiratory chain components

From DiMauro et al. (1987)

muscle disorder may also be neurogenic. For instance, in Kearns-Sayre syndrome, all autopsied cases have shown spongy degeneration of the white matter, even when limb-muscle biopsies showed myopathic changes.

The diagnosis of ocular myopathy is not difficult when the onset is in infancy or early childhood, or when the disorder has already affected other members of the family. Refsum syndrome should be excluded by determination of phytanic acid. Cases of late onset must be differentiated from myasthenia gravis and the exophthalmic ophthalmoplegia of Graves disease.

Relation to Mitochondrial Myopathies and Encephalomyopathies

Mitochondrial myopathies have been defined in two ways, by demonstrated biochemical abnormality and by observation of ragged red fibers in muscle biopsy. Identified abnormalities of mitochondrial enzymes (Table 105–2) are discussed in other chapters; some of these disorders are not associated with ragged red fibers. On the other hand, ragged red fibers are found in many syndromes—not only the Kearns-Sayre syndrome and other forms of progressive external ophthalmoplegia but also syndromes that have been assigned descriptive acronyms: *MERRF* (for *myoclonus epilepsy* and *ragged red fibers*) or *Fukuhara disease*, and *MELAS* (*mitochondrial encephalomyopathy, lactic acidosis,* and *stroke*). Patients with MERRF or MELAS do not have

ophthalmoplegia, cardiac disorder, or retinopathy.

1988 was a year of changing concepts in this field. Holt, Harding, and Morgan-Hughes first reported deletions of human mitochondrial DNA. Then Zeviani et al. indicated that deletions are found in almost all Kearns-Sayre patients and in many patients with other forms of progressive ophthalmoplegia, but not in those with MERRF or MELAS. Thus far, all patients with deletions of mitochondrial DNA have had ophthalmoplegia, with or without clinical disorders. These findings suggest a causal link between the deletions and clinical manifestations, but there are still problems to be resolved.

References

Allen RJ, DiMauro S, Coulter DL, Papadimitriou A, Rothenberg SP. Kearns-Sayre syndrome with reduced plasma and CSF folate. Ann Neurol 1983; 13:679–682.

Berenberg RA, Pellock JM, DiMauro S, et al. Lumping or splitting? "Ophthalmoplegia-Plus" or Kearns-Sayre syndrome? Ann Neurol 1977; 1:37–54.

Bril V, Rewcastle NB, Humphrey J. Oculoskeletal myopathy with abnormal mitochondria. Can J Neurol Sci 1984; 11:390–4.

Curless RG, Flynn J, Bachynski B, et al. Fatal metabolic acidosis, hyperglycemia, and coma after steroid therapy for Kearns-Sayre syndrome. Neurology 1986; 36:872–873.

DiMauro S, Bonilla E, Zeviani M, Servidei S, DeVivo DC, Schon EA. Mitochondrial myopathies. J Inher Metab Dis 1987; 10 (Supp 1):113–128.

Drachman DA. Ophthalmoplegia-plus; a classification of the disorders associated with progressive external ophthalmoplegia. In: Vinken PJ, Bruyn GW, eds. Handbook of Clinical Neurology (vol 22). New York: Elsevier-North Holland, 1975:203–216.

Dubrovsky A, Tarabuto AL, Martino R. Distal spinal muscular atrophy and ophthalmoparesis. Arch Neurol 1981; 38:594–596.

Gallastequi J, Hariman RJ, Handler B, et al. Cardiac involvement in the Kearns-Sayre syndrome. Am J Cardiol 1987; 60:385–388.

Holt IJ, Harding AE, Morgan-Hughes JA. Deletions of mitochondrial DNA in patients with mitochondrial myopathies. Nature 1988; 331:717–719.

Little BW, Perl DP. Oculopharyngeal muscular dystrophy: An autopsied case from the French-Canadian kindreds. J Neurol Sci 1982; 53:145–158.

Mullie MA, Harding AE, Petty RKH, Ikeda H, Morgan-Hughes JA, Sanders MD. The retinal manifestations of mitochondrial myopathy. Arch Ophthalmol 1985; 103:1825–1830.

Ogasahara S, Nishikawa Y, Yorifuji, et al. Treatment of Kearns-Sayre syndrome with coenzyme Q10. Neurology 1986; 36:45–53.

Pavlakis SG, Rowland LP, DeVivo DC, Bonilla E, DiMauro S. Mitochondrial myopathies and encephalomyopathies. In: Plum F, ed. Advances in Contemporary Neurology. Philadelphia: FA Davis, 1988:95–134.

Petty RKH, Harding AE, Morgan-Hughes JA. The clinical

features of mitochondrial myopathy. Brain 1986; 109:915–938.

Rowland LP. Progressive external ophthalmoplegia. In: Vinken PJ, Bruyn GW, eds. Handbook of Clinical Neurology (vol 22). New York: Elsevier-North Holland, 1975: 177–202.

Rowland LP, Hays AP, DiMauro S, DeVivo DC, Behrens MB. Diverse clinical disorders associated with morphological abnormalities of mitochondria. In: Scarlato G, Cerri CG, eds. Mitochondrial Pathology in Muscle Diseases. Padua, Italy: Piccin Medical Books, 1983:141–158.

Rowland LP, Hausmanowa-Petrusewicz I, Barurska B, et al. Kearns-Sayre syndrome in identical twins. Lethal dominant inheritance or acquired disease? Neurology 1988; 38:1399–1402.

Schmitt HP, Krause KH. Autopsy study of familial oculopharyngeal muscular dystrophy with distal spread and neurogenic involvement. Muscle Nerve 1981; 4:296–305.

Schnizler ER, Robertson WC Jr. Familial Kearns-Sayre syndrome. Neurology 1979; 29:1172–1174.

Seigel RS, Seeger JF, Gabrielsen TO, Allen RJ. Computed tomography in oculocraniosomatic disease (Kearns-Sayre syndrome). Radiology 1979; 130:159–164.

Tome FMS, Fardeau M. Ocular myopathies. Pathol Res Pract 1985; 180:19–27.

Wall JR, Henderson J, Strakosek CR, Joyner DM. Graves' ophthalmopathy. Can Med Assoc J 1981; 124:855–863.

Wallace DC, Zheng X, Lott MT et al. Familial mitochondrial encephalomyopathy (MERRF): Genetic, pathophysiological, and biochemical characterization of a mitochondrial DNA disease. Cell 1988; 55:601–610.

Zeviani M, Moraes CT, DiMauro S, Nakase H, Bonilla E, Schon EA, Rowland LP. Deletions of mitochondrial DNA in Kearns-Sayre syndrome. Neurology 1988; 38:1339–1346.

Chapter XII

Peripheral Neuropathies

106. GENERAL CONSIDERATIONS
David E. Pleasure
Donald L. Schotland

Peripheral neuropathy and *polyneuropathy* are terms that describe the clinical syndrome of weakness, sensory loss, and impairment of reflexes caused by diffuse lesions of peripheral nerves. *Mononeuropathy* indicates a disorder of a single nerve, and is often due to a local cause such as trauma or entrapment. *Mononeuropathy multiplex* signifies focal involvement of two or more nerves, usually due to a generalized disorder such as diabetes mellitus or vasculitis. *Neuritis* should be reserved for inflammatory disorders of nerve (i.e., leprous neuritis).

Symptoms and Signs. Polyneuropathy occurs at any age. Symptoms may progress for weeks or months, but onset is more acute in the *Guillain-Barré syndrome* (acute idiopathic polyradiculoneuritis), arsenic or thallium poisoning, tick paralysis, or porphyria. Most polyneuropathies affect both motor and sensory functions. A predominantly motor polyneuropathy is seen in motor neuron disease, dapsone or hexane intoxication, tick paralysis, porphyria, and in some cases of the Guillain-Barré syndrome. Sensory neuropathy, often with concomitant autonomic dysfunction, is seen in thallium poisoning, acute idiopathic sensory neuronopathy, the inherited sensory neuropathies, primary biliary cirrhosis, and occasionally with diabetes mellitus, amyloidosis, carcinoma, or lepromatous leprosy. Pure sensory neuropathy without autonomic dysfunction is seen in chronic pyridoxine (vitamin B_6) intoxication.

Symptoms of polyneuropathy include acral (distal) pain, paresthesias, weakness, and sensory loss. Pain may be spontaneous or elicited by stimulation of the skin, and may be sharp or burning. The paresthesias are usually described as numbness, tingling, or a feeling of constriction. Lack of nociception may result in degeneration of joints and in chronic ulcerations. Weakness is greatest in distal limb muscles in most cases; there may be paralysis of the intrinsic foot and hand muscles with foot or wrist drop. Tendon reflexes may be lost. In severe polyneuropathy, the patient may be quadriplegic and respirator-dependent. The cranial nerves may be affected, particularly in both Guillain-Barré syndrome and diphtheritic neuropathy. Cutaneous sensory loss has a stocking-and-glove distribution. All modes of sensation may be affected, or there may be selective impairment of "large fiber" functions (position and vibratory sense) or "small fiber" functions (pain and temperature perception). Often, there is a rise in the threshold to perception of painful stimuli, but with a delayed and greater than normal reaction. Palpation of nerves may induce pain and muscles may be tender.

Involvement of autonomic nerves may cause miosis, anhydrosis, orthostatic hypotension, sphincter symptoms, impotence, and vasomotor abnormalities; these may occur without other evidence of neuropathy, but *autonomic neuropathy* is more commonly seen in association with symmetric distal polyneuropathy. The most common causes of predominantly autonomic neuropathy in the United States are diabetes mellitus and amyloidosis. Tachycardia, rapid alterations in blood pressure, flushing and sweating, and abnormalities in gastrointestinal motility are sometimes prominent in patients with thallium poisoning, porphyria, and the Guillain-Barré syndrome.

In mononeuropathy or mononeuropathy multiplex, focal motor, sensory, and reflex deficits are restricted to areas of specific nerves. When multiple distal subcutaneous nerves are affected in mononeuropathy multiplex, the stocking-and-glove pattern of symmetric distal sensory loss may suggest polyneuropathy. The most frequent causes of mononeuropathy multiplex are diabetes mellitus, periarteritis nodosa, rheumatoid arthritis, brachial neuropathy, leprosy, and nerve trauma or sarcoid compression.

Superficial cutaneous nerves may be thickened and visibly enlarged due to Schwann cell proliferation and collagen deposition, which result from repeated episodes of segmental demyelination and remyelination, or to deposition of foreign substances (e.g., amyloid) in nerve. Hypertrophic nerves may be observed in the demyelinating form of Charcot-Marie-Tooth syndrome, Dejerine-Sottas neuropathy, Refsum disease, von Recklinghausen disease (neurofibromatosis), leprous neuritis, amyloidosis, chronic demyelinative polyneuritis, and acromegaly.

Fasciculations, which are spontaneous contractions of individual motor units, are visible as brief twitches under the skin or tongue. They are especially frequent in anterior horn cell disease, but are occasionally seen in chronic peripheral nerve disorders.

Etiology. Peripheral nerve disorders may be divided into hereditary and acquired forms. The most common hereditary disorder is Charcot-Marie-Tooth syndrome (peroneal muscular atrophy). Other inherited neuropathies are Dejerine-Sottas disease, Refsum disease, adrenoleukodystrophy, and other genetically determined abnormalities of lipid metabolism, familial predilection to pressure palsies, hereditary sensory neuropathy, hereditary amyloid neuropathy, familial brachial neuropathy, and the hepatic porphyrias. A careful family history and examination of blood relatives, including electrodiagnostic tests, are useful in diagnosis of genetic neuropathies.

The most common acquired neuropathies in the United States are those associated with diabetes mellitus or alcoholism and the Guillain-Barré syndrome. Other acquired neuropathies include chronic demyelinating polyneuropathy, acute idiopathic sensory and pandysautonomic neuropathies, tick paralysis, brachial neuropathy, and neuropathies related to hypothyroidism, acromegaly, vasculitic disorders, uremia, diphtheria, sarcoidosis, malignancies, or exposure to neurotoxins. A detailed social history and full diagnostic workup are helpful in diagnosing these acquired neuropathies.

Nerve trauma and entrapment syndromes are discussed in Section 59. It is important, however, to consider trauma and entrapment in the differential diagnosis of mononeuropathies and of mononeuropathy multiplex, particularly if the median nerve is affected at the wrist, the ulnar nerve at the elbow, or the peroneal nerve at the knee. Patients with any form of polyneuropathy are considered more vulnerable to mechanical injury to nerves than normal; in some patients with disease causing cachexia and immobility neuropathy may result from trauma rather than from underlying disease.

Electromyography and Nerve Conduction Studies. Electromyographic examination is carried out with needle electrodes inserted into the muscle. Denervation is indicated by the presence of fibrillation potentials, positive waves at rest, and reduced numbers of motor unit potentials, which are of normal or increased amplitude and duration. Giant polyphasic motor unit potentials may be seen in longstanding neuropathies and are attributed to collateral reinnervation of denervated muscle fibers by sprouting of axonal processes from surviving axons. *Nerve conduction velocity* studies usually can distinguish segmental demyelination from axonal degeneration and also provide information about the distribution of nerve lesions, including areas of focal nerve compression. In *segmental demyelination,* nerve conduction velocities are at least 30% slower than normal, and are often reduced more than 60%. Other features of segmental demyelination include conduction block, dispersion of evoked responses, prolonged distal latencies, and marked slowing of F-wave velocities. In patients with a *demyelinating neuropathy,* clinical severity correlates more with conduction block than with degree of conduction slowing. Nerve conduction studies in *axonal diseases (Wallerian degeneration)* show normal or near normal nerve conduction velocities, low-amplitude evoked responses, normal distal latencies, and slowing of F-wave responses proportional to the reduction of nerve conduction velocity. Evaluation of sensory evoked responses is a sensitive tool for evaluating neuropathy that affects sensory fibers. The amplitude potentials may be diminished even when there is no clinical sensory loss. The usual clinical and electrophysiologic studies provide no information on the status of autonomic and small unmyelinated sensory fibers, but specialized

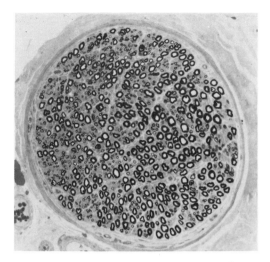

Fig. 106–1. Normal nerve in transverse semithin section. Well myelinated fibers are prominent. (Courtesy of Dr Arthur Asbury.)

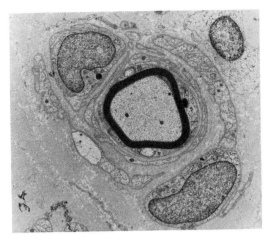

Fig. 106–3. Electron micrograph of onion bulb formation. (Courtesy of Dr. Arthur Asbury.)

techniques are now becoming available for their assessment.

Pathology. Cutaneous nerve biopsy, usually of the sural nerve, provides information about the extent of both axonal degeneration and of segmental demyelination. Semithin plastic embedded sections are necessary to evaluate the number and distribution of myelinated and nonmyelinated fibers and the pathologic changes in nerve components (Fig. 106–1). In mild chronic axonal neuropathy, there is a decrease in myelinated fibers (Fig. 106–2). Repeated cycles of segmental demyelination and remyelination produce concentric layering of Schwann cell processes and collagen that is easily seen by light and electron microscopy (Fig. 106–3). Paraffin-embedded sections are useful to detect inflammatory infiltrates, amyloid, and alterations in blood vessels. Occasionally, teased fiber preparations are needed to determine whether myelin abnormalities exist.

Nerve biopsy is especially helpful in the diagnosis of leprous, vasculitic, and amyloid neuropathies. The findings in Guillain-Barré syndrome and chronic demyelinating polyneuritis are also distinctive. Nerve biopsy is least informative in acute or subacute symmetric distal polyneuropathies due to toxins or metabolic disorders. Complications of sural nerve biopsy include persistent sensory loss in the cutaneous area innervated by the nerve (common), local infection (rare), and persistent pain due to formation of neuromas (rare). Fascicular biopsy diminishes the incidence of persistent sensory loss.

Other Studies. These may include complete blood count, erythrocyte sedimentation rate, antinuclear antibody, rheumatoid factor, blood glucose, blood urea nitrogen, phosphate, cholesterol, triglycerides, cryoglobulins, electrophoresis of serum and urine immunoproteins, tests for porphobilinogen and delta aminolevulinic acid, urinary porphyrins and heavy metals, serum phytanic and long chain fatty acid levels, leukocyte arylsulfatase, chest radiographs, sputum cytology, stool guaiac, and cerebrospinal fluid (CSF) examination for cells, protein, sugar, and serology. CSF protein content is increased in Guillain-Barré syndrome, and often also in chronic demyelinating polyneuritis, hypothyroidism, diabetic neuropathy, paraproteinemias, neuropathies associated with malignancy, Refsum disease, Charcot-Marie-Tooth

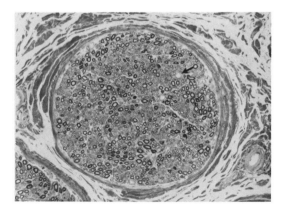

Fig. 106–2. Mild chronic neuropathy. Note slight decrease in number of myelinated fibers and occasional fiber with thinning of myelin sheath *(arrow)*. (Courtesy of Dr. Arthur Asbury.)

syndrome Type I, Dejerine-Sottas disease, and childhood leukodystrophies.

Differential Diagnosis and Treatment. Treatment of patients with peripheral nerve disorders can be divided into two phases: removal or treatment of the condition that is responsible for the disorder and symptomatic therapy. The former will be considered in the discussion of the individual peripheral nerve disorders. Symptomatic treatment of polyneuropathy consists of general supportive measures and physiotherapy. It is customary to supplement the diet with vitamins. This is essential when the polyneuropathy is due to dietary and vitamin deficiency but there is no evidence that vitamin therapy in excess of that contained in a well-balanced diet has any appreciable beneficial effect on other forms of polyneuropathy, and excessive vitamin B_6 ingestion can itself cause sensory neuropathy. Tracheal intubation may be required to prevent aspiration when oropharyngeal muscles are paralyzed, and respiratory support is needed if there is weakness of thoracic muscles and the diaphragm The corneas should be protected if there is weakness of eye closure. The patient's bed should be kept clean and the sheets smooth to prevent injury to the anesthetic skin. Chronic compression of vulnerable nerves (ulnar at elbow, common peroneal at knee) should be avoided. Paralyzed limbs should be splinted to prevent contractures. Physiotherapy should include massage of all weak muscles and passive movements of all joints to their fullest extent. When voluntary movements begin to return, muscle training exercises should be done daily. Patients should not attempt to walk before muscle testing indicates they are prepared. In chronic polyneuropathy with foot drop, bracing is helpful in improving walking. The patient with postural hypotension due to autonomic dysfunction should be instructed to arise gradually. Treatment should include the use of body stockings to minimize blood pooling in the legs and, if necessary, dietary salt supplementation or mineralocorticoid therapy to expand blood volume.

Course. The course of the polyneuropathy depends on the extent to which the destruction of nerves has progressed before treatment begins. With removal of the toxic agent or correction of the metabolic defects, recovery may be rapid if the macroscopic continuity of the nerves has not been interrupted. Recovery is delayed for months if axons are destroyed. Axonal regeneration proceeds at 1 to 2 mm/day, and there are often considerable delays in penetration by axons through focally damaged segments of nerve. Aberrant growth of axonal sprouts may lead to formation of persistent neuromas. After severe Wallerian degeneration, there may be permanent weakness, muscular wasting, diminution of reflexes, and sensory loss. In those neuropathies in which myelin damage is the basic pathologic event, recovery is usually more rapid and complete.

References

Asbury AK, Gilliatt RW. Peripheral Nerve Disorders: A Practical Approach. London: Butterworths, 1984.

Dawson DM, Hallet M, Millender LH. Entrapment Neuropathies. Boston: Little Brown, 1983.

Dyck PJ, Oviatt KF, Lambert EH. Intense evaluation of referred unclassified neuropathies yields improved diagnosis. Ann Neurol 1981; 10:222–226.

Dyck PJ, Thomas PK, Lambert EH, Bunge R. Peripheral Neuropathy. 2nd ed. Philadelphia: W.B. Saunders, 1984.

Feasby TE, Brown WF, Gilbert JJ, Hahn AF. The pathological basis of conduction block in human neuropathies. J Neurol Neurosurg Psychiatry 1985; 48:239–244.

Hallett M, Tandon D, Berardelli A. Treatment of peripheral neuropathies. J Neurol Neurosurg Psychiatry 1985; 48:1193–1207.

Kimura J. Principles and pitfalls of nerve conduction studies. Ann Neurol 1984; 16:415–429.

McLeod JG, Tuck RR, Pollard JD, Cameron J, Walsh JC. Chronic polyneuropathy of undetermined cause. J Neurol Neurosurg Psychiatry 1984; 47:530–535.

Powell HC, Myers RR. Pathology of experimental nerve compression. Lab Invest 1986; 55:91–100.

Schaumberg HH, Spencer PS, Thomas PK. Disorders of Peripheral Nerves. Philadelphia: F.A. Davis, 1983.

Shahani BT, Halperin JJ, Boulu P, Cohen J. Sympathetic skin response—a method of assessing unmyelinated axon dysfunction in peripheral neuropathies. J Neurol Neurosurg Psychiatry 1984; 47:536–542.

Shields RW Jr, Root KE Jr, Wilbourn AJ. Compression neuropathies in coma. Neurology 1986; 36:1370–1374.

Sumner AJ. The Physiology of Peripheral Nerve Disease. Philadelphia: W.B. Saunders, 1980.

---

107. HEREDITARY NEUROPATHIES

David E. Pleasure
Donald L. Schotland

Peroneal Muscular Atrophy

Peroneal muscular atrophy (Charcot-Marie-Tooth syndrome) includes several genetic disorders of the peripheral nervous system that most severely affect the peroneal and other distal muscles of the legs. Inheritance is usually autosomal dominant; less frequently, it is X-linked or autosomal recessive. Foot deformities are frequent and may be the only apparent manifestation in mildly affected family members. Sensation is usually impaired in a stocking-and-glove distribution, but sensation is preserved in some families. Achilles reflexes are absent; other tendon reflexes may be diminished.

Electrophysiology and Pathology. Measurement of nerve conduction velocities and sural nerve biopsy permit recognition of two distinct forms of Charcot-Marie-Tooth syndrome. In the demyelinating form (Type I), motor and sensory nerve conduction velocities are less than 65% of normal, and distal latencies are prolonged. Nerve biopsy shows segmental demyelination, partial remyelination, and Schwann cell proliferation. There are excess collagen fibrils and redundant loops of Schwann cell basement membrane. In the axonal form (Type II), motor and sensory nerve conduction velocities exceed 65% of normal, but the amplitude of evoked responses is reduced. Nerve biopsy shows Wallerian degeneration which is most severe in distal nerve segments.

Clinical Manifestations. In Type I Charcot-Marie-Tooth syndrome, symptoms begin in the first or second decade of life with foot drop and steppage gait. Distal muscle atrophy produces a "stork leg" deformity; intrinsic hand muscle atrophy appears later. Ankle jerks are lost and there is stocking-and-glove sensory impairment. Scoliosis and high pedal arches or club feet are common. Peripheral nerves are often palpably enlarged. Tremor is prominent in some patients; the clinical constellation of Charcot-Marie-Tooth syndrome with tremor is termed the Roussy-Levy syndrome.

In Type II Charcot-Marie-Tooth syndrome, the first symptoms of peroneal muscular atrophy often appear in adult life, but foot deformities may be evident in childhood. Atrophy and weakness of distal muscles, stocking-and-glove sensory impairment, and loss of tendon reflexes are similar to Type I Charcot-Marie-Tooth syndrome, but abnormalities are usually less severe, and nerves are not palpably enlarged.

Laboratory Data. Cerebrospinal fluid (CSF) protein content is frequently elevated in Type I Charcot-Marie-Tooth syndrome, but is normal in Type II. The CSF is otherwise normal, as are routine blood and urine studies.

Differential Diagnosis. Peroneal muscular atrophy is considered in patients with atrophy of the peroneal muscles, foot deformity,

and a positive family history. Even if family history is reported as negative, relatives should be examined because some affected individuals are asymptomatic or deny mild symptoms. Friedreich ataxia should be considered if distal neuropathy is accompanied by nystagmus, dysarthria, ataxia, or Babinski signs, especially if other members of the family are affected. Adrenoleukodystrophy should be considered in boys or men with peripheral neuropathy, adrenal insufficiency, and signs of cerebral or spinal cord degeneration. Familial amyloidosis may also resemble peroneal muscular atrophy, and can be recognized by sural nerve biopsy, or by DNA analysis indicating a mutation in the transthyretin gene. Dejerine-Sottas syndrome also resembles peroneal muscular atrophy, but onset is earlier, nerve hypertrophy is more prominent, CSF protein content is greater, and nerve conduction rates are slower than in Type I Charcot-Marie-Tooth syndrome. The distal motor and sensory abnormalities of Refsum disease are associated with deafness, retinitis pigmentosa, scaly skin, and elevated serum phytanic acid.

Lipomas and other masses in the lumbosacral canal may cause neurogenic foot deformities and distal weakness, but sensory loss is in a radicular pattern, the arms are spared, and the family history is usually negative. Patients with neurofibromatosis occasionally demonstrate hypertrophic neuropathy, but this is almost always more focal than in Type I Charcot-Marie-Tooth syndrome. Myotonic muscular dystrophy may include a similar pattern of distal muscle wasting and it is also dominantly inherited, but is unlike Charcot-Marie-Tooth syndrome. The disorder includes myotonia, cataracts, and frontal balding. There is normal sensation. EMG studies show nystagamus; conduction velocities are normal.

Course and Treatment. The progression of disability is slow in Type I Charcot-Marie-Tooth syndrome and even slower in Type II. Death does not occur because of this syndrome and incapacitation is rare. There is no specific treatment; reportedly beneficial response to vitamin E therapy has not been confirmed. Braces for correction of the foot drop enable most patients to remain ambulatory.

Dejerine-Sottas Disease

Recessively inherited Dejerine-Sottas disease begins in childhood with progressive limb weakness, stocking-and-glove impairment of sensation, and loss of tendon re-flexes. Peripheral nerves are enlarged. Ophthalmoparesis and impaired pupillary response to light are occasionally seen. Nerve conduction velocities are usually below 10 meters/second. Sural nerve biopsy shows enlarged fascicles that contain demyelinated and partially remyelinated axons surrounded by excess Schwann cells and collagen fibrils. These Schwann cells and collagen fibrils are arranged concentrically around axons, forming lamellar "onion bulbs." CSF protein content is often more than 100 mg/dl. No specific treatment is available; progression may be more rapid and disability more severe than in peroneal muscular atrophy.

Refsum Disease

This autosomal recessive disease is characterized by neurogenic weakness, stocking-and-glove sensory loss, areflexia, and enlarged nerves. In these respects, it resembles Dejerine-Sottas disease. But Refsum disease also has retinitis pigmentosa, causing impaired peripheral and night vision, progressive neurogenic hearing loss, and scaly skin. Nerve conduction rates are slow; sural nerve biopsy shows changes like those in Dejerine-Sottas disease. Refsum disease is caused by impairment of peroxisomal α-oxidation of branched chain fatty acids derived from the diet. As a result, serum phytanic acid content is markedly elevated. Treatment by plasmapheresis and restriction of phytol intake reduces serum phythanic acid concentrations and often improves neurologic function.

Hereditary Sensory Neuropathy

These genetic disorders affect sensory fibers in peripheral nerves and sometimes in autonomic fibers as well. Dominantly inherited, or Type I, hereditary sensory neuropathy is characterized by progressive sensory loss beginning in the first or second decade. There is progessive loss of pain, thermal sensibility, light touch, and proprioception. Tendon reflexes are lost. Ulcerations may appear on the feet and fingers owing to unperceived injuries. The disorder is caused by selective degeneration of sensory neurons in dorsal root ganglia. Other types of hereditary sensory neuropathy include an autosomal recessive form that resembles the dominantly inherited disorder, congenital sensory neuropathy with anhydrosis, hereditary sensory neuropathy with spastic paraparesis, and familial dysautonomia (Riley-Day syndrome).

Familial dysautonomia is an autosomal recessive condition seen most commonly in Jews. It starts in infancy with lack of pain and temperature sensibilities, gastrointestinal dysfunction, poor regulation of blood pressure, and absence of fungiform papillae on the tongue.

Porphyric Neuropathy

Porphyric neuropathy is an acute or subacute symmetric disorder, principally of the motor nerves, that occurs in the three dominantly inherited hepatic porphyrias, acute intermittent porphyria, hepatic coproporphyria, and variegate porphyria. The motor disorder is usually most severe, but sensory and autonomic symptoms may occur, and cardiac dysfunction may cause death.

Electrophysiology and Pathology. Motor nerve conduction velocities are normal or slightly diminished, but motor nerves may become electrically inexcitable in severe attacks. Sensory nerves are less severely affected. Porphyric neuropathy is characterized histologically by axonal degeneration.

Clinical Manifestations. Acute intermittent porphyria is characterized by recurrent crises of abdominal pain, psychiatric disturbances, delirium, and seizures. The crisis is sometimes precipitated by administration of barbiturates or other drugs. Variegate porphyria causes cutaneous hypersensitivity to sunlight with blistering and pigmented scars. Fulminant, primarily motor, polyneuropathy may occur in conjunction with other evidence of activity of the underlying disease and may progress rapidly to flaccid quadriplegia with respiratory and oropharyngeal paralysis. There may be tachycardia, swings in blood pressure, and other evidence of autonomic dysfunction.

Laboratory Data. Urinary excretion of Δ-aminolevulinic acid and porphobilinogen increases during attacks. Between attacks, the diagnosis can be made by assay for uroporphyrinogen-I synthetase in erythrocytes or cultured skin fibroblasts.

Differential Diagnosis. Porphyric neuropathy resembles the Guillain-Barré syndrome in acute onset and symmetric motor deficits. Onset with encephalopathy and visceral symptoms resembles the neuropathies associated with vasculitis.

Course and Teatment. Porphyric crises are treated with intravenous infusions of hyperosmolar D-glucose and hematin to repress Δ-aminolevulinic acid synthetase. Autonomic dysfunction may require therapy with a β-adrenergic blocking agent.

Hereditary Predisposition to Pressure Palsies

This dominantly inherited disorder is characterized clinically by recurrent mononeuropathy or mononeuropathy multiplex precipitated by minor trauma. Symptoms may begin in childhood or later, and nerves may become enlarged. Nerve conduction velocities are focally slowed in clinically affected nerves and frequently in segments of nerve that are not overtly involved. Nerve biopsy shows segmental demyelination and characteristic regions of very thick myelin.

Other Inherited Neuropathies

Hereditary amyloid neuropathies are discussed together with acquired forms later in this chapter. Inherited neuropathies in which there is an abnormality in lipid metabolism include, in addition to Refsum disease, conditions discussed in other chapters, hereditary abeta- and analphalipoproteinemias, Fabry disease, Neimann-Pick disease (sphingomyelin lipidosis), sialidosis Type I, chronic GM$_2$-gangliosidosis, adrenomyeloneuropathy, and sulfatide lipidosis (metachromatic leukodystrophy), and galactocerebroside lipidosis (globoid cell leukodystrophy or Krabbe disease). Two other inherited neuropathies mentioned in this section, ataxia telangiectasia and giant axonal neuropathy, are of unknown cause.

Abetalipoproteinemia (Bassen-Kornzweig disease) is an autosomal recessive condition that presents in the first decade of life with steatorrhea, distal sensorimotor neuropathy, and retinitis pigmentosa. Central nervous system dysfunction resembling Friedreich ataxia usually develops. Serum cholesterol is low, plasma betalipoprotein is absent, and erythrocytes have an acanthocytic or spicular deformity. The patients are vitamin E deficient, and vitamin E therapy may prevent progression of neurologic disability.

Analphalipoproteinemia (Tangier disease) is an autosomal recessive condition that presents with purely sensory, purely motor, or a mixed sensorimotor neuropathy in children or adults. Tonsils are enlarged and orange as a result of storage of cholesterol esters. Serum cholesterol is low because of near total absence of alphalipoprotein.

Fabry disease is an X-linked disorder due to deficiency of lysosomal ceramide trihexosidase. Although renal disease is the principal feature and telangiectasias are often present, some patients have recurrent attacks of distal burning pain and show loss of small peripheral sensory neurons.

Sialidosis Type I or the *cherry-red-spot myoclonus syndrome* begins in childhood or early adult life with retinal degeneration, myoclonus, distal hyporeflexia, and paresthesias. Nerve conduction velocities are reduced by 20 to 40%. Nerve biopsy shows segmental demyelination, remyelination, and Schwann cell vacuoles that contain electron-dense material. The disease is caused by deficiency of lysosomal neuraminidase.

Chronic GM$_2$ gangliosidosis is an autosomal recessive disease of Ashkenazi Jews resulting from deficient lysosomal hexosaminidase-A activity. The phenotypic expression resembles Friedreich ataxia, with early cerebellar signs and later appearance of upper and lower motor neuron deficits, dysarthria, and psychosis. Clinically apparent symmetric polyneuropathy was noted in one family.

Adrenoleukodystrophy is an X-linked disease of childhood characterized by mental retardation, loss of vision, spastic quadriplegia, and adrenal insufficiency. In a variant form called adrenomyeloneuropathy, symptoms begin in adult life and include symmetric distal neuropathy. Nerve biopsy shows both axonal degeneration and segmental demyelination, with evidence of lipid storage in Schwann cells. The disease is a consequence of deficient peroxisomal oxidation of long chain fatty acids.

Two recessively inherited lysosomal enzyme deficiencies, *sulfatide lipidosis (metachromatic leukodystrophy)* and *galactocerebroside lipidosis (Krabbe disease)* manifest with demyelinating neuropathy and severe encephalopathy. Galactocerebroside lipidosis appears in infancy and generally leads to death by age 1 year. Sulfatide lipidosis may become symptomatic at any age from infancy to adulthood. Occasionally, sulfatide lipidosis is first manifest by neuropathy. Nerve conduction velocities are slowed, and stored sulfatide can be seen as metachromatically staining material in sural nerve biopsies. Sulfatide excretion in the urine is elevated. Both these disorders can be diagnosed by assay of enzyme levels in leukocytes.

Ataxia telangiectasia is a recessively inherited disorder characterized by childhood onset of

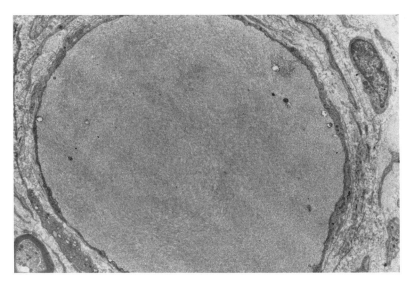

Fig. 107–1.   Giant axonal neuropathy. Electron micrograph of giant axon filled with masses of interweaving neurofilaments. (Courtesy of Dr. Arthur Asbury.)

conjunctival telangiectases, ataxia, impaired intellectual function, and immunologic deficiency. Mild distal sensorimotor axonal polyneuropathy is often present.

Giant axonal neuropathy is a disease of childhood characterized by symmetric distal polyneuropathy, mental retardation, and tightly coiled, kinky hair. It is presumed to be recessively inherited and is characterized pathologically by segmental axonal dilatations (Fig. 107–1) packed with 10 nm neurofilaments both in biopsy specimens of peripheral nerve and throughout the central nervous system.

References

Peroneal Muscular Atrophy

Dyck PJ. Inherited neuronal degeneration and atrophy affecting peripheral motor, sensory, and autonomic neurons. In: Dyck PJ, Thomas PK, Lambert EH, Bunge R, eds. Peripheral Neuropathy. Philadelphia: W.B. Saunders, 1984:1600–1655.

Fischbeck KH, ar-Rushi N, Pericak-Vance M, Roses AD, Fryns JP. X-linked neuropathy: Gene localization with DNA probes. Ann Neurol 1986; 20:527–532.

Harding AE, Thomas PK. The clinical features of hereditary motor and sensory neuropathy types I and II. Brain 1980; 103:259–280.

Williams LL, O'Dougherty MM, Wright FS, Bobulski RJ, Horrocks LA. Dietary essential fatty acids, vitamin E, and Charcot-Marie-Tooth disease. Neurology 1986; 36:1200–1205.

Dejerine-Sottas Disease

Dyke PJ, Lambert EH, Sanders K, O'Brien PC. Severe hypomyelination and marked abnormality of conduction in Dejerine-Sottas hypertrophic neuropathy: Myelin thickness and compound action potential of sural nerve in vitro. Mayo Clin Proc 1971; 46:432–436.

Refsum Disease

Refsum S, Stokke O, Eldjarn L, Fardeau M. Heredopathia atactica polyneuritiformis (Refsum's disease). In: Dyck PJ, Thomas PK, Lambert EH, Bunge R, eds. Peripheral Neuropathy. Philadelphia: W.B. Saunders, 1984:1680–1703.

Hereditary Sensory Neuropathy

Danon MJ, Carpenter S. Hereditary sensory neuropathy: Biopsy study of an autosomal dominant variety. Neurology 1985; 35:1226–1229.

Dyck PJ, Mellinger JF, Reagan TJ, et al. Not "indifference to pain", but varieties of hereditary sensory and autonomic neuropathies. Brain 1983; 106:373–390.

Schoene WC, Asbury AK, Astrom KE, Masters R. Hereditary sensory neuropathy. A clinical and ultrastructural study. J Neurol Sci 1970; 11:463–487.

Porphyric Neuropathy

Becker DM, Kramer S. The neurological manifestations of porphyria: A review. Medicine 1977; 56:411–423.

Kappas A, Sassa S, Anderson KE. The porphyrias. In: Stanbury JB, Wyngaarden JB, Fredrickson DS, Goldstein JL, Brown MS, eds. The Metabolic Basis of Inherited Disease, 5th ed. New York: McGraw-Hill, 1983:1301–1384.

Ridley A. Porphyric neuropathy. In: Dyck PJ, Thomas PK, Lambert EH, Bunge R, eds. Peripheral Neuropathy. Philadelphia: W.B. Saunders, 1984:1704–1715.

Hereditary Predisposition to Pressure Palsies

Behse F, Buchthal F, Carlsen F, Knappeis GG. Hereditary neuropathy with liability to pressure palsies. Electrophysiological and histological aspects. Brain 1972; 95:777–794.

Madrid R, Bradley WG. The pathology of neuropathies with focal thickening of the myelin sheath (tomaculous neuropathy). Studies on the formation of the abnormal myelin sheath. J Neurol Sci 1975; 25:415–448.

Staal A, deWeerdt CJ, Went LN. Hereditary compression syndrome of peripheral nerves. Neurology 1965; 15:1008–1017.

Windebank AJ. Inherited recurrent focal neuropathies. In: Dyck PJ, Thomas PK, Lambert EH, Bunge R, eds. Peripheral Neuropathy. Philadelphia: W.B. Saunders, 1984:1656–1679.

Other Inherited Neuropathies

Asbury AK, Johnson PC. Pathology of Peripheral Nerve. Philadelphia: W.B. Saunders, 1978.

Brin MF, Pedley TA, Lovelace RE, et al. Electrophysiologic features of abetalipoproteinemia: Functional consequences of vitamin E deficieny. Neurology 1986; 36:669–673.

Desnick RJ, Sweeley CC. Fabry's disease (alpha-galactosidase A deficiency). In: Stanbury JB, Wyngaarden JB, Fredrickson DS, Goldstein JL, Brown MS, eds. The Metabolic Basis of Inherited Disease, 5th ed. New York: McGraw-Hill, 1983: 905–944.

Griffin JW, Goren E, Schaumburg HH, Engel WK, Loriaux L. Adrenomyeloneuropathy: A probable variant of adrenoleukodystrophy. I. Clinical and endocrinologic aspects. Neurology 1977; 27:1107–1113.

Kolodny EH, Moser HW. Sulfatide lipidosis: Metachromatic leukodystrophy. In: Stanbury JB, Wyngaarden JB, Fredrickson DS, Goldstein JL, Brown MS, eds. The Metabolic Basis of Inherited Disease, 5th ed. New York: McGraw-Hill, 1983: 881–905.

Kumamoto T, Fukuhara N, Ohno T, Wakabayashi M, Miyatake T. Morphological studies of peripheral nerves and skeletal muscles of an adult case with adrenoleukomyeloneuropathy. Eur Neurol 1985; 24:229–236.

Martin JJ, Ceuterick C, Libert J. Skin and conjunctival nerve biopsies in adrenoleukodystrophy and its variants. Ann Neurol 1980; 8:291–295.

Martin JJ, Ceuterick C, Mercelis R, Joris C. Pathology of peripheral nerves in metachromatic leukodystrophy. A comparative study of ten patients. J Neurol Sci 1982; 53:95–112.

Moser HW, Moser AB, Powers JM, et al. The prenatal diagnosis of adrenoleukodystrophy. Demonstration of increased hexacosanoic acid levels in cultured amniocytes and fetal adrenal gland. Pediatr Res 1982; 16:172–175.

Ohnishi A, Dyck PJ. Loss of small peripheral sensory neurons in Fabry disease. Arch Neurol 1974; 31:120–127.

Said G, Marion MH, Selva J, Janet C. Hypertrophic and dying-back nerve fibers in Friedreich's ataxia. Neurology 1986; 36:1292–1299.

Schaumburg HH, Powers JM, Raine CS, et al. Adrenomyeloneuropathy: A probable variant of adrenoleukodystrophy. II. General pathologic, neuropathologic and biochemical aspects. Neurology 1977; 27:1114–1119.

Sheth KJ, Swick HM. Peripheral nerve conduction in Fabry's disease. Ann Neurol 1980; 7:319–323.

Steinman L, Tharp BR, Dorfman LJ, et al. Peripheral neuropathy in the cherry-red spot-myoclonus syndrome (Sialidosis type I). Ann Neurol 1980; 7:450–456.

Suzuki H, Suzuki Y. Galactosylceramide lipidosis: Globoid cell leukodystrophy (Krabbe's disease). In: Stanbury JB, Wyngaarden JB, Fredrickson DS, Goldstein JL, Brown MS, eds. The Metabolic Basis of Inherited Disease, 5th ed. New York: McGraw-Hill, 1983:857–880.

Wichman A, Buchthal F, Pezeshkpour GH, Gregg RE. Peripheral neuropathy in abetalipoproteinemia. Neurology 1985; 35:1279–1289.

Willner JP, Grabowski GA, Gordon RE, Bender AN, Desnick RJ. Chronic GM2 gangliosidosis masquerading as atypical Friedreich ataxia: Clinical , morphologic, and biochemical studies of nine cases. Neurology 1981; 31:787–798.

108. ACQUIRED NEUROPATHIES

David E. Pleasure
Donald L. Schotland

Guillain-Barré Syndrome

The Guillain-Barré syndrome is characterized by an acute onset of peripheral and cranial nerve dysfunction. Viral upper respiratory or gastrointestinal infection, immunization, or surgery often precedes neurologic symptoms by 5 days to 3 weeks. Rapidly progressive symmetric weakness, loss of tendon reflexes, facial diplegia, oropharyngeal and respiratory paresis, and impaired sensation in the hands and feet are frequent. The patient's condition worsens for several days to 3 weeks, then gradually improves, usually to normal or nearly normal function. Early plasmapheresis accelerates recovery and diminishes the incidence of long-term neurologic disability.

Etiology. The cause of Guillain-Barré syndrome is unknown. A disease with a similar clinical course (i.e., similar pathologic, electrophysiologic and cerebrospinal fluid (CSF) alterations) can be induced in experimental animals by immunization with whole peripheral nerve, peripheral nerve myelin or, in some species, peripheral nerve myelin P_2 basic protein or galactocerebroside. While there is no evidence of sensitization to these antigens in humans with spontaneous Guillain-Barré syndrome, activity of the disease seems to correlate with the appearance of serum antibodies to peripheral nerve myelin. Although Guillain-Barré syndrome is frequently preceded by a viral infection, there is as yet no evidence of viral invasion of peripheral nerves or nerve roots.

Electrophysiology and Pathology. Nerve conduction velocities are reduced in Guillain-Barré syndrome, but studies may be normal early in the course. Distal sensory and motor latencies are prolonged. Owing to demyelination of nerve roots, F-wave conduction velocity is often slowed. Conduction slowing may persist for months or years after clinical recovery. In general, severity of neurologic abnormality correlates poorly with the degree of slowing of nerve conduction velocities but well with the extent of electrophysiologically demonstrable nerve conduction block. Long-standing weakness is most apt to occur when there is electromyographic evidence of muscle denervation early in the course.

Guillain-Barré syndrome is characterized histologically by focal segmental demyelination (Fig. 108–1) associated with perivascular and endoneurial infiltrates of lymphocytes and monocytes or macrophages (Fig. 108–2). These lesions are scattered throughout the peripheral nerves, nerve roots, and cranial nerves. In particularly severe lesions, there is axonal degeneration plus segmental demyelination. During recovery, remyelination occurs but the lymphocytic infiltrates may persist.

Incidence. The Guillain-Barre syndrome is the most frequent acquired demyelinating neuropathy, with an incidence of 0.6 to 1.9 cases/100,000. The incidence increases gradually with age, but the disease may occur at any age. The genders are equally affected. The incidence of Guillain-Barré syndrome is increased in patients with Hodgkin disease and by pregnancy or general surgery.

Symptoms and Signs. The Guillain-Barré syndrome often appears days to weeks after symptoms of a viral upper respiratory or gastrointestinal infection. Usually the first neurologic symptoms are due to symmetric limb weakness, often with paresthesias. Unlike

most other neuropathies, proximal muscles are sometimes affected more than distal muscles in the early phases. Occasionally, facial, ocular, or oropharyngeal muscles may be affected first; more than half the patients have facial diplegia and a similar number develop dysphagia and dysarthria. Some patients require mechanical ventilation. Tendon reflexes may be normal for the first few days, but are then lost. The degree of sensory impairment is variable. In some patients, all sensory modalities are preserved; others have marked diminution in perception of joint position, vibration, pain, and temperature in stocking-and-glove distribution. Patients occasionally develop papilledema, sensory ataxia, transient extensor plantar responses, or evidence of autonomic dysfunction (e.g., orthostatic hypotension, transient hypertension, cardiac arrhythmia). Many have muscle tenderness and nerves are sensitive to pressure, but there are no signs of meningeal irritation such as nuchal rigidity.

A variant form of Guillain-Barré syndrome (Miller-Fisher syndrome) is characterized by gait ataxia, areflexia, and ophthalmoparesis. It is sometimes associated with pupillary abnormalities, but without limb weakness. Recovery from this form of Guillain-Barré syndrome is almost always complete.

Laboratory Data. Cerebrospinal fluid protein content is elevated in most patients, but

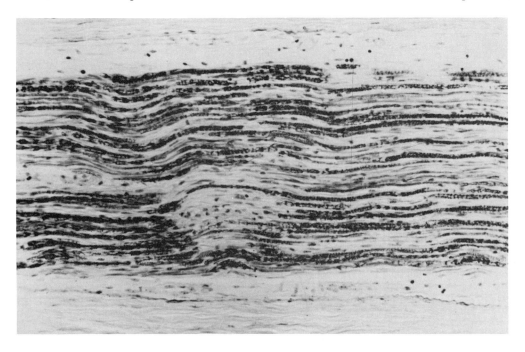

Fig. 108–1.   Focal demyelination in acute Guillain-Barré syndrome. (Courtesy of Dr. Arthur Asbury.)

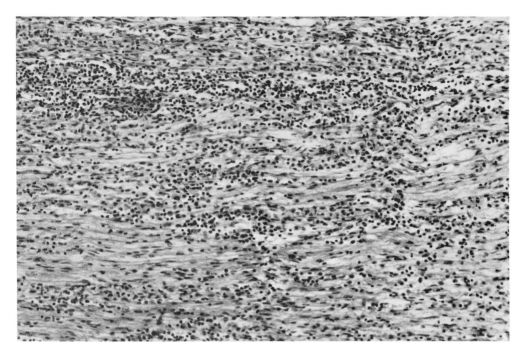

Fig. 108–2. Diffuse mononuclear infiltrate in peripheral nerve in Guillain-Barré syndrome. (Courtesy of Dr. Arthur Asbury.)

may be normal in the first few days after onset. The CSF cell count is usually normal, but some patients with otherwise typical Guillain-Barré syndrome have 10 to 100 mononuclear cells/microliter of CSF. Antecedent infectious mononucleosis, cytomegalovirus infection, viral hepatitis, HIV infection, or other viral disease may be documented by serologic studies.

Course and Prognosis. Symptoms are usually most severe within 1 week of onset, but may progress for 3 weeks or more. Death is unusual but may be due to aspiration pneumonia, pulmonary embolism, intercurrent infection, or autonomic dysfunction. The rate of recovery varies. In some, it is rapid with restoration to normal function within a few weeks. In most, recovery is slow and not complete for many months. Recovery is accelerated by early institution of plasmapheresis. In untreated series, about 35% of patients have permanent residual hyporeflexia, atrophy, and weakness of distal muscles, or facial paresis. A biphasic course of illness, with partial recovery followed by relapse, occurs in less than 10% of patients with the Guillain-Barré syndrome. Recurrence of the illness after full recovery occurs in about 2%.

Diagnosis and Differential Diagnosis. The characteristic history of subacute develop-

ment of symmetric motor or sensorimotor neuropathy after a viral illness, delivery, or surgery, together with electrophysiologic findings consistent with segmental demyelination and the high CSF protein content with normal CSF cell count provide strong presumptive evidence for the diagnosis of Guillain-Barré syndrome.

In the past, the principal diseases to be differentiated from Guillain-Barré syndrome were diphtheritic polyneuropathy and acute anterior poliomyelitis. Both are now rare in the United States. Diphtheritic polyneuropathy can usually be distinguished by the long latent period between the respiratory infection and onset of neuritis, the frequency of paralysis of accommodation, and the relatively slow evolution of neuritic symptoms. Acute anterior poliomyelitis can usually be distinguished by the asymmetry of the paralysis and by the presence of meningeal irritation, fever, and CSF pleocytosis early in the course. Occasional patients with acquired imunodeficiency syndrome (AIDS) or AIDS-related complex develop a relatively rapidly progressive demyelinating polyneuropathy, and HIV virus has been isolated from peripheral nerve or CSF from some such patients. Porphyric neuropathy resembles Guillain-Barré syndrome clinically, but is differentiated by history of recurrent abdominal crisis, mental symptoms, and onset after exposure to barbiturates or other drugs. Laboratory tests reveal high urinary levels of Δ-amino-levulinic acid and porphobilinogen in the urine. CSF protein content is not increased. Development of a Guillain-Barré-like syndrome during prolonged parenteral feeding should raise the possibility of *hypophospha-temia*-induced neural dysfunction. Toxic neuropathies due to hexane inhalation or thallium or arsenic ingestion occasionally begin acutely or subacutely. These can be distinguished from Guillain-Barré syndrome by history of toxin exposure or, in thallium or arsenic intoxication, by subsequent development of alopecia. Botulism may be difficult to discriminate on clinical grounds from purely motor forms of Guillain-Barré syndrome, but electrophysiologic tests in botulism reveal normal nerve conduction velocities and a facilitating response to repetitive nerve stimulation. Tick paralysis should be excluded by careful examination of the scalp.

Treatment. Early plasmapheresis has proven useful in patients with severe Guillain-Barré syndrome. The place for such therapy in milder cases has not yet been ascertained. Glucocorticoid administration does not shorten the course or affect the prognosis. Mechanically assisted ventilation is sometimes necessary, and precautions against aspiration of food or stomach contents must be taken if oropharyngeal muscles are affected. Exposure keratitis must be prevented in patients with facial diplegia.

Chronic Demyelinating Polyneuritis

This condition resembles Guillain-Barré syndrome in propensity for onset after nonspecific viral infection, presence of segmental demyelination, and lymphocytic infiltrates in peripheral nerve. While CSF protein content is increased, this is less consistent than in Guillain-Barré. Chronic idiopathic polyneuritis differs from the Guillain-Barré syndrome in that symptoms are less acute in onset and much more prolonged in course. Recurrent attacks are frequent. Weakness may be asymmetric. An infantile form begins with hypotonia and delayed motor development. In one reported adult case, chronic demyelinating polyneuritis was associated with ulcerative colitis, and selective inflammation of perineurium was observed. Optic neuritis has been noted in some patients. Nerves may become enlarged because of Schwann cell prolifera-

tion and collagen deposition after recurrent segmental demyelination and remyelination. In contrast to the Guillain-Barré syndrome, glucocorticoid therapy is often of benefit in speeding recovery and preventing relapse. Plasmapheresis is beneficial in some cases. Serologic tests for HIV should be carried out in patients with chronic idiopathic polyneuritis, because increasing numbers of patients with this complication of AIDS or AIDS-related syndrome are being recognized.

Acute Idiopathic Sensory Neuronopathy

This condition is acute or subacute in onset and is characterized by numbness and pain over the entire body and face. All sensory modalities are severely affected. Autonomic dysfunction may also be noted. Tendon reflexes are absent, but strength is normal. The syndrome has been reported in adults after administration of penicillin for diverse febrile illnesses. Motor-nerve conduction velocities are normal or near normal, but sensory potentials are reduced in amplitude or not recordable. In contrast to the Guillain-Barré syndrome, prognosis for recovery in acute idiopathic sensory neuronopathy is poor.

Chronic Idiopathic Sensory Neuropathy

Occasional elderly patients demonstrate a slowly progressive symmetric large fiber sensory neuropathy, often with sensory ataxia of the upper limbs. Carcinoma or paraproteinemic neuropathy should be suspected (see below), but idiopathic cases also occur. These patients fail to respond to plasmapheresis or to immunosuppressive therapy.

Acute Pandysautonomia

This condition is characterized by the acute or subacute onset of hypofunction of sympathetic and parasympathetic pathways. Symptoms include postural syncope, diminished tear and sweat production, impaired bladder function, constipation, and diminished sexual potency. Pharmacologic evidence of denervation hypersensitivity suggests that the defect is in the peripheral nervous system, but the pathologic basis for the syndrome is not clear. Gradual partial or complete recovery occurs without specific therapy.

Tick Paralysis

Tick infestation of the scalp may cause an acute ascending motor neuropathy that resembles the Guillain-Barré syndrome. The patient is ataxic and hyporeflexic or areflexic, but there is no impairment of sensation. Electrophysiologic examination suggests dysfunction of terminal branches of motor axons without evidence by repetitive stimulation studies of a neuromuscular junction defect. Removal of the tick results in rapid return of normal function.

Brachial Neuropathy

Brachial neuropathy *(neuralgic amyotrophy)* is an acute idiopathic mononeuropathy multiplex that affects the nerves of the arms. The first symptom is severe localized pain in either or both arms. As the pain subsides, atrophy and weakness of muscles innervated by one or more nerves in one or both arms appears, often with hyporeflexia and sensory loss in the distribution of the affected nerves.

The incidence of brachial neuropathy has not been determined, but it is probably nearly as frequent, though less dramatic, as Guillain-Barré syndrome. The syndrome is usually sporadic, but dominant inheritance has been reported. In occasional cases, symptoms follow immunization, particularly with tetanus toxoid, or unaccustomed vigorous exercise. Brachial neuropathy may also occur in small epidemics among military recruits or other groups. Neurologic features consistent with brachial plexus involvement are common in serum sickness and in the tick-borne disorder, Lyme disease. Brachial neuropathy is also a complication of intravenous heroin administration.

Electrophysiology and Pathology. EMG studies show denervation in affected muscles. Nerve conduction studies are generally normal or show nerve potentials of decreased amplitude but normal velocity. Relatively little is known about the pathology of brachial neuritis. Wallerian degeneration rather than segmental demyelination has been described in the few reported nerve biopsies.

Clinical Manifestations. Pain is the first symptom and is usually localized to one or more small areas of the arms. In general, the pain does not radiate like radicular pain; because of its point-like local character, it is often ascribed to bursitis or tendonitis. Usually, the pain subsides within a few days or weeks, just as the patient becomes aware of unilateral or bilateral arm weakness. If bilateral, the pattern of weakness is usually asymmetric. Proximal or distal muscles may be predominantly involved and examination often suggests dysfunction in discrete nerves or parts of the bra-

chial plexus. Sensory loss is usually seen and may either conform in distribution to the nerves showing motor dysfunction or involve other nerves. Sensory loss in an axillary nerve distribution is common. Biceps or triceps reflexes may be lost. There is often rapid atrophy of affected muscles. A similar disorder may affect the lumbosacral plexus, but is less common and even less well documented. In general, lumbosacral plexopathy suggests diabetic vasculopathy or invasion of the plexus by carcinoma.

Laboratory Data. No abnormalities in blood, urine, or CSF are noted.

Differential Diagnosis. Similar neurologic signs may follow hemorrhage into the axillary area or invasion of brachial plexus by tumor. The Horner syndrome is common when carcinoma involves the apex of the lung and first thoracic root (Pancoast syndrome) but is unusual in brachial neuropathy. Compression of cervical or high thoracic nerve roots by cervical spondylosis may cause arm pain and weakness, but both the pain and the weakness are radicular in distribution. Thoracic outlet syndromes may include pain and weakness like that of brachial neuropathy, but can be distinguished by tests that demonstrate vascular occlusion with maneuvers of the neck, shoulders, and arms.

Course and Treatment. Symptomatic treatment for pain is sometimes necessary early in the course. Most patients with weakness that involves predominantly proximal muscles recover fully in a few months without specific treatment. Those with severe distal weakness may require more than a year to recover and there may be some permanent distal weakness and atrophy.

Radiation Neuropathy

External irradiation of the axilla for treatment of breast carcinoma may cause delayed sensory loss in the hand, with or without weakness. Computed tomography and other imaging techniques aid in distinguishing radiation-induced dysfunction from invasion of the plexus by the carcinoma. Pathologic examination in radiation neuropathy reveals axonal degeneration and fibrosis. Radiation may also cause benign of malignant peripheral nerve tumors, particularly in patients with neurofibromatosis.

Neuropathy Induced by Cold

Frostbite and immersion foot cause local nerve injury and sensory and motor abnormalities. Neurologic symptoms usually clear slowly over months. Pathologic examination shows axonal degeneration, which most prominently affects the largest nerve fibers.

Neuropathy Associated with Cryoglobulins

Symmetric or asymmetric sensorimotor neuropathy occurs as a complication of cryoglobulinemia. Affected patients frequently have purpuric lesions and leg ulcerations. Symptoms of Raynaud syndrome and exacerbation of the neuropathy are common in cold weather. Nerve conduction studies show normal velocity and diminished amplitude of evoked responses, suggesting an axonal disorder.

Diabetic Neuropathy

Diabetes mellitus is the most frequent cause of neuropathy in the United States. There are three types of diabetic neuropathy: symmetric distal polyneuropathy, autonomic neuropathy, and mononeuropathy or mononeuropathy multiplex. *Symmetric distal polyneuropathy* is characterized by foot pain or paresthesias and loss of ankle reflexes. The most common motor sign is weakness of toe and foot extensors; in more severe cases, weakness also affects the hands. Foot ulcers and trophic degeneration of small joints of the feet may develop. *Diabetic autonomic neuropathy* is insidious in onset and is manifested by orthostatic hypotension, impotence, diarrhea or constipation, denervation of the heart, and impaired pupillary light reflexes. *Diabetic mononeuropathy* and *mononeuropathy multiplex* are often acute, most frequently affecting the lumbosacral plexus, sciatic, femoral, median, and ulnar nerves, and the third and seventh cranial nerves.

Etiology. The causes of diabetic neuropathies are unknown. Peripheral vascular disease is common in diabetics, but there is no direct correlation between the severity of the vascular disease and either polyneuropathy or autonomic neuropathy. Occasionally, autopsies of patients with diabetic mononeuropathy or mononeuropathy multiplex have revealed occlusion of the vasa nervorum with infarction of nerve fascicles; some diabetic patients with a clinical pattern of symmetric distal neuropathy in the legs had multiple small infarctions in the lumbosacral plexus. Hyperglycemia may play a role in the pathogenesis of symmetric distal diabetic polyneuropathy. Maintenance of blood sugar in the normal range improves motor nerve conduction velocities, slows progression of the neuropathy, and sometimes reverses neuropathic signs.

Electrophysiology and Pathology. Nerve conduction velocities are mildly reduced in symmetric distal diabetic polyneuropathy and sensory nerve potentials are often diminished in amplitude. Segments of nerve distal to nerve infarcts may be electrically inexcitable. Focal slowing of conduction velocity often is demonstrable in patients with longstanding diabetes mellitus, particularly in regions susceptible to trauma (e.g., the median nerve at the wrist, the ulnar nerve at the elbow, the peroneal nerve at the fibular head). Of diabetics, 5% have slowing of median nerve conduction at the wrist, usually without clinical evidence of the carpal tunnel syndrome. Because clinical electrophysiologic examination does not record conduction in autonomic fibers, nerve conduction studies in patients with purely autonomic diabetic neuropathy may be normal. EMG studies show denervation in distal muscles in most patients with symmetric distal diabetic neuropathy and in muscles innervated by nerves affected by diabetic mononeuropathy or mononeuropathy multiplex.

Distal nerve segments from patients with symmetric distal diabetic neuropathy show scattered axonal degeneration, often with regenerating nerve sprouts, and occasional segmental demyelination. The pathology of diabetic autonomic neuropathy is not well characterized.

Incidence. Diabetic neuropathy is uncommon in childhood, although nerve conduction velocities may be mildly reduced. The incidence of symmetric distal neuropathy or autonomic neuropathy increases with the duration of the diabetes mellitus; signs of both are usually present in longstanding diabetics who have not carefully controlled blood sugar. Diabetic mononeuropathy or mononeuropathy multiplex may begin shortly after adult-onset diabetes mellitus is recognized; sometimes it is an initial symptom of the disease in adults.

Symptoms and Signs. Paresthesias or pain in the soles of the feet are frequent initial symptoms of symmetric distal diabetic neuropathy. Distal weakness of the legs may also occur; the hands may be affected later. Ankle jerks are usually absent. Cutaneous sensation is often diminished in a stocking distribution and vibratory and position sense are impaired in the feet. When sensation is severely compromised, penetrating skin ulcers and trophic changes in the joints of the feet (Charcot joints) may develop after repeated trauma.

Diabetic autonomic neuropathy usually presents with orthostatic hypotension and, in men, with impotence. Loss of the normal tachycardic response to insulin-induced hypoglycemia may result from adrenergic denervation of the heart. Diarrhea, constipation, recurrent abdominal distention, and impaired micturition and pupillary responses are other signs of diabetic autonomic neuropathy.

Mononeuropathy multiplex localized to the lumbosacral plexus may occur early in the course of adult-onset diabetes mellitus, usually after rapid weight loss due to poor diabetic control (diabetic cachexia). Localized pain in the quadriceps or other proximal leg muscle is followed by asymmetric proximal leg weakness and atrophy. Patellar reflexes may be lost and cutaneous sensation is often diminished in the distribution of one or more cutaneous nerves of the thigh. More gradually progressive proximal leg weakness, without pain or sensory loss, has also been described in diabetes mellitus, but there is no evidence of a spinal cord disorder that would warrant the label *"diabetic amytrophy."* Diabetic *third-nerve palsy* presents with ptosis, weakness of adduction, and elevation of the eye. However, in contrast to the third-nerve palsy associated with enlarging or ruptured congenital aneurysm of the posterior communicating artery, the pupil is usually spared. Recovery after diabetic third-nerve palsy is the rule.

Course. Symmetric distal diabetic neuropathy and diabetic autonomic neuropathy are slowly progressive or static conditions. Diabetic mononeuropathy or mononeuropathy multiplex is usually acute or subacute and often clears without treatment.

Laboratory Data. Blood and urinary findings are those associated with diabetes mellitus. CSF protein content is increased about 65% of cases; values above 100 mg/dl are found in 15%. If blood glucose is increased, CSF glucose is also.

Diagnosis. The diagnosis of diabetic neuropathy is easy when diabetes mellitus is present and no other cause of neuropathy is discovered. Tabes dorsalis is rare, but may simulate severe symmetrc distal diabetic neuropathy; it can be diagnosed serologically. Amyloid neuropathy may resemble diabetic autonomic neuropathy and should be suspected if there is a family history of amyloi-

dosis or if paraprotein is found in blood or urine. Compression neuropathies and invasion of lumbosacral plexus by tumors may simulate diabetic mononeuropathy or mononeuropathy multiplex.

Treatment. Careful control of blood sugar is helpful in preventing progession of symmetric distal diabetic neuropathy. The patient should avoid injuring the anesthetic areas to prevent perforating ulcers and trophic degeneration of joints. Pain in the feet is sometimes relieved by treatment with a tricyclic antidepressant drug.

Hypothyroid Neuropathy

Burning or lancinating limb pains or paresthesias are common in patients with untreated severe hypothyroidism. Some of these patients are hyporeflexic and have distal sensory loss and mild distal weakness. Nerve conduction velocities are slowed. Nerve biopsy shows segmental demyelination and excessive glycogen within Schwann cells. The polyneuropathy clears rapidly with thyroid replacement therapy. Carpal tunnel syndrome and other compressive mononeuropathies are also frequent in patients with hypothyroidism. In these patients, nerve conduction studies demonstrate focal slowing at the compression site.

Acromegalic Neuropathy

Symmetric distal sensorimotor neuropathy has been reported in acromegalics. Nerves may be enlarged and nerve biopsy may show segmental demyelination. More common in such patients are entrapment neuropathies, especially of the median nerve at the wrist.

Vasculitic Neuropathies

The most common clinical picture of vasculitic neuropathy is subacute mononeuropathy multiplex; a distal motor-sensory neuropathy may also occur. Periarteritis nodosa should be suspected in the patient with mononeuropathy multiplex who also has weight loss, fever and evidence of vasculopathy affecting the kidneys, lungs, or other tissues. However, mononeuropathy or mononeuropathy multiplex may be the first sign of periarteritis nodosa, followed only later by involvement of other organs.

Nerve conduction studies may show electrical inexcitability of nerve segments distal to infarction caused by vascular occlusion. If some fascicles in the nerve are spared, these conduct at a normal rate, but the amplitude of the evoked response is diminished. The diagnosis of peripheral nerve involvement may be established by nerve biopsy (Fig. 108–3). However, the biopsy may show only axonal degeneration if vasculitis has caused a nerve infarction more proximally and if no affected vessels are in the specimen. Vasculitic neuropathy may also occur as a complication of intravenous amphetamine administration and in systemic lupus erythematosus, rheumatoid arthritis, scleroderma, hepatitis B, and hypersensitivity angiitis. Treatment is by glucocorticoids or other immunosuppressive agents.

Uremic Neuropathy

Uremic neuropathy is a symmetric distal mixed motor and sensory disorder that appears in patients with chronic renal failure. Early symptoms are calf cramps, subjective need to move the legs ("restless legs") and foot dysesthesias indistinguishable from those in diabetic and alcoholic symmetric distal polyneuropathies. Earliest signs of uremic neuropathy are loss of ankle tendon reflexes and a stocking distribution of sensory loss. Later, distal weakness appears in the legs and may progress proximally to the thighs; the intrinsic hand muscles may also be affected.

Nerve conduction studies show mild to moderate slowing. Nerve biopsy reveals scattered segmental demyelination in addition to fiber loss. The diameters of axons in the distal parts of limb nerves are reduced from those in normal controls.

Although accumulation of a toxic metabolite is the most likely cause of uremic neuropathy, the nature of this toxin has yet to be established. Dialysis ameliorates the neuropathy and after return of normal kidney function or successful renal transplantation, all neuropathic signs resolve.

Neuropathy Associated with Hepatic Diseases

Sensory polyneuropathy occurs in women with primary biliary cirrhosis and seems to be caused by xanthoma formation in and around nerves. Polyneuropathy in patients with cirrhosis induced by ethanol abuse is generally due to coincident thiamine deficiency and responds to thiamine therapy. Mononeuropathy multiplex occasionally occurs in patients with angiitis associated with hepatitis B. Polyneuropathy is a feature of many inherited diseases in which hepatic synthetic processes are abnormal. These include the hepatic porphyrias, analphalipoproteinemia, and abetalipoproteinemia.

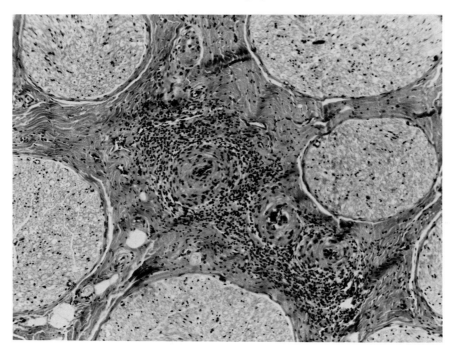

Fig. 108–3. Polyarteritis in large proximal nerve trunk. Three small epineurial arteries show inflammation in vessel wall and adventitia also luminal narrowing and fibrosis. Surrounding nerve fascicles are not involved in this section. (Courtesy of Dr. Arthur Asbury.)

Neuropathies Associated with Infection

LEPROSY

Leprosy is caused by infection with the acid-fast rod Mycobacterium leprae (Hansen bacillus). There are thought to be more than 10 million cases in the world. Although rare in the United States, it has been seen in recent immigrants in Florida, Louisiana, Texas, and New York.

Peripheral nerves are affected differently in the tuberculoid and lepromatous forms. In tuberculoid leprosy, nerve trunks, such as the ulnar, are injured by inclusion in regions of granuloma formation and scarring. Endoneurial caseation necrosis may occur. The clinical picture is one of mononeuritis or mononeuritis multiplex. In lepromatous leprosy, Hansen bacilli proliferate in large numbers within Schwann cells and macrophages in the endoneurium and perineurium of subcutaneous nerve twigs (Fig. 108–4), particularly in cool areas of the body. Loss of cutaneous sensibility is observed in affected patches; these may later coalesce to cover large parts of the body. Position sense may be preserved in affected areas, whereas pain and temperature sensibility is lost, a dissociation similar to that in syringomyelia. Acute mononeuritis multiplex may appear during chemotherapy of lepromatous leprosy in conjunction with erythema nodosum; this complication is treated with thalidomide. Treatment is designed to eradicate the causative bacteria and to prevent secondary immune reactions, which may damage nerves. To prevent mutilating injuries, it is important to avoid trauma to anesthetic areas.

DIPHTHERIA

Diphtheria and diphtheritic neuropathy are now rare in the United States. Corynebacterium diphtheriae infects the larynx, pharynx, or occasionally, a cutaneous wound. The organisms release an exotoxin that causes myocarditis and, later, symmetric neuropathy. The neuropathy often begins with impaired visual accommodation and paresis of ocular and oropharyngeal muscles, and is followed by quadriparesis. Nerve conduction studies show slowing of conduction reflecting the underlying demyelination although, as in Guillain-Barré syndrome, conduction may be normal early in the course. Diphtheritic neuropathy can be prevented by immunization of susceptible persons and by prompt antibiotic therapy if infection occurs.

BACTERIAL ENDOCARDITIS

Septic emboli to peripheral nerves occur in about 2% of patients with bacterial endocarditis. The neurologic syndrome is that of

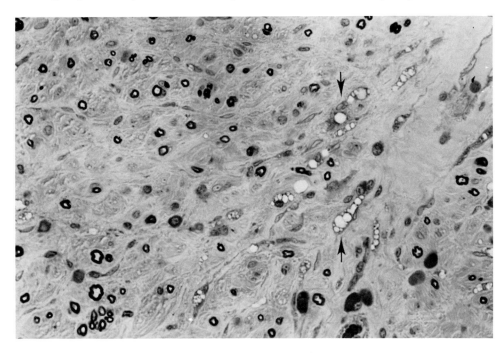

Fig. 108–4. Lepromatous leprous neuritis. Few myelinated fibers are scattered in fibrotic endoneurium. Abundant foam cells *(arrows)* contain M. Leprae bacilli when viewed at higher magnification. (Courtesy of Dr. Arthur Asbury.)

mononeuropathy or mononeuropathy multiplex.

ACQUIRED IMMUNODEFICIENCY SYNDROME (AIDS) AND AIDS-RELATED COMPLEX

Patients infected with the retrovirus HIV sometimes develop an acute or chronic demyelinating neuropathy. In CSF, both protein and cell count are sometimes elevated. Findings on nerve biopsy resemble those in idiopathic demyelinating polyneuritis with evidence of Wallerian degeneration in some cases. Vacuolation of perineurial cells is also seen occasionally. The HIV has been detected in peripheral nerves, as has evidence of cytomegalovirus infection. Favorable clinical responses to prednisone and plasmapheresis have been observed.

LYME NEUROPATHY

Radiculoneuritis, cranial neuritis, and meningitis are neurologic complications of spirochete infection. Borrelia burgdorferi is transmitted by bites of ioxodid ticks. This disorder should be suspected in patients with histories of erythema chronicum migrans, but can occur in the absence of this cutaneous lesion. The diagnosis may be suspected if the patient has arthralgia, nuchal rigidity, and has been in a tick-infested area; confirmation is by serologic tests. Cerebrospinal fluid pleocytosis and oligoclonal IgG bands are common. While Lyme neuropathy is most common on the east coast of the U.S., a similar disorder (Bannwarth syndrome) occurs in Europe. Treatment is with high doses of parenteral penicillin.

HERPES ZOSTER

Varicella viral infection of dorsal root ganglia produces radicular pain, which may precede or follow appearance of cutaneous lesions. The fifth and seventh nerve ganglia are also sometimes involved. Although seen most commonly exclusively with pain only, there may be paresis in a radicular pattern. Facial paresis with zoster infection of the seventh nerve ganglion is termed the Ramsay Hunt syndrome.

Sarcoid Neuropathy

Some 4% of patients with sarcoidosis have involvement of the nervous system, most commonly single or multiple cranial nerve palsies that fluctuate in intensity. Of the cranial nerves, the seventh is most commonly affected and, as in diabetes mellitus, the facial nerve syndrome of sarcoidosis is indistinguishable from idiopathic Bell palsy. In some instances, cranial neuropathies in patients with sarcoid neuropathy result from basilar meningitis. Patients with sarcoidosis occasionally develop symmetric polyneuropathy. Nerve biopsy shows a mixture of Wallerian degeneration and segmental demyelination with sarcoid granulomas in endoneurium and epineurium. Sarcoid neuropathy generally responds well to glucocorticoid therapy.

Symmetric Neuropathy Associated with Carcinoma (Paraneoplastic Neuropathy)

The occurrence of a mild symmetric distal neuropathy in the terminal stages of cancer has been recognized for many years. While most common with carcinoma of the lung, this may occur with carcinoma of any organ or with other malignant processes (e.g., multiple myeloma, lymphoma, Hodgkin disease, leukemia). Symptoms of polyneuropathy may also appear before clinical evidence of the primary tumor.

Both direct and indirect effects of malignant neoplasms on the peripheral nervous system are recognized. In some patients, the nerves or nerve roots are compressed or infiltrated by neoplastic cells. In others, there is no evidence of damage to the nerves by the neoplasm and dietary deficiency, metabolic, toxic, or immunologic factors may be responsible.

The clinical picture is variable. The neuropathy that is most characteristic of an associated carcinoma is a severe sensory ataxia of subacute onset, particularly of the arms. In this syndrome, electrodiagnostic studies reveal loss of evoked sensory responses. Autoantibodies directed against neuronal nuclei are found in the serum of these patients, and deposition of antibodies in dorsal root ganglia has been found at postmortem examination. Less reliably associated with carcinoma is a distal sensorimotor polyneuropathy without specific features. Occasionally, the protein content of the CSF is increased. Nerve biopsy may reveal infiltration by tumor cells, axonal degeneration, or demyelination. A primarily motor syndrome of subacute onset occurs in Hodgkin disease and other lymphomas. In these patients, the predominant lesion is degeneration of anterior horn cells, but demyelination, perivascular mononuclear cell infiltrates, and alterations in Schwann cell morphology in ventral roots are also observed.

The diagnosis of malignancy should be suspected in a middle-aged or elderly patient with a subacute sensory neuropathy, symmetric neuropathy, or polyradiculopathy of obscure cause. Remission of symptoms may occur, but the course is usually progressive until the primary malignancy causes death. Examination of the CSF for malignant cells is of value in the diagnosis of infiltration of the meninges by cancer. In some instances where such tumor infiltration occurs, radiotherapy or intrathecal chemotherapy may be of value.

Amyloid Neuropathy

Amyloid is an insoluble extracellular aggregate of protein sheets. Amyloid forms in nerve or other tissues when any of many proteins is produced in excess. The two principal forms of amyloid protein are immunoglobulin light chains (in patients with plasma cell dyscrasias) and a mutant form of transthyretin (in patients with inherited amyloid neuropathies). Clinical presentations of amyloid neuropathy include gradually progressive autonomic neuropathy, symmetric loss of pain and temperature sensation with spared position and vibratory senses, carpal tunnel syndrome, or some combination of these. The diagnosis of amyloid neuropathy can be established by histologic demonstration of amyloid in nerve (Fig. 108–5) or by detection of a transthyretin mutation by immunochemistry or DNA analysis. Electrophoresis of serum and urine with immunofixation can assist in the diagnosis of amyloid neuropathy secondary to plasma cell dyscrasia.

Neurologic symptoms are rare in seondary amyloidosis associated with chronic suppurative or inflammatory processes.

Nonamyloid Polyneuropathies Associated with Plasma Cell Dyscrasia

Symmetric neuropathy occurs in some patients with osteosclerotic myeloma and often remits when the myeloma is treated. A syndrome of severe polyneuropathy has been described in some patients with myeloma. Findings include hyperpigmentation of the skin, edema, excessive hair growth, papilledema, elevated spinal fluid proteins, hypogonadism, and hypothyroidism. Termed *POEMS syndrome* or *Crow-Fukase syndrome,* it is found most commonly in Japan. IgM paraproteinemia with symmetric neuropathy has been described in the elderly, especially in men.

Some of these patients have a syndrome characterized more by sensory than by motor polyneuropathy. They also have hand tremor and the presence in plasma of an IgM paraprotein that binds to myelin-associated glycoprotein and to specific glycolipids of peripheral nerves.

Polyneuropathy with Dietary Deficiency States

Dietary deficiency is generally considered the cause of the symmetric distal sensorimotor polyneuropathies associated with beriberi, alcoholism, pellagra, chronic malnutrition, and nontropical sprue. There is no evidence of a direct toxic effect of ethanol on nerves. Vitamin E deficiency contributes to neuropathy in fat malabsorption syndromes such as in chronic cholestasis.

Beriberi is endemic in hot climates, less common in temperate zones. It is subdivided into wet and dry forms, according to the presence or absence of edema and serous effusions. The edema and serous effusions in the wet form are due to cardiac failure; these symptoms respond to treatment with thiamine. Such patients usually have deficiencies of pyridoxine, pantothenic acid, and thiamine.

The symptoms and signs of alcoholic polyneuropathy and beriberi polyneuropathy are similar. Pains and paresthesia are present for several days or weeks before the onset of limb weakness, which may be severe with paralysis of the distal leg muscles and, in advanced stages, paralysis of the hands. There is cutaneous sensory loss below the wrists and knees, loss of ankle reflexes, and hypoactivity of other tendon reflexes. Nerve conduction velocities are normal or mildly slowed, but evoked responses are reduced in amplitude. Pathologic examination of peripheral nerves in thiamine deficiency reveals scattered degeneration and loss of axons, particularly in distal nerve segments. Treatment of both beriberi and alcoholic thiamine-deficiency neuropathy should be initiated with parenteral B-complex vitamins followed by oral thiamine. Recovery is slow; there may be residual muscular weakness and atrophy. The polyneuropathy of pellagra is clinically indistinguishable from thiamine-deficiency neuropathy and, in most cases, associated with deficiency of other B vitamins. Symmetric distal polyneuropathy is also seen in patients with vitamin B_{12} deficiency, but this is usually overshadowed by symptoms and signs of

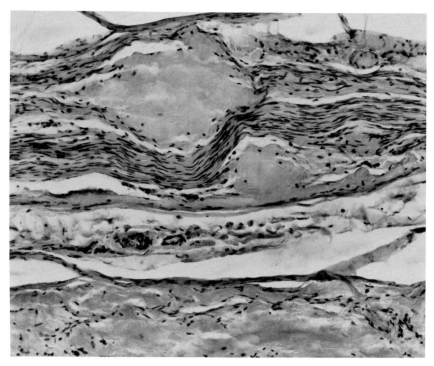

Fig. 108–5. Amyloid neuropathy. Massive deposits of endoneurial amyloid compress nerve fiber bundles. (Courtesy of Dr. Arthur Asbury.)

myelopathy. Vitamin B_6 deficiency is common in patients on long-term isoniazid therapy; it may cause symmetric distal polyneuropathy, primarily of the sensory nerves, and can be prevented by B_6 administration. Isoniazid also can occasionally elicit a vasculitic mononeuropathy multiplex.

Sensorimotor axonal polyneuropathy may complicate sepsis and multiorgan failure in gravely ill patients. This polyneuropathy usually clears with adequate parenteral supply of nutrients and vitamins.

Neuropathy Produced by Metals

ARSENIC

Damage to the peripheral nerves may follow chronic exposure to small amounts of arsenic or ingestion or parenteral administration of a large amount of the metal. Gastrointestinal symptoms, vomiting, and diarrhea occur when a toxic quantity of arsenic is ingested, but these symptoms may be absent if the arsenic is given parenterally or taken in small amounts over long periods. In acute arsenic poisoning, the onset of polyneuropathy is delayed 4 to 8 weeks; once symptoms develop, they reach maximum intensity within a few days. The evolution of polyneuropathy is much slower in patients with chronic arsenic poisoning. Sensory symptoms are prominent in the early stages. Pain and paresthesias in the legs may be present for several days or weeks before onset of weakness. The weakness progresses to complete flaccid paralysis of the legs and sometimes the arms. Cutaneous sensation is impaired in a stocking-and-glove distribution. Tendon reflexes are lost. Pigmentation and hyperkeratosis of the skin and changes in the nails ("Mees lines") are frequently present. Arsenic is present in the urine in the acute stages of poisoning and in the hair and nails in the late stages. Nerve conduction velocities may be normal or mildly diminished; the amplitude of evoked responses may be reduced. Pathologic examination of nerves shows axonal degeneration. Treatment of arsenic polyneuropathy should be with a chelating agent. Effectiveness of chelation therapy can be monitored by measuring arsenic excretion rates in 24-hour urine samples.

LEAD

In contrast to most other toxic neuropathies, lead poisoning causes focal weakness of the extensor muscles of the fingers and wrist. Lead neuropathy occurs almost exclusively in adults; infants poisoned with lead usually develop encephalopathy. Lead may enter the body through the skin, lungs, or gut. Occupational lead poisoning is encountered in battery workers, painters, and pottery glazers. Accidental lead poisoning follows ingestion of lead in food or beverages or in children who ingest lead paint. Lead poisoning may cause abdominal distress (lead colic). By its effect on renal tubules, lead poisoning often causes urate retention and "saturnine gout." Weakness usually begins in distal muscles innervated by the radial nerve, sparing the brachioradialis; it is often bilateral. Later, the weakness may extend to other muscles in the arms and occasionally to the legs. Sensory symptoms and signs are usually absent. Rarely, upper motor-neuron signs may occur with the lower motor-neuron disorder and mimic amyotrophic lateral sclerosis. Laboratory findings include anemia with basophilic stippling of the red cells, increased serum uric acid, and slight elevation of CSF protein content. Nerve conduction velocities are usually normal, raising the possibility that the disorder may be an anterior horn cell disease rather than a neuropathy. Urinary lead excretion is elevated, particularly after administration of a chelating agent. Urinary porphobilinogen excretion is also elevated, but delta-aminolevulinic acid is normal. The primary therapy is prevention of further exposure to lead. When exposure ceases, recovery is gradual over several months.

MERCURY

Mercury is used in the electrical and chemical industries. The alkylmercuries, particularly methylmercury, damage both central and peripheral nervous systems, causing ataxia, constricted visual fields or blindness, and symmetric distal polyneuropathy. Treatment with vitamin E or selenium may be of benefit.

THALLIUM

This element is used as a rodenticide and in some industrial processes. As with lead, children exposed to thallium are more likely to develop encephalopathy, whereas adults often develop neuropathy. In contrast to lead poisoning, however, thallium neuropathy is primarily sensory and autonomic. Severe distal dysesthesias appear acutely, and the course is complicated in many patients by tachycardia and hypertension. Quadriplegia, dysphagia, and dysarthria may occur in se-

vere cases. Most patients develop partial or total alopecia after onset of the neuropathic symptoms. The diagnosis is by history of thallium exposure. The typical syndrome of acute dysesthesias, autonomic dysfunction and subsequent alopecia, and identification of thallium in the urine are also of diagnostic value. Nerve conduction velocities are usually normal. Nerve biopsy or autopsy shows axonal degeneration. Thallium excretion can be accelerated by potassium administration, but potassium therapy may transiently worsen the pain and autonomic signs. Complete recovery usually occurs after exposure to thallium ends.

Neuropathy Produced by Drugs

ANTINEOPLASTIC DRUGS

The two most commonly used neurotoxic chemotherapeutic agents are vincristine and cisplatin. The vinca alkaloids produce distal or generalized hyporeflexia that may progress to symmetric distal sensorimotor or cranial neuropathy if the drug is continued. Neuropathy gradually disappears after therapy stops. Nerve biopsy shows axonal degeneration. Nerve conduction velocities are normal or mildly diminished. Cisplatin produces a sensory neuropathy attributable to loss of dorsal root ganglion neurons. Deficits may continue to worsen for a time after cessation of therapy and are sometimes irreversible. Adriamycin may also cause neuropathy.

OTHER DRUGS

Nitrofurantoin may cause a severe symmetric distal sensorimotor neuropathy, especially in patients with impaired renal function. A similar sensorimotor polyneuropathy is induced by chronic administration of amiodarone. Long-term isoniazid therapy is sometimes associated with a predominantly sensory neuropathy that can be prevented by vitamin B_6 therapy. Chronic ingestion of high doses of vitamin B_6 causes a pure sensory neuropathy. Long-term phenytoin administration occasionally causes hyporeflexia and distal diminution in sensation. Disulfiram, perhexiline maleate, and dapsone cause a predominantly motor disorder.

Neuropathy Produced by Aliphatic Chemicals

SOLVENTS

Carbon disulfide, hexane, and methyl N-butyl ketone are industrial solvents. Carbon disulfide toxicity was once frequent in rayon workers but is now rare. Hexane and methyl N-butyl ketone are inhaled for pleasure by some adolescents and cause subacute or chronic symmetric neuropathy, frequently with prominent weakness of proximal and distal limb muscles. Symptoms may worsen for several weeks after exposure is discontinued, but recovery eventually occurs. Nerve biopsy shows focal dilatations of axons that are filled with neurofilaments. Paranodal retraction of myelin caused by these "axonal balloons" is believed responsible for the considerable slowing of nerve conduction velocities.

OTHER CHEMICALS

Tri-ortho-cresyl phosphate ("ginger jake"), an adulterant used in illegal liquor (moonshine) and as a cooking oil contaminant, has been responsible for epidemics of neuropathy. Symmetric distal polyneuropathy is seen early, and weakness is often more prominent than sensory loss. Nerve biopsy shows distal axonal fragmentation. As the neuropathy clears, evidence of previously unrecognized irreversible damage to corticospinal tracts may become apparent, and late spasticity is common.

Acrylamide monomer is used to prepare polyacrylamide. It is used in chemical laboratories and to treat liquid sewage. Exposure produces a distal sensorimotor neuropathy that may be associated with trophic skin changes and a mild organic dementia. Nerve biopsy shows axonal degeneration with accumulations of neurofilaments in affected axons.

References

Guillain-Barré Syndrome

Arnason BGW. Acute inflammatory demyelinating polyradiculoneuropathies. In: Dyck PJ, Thomas PK, Lambert EL, Bunge R, eds. Peripheral Neuropathy. Philadelphia: W.B. Saunders, 1984:2050–2100.

Asbury AK. Diagnostic considerations in Guillain-Barré syndrome. Ann Neurol 1981; 9(suppl):1–5.

Asbury AK, Arnason BGW, Adams RD. The inflammatory lesion in idiopathic polyneuritis; its role in pathogenesis. Medicine 1969; 48:173–215.

Beghi E, Kurland LT, Mulder DW, Wiederholt WC. Guillain-Barré syndrome. Clinicoepidemiologic features and effect of influenza vaccine. Arch Neurol 1985; 42:1053–1057.

Brown WF, Feasby TE. Conduction block and denervation in Guillain-Barré syndrome. Brain 1984; 107:219–239.

Dowling PC, Cook SD. Role of infection in Guillain-Barré syndrome: Laboratory confirmation of herpes viruses in 41 cases. Ann Neurol 1981; 9(suppl):44–55.

Fisher CM. An unusual variant of acute idiopathic polyneuritis (syndrome of ophthalmoplegia, ataxia and areflexia). N Engl J Med 1956; 255:57–65.

The Guillain-Barré Study Group: Plasmapheresis and acute Guillain-Barré syndrome. Neurology 1985; 35:1095–1104.

Koski CL, Gratz E, Sutherland J, Mayer RF. Clinical correlation with antiperipheral nerve myelin antibodies in Guillain-Barré syndrome. Ann Neurol 1986; 19:573–577.

Lisak RP, Mitchell M, Zweiman B, Orrechio E, Asbury AK. Guillain-Barré syndrome and Hodgkin's disease: Three cases with immunological studies. Ann Neurol 1977; 1:72–78.

McLeod JG, Walsh JC, Prineas JW, Pollard JD. Acute idiopathic polyneuritis. A clinical and electrophysiological follow-up study. J Neurol Sci 1976; 27:145–162.

Pleasure D, Lovelace R, Duvoisin R. Prognosis of acute polyradiculoneuritis. Neurology 1968; 18:1143–1148.

Prineas JW. Pathology of the Guillain-Barré syndrome. Ann Neurol 1981; 9(suppl):6–19.

Schonberger LB, Hurwitz ES, Katona P, Holman RC, Bregman DJ. Guillain-Barré syndrome: Its epidemiology and associations with influenza vaccination. Ann Neurol 1981; 9(suppl):31–38.

Weintraub M. Hypophosphatemia mimiking acute Guillain-Barré-Strohl syndrome. A complication of parenteral hyperalimentation. JAMA 1976; 235: 1040–1041.

Chronic Demyelinating Polyneuritis

Austin JH. Observations on the syndrome of hypertrophic neuritis (the hypertrophic interstitial radiculoneuropathies). Medicine 1956; 35:187–237.

Chad DA, Smith TW, DeGirolamiu, Hammer K. Perineuritis and ulcerative colitis. Neurology 1986; 36:1377–1379.

Dalakis MC, Engel WK. Chronic relapsing (dysimmune) polyneuropathy: Pathogenesis and treatment. Ann Neurol 1981; 9(suppl):134–145.

Dyck PJ, Daube J, O'Brien P, et al. Plasma exchange in clinic inflammatory demyelinating polyradiculoneuropathy. N Engl J Med 1986; 314:461–465.

Dyck PJ, O'Brien PC, Oviatt KF, et al. Prednisone improves chronic inflammatory demyelinating polyradiculoneuropathy more than no treatment. Ann Neurol 1982; 11:136–141.

Lewis RA, Sumner AJ, Brown, MJ, Asbury AK. Multifocal demyelinating neuropathy with persistent conduction block. Neurology 1982; 32:958–964.

McCombe PA, Pollard JD, McLeod JG. Chronic inflammatory demyelinating polyradiculoneuropathy. A clinical and electrophysiological study of 92 cases. Brain 1987; 110:1617–1630.

Prineas JW, McLeod JG. Chronic relapsing polyneuritis. J Neurol Sci 1976; 27:427–458.

Sladky JT, Brown MJ, Berman PH. Chronic inflammatory demyelinating polyneuropathy of infancy: A corticosteroid-responsive disorder. Ann Neurol 1986; 20:76–81.

Acute Idiopathic Sensory Neuropathy

Colon RV, Snead OC, Oh SJ, Kashlan MB. Acute autonomic and sensory neuropathy. Ann Neurol 1980; 8:441–444.

Sterman AB, Schaumburg HH, Asbury AK. The acute sensory neuronopathy syndrome: A distinct clinical entity. Ann Neurol 1980; 7:354–358.

Chronic Idiopathic Sensory Neuropathy

Dalakis MC. Chronic idiopathic ataxic neuropathy. Ann Neurol 1986; 19:545–554.

Acute Pandysautonomia

Appenzeller O, Kornfeld M. Acute pandysautonomia. Arch Neurol 1973; 29:334–339.

Young RR Asbury AK, Adams RD, Corbett JL. Pure pandysautonomia with recovery. Description and discussion of diagnostic criteria. Brain 1975; 98:613–636.

Tick Paralysis

Swift TR, Ignacio OJ. Tick paralysis: Electrophysiologic signs. Neurology 1975; 25:1130–1133.

Brachial Neuropathy

Beghi E, Kurland LT, Mulder DW, Nicolosi A. Brachial plexus neuropathy in the population of Rochester, Minnesota, 1970–1981. Neurology 1985; 18:320–323.

Cosimano MD, Bilbao JM, Cohen SM: Hypertrophic brachial neuritis: Pathologic study of two cases. Ann Neurol 1988; 24:615–622.

Evans BA, Stevens JC, Dyck PJ. Lumbosacral plexus neuropathy. Neurology 1981; 31:1327–1330.

Flaggman PD, Kelly JJ. Brachial plexus neuropathy. An electrophysiologic evaluation. Arch Neurol 1980; 37:160–164.

Magee KR, DeJong RN. Paralytic brachial neuritis. JAMA 1960; 174:1258–1262.

Richter RW, Pearson J, Bruun B, Challenor YB, Brust JCM, Baden MB. Neurological complications of addiction to heroin. Bull NY Acad Med 1973; 19:3–21.

Tsairis P, Dych PJ, Mulder DW. Natural history of brachial plexus neuropathy, report on 99 patients. Arch Neurol 1972; 27:109–117.

Radiation Neuropathy

Foley KM, Woodruff JM, Ellis FT, Posner JB. Radiation induced malignant and atypical peripheral nerve sheath tumors. Ann Neurol 1980; 7:311–318.

Stoll BA, Andrews JT. Radiation induced peripheral neuropathy. Br Med J 1966; 1:834–837.

Neuropathy Induced by Cold

Thomas PK, Holdorff B. Neuropathy due to physical agents. In: Dyck PJ, Thomas PK, Lambert EL, Bunge R, eds. Peripheral Neuropathy. Philadelphia: W.B. Saunders, 1984:1479–1511.

Neuropathy Associated with Cryoglobulins

Garcia-Bragado F, Fernandez JM, Navarro C et al. Peripheral neuropathy in essential mixed myoglobulinemia. Arch Neurol 1988; 45:1210–1216.

Logothetis J, Kennedy WR, Ellington A, Williams RC. Cryoglobulinemic neuropathy. Incidence and clinical characteristics. Arch Neurol 1968; 19:389–397.

Diabetic Neuropathy

Archer AG, Watkins PJ, Thomas PK, Sharma AK, Payan J. The natural history of acute painful neuropathy in diabetes mellitus. J Neurol Neurosurg Psychiatry 1983; 46:491–499.

Asbury AK. Proximal diabetic neuropathy. Ann Neurol 1977; 2:179–180.

Asbury AK, Aldredge H, Hershberg R, Fisher CM. Oculomotor palsy in diabetes mellitus: A clinico-pathological study. Brain 1970; 93:555–566.

Behse F, Buchthal F, Carlsen F. Nerve biopsy and conduction studies in diabetic neuropathy. J Neurol Neurosurg Psychiatry 1977; 10:1072–1082.

Bradley WE, ed. Aspects of diabetic autonomic neuropathy [symposium]. Ann Intern Med 1980; 92:289–342.

Brown MJ, Asbury AK. Diabetic neuropathy. Ann Neurol 1984; 15:2–12.

Brown MJ, Martin JR, Asbury AK. Painful diabetic neuropathy. A morphometric study. Arch Neurol 1976; 33:164–171.

Committee on Health Care Issues, American Neurological Association. Does improved control of glycemia prevent or ameliorate diabetic polyneuropathy? Ann Neurol 1986; 19:288–290.

Dyck PJ, Lais A, Karnes JL, O'Brien P, Rizza R. Fiber loss is primary and multifocal in sural nerves in diabetic polyneuropathy. Ann Neurol 1986; 19:425–439.

Dyck PJ, Sherman WR, Hallcher LM, et al. Human diabetic endoneurial sorbitol fructose, and myo-inositol related to sural nerve morphometry. Ann Neurol 1980; 8:590–596.

Dyck PJ, Thomas PK, Asbury AK, Winegrad AI, Porte D Jr. Diabetic Neuropathy. Philadelphia: W.B. Saunders, 1987.

Harati Y. Diabetic peripheral neuropathies. Ann Int Med 1987; 107:546–559.

Johnson PC, Doll SC, Cromey DW. Pathogenesis of diabetic neuropathy. Ann Neurol 1986; 19:450–457.

Low PA, Walsh JC, Huang CY, McLeod JG. The sympathetic nervous system in diabetic neuropathy. A clinical and pathological study. Brain 1975; 98:341–356.

Raff MC, Asbury AK. Ischemic mononeuropathy and mononeuropathy multiplex in diabetes mellitus. N Engl J Med 1968; 279:17–22.

Hypothyroid Neuropathy

Crevagge LE, Logue RB. Peripheral neuropathy in myxedema. Ann Intern Med 1959; 50:1133–1137.

Dyck PJ, Lambert EH. Polyneuropathy associated with hypothyroidism. J Neuropathol Exp Neurol 1970; 29:631–658.

Fincham RW, Cape CA. Neuropathy in myxedema. A study of sensory nerve conduction in the upper extremities. Arch Neurol 1968; 19:464–466.

Acromegalic Neuropathy

Low PA, McLeod JG, Turtle JR, Donnelly P, Wright RG. Peripheral neuropathy in acromegaly. Brain 1974; 97:139–152.

Pickett JBE III, Layzer RB, Levin SR, Schneider V, Campbell MJ, Sumner AJ. Neuromuscular complications of acromegaly. Neurology 1975; 25:638–645.

Stewart BM. The hypertrophic neuropathy of acromegaly: A rare neuropathy associated with acromegaly. Arch Neurol 1966; 14:107–110.

Vasculitic Neuropathies

Caselli RJ, Daube JR, Hunder GG et al. Peripheral neuropathic syndromes in giant cell (temporal) arteritis. Neurology 1988; 38:685–689.

Conn DL, Dyck PJ. Angiopathic neuropathy in connective tissue diseases. In: Dyck PJ, Thomas PK, Lambert EH, Bunge R, eds. Peripheral Neuropathy. Philadelphia: W.B. Saunders, 1975; 1149–1165.

Ford RF, Siekert RG. Central nervous system manifestations of periarteritis nodosa. Neurology 1984: 34:2027–2043.

Johnson RT, Richardson EP. The neurological manifestations of systemic lupus erythematosus: A clinical pathological study of 24 cases and review of the literature. Medicine 1968; 47:337–369.

Kissel JT, Sliuka AP, Walmolts JR, Mendell JR. The clinical spectrum of necrotizing angiopathy of the peripheral nervous system. Ann Neurol 1985: 18:251–257.

Moore PM, Fauci AS. Neurologic manifestations of systemic vasculitis. Am J Med 1981; 71:517–524.

Said G, Lacroix-Ciaudo C, Fujimura H, Blas C, Faux N. The peripheral neuropathy of necrotizing arteritis: A clinicopathological study. Ann Neurol 1988; 23:461–465.

Scott DGI, Bacon PA, Tribe CR. Systemic rheumatoid vasculitis: A clinical and laboratory study of 50 cases. Medicine 1981; 60:288–297.

Stafford CR, Bogdanoff BM, Green L, Spector HB. Mononeuropathy multiplex as a complication of amphetamine angiitis. Neurology 1975; 25:570–572.

Teasdall RD, Frayha RA, Shulman LE. Cranial nerve involvement in systemic sclerois (scleroderma): A report of 10 cases. Medicine 1980; 59:149–159.

Warrell DA, Godfrey S, Olsen EGJ. Giant cell arteritis with peripheral neuropathy. Lancet 1968; 1:1010–1013.

Weller RO, Bruckner FE, Chamberlain MA. Rheumatoid neuropathy: A histological and electrophysiological study. J Neurol Neurosurg Psychiatry 1970; 33:592–594.

Uremic Neuropathy

Asbury AK. Uremic neuropathy. In: Dyck PJ, Thomas PK, Lambert EH, Bunge R, eds. Peripheral Neuropathy. Philadelphia: W.B. Saunders, 1984:1811–1825.

Dyck PJ, Johnson WJ, Lambert EH, O'Brien PC. Segmental demyelination secondary to axonal degeneration in uremic neuropathy. Mayo Clin Proc 1971; 46:400–431.

Said G, Boudier L, Selva J, Zingraff J, Drueke T. Different patterns of uremic polyneuropathy: Clinicopathologic study. Neurology 1983; 33:567–574.

Neuropathy Associated with Hepatic Diseases

Thomas PK, Walker JC. Xanthomatous neuropathy in primary biliary cirrhosis. Brain 1965; 88:1079–1088.

Neuropathies Associated with Infection

Leprosy

Pedley JC, Harman DJ, Waudby H, McDougall AC. Leprosy in peripheral nerves: Histopathlogical findings in 119 untreated patients in Nepal. J Neurol Neurosurg Psychiatry 1980; 43:198–204.

Rosenberg RN, Lovelace RE. Mononeuritis multiplex in lepromatous leprosy. Arch Neurol 1968; 19:310–314.

Sunderland S. The internal anatomy of nerve trunks in relation to the neural lesions of leprosy: Observations on pathology, symptomatology and treatment. Brain 1973; 95:865–888.

Diphtheria

Kurdi A, Abdul-Kader M. Clinical and electrophysiological studies of diphtheritic neuritis in Jordan. J Neurol Sci 1979; 42:243–250.

McDonald WI, Kocen RS. Diphtheritic neuropathy. In: Dyck PJ, Thomas PK, Lambert EH, Bunge R, eds. Peripheral Neuropathy. Philadelphia: W.B. Saunders, 1984: 2010–2017.

Acquired Immunodeficiency Syndrome (AIDS) and AIDS-Related Complex

Bailey RO, Baltch AL, Venkatesh R et al. Sensory motor neuropathy associated with AIDS. Neurology 1988; 38:886–891.

Cornblath DR, McArthur JC, Kennedy PGE, Witte AS, Griffin JW. Inflammatory demyelinating peripheral neuropathies associated with human T-cell lymphotropic virus type III infection. Ann Neurol 1987; 32–40.

Eidelberg D, Sotrel A, Vogel H, Walker P, Kleefield J, Crunpacker CS. Progressive polyradiculopathy in acquired immunodeficiency syndrome. Neurology 1986; 36:912–916.

Ho DD, Rota TR, Schooley RT, et al. Isolation of HTLV-III from cerebrospinal fluid and neural tissues of patients with neurological syndromes related to the acquired immunodeficiency syndrome. New Engl J Med 1985; 313:1493–1497.

So YT, Holtzman DM, Abrams DI, Olney RK. Peripheral neuropathy associated with AIDS, prevalence and clinical features from a population-based survey. Arch Neurol 1988; 45:945–948.

Bacterial Endocarditis

Pruitt AA, Rubin RH, Karchmer AW, Duncan GW. Neurologic complications of bacterial endocarditis. Medicine 1978; 57:329–343.

Herpes Zoster

Kendall D. Motor complications of herpes zoster. Br Med J 1957; 2:616–618.

Lyme Neuropathy

Henriksson A, Link H, Cruz M, Stiernstedt G. Immunoglobulin abnormalities in cerebrospinal fluid and blood over the course of lymphocytic meningoradiculitis (Bannworth's syndrome). Ann Neurol 1986; 20:337–345.

Pachner AR, Steere AC. The triad of neurologic manifestations of Lyme disease: Meningitis, cranial neuritis, and radiculoneuritis. Neurology 1985; 35:47–53.

Reik L Jr, Burgdorfer W, Donaldson JO. Neurologic abnormalities in Lyme disease without chronicum migrans. Am J Med 1986; 81:73–78.

Sarcoid Neuropathy

Challenor YB, Felton CP, Brust JCM. Peripheral nerve involvement in sarcoidosis: an electrodiagnostic study. J Neurol Neurosurg Psychiatry 1984; 46:1219–1222.

Matthews WB. Sarcoid neuropathy. In: Dyck PJ, Thomas PK, Lambert EH, Bunge R, eds. Peripheral Neuropathy. Philadelphia: W.B. Saunders, 1984: 2018–2026.

Nemni R, Galassi G, Cohen M, et al. Symmetric sarcoid polyneuropathy: Analysis of a sural nerve biopsy. Neurology 1981; 31:1217–1223.

Polyneuropathy Associated with Carcinoma

Croft PB, Wilkinson M. The course and prognosis on some types of carcinomatous neuromyopathy. Brain 1969; 92:1–8.

Dalakas MC, Engel WK. Polyneuropathy with monoclonal gammopathy: Studies of 11 patients. Ann Neurol 1981; 10:45–52.

Driedger H, Pruzanski W. Plasma cell neoplasia with peripheral polyneuropathy. A study of five cases and a review of the literature. Medicine 1980; 59:301–310.

Graus F, Elkon KB, Cordon-Cardo C, Posner JB. Sensory

neuronopathy and small cell lung cancer. Antineu-ronal antibody that also reacts with the tumor. Am J Med 1986; 80:45–52.

Hawley RJ, Cohen MH, Saini N, Armbrustmacher VW. The carcinomatous neuromyopathy of oat cell lung cancer. Ann Neurol 1980; 7:65–72.

Horwich MS, Cho L, Porro RS, Posner JB. Subacute sensory neuropathy: A remote effect of carcinoma. Ann Neurol 1977; 2:7–19.

Olson ME, Chernik NL, Posner JB. Infiltration of the leptomeninges by systemic cancer: A clinical and pathologic study. Arch Neurol 1974; 30:122–137.

Schold SC, Cho ES, Somasundaram M, Posner JB. Subacute motor neuropathy: A remote effect of lymphoma. Ann Neurol 1979; 5:271–287.

Victor M, Banker BQ, Adams RD. The neuropathology of multiple myeloma. J Neurol Neurosurg Psychiatry 1958; 21:73–88.

Amyloid Polyneuropathy

Andrade A, Araki S, Block WD, et al. Hereditary amy-loidosis. Arthritis Rheum 1970; 13:902–915.

Battle WM, Rubin MR, Cohen S, Snape WJ. Gastroin-testinal-mobility dysfunction in amyloidosis. N Engl J Med 1979; 301:24–25.

French JM, Hall G, Parish DJ, Smith WT. Peripheral and autonomic nerve involvement in primary amyloi-dosis associated with uncontrollable diarrhea and steatorrhea. Am J Med 1965; 39:277–284.

Kelly JJ Jr, Kyle RA, O'Brien PC, Dyck PJ. The natural history of peripheral neuropathy in primary systemic amyloidosis. Ann Neurol 1979; 6:1–7.

Koeppen AH, Mitzen EJ, Hans MB, Peng SK, Bailey RO. Familial amyloid polyneuropathy. Muscle Nerve 1985; 8:733–749.

Saraiva MJM, Costa PP, Goodman DS. Genetic expression of a transthyretin mutation in typical and late-onset Portuguese families with familial amyloidotic poly-neuropathy. Neurology 1986; 36:1413–1417.

Wallace MR, Dwulet FE, Conneally PM, Benson MD. Biochemical and molecular genetic characterization of a new variant prealbumin associated with hered-itary amyloidosis. J Clin Invest 1986; 78:6–12.

Nonamyloid Polyneuropathies Associated with Plasma Cell Dyscrasias

Bardwick PA, Zvaifler NJ, Gill GN, Newnow D, Green-way GD, Resnick DL. Plasma cell dyscrasia with polyneuropathy, organomegaly and M proteins and skin changes: The POEMS syndrome. Medicine 1980; 59:311–322.

Chou DKH, Ilyas AA, Evans JE, Costello C, Quarles RH, Jungalwala FB. Structure of sulfated glucuronyl gly-colipids in the nervous system reacting with HNK-1 antibody and some IgM paraproteins in neurop-athy. J Biol Chem 1986; 251:11717–11725.

Kelly JJ Jr, Kyle RA, Latov N (eds). Polyneuropathies associated with plasma cell dyscrasias. Boston: Mar-tinus-Nijhoff, 1988.

Latov N, Braun P, Gross RB, Sherman WH, Penn AS, Chess L. Plasma cell dyscrasia and peripheral neu-ropathy: Identification of the myelin antigens that react with human paraproteins. Proc Natl Acad Sci USA 1981; 78:7139–7142.

Latov N, Hays AP, Sherman WH. Peripheral neuropathy and anti-MAG antibodies. CRC Crit Rev Neurobiol 1988; 3:301–332.

Nobile-Orazio E, Vietorisz T, Messito MJ, Sherman WH, Latov N. Anti-MAG antibodies in patients with neu-ropathy and IgM-Proteins: Detection by ELISA. Neurology 1983; 33:939–942.

Neuropathy Associated with Deficiency States

Bolton CF, Gilbert JJ, Hahn AF, Sibbald WJ. Polyneu-ropathy in critically ill patients. J Neurol Neurosurg Psychiatry 1984; 47:1223–1231.

Cooke WT, Smith WE. Neurological disorders associated with adult coeliac disease. Brain 1966; 89:683–722.

Hillbom M, Weinberg A. Prognosis of alcoholic periph-eral neuropathy. J Neurol Neurosurg Psychiatry 1984; 47:699–703.

Kaplan JG, Pack D, Horoupian D et al. Distal axonopathy associated with chronic gluten enteropathy: A treat-able disorder. Neurology 1988; 38:642–645.

Sokol RJ, Guggenheim MA, Iannaccone ST, et al. Im-proved neurologic function after long-term correc-tion of vitamin E defciency in children with chronic cholestasis. New Engl J Med 1985; 313:1580–1586.

Tredici G, Minazzi M. Alcohol neuropathy: An electron-microscopic study. J Neurol Sci 1975; 25:333–346.

Victor M, Adams RD, Collins GH. The Wernicke-Kor-sakoff Syndrome. Philadelphia: FA Davis, 1971.

Toxic Neuropathies

Albers JW, Kallenbach LR, FIne LJ et al. Neurologic ab-normalities with remote occupational elemental mer-cury exposure. Ann Neurol 1988; 24:651–659.

poisoning. Arch Neurol 1972; 26:289–301.

Bradley WG, Lassman LP, Pearce GW, Walton JN. The neuromyopathy of vincristine in man. Clinical, elec-trophysiological and pathological studies. J Neurol Sci 1970; 10:107–131.

Davis LE, Standefer JC, Kornfeld M, Abercrombie DM, Butler C. Acute thallium poisoning: Toxicological and morphological studies of the nervous system. Ann Neurol 1981; 10:38–44.

Feldman RG, Niles CA, Kelly Hayes M, et al. Peripheral neuropathy in arsenic smelter workers. Neurology 1979; 939–944.

Laquery A, Ronnel A, Vignolly B, et al. Thalidomide neuropathy: An electrophysiologic study. Muscle Nerve 1986; 9:837–844.

LeQuesne PM, McLeod JG. Peripheral neuropathy fol-lowing a single exposure to arsenic. Clinical course in four patients with electrophysiological and his-tological studies. J Neurol Sci 1977; 32:437–451.

Ochoa J. Isoniazid neuropathy in man: quantitative elec-tron microscope study. Brain 1970; 93:831–850.

Parry GJ, Bredeson DE. Sensory neuropathy with low-dose pyridoxine. Neurology 35:1466–1468, 1985.

Ramirez JA, Mendell JR, Warmolts JR, Griggs RC. Pheny-toin neuropathy: Structural changes in the sural nerve. Ann Neurol 1986; 19:162–167.

Said G. Perhexiline neuropathy: A clinicopathological study. Ann Neurol 1978; 3:259–266.

Schaumberg HH, Kaplan J, Windebank A, et al. Sensory neuropathy from pyridoxine abuse. A new mega-vitamin syndrome. N Engl J Med 1983; 309:445–448.

Spencer PS, Schaumberg HH. Experimental and Clinical Neurotoxicology. Baltimore: Williams & Wilkins, 1980.

Windebank AJ, McCall JT, Dyck PJ. Metal neuropathy. In: Dyck PJ, Thomas PK, Lambert EH, Bunge R, eds. Peripheral Neuropathy. Philadelphia: W.B. Saun-ders, 1984:2133–2161.

Chapter XIII

Ataxias and Dementia

109. HEREDITARY ATAXIAS
Roger N. Rosenberg

The cerebellum and its connections are the primary site of disease in chronic progressive disorders that often occur in a familial or hereditary pattern. There is no satisfactory means of classifying these disorders owing to our limited knowledge of etiologic factors, variability of clinical manifestations, and the difficulty of correlating clinical signs with postmortem changes. The salient clinical feature in these disorders is a chronic, slowly progressive ataxia that usually begins in the legs. In addition, there may be signs and symptoms of lesions in posterior columns, pyramidal tracts, pontine nuclei, basal ganglia, and other regions of the brain. As a rule, the clinical picture is constant in a given kindred, but muscular dystrophy, optic atrophy, or spastic paraplegia is occasionally found in relatives.

On histologic study, there is selective neuronal system degeneration with reactive gliosis and demyelination. Current nosologic concepts rest primarily on the distribution of these degenerative changes. In individual cases, precise diagnosis is often possible only on postmortem study. Even then, classifying intermediate or mixed cases may be difficult. For present descriptive purposes, we may arbitrarily divide degenerations of the cerebellar system into several large groups on clinical and pathologic grounds as follows:

1. Hereditary spinocerebellar ataxia of Friedreich
2. Hereditary ataxia with muscular atrophy (Lévy-Roussy syndrome)
3. Hereditary cerebellar ataxia
   a) resembling olivopontocerebellar atrophy
   b) cerebello-olivary degeneration (Holmes)
4. Olivopontocerebellar atrophy (Dejerine-Thomas)
5. Parenchymatous cerebellar degeneration
6. Autosomal dominant ataxia of the Portuguese (Joseph disease)
7. Other forms of cerebellar ataxia

Friedreich Ataxia

Friedreich ataxia is a familial and hereditary disease with degenerative changes that are localized chiefly to the dorsal half of the spinal cord and the cerebellum. It is characterized clinically by the appearance of ataxia of the limbs and trunk, absence of tendon reflexes, loss of proprioceptive sensations in the limbs, and extensor plantar responses. This condition usually occurs in the first or second decade of life. Clubfoot and scoliosis are present in many cases. Dysarthria, muscle atrophy, and degeneration of the optic nerve may occur late in the course of the disease. Cardiomyopathy has often been reported, and diabetes mellitus is present in over 10% of the patients.

Pathology. On gross inspection, the spinal cord and cerebellum may appear normal or the cord may be thinner than normal; the cerebellum may be somewhat shrunken. The characteristic histologic changes in the cord are degeneration of the posterior funiculi, lateral corticospinal tracts, and the dorsal and ventral spinocerebellar tracts. These degenerative changes are most intense in the dorsal funiculi where gliosis is extensive. Degeneration also involves the dorsal roots, ganglia, and peripheral nerves. There is loss of cells in Clarke's column and, to a lesser extent, in the substantia gelatinosa and other cell masses of the posterior horn. Ventral horn cells are usually preserved.

The cerebellum and brain stem are usually normal, but shrinkage of the pons and the medulla has been reported. Atrophy of the Purkinje cells and those of the dentate nuclei has been found in some cases. No significant changes occur in the cerebral cortex; degeneration in the corticospinal tracts rarely extends above the medulla.

Activity of the enzyme lipoamide dehydrogenase has been reported to be about half normal in muscle and skin fibroblast homogenates from patients, but this has been a controversial finding. Mitochondrial malic enzyme has also been reported to be abnormal in some patients but, in most cases, no consistent biochemical abnormality has been defined.

Incidence. Friedreich ataxia is one of the more common hereditary diseases of the nervous system. All races are affected and it is slightly more common in males. It is usually inherited as an autosomal recessive disorder, but many patients have no family history of similar disease. The gene has been assigned to two chromosomes, 9 and 11; the syndrome may therefore be genetically heterogeneous.

The onset is usually in the first or second decade of life. Most commonly, it is between the seventh and thirteenth years. Symptoms may be present in infancy; occasionally, they do not appear until the third decade. Abortive forms, in which only one or two features of the disease are present (e.g., clubfeet, slight ataxia, absent knee jerks) are not uncommon.

Symptoms and Signs. Ataxia, sensory loss, nystagmus, alterations in the reflexes, clubfeet, and kyphoscoliosis are the characteristic features of the disease. Optic atrophy, cranial nerve palsies, mental deficiency, and dementia are less common.

Motor System. Ataxia of gait, the most common symptom, is usually the first to appear. The gait disorder may be seen in the latter half of the first decade in children who had apparently been able to walk normally, but more commonly it is noted that the children were slow in learning to walk, that gait was always clumsy and awkward, and that they were not as agile as other children. Within a few years after the onset of frank difficulty in locomotion, ataxia appears in the movements of the arms and then the trunk. The impairment of movement is the result of the combination of cerebellar asynergia and ataxia due to the loss of proprioceptive sense. Movements are jerky, awkward, and poorly controlled. Intention tremor, which is most common in the arms, may occasionally affect the muscles of the trunk (cerebellar titubation).

The muscles of articulation are involved in advanced cases, with explosive or slurred speech or finally such severe dysarthria that speech is unintelligible. Pseudoathetoid and choreic movements of the limbs may also be seen.

Weakness of the muscles is common, in some cases amounting to a complete or almost complete paralysis of the legs with paraplegia in flexion. As a rule, the muscles are flabby and disuse atrophy is common in the late stages of the disease. Localized atrophy may occur in the late stage, especially in distal limb muscles, but girdle and trunk muscles are also occasionally involved.

Sensory System. Evidence of involvement of the posterior funiculi is present in almost all patients. Loss of the appreciation of vibration is an early sign. Some impairment of position sense in the legs and later in the arms is almost always present. Occasionally, the loss of proprioceptive sense in trunk muscles confines the patient to bed or makes it necessary for the patient to have special support when sitting in a chair. Loss of two-point discrimination, partial or complete astereognosis, and some impairment of the appreciation of pain, temperature, and tactile sensation are occasionally seen in advanced cases.

Reflexes. Tendon reflexes in the legs are almost always absent. Rarely, in otherwise typical cases, they are preserved throughout the course of the disease. The reflexes are usually present in the arms at first, but may be absent later. The plantar responses are extensor in practically all patients. Occasionally, an extensor response may be found on only one side; the plantar responses may occasionally be flexor. The abdominal and cremasteric reflexes are preserved in most patients.

Other Neurologic Signs and Symptoms. Nystagmus usually develops at some stage of the disease. It is commonly of the fixation type (i.e., oscillatory movements of the eyes on movement before coming to rest), but horizontal nystagmus and vertical or rotary nystagmus have been reported. Optic atrophy is an inconstant feature. Oculomotor paralysis with diplopia and deafness or loss of labyrinthine reactions are rare manifestations. Impairment of the sphincters is uncommon except when the patients are bedridden. It is often difficult to determine whether incontinence is due to organic damage or inattention. Mental retardation, dementia, or psychosis occur in a few cases. The condition is not incompatible with a high degree of intellectual development. The incidence of convulsive sezures is greater than in the general population.

Skeletal Abnormalities. Clubfeet and kyphoscoliosis are the characteristic skeletal deformities. The abnormality in the shape of the foot usually takes the form of a double pes cavus, conjoined with talipes varus or equinovarus. Although not a constant feature of the disease, the foot deformity is present in almost 75% of individuals, and it is occasionally found in other members of the family as the only sign of the disease. The abnormality of the feet may be present from early infancy or it may not develop until late in the course of the disease. Deformity of the head is a rare finding. Kyphosis or scoliosis, usually in the upper thoracic regions, is present in over 80% of the patients. The spinal deformity usually develops late and progresses slowly.

Heart. Enlargement of the heart, cardiac murmurs, abnormalities in the EKG, and other signs of heart disease are not uncommon. Boyer and also Hewer found that cardiac involvement in the form of diffuse myocardial fibrosis with coronary thrombosis was a common cause of death.

Laboratory Findings. The laboratory findings are usually normal. Occasionally, there is a slight increase in the protein content and, rarely, a slight pleocytosis in the CSF. Abnormalities in the EKG, related to involvement of the heart muscle, are common.

Diagnosis. The characteristic spinal cord and cerebellar signs in combination with the abnormalities of the feet and spine make the diagnosis relatively simple in classic cases. In sporadic cases with no skeletal deformities, the differential diagnosis between Friedreich ataxia and multiple sclerosis may be difficult. The onset of symptoms at an early age and the progressive course of Friedreich ataxia, as well as the relative infrequency of the loss of tendon reflexes in multiple sclerosis, are important factors in the differential diagnosis.

Abortive or atypical forms of Friedreich ataxia are difficult to distinguish from other heredodegenerative diseases unless the typical syndrome is present in other members of the family.

Clinical Course. There are numerous instances in which the disease assumes an abortive form that may be compatible with a relatively normal life span without serious disability. In most patients, however, onset is in the early years of life, and the disease progresses to complete incapacity by the age of 20. Death usually occurs as the result of intercurrent infections, but may result from the cardiomyopathy.

Treatment. No specific treatment influences the course of Friedreich ataxia. Tenotomies or other orthopedic operations are indicated for the relief of the foot deformity. Muscle training and re-education are of value in the abortive forms and in the rare cases with spontaneous remissions.

Lévy-Roussy Syndrome

In 1926 Lévy and Roussy described a syndrome characterized by impairment of the equilibrium in walking and standing, loss of knee and ankle jerks, wasting of the muscles of the legs, and kyphoscoliosis. Typical cerebellar signs and nystagmus are not present. The symptoms develop early in childhood. They progress slowly and may arrest before the development of severe disabilities. The disorder is regarded as intermediate phenotypically between Friedreich ataxia and Charcot-Marie-Tooth disease. Harding and Thomas include it as a form of hereditary motor and sensory neuropathy type 1 (slow conduction velocities) and type 2 (normal conduction velocities). The occurrence of typical Friedreich ataxia, the syndrome of Lévy-Roussy, and Charcot-Marie-Tooth disease in different members of the same family has been reported. It is transmitted in an autosomal dominant pattern.

Hereditary Cerebellar Ataxia

In 1893, Marie applied the term *hereditary cerebellar ataxia* to cases in which the clinical picture differed from that of Friedreich ataxia in late onset of symptoms, more definite hereditary character, exaggeration of reflexes, and the frequent occurrence of optic atrophy and oculomotor palsies. Scoliosis, pes cavus, muscle atrophy, Romberg sign, and other signs of spinal cord involvement were said to be lacking, although spasticity was sometimes present. A kindred described by Sanger Brown in 1892 was considered an example of the disorder. The term "Marie's hereditary cerebellar ataxia" was subsequently widely employed to designate such cases.

The original nosologic concept has been considerably altered in the light of more recent clinical and pathologic observations. Some of the cases on which Marie's concept was based were later found on postmortem study to have a spinocerebellar degeneration and would now be classified as variants of

Friedreich ataxia. The hereditary cases with pathologically verified cerebellar degeneration seem to be a heterogeneous group of disorders. Greenfield classified them on the basis of the anatomic distribution of degenerative changes into two major groups: *type A*, presenting the features of olivopontocerebellar atrophy; and *type B*, the relatively rare cerebello-olivary degeneration of Holmes. Konigsmark and Weiner have further subdivided the olivopontocerebellar type into five groups. However, there is considerable clinical and pathologic variability, even within the same kindred. For example, in a large, dominantly inherited American family with 53 affected persons described by Schut in 1950 and by Landis and associates in 1974, one affected individual had a spinocerebellar degeneration that resembled Friedreich ataxia, one had a spastic paraplegia with minimal ataxia, and the others had cerebellar ataxia, many with pyramidal tract signs.

Pathology. In the more common type A, there is atrophy of the middle cerebellar peduncle, pontine nuclei, medullary olives, cerebellar cortex, and white matter. The cranial motor nerves, especially the oculomotor and hypoglossal nerves, and the anterior horn cells are sometimes affected. Degeneration is frequently seen in the long tracts of the spinal cord, but it is not of the severity found in Friedreich ataxia. Degenerative changes are rarely found in the dentate nuclei. In type B, the cortex of the superior surface of the cerebellum and the vermis is particularly affected. The inferior olives are also degenerated. In both types, there is profound loss of Purkinje cells, reduction in the number of cells in the molecular and granular layers, and degeneration of the fibers in the folia and white matter of the cerebellum. Ultrastructural studies in the Schut family have shown striking proliferation of membranous tubules in some Purkinje cells and aberrant axons in the molecular layer. Vermiform tubules that resembled paramyxovirus nucleocapsids were also observed.

Incidence. Hereditary cerebellar ataxia is much less common than Friedreich ataxia. The age of onset is later, usually in the fourth to sixth decades, but onset as early as the second and as late as the seventh decade has been recorded. In most of the kindreds studied, autosomal dominant transmission has been observed. Occasional sporadic cases may occur.

Symptoms and Signs. The initial symptom is usually an ataxia of gait. Frequent sudden falls are common. Later, there is incoordination of the arms, tremor of the hands, and dysarthria. In advanced stages, there may be weakness of the legs, rigidity, nystagmus, and oculomotor palsies. Optic atrophy occurs frequently in some families, but is lacking in others. The reflexes may be reduced or hyperactive. Ankle clonus and extensor plantar responses are found in some patients. Mental deterioration may occur late. Parkinsonism occurs in some cases of the olivopontocerebellar type.

Diagnosis. The development of a chronic progressive ataxia in an adult known to have affected relatives suggests the diagnosis of hereditary cerebellar ataxia. However, the absence of clinical signs of spinal cord involvement does not necessarily exclude a spinocerebellar degeneration. The differential diagnosis among the several forms of cerebellar ataxia and from atypical forms of Friedreich ataxia is difficult on clinical grounds alone. Sporadic cases do not differ in any consistent manner.

Course and Treatment. The course of the disease is progressive, but progress may be so slow that incapacitation does not occur for several or many decades. There is no specific therapy. Cases with rigidity or other features of parkinsonism may benefit from symptomatic treatment with levodopa.

Olivopontocerebellar Atrophy

In 1900, Dejerine and Thomas gave the descriptive name *olivopontocerebellar atrophy* to a form of chronic progressive ataxia that begins in middle age, in which atrophy of the cerebellum, pons, and inferior olives are conspicuous findings on postmortem study. Most cases encountered in clinical practice are sporadic and present a distinctive and generally more consistent clinical picture than the hereditary cases included previously among the hereditary cerebellar ataxias. However, Konigsmark and Weiner suggest that many sporadic cases probably reflect an unrecognized recessive heredity.

Pathology. Marked shrinkage of the ventral half of the pons, disappearance of the olivary eminence on the ventral surface of the medulla, and atrophy of the cerebellum are evident on gross postmortem inspection of the brain. Variable loss of Purkinje cells, reduction in the number of cells in the molecular and granular layer, demyelination of the middle cerebellar peduncle and the cerebellar hemispheres, and severe loss of cells in the pontine nuclei and olives are found on histologic examination. The vermis, the dentate and other cerebellar nuclei, the tegmentum of the pons, the corticospinal tracts, and the restiform body are usually well preserved. Degenerative changes in the striatum, especially the putamen, and loss of the pigmented cells of the substantia nigra may be found in cases with extrapyramidal features. More widespread degeneration in the CNS, including involvement of the posterior columns and the spinocerebellar fibers, is often present, especially in the autosomal dominant cases.

Symptoms and Signs. The clinical syndrome of olivopontocerebellar atrophy is characterized by the development in adult or late middle life of progressive cerebellar ataxia of the trunk and limbs, impairment of equilibrium and gait, slowness of voluntary movements, scanning speech, nystagmoid jerks, and oscillatory tremor of the head and trunk. Dysarthria, dysphagia, and oculomotor and facial palsies may also occur. Extrapyramidal symptoms include rigidity, immobile facies, and parkinsonian tremor. The reflexes are usually normal, but knee and ankle jerks may be lost and extensor responses may occur. Dementia is not rare, but is usually mild. Impairment of sphincter function commonly occurs with urinary and sometimes fecal incontinence.

Diagnosis. Olivopontocerebellar atrophy is differentiated from Friedreich ataxia by the relatively late onset and the absence of signs and symptoms of spinal cord disease. In familial cases, the differentiation from hereditary cerebellar ataxia is more difficult in view of persisting uncertainties regarding the classification of the hereditary ataxias. The family history is of primary importance. Posterior fossa tumor and cerebellar degeneration occurring as a remote effect of carcinoma should be considered in the differential diagnosis. Some cases with rigidity and tremor may initially be mistaken for Parkinson disease. Pneumoencephalography or CT usually shows enlargement of the prepontine cistern and fourth ventricle. Plaitakis and co-workers described a significant reduction in the activity of the enzyme glutamate dehydrogenase in several patients with recessively inherited olivopontocerebellar degeneration. The activity of this enzyme is normal in most patients with dominantly inherited olivopontocerebellar degeneration. One dominantly inherited family has had the primary mutation mapped to chromosome 6 near the HLA com-

plex. If this finding is confirmed, it would provide a means to identify a subgroup of patients and offer a marker for genetic counseling. Johnson and associates described juvenile patients with a progressive, recessively inherited form of ataxia and an associated deficiency of hexosaminidase.

Other Forms of Cerebellar Ataxia

ACUTE CEREBELLAR ATAXIA IN CHILDREN

Acute cerebellar ataxia is occasionally seen in young children without any obvious cause. The neurologic symptoms usually have a sudden onset and are preceded in more than half the cases by a nonspecific, undiagnosed illness of the respiratory or gastrointestinal tract. Most affected children are younger than 5. Boys and girls are affected equally often. The usual symptoms are ataxia of the trunk and limbs, disorders of eye movements, tremors of the head and trunk, hypotonia, and irritability. The disease is usually benign, with complete recovery within 6 months. Multiple sclerosis or other demyelinating disease seems unlikely because of the age of the patients and the lack of recurrence. Infection with poliomyelitis or echoviruses has been suggested as the cause.

ATAXIA TELANGIECTASIA

In recent years, many cases have been described in which telangiectases are most prominent in the bulbar conjunctivae (Fig. 109–1), and are associated with cerebellar degeneration and sinopulmonary infections. The syndrome may be regarded as a fifth form of phakomatosis. The disease was first reported by Madame Louis-Bar in 1941; since then more than 100 cases have been reported. The pathologic changes include degeneration of the Purkinje and basket cells and neurons of the dentate nucleus and inferior olives, granular cells of the cerebellum, demyelination of the posterior columns of the spinal cord, and degenerative changes in the ventral horn cells and spinal ganglia.

Other pathologic findings include respiratory tract infections, hypoplasia or absence of the thymus, reticuloendothelial malignancies, hypoplasia of lymphoid tissue, and telangiectases in the conjunctivae, skin, and nervous system.

The clinical symptoms vary considerably. Ataxia of gait beginning in infancy is the most common symptom. Other symptoms and signs include nystagmus, dysarthria, loss of

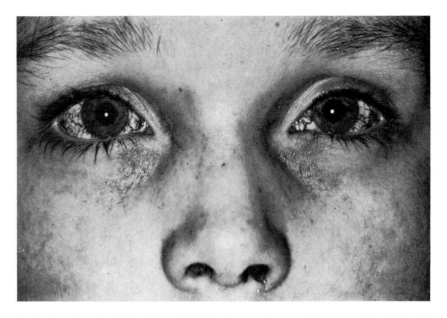

Fig. 109–1. Ataxia telangiectasia. Telangiectases in the bulbar conjunctiva. (Courtesy of Dr. G. Gaull.)

reflexes, retardation of development, and changes in the skin and hair.

There is a deficiency of IgA and IgE globulin in the serum.

The course of the disease is relentlessly progressive with death in childhood, but survival to age 25 has been reported. Death is usually due to pulmonary infections or malignant tumors of lymphatic or reticuloendothelial origin.

MARINESCO-SJÖGREN SYNDROME

A syndrome characterized by cerebellar ataxia, bilateral cataracts, and physical and mental retardation was reported in 1931 by Marinesco, Draganesco, and Vasilu. Fourteen cases were reported in 1950 by Sjögren, and since then about 50 cases have been reported.

The symptoms of cerebellar involvement and cataracts are evident early in life. Mild retardation of physical growth is present in most patients. The degree of mental retardation is variable, but most of the patients are imbeciles.

The disease does not affect the length of life. The cataracts can be removed by surgery; however, the patients may be greatly handicapped by their mental retardation.

MITOCHONDRIAL ENCEPHALOPATHY WITH LACTIC ACIDOSIS AND STROKE (MELAS)

Rowland and others have described a syndrome with normal development in early life with symptoms starting between 3 and 11 years. These patients were short-statured and developed seizures, stroke-like manifestations with hemiparesis, hemianopia, or cortical blindness. Nine of eleven patients had hemiparesis or hemianopsia, and six had episodes of cortical blindness. Nine patients developed dementia. Vomiting and sensory neural hearing loss were present in several. Two pairs of siblings were affected. Cerebellar signs were uncommon. NADH-CoQ reductase (complex 1) deficiency has been found in one patient.

RAMSAY HUNT SYNDROME

The combination of myoclonus with chronic progressive ataxia first described by Ramsay Hunt and termed *dyssynergia cerebellaris myoclonica* is a distinctive clinical syndrome. Atrophy of the dentate nucleus with demyelination of the superior cerebellar peduncles, degeneration of the posterior columns of the spinal cord and, to a lesser extent, of the spinocerebellar tracts are the major pathologic alterations. Hunt ascribed the myoclonus to the dentate atrophy, but this may be questioned because dentate lesions are often present in cerebellar degeneration without myoclonus and, conversely, cases have been described in which the dentate was spared. The clinical manifestations of dyssynergia cerebellaris myoclonica have been described in patients with different disease (e.g., Pallis' case of diffuse lipofuscinosis). Thus, the condition must be regarded as a syndrome rather than a specific entity. Some cases are associated with abnormal mitochondria in muscle *(ragged red fibers)*, as described by Fukuhara and Rowland. It has been referred to as the myoclonus epilepsy with ragged red fiber syndrome (MERRF syndrome).

A deficiency of the enzyme CoQ-cytochrome reductase (complex III) has been reported in a single patient with ataxia, proximal weakness, myoclonus, and dementia. The patient had a low oxygen uptake with NADH and flavin-linked substrates and normal oxygen uptake with ascorbate. One family had a pattern of maternal inheritance consistent with a mitochondrial DNA mutation.

JOSEPH DISEASE

Joseph disease or striatonigral degeneration was described for the first time in 1976 by Rosenberg and Nyhan and associates as a form of autosomal dominant motor system degeneration occurring in a large family of Portuguese ancestry numbering in excess of 329 persons in eight generations (Fig. 109–2). The neuropathologic findings were those of striatonigral degeneration with additional abnormal findings in the dentate nucleus of the cerebellum.

The patients differed clinically from previously described patients with striatonigral degeneration in that the elements of parkinsonian rigidity were minor relative to the marked degree of spasticity. In this variant, an autosomal dominant mode of inheritance was clearly documented. Subsequently, this form of degeneration inherited in a dominant manner has been encountered in at least 70 families, most of which are of Portuguese ancestry. It is not known whether these families are directly related. The disease has now been well described in the inhabitants of the Azores Islands, Portugal, the United States, and Japan. The median age at onset of symptoms was 25.

Neurologic deficits increase progressively in all affected members and usually result in death from pneumonia within 15 years. An early neurologic symptom is a lurching unsteadiness of gait. Rigidity is present early and is replaced by progressive spasticity. The legs become progressively stiff and spastic and are held in extension with adductor hypertonicity. Speech subsequently becomes slow and indistinct. Patients remain ambulatory for 10 years after the onset of gait instability. Urinary and bowel incontinence are minimal. Intellectual function remains intact.

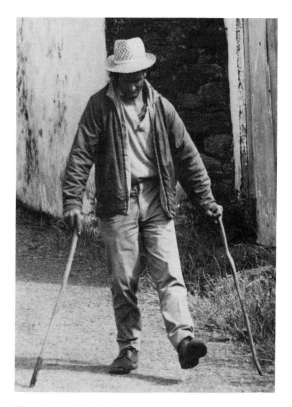

Fig. 109–2. Joseph disease. Patient has leg spasticity requiring the use of canes for walking. He also manifests neck dystonia, ophthalmoparesis, and facial fasciculations.

On examination, the main findings are weakness of the arms and legs and spasticity, especially of the legs. Patellar and ankle clonus are common, as are Babinski signs. The gait is slow with a slight increase in base and lurching from side to side due to spasticity. Pharyngeal weakness and spasticity cause difficulty with speech and swallowing. Horizontal and vertical nystagmus are prominent with hypermetric and hypometric saccades and impairment of vertical gaze. Facial fasciculations, facial myokymia, and lingual fasciculations without atrophy are common early manifestations. The CSF concentration of homovanillic acid is sometimes reduced.

True cerebellar ataxia has been seen in some segments of several affected families, establishing a linkage with the spinocerebellar degenerations. Significant progressive peripheral neuropathy similar to Machado disease has also been seen in some family members. Thus, a spectrum of involvement with prominent spasticity and pure extrapyramidal signs is seen at one end with true cerebellar disorders and amyotrophy at the other end.

There is no specific form of treatment, but several patients with prominent spasticity and choking due to pharyngeal involvement have been temporarily improved with dantrolene or levodopa. The basic molecular defect is not known, but brain protein abnormalities have been described on two-dimensional acrylamide gels. The activities of brain glutamate dehydrogenase and malate dehydrogenase are normal compared to those of control subjects. The neuropathology is that of a progressive neuronal loss and glial replacement in the striatum, substantia nigra, and basis pons with similar but less intense neuronal loss in the dentate nucleus of the cerebellum. The thoracic cord shows demyelination and atrophy of the spinocerebellar tacts and loss of anterior horn cells.

References

Friedreich Ataxia

Blass JP. Disorders of pyruvate metabolism. Neurology 1979; 29:280–286.

Boyer SH, Chisholm AW, McKusick VA. Cardiac aspects of Friedreich's ataxia. Circulation 1962; 25:493–505.

Chamberlain S, Shaw J, Rowland A et al. Mapping of mutation causing Friedreich's ataxia to human chromosome 5. Nature 1988; 324:248–250.

Friedreich N. Über Ataxie mit besonderer Berücksichtigung der hereditären Formen. Virchows Arch Path Anat 1876; 68:145–245.

Gatti RA, Berkel I, Boder E et al. Localization of an ataxia telangiectasia gene to chromosome 11q22-23. Nature 1988; 336:577–580.

Harding AE. The Hereditary Ataxias and Related Disorders. Edinburgh, Churchill Livingstone, 1984.

Hewer RL. Study of fatal cases of Friedreich's ataxia. Br Med J 1968; 3:649–652.

Hughes JT, Brownell B, Hewer RL. The peripheral sensory pathways in Friedreich's ataxia. Brain 1968; 91:803–817.

Kark RAP, Rodriguez-Budelli M, Perlman S, Gulley WF, Tarok K. Preclinical diagnosis and carrier detection in ataxia associated with abnormalities of lipoamide dehydrogenase. Neurology 1980; 30:502–508.

Rodriguez-Budelli M, Kark P. Kinetic evidence for a structural abnormality of lipoamide-dehydrogenase in two patients with Friedreich's ataxia. Neurology 1978; 28:1283–1286.

Skre H, Löken AC. Myoclonus epilepsy and subacute presenile dementia in heredo-ataxia. Acta Neurol Scand 1970; 46:18–42.

Stumpf DA, Parks JK, Eguren LA, Haas R. Friedreich ataxia. III. Mitochondrial malic enzyme deficiency. Neurology 1982; 32:221–227.

Thilenius OG, Grossman BJ. Friedreich's ataxia with heart disease in children. Pediatrics 1961; 27:246–254.

Urich H, Norman RM, Lloyd OC. Suprasegmental lesions in Friedreich's ataxia. Confin Neurol 1957; 17(suppl): 360–371.

Levy-Roussy Syndrome

Harding AE, Thomas PK. The clinical features of hereditary motor and sensory neuropathy type I and II. Brain, 103:259–280, 1980.

Oelschlager R, White HH, Schimke RN. Roussy-Levy syndrome: report of a kindred and discussion of the nosology. Acta Neurol Scand 1971; 47:80–90.

Rombold CR, Riley HA. The abortive type of Friedreich's ataxia. Arch Neurol Psychiatry 1926; 16:301–312.

Roussy G, Levy G. Sept cas d'une maladie familiale particuliére: troubles de la marche, pieds bots et aréflexie tendineuse généralisée, avec accessoirement, légère maladresse des mains. Rev Neurol 1926; 33:427–450.

Herditary Cerebellar Ataxia

Brown S. Hereditary ataxy. Brain 1892; 15:250–263.

Gilman S, Bloedel J, Lechtenberg R. Disorders of the Cerebellum. Philadelphia: FA Davis, 1981.

Greenfield J. The Spinocerebellar Degenerations. Springfield: Charles C Thomas, 1954.

Hoffman PM, Stuart WH, Earle KM, Brody JA. Hereditary late-onset cerebellar degeneration. Neurology 1971; 21:771–777.

Holmes G. A form of familial degeneration of the cerebellum. Brain 1907; 30:466–489.

Konigsmark BW, Weiner LP. The olivopontocerebellar atrophies; a review. Medicine 1970; 49:277–341.

Landis DMD, Rosenberg R, et al. Olivopontocerebellar degeneration: clinical and ultrastructural abnormalities. Arch Neurol 1974; 31:295–307.

Schut JW. Hereditary ataxia. Arch Neurol Psychiatry 1950; 63:535–568.

Sorbi S, Blass JP. Hereditary ataxias. Curr Neurol 1982; 4:37–54.

Taylor AMR, Flude E, Laher B, et al. Variant forms of ataxia telangiectasia. J Med Genet 1987; 24:669–677.

Olivopontocerebellar Atrophy

Critchley M, Greenfield JG. Olivo-ponto-cerebellar atrophy. Brain 1948; 71:343–364.

Déjerine J, Thomas A. L'atrophie olivo-ponto-cérébelleuse. Nouv Iconog Salpêtrière 1900; 13:330–370.

Francois J, Descamps L. Hérédo-ataxie par dégénérescence spino-ponto-cérébelleuse avec manifestations tapéto-rétiniennes et cochléo-vestibulaires. Monatsschr Psychiatrie Neurol 1951; 121:23–38.

Geary JR, Earle KM, Rose AS. Olivopontocerebellar atrophy. Neurology 1956; 6:218–224.

Johnson WG, Chutorian A, Miranda A. A new juvenile hexosaminidase deficiency disease presenting as cerebellar ataxia: clinical and biochemical studies. Neurology 1977; 27:1012–1018.

Klawans HL, Zeitlin E. L-dopa in parkinsonism associated with cerebellar dysfunction (probable olivopontocerebellar degeneration). J Neurol Neurosurg Psychiatry 1971; 34:14–19.

Plaitakis A, Nicklas WJ, Desnick RJ. Glutamate dehydrogenase deficiency in three patients with spinocerebellar ataxia: a new enzymatic defect? Trans Am Neurol Assoc 1979; 104:54–57.

Plaitakis A, Nicklas WJ, Desnick RJ. Glutamate dehydrogenase deficiency in three patients with spinocerebellar syndrome. Ann Neurol 1980; 7:297–303.

Other Forms of Cerebellar Ataxia
Acute Cerebellar Ataxia in Children

Siekert RG, Keith HM, Dion FR. Ataxia-telangiectasia in childhood. Proc Mayo Clin 1959; 34:581–587.

Weiss S, Carter S. Course and prognosis of acute cerebellar ataxia in children. Neurology 1959; 9:711–721.

Ataxia Telangiectasia

Aguilar MJ, Kamoshita S, Landing BH, Bader E, Sedgwick RP. Pathological observations in ataxia-telangiectasia. J Neuropath Exp Neurol 1968; 27:659–676.

Ammann AJ, Cain WA, Ishizaka K, Hong R, Good RA. Immunoglobulin E deficiency in ataxia-telangiectasia. N Engl J Med 1969; 281:469–472.

DiMauro S, Bonilla E, Zeuiani M, Nakagawa M, DeVivo D. Mitochondrial myopathies. Ann Neurol 17:521–538, 1985.

Harley RD, Baird HW, Craven EM. Ataxia telangiectasia. Report of seven cases. Arch Ophthalmol 1967; 77:582–592.

Hosking G. Ataxia telangiectasia. Dev Med Child Neurol 1982; 24:77–80.

Louis-Bar D. Sur un syndrome progressif comprenant des télagiectasies capillaires cutanées et conjonctivales symétriques, à disposition naevoide et des troubles cérébelleux. Confinîa Neurol 1941; 4:32–42.

McFarlin DE, Strober W, Waldman TA. Ataxia telangiectasia. Medicine 1972; 51:275–292.

Painter RB. Structural changes in chromatin as the basis for radiosensitivity in ataxia telangiectasia. Cytogenet Cell Genet 1982; 33:139–144.

Pavlakis S, Phillips P, DiMauro S, DeVivo D, Rowland LP. Mitochondrial myopathy, encephalopathy, lactic acidosis and stroke like episodes. Ann Neurol 1984; 16:481–488.

Rowland LP, Hays AP, DiMauro S, DeVivo D, Behrens M. Diverse clinical disorders associated with morphological abnormalities of mitochondria. In: Scarlato G, Cerri CG, eds. Mitochondrial Pathology in Muscle Disease. Padua Italy: Piccin Medical Books, 1983:141–158.

Waldmann TA, Misiti J, Nelson OL, Kraemer KH. Ataxia telangiectasia: a multisystem hereditary disease with immunodeficiency, impaired organ maturation, x-ray hypersensitivity, and a high incidence of neoplasia. Ann Intern Med 1983; 99:367–379.

Marinesco-Sjögren Syndrome

Anderson B. Marinesco-Sjögren syndrome, spinocerebellar ataxia, congenital cataract, somatic and mental retardation. Dev Med Child Neurol 1965; 7:249–257.

Todorov A. Le syndrome de Marinesco-Sjögren. Première étude anatomo-clinique. J Genet Hum 1965; 14:197–233.

Ramsay Hunt Syndrome

Bonduelle M, Escourolle R, Bouygues P, Lormeau G, Gray E. Atrophie olivo-ponto-cérébelleuse familiale avec myoclonies. Rev Neurol 1976; 132–113–124.

Critchley M. Dyssynergia cerebellaris progressive. Trans Am Neurol Assoc 1962; 87:81–85.

Fukuhara N. Myoclonus, epilepsy, and mitochondrial myopathy. In: Scarlato G, Cerri C, eds. Mitochondrial Pathology in Muscle Diseases. Padua, Italy: Piccin Medical Books, 1983: 87–110.

Hunt JR. Dyssynergia cerebellaris myoclonica. Brain 1921; 44:490–538.

Pallis CA, Duckett S, Pearse AGE. Diffuse lipofuscinosis of the central nervous system. Neurology 1967; 17:381–394.

Rosing H, Hopkins L, Wallace D, Epstein C, Weidenheim K. Maternally inherited mitochondrial myopathy and myoclonic epilepsy. Ann Neurol 1985; 17:228–237.

Rowland L, Hays AP, DiMauro S, DeVivo D, Behrens M. Diverse clinical disorders associated with morphological abnormalities of mitochondria. In: Mitochondrial Pathology in Muscle Disease. Scarlato G, Cerri CB, eds. Padua, Italy: Piccin, Medical Books, 1983: 141–158.

Joseph Disease

Rosenberg RN, Nyhan WL, Bay C, Shore P. Autosomal dominant striatonigral degeneration. A clinical, pathological and biochemical study of a new genetic disorder. Neurology 1976; 26:703–714.

Rosenberg RN, Nyhan WL, Coutinho P, Bay C. Joseph's disease: an autosomal dominant neurological disease in the Portuguese of the United States and the Azore Islands. Adv Neurol 1978; 21:33–57.

Rosenberg RN, Thomas L, Baskin F, Kirkpatrick J, Bay C, Nyhan WL. Joseph disease: protein patterns in fibroblasts and brain. Neurology 1979; 29:917–926.

Rosenberg RN, Ivy N, Kirkpatrick J, Bay C, Nyhan WL, Baskin F. Joseph disease and Huntington disease: protein patterns in fibroblasts and brain. Neurology 1981; 31:1003–1014.

110. PARENCHYMATOUS CEREBELLAR DEGENERATION
Sid Gilman

Parenchymatous cerebellar degeneration (secondary cerebellar degeneration, intracerebellar atrophy, lamellar atrophy of Purkinje cells, parenchymatous cortical cerebellar atrophy) is a pathologic condition of the cerebellum that causes symptoms of cerebellar dysfunction in middle age. The condition results from the nutritional disorder of alcoholism or the remote effects of neoplasms.

Pathology. The pathologic changes depend on the causative factors. In alcoholic cerebellar degeneration, gross inspection reveals obvious atrophy of the folia in the anterior and superior aspects of the vermis and in the anterior part of the anterior lobe of the cerebellum (Fig. 110–1). Microscopically, all cellular elements of the cerebellar cortex are degenerated in these regions, particularly the Purkinje cells. The olivary nuclei are involved regularly; the fastigial, interposed, and vestibular nuclei are affected less consistently. Other cerebellar and brain stem nuclei are unaltered.

In patients with cerebellar degeneration due to the remote effects of neoplasms, striking generalized changes appear in the cerebellum. With carcinomas, there is widespread loss of Purkinje cells, with no greater involvement of one site than another. The molecular layer is thinned and shows microglial proliferation. The granular layer is narrow and granule cells are sparse. The intracerebellar

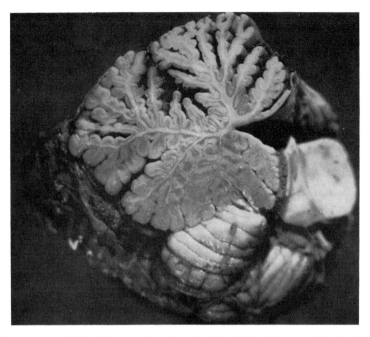

Fig. 110–1. Parenchymatous cerebellar degeneration. Atrophy of cerebellar foliae associated with chronic alcoholism. (Courtesy of Dr. Maurice Victor.)

nuclei usually show no change, but there may be demyelination of the superior cerebellar peduncles, along with gliosis in cerebral white matter, demyelination in the spinal cord, and degeneration of the pyramidal tract, oculomotor and other cranial nerve nuclei, and anterior horn cells. In cerebellar degeneration associated with neuroblastoma, scattered loss of Purkinje cells occurs, with demyelination and gliosis about and within the dentate nuclei.

Incidence. Parenchymatous cerebellar degeneration occurs rarely as judged from the number of reported cases with autopsy examination, but clinical experience indicates that it is a common form of cerebellar disorder in adults. No clear hereditary or familial incidence has been established. Alcoholic cerebellar degeneration appears three or four times more commonly in men than in women. Cerebellar degeneration from the remote effects of carcinoma occurs with an approximately equal incidence in men and women.

Pathogenesis. Alcoholic cerebellar degeneration probably results from nutritional deficiencies and not the toxic effects of alcohol. The cause of cerebellar degeneration as a remote effect of neoplasms outside the CNS has not been determined, but may be an autoimmune disorder since antibodies to cerebel-

lar antigens have been found in some cases. No single type of tumor occurs in association with cerebellar degeneration. In adults, lung, breast, uterine and ovarian carcinomas are associated with cerebellar degeneration. Neuroblastomas are associated with cerebellar degeneration in children. Hodgkin disease can produce a rapidly progressive cerebellar degeneration.

The symptoms of parenchymatous cerebellar degeneration usually begin in the fifth to seventh decades of life, but occasionally appear in the fourth decade. Alcoholic cerebellar degeneration occurs in patients with a background of excessive drinking and malnutrition for many years. The patient usually has an associated peripheral neuropathy and signs of nutritional deficiency. The remote effects of carcinoma in the adult generally occur between the fourth and seventh decade. The symptoms of cerebellar degeneration may appear before the neoplasm is detected.

Symptoms and Signs. The initial sign of alcoholic cerebellar degeneration is a gait disorder (i.e., staggering, stumbling, unsteadiness and, often, fear of walking). Other symptoms may develop later, including incoordination, tremor of the arms, and dysarthria. On examination, the patient has a broad-based stance and gait, often with instability of the trunk and, at times, an independent rhythmic tremor of the trunk or head. The patient walks slowly with small, ataxic steps while looking at the ground. The gait disorder worsens markedly when the patient attempts to walk in tandem. Apart from walking, coordinated movements of the legs are often performed surprisingly well. The arms are affected much less than the legs and nystagmus occurs infrequently. Tendon reflexes are usually normal, but the ankle jerks may be absent owing to concurrent peripheral neuropathy. The plantar responses are usually normal. The greater disorder of gait and of the coordinated muscular function of the legs corresponds to the location of the disease in the anterior portion of the cerebellar vermis.

Patients with cerebellar degeneration from the remote effects of carcinoma also have symptoms of unsteadiness in standing and walking, but they develop severe dysarthria, truncal titubation, and limb dysmetria. Opsoclonus and myoclonus can occur. The symptoms often progress rapidly and the ataxia may become so severe that the patient cannot even sit up in bed. Dysarthria may be so severe that speech becomes unintelligible. Tendon reflexes may be diminished, normal, or exaggerated, and extensor plantar responses can be seen. Dementia may occur.

Differential Diagnosis. Cerebellar degeneration secondary to alcoholism or the remote effects of neoplasms must be differentiated from other diseases of the cerebellum, including neoplasms, degenerative or toxic processes, congenital abnormalities, metabolic disorders, and demyelinating diseases. Olivopontocerebellar atrophy, Creutzfeldt-Jakob disease, the Dandy-Walker malformation, and the Chiari malformations may present with symptoms of cerebellar disease in the adult. Thallium poisoning can cause signs of cerebellar dysfunction, although alopecia and peripheral neuropathy with dysautonomia more commonly indicate this diagnosis. Phenytoin intoxication may explain signs of cerebellar disease and hypothyroidism may cause a disorder of cerebellar function that can be reversed by replacement therapy. Positron emission tomography may prove to be helpful in the diagnosis of parenchymatous cerebellar degeneration.

Course and Treatment. In alcoholic cerebellar degeneration, the cerebellar disorder usually evolves subacutely for weeks or months, but sometimes the onset is more abrupt. Once established, the disorder may remain un-changed for many years. With abstinence from alcohol and improved nutritional status, the symptoms usually remain static, improving only slightly. The symptoms of cerebellar degeneration from the remote effects of carcinoma can also evolve for months either before or after the discovery of the tumor. Removal of the carcinoma or radiation therapy of a neuroblastoma does not usually relieve the cerebellar symptoms. There is no specific therapy for the cerebellar dysfunction.

References

Anderson NE, Rosenblum MK. Paraneoplastic cerebellar degeneration: Clinical-immunologic correlations. Ann Neurol 1988; 24:559–567.

Brain WR, Wilkinson M. Subacute cerebellar degeneration associated with neoplasms. Brain 1965; 88:465–478.

Bray PF, Ziter FA, Lahey ME, Myers GG. The coincidence of neuroblastoma and acute cerebellar encephalopathy. J Pediatr 1969; 75:983–990.

Cunningham J, Graus F, Anderson N, Posner JB. Partial characterization of the Purkinje cell antigens in paraneoplastic cerebellar degeneration. Neurology 1986; 36:1163–1168.

Gilman S, Bloedel JR, Lechtenberg R. Disorders of the cerebellum. Philadelphia: FA Davis, 1981.

Gilman S, Adams K, Koeppe RA, Berent S. Cerebellar hypometabolism in alcoholic cerebellar degeneration studied with FDG and PET. Neurology 1988; 38:365.

Greenlee JR, Brashear HR. Antibodies to cerebellar Purkinje cells in patients with paraneoplastic cerebellar degeneration and ovarian carcinoma. Ann Neurol 1983; 14:609–613.

Henson RA, Urich H. Cancer and the nervous system. The neurological complications of systemic malignant diseases. Oxford: Blackwell, 1982.

Jaeckle KA, Graus F, Houghton A, Cordon-Cardo C, Nielsen SL, Posner JB. Autoimmune response of patients with paraneoplastic cerebellar degeneration to a Purkinje cell cytoplasmic protein antigen. Ann Neurol 1985; 18:592–600.

Nabatame H, Fukuyama H, Akiguchi I, Kameyama M, Nishimura K, Nakano Y. Spinocerebellar degeneration: Qualitative and quantitative MR analysis of atrophy. J Comput Assist Tomogr 1988; 12:298–303.

Vicor M, Adams RD, Collins GH. The Wernicke-Korsakoff Syndrome. Philadelphia: FA Davis, 1971.

Victor M, Adams RD, Mancall EL. A restricted form of cerebellar cortical degeneration occurring in alcoholic patients. Arch Neurol 1959; 1:579–688.

Wessel K, Diener HC, Schroth G, Dichgans J. Paraneoplastic cerebellar degeneration associated with Hodgkin's disease. J Neurol 1987; 235:122–124.

111. THE DEMENTIAS
Robert Katzman

Alzheimer Disease

One of the most common degenerative diseases of the brain is named after Alois Alzheimer, who described the major pathologic changes. For many years, the term *Alzheimer disease* was limited to the description of cases with an onset in the presenium, that is, before the age of 65. Clinical, pathologic, ultrastructural, and biochemical analyses indicate that Alzheimer disease and senile dementia are a single process; there is now a consensus to consider them a single disease. Community surveys in Northern Europe and the United States indicate that about 4% of persons over age 65 are incapacitated by an organic dementia. About 10% have progressive mental deterioration but can still function in the community. Pathologic studies in the same communities indicate that between 50 and 60% of the brains of patients with organic dementia have Alzheimer disease. Extrapolating these numbers, there may be as many as 700,000 individuals severely incapacitated by Alzheimer disease in the United States today and as many as 1.6 million with an earlier or milder form of this disorder.

Pathology. Alzheimer disease is characterized by atrophy of the cerebral cortex that is usually diffuse, although it may be more severe in the frontal and temporal lobes (Fig. 111–1). The degree of atrophy is variable. Brains of affected individuals weigh between 850 and 1,250 g at autopsy. Normal aging of the brain is also accompanied by atrophy; there is an overlap in the degree of atrophy of brains obtained from elderly Alzheimer patients and unaffected patients of the same age (Table 111–1). On microscopic examination, there is loss of both neurons and neuropil in the cortex and, sometimes, secondary demyelination in subcortical white matter. With quantitative morphometry, it has been shown that the greatest loss is that of large cortical neurons (i.e., neurons more than 90 μm^2 in cross-sectional area). The most characteristic findings are the argentophilic *senile plaques* and *neurofibrillary tangles*. The senile plaque (Fig. 111–2) is found throughout the cerebral cortex and hippocampus, and the number of plaques per microscopic field has been correlated with the degree of intellectual loss. The senile plaque is composed of enlarged, degenerating axonal endings surrounding a core composed mainly of extracellular amyloid. Amyloid is also found in the walls of some meningeal and cerebral arterioles. A unique peptide appears to be the major constituent of both the vascular and plaque amyloid. The degenerating axonal boutons contain lysosomes, degenerating mitochondria, and paired helical filaments. These paired hel-

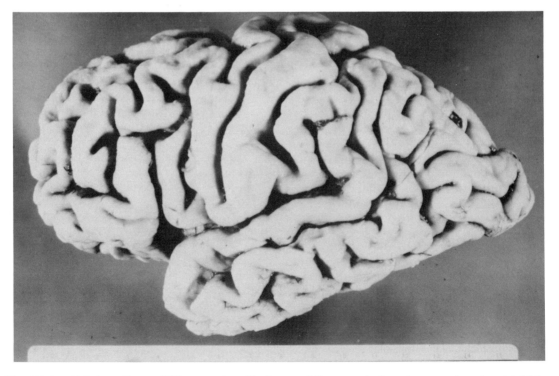

Fig. 111–1. Alzheimer disease. Diffuse atrophy of brain; especially severe in frontal, temporal, and parietal lobes with relative sparing of pre- and postcentral gyri. (Courtesy of Dr. Robert Terry.)

Table 111–1. Changes in Brain Weights and Cortical Thickness in Alzheimer Disease

Group	Weight (g)		
	Range	Mean + SEM	
Age-matched normals (N = 10)	930–1350	1152 ± 45	} p > 0.05
Alzheimer disease (N = 14)	918–1150	1055 ± 20	
Area	Cortical Thickness (mm)		
	Range	Mean ± SEM	
Midfrontal			
Age-matched normals (N = 12)	1.71–3.07	2.43 ± 0.10	} NS
Alzheimer disease (N = 18)	1.57–2.77	2.19 ± 0.08	
Superior temporal			
Age-matched normals (N = 12)	2.05–3.09	2.49 ± 0.10	} NS
Alzheimer disease (N = 18)	1.44–2.70	2.26 ± 0.08	

SEM = standard error of the mean
NS = not significant
(From Terry RD, et al. Ann Neurol 1981; 10:184–192.)

ical filaments, which are about 20 nm wide with a twist every 80 nm along their length, constitute the chief element found in the Alzheimer neurofibrillary tangle. These tangles consist of accumulation of these filaments within the body of a swollen neuron. Neurofibrillary tangles first occur in the hippocampus, particularly in region CA1 and subiculum; later, neurofibrillary tangles may be found throughout the cerebral cortex (Table 111–2). Other less prominent but still common features of Alzheimer disease include granulovacuolar degeneration of pyramidal cells of the hippocampus and congophilic angiopathy. The Hirano body, a rod-like body containing actin in a paracrystalline array, first described in the Guam-parkinsonism-dementia complex, is also found in Alzheimer disease.

Arteriosclerotic changes are absent or are present only to a minor degree in most cases.

Etiology. The cause of Alzheimer disease is unknown. Evidence of a genetic or familial predisposition is established. The risk of de-

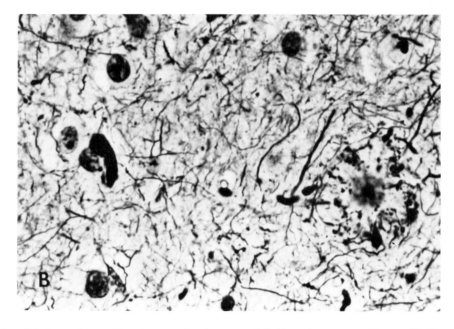

Fig. 111–2. Alzheimer disease. Prominent senile plaques on left. Several neurons with neurofibrillary tangles on right. Note also disruption of cortical organization. (Courtesy of Dr. Robert Terry.)

Table 111–2.   Selective Distribution of Lesions in Brain in Alzheimer Disease

Cell loss, plaques, and tangles occur regularly in:
    Neocortex, especially association areas
    Hippocampus, including entorhinal cortex
    Amygdala
    Basal nucleus

Sometimes in:
    Medial nucleus of thalamus
    Dorsal tegmentum
    Locus ceruleus
    Paramedian reticular area
    Lateral hypothalamic nuclei

veloping the disease at any given age is increased four- to fivefold among first-degree relatives of Alzheimer probands. There are many cases of Alzheimer disease in several generations, which is consistent with autosomal dominant inheritance; however, most cases occur sporadically. Concordance in identical twins is less than 60%, indicating that nongenetic factors play an important role in the pathogenesis of the disease.

Individuals with Down syndrome who live past the age of 40 develop pathologic and biochemical features identical to those of Alzheimer disease. Because cognitive function often cannot be tested in these individuals, dementia may not be apparent; however, an associated change in behavior usually occurs. This finding has raised the question of whether chromosomal changes play a role in the development of Alzheimer disease, but no chromosomal abnormality has been consistently demonstrated yet. Attempts to identify a toxic or viral etiology have been unsuccessful.

Biochemical Changes. Despite the devastating clinical changes that occur in Alzheimer disease, relatively few biochemical changes differentiate postmortem Alzheimer brain tissue from that of age-matched normal individuals (Table 111–3). The most consistent change is a 50 to 90% reduction of the activity of choline acetyltransferase in the cerebral cortex and hippocampus. Because choline acetyltransferase, which is the biosynthetic enzyme for acetylcholine, is found only in cholinergic neurons, it appears likely that there is selective loss of cholinergic neurons, particularly of the cholinergic projection pathway from deep neuclei located in the septum near the diagonal band of Broca to the hippocampus, and from the nearby basal nucleus of Meynert to the cerebral cortex. The apparent specificity of this loss is shown by the presence in the cortex and hippocampus of a normal complement of postsynaptic muscarinic receptors. Moreover, the degree of cognitive deficit measured during life is roughly proportional to the loss of choline acetyltransferase.

Significant reductions occur in the neuropeptides CRF (corticotropin releasing factor) and somatostatin, both of which have been identified within degenerating neurites of the

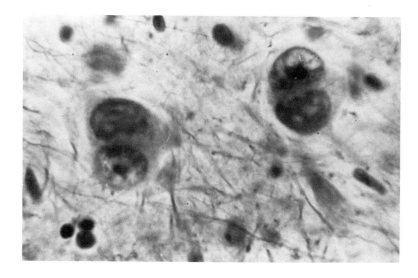

Fig. 111–3.   Intraneuronal inclusions in Pick disease. Silver stain. (Courtesy of Dr. Asao Hirano.)

Table 111–3. Neurotransmitter-Related Enzymes in Alzheimer Disease

Enzyme	Brain Region	Percentage of Activity in Age-Matched Normals
Choline acetyltransferase	Frontal cortex	10–30
	Hippocampus	10–30
	Caudate	40–80
Acetyl cholinesterase	Frontal cortex	10–50
	Hippocampus	10–50
	Caudate	30–60
Pseudocholinesterase	Frontal cortex	130–180
Glutamic acid decarboxylase	Frontal cortex	60–130
	Hippocampus	60–120
	Caudate	60–110
Tyrosine hydroxylase	Frontal cortex	80–100
	Hippocampus	80–100
Aromatic amino acid decarboxylase	Frontal cortex	100 ± 20
	Whole temporal lobe	100 ± 20
Dopamine-β-hydroxylase	Frontal cortex	90–130
Monoamine oxidase	Frontal cortex	80–150

(From Terry RD, Davies P. Annu Rev Neurosci 1980; 3:77–95.)

neuritic plaque. Evidence suggests involvement of glutaminergic neurons, which account for many of the large neurons lost in cerebral cortex and hippocampus, and variable involvement of ascending and descending serotonergic and adrenergic systems.

Symptoms and Signs. Alzheimer disease presents as a progressive dementia with increasing loss of memory, intellectual function, and disturbances in speech. In the initial stages, a slight dulling of intellectual faculties occurs. Thought processes are slowed, ability to perform in the social and economic spheres is impaired, and memory is defective. Disturbance of speech functions is a common early symptom (e.g., anomia, echolalia, difficulty in comprehending written and oral speech). To these may be added various apraxias and various types of agnosias.

If the patient has insight into the deterioration, he may become depressed, and depression is seen in about 25% of the patients. Agitation and restlessness are also common. Motor signs are uncommon early in the course, but as the disease progresses, reflex changes may be noted and a slow, shuffling gait develops. Myoclonus and convulsive seizures occur in some patients late in the course. Myoclonus has occasionally been reported early in the course as well. The clinical picture in the terminal stages is strikingly consistent. Intellectual activity ceases and the patient becomes meek and is reduced to a vegetative condition. Generalized weakness and

contractions may develop. Control of bowel and bladder functions is lost.

Laboratory Data. There are no significant changes in the usual laboratory examinations. CSF findings are typically normal. A slight increase in the protein content of the fluid has been noted in a few patients. Generalized slowing is regularly seen in the EEG. Psychometric or neuropsychologic examination is useful in following the progress of the disease. Cerebral blood flow falls as neurons cease functioning and oxygen demand is reduced. Dilatation of the lateral ventricles and widening of the cortical sulci, particularly in the frontal and temporal regions, are common CT findings, especially in the late stage of the disease. However, mild cortical atrophy is seen in some older individuals who are functioning normally by clinical and psychologic testing.

Differential Diagnosis. The diagnosis of *probable* Alzheimer's disease can be made with a higher degree of accuracy if the presence of dementia is established by clinical examination and confirmed by mental status and neuropsychologic tests with evidence that there is loss in two or more areas of cognition; if the history is that of insidious onset and progressive worsening; if focal neurologic findings such as hemiparesis, sensory loss, gait disturbance, and visual field deficits are absent in the early course of the illness; and if the patient is alert and awake. The diagnosis of *possible* Alzheimer's disease should be made if most of the aforementioned criteria are met with an exception, such as a variation in onset, presentation, or clinical course, or if a second systemic or brain disorder that could cause dementia is present, but is not the likely cause in an individual subject.

Documentation of the progression of the dementia by reexamination after several months is useful. Ordinarily, it is easy to differentiate Alzheimer disease from Korsakoff psychosis because, in the latter, there is a history of alcoholism, the memory defect is static, and other intellectual functions are intact. However, in some nonalcoholic patients, confusion arises when a history of progressive memory defect is given and CT shows mild atrophy. The condition of *pseudodementia* must be suspected when a history of depression preceded the onset of intellectual deterioration. The term pseudodementia is used to describe depressed patients in whom cognitive function is temporarily impaired on a functional basis; intellectual function improves when the depression is treated. In such instances, reexamination of the patient after several months may clarify the diagnosis.

Myxedema or pernicious anemia occasionally presents with intellectual deterioration as the primary symptom. These diseases can be ruled out by appropriate testing of thyroid function and determination of vitamin B_{12} levels. The dementia of acquired immunodeficiency syndrome (AIDS) is excluded by appropriate tests for the presence of virus and the state of the immune system. Dementia paralytica is excluded by the normal CSF. Huntington disease is excluded by the absence of the characteristic choreic movements and family history of the disease. Brain tumor is excluded by the absence of signs of increased intracranial pressure, focal changes on neurologic examination, or EEG, and the absence of a mass lesion on CT. Alzheimer disease is usually differentiated from the subacute progressive dementias such as Jakob-Creutzfeldt disease by the absence of myoclonus and other motor abnormalities early in the course as well as the absence of the periodic EEG. The rare occurrence of myoclonus as an early event in Alzheimer disease may make diagnosis difficult at first, but the differences in progression of the two diseases clarifies the situation in a few months. Dementia secondary to multiple cerebral infarcts usually occurs in the presence of hypertension, diabetes, or other factors predisposing to vascular disease. It has a step-like progression. Particularly in patients with a lacunar state, the early presence of a gait disturbance and later pseudobulbar signs, in addition to the dementia, help establish the diagnosis.

The differentiation of Alzheimer disease from chronic communicating hydrocephalus is important because the latter condition may be treated operatively. Most patients with chronic communicating hydrocephalus have a preceding history of subarachnoid hemorrhage, head trauma, or meningitis. In cases without an apparent cause, the patients who respond to shunt therapy are those with a history of the onset of progressive unsteadiness of gait with psychomotor retardation, mild intellectual loss and, occasionally, urinary incontinence. Confirmatory tests for chronic communicating hydrocephalus include marked enlargement of the ventricles with minimal cortical atrophy on CT and abnormal CSF flow determined by RISA cisternography or the CSF infusion test. However, in the absence of a typical clinical history, these laboratory findings by themselves are not sufficient for the diagnosis because about 10% of patients with Alzheimer disease have markedly enlarged ventricles together with some evidence of abnormal CSF flow. If Alzheimer patients are operated on, they usually show marked post-operative deterioration.

Course. The clinical course is progressive, terminating inevitably in complete incapacity and death. Plateaus sometimes occur during which cognitive impairment does not change for a year or two, but the progression of the disease then resumes. The duration of the disease is usually between 4 and 10 years, with extremes varying from less than 1 year to more than 20 years.

Treatment. Drugs designed to increase the function of the remaining cholinergic neurons are under experimental trial; however, at present, there is no proven effective therapy. Although custodial care is required in the terminal stage of the disease, it is often possible to maintain some degree of socialization despite marked cognitive impairment.

Pick Disease

Pick disease is a rare degenerative disease that occurs almost entirely in the presenium. Within this age group, the incidence of Pick disease is less than 2% that of Alzheimer disease. Pathologically, Pick disease is characterized by severe atrophy of the frontal and temporal poles with sparing of the motor and sensory cortex and the first temporal convolution. On microscopic examination, Pick disease is characterized by a diffuse loss of neurons, particularly in the outer layer of the cortex. Many of the preserved neurons are swollen and have a pale cytoplasm. Glial proliferation is prominent in both the gray and white matter. The basal ganglia are also involved in a high percentage of the cases. Some remaining neurons contain argentophilic intraneuronal inclusions known as *Pick bodies* (Fig. 111–3). The inclusions contain many 10-nm neurofilaments, vesicles, and complex lipid bodies. Alzheimer neurofibrillary tangles and senile plaques are not present.

The presentation of Pick disease is similar to that of Alzheimer disease. Although in some cases of Pick disease, personality, orientation, and attention span are more affected than memory early in the course (unlike Alzheimer disease), the consensus of opinion is that the differential diagnosis can be made only at biopsy and necropsy. Although CT sometimes demonstrates the localized atrophy of Pick disease, focal atrophy is also sometimes seen in Alzheimer disease. The finding of severe frontal and partial temporal atrophy alone may suggest, but would not prove, the diagnosis in the absence of histologic confirmation.

The course is similar to that of Alzheimer disease. There is no effective treatment.

References

Alzheimer Disease

Alzheimer A. Über eine eigenartige Erkrankung der Hirnrinde. Zbl Nervenheilk 1907; 30:177–179.

Armstrong DM, Terry RD. Somatostatin immunoreactivity within neuritic plaques. Brain Res 1985; 338:71–79.

Blessed G, Tomlinson BE, Roth M. The association between quantitative measures of dementia and of senile change in the cerebral gray matter of elderly subjects. Br J Psychiatry 1968; 114:797–818.

Faden AI, Townsend JJ. Myoclonus in Alzheimer disease: a confusing sign. Arch Neurol 1976; 33:278–280.

Feldman RG, Chandler KA, Levy LL, Glaser GH. Familial Alzheimer disease. Neurology 1963; 13:811–824.

Friedland RP, Brun A, Budinger TF. Pathological and positron emission tomographic correlations in Alzheimer's disease. Lancet 1985; 1:228.

Glenner GC, Wong CW. Alzheimer's disease: initial report of the purification and characterization of a novel cerebrovascular amyloid protein. Biochem Biophys Res Commun 1984; 120:885–890.

Goldman JE. The association of actin with Hirano bodies. J Neuropathol Exp Neurol 1983; 42:146–152.

Heston LL, Mastri AR, Anderson VE, White J. Dementia of the Alzheimer type: clinical genetics, natural history and associated conditions. Arch Gen Psychiatry 1981; 38:1085–1090.

Katzman R. Alzheimer's disease. N Engl J Med 1986; 314:964–973.

Katzman R. Differential diagnosis of dementing illnesses. In: Hutton JT, ed. Neurologic Clinics. Philadelphia: W.B. Saunders Co., 1986; 329–340.

Katzman R. The prevalence and malignancy of Alzheimer disease: a major killer. Arch Neurol 1976; 33:217–218.

Katzman R, Terry RD, Bick K, eds. Alzheimer's Disease: Senile Dementia and Related Disorders. New York: Raven Press, 1978.

Kiloh LG. Pseudo-dementia. Acta Psychiatry Scand 1961; 37:336.

Larsson T, Sjögren T, Jacobson G. Senile dementia. Acta Psychiatry Scand 1963; 39 (Suppl 167):1–259.

McKhann G, Drachman D, Folstein M, Katzman R, Price D, Stadlar EM. Clinical diagnosis of Alzheimer's disease: Report of the NINCDS-ADRDA Work Groups under the auspices of Department of Health and Human Services Task Force on Alzheimer's Disease. Neurology 1984; 34:939–944.

Price DL, Whitehouse PJ, Struble RG, et al. Basal forebrain cholinergic systems in Alzheimer's disease and related dementias. Neurosci Comment 1982; 1:84–92.

Selkoe DJ, Abraham C. Plaque amyloid in Alzheimer's disease (AD): purification of flow cytometry and protein characterization. Neurology (NY) 1985; 35(Suppl 1):217.

Sulkava R, Haltia M, Paetau A, Wikstrom J, Palo J. Accuracy of clinical diagnosis in primary degenerative dementia: correlation with neuropathological findings. J Neurol Neurosurg Psychiatry 1983; 46:9–13.

Terry RD, Davies P. Dementia of the Alzheimer type. Annu Rev Neurosci 1980; 3:77–95.

Terry RD, Gonatas NK, Weiss M. Ultrastructural studies in Alzheimer's in presenile dementia. Am J Pathol 1964; 44:269–297.

Terry RD, Katzman R. Senile dementia of the Alzheimer's type. Ann Neurol 1983: 14:497–506.

Terry RD, Peck A, DeTeresa R, Schecter R, Horoupian DS. Some morphometric aspects of the brain in senile dementia of the Alzheimer type. Ann Neurol 1981; 10:184–192.

Tomlinson BE, Blessed G, Roth M. Observations of the brains of demented old people. J Neurol Sci 1970; 11:205–242.

Whitehouse PJ, Price DL, Struble RG, et al. Alzheimer's disease and senile dementia: loss of neurons in basal forebrain. Science 1982; 215:1237–1239.

Yen SH, Horoupian DS, Terry RD. Immunocytochemical comparison of neurofibrillary tangles in senile dementia of Alzheimer type, progressive supranuclear palsy, and postencephalitic parkinsonism. Ann Neurol 1983; 13:172–175.

Pick Disease

Cummings JL, Duchen LW. Kluver-Bucy syndrome in Pick disease: clinical and pathologic correlations. Neurology 1981; 31:1415–1422.

Groen JJ, Endtz LJ. Hereditary Pick's disease. Second reexamination of a large family and discussion of other hereditary cases, with particular reference to electroencephalography and computed tomography. Brain 1982; 105:443–459.

Johannesson G, Hagber GB, Gustavson L, Ingvar DH. EEG and cognitive impairment in presenile dementia. Acta Neurol Scand 1979; 59:225–240.

McGeachie RE, Fleming JO, Sharer LR, Hyman RA. Diagnosis of Pick's disease by computed tomography. J Comput Assist Tomogr 1979; 3:113–115.

Pick A. Über die Beziehungen der senilen Hirnatrophie zur Aphasie. Prog Med Wochenshr 1892; 17:165–167.

Terry RD. Dementia: a brief and selective review. Arch Neurol 1976; 33:1.

Weschler AF, Verity A, Rosenchein S, Fried I, Scheibel AB. Pick's disease. A clinical, computed tomographic, and histologic study with Golgi impregnation observations. Arch Neurol 1982; 39:287–290.

Wisniewski HM, Coblentz JM, Terry RD. Pick's disease: a clinical and ultrastructural study. Arch Neurol 1972; 26:97.

Yates CM, Simpson J, Maloney AF, Gordon A. Neurochemical observations in a case of Pick's disease. J Neurol Sci 1980; 48:257–263.

Chapter XIV

Movement Disorders

112. SYDENHAM CHOREA
Sidney Carter

Sydenham chorea (acute chorea, St. Vitus dance, chorea minor, rheumatic chorea) is a disease of childhood characterized by rapid, irregular, aimless, involuntary movements of the muscles of the limbs, face, and trunk; there is also muscular weakness, hypotonia, and emotional lability. The cause is unknown, but it is considered a manifestation of rheumatic fever. The course is self-limited and fatalities are rare except as a result of cardiac complications.

Etiology and Pathology. Numerous reports have implicated a streptococcus or diplococcus as the causative organism of acute chorea, but these claims have not received general credence. The close relationship of chorea to rheumatic fever is shown by the large number of patients (approximately 75%) who show evidence at some time before, during, or after the attack of chorea of other manifestations of the disease in the form of arthritis, myocarditis, endocarditis, or pericarditis. Patients with rheumatic chorea have antibodies that react with subthalamic and caudate nuclei neurons in immunofluoresence assays. These antibodies also react with antigens shared by Group A streptococcal membranes.

Because uncomplicated acute chorea is rarely fatal, the pathologic changes in the brain have not been elucidated. Many of the changes reported in fatal cases can be attributed to embolic phenomena and terminal changes. Degenerative changes in the nerve cells of the cortex, basal ganglia, and cerebellum, ameboid changes in the glia, and proliferative changes in the meningeal and cortical vessels have been reported. A mild degree of inflammatory reaction has been found in a few patients.

Incidence. Acute chorea is almost exclusively a disease of childhood; over 80% of the cases occur in patients between the ages of 5 and 15. Onset before the age of 5 is rare and the occurrence of the first attack after the age of 15 is uncommon, except during pregnancy or the use of oral contraceptives in the late teens and early twenties. All races are affected. Girls are affected more than twice as frequently as boys. The disease occurs at all times of the year but is less common in summer.

Symptoms and Signs. The characteristic features are involuntary movements, incoordination, muscular weakness, and psychologic manifestations. The symptoms may be of gradual onset or may appear suddenly after an emotional upset. The adverse influence of all external stimuli on the symptoms makes it probable that the emotional upset only serves to call attention to pre-existing symptoms of a milder degree.

The severity of symptoms is subject to a great deal of variation. In mild cases, there may be only a general restlessness, facial grimacing, and a slight degree of incoordination in the performance of willed movements. In severe cases, the range and extent of the involuntary movements may incapacitate the child.

The involuntary movements are quick and are similar to normal willed movements, but they are not performed for any useful purpose. Jerking movements of the arm and flinging movements of the legs may interfere with normal use of the arms and make walking difficult or impossible. Involuntary movements of the facial muscles, tongue, and palate cause dysarthria, which may be so severe that the child ceases to try to talk. Involuntary movements of the abdominal and trunk muscles may alter the respiratory rate. The involuntary movements are generalized, but they are usually more severe in the arms than in the legs or face. In about 35% of the cases, the movements are greater on one side of the body and, rarely, they may appear to be entirely confined to that side (hemichorea). The severity of the involuntary movements is greatly influenced by emotional factors and external stimuli. The child may lie quietly in bed when undisturbed, but the movements may become severe when the child is emotionally excited or subjected to a prolonged examination. The involuntary movements disappear entirely when the patient is asleep, and they can be reduced in the waking state by administration of sedative drugs.

Weakness of voluntary movements and an inability to maintain any sustained effort occur. The occurrence of involuntary movements in antagonist muscles during the attempt to make voluntary movements causes incoordination, dropping or throwing of objects held in the hand, or an awkward stumbling gait. The inability to sustain contractions of the muscles can be demonstrated by increasing and decreasing the force of the pressure when the child grips the hand of the examiner. The weakness may occasionally be so great that one or more limbs appear to be paralyzed (paralytic chorea). There are no muscular atrophies, contractures, or fixation in abnormal postures. The appearance of the hands when the arms are held extended in front of the body is, however, quite characteristic. The wrist is sharply flexed and the fingers are hyperextended at the proximal and terminal phalanges. This posture of the hand (Warner hand) can be imitated only with difficulty by a normal person. Pronation of the forearm when the arms are extended (pronator sign) is also commonly seen. Voluntary movements are often performed rapidly in order to prevent their interruption by involuntary movements. On command, the tongue is protruded quickly, but is rapidly withdrawn to prevent biting of the tongue by involuntary movements of the jaw muscles.

The cranial nerves are unaffected except for the involuntary movements of the facial, jaw, tongue, and palatal muscles. There are no sensory changes. The tendon reflexes may be increased, decreased, or temporarily absent. Occasionally, the knee jerks are pendular in character, but more commonly the contraction of the quadriceps muscle on tapping the patellar tendon is maintained for a short interval, causing the leg to remain extended ("caught-up" or "hung-up" reflex). The plan-

tar response is usually flexor, but occasionally an extensor plantar response is obtained.

Mental changes of a mild or severe degree are frequently present. The child is fretful, irritable, or emotionally unstable. Apathy is not uncommon. The involuntary movements may prevent sleep and sleep may be interrupted by nightmares or unpleasant dreams. In severe cases, mental confusion, agitation, hallucinations, and delusions (chorea insaniens) may occur.

Chorea may recur or develop for the first time in young women during pregnancy (chorea gravidarum) or while taking oral contraceptives. The disease is apt to be more severe during pregnancy and mental symptoms are common.

Laboratory Data. Temperature and pulse are normal unless complications develop. The results of the examination of urine and blood, including the erythrocyte sedimentation rate and C-reactive protein, are often normal. Eosinophilia has been reported and a mild or moderate degree of anemia is not infrequent. The CSF is usually normal, but slight pleocytosis has been reported in a few cases. Nonspecific changes may be found in the EEG. Decrease in the percentage time of the alpha rhythm and the presence of continuous slow wave activity of increased amplitude have been reported.

Complications. Other manifestations of the rheumatic infection may occur during the course of the chorea or may precede or follow it. Cardiac complications, usually endocarditis, occur in approximately 20% of patients. Myocarditis and pericarditis are less common. Vegetative endocarditis and embolic phenomena may occur, but are rare. A previous history of rheumatic polyarthritis is common, but involvement of the joints during the course of the chorea is rare. Other infrequent complications include subcutaneous rheumatic nodules, erythema nodosum, and purpura.

Diagnosis. The diagnosis is made without difficulty from the appearance of the characteristic choreic movements in a child. Tics and habit-spasms may offer some difficulty, but these movements are stereotyped and localized always to the same muscle or groups of muscles.

Some difficulty in diagnosis may be encountered in the individual with apparent limb paralysis, but the previous existence or the subsequent development of choreic movements should clarify the diagnosis.

The age of onset, clinical course, and the character of the voluntary movements readily differentiate acute chorea from other diseases of the basal ganglia.

Prochlorperazine, haloperidol and, rarely, phenytoin can produce choreic movements or other basal ganglia manifestations. There are a few uncommon and ill-defined disorders that give rise to abnormal involuntary movements in children. *Familial benign chorea* is characterized by chorea and a combined resting and intention tremor. *Paroxysmal choreoathetosis* is an episodic disorder in which the choreic movements are sudden in onset but brief in duration with no abnormal movements between attacks.

Chorea is a rare but recognized neurologic complication of systemic lupus erythematosus and it may be the first and only sign before the diagnosis is established.

Course and Prognosis. Acute chorea is a benign disease and complete recovery is the rule in uncomplicated cases. The mortality rate of approximately 2% is due to associated cardiac complications. The duration of the symptoms is quite variable. In the average case, they persist for 3 to 6 weeks. Occasionally, the course may be prolonged for several months, and it is not unusual for involuntary movements of a mild degree to persist for many months after recrudescence of the more severe movements. Recurrences after months or several years are reported in approximately 35% of the cases.

Treatment. There is no specific treatment for the disease. Symptomatic therapy may be of great value in the control of the movements. In the mild form, bed rest during the period of active movements is sufficient. The room should be quiet and all external stimuli should be reduced to a minimum. When the severity of the movements interferes with proper rest, sedatives in the form of barbiturates, chloral hydrate, or paraldehyde may be needed. Phenothiazines, valproic acid, and haloperidol are of value in reducing the severity of the movements. There is no good evidence to show that the termination of pregnancy exerts any influence on the course of chorea of pregnancy.

Prophylactic administration of penicillin for many years is recommended to prevent other manifestations of rheumatic fever.

References

Alvarez LA, Novak G. Valproic acid in the treatment of Sydenham's chorea. Pediat Neurol 1985; 1:317–319.

Aron AM, Freeman JM, Carter S. The natural history of Sydenham's chorea. Am J Med 1965; 38:83–95.

Bird MT, Palkes H, Prensky AL. A follow-up study of Sydenham's chorea. Neurology 1976; 26:601–606.

Dhanaraj M, Radhabreshnan AR, Srenivas IT, Sayeed ZA. Sodium valproate in Sydenham's chorea. Neurology 1985; 35:114–115.

Greenfield JG, Wolfsohn JM. The pathology of Sydenham's chorea. Lancet 1922; 2:603–606.

Groothuis JR, Groothuis DR, Mukhopadhyay D, Grossman BJ, Altemeier WA. Lupus-associated chorea in childhood. Am J Dis Child 1977; 131:1131–1134.

Husby G, Van de Rijn I, Zabriskie JB, et al. Antibodies reacting with cytoplasm of subthalamic and caudate nuclei in chorea and acute rheumatic fever. J Exp Med 1976; 144:1094.

Jones TD, Bland EF. Clinical significance of chorea as manifestation of rheumatic fever. JAMA 1935; 105:571–577.

Massell BF. Prophylaxis of streptococcal infections and rheumatic fever. JAMA 1979; 241:1589–1594.

Nausieda PA, Bieliauskas LA, Bacon LD, Hagerty M, Koller NC, Glantz RN. Chronic dopaminergic sensitivity after Sydenham's chorea. Neurology 1983; 33:750–755.

Pincus JH, Chutorian A. Familial benign chorea with intention tremor: a clinical entity. J Pediatr 1967; 70:724–729.

Roig M et al. Carbamazepine: An alternative drug for the treatment of nonhereditary chorea. Pediatrics 1988; 82:492–495.

Willson P, Preece AA. Chorea gravidarum. Arch Intern Med 1932; 49:471, 671.

113. HUNTINGTON DISEASE AND OTHER FORMS OF CHOREA
Stanley Fahn

Choreic movements can be associated with a large number of disorders; the most common ones are listed in Table 113–1.

Huntington Disease

Huntington disease is a progressive hereditary disorder that usually appears in adult life. It is characterized by a movement disorder (usually chorea), dementia, and personality disorder. It was first recognized clinically by Waters in 1842 and became accepted as a clinical entity with the comprehensive description and interpretation of the mode of transmission by George Huntington in 1872.

Pathology. At postmortem examination, the brain appears shrunken and atrophic; the cerebral cortex and caudate nucleus are most affected (Fig. 113–1). Histologically, the cerebral cortex shows loss of neurons, especially in layer 3. The caudate nucleus and putamen are severely involved, with loss of neurons, particularly the medium-sized, spiny neurons and their GABAergic striatal efferents. As a result, there is atrophy of the striatopallidal

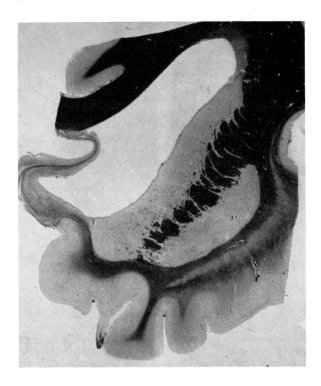

Fig. 113–1. Huntington chorea. Atrophy of caudate nucleus and dilatation of lateral ventricle. Myelin sheath stain.

Table 113–1.   Common Causes of Chorea

Hereditary
   Huntington disease
   Hereditary nonprogressive chorea
   Neuroacanthocytosis
   Wilson disease
   Ataxia-telangiectasia
   Lesch-Nyhan syndrome

Secondary
   Infections/immunologic
      Sydenham chorea
      Encephalitis
      Systemic lupus erythematosus
   Drug-induced
      Levodopa
      Anticonvulsants
      Anticholinergics
      Antipsychotics
   Metabolic and endocrine
      Chorea gravidarum
      Hyperthyroidism
      Birth control pills
      Hyperglycemic nonketotic encephalopathy
   Vascular
      Hemichorea/hemiballism with subthalamic nucleus lesion
      Periarteritis nodosa

Unknown Etiology
   Senile chorea
   Essential chorea

For a complete listing of causes of chorea, see Shoulson I. Clin Neuropharmacol 1986; 9(Suppl 2):585–599.

and striatonigral nerve fiber bundles. Less marked changes occur in other structures such as the thalamus and brain stem. A reactive gliosis is apparent in the affected areas. The striatal cell loss is associated with the movement disorder, whereas the dementia is attributed to changes in both the cerebral cortex and deep nuclei (i.e., subcortical dementia). In advanced cases the striatum may be completely devoid of cells and replaced by a gliotic process, at which time choreic movements abate and are replaced by dystonia and an akinetic-rigid state. The pathogenesis of this disorder remains unknown. The cellular loss in the striatum is held responsible for the following neurochemical changes: loss of striatal and nigral GABA and its synthesizing enzyme glutamic aid decarboxylase; decline in the striatal activity of the acetylcholine-synthesizing enzyme choline acetyltransferase; and reduced numbers of striatal receptors for dopamine and acetylcholine. These defects can be duplicated experimentally in animals by striatal injection of the excitotoxin kainic acid. The neurochemical changes have not yet been translated into effective therapy because trials with GABA and acetylcholine agonists have not been beneficial.

Prevalence and Hereditary Factors. Huntington chorea occurs worldwide and in all ethnic groups, especially whites. The prevalence rate in the United States and Europe ranges from 4 to 8/100,000, whereas in Japan the rate is 10% of this figure. The highest incidence rates have been reported from geographic regions where affected families have resided for many generations (e.g., the Lake Maracaibo region in Venezuela). The disease is transmitted from parent to offspring in autosomal dominant fashion with full penetrance. Hence each child of an affected parent has a 50% chance of being affected. New mutations are rare and no one has yet been definitely proven to be a spontaneous mutation. Cases without a positive family history can usually be attributed to early death or disappearance of a parent, inadequately examined parents, or unproven paternity.

The abnormal gene has been linked to the tip of the short arm of chromosome 4. Although the gene has not yet been identified or cloned, it is near a segment of DNA distinguished as a restriction fragment length polymorphism that can serve as a linkage marker for the Huntington gene. Individuals carrying the abnormal gene are now being identified through research protocols. Ethical questions have been raised regarding the use of this predictive test in a disease with as much variability in age at onset, and for which there is no satisfactory treatment.

Signs and Symptoms. Symptoms usually appear between 35 and 40 years of age. However, the range of age at onset is broad, with cases recorded as early as age 5 and as late as age 70. The three characteristic manifestations of the disease are movement disorder, personality disorder, and mental deterioration. The three may occur together at onset or one may precede the others by a period of years. In general, the onset of symptoms is insidious, beginning with clumsiness, dropping of objects, fidgetiness, irritability, slovenliness, and neglect of duties progressing to frank choreic movements and dementia. Overt psychotic episodes, depression, and irresponsible behavior may occur. The disease tends to run its course over a period of 15 years, more rapidly in those with an earlier age of onset.

Choreic Movements. The most striking and diagnostic feature of the disease is the appearance of involuntary movements that seem purposeless and abrupt but less rapid and lightning-like than those seen in myoclonus. The somatic muscles are affected in a random manner, and choreic movements flow from one part of the body to another. Proximal, distal, and axial muscles are involved. In the early stages and in the less severe form, there is slight grimacing of the face, shrugging of the shoulders, and jerking movements of the limbs. Pseudopurposeful movements are common in attempts to mask the involuntary jerking. As the disease progresses, walking is associated with more intense arm and leg movements, which cause a dancing, prancing, stuttering type of gait, an abnormality that is particularly characteristic of Huntington disease. Motor impersistence or inhibitory pauses during voluntary contraction probably account for "milkmaid grips" and inability to keep the tongue steadily protruded. Ocular movements become impaired with reduced saccades and loss of smooth pursuit. The choreic movements are increased by emotional stimuli, disappear during sleep, and become superimposed on voluntary movements to the point that they make volitional activity difficult. With increased severity, the routine daily activities of living become difficult, as do speech and swallowing. Terminally, choreic movements may disappear and be replaced by muscular rigidity and dystonia.

Mental Symptoms. Characteristically, there is an organic dementia with progressive impairment of memory, loss of intellectual capacity, apathy, and inattention to personal hygiene. Early in the disease, less profound abnormalities consist of irritability, impulsive behavior, and bouts of depression or fits of violence; these are not infrequent. In some patients, frank psychotic features that are schizophrenic predominate, and the underlying cause is not evident until choreic movements develop. The dementing and psychotic features of the disease usually lead to commitment to a mental institution.

Other Neurologic Manifestations. Cranial nerves remain intact except for rapid eye movements, which are impaired in a large percentage of patients. Sensation is usually unaffected. Tendon reflexes are usually normal, but may be hyperactive; the plantar responses may be abnormal.

Muscle tone is hypotonic in most patients except for those with the so-called "akinetic-rigid variety" *(Westphal variant)*. With childhood onset (approximately 10% of cases), the akinetic-rigid state usually occurs instead of chorea and in conjunction with mental abnormalities and convulsive seizures. This form of the disease is rapidly progressive with a fatal outcome in less than 10 years. The observation that 90% of all patients with childhood onset inherit the disease from their father is unexplained. In the terminal stages of the more classic form of Huntington disease, muscular rigidity and seizures are not unusual.

Laboratory Data. Routine studies of blood, urine, and CSF show no abnormalities. Diffuse abnormalities are seen in the EEG. Radiographs of the skull are normal, but CT shows enlarged ventricles with characteristic butterfly appearance of the lateral ventricles, a result of degeneration of the caudate nucleus (Fig. 113–2). Positron emission tomography using fluorodeoxyglucose has shown hypometabolism in the caudate and the putamen in affected patients and in some of their offspring prior to the appearance of symptoms.

Diagnosis and Differential Diagnosis. Huntington disease can be diagnosed without difficulty in an adult with the clinical triad of chorea, dementia and personality disorder, and a family history of the disease. Difficulties arise when the family history is lacking. The patient may be ignorant of the family history, or may deny that history. However, subsequent developments usually allow for the establishment of a firm diagnosis.

Other conditions in which choreic movements are a major manifestation can be excluded on clinical grounds. Sydenham chorea has an earlier age of onset, is self-limited, and lacks the characteristic mental disturbances. Chorea and mental disturbances occurring as a manifestation of lupus erythematosus are usually more acute in onset, the chorea is more localized and often periodic, and there are characteristic serologic and clinical abnormalities. Involuntary movements occurring in psychiatric patients on long-term treatment with neuroleptic agents (the so-called *tardive dyskinesia*) occasionally pose a diagnostic problem. However, such movements are usually repetitive (stereotypy), in contrast to the nonrepetitive and slowing nature of chorea. Oral-lingual-buccal dyskinesia is the most common feature of tardive dyskinesia. Gait is usually normal in tardive dyskinesia and is abnormal in Huntington disease. The presenile dementias (Alzheimer and Pick diseases) are similar in the mental disorder, but language is more often involved; aphasic abnormalities are not seen early in Huntington disease. Myoclonus, rather than chorea, occasionally occurs. The peculiarities of the childhood disorder with rigidity, convulsive seizures, and mental retardation require differentiation from other hereditable disorders such as the leukodystrophies and gangliosidosis. Tics, particularly those of the Gilles de la Tourette syndrome, usually pose little problem in view of the complex nature of the involuntary movements, the characteristic vocalizations, and their suppressibility. The hereditary disorder known as neuroacanthocytosis or chorea-acanthocytosis is manifested by mild chorea, tics, tongue-biting, peripheral neuropathy, increased serum creatine phosphokinase, and red-cell acanthocytes. Hereditary nonprogressive chorea begins in childhood, does not worsen, and is not associated with dementia or personality disorder.

Treatment. There is at present no known means of altering the disease process or the fatal outcome. Attempts to replace the deficiency in GABA by using GABA-mimetic agents or inhibitors of GABA metabolism have been unsuccessful. The choreic movements can be controlled by the use of neuroleptic agents, including dopamine receptor blockers such as haloperidol and perphenazine, and presynaptic dopamine depletors

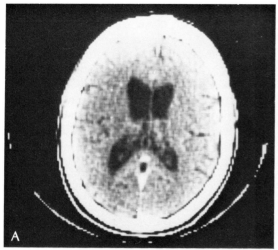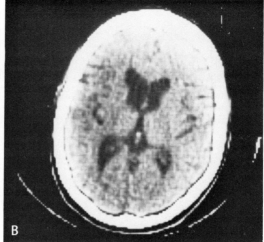

Fig. 113–2. CT scans at two axial levels showing ventricular enlargement with atrophy of the caudate nucleus, particularly the head of the caudate.

such as reserpine and tetrabenazine. Using these drugs combined with supervision of the patient's daily activities allows for management at home during the early stages of the disorder. However, as the disease advances, confinement to a psychiatric facility becomes necessary.

Senile Chorea

Choreic movements may begin and occur as an isolated symptom in individuals older than 60. As a rule, the movements begin insidiously, are mild, and usually involve the limbs. However, more complex movements of the lingual-facial-buccal regions are on occasion encountered. Slow progression in the intensity and extent of the movements may occur. There are no associated mental disturbances, nor is a family history of Huntington disease obtained. Pathologically, changes are found in the caudate nucleus and putamen, which show cellular loss, but not to the degree seen in Huntington disease. Significantly, degenerative changes in the cerebral cortex are absent. Though some have considered senile chorea to be a variant of Huntington disease, it seems more likely that it is a distinct pathologic entity. The cause of this degenerative process remains unknown, but it may well have several different causes. In general, the symptoms are mild and there is little need to resort to therapeutic measures. However, in those instances in which oral-facial and neck muscle involvement occurs, drugs used to control chorea as indicated previously may prove useful.

Hemichorea and Hemiballism

Choreic movements confined to the arm and leg on one side of the body may develop abruptly in middle-aged or elderly patients. Ballistic movements are a more violent form of chorea and are characterized by continuous uncoordinated activity of the axial and proximal appendicular muscles, so vigorous that the limbs are forcefully and aimlessly thrown about. The sudden onset suggests a vascular basis; indeed they may be preceded by hemiplegia or hemiparesis. In such instances, the choreic or ballistic movements appear when return of motor function occurs. This type of movement disorder, *hemiballism*, is the result of a destructive lesion of the contralateral subthalamic nucleus or its connections. It has also been seen with scattered encephalomalacic lesions involving the internal capsule and basal ganglia. Vascular lesions, hemorrhagic or occlusive in nature, are the most common cause, but hemiballism has been found in association with tumors in the subthalamic nucleus and has occasionally followed attempted thalamotomy when the target was missed.

In general, the movements tend to diminish over time, but they may be persistent and require therapeutic intervention. The agents noted previously for the control of choreic movements in general have proven effective.

References

Huntington Disease

Gusella JF, Wexler NS, Conneally PM, et al. A polymorphic DNA marker genetically linked to Huntington's disease. Nature 1983; 306:234–238.

Haerer AF, Currier RD, Jackson JF. Hereditary nonprogressive chorea of early onset. N Engl J Med 1967; 276:1220–1224.

Hayden MR. Huntington's Chorea. New York: Springer-Verlag, 1981.

Hayden MR, Hewitt J, Stoessl AJ, Clark C, Ammann W, Martin WRW. The combined use of positron emission tomography and DNA polymorphisms for preclinical detection of Huntington's disease. Neurology; 37:1441–1447, 1987.

Levine IM, Estes JW, Looney JM. Hereditary neurological disease with acanthocytosis. A new syndrome. Arch Neurol 1968; 19:403–409.

Martin JB. Huntington's disease: New approaches to an old problem. Neurology 1984; 34:1059–1072.

Sakai T, Manatari S, Iwashita H, Goto I, Kuroiwa Y. Chorea-acanthocytosis: clues to clinical diagnosis. Arch Neurol 1981; 38:335–338.

Shoulson I. On chorea. Clin Neuropharmacol 1986; 9(Suppl 2):S85–S99.

Suchowersky O, Hayden MR, Martin WRW, Stoessl AJ, Hildebrand AM, Pate BD. Cerebral metabolism of glucose in benign hereditary chorea. Movement Disorders 1986; 1:33–44.

Senile Chorea, Hemichorea, and Hemiballism

Alcock NS. A note on the pathology of senile chorea (non-hereditary). Brain 1936; 59:376–387.

Johnson WG, Fahn S. Treatment of vascular hemiballism and hemichorea. Neurology 1977; 27:631–636.

Klawans HL, Moses H, Nausieda PA, Bergen D, Weiner WJ. Treatment and prognosis of hemiballismus. N Engl J Med 1976; 295:1348–1350.

---

114. MYOCLONUS
Stanley Fahn

The term *myoclonus* refers to brief, "lightning-like" muscle jerks. They are usually due to positive muscle contractions, but can also be due to sudden, brief lapses of contraction (i.e., so-called negative myoclonus) such as is seen in *asterixis*. Asterixis is a tremor-like phenomenon of the extended wrists due to brief lapses of muscle contraction. It is usually encountered in the metabolic encephalopathies that accompany severe hepatic, renal, and pulmonary disorders.

Clinically, there is a wide expression of myoclonus. The jerks may occur singly or repetitively. They may be focal, segmental, or generalized. The amplitude ranges from mild contractions that do not move a joint to gross contractions that move limbs, the head, or the trunk. Myoclonic jerks range in frequency from rare, isolated events to many events each minute; they may occur at rest, with action, or with intention movements. Commonly, myoclonic jerks are stimulus-sensitive; they can be induced by sudden noise,

movement, light, or visual threat. Finally, these jerks can occur irregularly and unpredictably. They can occur in bursts of oscillations or they can be very rhythmic as in palatal myoclonus. They resemble tremor in such situations.

Myoclonus can be classified into the following etiologic categories: physiologic myoclonus, essential myoclonus, epileptic myoclonus, and symptomatic myoclonus. Examples of physiologic myoclonus include sleep jerks and hiccough. Essential myoclonus is abnormal, may be familial or sporadic, is not associated with other neurologic abnormalities, and does not have a progressive course. Periodic movements of sleep, previously called "nocturnal myoclonus," can be considered a form of essential myoclonus and are sometimes accompanied by the restless-legs syndrome. Epileptic myoclonus occurs in patients whose main complaint is epilepsy but who also have myoclonus. Symptomatic myoclonus occurs as part of a more widespread encephalopathy, including storage diseases, spinocerebellar degenerations, dementias, viral encephalopathies, metabolic encephalopathies, toxic encephalopathies, physical encephalopathies (e.g., posthypoxic and posttraumatic), and with focal brain damage. Myoclonus can sometimes be controlled with the anticonvulsants, clonazepam and valproic acid, and with the serotonin precursor, 5-hydroxytryptophan.

References

Aigner BR, Mulder DW. Myoclonus: clinical significance and an approach to classification. Arch Neurol 1960; 2:600–615.

Fahn S, Marsden CD, Van Woert NH, eds. Myoclonus. Adv Neurol. New York: Raven Press, 1986.

Jankovic J, Pardo R. Segmental myoclonus: clinical and pharmacologic study. Arch Neurol 1986; 43:1025–1031.

Lance JW, Adams RD. The syndrome of intention or action myoclonus as a sequel to hypoxic encephalopathy. Brain 1963; 86:111–136.

Lott I, Kinsbourne M. Myoclonic encephalopathy of infants. Adv Neurol 1986; 43:127–136.

Marsden CD, Hallett M, Fahn S. The nosology and pathophysiology of myoclonus. In: Marsden CD, Fahn S, eds. Movement Disorders. London: Butterworths, 1982: 196–248.

Van Woert MH, Rosenbaum D, Chung E. Biochemistry and therapeutics of posthypoxic myoclonus. Adv Neurol 1986; 43:171–181.

Young RR, Shahani BT. Asterixis: One type of negative myoclonus. Adv Neurol 1986; 43:137–156.

115. GILLES DE LA TOURETTE SYNDROME
Stanley Fahn

Tics range from simple myoclonic jerks to a complex pattern of rapid, coordinated, involuntary movements. The presence of vocal tics (vocalizations) has been used as a criterion to define a subset of tics, namely the Gilles de la Tourette syndrome. Onset is in childhood (2 to 15 years of age). Tics usually begin in the face (eye-blinking, grimacing) and neck (head-shaking). Later they spread to involve the limbs and are accompanied by explosive sounds (barking, throat clearing) and sometimes by foul utterances (coprolalia). The tics are not infrequently associated with compulsive ideation and hyperactive behavior. EEG abnormalities, though nonspecific, are frequently demonstrated. It appears to be inherited with autosomal dominant transmission. In patients who have come to necropsy, no specific morphologic changes in the brain have been noted. The disorder increases in severity during childhood, but seems to spontaneously resolve by adult life in many cases. It can be differentiated from other dyskinesias of childhood. Sydenham chorea differs in the type of movement disorder and is self-limited. Essential myoclonus, however, resembles simple tics, and the two conditions are difficult to distinguish. The motor and vocal tics of Gilles de la Tourette syndrome can be reduced with the use of haloperidol in doses from 5 to 20 mg/day, clonidine in doses from 0.3 to 2 mg/day, or clonazepam in doses from 2 to 8 mg/day.

References

Cohen DJ, Bruun RD, Leckman JF, editors. Tourette's Syndrome & Tic Disorders: Clinical Understanding and Treatment. John Wiley & Sons, New York, 1988.

Friedhoff AJ, Chase TN, eds. Gilles de la Tourette syndrome. Advances in Neurology, vol 36. New York: Raven Press, 1982.

Jankovic J. The neurology of tics. In Marsden CD, Fahn S, eds. Movement Disorders 2. London: Butterworths, 1987; 38:383–405.

Kurlan R, Behr J, Medved L, Shoulson I, Pauls D, Kidd JR, Kidd KK: Familial Tourette's syndrome: Report of a large pedigree and potential for linkage analysis. Neurology 1986; 36:772–776.

Shapiro AK, Shapiro ES, Young JG, Feinberg TE. Gilles de la Tourette Syndrome. 2nd ed. Raven Press, New York, 1988.

116. DYSTONIA
Stanley Fahn

Dystonic movements, spasms, and postures can occur from various causes. When a known pathologic process is present, the disorder is referred to as symptomatic torsion dystonia. Separable are cases in which clinical characteristics, genetic background, and natural history constitute a nosologic entity, often referred to as idiopathic or hereditary *torsion dystonia* or *dystonia musculorum deformans.*

Dystonic movements are sustained contractions that are typically twisting in nature and usually increase with action. The spasms can be rapid and the repetitive recurring pattern may give the appearance of rhythmicity. With childhood onset, the legs are the most affected site. The dystonic movement of action results in a peculiar twisting of the leg when the child walks forward, even though walking backward, running, or dancing can still be done normally. As the disorder progresses, the movements appear when the child is at rest; the foot becomes plantar flexed and turned inward. With progression, there is involvement of other limbs and axial muscles of the trunk (scoliosis, lordosis, and tortipelvis) or neck (torticollis, retrocollis). When the arms are involved, the forearm and the wrist often show hyperpronation and the arm moves backward (behind the body) when the patient walks. With more advanced disease, the contractions become constant so that, instead of moving, the body part remains in a fixed dystonic posture.

Adult-onset dystonia usually begins in the arms *(writer's cramp)*, neck *(torticollis)*, or face and jaw *(Meige syndrome—*blepharospasm and oromandibular dystonia). Involvement of the vocal cords *(spastic dysphonia)* is less common. With adult onset, the disease tends to remain limited as focal or segmental dystonia and does not usually become generalized.

Pathology and Pathogenesis. The pathology of torsion dystonia is unknown. Gross examination of the brain and histologic studies by light microscopy have failed to reveal any consistent morphologic changes. In view of this, considerable emphasis has been given to the possibility that a biochemical abnormality of the basal ganglia, genetically determined, may underlie the disorder.

That dystonic symptoms arise from dysfunction within the basal ganglia seems most likely because, in those conditions with symptomatic dystonia such as Wilson disease, encephalitis lethargica, and Hallervorden-Spatz disease, characteristic pathologic changes are found in this region. Furthermore, in traumatic hemidystonia, infarction of the contralateral caudate and putamen has been encountered. In support of a biochemical abnormality are the documented instances of dystonic reactions occurring with the use of pharmacologic agents, particularly those that affect striatal amine function such as the phenothiazines and levodopa. Recent evidence suggests that norepinephrine and serotonin levels are altered in some brain stem and basal ganglia structures.

An autosomal dominant mode of inheritance has been established. The suggestion that torsion dystonia among Ashkenazi Jews, the most commonly affected ethnic group, is inherited as an autosomal recessive pattern is being questioned.

Symptomatic dystonia has occurred with a variety of cerebral disorders, including Wilson disease, postencephalitic states, head trauma, perinatal birth injuries such as kernicterus, and brain tumors. It has been induced by a variety of pharmacologic agents, particularly the phenothiazines and butyrophenones, and by levodopa in parkinsonian patients. When a history of any of these known disorders is lacking and the sole manifestation is dystonic movement or posture, it is reasonably certain that the disorder is idiopathic. Two major forms of this type of dystonia have been recognized based on age of onset, clinical characteristics, and genetic background.

Signs and Symptoms. Childhood-onset dystonia generally begins between the ages of 5 and 15 years and though mode of onset may be variable, the most frequent initial symptoms involve the legs; intermittent spasmodic inversion of the foot is usually apparent on walking. Bizarre stepping or a bowing gait may be noted when the dystonic movements affect proximal muscles of the leg. Difficulty in placing the heel on the ground is evident when distal muscles are involved (Fig. 116–1). As the movements become more intense and the proximal muscles more prominently involved, lordosis and tortipelvis appear (Fig. 116–2). As the disease progresses, the neck and shoulder girdle become involved and torticollis becomes apparent. Facial grimacing and difficulties in speech become evident as the muscles subserving these functions become impaired. The continuous spasms result in marked distortion of the body to a degree rarely seen in any other disease process. Although muscle tone and power appear to be normal, the involuntary movements interfere with function and make voluntary activity extremely difficult. In gen-

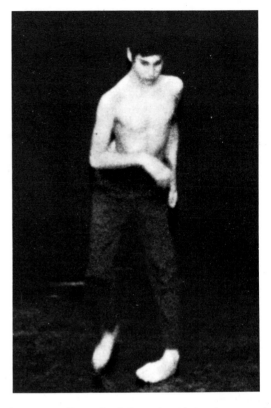

Fig. 116–1. Generalized dystonia with involvement of the legs, trunk, and arms. Patient is still able to walk.

eral, mental activity remains normal and no alterations in tendon reflexes or sensation occur. The rate of progression of this type of dystonia is extremely variable, although in most cases it is greatest within the first 5 to 10 years after onset, following which the disease may enter a quiescent static phase.

Adult-onset dystonia is three times more common and runs a more benign course. It frequently begins with movements in the neck, face, jaw, or arm, and rarely involves the leg. It tends to remain restricted to the initial body area for extended periods of time; progression to more segmental symptoms of dystonia may occur, but is of a less disabling nature.

Diagnosis and Differential Diagnosis. The diagnosis of idiopathic torsion dystonia is tenable when typical dystonic movements and postures begin in childhood or young adult life, when perinatal and developmental history is normal, when there is no antecedent illness or drug ingestion that can be implicated as a cause of the symptoms, when no other neurologic deficits are found, when no abnormalities of copper metabolism are un-

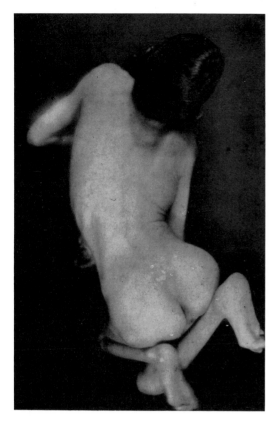

Fig. 116–2. An advanced state of generalized dystonia with fixed postures: torticollis, scoliosis, tortipelvis, and limb dystonia.

covered, and when CT and MR scans are normal.

The bizarre nature of the initial symptoms and their exaggeration in periods of stress, as well as their variability in certain settings, not infrequently lead to a diagnosis of hysteria. This diagnosis often leads to a long delay in identification of the nature of the disorder, and to prolonged periods of needless psychotherapy. Awareness of the capricious nature of the disorder and serial observation of patients can avoid this pitfall. Differentiation from symptomatic forms of dystonia may be difficult during the early phases, but the occurrence of additional neurologic deficits usually resolves the issue.

Treatment. The extreme variability of the natural history of this disorder makes evaluation of the effects of various treatment measures difficult to assess. Dystonic movements have been reported to be effectively controlled for varying periods by drugs, surgical intervention, or biofeedback techniques. Drugs that have proven useful are those that produce a degree of muscle relaxation such

as diazepam and high-dosage anticholinergics (e.g., trihexiphenidyl hydrochloride, ethopropazine hydrochloride). Stereotoxic thalamotomy may be useful in unilateral dystonia, but bilateral thalamotomy carries the risk of additional neurologic deficit, particularly speech disturbance.

For local dystonias, such as blepharospasm and spastic dysphonia, local injections of botulinum toxin have been beneficial.

Spasmodic Torticollis (Wry Neck)

The restriction of dyskinetic neck muscle movement that causes abnormal head posture is the distinguishing characteristic of this symptom complex. Involuntary activity involves the sternocleidomastoid, trapezius, and scalenus muscles in sustained contractions that result in slow, twisting, turning movements of the head (torticollis—Fig. 116–3) or, less often, forward flexion (anterocollis) or forceful extension (retrocollis). In most instances, there is bilateral involvement, and the resultant postural deformity is maintained for varying lengths of time. The muscles of the neck seem tense, and the continual muscular activity may lead to some degree of hypertrophy, especially evident in the sternocleidomastoid. The amount of active motion or static postural deformity is extremely

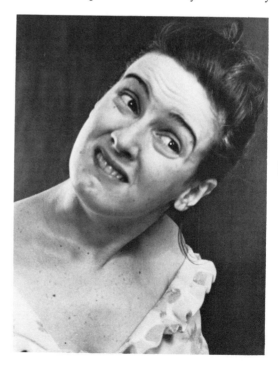

Fig. 116–3. Spasmodic torticollis with some dystonia of facial muscles (segmental dystonia).

variable. Similar activity may spread to facial and brachial musculature. Some long-term observations indicate that about 65% of patients develop additional dystonic features within 10 years of onset.

Spasmodic torticollis may be an acute or tardive complication of treatment with antipsychotic drugs, a fragment of dystonia musculorum deformans, or a compensatory postural defect in persons with congenital ocular muscle imbalance or defects of the cervical spine or musculature. Hyperthyroidism has been present in a few cases. In some instances, it has occurred as part of a wide spectrum of extrapyramidal symptoms that follow encephalitis lethargica. The pathophysiology and pathology are unknown. It occurs in patients of all ages, but usually during the third to sixth decades. The course is variable, being transitory and remitting after a few months in some patients and relentlessly progressive to incapacity in others. Most cases plateau at a certain level of severity.

The evaluation of torticollis should include a history of drug ingestion, a search for ocular and bony vertebral abnormalities, and other neurologic conditions with which it may be associated. Definable conditions account for only a small percentage of cases. In most cases, no known cause is uncovered.

There is no specific therapy for torticollis except when an underlying correctable disease process is found. Many measures have been recommended to ameliorate the symptoms. Sensory biofeedback techniques have been used. Of the number of pharmacologic agents, diazepam and anticholinergics have been reported to be effective in some patients. In more severely affected patients, a variety of surgical measures have been attempted with inconsistent results. Selective denervation of the affected muscles by section of the extradural fibers of the anterior cervical root or the spinal accessory nerve has been used. Although the movements decrease on the operated side, they frequently recur in the contralateral group of muscles. Bilateral procedures may result in extensive disability; a procedure of this magnitude should be performed only in extreme situations. Botulinum toxin injections are being investigated.

BLEPHAROSPASM

The second most common form of focal dystonia is blepharospasm. Due to contractions of the orbicularis oculi muscles, this condition is usually accompanied by co-contrac-

tions of other muscles innervated by the facial nerve. It is common for patients to have an extension of involvement to the jaw, tongue, and vocalis and neck muscles, forming a cranial segmental dystonia, often referred to as Meige syndrome. Blepharospasm occurs more often in women than in men. The usual age at onset is over 50 years, although younger individuals are sometimes affected. It often begins with increased frequency of blinking; then there is sustained eyelid closure before more forceful contractions of the orbicularis oculi develop. Abnormalities of the blink reflex have been found in patients with blepharospasm. Injections of botulinum toxin in the subcutaneous tissues of the upper and lower lids have markedly lessened the symptoms in over 70% of patients.

References

Berardelli A, Rothwell JC, Day BL, Marsden CD. Pathophysiology of blepharospasm and oromandibular dystonia. Brain 1985; 108:593–609.

Bertrand CM, Molina-Negro P. Selective peripheral denervation in 111 cases of spasmodic torticollis. Adv Neurol 1987; 50:637–643.

Burke RE, Brine MF, Fahn S, Bressman SB, Moskowitz C. Analysis of the clinical course of non-Jewish, autosomal dominant torsion dystonia. Movement Disorders 1986; 1:163–178.

Burke RE, Fahn S, Gold AP. Delayed-onset dystonia in patients with "static" encephalopathy. J Neurol Neurosurg Psychiatry 1980; 43:789–797.

Cooper IS. 20-year follow up study of the neurosurgical treatment of dystonia musculorum deformans. Adv Neurol 1976; 14:423–447.

Eldridge R, Fahn S, eds. Dystonia. Adv Neurol 1976; 14.

Fahn S. High dosage anticholinergic therapy in dystonia. Neurology 1983; 33:1255–1261.

Fahn S. The varied clinical expressions of dystonia. Neurol Clin 1984; 2:541–552.

Fahn S, Marsden CD. The treatment of dystonia. In: Marsden CD, Fahn S, eds. Movement Disorders 2. London: Butterworths, 1987: 359–382.

Fahn S, Marsden CD, Calne DB. Classification and investigation of dystonia. In: Marsden CD, Fahn S, eds. Movement Disorders 2. London: Butterworths, 1987; 332–358.

Fahn S, Marsden CD, Calne DB, editors. Dystonia 2. Adv Neurol. vol. 50, New York: Raven Press, 1988.

Friedman A, Fahn S: Spontaneous remissions in spasmodic torticollis. Neurology 1986; 36:398–400.

Herz E. Dystonia. I. Historical review: analysis of dystonic symptoms and physiologic mechanics involved. II. Clinical classification. Arch Neurol Psychiatry 1944; 51:305–355.

Hornykiewicz O, Kish SJ, Becker LE, et al. Brain neurotransmitters in dystonia musculorum deformans. N Engl J Med 1986; 315:347–353.

Jankovic J, Ford J: Blepharospasm and orofacial-cervical dystonia: clinical and pharmacological findings in 100 patients. Ann Neurol 1983; 13:402–411.

Scott AB, Kennedy RA, Stubbs HA. Botulinum toxin injection as a treatment for blepharospasm. Arch Ophthalmol 1985; 103:347–350.

117. BENIGN ESSENTIAL TREMOR
Roger C. Duvoisin

Benign essential tremor, the most common of the movement disorders, is characterized by a postural tremor that usually affects both hands symmetrically. It often involves the head, and frequently, the voice. *Essential tremor, familial tremor,* and *senile tremor* refer to the same disorder. It usually occurs in families and seems to be transmitted as an autosomal dominant trait with variation in age at onset and severity, even within a kindred. There is no known pathology and the pathophysiology is not fully understood. Population surveys have shown prevalences varying from 0.41 to 5.6% of adults over age 40 in different populations. Prevalence is somewhat higher in women and in whites.

The onset is usually in adult life. Initially, the tremor may only be apparent during periods of stress when it is felt as transient "nervousness." At first, the tremor is perhaps best described as tremulousness with a frequency of 8 to 10 Hz, appearing symmetrically in both hands. The tremor is most prominent when the arms are held outstretched and diminishes at rest and during movement, in contrast to the tremor of Parkinson disease and of cerebellar disorders. The tremor occasionally appears in childhood or adolescence; it may not be seen until advanced age when it may be designated *senile tremor.*

The condition may remain static for many years, even decades, but usually increases gradually in severity and often spreads to involve the head in a rhythmic bobbing that may be either vertical or horizontal. Not infrequently, it then spreads to the thorax and diaphragm, causing a characteristic vocal tremor. The tremor also occasionally involves the abdominal muscles and rarely the legs. Tremor of the trunk on standing, "orthostatic tremor," may also occur. Patients often report that the tremor is more severe on first arising in the morning. Many patients note that tremor is temporarily suppressed by drinking alcoholic beverages, but there is usually a rebound exacerbation.

Patients with head tremor often tilt the head slightly to one side in a "position of comfort" that seems to minimize the tremor. The effort of maintaining this position sometimes results in muscle-tension headaches. Mild facial hypomimia commonly accompanies the tremor.

Treatment. The most effective pharmacologic therapy is the use of beta-blockers. Propranolol in doses up to 120 mg daily may significantly reduce the amplitude of the tremor, but it is rarely, if ever, completely abolished. Stereotactic thalamotomy can abolish essential tremor in the contralateral limbs, but the condition is rarely sufficiently disabling to warrant brain surgery. Primidone, diazepam, clonazepam, and related agents may also prove useful in some cases.

Differential Diagnosis. Essential tremor is frequently misdiagnosed as parkinsonism, especially in the elderly. Differentiation may readily be made, however, by the absence of muscular rigidity, bradykinesia, and the postural features of parkinsonism. The patient's handwriting is large, irregular, and tremulous in striking contrast to the micrographia of parkinsonism. Head tremor rarely, if ever, occurs in parkinsonism; instead there is tremor of the lips, tongue, and jaw. The absence of any other neurologic manifestation after many years of tremor in both hands usually suffices to exclude parkinsonism. Patients with a long history of tremor of both hands occasionally develop signs and symptoms of Parkinson disease. The clinical features of these cases and the prevalence of both disorders in the population at large suggest that most such occurrences are coincidental.

Severe tremor of the hands, head, and diaphragm, and the positive family history, may occasionally suggest Huntington disease. Hyperthyroidism, lithium intoxication, chronic alcoholism, drug addiction, and anxiety tremor are usually excluded by the absence of associated features and the clinical setting. Postural tremor similar to essential tremor occurs in many patients with primary torsion dystonia.

References

Haerer AF, Anderson UW, Schoenberg BS. Prevalence of essential tremor. Arch Neurol 1982; 39:750–752.

Koller WC, Royse VL. Efficacy of primidone in essential tremor. Neurology 1986; 36:121–124.

Larsen TA, Calne DB. Essential tremor. Clin Neuropharmacol 1983; 6:185–206.

Leigh PN, Jefferson D, Twomey A, Marsden CD. Beta-adrenoreceptor mechanisms in essential tremor; a double-blind placebo controlled trial of metoprolol, sotalol, and atenolol. J Neurol Neurosurg Psychiatry 1983; 46:710–715.

Wee, AS, Subramony SH, Currier RD. 'Orthostatic tremor' in familial-essential tremor. Neurology 1986; 36:1241–1244.

Winkler GF, Young RR. Efficacy of chronic propranolol therapy in action tremors of the familial, senile or essential varieties. N Engl J Med 1974; 290:984–988.

118. PARKINSONISM
Melvin D. Yahr

In 1817, James Parkinson first described the major manifestations of a syndrome that is characterized by tremor, muscular rigidity, and loss of postural reflexes. Not only is it one of the most frequently encountered of all the basal ganglia disorders, but parkinsonism is a leading cause of neurologic disability in individuals older than 60. Though the exact frequency is unknown, it has been estimated to have a prevalence rate of 100 to 150/100,000 population with an annual incidence of 20 cases/100,000. As a symptom complex, parkinsonism has been noted in several diseases as the sole manifestation or with other signs and symptoms. However, no definable cause has been uncovered in most patients. Because most cases appear to have many features in common, particularly in regard to age of onset and evolution of symptoms, they have been designated as *Parkinson disease* or *primary parkinsonism*. The cases with definable diseases are classified as *secondary* or *symptomatic parkinsonism*. This separation into clinical groups cannot be construed as indicative of a difference in pathophysiology or even pathogenetic mechanisms; the underlying basis of symptoms for all parkinsonism may have a common origin. Sufficient evidence now exists that the loss of pigmented neurons, particularly in the substantia nigra, locus ceruleus, and brain-stem nuclei, is a common feature in all forms of parkinsonism.

The significance of these morphologic changes has become evident since the demonstration that dopamine, a neurotransmitter substance, is found in high concentration in the neostriatum (i.e., the caudate nucleus, putamen, and pallidum). In parkinsonism, selective depletion of dopamine occurs in these structures and can be correlated with the degree of degeneration of the substantia nigra. Not only has this been shown in humans, but it has been produced experimentally in animals. The greater the cell loss in the substantia nigra, the lower the concentration of dopamine in the striatum and the more severe the degree of clinical parkinsonism. However, the exact mechanism by which selective damage to the substantia nigra occurs is unknown.

In light of these findings, parkinsonism may be defined in biochemical terms as a dopamine deficiency state resulting from disease, injury, or dysfunction of the dopaminergic neuronal system. The physiologic role of this system appears to be one of inhibitory modulation of the striatum, which it produces by counterbalancing the excitatory cholinergic activity in this region. Acetylcholine, the neurotransmitter of this latter system, is abundant in the striatum, and its concentration has been shown to be unaltered in parkinsonism. In the normal healthy state, a balance exists between the effects of acetylcholine and dopamine. With loss of the latter, the balance is disturbed and cholinergic activity predominates. It is not yet completely certain whether the loss of dopamine is the only defect or whether it is responsible for all the manifestations of the disorder. Indeed it has been suggested that other neurotransmitters such as noradrenalin, GABA, and serotonin may be either primarily or secondarily involved. Neuropeptides may play a role in parkinsonism because some have been found in high concentrations in the basal ganglia and even within the same cells that contain neurotransmitter agents. If, as suggested, this is true in nigral cells, neuropeptide deficiency may also be involved in causing parkinsonism. The only established approach to the treatment of parkinsonism that has a beneficial effect on the symptoms is the restoration of normal striatal dopamine activity.

Paralysis Agitans (Shaking Palsy)

The largest number of cases of parkinsonism falls into the category of paralysis agitans *(Parkinson disease)*. The disease usually begins between the ages of 50 and 65, though a rarely encountered juvenile form has also been described. Parkinson disease occurs in both sexes and in all races throughout the world. Although there is no evidence to indicate a hereditary factor, a familial incidence is claimed by some authorities.

The characteristic pathologic findings are neuronal loss and depigmentation in the substantia nigra, particularly the zona compacta (Fig. 118–1). Similarly, loss of cells and pigment occurs in the locus ceruleus and in the dorsal vagal nucleus of the brain stem. Characteristically, these areas also show an eosinophilic intraneuronal inclusion body (the *Lewy body*), which is the pathologic hallmark of Parkinson's disease. Neither the pathogenesis of these morphologic changes nor the etiology of Parkinson's disease has as yet been elucidated. Consideration has been

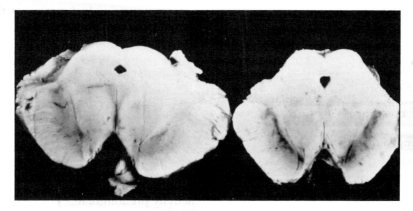

Fig. 118–1. Parkinson pathology. Depigmentation of substantia nigra of a Parkinson patient (left) in contrast to that of a normal patient (right).

given to a number of possibilities including the following: a defect in synthesis or transport of neurofilaments due to a viral or subviral agent or an abnormality in DNA repair mechanisms either acquired or inherited. To date, however, no infectious agent or specific pattern of inheritance has been identified.

The recent finding of a parkinsonian disorder with clinical and neuropathologic findings similar to those of Parkinson disease, in individuals who had unknowingly self-injected the pyridine derivative MPTP (n-methyl 4-phenyl-1236-tetrahydropyridine), has aroused interest in environmental toxins, particularly industrial pollutants of allied chemical structure. To account for the late age of onset, a combined process of cell damage is proposed in which exposure to the toxin occurs at an early age in subclinical fashion with symptoms delayed until age-related neuronal loss becomes superimposed. This concept has yet to take into consideration that Parkinson disease has been recognized for more than a century, long antedating modern pollutants, and that epidemiologic studies show its incidence and prevalence rates as well as worldwide distribution to be relatively stable over this time.

In contrast to considering exposure to an exogenous toxic factor, researchers have investigated an endogenous source related to an accumulation of toxic products of dopamine metabolism. Hydrogen peroxide is a by-product of dopamine metabolism and normally catabolized by catalase or peroxidase. These enzymes occur in reduced amounts in the nigral region of those suffering from Parkinson's disease. It is postulated that this enzyme deficiency leads to a failure of the detoxifying system for H_2O_2, which exerts a cytotoxic effect on the amine-forming neurons by way of free hydroxy radicals, superoxide radicals, or lipid peroxide. This theory embraces the concept that some type of premature or accelerated aging process is operative since similar but less severe changes occur in nigral cells in aged individuals. It does not, however, address the issue of the triggering factor for this process and is hence an explanation more of a pathogenetic mechanism than of an etiologic one.

The classic triad of symptoms includes *tremor, rigidity,* and *akinesia.* Disturbances of *posture, equilibrium,* and *autonomic* function occur equally frequently. The early symptoms are often so subtle that it is difficult to ascertain the time of onset. Because the disease tends to occur in the middle years of life, a sense of slowness, loss of agility, feelings of tremulousness, or even depression with attendant psychomotor retardation may be attributed to advancing years. It is only when one of the cardinal symptoms becomes evident that the situation becomes clear and the appropriate diagnosis is reached. Early valuable signs, usually present for years before other more obvious symptoms appear, are lack of mobility of facial expression with infrequent blinking of the eyelids, fixed or tilted postures of the trunk, a hesitant rise from a chair in assuming the erect position, and an inability to sit down with ease. A poverty of movement with a tendency to maintain a single position for unusually long intervals is another early sign. These heralding events all appear to be less well remembered by the patient than the first instance in which tremor or difficulty in the use of the limbs appears and for which medical attention is sought. As indicated in Table 118–1, tremor was the initial complaint in more than 70% of patients. However, it was readily evident on questioning that many could recall one of the aforementioned ill-defined symptoms as being present for years preceding tremor.

The *tremor* of Parkinson disease has often been described as having distinctive characteristics. It is typically referred to as "pill-rolling," involving the thumb and forefinger, alternatingly evident at rest with a frequency of 4 to 7 Hz. However, it is variable. The rhythmic alternating nature is a constant characteristic, but the rate, amplitude, and areas of bodily involvement are not. There may be tremor of the so-called action variety, postural or intentional, of variable frequencies with either minimal or extensive movement of the involved segments of the body, proximal or distal. The tremor, once it occurs, tends to spread and involve other segments, but not invariably. Sometimes the tremor remains localized to the initial site, whereas other features of the disorder may become more widespread. Tremor is an unsettling symptom to patients because it is so visible and carries with it undesirable connotations about the emotional stability of the individual. However, it contributes less to the disability of the patient than do other manifestations.

Rigidity of the muscles (i.e., resistance to passive movement) is present in almost all cases of Parkinson disease. Initially, it may be mild and restricted to a few groups of muscles, but it invariably progresses to involve more areas of the body. In its early stages

Table 118–1.   Initial Symptoms in Parkinson Disease

	No. of Cases (183)	(%)
Tremor	129	70.5
Stiffness or slowness of movement	36	19.7
Loss of dexterity and/or handwriting disturbance	23	12.6
Gait disturbance	21	11.5
Muscle pain, cramps, aching	15	8.2
Depression, nervousness, or other psychiatric disturbance	8	4.4
Speech disturbance	7	3.8
General fatigue, muscle weakness	5	2.7
Drooling	3	1.6
Loss of arm swing	3	1.6
Facial masking	3	1.6
Dysphagia	1	0.5
Paresthesia	1	0.5
Average number of initial symptoms per patient	1.4	

when it is not readily obtainable by passive movements to a limb, it can be induced by having the patient perform active synkinetic movements of the contralateral limb. Rigidity contributes to the limited range and slowness of movement that characterize Parkinson disease, but less so than akinesia. It is also, to a limited extent, a cause of the sense of muscle weakness that many patients experience. This symptom, however, is more apparent than real because the Parkinson patient can usually carry out an initial forceful contraction, but may not be able to maintain or repeat it. Rigidity has also been implicated as a cause of the postural deformities of the limbs and trunk that are characteristic. The sustained forceful contraction of rigid muscles can conceivably produce such abnormalities; however, their early occurrence in parkinsonism when rigidity is barely demonstrable and their experimental production in animals without rigidity, in whom the nigrostriatal pathway is interrupted, suggest that it is a real symptom. Indeed, accumulated evidence indicates that striatal imbalance resulting from dopamine deficiency underlies the postural abnormalities.

The *body posture* of the individual with established Parkinson disease is readily recognizable (Fig. 118–2). In the erect position, the head is bowed, the trunk is bent forward, the shoulders are drooped, the arms are flexed at the elbows with the hands held in front of the body, and the knees assume a flexed posture. The center of gravity appears to be displaced forward, leading to the patient's inability to stand erect without toppling and the tendency to be propulsive when walking. The small-stepped *festinating gait* is a distinctive feature and results from a combination of akinesia, rigidity, and the postural abnormality. Less profound postural abnormalities can be detected in the early stages of parkinsonism. The most common are seen in the upper limbs. A tendency for the hand to assume an ulnar deviated position with flexion of the fingers at the metacarpal phalangeal joints, the so-called *"striatal hand,"* is often encountered. Tilting of the trunk, usually to the side opposite that of initial limb involvement, and equinovarus posture of the foot are other postural abnormalities.

The most disabling feature of Parkinson disease is the inability to rapidly and easily perform the most ordinary volitional motor activities. The terms *bradykinesia, hypokinesia,* and *akinesia* aptly describe the degrees of im-

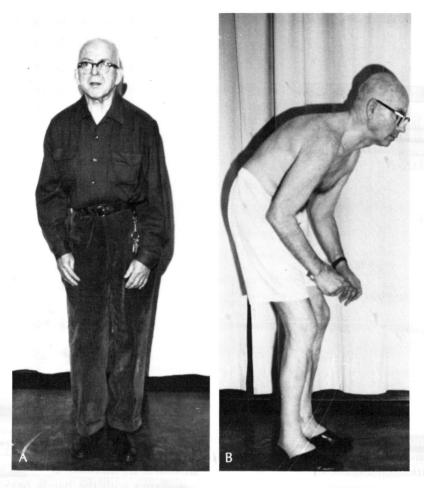

Fig. 118–2. Parkinson patient body posture. *A,* Front view. *B,* Side view.

paired movement that occur without any disturbance in muscle power or coordination. In all the acts of daily living, there is a delay in execution, which at times may reach a total standstill. A meal normally consumed in 20 minutes may be only half eaten in an hour or more. Dressing and washing may require the better part of a morning; walking may be interrupted with the patient coming to a complete halt and being "frozen" in place. The poverty of movement that results from the bradykinetic and akinetic state is apparent in a broad variety of reflex motor activities that normally occur with little or no conscious awareness. Periodic eyeblinking, mimetic facial movements, associated movements of the arms when walking, shifting of weight when standing or sitting, and assuming a relaxed posture when sitting are all impaired and rarely occur except with conscious effort. In fact, the patient with Parkinson disease is under constant stress to voluntarily perform ac-

tions that normally come naturally and involuntarily. Akinetic mechanisms play a role in the voice disturbance (i.e., its reduced amplitude and monotonous quality), the gait disorder, which is shuffling in nature and difficult to start, maintain, or alter in tempo on command, and in the use of the arms, especially in writing. With advancing akinesia, patients with Parkinson disease can rarely maintain the continuous motor activity required in script writing; they resort to printing individual letters. The capricious nature of akinesia adds greatly to the misery that the patient experiences. Its intermittent paradoxic nature leads to accusatory remarks by those involved in his daily care; they may question the patient's motivation and sense of dependency. The literature on parkinsonism is replete with descriptions of patients who, though totally immobile and in need of assistance for any and every act, suddenly rise and move normally; this is the so-called *"paradoxic akinetic reaction.''* Family members, nurses, and attendants are likely to say, ''he can do it when he wants to, five minutes ago he couldn't move a muscle, now he can do anything he wants,'' as if the phenomenon were willed or strictly a matter of motivational nature. Psychologic factors undoubtedly play a role in chronic illness, and Parkinson disease is no exception, but this profound disturbance in motor activity is without question primarily based on organic neural factors involving the integrative functions of the nervous system at a high level.

Many symptoms referable to *autonomic dysfunction* are encountered in Parkinson disease: thermal paresthesias undoubtedly related to alterations in vasomotor control of peripheral blood vessels; hyperhidrosis indicating overactivity of sweat gland innervation; and a tendency to hypotension with poor baroreceptor mechanisms, sometimes causing orthostatic syncope and bowel and bladder dysfunction, the former as a result of poor lower-bowel contraction and the latter as a result of inadequate bladder emptying (a result of decreased action of the detrusor muscle). Skin changes with eczematous eruption, especially over the forehead and sialorrhea, are not fully explained and may not be a direct expression of autonomic dysfunction. More likely, eczematous eruption relates to the attendant difficulties in personal hygiene.

Considerable comment has been made about the *intellectual capacity* of those with Parkinson disease. There are some who feel that dementia is an intrinsic characteristic of the disease, increasing in severity as it progresses. Others have implied that intellectual deterioration occurs in those patients with specific manifestations of the disease, particularly akinesia. Contrary to these reports are those that contend, as did James Parkinson, that the senses are unaffected. However, when testing is carried out so that motor activities play only a minor role in test performance (hence akinetic and rigid aspects of the disease are not a factor), it does appear that a number of cognitive, perceptual, and memory deficits are present. To some extent, the cognitive and perceptual deficits relate to cerebral dominance; patients with minor hemisphere involvement are more seriously affected. These findings suggest that the striatum, in addition to the cerebral cortex, plays a role in cerebral dominance. Striatal abnormalities may cause a modest degree of intellectual deficit; striatal abnormalities cannot, however, explain frank dementia, for which another explanation must be sought. In some cases, the dopamine deficit of Parkinson disease may not be limited to the striatum but could involve mesocortical projections as well; the degree of intellectual loss could be due to an interaction of the disease and the normal decline of intellect with age. There may also be different types of Parkinson disease—one form with intellectual deterioration, and the other form without changes in intellect. CT scans of patients with Parkinson disease are more often abnormal than those of age-matched controls; most of the patients with abnormal CT scans have organic mental syndromes. It can be concluded that parkinsonism patients with definite dementia are a separate or distinct subset of parkinsonism patients. This nosologic concept is important; if a potentially heterogeneous group of diseases is not split, there is a strong possibility not only of overlooking some important etiologic aspects but also of distorting the clinical understanding of the disease.

Tendon reflexes are usually unimpaired in Parkinson disease, although an abnormal extensor plantar response may occasionally be elicited. A hyperactive or exaggerated *glabellar reflex* (Myerson sign) is present in most patients, and palmomental reflexes are usually positive.

Symptomatic or Secondary Parkinsonism

Parkinsonism has occurred as the predominate manifestation in a variety of diseases and conditions of the nervous system, including poisoning with carbon monoxide, manganese, or other heavy metals, brain tumors in the region of the basal ganglia, cerebral trauma, intoxication with neuroleptic agents, infectious processes such as encephalitides, and multineuronal degenerative disorders of unknown cause (Table 118–2). It also occurs in association with cerebral arteriosclerosis and endocrine dysfunction such as hypoparathyroidism. In most instances, the associated neurologic deficits, atypical features of the symptoms, or other systemic manifestations of the related disease arouse suspicion that the disorder is not primary parkinsonism.

Postencephalitic Parkinsonism

One of the most prominent sequelae of the epidemic of encephalitis lethargica (von Economo disease) that occurred between 1919 and 1926 was the parkinsonian syndrome. The

Table 118-2. Causes of Secondary Parkinsonism

Infectious: Postviral encephalitis	Tumors: basal ganglia
Atherosclerotic (pseudoparkinsonism)	Cerebral arteriovenous malformations
Drug-induced	Head trauma
Phenothiazines	"Degenerative"
Thioxanthenes	Parkinson-dementia complex (Guam)
Butyrophenones	Striatonigral degeneration
Toxic agents	Progressive supranuclear palsy
Carbon monoxide	Olivopontocerebellar atrophy
Carbon disulfide	Parkinsonism with autonomic dystrophy
Manganese	(Shy-Drager, multisystem atrophy)
MPTP (Meperidine analogue)	Senile and presenile states
Metabolic	Neuroaxonal dystrophy
Parathyroid dysfunction—hypoparathyroid	
Anoxic states	

syndrome developed after mild as well as severe encephalitis lethargica. Although in most instances prominent symptoms immediately followed the acute infectious process, in some patients they were not evident for up to 10 years. The causative agent of encephalitis lethargica was never established. However, studies suggest that it may have been produced by a virus of the influenza A variety. Parkinsonism appears to have been a unique sequela of this form of encephalitis because it rarely follows any other viral encephalitides. Pathologically, postencephalitic parkinsonism differs from the idiopathic parkinsonism in that cellular loss of the melanin-containing neurons is greater, neurofibrillary changes occur in many of the remaining nerve cells, and no Lewy bodies are present. Persistent inflammatory changes are occasionally found even years after the initial infections. Multifocal areas of glial scarring may be found throughout the nervous system.

Postencephalitic parkinsonism has a number of distinctive or unique features, including the following: (1) because the pandemic of influenza of 1918 to 1919 occurred concurrently with encephalitis, careful documentation must be undertaken to differentiate these two infectious processes; (2) in addition to any or all of the aforementioned parkinsonian symptoms, one or more neurologic deficits may occur (e.g., hemiplegia, bulbar or ocular palsies, dystonic phenomena, tics, behavioral disorders); (3) secondary parkinsonism generally develops incompletely and is static or slowly progressive for years; and (4) oculogyric crises (i.e., spasms of conjugate eye muscles) occur so that the eyes are deviated upward, downward, or to one side for minutes or hours at a time.

The response of postencephalitic parkinsonism to treatment with pharmacologic agents differs from that of Parkinson disease. Although improvement of symptoms occurs with levodopa, tolerance is limited. Most patients must be treated cautiously with less than half the usual therapeutic dose (2 to 3 g/day) because they rapidly develop abnormal involuntary movements and are prone to abnormal behavioral reactions. However, most postencephalitic patients can tolerate large doses of anticholinergic agents.

Arteriosclerotic Parkinsonism

Atherosclerotic involvement of the cerebral vessels has been implicated as a cause of parkinsonism. Although the symptoms produced by both disorders appear on superficial examination to resemble each other, there are distinctive differences. Critchley first proposed the term *arteriosclerotic parkinsonism* in 1929 and later re-emphasized the differing nature of the two disorders, suggesting that when there is an underlying cerebrovascular disease, it should be considered *pseudoparkinsonism*. It has been suggested that the term arteriosclerotic parkinsonism should be abandoned.

Pathologically, multiple small cerebral infarctions (lacunes) secondary to small vessel occlusion are not infrequently found throughout the brain in these patients. The neuronal cell loss, which is diffuse, may involve the substantia nigra, but is rarely of an extensive degree when compared to other changes in the CNS. In fact, the globus pallidus may be more severely affected, and there are lesions in the brain stem and cerebral cortex.

Signs and Symptoms. As a rule, the onset of symptoms is insidious, with most cases beginning in the seventh decade of life, although pseudoparkinsonism has been seen in younger patients in their fourth decade. Only rarely is there a history of a major stroke preceding onset, although symptoms referable to so-called minor strokes may be elicited. Early symptoms usually center around impaired mobility; gait disturbance is the most common initial complaint. Other presenting complaints may refer to pseudobulbar phenomena with dysarthria, some degree of dysphasia, and emotional incontinence. On occasion, patients present with progressive dementia and poverty of movement. Tremor is rare, but alteration in muscle tone does occur. It differs from the cogwheel type that is characteristic of Parkinson disease in that there is a stiffening of the limb in response to contact and a sense of resistance with attempted change of position. This type of alteration in muscle tone is known as *gegenhalten*. Hyperactive reflexes, abnormal plantar responses, and palmomental and snouting reflexes are all usually found.

The disease usually progresses in steps more rapid than those of Parkinson disease. Tolerance for the usual antiparkinson drugs, whether anticholinergic or dopaminergic, is poor.

Striatonigral Degeneration

Striatonigral degeneration is an uncommon form of parkinsonism that was first identified as a separate entity by Adams and co-workers in 1961. Clinically, it is difficult to distinguish these patients from those with primary parkinsonism, although they have a tendency to show a greater degree of rigidity, a more rapid course, and a poor response to pharmacologic agents. Pathologically, however, these cases are characterized by neuronal degeneration of the striatum, particularly the putamen, whereas the substantia nigra is only mildly affected. Neuronal loss occurs in the putamen, which is replaced by a dense gliosis with scattered pigment accumulation that may extend into the globus pallidus.

Drug-Induced Parkinsonism

The use of neuroleptics as psychotherapeutic or antiemetic agents has resulted in a number of extrapyramidal syndromes. Symptoms include the parkinsonian triad, dystonic movements involving the tongue and face, and *akathisia*, which is a restless fidgety state in which the patient feels a desire to be in constant motion. Adults are more likely to develop parkinsonism and akathisia, whereas dystonic movements predominate in children. In some instances, these reactions are dose-dependent; in others they are related to individual susceptibility. The symptoms usually disappear within a few days when the drugs are withdrawn, but occasionally persist for months. In some subjects, permanent remnants of parkinsonian symptoms have been found years after elimination of the drugs. Paradoxically, involuntary movements may first appear after withdrawal of neuroleptic agents. This condition, termed *tardive dyskinesia*, tends to occur in older patients who have been on phenothiazine drugs for extended periods, during which they have shown signs of parkinsonism. Stereotyped repetitive movements of lips, tongue, and mouth and choreic movements of limbs and trunk characterize this disorder. It may diminish in intensity or disappear spontaneously after weeks or months, but in some patients it has persisted indefinitely. Basal ganglia symptoms, particularly parkinsonism, can usually be minimized by the simultaneous administration of one of the centrally active anticholinergic agents, such as benzotropine or trihexyphenidyl hydrochloride. Cautious use of neuroleptics, employing restricted doses and scheduled drug abstention in those requiring long-term treatment, may be the best preventive measure.

MPTP-Induced Parkinsonism

The development of a Parkinson syndrome following inadvertent exposure or unknowing use of MPTP (n-methyl 4 phenyl 1236-tetrahydropyridine) has recently been uncovered. Not only is it of clinical interest, but it has provided a means of producing an animal model of the disorder that may hold clues to the pathogenesis and etiology of Parkinson disease. The exact mechanism of MPTP toxicity has not been fully elucidated, but it is known to be rapidly oxidized by monoamine oxidase to MPP+ (1-methyl-4-phenyl pyridine). Inhibiting the conversion by an MAO-B inhibitor, such as deprenyl, prevents the formation of this charged molecule and the neurotoxic effects. Hence, either MPP+ or some product released as a result of the oxidative metabolic process involved in its formation may be the toxic factor. These findings have stimulated a search for a similar toxin to MPTP or a metabolic process of like nature and by-products as the etiologic factor in primary Parkinson disease. They have also aroused interest in utilizing deprenyl as a means of prevention.

To date, MPTP-induced parkinsonism has been described in a group of drug abusers who have used it intravenously and in laboratory workers exposed by either inhalation or skin contact. The clinical syndrome is indistinguishable from primary Parkinson disease and is responsive to the use of levodopa. It is, however, not established as yet whether the induced Parkinson state is progressive or static or whether minimal exposure with subclinical effects may predispose to the future development of parkinsonism.

Parkinson-Dementia Complex of Guam

Parkinsonism occurs in association with a severe progressive dementia and motor neuron disease among the indigenous Chamorro population of Guam and the Mariana Islands. The syndrome predominantly affects males and begins between ages 50 and 60; death usually occurs within 5 years. The syndrome is responsible for about 7% of deaths among the adult Chamorro population. The disorder tends to run in families. Motor neuron signs may be upper or lower in nature, resembling ALS, which is also common among the Chamorro people (approximately 10% of adult deaths).

Pathologically, the syndrome has features of both parkinsonism and Alzheimer disease. Depigmentation of the substantia nigra and locus ceruleus occurs, as do Alzheimer neurofibrillary tangles and severe cortical atrophy. Lewy bodies and senile plaques are absent. Motor neuron loss and pyramidal tract degeneration also occur.

Levodopa therapy alleviates the extrapyramidal symptoms in this syndrome; the dementia and motor neuron involvements are unaffected. The cause is unknown. It does not appear to be postencephalitic, nor is there evidence to suggest a viral cause.

Laboratory Studies. Routine examination of blood, CSF, and urine is normal in all forms of parkinsonism. In primary parkinsonism and the more frequently encountered secondary forms (postencephalitic, progressive supranuclear palsy), the deficiency of dopamine in the striatum causes a decrease of its acid metabolite, homovanillic acid (HVA), in the CSF. The EEG is usually normal, although diffuse slowing may occur. A greater degree of abnormalities, usually nonspecific, is seen in secondary forms of parkinsonism. Skull radiographs and routine isotope brain scanning show no abnormalities. CT reveals normal findings in parkinsonism but is useful in eliminating disorders with similar symptoms such as arteriosclerotic pseudoparkinsonism.

Management of Parkinsonism

The treatment of parkinsonism is symptomatic, supportive, and palliative. Only in the exceptional case of secondary parkinsonism resulting from the use of drugs or occurring in association with a specific disease does treatment of the causative factor result in eradication of symptoms. Parkinsonism patients require lifelong treatment with specific medications, supportive psychotherapeutic measures, and physical therapy.

Predefined, unalterable rules regarding treatment, when applied indiscriminately to all patients, give less than optimal results. Treatment programs should be personalized, using as a guide the patient's symptoms, the degree of functional impairment, and the expected benefits and risks of available therapeutic agents. Judicious treatment may control the symptoms of parkinsonism for extended periods. In most patients, it allows relatively normal activities during most phases of the disorder. The introduction of new pharmacologic approaches to its treatment has markedly forestalled the disabling progression of parkinsonism.

The rate of progression roughly corresponds to the degree of dopamine deficiency in the brain; it also helps determine the type of drugs used. During the initial phase of parkinsonism, dopamine deficiency is minimal despite damage to the nigral cells. Surviving cells are able to compensate for those that have been lost by an increasing activity and by synthesizing and releasing more dopamine per unit of time than normally. This phase of parkinsonism may be considered a partially compensated one best treated by agents that can enhance the existing state of striatal dopaminergic activity. As the disease progresses due to continued degeneration of dopaminergic cells in the nigra (with increasing dopamine deficiency), a decompensated phase of parkinsonism ensues. The goal of treatment is to promote the production of dopamine in the striatum by administration of its immediate precursor, levodopa, or by direct stimulation of dopamine receptor mechanisms by ergoline derivatives.

Compensated Phase Treatment. The decision to use drug therapy is determined by the patient's symptoms and functional impairment; when these are mild and there is little if any function impairment, reassurance and periodic examination may suffice. This approach is applicable when there is mild tremor at rest in one limb. When some degree of akinesia and rigidity develops with minimally impaired coordinated movements, the use of the following, either alone or in combination, is indicated.

Anticholinergic Agents. Several drugs, closely allied in chemical structure, have a primary action of counteracting the muscarinic effects of acetylcholine in the CNS. There is little reason aside from personal preference for choosing one rather than another. When used in appropriate dosage, they can produce a moderate degree of improvement in all symptoms of parkinsonism. However, their usefulness is restricted by side effects that prevent administration in full dosage. The most common side effects are dryness of the mouth, blurred vision, urinary retention, obstipation, and psychic phenomena ranging from mild behavioral abnormalities to overt psychotic episodes.

The order of presentation of these compounds is not necessarily the sequence in which they are used. A rule of thumb is that for mild cases and for those patients in older age groups, the less potent agents may be preferred. For example, diphenhydramine is often used in preference to one of the piperidyls or benztropine because it is less likely to cause disturbing side effects. Improvement may be less than optimal, but this is more acceptable than annoying side effects. In general, initiating therapy with one of the piperidyl compounds, preferably trihexyphenidyl, and adding an agent from one of the other groups is the more desirable form of therapy.

Piperidyl Compounds. Trihexyphenidyl (Artane) is the oldest but still the drug of choice in this group of compounds. It should be started in a dosage of 2 mg given 3 times daily and slowly increased to tolerance. Most patients tolerate up to 10 mg per day with only minor annoying side effects. Some patients may tolerate 20 mg per day. A modest decrease in all symptoms of parkinsonism can be expected from its use.

Similar effects may be obtained from cycrimine (Pagitane), which is begun in a dosage of 1.25 mg 3 times daily and increased to a total daily dose of 20 mg; procyclidine (Kemadrin), begun in a dosage of 5 mg twice daily and increased to 30 mg; or biperiden (Akineton), beginning with 2 mg 3 times daily and increasing to a total daily dosage of 20 mg.

Tropane. Benztropine mesylate (Cogentin) is a potent anticholinergic compound with pharmacologic actions that closely mimic those of atropine. Because of this, it cannot be used in full dosage without producing undesirable side effects. It is extremely useful in treating patients who are receiving full dosage of one of the piperidyl compounds or levodopa. When this drug is given in 1-mg or 2-mg doses at bedtime, the long duration of action eases symptoms during the night and when the patient wakes in the morning. It is also available as a parenteral preparation and can be used in 1-mg doses to reverse the symptoms of parkinsonism caused by the use of neuroleptics.

Antihistamines. These agents have a mild degree of antiparkinsonism action as a result of anticholinergic properties. They are useful in patients who cannot tolerate the more potent drugs; they may also be given in combination with the more potent agents. They are frequently started simultaneously with, or soon after, levodopa or one of the piperidyls.

Diphenhydramine (Benadryl) is preferred because it is well tolerated. It is administered in a starting dosage of 25 mg 3 times daily and can be increased to 50 mg 4 times daily. A major limiting side effect is its soporific action.

Orphenadrine (Disipal), 50 mg, phenindiamine (Thephorin), 25 mg, or chlorphenoxamine (Phenoxene), 50 mg, each given 3 times a day can be used instead of diphenhydramine.

Amantadine. Introduced as an antiviral agent, amantadine (Symmetrel) was accidentally found to have beneficial effects on the symptoms of parkinsonism. The mechanism of action is controversial; some investigators believe that it acts directly on striatal dopaminergic mechanisms, but others consider blockage of cholinergic action more important. When it is used alone in doses of 100 mg 2 or 3 times per day, therapeutic effects (i.e., mild reversal of parkinsonism symptoms) are evident within 48 to 72 hours. More effective action can be achieved when it is combined with an anticholinergic agent such as trihexyphenidyl. The effects of amantadine are short-lived, tending to diminish after a few months. Many of its side effects are similar to those of the anticholinergic agents, particularly the induction of confusional and delusional states. After long-term use, edema and a form of livedo reticularis develop over the limbs in some patients.

Tricyclic Compounds. The antidepressants imipramine (Tofranil) and amitryptyline (Elavil) are useful in the early phases of parkinsonism. Not only do they block the reuptake and storage of dopamine, making it more available at the synaptic cleft in the striatum, but they have anticholinergic action. Used alone or in combination with levodopa or other drugs, antidepressants may improve akinesias, rigidity, and the depressive symptoms of early parkinsonism. Imipramine (10 mg) or amitryptyline (25 mg), given 3 or 4 times per day, may be administered safely for extended periods without untoward side effects.

Decompensated Phase Treatment. Patients in this category have established signs and symptoms of parkinsonism. They have difficulty with the routines of daily living, including business or social obligations. They are best treated initially with agents capable of replenishing striatal dopamine. As the disease progresses, drugs that modify the catabolism of striatal dopamine or that mimic its pharmacologic effect should be added.

Levodopa/Carbidopa (Sinemet). The best means for making levodopa available to the brain for conversion to dopamine is its administration with a peripheral decarboxylase inhibitor (i.e., carbidopa). The combination tablet contains fixed ratios of carbidopa (10 or 25 mg) to levodopa (100 or 250 mg). Treatment is best started with low doses of Sinemet 10/100 given 3 times per day and increased by one tablet every 3 days. The dosage at which therapeutic responses occur is variable. In general, patients begin to show some improvement when a total daily dose of Sinemet 50/500 mg is reached. Further increases are then made at monthly intervals with the goal of finding the minimal dosage that gives an acceptable degree of functional improvement. In most instances, this will be between 70/700 mg and 100/1000 mg; exceptional patients require 150/1500 mg daily. Sinemet is best administered in four equally divided doses during the waking hours; occasionally, more frequent doses are desirable.

At onset of treatment with Sinemet, side effects are infrequent. Some patients experience nausea and vomiting, which may be avoided by using the combination tablet that contains 25 mg carbidopa and 100 mg of levodopa. Alternately, reducing the dosage by half may be effective. Those in the older age groups may experience confusional states, which are primarily nocturnal, requiring lower doses or discontinuation of the drug. Toxic psychosis may occur at any time in patients taking this drug; the reaction must be recognized and the dosage must be readjusted.

The most frequent and therapeutically limiting side effect of levodopa is the appearance of abnormal *involuntary movements.* These may be mild, choreic movements limited to a bodily segment or they may be severe, generalized, and dystonic. These involuntary movements are dose- as well as time-related. They occur more frequently in patients taking high doses of levodopa and in those who have been taking levodopa for extended periods. Indeed, abnormal movements may be induced in patients on long-term therapy at daily dosage levels that were previously tolerated without such side effects. The only effective measure for their control is reduction of the dosage of Sinemet. In general, the daily dosage is reduced until a dosage is found at which the movements are tolerable and a degree of control of parkinson symptoms is possible.

Equally difficult to manage are the erratic and variable responses to therapy, the so-called *"on-off" phenomena.* These consist of episodes in which patients alternate between having full-blown parkinson symptoms and having no symptoms. These on-off phenomena may occur precipitously and in random fashion or they may be gradual and predictable in onset, related to a shortened duration of action of a given dose of Sinemet. The latter variety, often termed an *end-dose "off" response,* may be controlled by rearranging the schedule so that intervals of 2 or 3 hours are used rather than intervals of 4 or 5 hours. More often than not, this regimen proves to be less than completely satisfactory and ancillary agents must be used. Those that have proved most effective are still considered investigative, and only a few are available for general use.

Ergoline Derivatives. At present, only one of these compounds has been validated for clinical use, but others are undergoing clinical trial and may prove more effective. These compounds act directly on dopamine receptors. Unfortunately, they are not specific for the postsynaptic striatal dopamine receptor and hence give less than the precise action desired.

Bromocriptine. This semisynthetic ergoline compound activates dopamine receptors and has antiparkinsonian properties. It is less potent than Sinemet or other levodopa preparations and many of its side effects are similar. Included are nausea, vomiting, and hypotension, which occur more frequently, particularly during the induction phase of treatment. With long-term usage or higher dosage, additional side effects such as limb edema, phlebitis, pleuropulmonary fibrosis, and toxic psychoses have been noted. Bromocriptine does have one advantage over other dopaminergic agents in that involuntary movements occur less frequently. Because bromocriptine may induce orthostatic hypotension, it should be introduced cautiously. Indeed, a test dose of 1.25 mg given after the noon meal is an appropriate way to begin treatment. If no syncopal phenomena are reported, it can then be increased by 1.25 mg every 3 to 4 days until the desired dosage is achieved.

Bromocriptine has been used most often as an adjunctive agent to levodopa when the latter begins losing its therapeutic effectiveness. Its addition, in divided doses totaling 10 to 30 mg a day, may improve the parkinsonian state. Particularly responsive are those in whom fluctuating responses (end-dose or on-off) are occurring. These patients may experience a decrease in their severity and frequency.

Bromocriptine, administered alone or in combination with Sinemet, has also been advocated as initial and primary therapy. In patients with minimal symptoms and in the early phase of the disease it has been used as monotherapy. Bromocriptine in doses as minimal as 1.25 mg three times a day is reported by some as effective, but such a response is only rarely encountered. In more advanced cases, beginning treatment with a combination of bromocriptine and Sinemet may have advantages over the use of either agent alone. Not only does this regimen allow for the administration of lower doses of each, but it has been reported in long-term follow-up to result in a lessened occurrence of fluctuating responses and hyperkinetic phenomena.

Monoamine Oxidase Inhibitors. In general, most of the agents available in this family of drugs act on both monoamine oxidases (MAO), A and B. They cannot be given concurrently with levodopa. L-deprenil is an exception and hence can be used to prevent the degradation of dopamine in the striatum.

L-Deprenyl. This compound is an inhibitor of MAO-B, the form in which this enzyme is present in the striatum. Dopamine is a major substrate for MAO-B and the pathways by which it is primarily metabolized. Inhibiting MAO-B allows dopamine to accumulate, enhancing and prolonging its action. In contrast to other MAO inhibitors such as tranylcypromine, which inhibit MAO-A and -B, deprenil can be administered in conjunction with Sinemet without fear of producing hypertensive crises. Its usefulness at present is as an adjunct to Sinemet in the control of "on-off" phenomena, especially the end-dose variety, as well as in patients who have lost the benefit from the current therapeutic program.

Deprenyl added in fixed dosage of 5 mg twice a day produces a pharmacologic response within a few days. In some the beneficial response is complicated by accentuating the side effects of levodopa and the dosage of the latter may need to be readjusted to a lower level. Few reports of the long-term usage of this combination of therapeutic agents are available. Although some report that the beneficial effects of deprenyl begin to wane after two to three years, one group of investigators has reported sustained effect in patients with resultant prolongation of life expectancy. They have interpreted these findings as indicative of the ability of deprenyl to retard or prevent further degeneration of the nigrostriatal pathway, thus halting progression of the disease. Controlled studies to determine the validity of these findings are in progress.

In summary, the patient with established parkinsonian symptoms is best treated with levodopa combined with carbidopa (Sinemet). The dosage should be individualized and limited to the lowest level that gives functional improvement; Sinemet should not be used in attempts to erase every vestige of the disease. When Sinemet is appropriately used, as many as 80% of those with Parkinson disease can expect to experience benefits. These are optimal during the first three years of use; later the effectiveness of the drug declines, but there are still substantial benefits. The incidence of side effects increases with the length of time the drug is used. At present, no completely satisfactory means of treatment exists for this phase of the disease, although ancillary agents show promise of being helpful.

Ancillary Therapeutic Measures. *Physical Therapy and Exercise.* The general tendency of patients with Parkinson disease to become inactive and dependent can in part be overcome by the judicious use of physiotherapy. This need not be extensive, nor is elaborate gadgetry required. The regimen should be individualized, with thoughtful attention given to the patient's abilities and disabilities and with specific programs established for each. By and large, physiotherapy is directed toward the maintenance of joint mobility, correction and prevention of postural abnormalities of trunk and limbs, and maintenance of normal gait. Passive stretching of the limbs, muscle massage, resistive exercises, and gait training are all used to accomplish this objective. As a rule, treatment is given anywhere from one to five times a week, depending on individual needs. In addition, all patients are advised to establish a daily program of exercises. Patients are encouraged to take long walks, use a stationary bicycle, and practice the exercises outlined by the physiotherapist. The patient should be constantly reminded that disability can be prevented or at least delayed by physical activity, and that much of this must be done by himself.

Supportive Psychotherapy. Few patients accept the diagnosis of parkinsonism with equanimity. The realization that one is suffering from this disorder usually evokes visions of total disability and confinement to a wheelchair or bed. The anxiety and depression in the early stages of the disease contribute as much to the disability as do the symptoms of parkinsonism. It is therefore of utmost importance that at the time of initial contact with the patient, the physician should emphasize the slowly progressive course of the disease, what can and cannot be done to control the symptoms, and that progressive periods are interwoven with periods when the disease is stationary. Much can be accomplished by dispelling fears about insanity and inheritance that are often acquired from hearsay rather than from reliable sources. Realistic goals for business and family life must be discussed. Every attempt must be made to maintain the patient as a social being because many parkinsonism patients tend to withdraw from interpersonal relations as a consequence of their altered outward appearance. The successful treatment of parkinsonism depends on the physician's ability and willingness to offer a total care program to the patient. When this is done, there are only rare instances when the need arises for referral of patients for specific psychiatric treatment.

Surgical Measures. Surgical attempts to alleviate parkinsonism are primarily directed to the interruption of one or more neural pathways, the integrity of which appears essential for the production of symptoms. Such interruption should be at a site where normal sensory and motor functions will not be affected. Lesions produced by electrocoagulation or freezing in the ventrolateral nucleus of the thalamus have relieved contralateral tremor and rigidity in the limbs. However, akinesia and disturbances in gait, posture, and voice are not appreciably improved; multiple lesions are necessary to relieve cervical, truncal, and bilateral limb symptoms. Because tremor and rigidity are bilateral in most cases, a good result on one side often encourages an attempt to do the same for the other. Most surgeons prefer to wait 6 months to 1 year before operating on the second side to minimize the complications that are likely to occur with bilateral procedures. Even so, the bilateral procedure frequently produces adverse effects on speech and, though recovery usually occurs, the patient may retain some degree of dysarthria and hypophonia. Because the manifestations become bilateral within a year or two of the onset in most cases, and because disability is eventually due not so much to tremor or rigidity but to akinesia and postural abnormalities, stereotactic surgery benefits only a limited number of patients. The best candidate for surgery is the patient whose chief manifestation is unilateral tremor and rigidity, preferably in the arm, and whose disease seems to progress slowly. These characteristics represent an early stage of the disease, and usually the patient is not yet seriously disabled. Thus, proponents of stereotactic surgery urge that thalamotomy be considered early in the course of Parkinson disease, although critics point out that surgery does not benefit the more advanced patients who most need help, nor does it prevent progression of the disease. The introduction of more effective pharmacologic therapy has diminished the enthusiasm for surgical intervention. A balanced judgment would be that thalamotomy be used for cases resistant to other forms of therapy and in which relief of upper limb tremor is desired.

An alternate surgical approach, still in the stage of development, has utilized adrenal medullary autografts or neonatal nigral cells transplanted to the striatum. These have been placed either within the caudate nucleus or putamen or on the surface of the former in direct contact with ventricular fluid. To date, only a limited number of patients have undergone the procedure, with reported results varying from dramatic reversal of the Parkinson state to only modest improvement. Because postoperative follow-up periods are relatively short, one cannot fully assess the value of this operative procedure. However, the feasibility of cell grafting in brain appears to have been established, but considerable investigation is still necessary to determine the optimal type of cell to be used, the most appropriate site of implantation, and the long-term survival, if any, of such grafts. Until such time as these issues are resolved, this operative procedure must be considered experimental and not an accepted mode of treatment for Parkinson disease.

Course. All forms of parkinsonism are progressive disorders leading over variable periods of time to considerable motor disability. The most progressive are those in which it is associated with other neurologic disorders such as progressive supranuclear palsy where a fatal outcome can be expected within five years. Postencephalitic parkinsonism has

been unique in that its evolution has been relatively slow and patients have remained functional for extended periods, some for 30 years or longer. Prior to treatment with levodopa, Parkinson disease, or what is now referred to as *primary parkinsonism,* could be expected to cause severe disablity or death in 25% of patients within 5 years of onset, which rose to 65% in the succeeding 5 years and to 80% in those surviving for 15 years. It had been estimated that those suffering from Parkinson disease had a mortality rate three times that of the general population matched for age, sex, and racial origin. Although there is no evidence to indicate that levodopa alters the underlying pathologic process or stems the progressive nature of the disease, there are indications of a major impact on survival time and functional capacity. Studies show that the added risk of mortality from Parkinson disease has been reduced by 50% and that longevity is extended by several years.

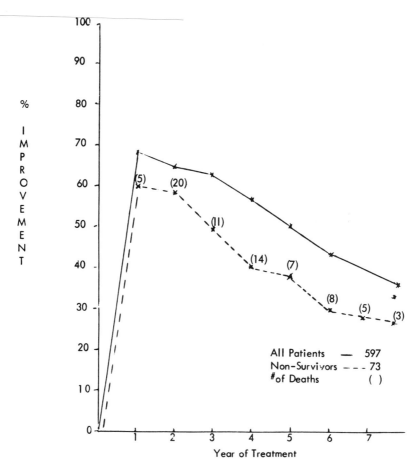

Fig. 118–3. Degree of improvement of Parkinson signs during each year of treatment with levodopa. Nonsurviving patients are compared with the total group treated.

As indicated early in this section, it has been suggested on theoretical grounds and limited clinical data that L-deprenil may be able to halt or retard the inexorable progressive nature of the disease. Although extensive controlled clinical trials are needed, these newer therapeutic agents have improved the quality of life for patients with parkinsonism. No longer do they suffer the severe incapacity and dependence that previously characterized this disorder.

However, the treatment of parkinsonism is still far from ideal. Follow-up studies covering periods of up to eight years of levodopa treatment reveal gradual loss of therapeutic efficacy. Optimal responses are obtained during the first three years of treatment with levodopa, regardless of duration of the disease, and then diminish (Fig. 118–3). It is not known at this time whether this pattern relates to intrinsic factors of the disease itself or to pharmacologic properties of the drug.

References

Ballard PA, Tetrud JW, Langston JW. Permanent human parkinsonism due to 1-methyl-4-phenyl-1,2,3,6-tetrahydropyridine (MPTP): seven cases. Neurology 1985; 35:949–957.

Barr A. The Shy-Drager syndrome. In: Vinken PJ, Bruyn GW, Klawans HL, eds. Handbook of Clinical Neurology, vol 38. New York: Elsevier-North Holland, 1979:233–256.

Cotzias CG. Modification of parkinsonism—chronic treatment with L-DOPA. N Engl J Med 1969; 280:337–345.

Duvoisin RC, Mendoza M, Yahr MD. A comparative study of bromocriptine and levodopa in Parkinson's disease. Adv Biochem Psychopharmacol 1980; 23:271–275.

Duvoisin RC, Yahr MD. Encephalitis and parkinsonism. Arch Neurol 1965; 12:227–239.

Fahn S. Secondary parkinsonism. In: Goldensohn ES, Appel SH, eds. Scientific Approaches to Clinical Neurology. Philadelphia: Lea & Febiger, 1977.

Fahn S, Calne DB, Shoulson I, eds. Experimental Therapeutics of Movement Disorders. New York: Raven Press, 1983.

Fahn S, Duffy P. Parkinson's disease. In: Goldensohn ES, Appel SH, eds. Scientific Approaches to Clinical Neurology. Philadelphia: Lea & Febiger, 1977.

Garruto RM, Gajdusek C, Chen K. Amyotrophic lateral sclerosis and parkinsonism-dementia among Filipino migrants to Guam. Ann Neurol 1981; 4:341–351.

Hoehn MM, Yahr MD. Parkinsonism: onset, progression and mortality. Neurology 1967; 17:427–442.

Hornykiewicz O. Neurohumoral interactions and basal ganglia dysfunction. Res Publ Assoc Res Nerv Ment Dis 1976; 55:269.

Kebabian JW, Calne DB. Multiple receptors for dopamine. Nature 1979; 297:93–96.

Kurlan R. International symposium on early dopamine agonist therapy of Parkinson's disease. Arch Neurol 1988; 45:204–208.

Lindvall O, Backlund E, Farde L, Sedvall G, Freedman R, Hoffer B, Nobin A, Seiger A, Olson L. Transplantation in Parkinson's disease: two cases of adrenal medullary grafts to the putamen. Ann Neurol 1987; 22:51.

Madrazo I, Drucker-Colin R, Diaz V, Martinez-Mata J, Torres C, Becerril JJ. Open microsurgical autograft of adrenal medulla to the right caudate nucleus in two patients with intractable Parkinson's disease. N Engl J Med 1987; 316:831–834.

Madrazo I, Leon V, Torres C, Aguilera M, Varela G, Alvarez F, Fraga A. Transplantation of fetal substantia nigra and adrenal medulla to the caudate nucleus in two patients with Parkinson's disease. Ann Neurol 1987; 22:51.

Marsden CD, Fahn S, eds. Movement Disorders. London: Butterworths, 1981.

Marsden CD, Parkes JD. "On-off" effects in patients with Parkinson's disease on chronic levodopa therapy. Lancet 1976; 1:292–295.

Parkinson J. An Essay on the Shaking Palsy. London: Neely and Jones, 1817.

Rinne UK. Early combination of bromocriptine and levodopa in the treament of Parkinson's disease: a 5-year follow-up. Neurology 1987; 37:826–829.

Snyder SH, D'Amato RJ. MPTP: a neurotoxin relevant to the pathophysiology of Parkinson's disease 1985, George C. Cotzias lecture. Neurology 1986; 36:250–258.

Steele JC, Richardson JC, Olszewski J. Progressive supranuclear palsy. Arch Neurol 1964; 10:333–359.

Ward CD, Duvoisin RC, Ince SE, Nutt JD, Eldridge R, Calne DB. Parkinson's disease in 65 pairs of twins and in a set of quadruplets. Neurology 1983; 33:815–825.

Yahr MD. Evaluation of long-term therapy in Parkinson's disease: mortality and therapeutic efficacy. In: Birkmayer W, Hornykiewicz O, eds. Advances in Parkinsonism. Basel: F Hoffman La Roche & Co., 1976:435–443.

Yahr MD. Overview of present day treatment of Parkinson's disease. J Neural Transm 1978; 43:227–238.

Yahr MD ed. Parkinsonism: current perspectives and new horizons. J Clin Neuropharmacol 1986; 9(Suppl 1).

Yahr MD, Bergmann KJ, eds. Parkinson's Disease. Advances in Neurology, vol 45. New York: Raven Press, 1986.

Yahr MD, Mendoza MR, Moros D, Bergmann KJ. Treatment of Parkinson's disease in early and late phases. Use of pharmacological agents with special reference to deprenyl (selegiline). Acta Neurol Scand 1983; 95(Suppl):95–102.

119. PROGRESSIVE SUPRANUCLEAR PALSY
Roger C. Duvoisin

In postmortem studies of patients who had a clinical syndrome of pseudobulbar palsy, supranuclear ocular palsy, chiefly affecting vertical gaze, extrapyramidal rigidity, gait ataxia, and dementia, Olszewski, Steele, and Richardson noted a consistent pattern of neuronal degeneration and neurofibrillary tangles, chiefly affecting the pons and midbrain. They termed this condition "heterogenous system degeneration" and, later, "progressive supranuclear palsy." Subsequent experience has confirmed these observations and progressive supranuclear palsy has gained wide recognition as a distinct entity.

Etiology. The cause of this disorder is unknown. The pathology is reminiscent of encephalitis lethargica, suggesting a chronic viral infection, although no infectious agent has been implicated and experimental attempts to transmit the disorder to primates have been unsuccessful. Familial cases have not been observed.

Pathology. Neuronal degeneration affects the substantia nigra, pontine tegmentum, the periaqueductal gray matter, and the pallidum. Degeneration of anterior horn cells in the spinal cord has been noted in some cases. The cerebral cortex is spared, although PET studies have shown reduced glucose metabolism in the frontal and temporal areas. Neurofibrillary tangles of the globose type are prominent in the affected areas. Ultrastructural studies have shown interlacing bundles of straight filaments 150 A in diameter.

Symptoms and Signs. Impairment of gait is usually the first sign of supranuclear palsy; there are transient episodes of unsteadiness in which the patient suddenly falls for no apparent reason, usually backward and after a brief retropulsion. Diplopia is also a common initial symptom. Later, there is a general slowness and stiffness of movement. Many patients have a mild resting tremor of one or both hands, which can lead to the erroneous diagnosis of parkinsonism. Treatment with levodopa may provide some improvement especially of the rigidity, tremor, and bradykinesia. However, other features that do not respond to this treatment subsequently develop. Most commonly, ocular movements are impaired and the coordination of head and eye movement is disturbed. A characteristic feature is the preservation of ocular movement on oculocephalic maneuvers, indicating that the ocular palsy is supranuclear in origin. Vertical gaze is usually more severely impaired than lateral gaze. The patient cannot look down or flex the neck to use head movement to compensate for the impaired ocular motility (Fig. 119–1). Sustained frontalis contraction, lid retraction, and infrequent eyeblink give the patient a surprised facial expression. Eyelid opening and closing apraxia are common. Progression of the gait disturbance and severe rigidity may confine the patient to bed and chair within a few years. Typically, the patient walks on a broad base, shuffling with short steps, and falls backward if unsupported. Progressive dysarthria ultimately renders speech unintelligible; dysphagia predisposes to aspiration pneumonitis. Dementia occurs in many patients. Pseudobulbar emotional incontinence develops in many later in the course. Convulsive seizures may occur. Intense rigidity of the posterior cervical muscles results in nuchal hyperextension. The patient eventually succumbs to intercurrent infection. Sleep disorders have been noted in advanced cases and sleep apnea may contribute to the patient's death. The course is one of inexorable deterioration culminating in death in 6 to 10 years.

Laboratory Data. Routine laboratory investigations are normal. The EEG may show some slowing and disorganization without localizing features. Atrophy of the pons and midbrain may be noted on CT. CSF examinations have been unremarkable.

Diagnosis. The triad of mental disorder, supranuclear ophthalmoplegia, and abnormal gait, present in 80% or more of the patients, should suggest this diagnosis. The chief differential diagnosis is Parkinson disease. Differentiation from olivopontocerebellar atrophy with ophthalmoplegia may be difficult; however, the ocular palsy in that condition preferentially affects horizontal movements. In the absence of the characteristic ocular palsy, diagnosis may be extremely difficult. Patients presenting with parkinsonian features are often diagnosed as having Parkinson disease until the characteristic ocular abnormalities appear. They comprise about 4 to 5% of patients classified as having Parkinson disease in clinical practice. Neuroimaging showing atrophy of the pontine and midbrain tegmentum but sparing the pons and cerebellum may help confirm the diagnosis of progressive supranuclear palsy.

Treatment. There is no specific treatment. Levodopa may be helpful in alleviating the parkinsonian features of rigidity, tremor, and bradykinesia, but benefit may be limited by toxic psychic effects, which tend to become prominent when dementia develops. Anticholinergic drugs administered in modest doses may be useful in controlling drooling. Tricyclic antidepressants may be used to combat depression and emotional incontinence. Cricopharyngeal myotomy may alleviate dysphagia, in some patients.

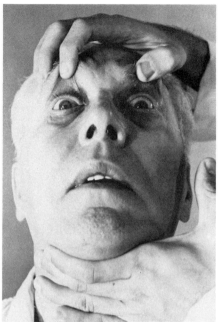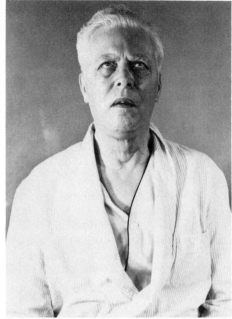

Fig. 119–1. Progressive supranuclear palsy. Oculocephalic maneuver demonstrates intact reflex downgaze in a patient unable to look down voluntarily.

References

Davis PH, Bergeron C, McLachlan DR. Atypical presentation of progressive supranuclear palsy. Ann Neurol 1985; 17:337–343.

Duvoisin RC, Golbe LI, Lepore FE. Progressive supranuclear palsy. Can J Neurol Sci 1987; 14:547–554.

Jackson JA, Jankovic J, Ford J. Progressive supranuclear palsy: clinical features and response to treatment in 16 patients. Ann Neurol 1983; 13:273–278.

Klawans HL Jr, Ringel SP. Observations on the efficacy of L-dopa in progressive supranuclear palsy. Eur Neurol 1971; 5:115–129.

Kristensen MO. Progressive supranuclear palsy—20 years later. Acta Neurol Scand 1985; 71:177–189.

Steele JC. Progressive supranuclear palsy. Brain 1972; 95:693–704.

Troost BT, Daroff RB. The ocular motor deficits in progressive supranuclear palsy. Ann Neurol 1977; 2:397–403.

120. TARDIVE DYSKINESIA

Stanley Fahn

Tardive dyskinesia is a drug-induced syndrome of persistent, abnormal, involuntary movements and commonly also of persistent *akathisia* (motor restlessness) due to chronic exposure to antipsychotic medications, such as the phenothiazines and butyrophenones, and certain other agents such as metoclopramide. These drugs block dopamine receptors and can also cause neurologic syndromes other than tardive dyskinesia. The following is a list of the adverse neurologic effects of antipsychotic drugs:

Acute Effects
    Acute idiosyncratic dystonia
    Acute akathisia
Toxic Effects
    Parkinsonism
Unexplained Effects
    Oculogyric crisis
    Neuroleptic malignant syndrome
Tardive Effects
    Classic tardive dyskinesia
Tardive akathisia
Tardive dystonia
Withdrawal emergent syndrome

Acute dystonic reactions tend to occur within the first two days of exposure to the dopamine receptor blocker and predominantly affect children and young adults. Severe twisting and uncomfortable postures of limbs, trunk, neck, tongue, and face are dramatic; these are easily reversible with parenteral administration of antihistamines (e.g., diphenhydramine 50 mg IV), anticholinergics (e.g., benztropine mesylate 2 mg IM), or diazepam (5 to 7.5 mg IM). Acute akathisia is an inner feeling of restlessness in which the patient has the urge to walk, pace, or run. It may develop as the dosage is being increased and can occur in subjects of any age. Occasionally, anticholinergics or higher dosages of antipsychotics relieve this symptom.

Drug-induced parkinsonism is a toxic reaction (i.e., a feature of overdosage). It resembles idiopathic parkinsonism in manifesting all the cardinal signs of the syndrome. Levodopa is not effective in reversing this complication probably because the dopamine receptors are blocked and occupied by the antipsychotic agent. Oral anticholinergic drugs and amantadine are effective. Upon withdrawal of the offending antipsychotic drug, the symptoms slowly disappear in weeks or months.

Oculogyric crisis is a form of dystonia in which the eyes are conjugately deviated in a fixed posture for minutes or hours. In contrast to acute dystonic reactions, oculogyric crisis can occur any time in the course of antipsychotic drug therapy and can develop in adults as well as in children. Although it may be a toxic state, it can be relieved by the same drugs that are used to treat acute idiosyncratic dystonia. The least understood neuroleptic complication is the *neuroleptic malignant syndrome*. It is characterized by a triad of fever, signs of autonomic dysfunction (e.g., pallor, diaphoresis, blood pressure instability, tachycardia, pulmonary congestion, tachypnea), and a movement disorder (e.g., akinesia, hypertonicity, or dyskinesia). Stupor, coma, and death are not uncommon. Withdrawal of antipsychotic medication and supportive therapy are the recommended treatment. The antipsychotic medication can later be restarted without recurrence of the syndrome.

Tardive dyskinesia, tardive akathisia, and tardive dystonia are the most feared complications of antipsychotic medications because the symptoms are frequently persistent and often permanent. *Tardive dyskinesia* consists of repetitive (stereotypic) rapid movements. The lower part of the face is most often involved; this orolingual-buccal dyskinesia resembles continual chewing movements, with the tongue intermittently darting out of the mouth ("fly-catcher" tongue). Movements of the trunk may cause a repetitive pattern of flexion and extension ("body-rocking"). The distal parts of the limbs may show incessant flexion-extension movements ("piano-playing" fingers and toes), whereas the proximal muscles are usually spared. When the patient stands, there may be repetitive movements of the legs ("marching-in-place"). Superficially, the gait may appear unaffected, but the arms tend to swing more than normal and the

stride may be lengthened. The patient may not be aware of the dyskinesia unless there is an associated *tardive akathisia*. In contrast to acute akathisia, the delayed type tends to become worse when antipsychotic medication is withdrawn, similar to the worsening of tardive dyskinesia on discontinuing these drugs. As with tardive dyskinesia, tardive akathisia tends to persist. Sometimes patients feel as if they are going to jump out of their skins. Akathisia can be a most distressing symptom.

The prevalence of tardive dyskinesia increases with age, and it is most common among elderly women. It is more likely to occur with exposure to high dosages and longer duration of treatment with antipsychotic drugs. The exact time of onset is difficult to discern because antipsychotic drugs mask the symptom. Reducing the dosage or discontinuing the drug can unmask the disorder. Reinstituting the drug hides the symptoms again. Dyskinesia is a complication of drugs that block and bind with the dopamine receptor, but it has not been reported as a complication of dopamine-depleting drugs, such as reserpine. Supersensitivity of dopamine receptors is probably an underlying feature of the disorder, but other unknown factors are also necessary.

Not all cases of oral *dyskinesia* are tardive dyskinesia. There are many other choreic and nonchoreic causes. Essential to the diagnosis of tardive dyskinesia is a history of exposure to dopamine receptor-blocking drugs. For this diagnosis, the symptoms should have started while the patient was still taking the drug or less than three months after discontinuing the drug. If oral dyskinesia is induced by other types of drugs, it is not, by definition, tardive dyskinesia. The following list outlines the classification of oral dyskinesia.

> Chorea (orolingual-buccal dyskinesia)
> > Encephalitis lethargica; postencephalitic
> > Drug-induced
> > > Tardive dyskinesia (antipsychotics)
> > > Levodopa
> > > Anticholinergic drugs
> > > Phenytoin intoxication
> > > Antihistamines
> > > Tricyclic antidepressants
> > Huntington disease
> > Hepatocerebral degeneration
> > Cerebellar infarction
> > Edentulous malocclusion
> > Idiopathic
> Dystonia

Meige syndrome
   Complete: oromandibular dystonia
      plus blepharospasm
   Incomplete syndromes
      Mandibular dystonia
      Orofacial dystonia
      Lingual dystonia
      Pharyngeal dystonia
      Essential blepharospasm
   Bruxism
   As part of segmental or generalized
      dystonic syndrome
Myoclonus and Tics
   Facial tics
   Facial myoclonus of central origin
   Facial nerve irritability
      Hemifacial spasm
      Myokymia
      Faulty regeneration; synkinesis
Tremor
   Essential tremor of neck and jaw
   Parkinsonian tremor of jaw, tongue,
      and lips
   Idiopathic tremor of neck, jaw, tongue,
      or lips

Huntington disease is the most common differential diagnosis of the oral choreic dyskinesias, and the dystonic oral dyskinesia referred to as *Meige syndrome* (oromandibular dystonia) is probably the most common form of spontaneous oral dyskinesia. Clinical features differentiating these disorders from classic tardive dyskinesia are presented in Tables 120–1 and 120–2. Patients with Huntington disease are frequently treated with antipsychotic drugs; a resulting tardive dyskinesia may be superimposed on the chorea.

Table 120–1. Clinical Features of Tardive Dyskinesia (TD) and Huntington Disease (HD)

Clinical Signs	TD	HD
Impersistent protrusion of tongue	–	+
Milk-maid grip	–	+
Postural instability	–	+
Forehead chorea	–	+
Oro-lingual-buccal dyskinesia	+	±
Repetitive choreic movements	+	–
Flowing choreic movements	–	+
Body-rocking movements	+	–
Marching in place	+	–
Stuttering-ataxic gait	–	+
Akathisia	+	–

+ present
– absent
± occasionally present

Table 120–2. Clinical Features of Tardive Dyskinesia (TD) and Meige Syndrome

Clinical Signs	Commonly Present In	
	TD	Meige
Type of involuntary movements	choreic	dystonic
Mouth/face	+ + +	+ + +
Blepharospasm	+	+ + +
Platysma	±	+ + +
Masticatory muscles	+ + +	+ + +
Nuchal muscles	+	+ +
Trunk, legs	+	–
Stereotypy	+ + +	–
Akathisia	+ +	–

– never seen
± may be seen
+ occasionally seen
+ + usually seen
+ + + always seen

The presence of akathisia or repetitive (stereotyped) involuntary movements suggests the additional diagnosis of tardive dyskinesia.

Efforts should be made to avoid tardive dyskinesia. Antipsychotic drugs should be given only when indicated, namely to control psychosis or a few other conditions where no other effective agent has been helpful, as in some choreic disorders or tics. These drugs should not be used indiscriminately and, when used, the dosage and duration should be as low and as brief as possible. If the psychosis has been controlled, the physician should attempt to reduce the dosage and even try to eliminate the drug, if possible. Once classic tardive dyskinesia or tardive akathisia has appeared, treatment depends on eliminating the causative agents, the antipsychotic drugs. Unfortunately, psychosis may no longer be under control if these drugs are withdrawn; the medication is required and increasing the dosage may suppress the dyskinesia and akathisia. If the antipsychotic drug can be safely tapered and discontinued, the dyskinesia and akathisia may slowly subside in months or years. If the dyskinetic or akathitic symptoms are too distressful, treatment with dopamine-depleting drugs may suppress them. Reserpine is the preferred drug; the dosage should be increased gradually to avoid the side effects of postural hypotension or depression. A dosage of 6 mg/day or more may be required. Addition of alpha-methyltyrosine may be necessary to relieve symptoms, but this combination is more likely to cause postural hypotension and parkinsonism. With time, these dopamine-depleting drugs may eventually be tapered and discontinued.

There are two clinical variations of tardive dyskinesia. One is the *withdrawal emergent syndrome*, in which the choreic movements that appear when the antipsychotic drug is suddenly discontinued resemble those of Sydenham chorea or Huntington disease. These are flowing, rather than repetitive, choreic movements. The withdrawal emergent syndrome is most common in children and is self-limiting. Reintroducing the antipsychotic drug and tapering it slowly may eliminate the choreic movements. The other variant is *tardive dystonia*, in which the involuntary movements are dystonic rather than rapid and repetitive. Tardive dystonia can occur in either children or in adults. The clinical picture resembles idiopathic or hereditary torsion dystonia, with leg as well as axial involvement in children and with face and neck involvement in adults. Tardive dystonia persists, but some patients may respond to do-pamine-depleting drugs and others to anticholinergic agents.

References

Burke RE, Fahn S, Jankovic J, Marsden CD, Lang AE, Gollomp S, Ilson J. Tardive dystonia: late-onset and persistent dystonia caused by antipsychotic drugs. Neurology 1982; 32:1335–1346.

Fahn S. The tardive dyskinesias. In: Matthews WB, Glaser GH, eds. Recent Advances in Clinical Neurology, vol 4. Edinburgh: Churchill Livingstone, 1984:229–260.

Fahn S. A therapeutic approach to tardive dyskinesia. J Clin Psychiatry 1985; 46:19–24.

Friedman J, Feinberg SS, Feldman RG. A neuroleptic malignant-like syndrome due to L-dopa withdrawal. Ann Neurol 1984; 16:126–127.

Henderson VW, Wooten GF. Neuroleptic malignant syndrome: A pathogenetic role for dopamine receptor blockade? Neurology 1981; 31:132–137.

Kang UJ, Burke RE, Fahn S. Natural history and treatment of tardive dystonia. Movement Disorders 1986; 1:193–208.

Smith JM, Baldessarini RJ. Changes in prevalence, severity and recovery in tardive dyskinesia with age. Arch Gen Psychiatry 1980; 37:1368–1373.

Tanner CM, Klawans HL. Tardive dyskinesia: prevention and treatment. Clin Neuropharmacol 1986; 9(Suppl 2):S76–S84.

Chapter XV

Spinal Cord Diseases

121. HEREDITARY SPASTIC PARAPLEGIA

Lewis P. Rowland

The term *hereditary spastic paraplegia* implies a condition that affects the corticospinal tracts alone. However, even in Strumpell's original report of a family in 1880, the spinocerebellar tracts were involved at autopsy. The term has continued to be applied to familial cases in which abnormal clinical signs are restricted to the corticospinal tracts or in which other neurologic abnormalities are relatively inconspicuous.

The syndrome is clearly heterogeneous. Some cases start in early life, some in adolescence, and some in middle life. Some are seriously disabling while others are less serious and compatible with a productive and full life. Some are inherited in autosomal dominant fashion, some are autosomal recessive, and some are X-linked.

Heterogeneity is also evident in associated signs. Although the essential feature should be a progressive gait disorder with upper motor neuron signs, other systems have been found to have been affected at autopsy or are implicated by abnormalities in visual or somatosensory evoked responses. Even clinically, some cases of spastic paraparesis are associated with distal wasting and amyotrophy, some with mild cerebellar signs, and some with proprioceptive sensory loss; if these signs were more evident, the disorder would be linked to inherited spinocerebellar degenerations. Other clinical variations include association with optic atrophy or retinitis pigmentosa. The *Sjögren-Larsson syndrome* combines congenital ichthyosis, spastic paraplegia, and mental retardation; about 35% of the cases also have retinitis pigmentosa.

No biochemical abnormality has been identified in any form of hereditary spastic para-

plegia except for adrenoleucodystrophy, which is discussed in Section 84. In one family, blood and urinary levels of glycine were abnormally high but the site of abnormal metabolism was not identified, and few other families have been so studied.

It is clear that many different disorders are subsumed by this title; it will probably take molecular DNA analysis to separate the fundamental types. Sporadic cases of spastic paraparesis could be new mutations, but most of them seem to be due to multiple sclerosis. The evaluation of any sporadic case of spastic paraplegia should include evoked potential studies, CSF examination (including gamma globulin and oligoclonal bands), and MRI to evaluate the possibility of multiple sclerosis, compressive lesions of the upper cervical spinal cord or region of the foramen magnum, Chiari malformation, and syringomyelia.

References

Baraitsen M. The Genetics of Neurological Disorders. Oxford: Oxford University Press, 1982: 200–210.

Beal MF, Richardson EP. Primary lateral sclerosis: a case report. Arch Neurol 1981; 38:30–33.

Boustany R, Fleischnick E, Alper C, et al. The autosomal dominant form of pure spastic paraplegia. Neurology 1987; 37:910–915.

Harding AE. The hereditary ataxias and related disorders. Edinburgh: Churchill Livingstone, 1984.

Holmes GL, Shaywitz BA. Strumpell's pure familial spastic paraplegia: case study and review of the literature. J Neurol Neurosurg Psychiatry 1977; 40:1007–1008.

Johnson AW, McKusick VA. A sex-linked recessive form of spastic paraplegia. Am J Hum Genet 1962; 14:83–94.

Kempster PA, Iansek, Balla JI, Dennis PM, Biegler B. Value of visual evoked response and oligoclonal bands in CSF in diagnosis of spinal multiple sclerosis. Lancet 1987; 1:769–771.

McLeod JG, Morgan JA, Reye C. Electrophysiological studies in familial spastic paraplegia. J Neurol Neurosurg Psychiatry 1970; 40:611–615.

Miller DH, McDonald WI, Blumhardt L, et al. Magnetic resonance imaging in isolated noncompressive spinal cord syndromes. Ann Neurol 1987; 22:714–723.

Noetzel MJ, Landau WM, Moser HW. Adrenoleuco-dystrophy carrier state presenting as a chronic non-progressive spinal cord disorder. Arch Neurol 1987; 44:566–568.

Pajunas KW, McQuillen MP. Cranial MRI in the evaluation of myelopathy of unknown origin. Neurology 1987; 37:840–843.

Pedersen L, Trojaborg W. Visual, auditory and somato-sensory involvement in hereditary cerebellar ataxia, Friedreich's ataxia, and familial spastic paraplegia. EEG Clin Neurophysiol 1981; 52:283–297.

Rothschild H, Happel L, Rampp D, Hackett E. Autosomal recessive spastc paraplegia: involvement above the spinal cord. Clin Genet 1979; 15:356–360.

Younger DS, Chou S, Hays AP et al. Primary lateral sclerosis—a clinical diagnosis re-emerges. Arch Neurol 1988; 45:1304–1307.

Zatz M, Penha-Serrano C, Otto PA. X-linked recessive type of pure spastic paraplegia in a large pedigree: absence of detectable linkage with Xg. J Med Genet 1976; 13:217–222.

122. SPINAL MUSCULAR ATROPHIES

Theodore L. Munsat

The spinal muscular atrophies are motor neuron diseases that affect only the lower motor neuron (alpha motoneuron). Other neurosystems and organ systems are spared. The spinal muscular atrophies differ from amyotrophic lateral sclerosis (ALS) because there are no upper motor neuron signs. In addition, spinal muscular atrophies usually begin in childhood, whereas ALS is a disease of late life. Some 50% of spinal muscular atrophies are inherited; ALS is rarely inherited. The spinal muscular atrophies constitute a clinically heterogeneous group. The degree of genetic heterogeneity remains to be demonstrated. The true incidence and clinical heterogeneity became apparent when histochemical techniques improved our ability to differentiate denervating conditions from myopathies. For example, more than 50% of patients previously diagnosed as having limb-girdle muscular dystrophy have, in fact, spinal muscular atrophy. On the other hand, some patients with what seems at first to be spinal muscular atrophy later develop evidence of a mixed motor-sensory peripheral neuropathy that evolves into the Charcot-Marie-Tooth syndrome.

Generalized Forms

The spinal muscular atrophies can best be classified by the topographic neuroanatomic distribution of damage and by the age of onset. The prototype spinal muscular atrophy is the infantile form *(Werdnig-Hoffmann disease).*

Werdnig-Hoffmann disease is usually evident within the first few weeks of life. It is one of the more common causes of the floppy infant syndrome (Fig. 122–1). Intrauterine movement may be depressed. Contractures at birth are uncommon but may be seen. The weakness is symmetric and involves all limbs, trunks, and respiratory muscles. Cardiac muscle is spared. The tendon reflexes are depressed or absent. Oropharyngeal muscles are almost always involved and tongue fasciculations can be seen in over 50%. The cry is weak and sucking is impaired. Aspiration is a constant threat and impaired coughing frequently leads to pneumonitis.

The weakness is progressive with a reduction in all voluntary motor activities. Death occurs within a few years. Although there is controversy about "benign" cases of longer survival, it is generally agreed that onset before age 6 months has a poor prognosis. Autosomal recessive inheritance occurs in about 50% of cases. As yet there is no reliable way to detect the heterozygote. Affected siblings usually have a similar course, although there are exceptions.

Later onset cases, with generalized involvement, evolve much more slowly and have a better prognosis *(Kugelberg-Welander syndrome*—Fig. 122–2). Onset may be in later childhood or even in adulthood. Unless fasciculation is seen in limb muscles, the syndrome is clinically indistinguishable from limb-girdle muscular dystrophy. The oropharyngeal muscles are usually spared in the late-onset cases and inheritance may be autosomal recessive or dominant, or even X-linked. Whether cases with intermediate age of onset warrant separate classification is unclear. The adequacy of respiratory function is the most important determinant of the course of Kugelberg-Welander syndrome.

In addition to the classic findings of denervation, the EMG in the more benign cases reveals spontaneous motor unit discharge at rates of 5 to 51 Hz, even during sleep. The serum creatine kinase may be two or three times the upper limit of normal. Muscle biopsy is helpful in making an accurate diagnosis, especially in late-onset forms. In Werdnig-Hoffmann disease, the changes are usually characteristic if an affected muscle is sampled. The histologic and histochemical changes do not correlate with severity or prognosis. Muscle fiber diameters tend to have a bimodal distribution with normal or even enlarged fibers and markedly atrophic

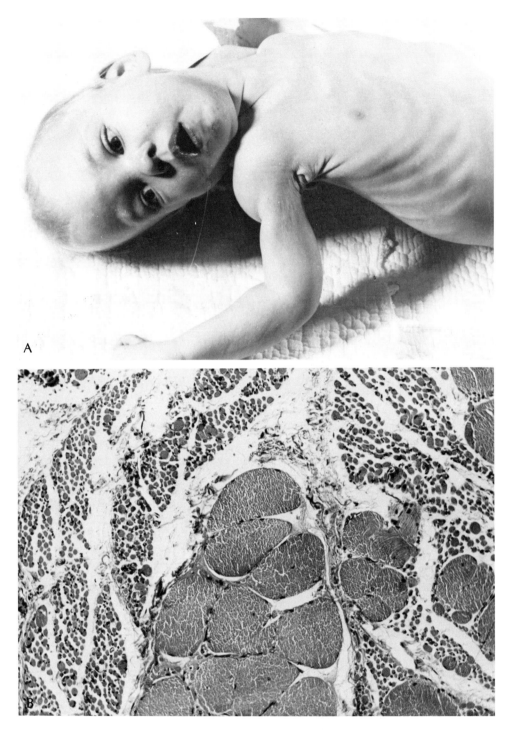

Fig. 122–1. *A.* Infantile, generalized, spinal muscular atrophy (Werdnig-Hoffmann disease). This baby was hypotonic and weak at birth and had difficulty swallowing and respiratory insufficiency. Progressive weakness caused death at 8 months. *B.* Muscle biopsy at 1 month revealed bimodal distribution of fiber diameters. The atrophic fibers were rounded and fetal in appearance. The others were hypertrophied but otherwise normal.

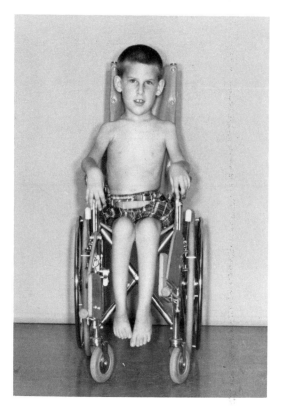

Fig. 122–2. This 6-year-old boy developed generalized weakness at 6 months. Motor milestones were delayed but he did walk for a few months before becoming wheelchair confined. No definite progression was ever noted. Muscle biopsy and EMG were consistent with a denervating process. An example of later onset generalized spinal muscular atrophy (Kugelberg-Hoffmann disease) with a much more favorable course than Werdnig-Hoffmann disease.

fibers that are 5 μm to 15 μm in diameter (see Fig. 122–1B). These atrophic fibers are rounded, without angulation, and are distributed in groups or large sheets. They are of both fiber types, although accurate identification of type is often difficult. Evidence of reinnervation (fiber-type grouping) may be extensive or it may be absent (Fig. 122–3).

In the chronic cases, particularly those lasting more than 10 years, biopsy features that are usually found in myopathies can be observed, which may lead to diagnostic confusion. These features include variation in fiber diameter, internally placed nuclei, degenerative changes such as necrosis and phagocytosis, and increased fat and connective tissue. The EMG may be diagnostically decisive in such cases.

Focal Forms

The advent of histochemical techniques and EMG provided evidence that many cases of focal atrophy and weakness were neurogenic. Some patients with slowly progressive weakness and wasting in *facioscapulohumeral* distribution have biopsy or EMG findings of a denervating disease. Some of these cases are inherited in an autosomal dominant fashion, as in facioscapulohumeral dystrophy. The course progresses slowly. Similarly, some patients with a *scapuloperoneal* or distal arm distribution of weakness may show signs of a denervating process. Prominent cranial nerve involvement in children is seen in the *Fazio-Londe syndrome.*

In some patients, slowly progressive anterior horn cell disease may be focal, involving only part of a large muscle, such as the quadriceps or gastrocnemius. The lesions may be symmetric or they may seem random and asymmetric (Fig. 122–4). The course is slowly progressive with no involvement of sensory pathways or upper motor neuron deficit. The term *benign focal amyotrophy* describes this syndrome.

Secondary Spinal Muscular Atrophy

Generalized spinal muscular atrophy of late onset may be associated with a definable underlying condition. It is important to identify these cases because treatment of the underlying disease may cause improvement or even cure of the anterior horn cell degeneration. Such cases can be seen in association with plasma cell dyscrasias. Lead toxicity may sometimes produce a similar clinical picture. Hexosaminidase deficiency may account for inherited forms of spinal muscular atrophy.

Postpolio Syndrome

Patients who had paralytic poliomyelitis early in life and whose neurologic deficit had been stable note increasing weakness years or decades after the initial attack. If these patients are observed long enough, they seem to be slowly losing strength—most likely from the additional loss of motor units that had become enlarged and functionally more important with reinnervation. This postpolio syndrome is not ALS; upper motor neuron signs do not develop (unless there is cord compression from scoliosis) and the evolution is extremely slow. The new motor neuron loss characteristically begins in muscles previously affected by polio, then spreads to homologous muscles on the other side of the

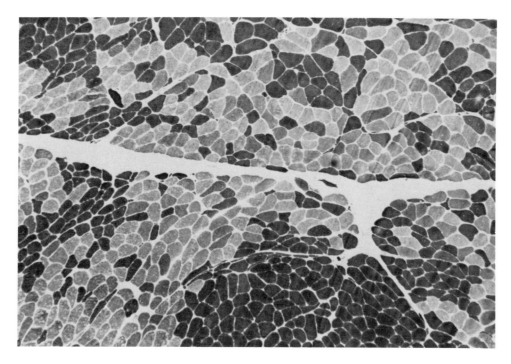

Fig. 122–3. Fiber type grouping is the most reliable indication of denervation-reinnervation. Groups of similarly reacting fibers are often demarcated by fascicular boundaries, which presumably guide the regenerating nerve. Reinnervated fibers may be of normal size. If histochemical studies are not done, diagnosis can easily be missed. ATPase at pH 9.6.

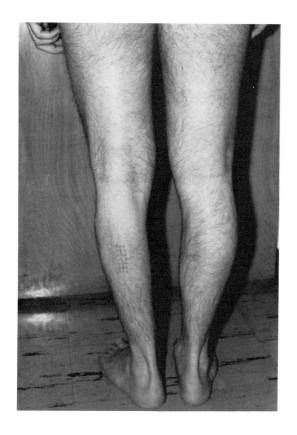

Fig. 122–4. This 24-year-old man first noticed painless, slowly progressive atrophy of his left calf at age 20. Examination revealed atrophy and weakness of the left gastrocnemius and left deltoid with no reflex or sensory change. The myelogram was normal. Biopsy and EMG revealed denervation with reinnervation. Example of benign focal amyotrophy.

body, and eventually to muscles that were presumably unaffected by the previous attack. The pathogenesis of this condition is not known, but could be the normal age-related loss of motor units. However, late progression can be observed in young adults. Reactivation of latent virus or late effects of earlier neuronal injury have also been considered, but poliomyelitis antibody titers do not increase during the period of progression.

Signs and Symptoms. Although the primary process in spinal muscular atrophy is one of denervation, overt fasciculations are seen in less than 50% of the cases. They are most easily seen in the tongue in affected children, and over the thorax in adults. Intramuscular administration of 1 mg neostigmine often brings out latent fasciculation. In the generalized form, weakness is often more marked proximally, but in many cases it is difficult to determine a proximal or distal gradient. The reflexes are depressed throughout, even in the focal forms. Intellect is not only spared, but children with slowly evolving or static disease seem to function at a higher level than controls. Secondary contractures and skeletal deformities are a major deterrent to functional performance and can be prevented.

Etiology. The etiology of the spinal muscular atrophies is uncertain. Some cases begin in the setting of an infection; others begin after immunization. Autosomal dominant, autosomal recessive, and X-linked recessive inheritance has been recorded. These observations suggest there are several different causes. Pathologic studies have been of little help, although gliosis in motor nerve roots suggests that the cell body may not always be the site of primary damage. Studies seeking to identify a defective gene by recombinant DNA techniques are in progress.

Treatment. Genetic counseling, psychosocial support, and prevention of damaging secondary effects of the denervation are the main therapies. In the late-onset and more benign forms, it is particularly important to recognize and prevent contractures and scoliosis because these patients often become productive individuals with satisfying lives. Scoliosis must be watched carefully; decompensation can occur rapidly with life-threatening cardiopulmonary compromise. Appropriately timed surgical release of contractures and vertebral fixation can be beneficial. Intrauterine diagnosis is not yet possible.

References

Albers JW, Zimmowodzki S, Lowrey CM, Miller B. Juvenile progressive bulbar palsy. Arch Neurol 1983, 40:351–353.

Dalakas MC, Elder G, Hallett M, et al. A long-term follow-up study of patients with post-poliomyelitis neuromuscular symptoms. N Engl J Med 1986; 314:959–963.

Furukawa T, Toyokura Y. Chronic spinal muscular atrophy of the facioscapulohumeral type. J Med Genet 1976; 13:285–289.

Harding AE, Bradbury PG, Murray NMF. Chronic asymmetrical spinal muscular atrophy. J Neurol Sci 1983; 59:69–83.

Hausmanowa-Petrusewicz I, Borkowska J, Janczewski Z. X-linked adult form of spinal muscular atrophy. J Neurol 1983; 229:175–188.

Howard RS, Wiles CM, Spencer GT. The late sequelae of poliomyelitis. Quart J Med 1988; 66:219–232.

Johnson WG, Wigger HJ, Karp HR, Glaubiger LM, Rowland LP. Juvenile spinal muscular atrophy: A new hexosaminidase deficiency phenotype. Ann Neurol 1982; 32:11–16.

Kugelberg E, Welander L. Familial neurogenic muscular atrophy simulating ordinary proximal dystrophy. Acta Psychiatr Scand 1954; 29:42–43.

Munsat TL, Woods RK, Fowler WM, Pearson CM. Neurogenic muscular atrophy of infancy with prolonged survival. The variable course of Werdnig-Hoffmann disease. Brain 1969: 92:9–24.

Parry GJ, Holtz S, Ben-Zeen D, Drori, JB. Gammopathy with proximal motor axonopathy simulating motor neuron disease. Neurology 1986; 36:273–276.

Pearn JH, Carter CO, Wilson J. The genetic identity of acute infantile spinal muscular atrophy. Brain 1973; 96:463–470.

Pearn J. Classification of spinal muscular atrophies. Lancet 1980; 1:919–922.

Peggs JE, Schochet SS Jr, Gutmann L. Benign focal amyotrophy. Arch Neurol 1984; 34:678–679.

Rowland LP, ed. Human Motor Neuron Diseases. New York: Raven Press, 1982.

Russman BS, Melchreit R, Drennan JC. Spinal muscular atrophy: the natural course of disease. Muscle Nerve 1983; 6:179–181.

123. ADULT MOTOR NEURON DISEASES
Theodore L. Munsat

The motor neuron diseases are characterized by selective damage to the neural systems that mediate voluntary movement. There is a striking lack of involvement of other pathways; sensation, cognition, autonomic function, and other organ systems are spared. These diseases represent a system degeneration in the purest sense. The subgroups may be defined clinically by the relative involvement of lower motor neuron or upper motor neuron function, topographical damage within the brain or spinal cord, and the patient's age at onset. Although still speculative, there is reason to believe that the causes of these conditions are multiple.

Amyotrophic Lateral Sclerosis

Credit for the first accurate description and clinicopathologic correlation of amyotrophic lateral sclerosis (ALS) should go to Charcot, although there were earlier descriptions of the disease. Charcot pointed out the unique involvement of lateral columns and anterior gray matter and noted that these two areas of the spinal cord were closely connected. Subsequently, a number of overlapping and confusing terms were used to describe the disorder because it lacked defined biochemical or clinical features.

ALS is confined to the voluntary motor system, with progressive degeneration of corticospinal tracts and alpha motoneurons. Clinical signs of both upper and lower motor neuron disease should be present for a definite diagnosis. Although upper motor neuron *(primary lateral sclerosis)* or lower motor neuron *(progressive muscular atrophy)* signs may predominate at the onset, both will be present within a few years in most cases. ALS is defined as much by the absence of other neurologic and organ system involvement as it is by the positive findings. Another important exclusion is the sparing of voluntary eye muscles and urinary sphincters. Within this constellation of clinical findings, there are at least four subgroups: familial, Guamanian, secondary, and sporadic.

FAMILIAL

ALS is familial and presumably inherited in 8 to 10% of cases. Inheritance is usually autosomal dominant, or less often, recessive. Intrafamilial variability is minor. In contrast to sporadic forms, in which the pathologic changes are limited to the lateral columns and anterior horn cells, pathologic changes may also be found in the spinocerebellar tracts and posterior columns, although there is no clinical evidence of these additional lesions. The biochemical abnormality is not known, but hexosaminidase is lacking in some autosomal recessive forms.

GUAMANIAN

The previously extraordinarily high incidence of ALS among the Chamorros on Guam (50–100 times the incidence anywhere else in the world) has attracted attention for many years. Recent evidence strongly suggests that an excitotoxin contained in the cycad nut was the responsible agent. The clinical disease is similar to sporadic ALS elsewhere. However, the pathologic changes are more widespread, as in the familial form. On Guam, ALS is often associated with components of the Parkinson-dementia complex.

SECONDARY

In older textbooks of neurology, there were frequent references to ALS as a result of syphilis, mercury toxicity, or hypoglycemia. With current advanced diagnostic technology and better clinical acumen, diagnostic errors are rarely made, but there are still a few conditions that may require consideration as secondary forms of ALS. A suspected association with carcinoma has not been substantiated, but motor neuron syndromes do occur with plasma cell dyscrasias such as multiple myeloma and macroglobulinemia, although upper motor neuron findings are sometimes minor or completely lacking in these cases. Occasionally, lead neurotoxicity can cause both upper and lower motor neuron signs. The most difficult differential diagnosis is between ALS and cervical spondylosis, especially if an element of lumbosacral root disease is also present. Cervical vertebral surgery may be indicated in these cases, even if the diagnosis is uncertain.

SPORADIC

This is the most common form of ALS seen in everyday practice. Except for the endemic areas in the Southwestern Pacific, there are remarkably constant prevalence (4–6/100,000) and incidence (0.8–1.2/100,000) rates with a death rate of about 50/100,000. There are no significant racial or ethnic patterns. Chamorros who emigrate from endemic to nonendemic areas early in life have an incidence lower than those who do not relocate, but higher than residents of the country to which they move. Searches to detect environmental determinants have revealed statistical correlations with animal-hide exposure, high milk consumption, heavy metals, and exercise, but the significance of these studies has been challenged.

Clinical Features. ALS is a disease of middle and late life and only rarely begins in patients in their 20s or 30s. The incidence may increase in a linear manner with advancing age.

The initial manifestations of ALS vary depending on the proportion of upper and lower motor neuron involvement and the site of the damage within the CNS. Gait disorder, limb weakness, dysarthria or dysphagia, and loss of muscle bulk are common initial complaints. If the deficit is asymmetric at onset, it rapidly becomes symmetric. Neurologic symptoms are often accompanied or preceded by unexplained weight loss, cramps, and fasciculations. Prominent fasciculation is seen in few diseases other than ALS. Dysarthria and dysphagia are most often caused by a combination of upper and lower motor neuron deficits. Tongue atrophy and fasciculations are common and tongue movements are slowed. Intellect, sphincter control, and sensation are spared. Reflexes are increased or depressed, depending on the balance between upper and lower motor neuron deficits. Respiratory impairment, present in all patients at some point, may occur early in an otherwise intact patient. Unlike the myopathies, respiratory decompensation often occurs rapidly.

Laboratory Data. Laboratory investigations are unremarkable except for the changes of a subacute denervating process. Routine radiologic and blood studies are normal, as are the EEG and cortical evoked potentials. The cerebrospinal fluid (CSF) may reveal a slight increase in protein, about 20 mg above that expected for the patient's age, but more often it is normal. Serum creatine kinase may be elevated as much as 50% if rapid denervation is occurring. EMG alterations vary with the stage of the disease and the amount and distribution of lower motor neuron damage. In advanced disease, fibrillations and positive sharp waves are easily found and are widespread. However, in the early stages, particularly if upper motor neuron signs predominate, these changes of acute denervation may not be prominent; biopsy of an apparently normal muscle may provide useful evidence of denervation.

Motor nerve conduction velocities are slightly reduced and even sensory conduction may be slow. F-waves are reported as normal or prolonged. Diagnostic workups for occult neoplasia are not indicated, but all patients should be screened for lead toxicity, paraproteinemia, and causes of multiple nerve root compression as in cervical spondylosis. If there is no evidence of involvement above the level of the foramen magnum, a myelogram or magnetic resonance scan usually should be carried out in patients with upper motor neuron signs in both legs. When there is evidence of both upper and lower motor neuron dis-

ease in the same limb, especially a leg, myelography is not necessary.

Pathology. In sporadic cases of ALS, the pathology is nonspecific, although highly stylized anatomically (Fig. 123–1). The large motor neurons of the anterior horn cells are reduced in number. Those remaining are shrunken and contain lipofuscin. The reduction in anterior horn cells reduces the size of the anterior roots when contrasted with the posterior roots. Similar changes are seen in the brain-stem motor nuclei, except for those nuclei that innervate the ocular muscles. There is a noticeable lack of cellular reaction around degenerating and absent cells. Occasional cell bodies may contain eosinophilic inclusions *(Bunina bodies)*. Degeneration of the corticospinal tracts is nonspecific. Demyelination is presumably seondary in nature, although direct evidence of a primary axonal degeneration is lacking. Axons in the motor root exit zone often demonstrate peculiar axonal swellings that are caused by neurofilamentous aggregates, which could impede axoplasmic transport. Similar changes have been seen in canine forms of motor unit disease or some experimental toxic neuropathy.

Etiology. Of the many theories about the cause of ALS that have been considered, none has withstood the test of time and none has led to successful therapy. The theory of defective pancreatic function (both endocrine and exocrine) led to treatment with pancreatic extracts. After initial enthusiasm, it was found to be ineffective. However, the issue of the presence and nature of a defect in carbohydrate metabolism remains unresolved.

Epidemiologic study negated reports that gastrectomy may lead to degeneration of anterior horn cells, but observations that amino acid absorption may be defective in ALS and that immune complexes are deposited in the jejunal mucosa suggest a possible absorptive defect.

Rarely, immune complexes have been demonstrated in blood and in kidney; however, the significance remains unclear. Cellular immunity seems to be impaired in Guamanian ALS but not in the sporadic form. Surveys of histocompatibility antigens have revealed contradictory results that cast doubt on the significance of the studies. CSF levels of cyclic AMP were depressed, but when these were returned to normal by using phosphodiesterase inhibitors, there was no change in clinical course.

If the incidence of ALS increases in a linear

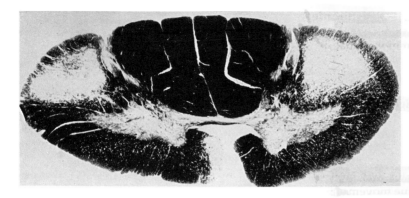

Fig. 123–1. ALS. Degeneration of lateral and anterior funiculi of spinal cord. Myelin sheath stain.

manner with age, new hypotheses may be tested; for example, age-related damage to DNA-initiated repair processes or deterioration of age-related neurotransmitter systems.

The possibility that ALS results from a slow viral infection has not been substantiated by attempts to recover the putative virus from postmortem tissue or to demonstrate poliovirus by hybridization techniques. Antiviral therapy has been unsuccessful. As attractive as the viral hypothesis may be, there is little evidence to support it.

Prognosis. ALS is a progressive disease, a feature that is often useful in making a diagnosis. Although more protracted cases can be seen, death usually occurs within 5 years of onset, especially when there are both upper and lower motor neuron signs. Cases of longer duration have few if any upper motor neuron signs, and are probably more appropriately regarded as spinal muscular atrophy. Although patients with oropharyngeal symptoms may have a shorter course, this is usually because of aspiration rather than because the disease is inherently more malignant; these patients are generally older and less able to tolerate the general stress of a chronic disease. If respiratory assistance is given and nutrition maintained, patients can live for many years in a totally dependent condition. Recent quantitation of strength change has revealed a remarkably linear rate of decline (Fig. 123–2). Although the rate of deterioration is equal in homologous parts of the body, different regions may deteriorate at different rates.

Treatment. No medical therapy alters the rate of deterioration. Many therapeutic agents have been tried, including pancreatic extracts, antiviral drugs, phosphodiesterase inhibitors, gangliosides, reptile venoms, and plasmapheresis, with and without immunosuppression. Initial enthusiasm was short-lived when further studies proved disappointing. Recently, therapeutic benefit with thyrotropin-releasing hormone has been reported, but this remains controversial.

However, much can be done for ALS patients to make their condition more tolerable. Difficult decisions must be made, including whether to make the patient as comfortable as possible or to prolong life at all costs.

Baclofen, a GABA derivative with anti-spasticity activity, can aid patients with prominent upper motor neuron signs. It may relieve both oropharyngeal and limb spasticity. Unfortunately, the response is often brief. Diazepam can also be used, but the hepatotoxicity of dantrolene precludes its use. Prominent sialorrhea can be an early and disturbing symptom. Trihexiphenidyl, amitriptyline, or atropine may be of benefit. Some patients show a modest response to neostigmine. Cramps, which can be very disturbing in the

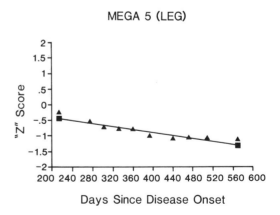

MEGA 5 (LEG)

Days Since Disease Onset

Fig. 123–2. Plot of combined strength of selected muscles in both legs (Mega 5) against time in a single ALS patient. "Z" score is standard deviation units of reference group of ALS patients. Note linearity of regression line. Although rates of deterioration vary between patients and in different regions of same patient, linearity of change is constant.

early phases of ALS, often respond to baclofen.

Vocal cord injections to reduce the risk of aspiration and cricopharyngeal myotomy to decrease dysphagia have been advocated. Tracheotomy should only be carried out if patient and family have been fully informed about the quality of prolonged life on a respirator. Feeding gastrostomy or esophagostomy may be useful.

A compassionate, understanding, and knowledgeable physician can make the difference between a family that decompensates under the stress of the diagnosis, and one that is able to weather the many crises in this difficult illness.

Primary Lateral Sclerosis and Familial Spastic Paraparesis

Primary lateral sclerosis is a neurologic illness of progressive upper motor neuron loss without clinical or pathologic damage to lower motor neurons. In the early stages, it is not possible to determine whether the syndrome will evolve into true ALS. If evidence of lower motor neuron deficit is not present within 2 years of the onset of symptoms, it is unlikely to develop subsequently. The patient can be considered to have primary lateral sclerosis. Symptoms most frequently begin in the legs with a progressive spastic gait disturbance. It evolves slowly but progressively for years or decades. The progression is linear, eventually spreading to involve the arms, then speech and swallowing. In contrast to ALS, upper motor neuron bladder dysfunction is common and posterior column loss may be seen.

The nature of this condition is unclear. Few complete autopsies have been performed in uncomplicated cases because longevity is not significantly affected. The damage is nonspecific and limited to corticobulbar and corticospinal tracts. If there is a positive family history, these cases are usually classified as related to the spinocerebellar degenerations (familial spastic paraparesis). Some cases may have the metabolic defect associated with adrenoleukodystrophy, while others appear to have a demyelinating disorder.

Most cases of spastic paraparesis in middle life are caused by demyelination that is manifested by abnormal visual evoked responses, CSF evidence of increased gamma globulin content, oligoclonal bands and especially abnormal cranial MRI. The compressive lesions of cervical spondylosis may also cause spastic paraparesis. Tropical spastic paraparesis has been recorded in association with HTLV I infection.

PROGRESSIVE MUSCULAR ATROPHY

Many patients with clinical evidence of lower motor neuron disease have upper motor neuron degeneration at autopsy. However, if upper motor neuron signs do not develop within 2 years, it seems unlikely that ALS will develop. These patients usually continue with a slowly evolving lower motor neuron disease that is more appropriately considered a spinal muscular atrophy.

PROGRESSIVE BULBAR PALSY

Some patients with ALS present with symptoms restricted to dysarthria and dysphagia. These cases are often first seen by otolaryngologists. The oropharyngeal dysfunction, as it progresses, is due to both upper and lower motor neuron disorders; tongue atrophy, fasciculations, and emotional lability are characteristic. Occasionally, the disseminated nature of the disease can be demonstrated by EMG or muscle biopsy, and within a few or several months, the limbs become clinically involved. Because of the important function of the involved muscles and the fact that patients with bulbar onset are older, the outlook is less favorable.

Progressive bulbar palsy in childhood has been called Fazio-Londe disease. The age of onset is between 2 and 12 years and the course may be rapidly progressive or evolve over several years, terminating in death from bulbar and respiratory insufficiency. The limbs are generally spared. Autosomal recessive inheritance has been reported.

References

Amyotrophic Lateral Sclerosis

Andres PL, Hedlund W, Finison L, et al. Quantitative motor assessment in amyotrophic lateral sclerosis. Neurology 1986; 36:937–941.

Bobowick AR, Brody JA. Epidemiology of motor neuron diseases. N Engl J Med 1975; 288:1047–1055.

Brahic M, Smith RA, Gibbs CJ, et al. Detection of picornoverus sequences in nervous tissue of amyotrophic lateral sclerosis and control patients. Ann Neurol 1985; 18:337–343.

Caroscio JT, Cohen JA, Zawodniak J, et al. A double-blind, placebo-controlled trial of TRH in amyotrophic lateral sclerosis. Neurology 1986; 36:141–145.

Chou SM. Pathognomy of intraneural inclusions in ALS. In Tsubaki T, Toyokura Y, eds. Amyotrophic Lateral Sclerosis. Tokyo: University of Tokyo Press, 1979; 135–176.

Engel WK, Siddique T, Nicoloff JT. Effect on weakness and spasticity in amyotrophic lateral sclerosis of thyrotropin-releasing hormone. Lancet 1983; 1:73–75.

Garruto RM, Yamagihara R, Gajdusek DC. Disappearance of high-incidence amyotrophic lateral sclerosis and parkinsonism dementia on Guam. Neurology 1985; 35:193–198.

Juergens SM, et al. ALS in Rochester, Minnesota, 1925–1977. Neurology 1980; 30:463–470.

Mulder DW, Kurland LT, Offord KP, Beard CM. Familial adult motor neuron disease: Amyotrophic lateral sclerosis. Neurology 1986; 36:511–517.

Munsat TL, Bradley WG. Amyotrophic Lateral Sclerosis. In Tyler HR, Dawson DM, eds. Current Neurology (vol 2). Boston: Houghton-Mifflin, 1979:79–103.

Munsat TL, Andres PL, Finison L, Conlon T, Thibodeau L. The natural history of motoneuron loss in amyotrophic lateral sclerosis. Neurology 1988; 38:409–413.

Oldstone MB, Wilson CB, Perrin LH. Evidence of immune-complex formation in patients with amyotrophic lateral sclerosis. Lancet 1976; 2:169–172.

O'Neil BP, Swanson JW, Brown FR, Griffin JW. Familial spastic paraparesis: An adrenoleukodystrophy phenotype? Neurology 1985; 35:1233–1235.

Rowland LP, ed. Human Motor Neuron Diseases. New York: Raven Press, 1982.

Salazar AM, Masters CL, Gajdusek CL, Gibbs CJ Jr. Syndromes of amyotrophic lateral sclerosis and dementia: relation to transmissible Creutzfeldt-Jakob disease. Ann Neurol 1983; 14:17–26.

Shy ME, Rowland LP, Smith T, et al. Motor neuron disease and plasma cell dyscrasia. Neurology 1986; 36:1429–1436.

Spencer PS, Nunn PB, Hugon J, Ludolph AC, Ross SM, Roy DN, Roberson RC. Guam amyotrophic lateral sclerosis—Parkinsonism—dementia linked to a plant excitant neurotoxin. Science 1987; 237:517–522.

Weiner LP, Stohlman SA, Davis RL. Attempts to demonstrate virus in amyotrophic lateral sclerosis. Neurology 1980; 30:1319–1322.

Primary Lateral Sclerosis

Bhaganiti S, Ehrlich C, Kula RW, Kwoh S, Eninsky J, Udani V, Poiesy BJ. Detection of human T-cell lymphoma/leukemia virus type I DNA and antigen in spinal fluid and blood of patients with chronic progressive myelopathy. N Engl J Med 1988; 318:1141–1147.

Miska RM, Pojunas W, McQuillen MP. Cranial magnetic resonance imaging in the evaluation of myelopathy of undetermined etiology. Neurology 1987; 37:840–843.

Progressive Muscular Atrophy

Johnson WG, Wigger HJ, Karp HR, Glaubiger LM, Rowland LP. Juvenile spinal muscular atrophy—a new hexosaminidase deficiency phenotype. Ann Neurol 1982; 11:11–16.

Norris FH Jr. Adult spinal motor neuron disease. Progressive muscular atrophy (Aran's Disease) in relation to amyotrophic lateral sclerosis. In: Vinken PJ, Bruyn GW, eds. Handbook of Clinical Neurology, (vol 22). New York: Elsevier-North Holland, 1975.

124. SYRINGOMYELIA
Elliott L. Mancall

Cavitation within the spinal cord was first described by Esteinne in 1546 in his "La Dissection Du Corps Humain." Charles P. Ollivier D'Angers first applied the term *syringomyelia* in 1827. In brief, the term connotes a chronic and progressive disorder that primarily involves the spinal cord. It is characterized clinically by amyotrophy, loss of pain and temperature sensibility with relative preservation of touch and proprioception, and paraparesis associated with skeletal defects such as scoliosis and neurogenic arthropathies. Although the exact incidence of syringomyelia is not known, it is considered rare. It occurs more frequently in men than in women. Familial cases have been described. The disease usually appears in the third or fourth decade of life, with a mean age at onset of about 30 years. It may develop, albeit rarely, in childhood or late adult years. Syringomyelia usually progresses slowly; the course extends over many years. An acute course may be evident when the brain stem is affected (i.e., *syringobulbia*).

Clinical Manifestations. The symptomatic presentation depends primarily upon the precise location of the lesion within the neuraxis. The syringomyelic cavity, or syrinx, is encountered most commonly in the lower cervical region, particularly at the base of the posterior horn and extending into the central gray matter and anterior commissure of the cord. By virtue of its location, the cyst interrupts the decussating spinothalamic fibers that mediate pain and temperature sensibility, resulting in loss of these sensations; light touch, vibratory sense, and position sense are relatively preserved, at least early in the course of the disease, by virtue of sparing of the posterior columns. This pattern of loss of cutaneous sensibility with preservation of posterior column sensory modalities is commonly referred to as *dissociated sensory loss.* Pain and temperature sensations typically are impaired in the arm on the involved side, sometimes in both arms or in a shawl-like distribution (*en cuirasse*) across the shoulders and upper torso anteriorly and posteriorly. When the cavity enlarges to involve the posterior columns, there is loss of position and vibratory sense in the feet, and astereognosis may be noted in the hands. Extension of the lesion into the anterior horns with resultant loss of motor neurons causes amyotrophy that begins in the small muscles of the hands, ascends to the forearms, and ultimately affects the shoulder girdle muscles. The hand may be strikingly atrophied, with the development of a claw-hand deformity (*main en* *griffe)*. Weakness appears in the hands, forearms, and shoulder girdle, and fasciculations may be seen. Because the syrinx is asymmetrically placed early in its development, manifestations in the arms and hands tend to be similarly asymmetric in distribution. Muscle stretch reflexes in the arms characteristically are lost early. As the syringomyelic cavity extends into the lateral columns of the cord, spasticity appears in the legs, symmetrically or asymmetrically, with paraparesis, hyperreflexia, and extensor plantar responses. Impairment of bowel and bladder functions occurs, usually as a late manifestation. Horner syndrome may appear, reflecting damage to the sympathetic neurons in the intermediolateral cell column.

Pain, generally deep and aching in quality, is sometimes experienced early in the course, and may be severe. When present, pain usually involves the neck and shoulders, but may follow a radicular distribution in the arms or trunk.

The syrinx sometimes ascends superiorly into the medulla, producing the syndrome of syringobulbia. This is evidenced by dysphagia, pharyngeal and palatal weakness, asymmetric weakness and atrophy of the tongue, sensory loss involving primarily pain and temperature sense in the distribution of the trigeminal nerve, and nystagmus. Signs of cerebellar dysfunction may appear. Rarely, the syrinx may extend even higher in the brain stem or into the centrum semiovale as a *syringocephalus.*

In addition to these purely neurologic signs, many other clinical abnormalities are manifest. Scoliosis is characteristically seen, and neurogenic arthropathies *(Charcot joints)* may affect the shoulder, elbow, or wrist. The disease may actually present with acute painful enlargement of the shoulder, which is associated with destruction of the head of the humerus. Painless ulcers of the hands are not infrequent. The hands are occasionally the site of remarkable subcutaneous edema and hyperhydrosis *(main succulente)*, presumably due to interruption of central autonomic pathways.

A cyst sometimes develops in the lumbar cord either in association with or independent of a cervical syrinx. Lumbar syringomyelia is characterized by atrophy of proximal and distal leg muscles with dissociated sensory loss in lumbar and sacral dermatomes. Stretch reflexes are reduced or lost in the legs; impairment of sphincter function is common. The plantar responses are ordinarily flexor.

Pathology and Pathogenesis. As emphasized by Greenfield, syringomyelia may be defined as a condition of tubular cavitation of the spinal cord, usually beginning within the cervical cord and generally extending ultimately over many segments. Syringomyelia should be looked upon as distinct from simple cystic expansion of the central canal of the cord; the term *hydromyelia* is more appropriately applied to the latter condition. The syringomyelic cavity may communicate with the central canal, and ependymal cells occasionally line the wall of the syrinx. The fluid within the cyst is similar to, if not identical with, the cerebrospinal fluid (CSF). The syrinx may be limited to the cervical cord or may extend the length of the cord; it tends to vary in transverse diameter from segment to segment, usually achieving maximal extent in the cervical and lumbosacral enlargements. Originally confined to the base of a posterior horn or to the anterior commissure of the cord, the cyst slowly enlarges to involve much of both gray and white matter; at times, only a narrow rim of cord parenchyma can be identified histologically. The cyst itself is surrounded by a dense glial fibril wall. Extension of the cavity into the medulla or, rarely, higher within the neuraxis may be noted. Developmental abnormalities in the cervical spine and at the base of the skull, such as in platybasia, are common. Features of the Arnold-Chiari malformation, such as displacement of the cerebellar tonsils into the cervical canal, are often identified. Hydrocephalus is frequent and cerebellar hypoplasia may be found. In a few cases, ependymoma or astrocytoma of the spinal cord is encountered, usually in juxtaposition with the syrinx itself.

The pathogenesis of syringomyelia remains uncertain. Following Gardner, it is widely held that most cases of syringomyelia are of a "communicating" variety. As such, dilatation of the central canal of the spinal cord is thought to be caused by CSF pulsations directed downward from the fourth ventricle because the foramina of exit is occluded by a developmental defect in the rhombic roof or other anomalies of the medullocervical junction. According to this hydrodynamic theory, obstruction or atresia of the normal outlets of the fourth ventricle is essential; in most cases, the ventricular obstruction is associated with features of the Arnold-Chiari malformation, and often with hydrocephalus. As a modification of Gardner's theory, Boulay and associates have emphasized systolic excursions of CSF in the basal cisterns in the formation of the cystic cavity.

In the more traditional nomenclature of Greenfield, however, distension of the central canal is designated *hydromyelia,* and the term syringomyelia is reserved for a noncommunicating cyst. From this perspective, the syringomyelic cavity cannot be considered part of the ventricular system in what is essentially a persistent embryonic configuration but, rather, an independent development. Noncommunicating syrinx has been attributed to several factors, including extension of CSF under pressure along the Virchow-Robin spaces, cystic degeneration of an intramedullary glioma, and ischemia with cyst formation secondary to arachnoiditis due to meningitis or subarachnoid hemorrhage with resultant insufficiency of blood flow in the anterior spinal artery. A syrinx may also develop after spinal cord trauma, either soon after resorption of an intramedullary hematoma *(hematomyelia)* or as a delayed phenomenon after cord contusion or compression with resultant microcystic cavitation. Birth trauma may be important in the development of syringomyelia.

The distinction between communicating and noncommunicating forms of syringomyelia may be an artificial one, and the term *syringohydromyelia* has been suggested as a more inclusive term. Most instances of syringomyelia seem to fall into the Gardner com-

municating variety, although the precise pathogenetic mechanisms remain incompletely understood. In some individuals the original communication with the fourth ventricle may have been obliterated with the passage of time, resulting in the spurious appearance of a noncommunicating configuration.

Laboratory Data. Examination of the CSF ordinarily demonstrates few abnormalities. CSF pressure is sometimes elevated and a complete subarachnoid block may be noted. The cell count is only rarely more than 10/mm³. A mild elevation of CSF protein content occurs in half the patients; in the face of subarachnoid block, CSF protein may exceed 100 mg/dl.

Several radiographic changes may be encountered. The cervical spinal canal is commonly widened, with erosion of the pedicles. Myelography usually reveals a wide cord, particularly in the cervical region, at times with complete subarachnoid block (Figs. 124–1 and 124–2). Metrizamide-CT myelography may demonstrate either an expanded or collapsed cord. Metrizamide injected by either the spinal subarachnoid route or by ventriculography may enter and outline the syringomyelic cavity. Also, radiographic studies may demonstrate features of basilar impression, craniovertebral anomalies, such as fusion of the atlas to the occiput, hydrocephalus, or the Arnold-Chiari malformation (Fig. 124–3).

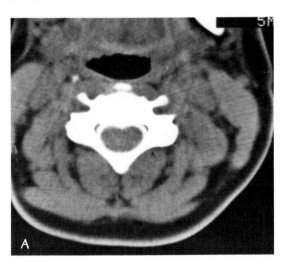 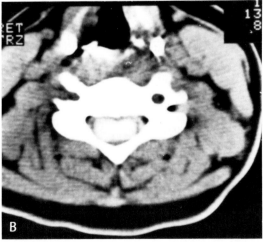

Fig. 124–1. Syringomyelia. *A.* CT myelogram showing enlarged cord and narrowed subarachnoid space. *B.* Delayed film (4 hours later) shows that contrast medium has penetrated spinal cord from subarachnoid space. (Courtesy of Drs. S.K. Hilal and M. Mawad.)

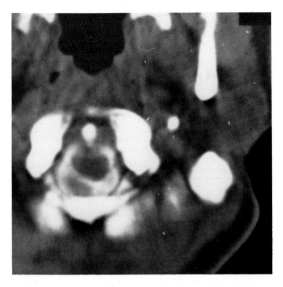

Fig. 124–2. Arnold-Chiari malformation with syringomyelia. Upper cervical cord is much enlarged. Below the shadow of the cord there are two lucent areas within the density of the contrast-filled subarachnoid space, which are cerebellar tonsils. These extend below the foramen magnum into the spinal canal. (Courtesy of Drs. S.K. Hilal and M. Mawad.)

Differential Diagnosis. Several disorders must be considered in the differential diagnosis of syringomyelia. Amyotrophic lateral sclerosis (ALS) commonly presents with weakness, atrophy, and reflex loss in the arms that is often asymmetric, with heightened reflexes and extensor plantar responses in the legs. Sensory loss, however, does not occur in ALS. Multiple sclerosis may mimic syringomyelia, particularly in its early stage. Early atrophy of hand muscles, however, does not occur in multiple sclerosis and the lack of evidence of dissemination of lesions elsewhere would argue against this diagnosis. Evaluation of visual evoked responses and of CSF for gamma globulin content, oligoclonal bands, and myelin basic protein are also helpful in identifying multiple sclerosis. Intrinsic tumors of the spinal cord may pursue a chronic course and produce clinical signs similar to those of syringomyelia. Myelography and metrizamide-CT myelography generally distinguish the two, but surgical exploration is sometimes necessary. Myelography is also important in differentiating syringomyelia from cervical spondylosis, another source of diagnostic confusion. Anomalies of the craniovertebral junction and cervical ribs may also cause symptoms reminiscent of syringomyelia; because both may be associated with true syringomyelia, identification of

these abnormalities is not sufficient to exclude cavitation within the spinal cord; thus, myelography may be important here as well. MRI (Fig. 124–3) has proven to be an excellent screening test for syringomyelia but has not yet completely replaced metrizamide-CT myelography.

Treatment. There is no specific therapy for syringomyelia. Radiation therapy to halt extension of the syringomyelic cavity is of doubtful benefit. Radiation is best used when syringomyelia is associated with an intramedullary tumor. The pain of syringomyelia may be dramatically relieved by radiation. Surgical therapy is widely advocated. Posterior fossa decompression with removal of the posterior rim of the foramen magnum and of the arches of the atlas and axis (with reduction of an associated Arnold-Chiari malformation) sometimes appears helpful, but long-term results have not been encouraging. Surgical decompression of the syrinx itself (syringotomy) may be beneficial in selected patients. When hydrocephalus is present, it should be treated with an appropriate ventricular shunting procedure. Excision of the filum terminale as a so-called "terminal ventriculostomy" has also been proposed. It is clear that no single mode of therapy is universally applicable, and none is entirely satisfactory.

References

Banerji NK, Millar JHD. Chiari malformation presenting in adult life. Its relationship to syringomyelia. Brain 1974; 97:157–168.

Barnett HJM, Foster JB, Hudgson P. Syringomyelia. Philadelphia: W.B. Saunders, 1973.

Berry RG, Chambers RA, Lublin FD. Syringoencephalomyelia (Syringocephalus). J Neuropathol Exp Neurol 1981; 40:633–644.

Bonafe A, Manelfe C, Espagno J, Guirard B, Rascola A. Evaluation of syringomyelia with metrizamide computed tomographic myelography. J Comput Tomogr 1980; 4:797–802.

duBoulay G, Shah SH, Curie JC, Logue V. The mechanism of hydromyelia in Chiari type 1 malformation. Br J Radiol 1974; 47:579–587.

Eggers C, Hamer J. Hydrosyringomyelia in childhood. Clinical aspects, pathogenesis and therapy. Neuropädiatrie 1979; 10:87–99.

Faulhauer K, Loew K. The surgical treatment of syringomyelia. Long-term results. Acta Neurochirurgica 1978; 44:215–222.

Foster NL, Wing SD, Bray PF. Metrizamide ventriculography in syringomyelia. Neurology 1980; 30:1323–1326.

Garcia-Uria J, Leunda G, Carrillo R, Bravo G. Syringomyelia: Long-term results after posterior fossa decompression. J Neurosurg 1981; 54:380–383.

Gardner WJ. Hydrodynamic mechanism of syringomyelia. Its relationship to myelocele. J Neurol Neurosurg Psychiatry 1965; 28:247–259.

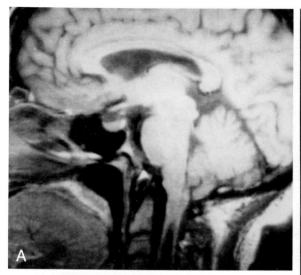
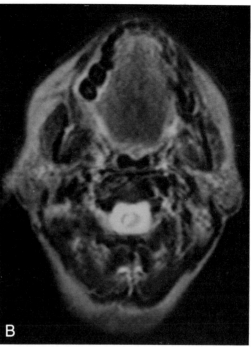

Fig. 124–3. Chiari malformation with syrinx. *A.* Sagittal T1-weighted MR scan shows intramedullary fluid intensity signal in high cervical region and tonsillar herniation. *B.* Axial T2-weighted MR scan at C2 level reveals high signal, representing CSF surrounding the cord in thecal sac and within cord in syrinx. (Courtesy of Drs. J.A. Bello and S.K. Hilal.)

Gardner WH, McMurry FG. "Non-communicating" syringomyelia: A nonexistent entity. Surg Neurol 1976; 6:251–256.

Giménez-Roldán S, Benito C, Mateo D. Familial communicating syringomyelia. J Neurol Sci 1978; 36:135–146.

Greenfield J. Syringomyelia and syringobulbia. In Blackwood W, ed. Greenfield's Neuropathology, 2nd ed. London: Arnold, 1963.

Haponik EF, Givens D, Angelo J. Syringobulbiamyelia with obstructive sleep apnea. Neurology 1983; 33:1046–1049.

Kan S, Fox AJ, Vinuela F, et al. Delayed CT metrizaroxide enhancement of syringomyelia secondary to tremor. AJNR 1983; 4:73–78.

Love JG, Olafson RA. Syringomyelia: A look at surgical therapy. J Neurosurg 1966; 24:714–718.

Martin G. Syringomyelia, a hypothesis and proposed method of treatment. J Neurol Neurosurg Psychiatry 1983; 46:365.

Poser CM. The Relationship Between Syringomyelia and Neoplasm. Springfield: Charles C Thomas, 1956.

Sackellares JC, Swift TR. Shoulder enlargement as the presenting sign in syringomyelia. JAMA 1976; 236:2878–2879.

Williams B. On the pathogenesis of syringomyelia: A review. J Roy Soc Med 1980; 73:798–806.

---

125. SUBACUTE COMBINED DEGENERATION OF THE SPINAL CORD

Elliott L. Mancall

The neurologic manifestations of pernicious anemia result from changes in both the central and peripheral nervous systems. The term *subacute combined degeneration of the spinal cord* is most appropriately used for this condition; less desirable synonyms include *combined system disease* and *funicular myelitis.* The clinical syndrome is characterized by paresthesias in the feet and sometimes the hands, loss of posterior column sensibility with sensory ataxia, and spasticity and weakness of the legs. Similar symptoms have been associated with other anemias or nutritional deficiencies (e.g., Jamaican neuropathy or Strachan syndrome). As with pernicious anemia itself, the symptoms in such conditions may be related to changes in either peripheral nerves or the spinal cord.

Etiology. Both the anemia and the neurologic disorder are due to deficiency of vitamin B_{12} (cyanocobalamin). Patients with pernicious anemia have a defect of gastric secretion that deprives them of intrinsic factor, a protein that binds vitamin B_{12} (extrinsic factor), that is specifically required for intestinal absorption of the vitamin. Vitamin B_{12} is present in low concentration in meat but not in vegetables. Failure to secrete intrinsic factor may be caused by an autoimmune disorder that involves both antibodies to gastric parietal cells and lymphocytic infiltration of the gastric mucosa, which destroys the gastric cells that secrete both acid and intrinsic factor. The same metabolic abnormality may occur when there is malabsorption of vitamin B_{12} from other causes, especially after gastrectomy. The neurologic lesions in pernicious anemia may be due to inactivity of the vitamin B_{12}-dependent enzyme, methionine synthetase, which impairs the biosynthesis of methionine.

Pathology. The pathologic changes in the spinal cord involve white matter much more than gray matter. Although peripheral nerves are often affected, the primary changes appear in the spinal cord. These consist of the symmetric loss of myelin sheaths and, to a lesser extent, of axons, most prominent in the posterior and lateral columns (Figs. 125–1 and 125–2). The lesions appear first in the posterior columns of the thoracic cord, subsequently spreading laterally, superiorly and inferiorly. At times, much of the white matter of the cord is involved. The anterior horn cells may show changes characteristic of axonal reaction when there is associated peripheral nerve degeneration. Patchy demyelination is often found in the cerebral white matter (Fig. 125–3). Rarely, axonal reaction is observed in cortical neurons. Demyelination of the optic nerves may be encountered. Inflammatory cells are absent.

Incidence. The incidence of subacute combined degeneration parallels that of pernicious anemia; the spinal cord is probably involved to some extent in many untreated cases. However, in most established cases of pernicious anemia, clinical neurologic abnormalities are minimal or lacking. The converse is of particular importance: the classic posterolateral syndrome of subacute combined degeneration may appear with only minimal

hematologic alterations. Neurologic symptoms usually appear shortly after the onset of the anemia, but may precede the hematologic disorder. Subacute combined degeneration due to deficiency of vitamin B_{12} is a clinical rarity today, because diagnosis is made so rapidly and because vitamin B_{12} is often administered indiscriminately in the treatment of many nonspecific illnesses.

Symptoms and Signs. Both sensory and motor symptoms are present in varying proportion, depending on the degree of damage to the individual tracts within the spinal cord or peripheral nerves, or both. Because the disease usually begins in the dorsal columns in the thoracic cord, the first symptoms typically include paresthesias of the feet, spreading up the legs and only later involving the hands and arms. Impairment or loss of vibratory and position sensation occurs in the legs; sensory ataxia appears, always with a positive Romberg sign. The legs are often weak and spastic and the tendon reflexes are exaggerated; however, the tendon reflexes are lost when polyneuropathy develops. Extensor plantar responses, indicating disease of the corticospinal tracts, are the rule.

The arms are affected as the disease progresses, but rarely as severely as the legs. Cranial nerve palsies are rare. Visual impairment, sometimes associated with optic atrophy, may reflect either severe anemia or development of demyelination within the optic nerves. Visual evoked responses are often abnormal even in the absence of overt visual failure.

Mental changes appear in some cases. Irritability, paranoia, and confusion are com-

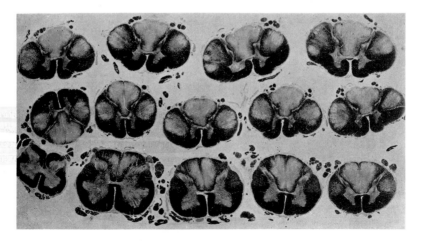

Fig. 125–1. Subacute combined degeneration. Sections of spinal cord at various levels showing segmental loss of myelin, which is most intense in the dorsal and lateral columns.

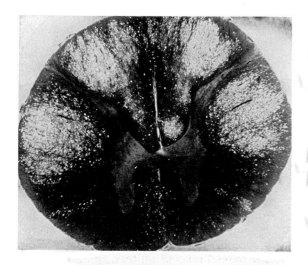

Fig. 125–2. Subacute combined degeneration. Destruction of myelin predominating in the posterior and lateral columns. Swelling of affected myelin sheaths cause spongy appearance.

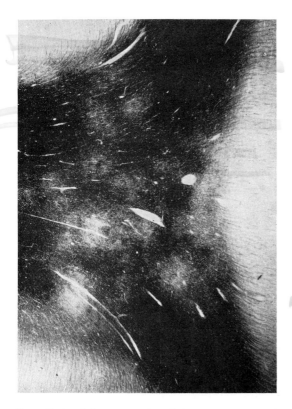

Fig. 125–3. Subacute combined degeneration. Partial loss of myelin of white matter of frontal lobe. (Courtesy of Dr. L. Roizin.)

mon, although frank psychotic episodes rarely occur. Impairment of memory is frequently observed, at times with other features of a dementing illness. These manifestations are attributed to the alterations of the cerebral white matter and should be looked upon as an integral part of the neurologic disease.

Laboratory Data. The laboratory findings are those of pernicious anemia. Of greatest diagnostic importance in terms of sensitivity is the level of serum vitamin B_{12} as determined by radioisotope dilution; red cell indices, in particular the mean corpuscular volume, and determination of the amount of hemoglobin are also important. The Schilling test, with and without intrinsic factor, is useful in determining the cause of an already documented vitamin B_{12} deficiency; search for histamine-fast achlorhydria is of similar aid. In most cases, there are antibodies to gastric parietal cells or to intrinsic factor. Additionally, clues to the presence of vitamin B_{12} deficiency may be found in the observation of a high lactic dehydrogenase level in serum or of an elevated unconjugated serum bilirubin; both of these abnormalities are nonspecific, but may provide an initial diagnostic lead in the laboratory investigation of these patients. The serum vitamin B_{12} content may be normal if the patient has received injections of vitamin B_{12}; if this is the situation, diagnosis depends on the Schilling test.

Diagnosis. Diagnosis of subacute combined degeneration of the cord is ordinarily made without difficulty when the characteristic posterolateral syndrome appears in association with psychological alterations, dementia, or visual impairment in a patient with low-serum vitamin B_{12}, gastric achlorhydria, and other typical laboratory features of pernicious anemia. When the outset of neurologic alterations precedes recognition of the hematologic changes, difficulties in diagnosis may be encountered; the features of anemia itself may be obscured by prior inadequate treatment with either folic acid or vitamin B_{12}. The appearance of neurologic symptoms, when macrocytic anemia has responded to treatment with folic acid alone, suggests that pernicious anemia is the basic disorder.

Peripheral neuropathy, particularly when associated with other nutritional deficiencies, may pose difficulties in making the differential diagnosis. The absence of convincing evidence of intrinsic disease of the spinal cord helps in distinguishing peripheral neuropathy from pernicious anemia.

Course. Although remissions are not infrequent in pernicious anemia, spontaneous improvement in the neurologic signs themselves, once fully established, is uncommon. Without specific treatment, neurologic abnormalities are inexorably progressive and fatal. With adequate therapy, the hematologic disorder ordinarily responds within a few days or weeks, but improvement in the neurologic manifestations tends to be much slower; noticeable improvement within 2 months of the start of treatment may be anticipated.

Treatment. The basic treatment is that for pernicious anemia. Vitamin B_{12} is injected intramuscularly daily or every other day for at least 3 weeks, then once or twice weekly for the next 2 months. Vitamin B_{12} should be continued parenterally thereafter for the duration of the patient's life, in a monthly dose of 1 mg. Premature cessation of treatment invariably results in recurrence of the symptoms after a delay of some months.

Treatment with folic acid is contraindicated in patients with pernicious anemia. The anemia itself responds to folic acid, but the neurologic symptoms may progress or even develop de novo in patients treated with this agent alone.

References

Baldwin JW, Dalessio DJ. Folic acid therapy and cord degeneration in pernicious anemia. N Engl J Med 1961; 264:1339–1342.

Carmel R. Pernicious anemia: Report of patients without the expected findings of very low serum cobalamin levels, anemia, and macrocytosis. Arch Int Med 1988; 148:1712–1714.

Fairbanks VF, Elenback LR. Tests for pernicious anemia. Serum vitamin B_{12} assay. Mayo Clin Proc 1983; 58:135–137.

Ferraro A, Arieti S, English WH. Cerebral changes in the course of pernicious anemia and their relationship to psychic symptoms. J Neuropathol Exp Neurol 1945; 4:217–239.

Freeman AG, Heaton JM. The aetiology of retrobulbar neuritis in Addisonian pernicious anemia. Lancet 1961; 1:908–911.

Lindenbaum J, Healton EB, Savage DG et al. Neuropsychiatric disorders caused by cobalamin deficiency in the absence of anemia or macrocytosis. New Engl J Med 1988; 318:1720–1728.

Pant SS, Asbury AK, Richardson EP Jr. The myelopathy of pernicious anemia. Acta Neurol Scand 1968; 44(suppl 35):1–36.

Robertson DM, Dinsdale HB, Campbell RJ. Subacute combined degeneration of the spinal cord. Arch Neurol 1971; 24:203–207.

Scott JM, Dinn JJ, Wilson P, Weir DG. Pathogenesis of subacute combined degeneration: A result of methyl group deficiency. Lancet 1981; 2:334–336.

Scott JM, Weir DG. Hypothesis: The methyl folate trap. Lancet 1981; 2:337–340.

Shorvon SD, Carney MWP, Chanarin I, Reynolds EH. The neuropsychiatry of megaloblastic anemia. Br Med J 1980; 281:1036–1038.

Sigal SH, Hall CA, Antel JP. Plasma R binder deficiency and neurologic disease. New Engl J Med 1987; 317:1330–1332.

Strachan RW, Henderson JG. Psychiatric syndromes due to avitaminosis B_{12} with normal blood and marrow. Q J Med 1965; 34:303–317.

Troncoso MD, Mancall EL, Schatz NJ. Visual evoked responses in pericious anemia. Arch Neurol 1979; 36:168–169.

Weir DG, Gatenby PBB. Subacute combined degeneration of the cord after partial gastrectomy. Br Med J 1963; 2:1175–1176.

Williams JA, Hall GS, Thompson AG, Cooke WT. Neurological disease after partial gastrectomy. Br J Med 1969; 3:210–212.

126. TROPICAL MYELONEUROPATHIES
Lewis P. Rowland
Elliott L. Mancall

The term *tropical myeloneuropathies* refers to several syndromes that are encountered in equatorial countries around the world. The syndromes are manifestations of lesions in spinal cord and peripheral nerves, separately or together. These disorders have been long-standing public health problems. However, in the past decade they have assumed major theoretical importance because specific syndromes have been assigned to specific etiologies, including infection with human T-cell lymphotropic virus type I (HTLV-I), and with chronic ingestion of cassava beans or lathyrinogenic agents. Other exogenous toxins may play a role. In the past and perhaps still today, similar syndromes have been ascribed to nutritional deprivation.

Among the numerous names for these disorders are: *Strachan syndrome, Jamaican neuropathy, tropical spastic paraparesis (TSP), tropical ataxic neuropathy,* and *lathyrism.* TSP has generated other acronyms: *RAM* (for *retrovirus-associated myelopathy*) and *HAM* (for *HTLV-I-associated myelopathy*).

History, Clinical Manifestations, and Pathology

Because the symptoms and signs of these disorders are similar, and because modes of pathogenesis are only now being identified with precision, it seems reasonable to describe the several conditions together.

STRACHAN SYNDROME (NUTRITIONAL NEUROPATHY)

Strachan is credited with the first description of these syndromes when, in 1897, he reported his observations of a disorder found on the Carribbean island of Jamaica. The symptoms included numbness and burning limbs, girdling pains, impairment of vision and hearing, muscle weakness and wasting, hyporeflexia, and sensory ataxia. Mucocutaneous lesions included angular stomatitis, glossitis, and scrotal dermatitis. Scott later described similar manifestations in Jamaican sugar-cane workers; identical cases were reported in World War II prisoner-of-war camps in the Middle East and Asia, in the malnourished populations of Africa, India, and Malaya, and among those beseiged in Madrid in the Spanish Civil War. Most patients so afflicted with *Strachan syndrome* have a predominantly sensory neuropathy, presumably a consequence of nutritional depletion. Neuropathologic studies have demonstrated symmetric ascending (secondary) degeneration in the posterior columns, spinocerebellar tracts, optic nerves, and peripheral nerves.

JAMAICAN NEUROPATHIES: TROPICAL ATAXIC NEUROPATHY AND TROPICAL SPASTIC PARAPARESIS

In 1964, Montgomery, Cruickshank, and colleagues described another group of patients in Jamaica. The dominant signs were spasticity and other evidence of corticospinal tract disease, sometimes with the peripheral manifestations of Strachan syndrome.

Two seemingly distinct varieties have been identified. Both are primarily diseases of adults. The ataxic form seems less common in Jamaica (but is more common in Nigeria). It evolves slowly and is generally less severe than the spastic type. Manifestations include sensory ataxia, numbness and burning of the feet, deafness, visual impairment with optic atrophy, and a central or paracentral scotoma, mild spasticity with occasional extensor plantar responses, and wasting and weakness of the legs, at times with footdrop. Although these patients appear chronically undernourished, few exhibit stigmata of nutritional disorder.

The other variety of Jamaican neuropathy is more common. This form is called tropical spastic paraparesis (TSP). It is a subacute neuropathy in which pyramidal tract signs predominate and are accompanied by impairment of posterior column sensibility, bladder dysfunction, and girdling lumbar pain. In both varieties, histamine-fast gastric achlorhydria and positive serologic tests for syphilis are frequent; in the more common subacute form, protein elevation and lymphocytic pleocytosis are found in the cerebrospinal fluid (CSF).

Antibodies to HTLV-I have been found in more than 80% of patients and the virus has been isolated from CSF. The serologic abnormalities are similar in type and degree in tropical countries throughout the world—Colombia, the Seychelles, Martinique, and the southernmost part of Japan around the city of Kagoshima.

The pathologic basis of tropical ataxic neuropathy (TAN) is not clear; it is presumed to be a myelopathy and the ataxia is attributed to sensory loss. The pathology of TSP also needs more study, but the early descriptions included symmetric and severe degeneration of the pyramidal tracts and posterior columns. The spinocerebellar and spinothalamic pathways are affected in some cases. Nerve cell loss is evident in Clarke's column and in the anterior horns. Demyelination appears in the posterior spinal roots and in the optic and auditory nerves. In more acute cases, inflammatory exudates are seen in cord and spinal roots.

LATHYRISM

The clinical manifestations of lathyrism are similar to those of TSP. It is mainly a disease of adults and the manifestations are primarily those of pyramidal tract dysfunction. It is slowly progressive but may ultimately cause paraplegia. Descriptions of the disease extend back to ancient Hindu writings and to Hippocrates. Lathyrism was once probably prevalent in Europe as well as tropical countries, but now seems restricted to India, Bangladesh, and Ethiopia.

Etiology

Malnutrition. Nutritional deprivation has long been recognized as a cause of peripheral neuropathy, optic neuropathy, and myelopathy. Avitaminosis and lack of other dietary necessities may account for some of the original cases of TSP and TAN, but other causes are now likely.

Persistent Viral Infection. The widespread evidence of HTLV-I infection in patients with TSP has had a major impact. Theoretically, this observation has been important because it again shows that chronic viral infection may cause chronic human disease. It has raised the possibility that viral infection may play a role in multiple sclerosis and perhaps even in amyotrophic lateral sclerosis. However, the virus has not yet been proven to cause the syndrome. Nor is it clear how the disease may spread. In Japan, many of the patients received blood transfusions shortly before the onset of neurologic symptoms. In other parts of the world, serologic tests for syphilis have been positive. Yaws is another treponemal disorder in those countries, raising the possibility of venereal transmission.

Dietary Toxins. The cause of lathyrism has long been ascribed to chronic ingestion of the chickling pea or vetch. Lathyrus sativus is a nourishing and inexpensive food that has been popular in impoverished countries. The active agent, isolated by Peter Spencer and his colleagues, has been found to be a simple amino acid: beta-(N)-oxalyl-amino-L-alanine (BOAA). (They have implicated a similar, but different, amino acid in the Parkinsonism-ALS-dementia complex of Guam.)

Another dietary constituent has been implicated in the African ataxic disorder, TAN. Among patients in Nigeria, ingestion of the cassava plant seems to be important. Although the essential ingredient has not been identified, some investigators suspect compounds that can generate cyanide.

Other Toxins. No other toxins have been shown to be important in TSP or TAN. However, another myelopathy closely resembles TSP clinically and was encountered in Japan until corrective measures were taken. That condition, called *subacute myelo-optic neuropathy (SMON)*, was attributed to use of iodochlorhydroxyquinoline to treat travelers' diarrhea. The drug was withdrawn and the syndrome seems to have disappeared.

Prevention and Treatment

These tropical diseases are widespread. They have been called the "hidden endemias." Prevention seems more likely to have an impact than treatment. Malnutrition ought to be preventable. Venereal transmission is amenable to control (though perhaps not easily). Exogenous toxins can be excluded from the environment.

Once there is neurologic damage, however, the task is more difficult. Antiviral drug therapy remains a goal but is not yet effective for these disorders. Even replacement therapy with vitamins may not restore function to normal. Thus, rehabilitation and adaptation remain important.

References

Cliff J, Lundqvist P, Martensson J, et al. Association of high cyanide and low sulphur intake in cassava-induced spastic paraparesis. Lancet 1985; 2:1211–1212.

Cruickshank EK. Neuromuscular disease in relation to nutrition. Fed Proc 1961; 20(supp 7):345–360.

Cuetter AC. Strachan's syndrome: a nutritional disorder of the nervous system. Proceedings of the weekly seminar in Neurology. Edward Hines Jr. Veterans Administration Hospital, Hines, IL. Vol. XVIII, No. 1, 1968.

Denny-Brown D. Neurological conditions resulting from prolonged and severe dietary restriction. Medicine 1947; 26:41–113.

Fisher M. Residual neuropathological changes in Canadians held prisoners of war by the Japanese. Can Serv-Med J 1955; 11:157–199.

Gordon JJ, Gordon JJ, Inns RH, Johnson MK, et al. The delayed neuropathic effects of nerve agents and other organophosphorus compounds. Arch Toxicol 1983; 52:71–82.

Montgomery RD, Cruickshank EK, Robertson WB, McMenemey WH. Clinical and pathological observations on Jamaican neuropathy. Brain 1964; 87; 3:425–462.

Osame M, Matsumoto M, Usuku K, et al. Chronic progressive myelopathy associated with elevated antibodies to human T-lymphotropic virus Type I and adult T-cell leukemialike cells. Ann Neurol 1987; 21:117–123.

Osuntokun BO. An ataxic neuropathy in Nigeria: a clinical, biochemical and electrophysiological study. Brain 1965; 91:215–248.

Roman GC. Retrovirus-associated myelopathies. Arch Neurol 1987; 44:559–663.

Roman GC, Spencer PS, Schoenberg BS. Tropical myeloneuropathies. The hidden endemias. Neurology 1985; 35:1158–1170.

Sever JL, Gibbs CJ Jr (eds). Retroviruses in the nervous system. Ann Neurol 1988; 23(supplement):S1–S217.

Spencer PS, Nunn PB, Ludolph AC, Ross SM, Roy DW, Robertson RC. Linkage of Guam amyotrophic lateral sclerosis-parkinsonism-dementia syndrome to a plant excitant neurotoxin? Science 1987; 237:517–520.

Spencer PS, Schaumberg HH. Lathyrism: A neurotoxic disease. Neurobehav Toxicol Teratol 1983; 5:625–629.

Strachan H. On a form of multiple neuritis prevalent in the West Indies. Practitioner 1897; 59:477.

Vernant JC, Maurs L, Gesain A, et al. Endemic tropical spastic paraparesis associated with human T-lymphotropic virus type I: A clinical and seroepidemiological study of 25 cases. Ann Neurol 1987; 21:123–131.

Chapter XVI

Neuromuscular Junction

127. MYASTHENIA GRAVIS

Audrey S. Penn
Lewis P. Rowland

Myasthenia gravis is caused by a defect of neuromuscular transmission due to an antibody-mediated attack upon nicotinic acetylcholine receptors (AChR). It is characterized by fluctuating weakness that is improved by inhibitors of cholinesterase.

Etiology and Pathogenesis. It is not known how myasthenia gravis starts. However, the pathogenesis is clearly related to antibodies to AChR. An experimental disease has been induced in several different species of animals by immunizing them with AChR purified from the electric organ of eels or torpedo fish, an organ that contains large amounts of AChR. In immunized animals, the weakness has all the essential clinical and physiologic characteristics of human myasthenia; endplates show identical amputation of the tips of synaptic folds with loss of AChR, and the weakness appears when antibodies to AChR appear in the blood. Antibodies have been localized at the neuromuscular junction in immunocytologic studies. Antibodies to human AChR have been demonstrated in almost all patients with generalized myasthenia gravis. In infants of myasthenic mothers, symptoms parallel the appearance and disappearance of these antibodies. These facts were established in a series of investigations by the collaboration of workers at the Salk Institute (Lindstrom, Seybold, Lennon) and at the Mayo Clinic (Engel, Lambert). Their findings were confirmed in several other laboratories in the mid-1970s. Drachman showed that injection of IgG from human patients can induce features of the disease in mice. Pinching subsequently found that symptoms were ameliorated by plasmapheresis.

The polyclonal IgG response to AChR is produced by B-lymphocytes in peripheral lymphoid organs and the thymus. The antibodies react with multiple determinants on AChR, and enough antibody circulates to saturate up to 80% of AChR sites on muscle. A small percentage of the antiAChR molecules interfere directly with the binding of acetylcholine (ACh), but the major damage to endplates seems to result from actual loss of receptors due to acceleration of normal degradative processes (internalization, endocytosis, lysosomal hydrolysis) with inadequate replacement by new synthesis and by complement-mediated lysis of the membrane. As a consequence of the loss of AChR and the erosion and simplification of the endplates, the amplitude of miniature end-plate potentials is about 20% of normal, and patients are abnormally sensitive to the competitive antagonist, curare. The characteristic decremental response to repetitive stimulation of the motor nerve reflects failure of endplate potentials to reach threshold so that progressively fewer fibers respond to arrival of a nerve impulse.

How the antibodies arise is not known, but as in many other autoimmune diseases, a persistent viral infection is suspected. The thymus gland is almost always abnormal, either because of prominent germinal centers, "hyperplasia," or because there is a thymoma. AChR-antibodies are synthesized by B-cells in cultures of thymic gland from patients with or without hyperplastic glands, but it is not known why the abnormal synthesis of antibodies begins. In the thymus, there are normally epithelioid or "myoid" cells that have histologic characteristics of muscle and that bear AChR; these cells could present the antigen to thymic lymphocytes. Antibody synthesis within thymus requires T-helper cells and antigen-presenting cells that share Class II DR HLA antigens with B cells, and which must be sensitized to AChR. Excessive and inappropriately prolonged synthesis of thymic hormones that normally promote differentiation of T-helper cells may contribute. (Significant loss of T-suppressor cells has not been documented.) Still another possible initiating factor is immunogenic alteration of the antigen, AChR, at end-plates, because D-penicillamine therapy of patients with rheumatoid arthritis may initiate a syndrome that is indistinguishable from myasthenia gravis except that it subsides when administration of the drug is stopped.

There are few familial cases of the disease, but disproportionate frequency of HLA haplotypes (B8, DR3) in myasthenic patients suggests that genetic predisposition may be important. Other autoimmune diseases also seem to occur with disproportionate frequency in patients with myasthenia, especally hyperthyroidism and other thyroid disorders, systemic lupus erythematosus, rheumatoid arthritis, amd pemphigus.

Although most antibodies seem directed against antigenic determinants on the AChR molecule other than the acetylcholine binding site, physiologic studies indicate impaired responsiveness to the agonist, thereby accounting for the physiologic abnormalities, clinical symptoms, and the beneficial effects of drugs that inhibit acetylcholinesterase.

Special Forms of Myasthenia Gravis

JUVENILE AND ADULT FORMS

Typical myasthenia gravis may begin at any age, but it is most common in the second to fourth decades. It is less common before age 10 or after age 65. Circulating AChR antibodies are demonstrated in about 85% of these patients. Patients without antibodies do not differ clinically. These are the typical forms of myasthenia; other forms are rare.

NEONATAL MYASTHENIA

About 12% of infants born to myasthenic mothers have a syndrome characterized by impaired sucking, weak cry, limp limbs, and sometimes respiratory insufficiency. Symptoms begin in the first 48 hours and may last several days or weeks, after which the children are normal. The mothers are usually symptomatic, but may be in complete remission; in either case, AChR antibodies are demonstrable in both mother and child. Symptoms disappear as the antibody titer in the infant declines.

CONGENITAL MYASTHENIA

It had long been recognized that children with congenital myasthenia, although rarely encountered, share several characteristics: unaffected mothers; ophthalmoplegia as the dominant sign in infancy; and a high incidence of affected relatives in a pattern suggesting autosomal recessive inheritance occurred in some. With the advent of assays for AChR-antibody, another characteristic has been added. AChR antibodies are not found in serum of these patients; however, decremental responses are found consistently. Cytochemical and physiologic studies have suggested several different pre- or postsynaptic abnormalities (e.g., impaired release or synthesis of ACh, an abnormal AChR ion channel and deficient end-plate cholinesterase). Thus, congenital myasthenia forms a heterogeneous group of synaptic disorders of nonimmune etiology.

DRUG-INDUCED MYASTHENIA

The best example of this occurs in patients who receive D-penicillamine for rheumatoid arthritis, scleroderma, or hepatolenticular degeneration. The clinical manifestations and AChR antibody titers are similar to typical adult myasthenia but both disappear when drug administration is discontinued. Cases attributed to trimethadione or phenytoin have been less thoroughly studied.

Pathology. The overt pathology of myasthenia is found primarily in the thymus gland. About 70% of thymus glands from adult myasthenia gravis patients are not involuted and weigh more than normal. The glands show lymphoid hyperplasia: numerous lymphoid follicles with germinal centers in the medulla of the gland. (In normal individuals, germinal centers are numerous in lymph nodes and spleen but are sparse in the thymus.) Immunocytochemical methods indicate that these thymic germinal centers contain B-cells, plasma cells, HLA Class II DR positive T cells near normal medullary cells, and interdigitating cells. Both normal and myasthenic glands contain α-thymosin, a thymic hormone that is important for T-cell maturation.

Another 10% of myasthenic thymus glands contain thymomas of the lymphoepithelial type. The cells in these tumors are T-cells. Benign thymomas may nearly replace the gland, with only residual glandular material at the edges, or they may rest within large hyperplastic glands. The tumors tend to occur in older patients, but in Castleman's series, 15% occurred in patients between the ages of 20 and 29. The tumor may invade contiguous pleura, pericardium, or blood vessels, but almost never spreads to other organs. In older patients without thymoma, thymus glands that appear involuted often show hyperplastic foci within fatty tissue on careful microscopic examination of multiple samples.

In about 50% of cases, there are lymphorrhages in muscle, which are focal clusters of lymphocytes near small necrotic foci without perivascular predilection. In a few cases, especially in patients with thymoma, there is diffuse muscle fiber necrosis with infiltration of inflammatory cells; similar lesions are rarely encountered in the myocardium. Lymphorrhages are not seen near damaged neuromuscular junctions (although inflammatory cells may be seen in necrotic endplates in rat experimental autoimmune myasthenia gravis), but morphometric studies have shown loss of synaptic folds and widened clefts. Some nerve terminals are smaller than normal and multiple small terminals are applied to the elongated simplified postsynaptic membrane; others are absent. Other endplates appear normal. On residual synaptic folds, immunocytochemical methods show Y-shaped antibody-like structures, IgG, and complement components 2 and 9, and complement membrane attack complex. These results suggest that the destructive lesion involves molecules bound to AChR in situ as well as complement-dependent injury.

Incidence. Myasthenia gravis is a common disease. An apparent increase in the incidence of the disease in recent years is probably due to improved diagnosis. According to Kurland, the prevalence rate is 3/100,000 (or about 6000 cases) in the United States. A similar prevalence rate was given by Garland and Clark for England. Before age 40, the disease is three times more common in women, but at older ages both sexes are affected equally.

Familial cases are rare; single members of pairs of fraternal twins and several sets of identical twins have been affected. Young women with myasthenia tend to have HLA B-8, DR3 haplotypes (young Japanese women HLA-A12), implying a linked immune response gene that codes for a protein involved in the autoimmune response. First-degree relatives show an unusual incidence of other autoimmune diseases (systemic lupus erythematosus, rheumatoid arthritis, thyroid disease) and HLA-B-8 haplotype.

Symptoms. The symptoms of myasthenia have three general characteristics that, together, provide a diagnostic combination. Formal diagnosis, until recently, depended on demonstration of the response to cholinergic drugs and electrophysiologic evidence of abnormal neuromuscular transmission. Now, demonstration of circulating antibodies to AChR is also part of routine diagnosis.

The fluctuating nature of myasthenic weakness is unlike any other disease. The weakness varies in the course of a single day, sometimes within minutes, and it varies from day to day, or over longer periods. Major prolonged variations are termed *remissions* or *exacerbations;* when an exacerbation involves respiratory muscles to the point of inadequate ventilation, it is called a *crisis*. Variations sometimes seem related to exercise; this and the nature of the physiologic abnormality have long been termed "excessive fatigability," but there are practical reasons to de-emphasize fatigability as a central characteristic of myasthenia. Patients with the disease almost never complain of fatigue or symptoms that might be construed as fatigue. Myasthenic symptoms are *always* due to weakness, not to rapid tiring. In contrast, patients who complain of fatigue, if they are not anemic or harboring a malignant tumor, almost always have emotional problems, usually depression.

The second characteristic of myasthenia is the distribution of weakness. Ocular muscles are affected first in about 40% of the cases and are ultimately involved in about 85%. Ptosis and diplopia are the symptoms that result. Other common symptoms affect facial or oropharyngeal muscles, resulting in dysarthria, dysphagia, and limitation of facial movements. Together, oropharyngeal and ocular weakness cause symptoms in virtually all patients with myasthenia. Limb and neck weakness is also common, but in conjunction with cranial weakness. Almost never are limbs affected alone.

Crisis seems most likely to occur in patients with oropharyngeal or respiratory muscle weakness. It seems to be provoked by respiratory infection in many cases, or by surgical procedures, including thymectomy, although it may occur with no apparent provocation. Systemic illness may aggravate myasthenic weakness for reasons that are not clear; in patients with oropharyngeal weakness, aspiration of secretions may occlude lung passages to cause rather abrupt onset of respiratory difficulty. Major surgery may be followed by respiratory weakness without aspiration, however, so this cannot be the entire explanation. "Spontaneous" crisis seems to be less common now than it once was.

The third characteristic of myasthenic weakness is the clinical response to cholinergic drugs. This occurs so uniformly that it has become part of the definition, but it may be difficult to demonstrate in some patients, especially those with purely ocular myasthenia.

Aside from the fluctuating nature of the weakness, myasthenia is not a steadily progressive disease. However, the general nature of the disease is usually established within weeks or months after the first symptoms. If myasthenia is restricted to ocular muscles for 2 years, certainly if it is restricted after 3 years, it is likely to remain restricted, and only in rare cases does it then become generalized. (Solely ocular myasthenia differs serologically from generalized myasthenia because AChR antibodies are found in lower incidence—50%—and in low titer.) Spontaneous remissions are also more likely to occur in the first 2 years.

Before the advent of respiratory care units and the introduction of positive pressure respirators in the 1960s, crisis was a life-threatening event and the mortality of the disease was about 25%. With improved respiratory care, however, it is now exceptional for patients to die of myasthenia, except when cardiac, renal, or other disease complicates the picture.

Signs. The vital signs and general physical examination are usually within normal limits, unless the patient is in crisis. The findings on neurologic examination depend on the distribution of weakness. Weakness of the facial and levator palpabrae muscles produces a characteristic expressionless facies with drooping eyelids. Weakness of the ocular muscles may cause paralysis or weakness of isolated muscles, paralysis of conjugate gaze, complete ophthalmoplegia in one or both eyes, or a pattern resembling internuclear ophthalmoplegia. Weakness of oropharyngeal or limb muscles, when present, can be shown by appropriate tests. Respiratory muscle weakness can be detected by pulmonary function tests, which include inspiratory and expiratory muscle pressures. Muscular wasting of variable degree is found in about 10%

of cases, but this is not focal, and is usually encountered only in patients with malnutrition due to severe dysphagia. Fasciculations do not occur, unless the patient has received excessive amounts of cholinergic drugs. Sensation is normal and the reflexes are preserved, even in muscles that are weak.

Laboratory Data. Routine examinations of blood, urine, and CSF are normal. The characteristic electrodiagnostic abnormality is progressive decrement in the amplitude of muscle action potentials evoked by repetitive nerve stimulation at 3 or 5 Hz. In generalized myasthenia, the decremental response can be demonstrated in about 90% of patients, if at least three nerve-muscle systems are used (median-thenar; ulnar-hypothenar; accessory-trapezius). In microelectrode study of intercostal muscle, the amplitude of miniature end-plate potentials is reduced to about 20% of normal. This is caused by a decrease in the number of AChR available to agonists applied by microiontophoresis. In single-fiber electromyography (SFEMG), a small electrode measures the interval between potentials of the muscle fibers in the same motor unit. This interval normally varies, a phenomenon called *jitter,* and the normal temporal limits of jitter have been defined. In myasthenia, the jitter is increased and an impulse may not appear at the expected time; this is called *blocking* and the number of blockings is increased in myasthenic muscle. All of these electrophysiologic abnormalities are characteristic of myasthenia, but blocking and jitter are also seen in disorders of acetylcholine release. The standard EMG is usually normal, occasionally shows a myopathic pattern, and almost never shows signs of denervation unless some other condition supervenes. Similarly, nerve conduction velocities are normal.

Antibodies to AChR are found in 85 to 90% of patients of all ages if human muscle is used as the test antigen. There have been no false-positive results except for rare patients with Eaton-Lambert syndrome, but antibodies may not be detected in patients with strictly ocular disease, in some patients in remission (or after thymectomy), or even in some patients with severe symptoms. The titer does not match the severity of symptoms; patients in complete clinical remission may have high titers. Antibodies to myofibrillar proteins (myosin, actin, actinin) are found in 85% of patients with thymoma and may be the first evidence of thymoma in some cases.

The different forms of congenital myasthenia can be identified only in a few special centers that are prepared to analyze intercostal muscle biopsies for miniature end-plate potentials, AChR numbers, and determination of bound antibodies.

Other serologic abnormalities are encountered with varying frequency, but in several studies, antinuclear factor, rheumatoid factor, and thyroid antibodies were encountered more often than in control populations. Laboratory (and clinical) evidence of hyperthyroidism occurs at some time in about 5% of patients with myasthenia. Radiographs of the chest (including 10° oblique films) provide evidence of thymoma in about 15% of patients, especially in those older than 40. Computed tomography (CT) of the mediastinum demonstrates all but microscopic thymomas. It remains to be seen whether magnetic resonance imaging is even more useful than CT.

Diagnosis. The diagnosis of myasthenia gravis can be made without difficulty in most cases from the characteristic history and physical examination. The dramatic improvement that follows the injection of neostigmine or edrophonium makes the administration of these drugs essential. Return of strength in weak muscles (Fig. 127–1) occurs so uniformly after the parenteral administration of 1.5 mg of neostigmine that the failure of such a response almost precludes the diagnosis of myasthenia gravis. However, the response of some patients with solely ocular myasthenia may be difficult to demonstrate. In special circumstances, the sensitivity of patients with myasthenia to d-tubocurarine can prove the diagnosis, but only with careful attention to published descriptions of the test and in the presence of skilled personnel and facilities to support respiration if necessary.

In the neostigmine test, 1.5 to 2 mg of this drug and 0.4 mg atropine sulfate are given intramuscularly. Objective improvement in muscular power is recorded at 20-minute intervals up to 2 hours. Edrophonium is given intravenously in a dosage of 1 to 10 mg. The initial dose is up to 2 mg followed in 30 seconds by an additional 3 mg, and then in another 30 seconds by 5 mg, to a maximum of 10 mg. Improvement is observed within 30 seconds and lasts a few minutes. Because of the immediate and dramatic nature of the response, edrophonium is preferred for evaluation of cranial muscle weakness and neostigmine is generally reserved for evaluation of limb or respiratory weakness, which may require more time. Placebo injections are sometimes useful in evaluating limb weakness, but placebos are not necessary in evaluating cranial muscle weakness because that abnormality cannot be simulated.

For all practical purposes, a positive response is diagnostic of myasthenia gravis.

Differential Diagnosis. The differential diagnosis includes all diseases that are accompanied by weakness of oropharyngeal or limb muscles such as the muscular dystrophies, amyotrophic lateral sclerosis, progressive bulbar palsy, ophthalmoplegias of other causes, and the asthenia of psychoneurosis or hyperthyroidism. There is usually no difficulty in differentiating these conditions from myasthenia gravis by the findings on physical and neurologic examination and by the failure of symptoms in these conditions to improve after parenteral injection of neostigmine or edrophonium.

The only other conditions in which clinical improvement has been documented after use of edrophonium are other disorders of neuromuscular transmission—botulinum intoxication, snake bite, organophosphate intoxication, or unusual cases that include features of both myasthenia and the Lambert-Eaton

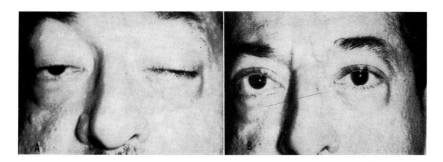

Fig. 127–1. Myasthenia gravis. *A.* Severe ptosis of the lids. *B.* Same patient one minute after intravenous injection of 10 mg of edrophonium. (From Rowland LP, Hoefer PFA, Aranow H Jr. Res Publ Assoc Res Nerv Ment Dis 1961; 38:548–600.)

syndrome. Denervating disorders, such as motor neuron disease or peripheral neuropathy, do not show a reproducible or unequivocal clinical response to edrophonium or neostigmine.

Treatment. Clinicians must choose the sequence and combination of five different kinds of therapy: anticholinesterase drug therapy and plasmapheresis are symptomatic treatments, whereas thymectomy, steroids, and other immunosuppressive drugs may alter the course of the disease.

It is generally agreed that anticholinesterase drug therapy should be given as soon as the diagnosis is made. Of the three available drugs (neostigmine, pyridostigmine, and ambenonium), pyridostigmine is most popular, but has not been formally assessed in controlled comparison with the other drugs. The muscarinic side-effects of abdominal cramps and diarrhea are the same for all three drugs, but are least severe for pyridostigmine treatment; none has more side-effects than another. The usual starting dose of pyridostigmine is 60 mg, given orally, every 4 hours while the patient is awake. Depending on clinical response, the dosage can be increased, but incremental benefit is not to be expected in amounts greater than 120 mg every 2 hours. If patients have difficulty eating, doses can be taken about 30 minutes before a meal. If patients have special difficulty on waking in the morning, a prolonged-release 180-mg tablet of pyridostigmine (Timespan) can be taken at bedtime. Muscarinic symptoms can be ameliorated by atropine, 0.4 mg, with each dose of pyridostigmine. Other drugs may be taken if diarrhea is prominent. There is no evidence that any one of the three drugs is more effective than the others in individual patients and there is no evidence that combinations of two drugs are better than any one alone.

Although cholinergic drug therapy sometimes gives impressive results, there are serious limitations. In ocular myasthenia, ptosis may be helped, but some diplopia almost always persists. In generalized myasthenia, patients may improve remarkably, but some symptoms usually remain. Cholinergic drugs do not return function to normal and the risk of crisis persists because the disease is not cured. Therefore, one of the other treatments is usually used promptly to treat generalized myasthenia.

Thymectomy was originally reserved for patients with serious disability because the operation had a high mortality. With advances in surgery and anesthesia, however, the operative mortality is now negligible in major centers. About 80% of patients without thymoma become asymptomatic or go into complete remission after thymectomy; although there has been no controlled trial of thymectomy, these results seem to diverge from the natural history of the untreated disease. Thus, thymectomy is now recommended for most patients with generalized myasthenia. Decisions made for children or patients older than 65 must be individualized. Although it is safe, thymectomy is a major operation and is not usually recommended for patients with ocular myasthenia. The beneficial effects of thymectomy are usually delayed for months or years. It is never an emergency measure and other forms of therapy usually are needed in the interim.

Prednisone therapy is used by some authorities to prepare patients for thymectomy, but that function is also served by plasmapheresis. Exchanges of about 5% of calculated blood volume may be given several times before the day of surgery to be certain that the patient is functioning as well as possible, and to ameliorate or avoid a postoperative respiratory crisis. Plasmapheresis is also used for other exacerbations; the resulting improvement, seen in most patients, may be slight or dramatic and may last only a few days or several months. Plasmapheresis is safe but expensive and is not convenient for many patients.

If a patient is still seriously disabled after thymectomy, most clinicians use prednisone in a dosage of 100 mg every other day. Once improvement is achieved, this should be tapered to 20 to 30 mg every other day. This has become a popular form of treatment for disabled patients, but there has been no controlled trial. If the patient does not improve in about 6 months, treatment with azathioprine or cyclophosphamide would be considered, in dosages of 150 to 200 mg daily for an adult. Whether steroids and immunosuppressive drugs have additive effects is uncertain and the relative risks are difficult to assess. The numerous side-effects of prednisone must be weighed against the possibilities of marrow suppression, susceptibility to infection, or delayed malignancy in patients who are taking immunosuppressives.

Prednisone, in dosages of 20 to 35 mg on alternate days, is also recommended by some clinicians for ocular myasthenia, weighing risks against potential benefit. For some patients in sensitive occupations, the risks of prednisone therapy may be necessary (e.g., actors, police officers, roofers or others who work on heights, or those who require stereoscopic vision). However, ocular myasthenia is not a threat to life; pyridostigmine may alleviate ptosis and an eye-patch can end diplopia. Thymectomy has become so safe that it might be considered for ocular myasthenia that is truly disabling.

Patients with thymoma are likely to have more severe myasthenia and are less likely to improve after thymectomy; nevertheless, many of these patients also improve if the surrounding thymus gland is excised in addition to the tumor.

Myasthenic crisis is defined as the need for assisted ventilation, a condition that arises in about 10% of myasthenic patients. It is more likely to occur in patients with dysarthria, dysphagia, and documented respiratory muscle weakness, presumably because they are liable to aspirate oral secretions, but crisis may also occur in other patients after respiratory infection or major surgery (including thymectomy). The principles of treatment are those of respiratory failure in general. Cholinergic drug therapy is usually discontinued once an endotracheal tube has been placed and positive pressure respiration started; this practice avoids questions about proper dosage or cholinergic stimulation of pulmonary secretions. Crisis is viewed as a temporary exacerbation that subsides in a few days or weeks. The therapeutic goal is to maintain vital functions and to avoid or treat infection until the patient spontaneously recovers from the crisis. Cholinergic drug therapy need not be restarted unless fever and other signs of infection have subsided, there are no pulmonary complications, and the patient is breathing without assistance.

The determination of whether plasma exchange actually shortens the duration of crisis would require a controlled trial, but the efficacy of pulmonary intensive care is now so good that crisis is almost never fatal and many patients remit. Because of advances in therapy, myasthenia is still serious, but not so grave.

References

Albuquerque EX, Rash JE, Mayer RG, Satterfield JR. Electrophysiological and morphological study of the neuromuscular junction in myasthenia gravis. Exp Neurol 1976; 51:536–563.

Bever CT Jr, Chang HW, Penn AS, Jaffe IA, Bock E. Penicillamine-induced myasthenia gravis effects of penicillamine on acetylcholine receptor. Neurology 1982; 32:1077–1082.

Donaldson JO, Penn AS, Lisak RP, Abramsky O, Brenner T, Schotland DL. Antiacetylcholine receptor antibody in neonatal myasthenia gravis. Am J Dis Child 1981; 135:222–226.

Drachman DB, ed. The immunology of myasthenia gravis. Ann NY Acad Sci 1987.

Eaton LM, Lambert EH. Electromyography and electric stimulation of nerves in diseases of motor unit: Observations in myasthenic syndrome associated with malignant tumors. JAMA 1957; 163:1117–1120.

Engel AG. Acquired autoimmune myasthenia gravis. In: Engel AG, Banker BQ, eds. Myology. New York: McGraw-Hill, 1986:1925–54.

Engel AG. Immune complexes at motor endplate in myasthenia gravis. Mayo Clin Proc 1977; 52:267–280.

Erb W. Zur Causistik der bulbären Lächmungen: über einem neuen, wahrscheinlich bulbären symptomen-complex. Arch Psychiatr Nervenkr 1879; 336–350.

Fon GT, Bein ME, Mancuso AA, Keesey JC, Lupetin AR, Wong WS. Computed tomography of the anterior mediastinum in myasthenia gravis. Radiology 1982; 142:135–146.

Goldflam S. Über einen scheinbar heilbaren bulbärparalytischen Symptomencomplex mit Beteiligungen der Extremitäten. Deutsche Z Nervenheilk 1893; 4:312–352.

Greer M, Schotland M. Myasthenia gravis in the newborn. Pediatrics 1960; 26:101–108.

Jolly F. Über Myasthenia Gravis pseudoparalytica. Berl Klin Wochenshr 1895; 1:1–7.

Kamo I, Furukawa S, Tada A, et al. Monoclonal antibody to acetylcholine receptor: Cell line established from thymus of patient with myasthenia gravis. Science 1982; 215:995–997.

Kurtzke J. Epidemiology of myasthenia gravis. Adv Neurol 1978; 19:545–564.

Levinson AI, Zweiman B, Lisak RM. Immunopathogenesis and treatment of myasthenia gravis. J Clin Immunol 1987; 7:187–197.

Lewis JE, Wick MR, Scheithauer BW, Bernatz PE, Taylor WF. Thymoma: A clinicopathologic review. Cancer 1987; 60:2727–2743.

Limburg PC, The TH, Hummel-Tappel E, Oosterhuis HJGH. Anti-acetylcholine receptor antibodies in myasthenia gravis. I. Relation to clinical parameters in 250 patients. J Neurol Sci 1983; 58:357–370.

Lindstrom J, Seybold M, Lennon VA, Whittingham S, Duane DD. Antibody to acetylcholine receptor in myasthenia gravis: Prevalence, clinical correlates, and diagnostic value. Neurology 1976; 26:1054–1059.

Lisak RP, Barchi RL. Myasthenia gravis. Philadelphia: W.B. Saunders, 1982.

Masaoka A, Monden Y, Seike Y, Tanioka T, Kagatoni K. Reoperation after transcervical thymectomy for myasthenia gravis. Neurology 1982; 32:83–85.

Melms A, Schalke BCG, Kirchner T. Thymus in myasthenia gravis: isolation of T-lymphocyte lines specific for AChR. J Clin Invest 1988; 81:902–908.

Mora M, Lambert EH, Engel AG. Synaptic vesicle abnormality in familial infantile myasthenia. Neurology 1987; 37:206–214.

Morel E, Eynard B, Vernet B, et al. Neonatal myastheia gravis: clinical and immunologic appraisal in 30 cases. Neurology 1988; 38:138–142.

Pachner AR. Myasthenia gravis. Immunol Allerg Clin No Am 1988; 8:277–293.

Patrick J, Lindstrom J. Autoimmune response to acetyl-choline receptor. Science 1973; 180:871–872.

Perez MC, Buot WL, Mercado-Danguilas C, Bagabaldo ZG, Renales LD. Stable remissions in myasthenia gravis. Neurology 1981; 31:32–37.

Rodriguez M, Gomez MR, Howard FM, Taylor WF. Myasthenia gravis in children: Long-term follow-up. Ann Neurol 1983:13:504–510.

Rosenberg M, Jauregui WO, Vega ME, Herrera MR, Roncoroni AJ. Recurrence of thymic hyperplasia after thymectomy in myasthenia gravis: A cause of failure of surgical treatment. Am J Med 1983; 74:78–82.

Rowland LP. Controversies about the treatment of myasthenia gravis. J Neurol Neurosurg Psychiatry 1980; 43:644–659.

Rowland LP, Hoefer PFA, Aranow H Jr, Merritt HH. Fatalities in myasthenia gravis. A review of 39 cases with 26 autopsies. Neurology 1956; 6:307–326.

Rowland LP, Hoefer PFR, Aranow H Jr. Myasthenic syndromes. Res Publ Assoc Res Nerv Ment Dis 1961; 38:548–600.

Scadding GK, Vincent A, Newsom-Davis J, Henry K. Acetylcholine receptor antibody synthesis by thymic lymphocytes: Correlation with thymic histology. Neurology 1981; 31:935–943.

Toyka KV, Drachman DB, Pestronk A, Kao I. Myasthenia gravis: Passive transfer from man to mouse. Science 1975; 190:397–399.

Vincent A. Immunology of acetylcholine receptors in relation to myasthenia gravis. Physiol Rev 1980; 60:757–824.

Vincent A, Cull-Candy SG, Newson-Davis J, Trautmann A, Molenaar PC, Polak RL. Congenital myasthenia end-plate acetylcholine receptors and electrophysiology in five cases. Muscle Nerve 1981; 4:306–318.

Wekerle H, Muller-Hermelink HK. The thymus in myasthenia gravis. In: Muller-Hermelink HK, ed. The Human Thymus. Histopathology and Physiology. Curr Top Pathol 1986; 75:179–206.

Witt NJ, Bolton CF. Neuromuscular disorders and thymoma. Muscle Nerve 1988; 11:398–405.

128. OTHER DISORDERS OF NEUROMUSCULAR TRANSMISSION

Audrey S. Penn

Eaton-Lambert Syndrome

The Eaton-Lambert syndrome is encountered in adults (mostly men) with oat-cell carcinoma of the bronchus; less commonly (and mostly in women), it occurs without associated neoplasm, with evidence of IgG-mediated autoimmunity. The abnormality of neurotransmission is due to inadequate release of acetylcholine from nerve terminals at both nicotinic and muscarinic sites and is related to abnormal voltage-dependent calcium channels. When IgG from affected patients is injected into mice, the number of ACh quanta released by nerve stimulation is reduced, and there is disarray of the active zone particles that are detected by freeze-fracture ultrastructural analysis.

The syndrome may be suspected in patients with symptoms of proximal limb weakness who have lost knee and ankle jerks and who complain of dry mouth or myalgia. Less common symptoms include paresthesias, impotence, hypohidrosis, and ptosis.

The disease is defined by, and the diagnosis is made by the characteristic *incremental response to repetitive nerve stimulation*, a pattern that is the opposite of myasthenia gravis. The first evoked potential has an abnormally low amplitude, which decrements even further at low rates of stimulation. At rates above 10 Hz, however, there is a marked increase in the amplitude of evoked response (2–20 times the original value). This incremental response results from facilitation of release of transmitter at high rates of stimulation; at low rates the number of quanta released per impulse (quantal content) is inadequate to produce end-plate potentials that achieve threshold. Similar abnormalities are found in preparations exposed to botulinum toxin or to a milieu low in calcium or high in magnesium.

Treatment includes therapy of the concomitant tumor. Drugs that facilitate release of ACh have been used with physiologic and symptomatic improvement, but are hazardous; guanidine (20–30 mg/kg/day) may depress bone marrow or cause severe tremors and cerebellar disorder; 4-amino pyridine causes convulsions, but 3, 4-diaminopyridine is as effective and is less toxic. Steroids, plasmapheresis, anticholinesterases, and immunosuppressive drugs have also been used beneficially in some cases.

Botulism

Botulism is a disease in which nearly total paralysis of nicotinic and muscarinic cholinergic transmission is caused by botulinum toxin acting on presynaptic mechanisms for release of acetylcholine in response to nerve stimulation. The toxin is produced by spores of Clostridium botulinum, which may contaminate foods grown in soil (Types A, B, F, and G) or fish (Type E). Intoxication results if contaminated food is inadequately cooked and the spores are not destroyed. Toxin can be produced in anaerobic wounds that have been contaminated by organisms and spores. Ingestion or inhalation of spores by infants may cause botulism when toxin is then produced in the gastrointestinal tract during periods of constipation. An analogous syndrome may occur in adults with persistent growth of C. botulinum in the intestine after surgery, from gastric achlorhydria, or from antibiotic therapy. The toxin causes destruction of the terminal twigs of cholinergic nerve endings, which require several months to regenerate and remodel after a single exposure.

Electrophysiologic evidence of severely disturbed neuromuscular transmission includes an abnormally small single muscle action potential evoked in response to a supramaximal nerve stimulus. When the synapse is driven by repetitive stimulation at high rates (20–50 Hz), the evoked response is potentiated up to 400%. In affected infants, unusually brief and low amplitude and overly abundant muscle action potentials have been detected. This is presumably related to involvement of terminal nerve twigs in endings of many motor units. In patients who have been treated for blepharospasm or other movement disorders by intramuscular injections of botulinum toxin, single fiber EMG shows increased jitter in muscles remote from those injected and the jitter is maximally increased at low firing rates. These abnormalities are not symptomatic but imply an effect of circulating toxin.

C. botulinum toxin may be the "most poisonous poison" (lethal dose for a mouse is 10^{-12} g/kg body weight). If the patient survives and reaches a hospital, symptoms include dry, sore mouth and throat, blurred vision, diplopia, nausea, and vomiting. Signs include hypohydrosis, total external ophthalmoplegia, and symmetric facial, oropharyngeal, limb, and respiratory paralysis. Pupillary paralysis, however, is not invariable. Not all patients are equally affected, suggesting variable toxin intake or variable individual responses. When cases occur in clusters, the diagnosis is usually suspected immediately.

Isolated cases in children and adolescents may be thought to be the Guillain-Barré syndrome, myasthenia gravis, or even diphtheria. Ptosis has responded to intravenous edrophonium in a few cases, but response to anticholinesterase drugs is neither sufficiently extensive nor prolonged to be therapeutic. Infants with botulism are usually younger than 6 months of age. They show generalized weakness, decreased or absent sucking and gag reflex, facial diplegia, lethargy, ptosis, and ophthalmoparesis. Diagnosis is made by the following characteristics: clustering of cases, symmetry of signs, dry mouth or absence of secretion, pupillary paralysis, and the characteristic incremental response to repetitive nerve stimulation. The Centers for Disease Control or appropriate state laboratories should be notified so that the toxin can be identified in refrigerated samples of serum. In suspected infantile botulism, feces should be evaluated for the presence of C. botulinum as well as toxin.

Patients should be treated in intensive care facilities for respiratory care. Specific therapy includes antitoxin (a horse serum product that may cause serum sickness or anaphylaxis) and guanidine hydrochloride, which promotes release of transmitter from residual spared nerve endings, but may depress bone marrow.

Antibiotic-Induced Neuromuscular Blockade

Aminoglycoside antibiotics (such as neomycin, streptomycin, and kanamycin) or polypeptide antibiotics (colistin and polymyxin B) may cause symptomatic block in neuromuscular transmission in patients without any known neuromuscular disease. Antibiotics may occasionally aggravate myasthenia gravis. The problem occurs when blood levels are excessively high, which usually occurs in patients with renal insufficiency, but levels may be within the therapeutic range. Studies of bath-applied streptomycin in nerve-muscle preparations disclosed inadequate release of ACh; the effect was antagonized by an excess of calcium ion. In addition, the sensitivity of the postjunctional membrane to ACh was reduced. Different compounds differed in relative effects on pre- and post-synaptic events. Neomycin and colistin produced the most severe derangements; the effects of kanamycin, gentamicin, streptomycin, tobramycin, and amikacin were moderate; tetracycline, erythromycin, vancomycin, penicillin-G, and clindamycin had negligible effects. Patients who fail to regain normal ventilatory effort after anesthesia or who show delayed depression of respiration after extubation and who are receiving one of the more potent agents should receive ventilatory support until the agent can be discontinued or another antibiotic substituted.

References

Eaton-Lambert Syndrome

Brown JC, Johns RJ. Diagnostic difficulties encountered in the myasthenic syndrome sometimes associated with carcinoma. J Neurol Neurosurg Psychiatry 1974; 37:1214–1224.

Engel AG. Myasthenic syndromes. In: Engel AG, Banker BQ, eds. Myology. New York: McGraw-Hill, 1986.

Lambert EH, Elmqvist D. Quantal components of endplate potentials in the myasthenic syndrome. Ann NY Acad Sci 1971; 183:183–199.

Lambert EH, Rooke ED, Eaton LM, Hodgson CH. Myasthenic syndrome occasionally associated with bronchial neoplasm: Neurophysiologic studies. In: Viets HR, ed. Myasthenia Gravis. Springfield: Charles C Thomas, 1961:362–410.

Lang B, Newsom-Davis J, Wray D, Vincent A, Murray N. Autoimmune etiology for myasthenic (Eaton-Lambert) syndrome. Lancet 1981; 2:224–226.

Lennon VA, Lambert EH, Whittingham S, Fairbanks V. Autoimmunity in the Lambert-Eaton myasthenic syndrome. Muscle Nerve 1982; 5:S21–S25.

Lundh H, Nilsson O, Rosen I. Treatment of Lambert-Eaton syndrome: 3,4-Diaminopyridine and pyridostigmine. Neurology 1984; 34:1324–1330.

O'Neill JH, Murray NMF, Newsom-Davis J. The Lambert-Eaton myasthenic syndrome: a review of 50 cases. Brain 1988; 111:577–596.

Roberts, A, Perera S, Lang B, Vincent A, Newson-Davis J. Paraneoplastic myasthenic syndrome IgG inhibits $^{45}Ca^{2+}$ flux in a small cell carcinoma line. Nature 1985; 2:737–739.

Botulism

Arnon SS, Midura TF, Clay SH, Wood RM, Chin J. Infant botulism; epidemiological, clinical and laboratory aspects. JAMA 1977; 237:1946–1951.

Chia JK, Clark JB, Ryan CA, Pollack M. Botulism in an adult associated with food-borne intestinal infection with Clostridium botulinum. N Engl J Med 1986; 315:239–241.

DeJesus PV, Slater R, Spitz LK, Penn AS. Neuromuscular physiology of wound botulism. Arch Neurol 1973; 29:425–431.

Hagenah R, Muller-Jensen H. Botulism: clinical neurophysiological findings. J Neurol 1978; 217:159–171.

MacDonald KL, Rutherford GW, Friedman SM, et al. Botulism and botulism-like illness in chronic drug abusers. Ann Intern Med 1985; 102:616–618.

MacDonald KL, Spengler RF, Hatheway CL, et al. Type A botulism from sauteed onions. Clinical and epidemiological observations. JAMA 1985; 253:1275–1278.

Pickett J. Infant botulism—the first five years. Muscle Nerve 1982; 5:S26–S28.

Pickett J, Berg B, Chaplin E, Brunstelter-Shafer M. Syndrome of botulism in infancy: Clinical and electrophysiologic study. N Engl J Med 1976; 295:770–772.

Terranova W, Palumbo JN, Breman JG. Ocular findings in botulism type B. JAMA 1979; 241:475–477.

Chapter XVII

Myopathy

129. IDENTIFYING DISORDERS OF THE MOTOR UNIT

Lewis P. Rowland

Muscle weakness may result from lesions of the corticospinal tract or the motor unit. Central disorders are accompanied by the distinctive and recognizable signs of upper motor neuron dysfunction. However, lesions of the motor unit (which includes the anterior horn cell, peripheral motor nerve, and muscle) are all manifested by flaccid weakness, wasting, and depression of tendon reflexes. Because the manifestations are so similar, there may be problems identifying disorders that affect one or another of the structures of the motor unit. In recent years, there has been controversy about the classification of individual cases as well as about some of the criteria used to distinguish the disorders. Nevertheless, for many reasons, it is still convenient to separate diseases of the motor unit according to the signs, symptoms, and laboratory data, as indicated in Table 129–1. It is necessary to oversimplify to prepare such a table; the reader must recognize that there are probably exceptions to each of the statements made in the table and individual cases may be impossible to define because of ambiguities or incongruities in clinical or laboratory data. Nevertheless, consistency between the different sets of data is usual. Some syndromes can be recognized clinically without recourse to laboratory tests, including typical cases of Duchenne dystrophy, Werdnig-Hoffmann disease, peripheral neuropathies, myotonic dystrophy, myotonia congenita, periodic paralysis, dermatomyositis, myasthenia gravis, and the myoglobinurias, to name a few. Controversies are mostly limited to syndromes of proximal limb weakness without clear signs of motor neuron disease

(fasciculation) or peripheral neuropathy (sensory loss, high CSF protein).

Because of the importance given to the laboratory tests, it is appropriate to describe them briefly. In a normal individual, the electromyogram (EMG), as recorded with concentric needle electrodes, is silent at rest. With voluntary innervation, motor unit potentials are recorded in numbers roughly proportionate to effort ("interference pattern"); the amplitude and duration of individual potentials have been defined quantitatively. In denervated muscle, fasciculations are seen in resting muscle, the number of motor units under voluntary control is decreased, and both duration and amplitude of individual potentials increase, presumably due to collateral sprouting of nerve fibers, so that the motor unit includes a greater than normal number of muscle fibers. In a typically myopathic disorder, there is no electrical activity at rest, the interference pattern is maintained, and individual potentials are smaller than normal (of reduced amplitude and duration).

Measurements of *nerve conduction velocity* help to distinguish disorders of the perikaryon (motor neuron diseases) from those of peripheral nerve (peripheral neuropathy). The speed of conduction in a motor nerve is determined by stimulating at one point on the nerve and measuring the time taken before the muscle responds, an interval attributed to the time for conduction in the nerve, nerve terminals, neuromuscular junctions, and muscle fibers. If the procedure is repeated at a second site, closer to the muscle, the interval is shorter because the impulse travels a shorter distance in the nerve. By subtracting one time from the other, it is possible to determine the time taken for the impulse to cover the measurable distance between the two sites of stimulation. The result is a rate of meters per second (mps). The velocity dif-

Table 129–1.   Identification of Disorders of the Motor Unit

	Anterior Horn Cell	Peripheral Nerve	Neuromuscular Junction	Muscle
Clinical				
Symptoms				
Persistent weakness	Yes	Yes	Yes	Yes
Variable weakness	No	No	Yes	No
Painful cramps	Often	Rare	No	Rare
Myoglobinuria	No	No	No	No
Paresthesias	No	Yes	No	No
Bladder disorder	Rare	Occasional	No	No
Signs				
Weakness	Yes	Yes	Yes	Yes
Wasting	Yes	Yes	No	Yes
Reflexes lost	Yes	Yes	No (MG)	Yes
Reflexes increased	Yes (ALS)	No	No	No
Babinski	Yes (ALS)	No	No	No
Acral sensory loss	No	Yes	No	No
Fasciculation	Common	Rare	No	No
Laboratory				
Serum enzymes ↑	No or mild	No	No	Yes
CSF protein ↑	Yes or mild	Yes	No	No
Motor nerve conduction				
Velocity slow	No or mild	Often	No	No
↑ or ↓ amplitude (repetitive stimulation)	No	No	Yes	No
EMG				
denervation	Yes	Yes	No	No
myopathic	No	No	No	Yes
Biopsy				
Neurogenic features	Yes	Yes	No	No
Myopathic features	No	No	No	Yes

fers in different nerves, is slower in cool limbs, and is influenced by age. Therefore normal values may differ, but rates are almost always more than 40 mps. (Similar methods have been developed to measure sensory conduction velocities.)

In the *muscle biopsy*, evidence of degeneration and regeneration affects fibers in a random pattern in a myopathy. Some fibers are unusually large, and fiber-splitting may be evident. In chronic diseases, there is usually little or no inflammatory cellular response; however, infiltration by white blood cells may be prominent in dermatomyositis and polymyositis. In the dystrophies, there may be infiltration by fat and connective tissue, especially as the disease advances. In denervated muscle, the major fiber change is simple atrophy, and groups of small fibers are typically seen adjacent to groups of fibers of normal size. In histochemical stains, fibers of different types are normally intermixed in a random checkerboard pattern, but in denervated muscle, fibers of the same staining type are grouped, presumably because of reinner-

vation of adjacent fibers, by one motor neuron. In denervated muscle, angular fibers may be the earliest sign. In other conditions, histochemical stains may give evidence of storage products, such as glycogen or fat, or may signify structurally specific abnormalities, such as nemaline rods, central cores or other unusual structures.

Slow conduction velocities imply demyelinating neuropathy; in motor neuron diseases, conduction is normal or only slightly delayed. However, conduction velocities are also normal in axonal forms of peripheral neuropathy. Therefore, slow conduction velocities indicate the presence of a peripheral neuropathy, but normal conductions may be seen in either peripheral neuropathy or motor neuron disease.

Serum enzyme determination is another important diagnostic aid. Creatine kinase (CK) is the most commonly used enzyme for diagnostic purposes; it is present in high concentration in muscle, and is not significantly present in liver, lung, or erythrocytes. To this extent, it is specific, and high serum content of CK is usually indicative of disease of the heart or skeletal muscle. The highest values are seen in Duchenne dystrophy, dermatomyositis, polymyositis, and attacks of myoglobinuria. In these conditions, other sarcoplasmic enzymes are also found in the serum, including serum glutamic-oxaloacetic transaminase (SGOT), serum glutamic-pyruvic transaminase (SGPT), and lactate dehydrogenase. However, CK may be increased in neurogenic diseases, too, especially Werdnig-Hoffmann disease, Kugelberg-Welander syndrome, and ALS, although not to the same extent as in the myopathies named. For instance, with a CK test in which the normal maximum is 50 units, values of about 3,000 are common in Duchenne dystrophy or dermatomyositis, and may reach 50,000 in myoglobinuria. In the denervating diseases, CK values greater than 500 would be unusual. In denervating diseases, the other sarcoplasmic enzymes are not increased in serum. In some individuals, CK may be increased inexplicably, with no other evidence of any muscle disease. Cardiologists have used isoenzyme analysis of CK to help differentiate between skeletal muscle and heart as the source of the increased serum activity; however, in the differential diagnosis of muscle disease, isoenzyme study has not been helpful, and the appearance of the "cardiac isoenzyme" of CK does not necessarily implicate the heart when there is limb weakness.

Definitions. It is useful to define some terms. *Atrophy* is used in three ways: to denote wasting of muscle in any condition, to denote small muscle fibers under the light microscope, and to name some diseases. By historical accident, all the diseases in which the word atrophy has been used in the name proved to be neurogenic (such as peroneal muscular atrophy or spinal muscular atrophy). Therefore, it seems prudent to use the word *wasting* in clinical description of limb muscles, unless it is known that the disorder is neurogenic. *Myopathies* are conditions in which the symptoms are due to dysfunction of muscle and in which there is no evidence of causal emotional disorder or of denervation on clinical grounds or in laboratory tests. The symptoms of myopathies are almost always due to weakness, but other symptoms include impaired relaxation (myotonia), cramps or contracture (in McArdle disease), or myoglobinuria. *Dystrophies* are myopathies with four special characteristics: (1) they are inherited; (2) all symptoms are due to weakness; (3) the weakness is progressive; and (4)

there are no histologic abnormalities in muscle other than degeneration and regeneration, or the reaction to those changes in muscle fibers (infiltration by fat and connective tissue). There is no storage of abnormal metabolic products. Some heritable myopathies are not called dystrophies because weakness is not the dominant symptom (as in familial myoglobinurias) or the syndrome is not usually progressive (as in periodic paralysis or static, presumably congenital, myopathies) and other names are assigned.

References

Brooke MM. A clinician's view of neuromuscular disease. 2nd Ed. Williams & Wilkins, Baltimore, 1986.

Engel AG, Banker BQ (eds.). Myology. McGraw-Hill, New York, 1986.

Walton JN (ed.). Disorders of Voluntary Muscle. 5th ed, 1988, Churchill Livingstone, Edinburgh.

130. PROGRESSIVE MUSCULAR DYSTROPHIES
Allen D. Roses

The progressive muscular dystrophies are inherited diseases that are distinguished from one another by clinical criteria. The pathogenesis of these diseases is unknown. The inherited biochemical defect has been identified in Duchenne dystrophy but is unknown in the other dystrophies. In those diseases, it is not known whether the fundamental biochemical abnormalities affect the motor neuron, muscle fiber, surface membrane, vascular supply, or other important structural component.

The most common muscular dystrophies are the *Duchenne, facioscapulohumeral* (FSH), and *myotonic* types. They are clearly differentiated by clinical presentation, mode of inheritance, and prognosis. The term *limb-girdle muscular dystrophy* is frequently used as a wastebasket diagnosis when there are transitional or borderline manifestations. Definite forms of limb-girdle muscular dystrophy are usually inherited as an autosomal recessive trait in segregated populations where relatives intermarry with relative frequency. These families are not encountered commonly, and detailed family histories are imperative. Autosomal dominant limb-girdle dystrophy has been verified in several pedigrees. As more information has accumulated about metabolic and inflammatory myopathies, some syndromes that were labeled as limb-girdle dystrophy proved later to be metabolic myopathies or polymyositis. The essential features of the three most common well-defined muscular dystrophies are shown in Table 130–1. No classification of the muscular dystrophies is satisfactory, but it is useful to list the disorders that appear to be distinct entities on genetic, clinical, and pathologic grounds. The following list is a slight modification of the classification of Walton and Gardner-Medwin:

X-linked muscular dystrophies
    Severe (Duchenne)
    Slower progression (Becker—a mutation of the same large gene as Duchenne)
    Scapuloperoneal
    Slow progression with early contracture (Emery-Dreifuss—different X locus from Duchenne/Becker)
Autosomal dominant muscular dystrophies
    Facioscapulohumeral
    Scapuloperoneal
    Limb-girdle
    Distal (adult-onset)
    Distal (infantile-onset)
    Ocular
    Oculopharyngeal
    Myotonic
Autosomal recessive muscular dystrophies
    Limb-girdle (with defined inheritance pattern)
    Childhood onset muscular dystrophy (resembling Duchenne)
    Congenital
    Scapulohumeral
    Limb-girdle and others that may have apparent sporadic onset

Duchenne Muscular Dystrophy

The estimated incidence of Duchenne muscular dystrophy is 1.9 to 4/100,000. These estimates have been similar in Europe, Australia, South America, and the United States.

The Duchenne type is virtually confined to boys, although rare cases of girls with Turner syndrome (XO genotype) or X translocations are known. Estimates of the mutation rate are high because affected males do not reproduce. However, there is no direct evidence that the mutation occurs in the ovary of the mother of an affected boy. Mothers of patients who have carried deletions also carry the deletion in one of their X chromosomes in most cases. Even when the deletion is absent in the mother, she still may transmit the deletion mutation to multiple offspring by an undefined mechanism, possibly a gonadal mosaic. A mutation in the sperm of an antecedent male or in meiosis of an antecedent female results in an unsuspected larger pool of carrier women who are not ascertained until the birth of an affected boy.

Clinical Features. The symptoms are due to muscular weakness or contractures and are usually evident before age 3 years, with gradual onset of difficulty walking or climbing stairs. Toe-walking and waddling gait are early manifestations; attempts to run result in much commotion but little progression because the boy cannot raise his knees properly. After unexpected falls, he may need help to rise and, in getting up from a chair, he braces his hands on his thighs or on the chair. A

Table 130–1. **Features of the Most Common Muscular Dystrophies**

	Duchenne	Facioscapulohumeral	Myotonic
Age of onset	Childhood	Adolescence	Birth through fifth decade
Sex	Male	Either	Either
Pseudohypertrophy	Common	Rare	Never
Initial clinical distribution	Pelvic girdle	Shoulder girdle	Distal limbs
Weakness of face	Rare and mild	Always	Common
Rate of progression	Relatively rapid	Slow (abortive)	Slow (variable)
Contractures and deformity	Common	Rare	Rare
Cardiac disorder	Usually late	Rare	Common
Inheritance	X-linked recessive	Dominant	Dominant
Expressivity	Full	Variable	Variable
Genetic heterogeneity	Multiple mutations at same locus for Duchenne and Becker	Documented (morphologic and EMG changes in muscles)	No evidence

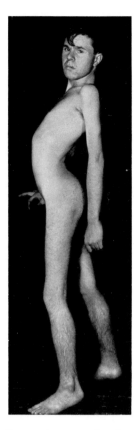

Fig. 130–1. Progressive muscular dystrophy. Lumbar lordosis. (Courtesy Dr. P.I. Yakovlev.)

straight back or lordotic posture is common. The calves are often visibly enlarged.

As the disease progresses, muscle wasting becomes more obvious. The gait may be precariously balanced with progressive lordosis, forward tilting of the pelvis, and protuberance of the abdomen. The upper trunk and head seem to brace back to achieve a center of gravity compatible with the waddling gait (Fig. 130–1). Iliofemoral or gastrocnemius contractures may interfere with gait.

Another feature of the disease is *Gowers sign*, which may be seen in spinal muscular atrophy or juvenile acid-maltase deficiency, but is almost universal in Duchenne dystrophy. In attempting to rise from a supine position, the patient first turns over onto the abdomen and raises the trunk to the crawling position. He then places the feet firmly on the floor with the aid of his arms and gradually elevates the upper part of the body by "climbing up his own trunk" with the arms (Fig. 130–2). As the disease progresses he may require a chair or fixed object to pull up to a standing position. Most boys cannot walk by

the time they are 11 years old; if a boy is still walking reasonably well at the age of 12, the disorder is usually called Becker dystrophy.

In most cases, the dystrophy is limited to the muscles of the trunk and limbs. The gastrocnemius, triceps, and deltoids are most frequently affected by the pseudohypertrophy. On palpation, the large muscles feel firm and rubbery while wasted muscles may be difficult to feel because of the overlying fat. There is symmetric involvement of the two sides. Spontaneous abnormal movements, fasciculations, or solely unilateral involvement are not seen.

Although no other cerebral symptoms are present, mild mental retardation seems to be common in Duchenne dystrophy. The children are usually not at the intellectual level of unaffected siblings. Sensation is normal and there are no sphincter disturbances. Tendon reflexes may be lost early but may persist even in wasted muscle. The knee jerks usually disappear before the ankle jerks, but contractures at the ankles may be present early. Cutaneous reflexes are preserved and the plantar responses are flexor.

Laboratory Data. Routine examinations of the blood, urine, and CSF are normal. Serum levels of creatine kinase (CK), aldolase, lactic dehydrogenase, and several other enzymes are much increased, particularly in young boys. High CK levels may be present at birth and continue to rise during the first year of life, even before overt symptoms are evident. Female relatives may have higher CK levels than age-matched controls. Definitely increased serum CK in a potential carrier makes it likely that she is a heterozygote. CK is a nonspecific test and normal CK activity does not exclude the carrier state. Definite carriers are mothers of an affected boy who also have some other affected male relative (e.g., brother, maternal uncle); 70 to 80% of these women have elevated CK levels. Therefore it is possible to identify carriers, but impossible to guarantee any women that she is *not* a carrier. This is true even using DNA probes (see below). Five to ten percent of carriers have demonstrable proximal limb weakness; mild changes have been found in muscle biopsy of some asymptomatic carriers.

EMG and muscle biopsy show the changes chacteristic of a myopathy. A tissue diagnosis of Duchenne dystrophy should be made by biopsy in the first known affected boy in a pedigree to exclude other less common diseases. There is excessive variation in the di-

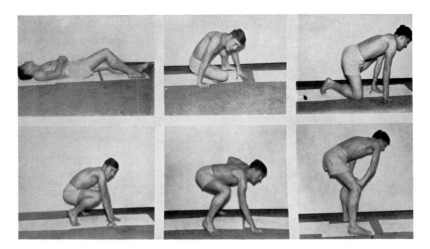

Fig. 130–2. Gowers sign in patient with Duchenne or Becker variety of muscular dystrophy. Postures assumed in attempting to rise from supine position.

ameter of rounded muscle fibers with prominent infiltration by fat and connective tissue. Enlargement of fibers (true hypertrophy) may add to the pseudohypertrophy caused by the increased fat and connective tissue. Establishing the diagnosis of Duchenne dystrophy with certainty gives the family the opportunity for female relatives to have genetic and family counseling and carrier testing.

DNA probes identifying deletions of coding sequences for the gene are being introduced for diagnostic purposes. A documented deletion would preclude the need for a diagnostic muscle biopsy.

Molecular genetic techniques have identified a very large, previously unknown protein, named dystrophin, as the site of the genetic defect. Most of the affected boys have a deletion of part of the gene (74% in our clinic). Immunocytologic studies have localized dystrophin to the muscle sarcolemma, where it appears to be associated with the inner side of the membrane. DNA sequencing studies have demonstrated actinin-type sequences and long stretches of spectrin-like sequences. The possible involvement of dystrophin in the integrity of the muscle membrane suggests that a spectrin (or now spectrin-like) molecular defect may prove relevant to pathogenetic mechanisms.

Course. The course of Duchenne dystrophy is predictable. Slower progression of symptoms and signs suggests the Becker form, which is more variable than Duchenne dystrophy. Becker dystrophy may present early and may seem indistinguishable from Duchenne dystrophy except that it progresses more slowly. Most Becker patients are still walking at age 12 years, when almost all Duchenne patients are in wheelchairs. Unless a previously diagnosed Becker case were present in a pedigree, it would be impossible to distinguish this form in childhood and the true proportion of Becker patients may therefore be underestimated. The ratio of Becker to Duchenne families is probably about 1:8. This differentiation is based on clinical criteria. Therefore, when one is counseling new families that have no history of progressive muscular dystrophy, it is helpful to present the possibility of the slow Becker form. Another subgroup currently classified as Becker dystrophy includes patients with onset of symptoms in the second decade and an even more favorable prognosis.

Both Duchenne and Becker dystrophy are due to defects of dystrophin. The exact nature of the heterogeneous mutations responsible for the more rapid progression of Duchenne dystrophy or the slower progression of Becker dystrophy is still being studied. Because both forms may be present in the same sibship, the possibility is suggested that some therapeutic intervention could slow the rate of the disease even in the situation in which a deletion causing a more rapid course is present.

Diagnosis. Duchenne dystrophy can be diagnosed by the onset of weakness in early childhood, pseudohypertrophy, characteristic distribution of weakness, family history, increased serum enzyme activity, and muscle biopsy or deletion analysis of the dystrophic gene. A few diseases mimic Duchenne dystophy: juvenile spinal musclar atrophy (Kugelberg-Welander), late-onset acid maltase deficiency, and juvenile glycogen debrancher deficiency may rarely affect young boys. However, these diseases are inherited as autosomal recessive traits and may therefore affect girls.

Girls rarely have a syndrome similar to Duchenne dystrophy. In documented pedigrees of Duchenne dystrophy, manifesting carriers or severely affected girls may be attributed to *lyonization*, the random inactivation of one of the X chromosomes that occurs in all female somatic cells. Every female is a mosaic for X-linked genes for which she is heterozygous and could theoretically express the Duchenne gene. Additional rare female cases are due to balanced X-autosomal translocations with the break point on the Xp21 areas of the short arm.

Confusion of Duchenne dystrophy with other diseases is uncommon, but the progressive dystrophies must be distinguished from polymyositis or dermatomyositis. The lack of family history, more rapid course, inflammatory response in muscle biopsy, and the characteristic rash of dermatomyositis are helpful. In polyneuritis, particularly the Guillain-Barré form, the weakness may be greatest in proximal muscles. The acute onset, lack of family history, sensory loss, and lack of flagrant elevations of serum enzyme activity usually do not lead to confusion with Duchenne or Becker dystrophy. EMG signs of denervation, high CSF protein content, and subsequent regression of symptoms establish the diagnosis of polyneuritis.

Treatment. There is no effective drug treatment for Duchenne dystrophy. Judicious and appropriately timed tendon-lengthening operations and sectioning of contractures may be helpful in medical centers where early postoperative ambulation is stressed. Use of light orthoses can stabilize the ankle or other joints.

Genetic Counseling. Recombinant DNA techniques have identified dystrophin as the genetic locus responsible for deletion mutations. The entire gene has been cloned and the exons identified. Deletions of dystrophin coding sequences in approximately 75% of the affected boys can be identified. At present only deletion or duplication mutants have been documented in Duchenne and Becker dystrophy. It is interesting that few (if any) point mutations lead to disease.

Deletion mutations in a family allow accurate genetic counseling to be performed. If a restriction fragment length polymorphism can be detected, it is possible to confirm sex and predict whether the deletion is present. Figure 130–3 illustrates the data from a prenatal diagnosis of a confirmed deletion carrier fetus. Figure 130–4 illustrates the pedigree of this female (IV-2). Her mother (III-4) is one of two daughters and an affected son who each carry the deletion mutation. Their mother does not carry the deletion and represents either a gonadal mosaic or an as yet undefined X chromosome mutation (such as a duplication) that she inherited or that became the first mutant. When a deletion is present, family counseling is very accurate. All affected males should be screened for deletions with coding sequences probes so that accurate genetic counseling is available for all female relatives.

Intragenic recombination, or cross-overs occurring within the large gene locus, have been documented with an estimated recombination frequency of 2 to 5%. Linkage markers in cases where deletions cannot be documented therefore are only 95 to 98% accurate. This accuracy is acceptable for carrier diagnosis, but is marginally acceptable for prenatal diagnoses. Rather than use linkage markers for prenatal diagnoses, one should try to identify a possible deletion mutation using genetic probes.

CK testing is still of considerable value in carrier testing in families where a deletion mutation has not been found. CK testing of fetal blood has no place in prenatal diagnosis.

Facioscapulohumeral (FSH) Muscular Dystrophy

FSH muscular dystrophy is inherited as an autosomal dominant trait and is variable in clinical expression, even in a single family. Although the symptoms and signs suggest a single disease entity, families with similar clinical manifestations may be separated by differing pathologic and EMG features. There seems to be a genetically heterogeneous group of distinct biochemical defects responsible for the phenotypic clinical expression of FSH muscular dystrophy.

Clinical Features. Facial or shoulder girdle weakness usually appears in adolescence, but signs may be apparent on examination in early childhood. Ocular and tongue muscles and muscles of mastication are spared, but facial weakness may be prominent. Difficulties in whistling, closing the eyes, or lifting the arms overhead are common initial symptoms. The lower lips may protrude and

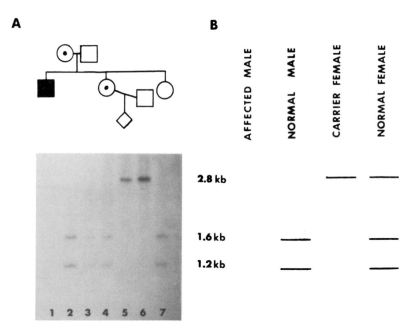

Fig. 130–3. Prenatal diagnosis in Duchenne muscular dystrophy. Panel *A,* Autoradiograph of Southern blot of 1% agarose gel with DNA samples from each individual digested with Xmnl and probed with pERT 87–15. The affected male is deleted (no signal). His sister who was pregnant has a deleted X and an X chromosome with the 1.6/1.2 allele. Her husband's X chromosome contains the 2.8 allele. The fetus contains the husband's X and the deleted X. Panel *B,* Diagram of the four possible outcomes of the prenatal diagnosis. The fetus is a carrier female.

winged scapulas or an enlarged supraclavicular triangle may be apparent. The clavicles may be parallel to the floor and the superior margins of the scapulas may be visible from the front. Lordosis may develop and anterior tibial weakness may occur. Gait may be impaired because of footdrop, but the ability to walk is rarely lost and then only late because the pelvic girdle is usually spared.

Diagnosis. FSH dystrophy may be confused with the scapuloperoneal syndromes, which are manifested by weakness of scapular, anterior tibial, and peroneal muscles. The facial weakness is the distinguishing feature of FSH dystrophy.

Distinct pathologic descriptions of muscle biopsies from families with apparently indistinguishable clinical disorders include dystrophic changes, inflammatory changes with type 2 fiber hypertrophy, small rounded type 1 fibers or angular fibers reminiscent of denervation, and structural abnormalities of muscle mitochondria. Thus FSH syndromes provide an example of an apparently homogeneous clinical phenotype with heterogeneous causes.

Myotonic Muscular Dystrophy

Myotonic muscular dystrophy (myotonia atrophica, dystrophia myotonica, Steinert disease) is inherited as an autosomal dominant trait. The highest incidence figures of 4.9 to 11/100,000 are undoubtedly underestimates. Pedigree analyses demonstrate many new cases for every newly presenting patient. Because the onset in individuals is variable, patients may consult medical specialists who are unfamiliar with myotonic dystrophy and therefore do not suspect it. Thus, many patients carrying the myotonic dystrophy gene are undiagnosed. The disease affects several organ systems and is characterized by myotonia, weakness and wasting of muscles, cataracts, cardiac abnormalities, and testicular atrophy. There is variable penetrance and expressivity; siblings may have different clinical manifestations. Myotonic dystrophy may be a cause of reproductive complications and aborted pregnancy in affected women; it may also present as a distinct syndrome of congenital myotonic dystrophy. Other members of the same family may have only cataracts with minimal symptoms or signs in other systems.

The biochemical abnormality is unknown, but physiologic studies of myotonia show that muscle relaxation is slow because of repetitive firing of fibers, which suggests that the gene affects membrane functions. Myotonia persists after spinal anesthesia, nerve block, or

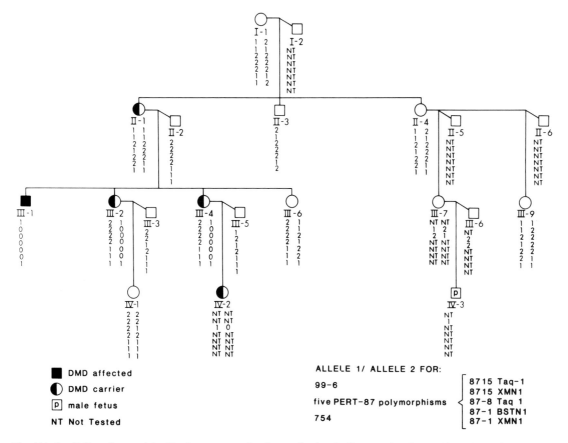

Fig. 130–4. Full pedigree of the Duchenne muscular dystrophy family illustrated in Figure 130–3. Note that II-1 does not have a deleted X in her blood DNA. Her son is deleted. This finding might be viewed as a new mutation in the absence of data from III-2 and III-4. II-1 may be a gonadal mosaic or there may be alternative explanations. In fact, she is functionally a carrier.

curarization and is therefore a property of the muscle membrane. An abnormality of chloride conductance has been associated with the myotonia of congenital myotonia (Thomsen disease) and goat myotonia, but is not present in muscle fibers from patients with myotonic dystrophy. The conditions listed below are characterized by myotonia:

Inherited Forms
  Congenital myotonia
    Autosomal dominant form
    Autosomal recessive form
  Myotonic muscular dystrophy (autosomal dominant)
  Adynamia episodica (hyperkalemic periodic paralysis) (autosomal dominant)
  Paramyotonia congenita (autosomal dominant)
  Chondrodystrophic myotonia (Schwartz-Jampel syndrome) (autosomal recessive)
  Syndrome of myotonia, myokymia, hyper-

hidrosis, muscle wasting (Isaacs syndrome) (? inheritance)
  Myotonia levior (? inheritance)
Acquired Forms
  Associated with carcinoma of the lung
  Induced by 20,25-diazacholesterol
  Induced by aromatic monocarboxylic acids such as 2,4-dichlorophenoxyacetate
  Induced by clofibrate
  Induced by other drugs or toxins
Conditions Resembling Myotonia
  Hypothyroidism
  Electrical myotonia of glycogen storage diseases (acid maltase deficiency and limit dextrinosis) and myositis

Abnormalities of membrane phosphorylation in both muscle and erythrocytes suggest that the biochemical defect affects other membranes too. Abnormalities in cation permeability and flux through membranes have been described, but the relationship of these data to the genetic defect remains unknown. Myotonia can be induced in animals by membrane-active drugs such as aromatic monocarboxylic acids or clofibrate, or by treatment of humans with an inhibitor of the final step of cholesterol synthesis, 20,25-diazacholesterol. The alteration of the lipid composition of muscle surface membranes may be responsible for the tendency of muscle fibers to fire repetitively. However, no consistent lipid abnormalities have been discovered in tissue from myotonic dystrophy patients.

Symptoms. The characteristic and diagnostic symptom is failure of the muscles to relax promptly after forceful contraction. The myotonia is most apt to appear when the muscle action is vigorous or abrupt. Myotonia of hand muscles, for example, may not be present when the patient fails to make a forceful contraction, but it may be evident when the patient grasps an object firmly. The distribution of the myotonia is variable. Rarely, all muscles of the body are affected, although symptoms are usually limited to the hands. The patients may become so well-adjusted to the difficulty in relaxing muscles that they may not complain of it or even realize that the symptoms are not normal. Frequently, myotonia is not a symptom but can be brought out by testing. The myotonia of myotonic dystrophy is usually not as prominent as that of myotonia congenita; most patients are not severely compromised by it.

Weakness and wasting of distal limb muscles is usually more disabling than the myotonia. Vision may be affected by cataracts. Abnormal cardiac arrhythmias may cause palpitations or dizzy spells. Abdominal cramps may accompany gastric or bowel dilatation. Swallowing difficulties are due to altered esophageal motility and dilatation. Hypersomnolence may also occur. Many of those who carry the gene never have any symptoms.

Infants of women with myotonic muscular dystrophy may have a special form of *congenital myotonic dystrophy* (Table 130–2). These floppy infants have difficulty sucking and nursing, although peripheral myotonia and limb weakness are lacking. Respiratory distress may be serious. Mental retardation is common and may be severe.

Signs. *Myotonia.* Myotonia can be demonstrated by the slow worm-like relaxation of grip after the patient forcefully grasps the examiner's fingers. It can also be shown by the prolonged contraction and slow relaxation of the thenar muscles when the base of the

Table 130–2. Manifestations of Congenital Myotonic Dystrophy

	Number of Cases	%
Total Studied	126	100.
Facial Weakness	108	85.7
Hypotonia	88	69.8
Delayed Motor Development	81	64.3
Mental Retardation	79	62.7
Talipes	66	52.4
Neonatal Respiratory Distress	60	47.6
Neonatal Feeding Difficulty	73	57.9
Hydramnios	32	25.4
Reduced Fetal Movement	28	22.2

(From Harper PS. Myotonic Dystrophy. Philadelphia: WB Saunders, 1977.)

thumb is struck with a percussion hammer. Myotonia of tongue muscles is manifested by a sustained localized contraction when a tongue depressor is placed under the tongue and the tongue is struck with a percussion hammer. A similar phenomenon can be demonstrated by percussing the muscles of the arm, leg, or trunk if they are affected by myotonia. The myotonia may disappear when wasting is advanced. Most patients with myotonia experience increased stiffness in cold weather, but there is a specific syndrome in which myotonia, especially of the orbicularis oculi, is characteristically brought out only by cold *(paramyotonia)*. This rare condition is also inherited in dominant fashion, but differs from other myotonic syndromes in that transient attacks of flaccid paralysis may be precipitated by cold. During the paralytic attack, the myotonia as abolished.

Weakness and Wasting. Although any muscles may be affected in late stages of the disease, wasting and weakness are commonly confined to the facial and neck muscles at first. Wasting of facial muscles gives the patient a characteristic long, lean, and expressionless appearance (Fig. 130–5). Voluntary and emotional movements are weak. The orbicularis oculi is often affected. The sternomastoid and intrinsic muscles of the neck are amost always small and weak. The patient cannot lift the head from the bed while in the supine position and turning movements of the head are weak. The muscles of deglutition are occasionally involved. Articulation or phonation is frequently impaired. The voice may be weak or nasal in quality. Wasting, with accompanying weakness, may extend to other muscles of the trunk or limbs. The wast-

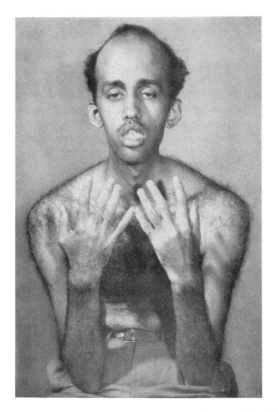

Fig. 130–5. Myotonic muscular dystrophy. Atrophy of facial, temporal, neck, and hand muscles.

ing is not preceded by hypertrophy and fasciculations do not occur. Smooth muscles of the gastrointestinal tract are occasionally affected. Cardiac abnormalities are more common. Sensation is normal and tendon reflexes are preserved unless the muscles are wasted.

Other Signs. Cataracts are present in most affected adult patients. The cataract starts in the posterior portion of the lens and frequently appears dust-like and iridescent under slit-lamp examination. It spreads slowly to involve other portions of the lens and may then interfere with vision. Development of lens opacity is related to age and is rarely seen in children. Slit-lamp examination is valuable in mapping myotonic dystrophy pedigrees. Cataracts may be the only sign in older individuals who have transmitted the gene.

Mental retardation is frequent and may not be directly related to the degree of myotonia or wasting. A personality pattern has been noted; some affected individuals seem to be unduly suspicious and uncooperative. Sociopathic personality disorders are common.

Gonadal atrophy may appear as early as the second decade, but is usually apparent in the third or fourth decade after the patient has already had children. In men, the testes are small and firm and there may be impotence. Women may have early menopause, although many patients have large families. Early baldness occurs commonly in men.

Laboratory Data. Routine examinations of blood, urine, and CSF do not show significant abnormalities, except for a reduction of the gamma globulin content of the serum because of rapid catabolism of IgG. Increased follicle-stimulating hormone levels may be seen in men with gonadal atrophy. About 35% of the patients show an abnormal response to glucose-loading with prolonged elevation of blood glucose and high serum insulin levels, but with normal growth hormone responses. "Insulin resistance" may also be seen in asymptomatic relatives in pedigree studies. Diabetes mellitus does not seem to be more common than in the general population. Serum CK activity is normal or only slightly increased. Diurnal cortisol levels are normal but 24-hour urine 17-ketosteroid levels may be decreased in patients wth gonadal atrophy.

In myotonic muscle, galvanic stimulation evokes a contraction that is sustained as long as the current flows and relaxes slowly after the stimulation is withdrawn (myotonic reaction). The EMG concomitant of myotonia is repetitive firing of muscle fibers, induced by movement of the needle, percussion, or voluntary contraction. Reduced duration of individual motor unit potentials is indicative of myopathy, as it is in other dystrophies.

The EKG is abnormal in most cases. Bradycardia and first-degree heart block are common; slowed or interrupted atrial-ventricular conduction is the most common sign. Progressive prolongation of the His-ventricular conduction time may lead to complete heart block. Patients may complain of nonspecific dizziness, and syncope can occur. There is often a history of sudden death in relatives and longitudinal family studies have documented sudden death in identified patients who had abnormal EKG, but no antecedent cardiac symptoms. Functional studies such as radionuclide angiography have documented myocardial asynergy and significantly decreased cardiac output with exercise.

Course. Myotonic dystrophy is progressive and symptoms refect the rate of progression and the systems involved. The course is frequently so slow that many patients live to old age without becoming incapacitated. When muscle wasting is extensive, patients may require a wheelchair or may become bedridden.

Limited or oligosymptomatic forms of the disease are common.

Diagnosis. The diagnosis can be made by the characteristic appearance (with wasting of the muscles of the neck and face) and the myotonia of limb muscles (see Fig. 130–5). Most patients are identified by the combination of myotonia, dystrophic weakness, and cataracts. Asymptomatic patients may be identified by combinations of physical signs or laboratory abnormalities such as hyperinsulin responses to glucose loads, abnormal esophageal motility, or increased IgG catabolism. There is no weakness, cataract, gonadal atrophy, or other multisystemic signs in congenital myotonia. Paramyotonia and hyperkalemic periodic paralysis are distinguished by myotonia only on exposure to cold or by repeated attacks of paralysis. *Chondrodystrophic myotonia (Schwartz-Jampel syndrome)* is distinguished by the combination of dwarfism, blepharophimosis, kyphoscoliosis, and flexion contractures of the limbs.

Differential Diagnosis. The unique clinical picture of myotonic dystrophy is not simulated by any other disease. Progressive muscular dystrophy may be considered in the few patients with myotonia that is inconspicuous or in those patients who have had myotonia but in whom it has disappeared. The history of previously symptomatic myotonia and the presence of other physical characteristics should establish the diagnosis. Myotonic dystrophy should be considered in the differential diagnosis of mental retardation, cataracts, dysphagia, cardiac arrhythmia, and hypothyroidism.

Treatment. The myotonia can be relieved or alleviated by the oral administration of quinidine or procaine amide. Because myotonia is rarely a major problem in myotonic dystrophy, treatment with these drugs should be judicious; both may increase heart block, and procaine amide may cause a syndrome of lupus erythematosus. Phenytoin may relieve myotonia without increasing atrioventricular block. In patients with complete heart block or when the His-ventricular conduction time exceeds 70 msec, insertion of a demand cardiac pacemaker is of value. Cataracts can be treated surgically, but macular degeneration or diabetic retinopathy should be excluded preoperatively as the cause of decreased vision. There is no effective treatment for the muscular weakness and wasting.

Genetic Counseling. The locus for the gene for myotonic dystrophy is on the proximal long arm of chromosome 19. No deletion mutations have been found. Tightly linked DNA restriction fragment-length polymorphisms are available for accurate diagnosis using linkage estimates. No new mutant with documented parentage has been described, so the use of linkage markers differs from Duchenne dystrophy in accuracy. DNA probes for apolipoprotein C2 are available and are 98% accurate in informative matings where the coinheritance of the polymorphic marker and the disease allele is known. An anonymous probe, LDR-152, is approximately 99% accurate in informative matings. It is anticipated that the gene will be delineated soon so that direct testing, without linkage markers, may be available in the future. The main clinical application in myotonic dystrophy is to assure young asymptomatic siblings of affected individuals that they do not carry the gene and can proceed with their families. Because of the personalities of many affected individuals, fewer prenatal diagnoses are requested than in other relatively common genetic diseases.

Myotonia Congenita

Myotonia congenita was described by Thomsen in 1876 and is characterized by generalized myotonia. Weakness is exceptional. The other stigmata of myotonic dystrophy are also missing. Myotonia congenita is distinct from myotonic dystrophy; cases in the early literature referred to as myotonia congenita plus one or another of the symptoms affected by myotonic dystrophy were undoubtedly patients with myotonic dystrophy. The myotonia of myotonia congenita is frequently more severe and symptomatic than in myotonic dystrophy. Myotonia congenita is most frequently inherited as an autosomal dominant trait, but families with autosomal recessive inheritance pattern have been reported.

Congenital Muscular Dystrophy

Congenital muscular dystrophy refers to genetically transmitted degenerative disease of muscle that is present clinically at birth. Because there are several distinct forms of this syndrome, it is probable that there are distinct congenital diseases. Since the gene defect for any of the congenital muscular dystrophies is unknown, the syndrome is classified clinically. Many cases appear sporadically, but it is suspected that most represent autosomal recessive traits.

The most recognizable form is that described by Fukayama and colleagues in Japanese families, but it has also been reported sporadically elsewhere. The mother is often aware of decreased fetal movements. A history of spontaneous abortions may be present. The infant cries and sucks poorly, is hypotonic, may have a funnel-chest abnormality, and has more proximal than distal limb weakness. Seizures are common, with or without associated fever. It is apparent as the child grows that mental retardation is prominent. Contractures at the knees, elbows, and hips develop and the child is virtually paralyzed by 10 years of age. Both sexes are affected and consanguineous marriages have been commonly encountered in the Japanese cases. EEGs are abnormal showing focal paroxysmal discharges wth spikes in the frontoparietal areas. CT reveals enlarged ventricles and a paucity of cortical gyri development. The EMG reveals myopathic abnormalities, and serum enzyme levels may be high. CK is frequently 10 to 50 times normal during the first six years, then gradually declines.

The other major group of congenital muscular dystrophy patients presents at birth with hypotonia and weakness. Contractures may occur in some forms of the syndrome, although not always when multiple children in the same family are affected. Progression of the disease is variable. Death can occur in the first year of life or the disease may appear to be relatively benign with delayed motor milestones. Within a family there appears to be a reasonable correlation between affected siblings. The diagnosis is usually made by muscle biopsy, ruling out other myopathies that may be morphologically distinguished, such as nemaline myopathy. Serum enzymes are usually mildly elevated but may be normal. The EMG is usually abnormal with brief, small-amplitude polyphasic potentials without fibrillation potentials.

As more is known about the potential gene product defects that can severely affect muscle early in life, the congenital muscular dystrophies will no doubt be characterized more specifically. Recognition is important for genetic counseling and differentiation from other neuropathic illnesses of similar clinical presentation that usually are not associated with retardation or other central nervous system abnormalities.

References

Duchenne Muscular Dystrophy

Banker BQ. Congenital muscular dystrophy. In: Engel AG, Banker BQ, eds. Myology. New York: McGraw-Hill, 1986; 1367–1382.

Bartlett RJ, Pericak-Vance MA, Koh J et al. Duchenne muscular dystrophy; high frequency of deletions. Neurology 1988; 38:1–4.

Bonilla E, Samitt CE, Miranda AF et al. Duchenne muscular dystrophy; deficiency of dystrophin at the muscle cell surface. Cell 1988; 54:447–452.

Brown RH Jr, Hoffman EP. Molecular biology of Duchenne muscular dystrophy. Trends Neurosci 1988; 11:480–483.

Carpenter S, Karpate G. Duchenne muscular dystrophy. Plasma membrane loss initiates muscle cell neurosis unless it is repaired. Brain 1979; 102:147–161.

Dubowitz V. The female carrier of Duchenne muscular dystrophy. Br Med J 1982; 1:1423–1424.

Emery AEH. Duchenne muscular dystrophy. Oxford University Press, Oxford, 1987.

Engel AG. Duchenne dystrophy. In: Engel AG, Banker BQ, eds. Myology. New York: McGraw-Hill, 1986; 1185–1240.

Fukuyama U, Kawazura M, Haruna H. A peculiar form of congenital progressive muscular dystrophy. Report of fifteen cases. Paediatr Univ Tokyo 1960; 4–5.

Hoffman EP, Fischbeck KH, Brown KH, Johnson M, et al. Characterization of dystrophin in muscle biopsy specimens from patients with Duchenne's or Becker's muscular dystrophy. New Engl J Med 1988; 318:1363–1368.

Hopkins SLC, Jackson JA, Elsas LJ. Emery-Dreifuss humeroperoneal muscular dystrophy: an X-linked myopathy with unusual contractures and bradycardia. Ann Neurol 1982; 10:230–237.

Koenig M, Hoffman EP, Bertelson CJ, Monaco AP, et al. Complete cloning of the Duchenne muscular dystrophy (DMD) cDNA and preliminary organization of the DMD gene in normal and affected individuals. Cell 1987; 50:509–519.

Koh J, Pericak-Vance MA, Yamaoka LH, Hung W-Y, et al. Inherited deletion at Duchenne dystrophy locus in normal male. Lancet 1987; 2:1155–1156.

Lanman J, Pericak-Vance MA, Bartlett RJ, Chen JC, Speer M, Hung WY, Roses AD. Familial inheritance of an DXS164 deletion mutation for a heterozygous female. Am J Hum Genet 1987; 41:138–144.

Mokri B, Engel AG. Duchenne dystrophy: Electron microscopic findings pointing to a basic or early abnormality in the plasma membrane of the muscle fiber. Neurology 1975; 25:1111–1120.

Monaco AP, Neve RL, Colletti-Feener C, Bertelson CJ, Kurnit DM, Kunkel LM. Isolation of candidate cDNAs for portions of the Duchenne muscular dystrophy gene. Nature 1986; 323:646.

Moser H, Emery AEH. The manifesting carrier in Duchenne muscular dystrophy. Clin Genet 1974; 5:271–284.

Prosser EJ, Murphy EG, Thompson MW. Intelligence and the gene for Duchenne muscular dystrophy. Arch Dis Child 1969; 44:221–230.

Roses AD. The impact of molecular genetics on clinical neurology. Arch Neurol 1988; 45:1366–1376.

Roses AD, Shile PE, Herbstreith MH, Balakrishnan CV. Identification of abnormally (^{32}P)-phosphorylated cyanogen bromide cleavage product of erythrocyte membrane spectrin in Duchenne muscular dystrophy. Neurology 1981; 31:1026–1030.

Rowland LP. Clinical concepts of Duchenne muscular dystrophy; the impact of molecular genetics. Brain 1988; 111:479–495.

Scott MO, Sylvester JE, Heiman-Patterson T, Shi YJ, et al. Duchenne muscular dystrophy gene expression in normal and diseased human muscle. Science 1988; 239:1418–1419.

Siddique T, Bartlett RJ, Pericak-Vance MA, Yamaoka L, Koh J, Chen, J, Hung WY, Kandt R, Roses AD. Update on the molecular genetics of Duchenne muscular dystrophy. Muscle Nerve 1989 (in press).

Watkins SC, Hoffman EP, Slayter HS, Kunkel LM. Immunoelectron microscopic localization of dystrophin in myofibres. Nature 1988; 333:863–866.

Facioscapulohumeral Muscular Dystrophy

Fitzsimons RB, Gurwin EB, Bird AC. Retinal vascular abnormalities in fascioscapulohumeral muscular dystrophy. Brain 1987; 110:631–648.

Hanson PA, Rowland LP. Mobius syndrome and facioscapulohumeral muscular dystrophy. Arch Neurol 1974; 24:31–39.

Mechler F, Fawcett PRW, Mastaglia FL, Hudgson P. Mitochondrial myopathy. A study of clinically affected and asymptomatic members of a six-generation family. J Neurol Sci 1981; 50:191–200.

Munsat TL. Facioscapulohumeral dystrophy and the scapuloperoneal syndrome. In: Engel AG, Banker BQ, eds. Myology. New York: McGraw-Hill, 1986: 1251–1266.

Thomas PK, Schott GD, Morgan-Hughes JA. Adult-onset scapuloperoneal myopathy. J Neurol Neurosurg Psychiatry 1975; 38:1008–1015.

Limb-Girdle Muscular Dystrophy

Gilchrest JM, Pericak-Vance MA, Silverman LM, Roses AD. Clinical and genetic investigation in autosomal dominant limb-girdle dystrophy. Neurology 1988; 38:5–9.

Shields RW. Limb girdle syndromes. In: Engel AG, Banker BQ, eds. Myology. New York: McGraw-Hill, 1986: 1349–1366.

Swash M, Heathfield KWG. Quadriceps myopathy: a variant of the limb-girdle dystrophy syndrome. J Neurol Neurosurg Psychiatry 1983; 46:355–357.

Myotonic Muscular Dystrophy

Aberfeld DC, Namba T, Vye MV, Grob D. Chondrodystrophic myotonia: Report of two cases. Myotonia dwarfism, diffuse bone disease and unusual ocular and facial abnormalities. Arch Neurol 1970; 22:455–462.

Bartlett RJ, Pericak-Vance MA, Gilbert J, Yamaoka L, Herbstreith M, Hung WY, Lee J, Mohandas T, Bruns G, Laberge C, Thibault MC, Ross DA, Roses AD. A new probe for the diagnosis of myotonic muscular dystrophy. Science 1987; 235:1648–1650.

Becker PE. Genetic approaches to the nosology of muscle disease: myotonias and similar diseases. Birth Defects 1971; 7:52–62.

Becker PE, Knussmann R, Kuhn E. Myotonia Congenita and Syndromes Associated with Myotonia. Stuttgart: Georg Thieme, 1977.

Davies KE, Jackson J, Williamson R, Harper PS, Ball S, Sarfarazi M, Meredith L, Fey G. Linkage analysis of myotonic dystrophy and sequences on chromosome 19 using a cloned complement 3 gene probe. J Med Genet 1983; 20:259–263.

Desnuelle C, Lombet A, Serratrice G, Lazdunski M. Sodium channel and sodium pump in normal and pathological muscles from patients with myotonic muscular dystrophy and lower motor neuron impairment. J Clin Invest 1982; 69:358–367.

Dodge PR, Gamstorp I, Byers RK, Russell P. Myotonic dystrophy in infancy and childhood. Pediatrics 1965; 35:3–19.

Fowler WM Jr, Layzer RB, Taylor RG, et al. The Schwartz-Jampel syndrome. Its clinical, physiological and histological expressions. J Neurol Sci 1974; 22:127–146.

Furman RE, Barchi RL. Diazacholesterol myotonia; an electrophysiological study. Ann Neurol 1981; 10:251–260.

Kuhn E, Fiehn W, Seiler D, Schroder JM. Autosomal recessive (Becker) form of myotonia congenita. Muscle Nerve 1979; 2:109–117.

Landouzy L, Déjèrine J. De la myopathie atropique progressive; myopathie hereditaire, sans neuropathie, debutant d'ordinaire dans l'enfance par la face. Paris: F Alcan, 1885.

Moxley RT III, Griggs RC, Goldblatt D. Muscle insulin resistance in myotonic dystrophy. Neurology 1980; 30:1077–1083.

Nguyen HH, Wolfe JT III, Holmes DR Jr, Edwards WD. Pathology of the cardiac conduction system in myotonic dystrophy; 12 cases. J Am Coll Cardiol 1988; 11:662–671.

Pericak-Vance MA, Yamaoka LH, Assinder BA, Hung WY, et al. Tight linkage of apolipoprotein C_2 to myotonic dystrophy on chromosome 19. Neurology 1986; 36:1418–1423.

Prystowsky EN, Pritchett ELC, Roses AD, Gallagher JJ. The natural history of conduction system disease in myotonic muscular dystrophy as determined by serial electrophysiologic studies. Circulation 1979; 60:1360–1364.

Roses AD. The impact of molecular genetics on clinical neurology. TINS 1986; 9:518–522.

Roses AD, Harper P, Bossen E. Myotonic muscular dystrophy (dystrophia myotonica, myotonia atrophy). In: Vinken PJ, Bruyn GW, eds. Handbook of Clinical Neurology (vol 40). New York: Elsevier-North Holland, 1979:485–532.

Roses AD, Hartwig GB, Mabry M, Wong P, Nagano Y, Miller SE. Red blood cell and fibroblast membranes in Duchenne and myotonic muscular dystrophy. Muscle Nerve 1980; 3:36–54.

Roses AD, Pericak-Vance MA, Bartlett RJ, Yamaoka L, Lee JE, Koh J, Chen JC, Gilbert JR, Ross DA, Herbstreith MH, Sirotkin-Roses MJ. Myotonic dystrophy—update on progress to define the gene. Aust Paediatr J (in press).

Watters GV, Williams TW. Early onset myotonic dystrophy. Arch Neurol 1967; 17:139–152.

Wintzen AR, Schipperheyn JJ. Cardiac abnormalities in myotonic dystrophy. J Neurol Sci 1987; 80:259–268.

Wong P, Roses AD. Isolation of an abnormally phosphorylated erythrocyte membrane band 3 glycoprotein from patients with myotonic muscular dystrophy. J Membr Biol 1979; 45:147–166.

131. FAMILIAL PERIODIC PARALYSIS
Lewis P. Rowland

Familial periodic paralysis is the name given to a group of familial diseases of unknown cause characterized by recurrent attacks of weakness or paralysis of the limb muscles, accompanied by loss of deep reflexes and failure of the muscles to respond to electrical stimulation. It was once thought that all cases were associated with a decrease in the potassium content of the serum at the onset of the attacks of weakness. It is now known that at least two types can be distinguished and there are probably more. *Hypokalemic* and *hyperkalemic* forms are the most clearly defined. *Adynamia episodica hereditaria* is another name for the hyperkalemic form. *Paramyotonia* (Eulenberg syndrome) is a form of myotonia that is clinically most evident in a cold environment. Families with paramyotonia usually, but not always, include individuals who are susceptible to hyperkalemic attacks. A "normokalemic" form has been proposed but is probably the same as the hyperkalemic form. Although there are clinical distinctions (Table 131–1), these differences are not always demonstrable; identification of the syndrome depends on the serum potassium content in a spontaneous or induced attack. All forms show clear evidence of autosomal dominant inheritance.

Vacuoles are found in the muscles in the early stages of both hypokalemic and hyperkalemic forms of the disease. These vacuoles seem to arise from both the terminal cisterns of the sarcoplasmic reticulum and from proliferation of the T-tubules. In the later stage, there may be degeneration of the muscle fibers, possibly related to mild weakness in the intervals between attacks.

Hypokalemic Periodic Paralysis

In this form of the disease, the potassium content decreases in a spontaneous attack to values of 3.0 mEq/L or lower. Attacks may be induced by the injection of insulin, epinephrine, flurohydrocortisone, or glucose, or they may follow ingestion of a meal high in carbohydrates. The potassium content of the urine is also decreased in an attack. The inherited abnormality has not been identified and it is not clear why potassium shifts into muscle to cause the attack. Layzer has suggested that the fault may be an altered surface membrane that abnormally reduces muscle permeability to potassium. Johnsen has suggested that increased insulin release may be important.

Incidence. The disease is rare. There are no large series reported in the literature and only one or two cases are seen each year in any of the large neurologic clinics in this country. Males are affected 2 to 3 times as frequently as females. The first attack usually occurs at about the time of puberty, but it may occur as early as the age of 4 or be delayed to the sixth decade.

Symptoms and Signs. The attack usually begins after a period of rest. It commonly develops during the night or is present on waking in the morning. The extent of the paralysis varies from slight weakness of the legs to complete paralysis of all the muscles of the trunk and limbs. The oropharyngeal and respiratory muscles are usually spared, even in severe attacks. There may be retention of urine and feces during a severe attack. The duration of the individual attack varies from a few hours to 24 or 48 hours. According to some patients, strength improves if they

Table 131–1. The Clinical Features of Low and High Serum Potassium Periodic Paralysis and Paramyotonia

	Low Serum Potassium Periodic Paralysis	High Serum Potassium Periodic Paralysis	Paramyotonia Congenita
Age of onset	Usually second or latter part of first decade	First decade	First decade
Sex	Male preponderance	Equal	Equal
Incidence of paralysis	Interval of weeks or months	Interval of hours or days	May not be present; otherwise, interval of weeks or months
Degrees of paralysis	Tends to be severe	Tends to be mild but can be severe	Tends to be mild but can be severe
Effect of cold	May induce an attack	May induce an attack	Tends to induce an attack of paralysis
Effect of food (especially glucose)	May induce an attack	Relieves an attack	Relieves an attack of paralysis
Serum potassium	Low	High	Tends to be high
Oral potassium	Prevents an attack	Precipitates an attack	Precipitates an attack

(Modified from Hudson AJ. Brain 1963; 86:811.)

move around and keep active ("walking it off"). The interval between attacks may be as long as a year, or one or more attacks of weakness may occur daily. Weakness is especially likely to be present on the morning after the ingestion of a high-carbohydrate meal before retiring on the previous night. Rarely, the disease may occur in association with peroneal muscular atrophy.

In the interval between attacks, the patients are usually strong and the potassium content of the serum is normal. In some patients, mild proximal limb weakness persists. In a mild attack, tendon reflexes and electrical reactions of the muscles are diminished in proportion to the degree of weakness. In severe attacks, tendon and cutaneous reflexes are absent and the muscles do not respond to electrical stimulation. Cutaneous sensation is not disturbed.

Course. Familial hypokalemic periodic paralysis is not accompanied by any impairment of general health. As a rule, the frequency of the paralytic attacks decreases with the passage of the years and they may cease altogether after the age of 40 or 50. Fatalities are rare, but death may occur from respiratory paralysis.

Diagnosis. The diagnosis can usually be made without difficulty on the basis of the familial occurrence of transient attacks of weakness. The diagnosis can usually be con-

Table 131–2. Potassium and Paralysis: Noninherited Forms

Hypokalemic
  Excessive urinary loss
    Hyperaldosteronism
    Drugs: glycyrrhizate (licorice), thiazides, furosemide, chlorthalidone, ethacrynic acid, amphotercin, duogastrone
    Pyelonephritis, renal tubular acidosis
    Recovery from diabetic acidosis
    Ureterocolostomy
  Excessive gastrointestinal loss
    Malabsorption syndrome
    Laxative abuse
    Diarrhea
    Fistulas, vomiting, villous adenoma
    Pancreatic tumor, diarrhea
  Thyrotoxicosis
Hyperkalemia
  Uremia
  Addison disease
  Spironolactone excess
  Excessive intake
    Iatrogenic
    Geophagia

firmed by finding low potassium and high sodium content in the serum during an attack, or by inducing an attack with an intravenous infusion of glucose (100 g) and regular insulin (20 units). In sporadic cases, the first attack has to be differentiated from other causes of hypokalemia (Table 131–2). Persistent hypokalemia from any cause may be manifested as an acute attack of paralysis or persistent limb weakness with high levels of serum creatine kinase (CK). Sometimes there are attacks of myoglobinuria.

Repeated attacks of hypokalemic periodic paralysis, identical clinically to the familial form, occur in patients with hyperthyroidism. Japanese and Chinese people seem to be especially susceptible to this disorder.

Treatment. Acute attacks, spontaneous or induced, may be safely and rapidly terminated by ingestion of 20 to 100 mEq of potassium salts. (Intravenous administration of potassium is usually avoided because of the hazard of inducing hyperkalemia.)

Prophylactic treatment was not satisfactory until recently and numerous regimens were devised in an attempt to reduce the number of attacks: diet supplementation with potassium salts; low-sodium low-carbohydrate diet; and spironolactone, triampterine, or dexamethasone to promote retention of potassium. The most effective prophylaxis, however, results from oral administration of acetazolamide in doses of 250 to 1,000 mg daily. Treatment with acetazolamide may also be followed by improvement of the fixed weakness between attacks that was formerly attributed to myopathic changes in the muscles.

Although most patients with either type of familial periodic paralysis respond to acetazolamide therapy, there are some failures. The mechanism of action of acetazolamide is uncertain; the beneficial effect may be related to the metabolic acidosis it induces. When acetazolamide fails or when there are adverse reactions in hypokalemic cases to the drug, it is necessary to use the aforementioned prophylactic measures in different combinations.

The treatment of other forms of hypokalemic paralysis depends on the nature of the underlying renal disease, diarrhea, drug ingestion, or thyrotoxicosis. Patients with thyrotoxic periodic paralysis are susceptible to spontaneous or induced attacks during the period of hyperthyroidism. When the patients become euthyroid, spontaneous attacks cease and they are no longer sensitive to infusion of glucose and insulin. Glucose and insulin are useful in the interim between treatment of hyperthyroidism by drugs or radioiodine, before the euthyroid state returns. Repeated attacks can be prevented by either acetazolamide or propanolol.

Hyperkalemic Periodic Paralysis

In 1951, Frank Tyler recognized a form of familial periodic paralysis in which the attacks were not accompanied by a decrease in the serum potassium content. In 1956, Gamstorp and Mjönes drew attention to several features of these cases that separated them from the usual cases of periodic paralysis. They proposed the term *adynamia episodica hereditaria* to describe these cases. The disease is transmitted by an autosomal dominant gene with almost complete penetrance.

In addition to the absence of hypokalemia in the attacks, the syndrome is characterized by the early age of onset (usually before age 10), the tendency of the attacks to occur in the daytime and to be shorter and less severe. Myotonia is usually demonstrable by EMG, but abnormalities of muscular relaxation are rarely symptomatic. Myotonic lid-lag (Fig. 131–1) and lingual myotonia may be the sole clinical evidence of the trait. The serum po-

tassium content and urinary excretion of potassium may be increased during an attack. This may be due to leakage of potassium from muscle. The attacks tend to be precipitated by hunger, rest, and cold and by administration of potassium chloride.

Attacks may be terminated by administration of calcium gluconate, glucose, and insulin. Acetazolamide, in oral doses of 250 mg to 1 g daily, has been effective in reducing the number of attacks or in abolishing them altogether. Other diuretics that promote urinary excretion of potassium are also effective. If acetazolamide therapy fails, thiazides or fludrocortisone may be beneficial.

Beta-adrenergic drugs may also be effective prophylactic agents. Epinephrine, albuterol, and metaproterenol have all been used. They presumably act by increasing the activity of Na,K-ATPase.

A variant of adynamia episodica hereditaria was reported by Poskanzer and Kerr. The disease in their cases (21 members of a family of 45) was characterized by relative infrequency and long duration of the attacks. In a few families with hyperkalemic periodic paralysis, persistent or intermittent arrhythmia and sudden death have occurred in young children; it is not clear whether this is a special form of the disease.

Paramyotonia Congenita

Whether this is truly a separate genetic entity is now uncertain. All forms of myotonia are aggravated by cold and the attacks of paralysis in Eulenberg's cases suggest that they were due to hyperkalemic periodic paralysis. It is possible, however, that there is a disease in which myotonia is detectable or symptomatic only in cold and in which there is no hyperkalemic periodic paralysis.

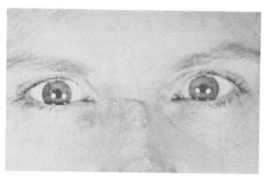

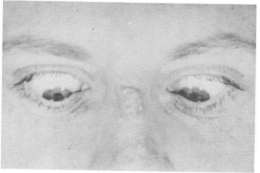

Fig. 131–1. Paramyotonia congenita. Myotonia of muscles of upper lids on looking downward. (Courtesy of Dr. Robert Layzer.)

References

Hypokalemic Periodic Paralysis

Comi G, Testa D, Cornelio F, Comola M, Canal N. Potassium depletion myopathy: a clinical and morphological study of six cases. Muscle Nerve 1985; 8:17–21.

Conway MJ, Seibel JA, Eaton RP. Thyrotoxicosis and periodic paralysis: improvement with beta blockade. Ann Intern Med 1974; 81:332–336.

Engel AG, Lambert EH, Rosevear JW, Tauxe WN. Clinical and electromyographic studies in a patient with primary hypokalemic periodic paralysis. Am J Med 1965; 38:626–640.

Griggs RC, Engel WK, Resnik JS. Acetazolamide treatment of hypokalemic periodic paralysis. Prevention of attacks and improvement of persistent weakness. Ann Intern Med 1970; 73:39–48.

Hofmann WW, Smith RA. Hypokalemic periodic paralysis studied in vitro. Brain 1970; 93:445–474.

Holtzapple GE. Periodic paralysis. JAMA 1905; 45:1224.

Hudson AJ. Progressive neurological disorder and myotonia congenita associated with paramyotonia. Brain 1963; 86:811–826.

Johnsen T. Familial periodic paralysis with hypokalemia. Dan Med Bull 1981; 28:1–27.

Johnsen T, Beck-Nielsen H. Insulin receptor, insulin secretion and glucose disappearance role in patients with periodic hypokalemic paralysis. Acta Endocrinol 1979; 90:272–282.

Knochel JP. Neuromuscular manifestations of electrolyte disorders. Am J Med 1982; 72:525–535.

Layzer RB, Goldfield E. Periodic paralysis caused by abuse of thyroid hormone. Neurology 1974; 24:949–952.

Layzer RB. Periodic paralysis and the sodium potassium pump. Ann Neurol 1982; 11:547–552.

Links TP, Zwarts MJ, Oosterhuis HJGH. Improvement of muscle strength in familial hypokalemic periodic paralysis with acetazolamide. J Neurol Neurosurg Psychiatry 1988; 51:1142–1145.

Martin AR, Levinson SR. Contribution of the Na,K pump to membrane potential in familial periodic paralysis. Muscle Nerve 1985; 8:359–362.

Minaker KL, Menelly GS, Flier JS, Rowe JW. Insulin-mediated hypokalemia and paralysis in familial hypokalemic periodic paralysis. Am J Med 1988; 84:1001–1006.

Riggs JE, Griggs RC. Diagnosis and treatment of periodic paralysis. Clin Neuropharmacol 1979; 4:123–138.

Roadma JS, Reidenberg MM. Symptomatic hypokalemia resulting from surreptitious diuretic ingestion. JAMA 1981; 246:1687–1689.

Rudel R, Ricker K. The primary periodic paralyses. TINS 1985; 8:467–470.

Van Horn G, Drosi JB, Schwartz FD. Hypokalemic myopathy and elevation of serum enzymes. Arch Neurol 1970; 22:335–341.

Vern BA, Danon MJ, Hanlon K. Hypokalemic periodic paralysis with unusual responses to acetazolamide and sympathetomimetics. J Neurol Sci 1987; 81:159–172.

Vroom FQ, Jarrell MA, Maren TH. Acetazolamide treatment of hypokalemic periodic paralysis. Probable mechanisms of action. Arch Neurol 1975; 32:385–392.

Waimsley RN, White GH. Occult causes of hypokalemia. Clin Chem 1984; 30:1406–1408.

Yazaki K, Kuribayashi T, Yamamura Y, Kurihara T, Araki S. Hypokalemic myopathy associated with 17X-hydroxylase deficiency: a case report. Neurology 1982; 32:94–97.

Hyperkalemic Periodic Paralysis

Bendheim PE, Reale EO, Berg BO. Beta adrenergic treatment of hyperkalemic periodic paralysis. Neurology 1985; 35:746–749.

Benstead TJ, Camfield PR, Ding DB. Treatment of paramyotonia congenita with acetazolamide. Can J Neurol Sci 1987; 14:156–158.

Bradley WG. Adynamia episodica hereditaria. Clinical, pathological, and electrophysiological studies in an affected family. Brain 1969; 92:345–378.

Danowski TS, et al. Clinical and ultrastructural observations in a kindred with normokalemic periodic paralysis. J Med Genet 1975; 12:20.

Gamstorp I, et al. Adynamia episodica hereditaria. Am J Med 1957; 23:385.

Gamstorp I. Adynamia episodica hereditaria and myotonia. Acta Neurol Scand 1963; 39:41.

Gelfand MC, Zarate A, Knepshield JH. Geophagia. A cause of life-threatening hyperkalemia. JAMA 1975; 234:738.

Layzer RB, Lovelace RE, Rowland LP. Hyperkalemic periodic paralysis. Arch Neurol 1967; 16:455–472.

Lisak RP, Lebeau J, Tucker SH, Rowland LP. Hyperkalemic periodic paralysis and cardiac arrhythmia. Neurology 1972; 22:810–815.

Magee KR. A study of paramyotonia congenita. Arch Neurol 1963; 8:461.

McArdle B. Adynamia episodica hereditaria and its treatment. Brain 1962; 85:121–148.

Perez G, Siegel L, Schreiner GE. Selective hypoaldosteronism with hyperkalemia. Ann Intern Med 1972; 76:757.

Ponce SP, Jennings AE, Madias NE, Harrington JT. Drug-induced hyperkalemia. Medicine 1985; 64:357–370.

Poskanzer DC, Kerr DNS. A third type of periodic paralysis with normokalemia and favorable response to sodium chloride. Am J Med 1961; 31:328.

Streeten DHP, Dalakos TG, Fellerman H. Studies on hyperkalemic periodic paralysis. Evidence of changes in plasma Na and Cl and induction of paralysis by adrenal glucocorticoids. J Clin Invest 1971; 50:142–155.

132. OTHER DISEASES OF MUSCLE

Lewis P. Rowland

Myoglobinuria

When necrosis of muscle is acute, myoglobin escapes into the blood and then into the urine. In the past, the term *myoglobinuria* was reserved for grossly pigmented urine, but modern techniques can detect amounts of this protein so minute that discoloration may not be evident. (Determination of serum myoglobin content by radioimmunoassay has the same significance as measurement of serum creatine kinase [CK] activity.) The clinically important syndromes, however, are associated with gross pigmenturia. Sometimes the disorder can be recognized without direct demonstration of myoglobin in the urine; for instance, in cases of acute renal failure with very high levels of serum CK activity. Inexplicably, *rhabdomyolysis* has become a popular term for these syndromes, although it is really a synonym for myoglobinuria.

No classification of the myoglobinurias is completely satisfactory, but Table 132–1 lists the most important causes. Many cases of inherited recurrent myoglobinuria are due to unidentified abnormalities. In six forms, however, the genetic defect has been recognized: lack of phosphorylase (McArdle), phosphofructokinase (Tarui), carnitine palmityl transferase (DiMauro-Bank), phosphoglyceralde-

Table 132–1. Classification of Human Myoglobinuria

I. *Hereditary Myoglobinuria*
  Phosphorylase deficiency (McArdle)
  Phosphofructokinase deficiency (Tarui)
  Carnitine palmityl transferase deficiency (DiMauro)
  Phosphoglycerate kinase (DiMauro)
  Phosphoglycerate mutase (DiMauro)
  Lactate dehydrogenase (Kanno)
  Incompletely characterized syndromes
    Excess lactate production (Larsson)
  Uncharacterized
    Familial; biochemical defect unknown
      Provoked by diarrhea or infection
      Provoked by exercise
    Familial susceptibility to succinylcholine or general anesthetics ("malignant hyperthermia")
    Repeated attacks in an individual; biochemical defect unknown
II. *Sporadic Myoglobinuria*
  Exertion in untrained individuals
    "Squat-jump" and related syndromes
    Anterior tibial syndrome
    Convulsions
    High-voltage electric shock, lightning stroke
    Agitated delerium, restraints
    Status asthmaticus
    Prolonged myoclonus or acute dystonia
  Crush syndrome
    Compression by fallen weights
    Compression by body in prolonged coma
  Ischemia
    Arterial occlusion
    Ischemia in compression and anterior tibial syndromes
    Coagulopathy in sickle cell disease or disseminated intravascular coagulation
    Ligation of vena cava
  Metabolic abnormalities
    Metabolic depression
      Barbiturate, carbon monoxide, narcotic coma
      Diabetic acidosis
      General anesthesia
      Hypothermia
    Exogenous toxins and drugs
      Haff disease
      Alcoholism
      Malayan sea-snake bite poison
      Plasmocid
      Succinylcholine
      Glycyrrhizate, carbenoxolone, amphotericin-B
      Heroin
      Phenylpropanolamine
      Lovastatin
      Malignant neuroleptic syndrome
    Chronic hypokalemia of any cause
    Heat stroke
    Toxic shock syndrome
  Progressive muscle disease ("polymyositis," "alcoholic myopathy")
  Cause unknown

hyde kinase (DiMauro), phosphoglycerate mutase (DiMauro), and lactate dehydrogenase (Kanno). Carnitine palmityl transferase (CPT) is important in lipid metabolism; the others are involved in glycogenolysis or glycolysis. In all these conditions, there is a disorder in the metabolism of a fuel necessary for muscular work; in all six, exercise is limited by painful cramps after exertion and myoglobinuria occurs after especially strenuous activity. There may be a subtle difference in the kinds of activity that provoke attacks, which are more prolonged in CPT deficiency than in the glycogen disorders. The glycogen disorders can be identified by a simple clinical test: a cramp is induced by ischemic exercise of forearm muscles for less than 1 minute and venous lactate fails to rise as it does in normal individuals or in those with CPT deficiency. Specific diagnosis requires histochemical or biochemical analysis of muscle homogenates. Five of the conditions are inherited in autosomal recessive pattern; phosphoglycerate kinase deficiency is X-linked.

Another important form of inherited myoglobinuria occurs in *malignant hyperthermia*, which seems to be due to succinylcholine in some cases and to halothane in others. The characteristic syndrome includes widespread muscular rigidity, a rapid rise in body temperature, myoglobinuria, and metabolic acidosis. In some cases, muscular rigidity is lacking. The syndrome seems to be transmitted by an autosomal dominant gene with incomplete penetrance in some families, but many cases are sporadic. The biochemical abnormality has not been identified, but may involve an unusual susceptibility of the sarcoplasmic reticulum to the offending drugs, impairing the ability of the sarcoplasmic reticulum to bind calcium. Heterogeneity of the syndrome is evident because some cases occur in patients with Duchenne muscular dystrophy, myotonia congenita, or central core disease. A closely related disorder is the *neuroleptic malignant syndrome*, which is similar in clinical manifestations, although the offending drugs are different and the disorder has not yet appeared in a family with malignant hyperthermia.

Most cases of *acquired myoglobinuria* occur in nonathletic individuals who are subjected to extremely vigorous exercise, a hazard faced primarily by military recruits. These individuals are otherwise normal. Even trained runners may experience myoglobinuria in marathon races. If muscle is compressed, as occurs in the crush syndrome of individuals pinned by fallen timber after bombing raids, or after prolonged coma in one position, myoglobinuria may ensue. Ischemia after occlusion of large arteries may also lead to necrosis of large amounts of muscle. Depression of muscle metabolism, especially after drug ingestion, may also be responsible in some cases. Hypokalemia from any cause may predispose to myoglobinuria, but especially after chronic licorice ingestion or abuse of thiazide diuretics. Alcoholics seem especially prone to acute attacks of myoglobinuria, which may punctuate or initiate a syndrome of chronic limb weakness ("alcoholic myopathy").

Whatever the cause, the clinical syndrome is similar: widespread myalgia, weakness, malaise, renal pain, and fever. Pigmenturia usually ceases within a few days, but the weakness may persist for weeks, and high concentrations of serum enzymes may not return to normal for even longer. The main hazard of the syndrome is heme-induced nephropathy with anuria, azotemia, and hyperkalemia. Hypercalcemia occurs in a few patients after anuria. Respiratory muscles may occasionally be symptomatically weakened.

Treatment of the acute episode is directed primarily toward the kidneys. Promotion of diuresis with mannitol seems desirable whenever there is oliguria. Dialysis and measures to combat hyperkalemia may be necessary. In recurrent cases due to defects of the glycolytic enzymes or to unknown cause, various therapeutic regimens have been tried, but the patients usually learn the limits of exercise tolerance. The treatment of malignant hyperthermia is unsatisfactory because the rigidity is not abolished by curare. Intravenous infusions of dantrolene may be beneficial because this drug inhibits the release of calcium from the sarcoplasmic reticulum, relaxing the hypercontracted muscle. The average dose in successfully treated patients is 2.5 mg/kg of body weight.

Glycogen Storage Diseases of Muscle

Muscle is involved in four syndromes of the seven major forms of glycogen storage disease in which the enzymatic defect has been identified. Muscle is also affected in three disorders of glycolysis. (Neurologic aspects of glycogen disorders are discussed in Chapter VIII.)

In *Pompe disease*, which is due to *infantile acid maltase deficiency*, glycogen accumulates in all tissues. The syndrome is evident in the first year of life and all typical cases have been fatal within two years. Quadriparesis is probably due to the combined effects of neuronal dysfunction and myopathy because glycogen distorts the architecture of both tissues. Cranial muscle function is also disturbed so that the neurologic disorder resembles Werdnig-Hoffmann syndrome. This could be fatal in itself, but glycogen accumulation in myocardial fibers leads to cardiomegaly and congestive heart failure. There is no treatment for this autosomal recessive disorder. The disease can be identified in utero because the enzyme is also lacking in amniotic cells and the pregnancy may be interrupted.

Glycogen accumulation and lack of acid maltase may also be found in older children and adults with syndromes that resemble limb-girdle dystrophy, polymyositis, or *juvenile* or *late-onset acid maltose deficiency*. There seems to be unusual propensity to affect respiratory muscles, so that this rare syndrome is probably one of the major myopathic causes of alveolar hypoventilation. Another unusual and unexplained feature is the presence of myotonia in the EMG, although this is not clinically evident. Histologically, there is vacuolar myopathy; on appropriate stains, the vacuoles are filled with glycogen. As in the infantile disease, lack of acid maltase can be demonstrated biochemically in muscle biopsies or by measuring the enzyme in urine. The late-onset cases lack the clinical homogeneity of the infantile cases and they are probably different genetic disorders, because infantile and late-onset cases have only once been reported in the same family.

In *type III glycogen storage disease (limit dextrinosis)*, which is due to *lack of the debrancher system*, the predominant syndrome is hepatomegaly, although some cases also show a myopathy that resembles limb-girdle dystrophy. Sometimes distal accentuation of weakness and wasting simulate a neurogenic disorder. Respiratory function is not affected. Recognition of the disease usually requires biochemical analysis of muscle biopsy.

Type IV storage disease (amylopectinosis or Andersen disease) is due to a lack of the branching enzyme. The dominant syndrome is cirrhosis of the liver in young children, but the abnormal polysaccharide is also stored in muscle. Weakness has been a symptom in most of the few reported cases.

The other five disorders cause recurrent myoglobinuria (lack of phosphorylase, phosphofructokinase, phosphoglycerate kinase, phosphoglycerate mutase, or lactate dehydrogenase).

Mitochondrial Myopathies and Encephalomyopathies

As histochemical and biochemical methods have been applied to the study of syndromes resembling congenital myopathies, limb-girdle dystrophy, and polymyositis, new abnormalities have been found, although the fundamental disorders are still unknown. Among these are the *mitochondrial myopathies,* appearing as ragged red fibers in the Gomori trichrome stain, and *lipid storage myopathies* in which droplets of fat are seen within muscle fibers with special stains. The two categories are linked because lactate acidosis may be found in both and because the histologic abnormalities are sometimes found together. Among the lipid storage disorders, some are associated with decreased content of carnitine in muscle alone *(muscle carnitine deficiency),* and some are associated with *systemic carnitine deficiency.* The clinical disorder of the restricted form is sporadic or familial proximal limb weakness, which may be punctuated by periods of exacerbation but has no other distinctive characteristics. Cramps and myoglobinuria are not found in this syndrome, although they are in the closely related carnitine palmityl transferase deficiency. The weakness may improve after oral administration of carnitine. In the systemic disease, a similar abnormality may be present in the liver; the disorder is then accompanied by episodic hepatic encephalopathy, which may be fatal. In many cases of lipid storage myopathy, as defined histologically, carnitine content is normal and the essential abnormality has yet to be identified.

Lactic acidosis may accompany lipid storage myopathy and is found in a variety of neurologic and myopathic syndromes, some including both sets of disorder. Ragged red fibers are seen in occasional cases of so many other recognized disorders that the abnormality may be an unexplained coincidence in patients with fixed myopathy (either familial or sporadic), ALS, hypothyroidism, periodic paralysis, or other disorders. However, the same mitochondrial abnormalities seem to be encountered regularly in ocular myopathies and the Kearns-Sayre syndrome. Additionally, ragged red fibers seem to occur regularly in four sets of emerging syndromes that have yet to be defined clearly: (1) *infantile encepha-*

lopathies with lactic acidosis (some due to lack of pyruvate dehydrogenase, cytochrome B, or cytochrome C oxidase; others of unknown origin); (2) a childhood syndrome of fixed myopathy, encephalopathy, lactic acidosis, and strokes *(MELAS)* that may cause cerebral blindness before a fatal outcome; (3) juvenile syndromes of fixed limb weakness or exercise intolerance and lactic acidosis; and (4) a juvenile syndrome that resembles the Ramsay Hunt syndrome with ataxia and myoclonus *(myoclonus epilepsy and ragged red fibers,* or *MERRF).* Ragged red fibers are regularly found in the syndromes listed below:

> Kearns-Sayre syndrome
> Familial ocular myopathies
> Sporadic ocular myopathies
> Juvenile myopathy and lactate acidosis
> Infantile encephalopathy and lactic acidosis due to lack of pyruvate dehydrogenase, cytochrome B or C, or unknown cause
> Juvenile myopathy, encephalopathy, lactic acidosis, and stroke (MELAS)
> Juvenile cerebellar degeneration and myoclonus (Fukuhara syndrome, MERRF)

Treatment of these mitochondrial disorders has not been satisfactory, but infantile cytochrome-C oxidase deficiency may be transient.

Congenital Myopathies

The use of histochemical techniques has led to the recognition of unusual structures in skeletal muscles of children with mild forms of myopathic weakness. Although these syndromes are not usually evident in the first or the second year of life (other than delayed walking), the persistent and relative static weakness suggests that the disorder is congenital. Sometimes there are symptoms in the neonatal period or later in infancy, especially if there is difficulty in nursing. The disorders have been named after the predominant structural abnormality.

In *central core disease,* an amorphous area in the center of the fiber stains blue with Gomori trichrome stain, in contrast with the red peripheral fibrils. The cores are devoid of enzymatic activity histochemically, and with the electronic microscope the area lacks mitochondria. In *nemaline disease,* small rods near the sarcolemma stain bright red with the modified trichrome stain. Ultrastructural and extraction experiments suggest that the rods originate from Z-band material. In *myotubular*

or *centronuclear myopathy,* the nuclei are situated centrally and are surrounded by a pale halo. In *pleoconial myopathy* there are too many mitochondria; in *megaconial myopathy,* the mitochondria are abnormally enlarged, and in some patients, the mitochondria contain abnormal crystalline inclusions. Other less clearly demarcated structural abnormalities have been recognized as well. (Although not a congenital myopathy, nonthyroidal hypermetabolism in adults may be associated with abnormal mitochondria in *Luft disease.)*

The common clinical syndrome for all these congenital myopathies is proximal limb weakness. Although usually mild and static, the weakness is occasionally progressive and may be fatal. There are other cases of congenital myopathy in which nonspecific myopathic changes are evident in the biopsy, with no characteristic structural abnormality. The term *congenital muscular dystrophy* has been used for some of these cases but if the word "dystrophy" is used to imply a progressive disease, *congenital myopathy* seems a better term for static disorders. Regardless of whether specific structural abnormalities are found, it is difficult to relate the morphologic changes in muscle to a specific clinical picture. Several skeletal abnormalities may be seen in centronuclear or nemaline myopathies or fiber-type disproportion. These include a long and lean face, kyphoscoliosis, deformities of the feet, and congenital dislocation of the hip. Central core disease seems to increase the risk of malignant hyperthermia. Centronuclear myopathy may be more likely than the others to include ptosis and ophthalmoplegia. Still another form of congenital myopathy warrants the name *arthrogryposis congenita multiplex* because of multiple congenital contractures; most cases of arthrogryposis prove by EMG and muscle biopsy to be neurogenic but some are myopathic. In the *Prader-Willi syndrome,* hypotonia, dysphagia, depressed myotatic reflexes, and cryptorchidism may be prominent in infancy, but there is no permanent weakness. The syndrome is later recognized by mental retardation, obesity, short stature, skeletal abnormalities, childhood diabetes, and a characteristic facial appearance with a triangular-shaped upper lip. Deletions on chromosome 15 seem to be responsible for most but perhaps not all cases of Prader-Willi syndromes.

References

Myoglobinuria

Araki M, Takagi A, Higuchi I, Sugita H. Neuroleptic malignant syndrome. Caffeine contracture of single muscle fibers and muscle pathology. Neurology 1988; 38:297–301.

Bank WJ, DiMauro S, Bonilla E, Capuzzi DM, Rowland LP. A disorder of lipid metabolism and myoglobinuria. Absence of carnitine palmityl transferase. N Engl J Med 1975; 292:443–449.

Britt BA, Kalow W. Malignant hyperthermia: a statistical review. Can Anaesth Soc J 1970; 17:293–315.

Corpier CL, Jones PH, Suki WN, Lederer ED, Quinones MA, Schmidt SW, Young JB. Rhabdomyolysis and renal injury with lovastatin use. Report of two cases in cardiac transplant patients. JAMA 1988; 260:239–241.

DiMauro S, DiMauro PMM. Muscle carnitine palmityl transferase deficiency and myoglobinuria. Science 1973; 182:929–931.

DiMauro S, Dalakas M, Miranda AF. Phosphoglycerate kinase deficiency: another cause of recurrent myoglobinuria. Ann Neurol 1983; 13:11–19.

Eiser AR, Neff MS, Slifkin RF. Acute myoglobinuric renal failure. A consequence of neuroleptic malignant syndrome. Arch Intern Med 1982; 142:601–603.

Frank JP, Harati Y, Butler IJ, Nelson TE, Scott CE. Central core disease and malignant hyperthermia syndrome. Ann Neurol 1980; 7:11–17.

Gabow PA, Kaehny WD, Kelleher SP. The spectrum of rhabdomyolysis. Medicine 1982; 61:141–152.

Knochel JP. Environmental heat illness. An eclectic review. Arch Intern Med 1974; 133:841.

Knochel JP. Rhabdomyolysis and myoglobinuria. Ann Rev Med 1982; 33:435–443.

Kolb ME, Horne ML, Matz R. Dantrolene in human malignant hyperthermia. A multicenter study. Anaesthesiology 1982; 56:254–262.

Melamed I, Romen Y, Keren G, Epstein Y, Dolev E. March myoglobinuria. A hazard to renal function. Arch Intern Med 1982; 142:1277–1279.

Nelson TE, Flewellen EH. Current concepts: the malignant hyperthermia syndrome. N Engl J Med 1983; 309:445–448.

Ording H. Diagnosis of susceptibility to malignant hyperthermia. Br J Anaesth 1988; 60:287–302.

Penn AS, Rowland LP, Fraser DW. Drugs, coma, and myoglobinuria. Arch Neurol 1972; 26:336.

Perkoff GT. Alcoholic myopathy. Ann Rev Med 1971; 23:125.

Rowland LP. Myoglobinuria, 1984. Can J Neurol Sci 1984; 11:1–13.

Willner JH, Nakagawa M. Controversies in malignant hyperthermia. Sem Neurol 1983; 3:275–284.

Glycogen Storage Diseases of the Muscle

DiMauro S. Metabolic myopathies. In: Vinken PJ, Bruyn GW, eds. Handbook of Clinical Neurology (vol 41). New York: Elsevier-North Holland, 1979:175–234.

DiMauro S, Bresolin N. Phosphorylase deficiency. In: Engel AG, Banker BQ, eds. Myology. New York: McGraw-Hill, 1986: 1585–1602.

DiMauro S, Bresolin N. Newly recognized defects in distal glycolysis. In: Engel AG, Banker BQ, eds. Myology. New York: McGraw-Hill, 1986: 1619–1628.

DiMauro S, Hartwig GB, Hays A, et al. Debrancher deficiency: neuromuscular disorder in five adults. Ann Neurol 1979; 5:422–436.

Engel AG, Acid Maltase deficiency. In: Engel AG, Banker BQ, eds. Myology. New York: McGraw-Hill, 1986: 1619–1625.

Rowland LP, DiMauro S. Glycogen storage diseases of the muscle. Res Publ Res Assoc Nerv Ment Dis 1983; 60:239–254.

Rowland LP, DiMauro S, Layzer RB. Phosphofructokinase deficiency. In: Engel AG, Banker BQ, eds. Myology. New York: McGraw-Hill, 1986: 1603–1618.

Rowland LP, Layzer RB, DeMauro S. Pathophysiology of metabolic muscle disorders. In: Asbury A, McDonald I, McKhann G, eds. Scientific Basis of Clinical Neurology. Philadelphia: W.B. Saunders Co., 197–207.

Servidei S, Shanske S, Zeviani M, Lebo R, Fletterick R, DiMauro S. McArdle's disease: biochemical and molecular genetic studies. Ann Neurol 1988; 24:774–781.

Mitochondrial Myopathies and Encephalomyopathies

Allen RJ, DiMauro S, Coulter DL, Papadimitriou A, Rothenberg SP. Kearns-Sayre syndrome with reduced plasma and cerebrospinal fluid folate. Ann Neurol 1983; 13:679–681.

DiMauro S. Metabolic myopathies. In: Vinken PJ, Bruyn GW, eds. Handbook of Clinical Neurology (vol 41). New York: Elsevier-North Holland, 1979:175–234.

DiMauro S. Mitochondrial myopathies. CRC Crit Rev 1988 (in press).

DiMauro S, Bonilla E, Zeviani M, Servidei S, DeVivo DC, Schon EA. Mitochondrial myopathies. J Inher Metabl Dis 1987: 10 Suppl 1:113–128.

DiMauro S, Trevisan C, Hays AP. Disorders of lipid metabolism in muscle. Muscle Nerve 1980; 3:369–388.

Engel AG, Angelini C. Carnitine deficiency of human skeletal muscle associated lipid storage myopathy. A new syndrome. Science 1973; 179:899–902.

Goda S, Hamada T, Ishimoto S, Kobayashi T, Goto I, Kuroiwa Y. Clinical improvement after administration of coenzyme Q10 in a patient with mitochondrial encephalomyopathy. J Neurol 1987; 234:62–63.

Holt IJ, Harding AE, Morgan-Hughes JA. Deletions of mitochondrial DNA in patients with mitochondrial myopathies. Nature 1988; 331:717–719.

Mitsumoto H, Aprille JR, Wray SH, Nemni R, Bradley WG. Chronic progressive external ophthalmoplegia (CPEO): clinical, morphologic, and biochemical studies. Neurology 1983; 33:452–462.

Morgan-Hughes JA, Hayes DJ, Clark JB, Landon DN, Swash M, Stark RJ, Rudge P. Mitochondrial encephalopathies. Biochemical studies in two cases revealing defects in the respiratory chain. Brain 1982; 105:553–582.

Ogasahara S, Nishikawa Y, Yorifuji S, et al. Treatment of Kearns-Sayre syndrome with coenzyme Q10. Neurology 1986; 36:45–53.

Pavlakis S, Phillips PC, DiMauro S, DeVivo DC, Rowland LP. Mitochondrial myopathy, encephalopathy, lactic acidosis, and strokelike episodes. Ann Neurol 1984; 16:481–488.

Pavlakis SG, Rowland LP, DeVivo DC, Bonilla E, DiMauro S. Mitochondrial myopathies and encephalomyopathies. In: Plum F, ed. Advances in Contemporary Neurology; Philadelphia: FA Davis, 1988, 95–134.

Petty RKH, Harding AE, Morgan-Hughes JA. The clinical features of mitochondrial myopathy. Brain 1986; 109:915–938.

Rowland LP, Hays AP, DiMauro S, DeVivo DC, Behrens MM. Diverse clinical disorders associated with morphological abnormalities of the mitochondria. In: Scarlato G, eds. Mitochondrial Pathology in Muscle Diseases. Padua, Italy: Piccin Medical Books, 1983:141–158.

Shy GM, et al. Two childhood myopathies with abnormal mitochondria. I. Megaconial myopathy. II. Pleoconial myopathy. Brain 1966; 89:133–158.

Wallace DC, Zheng X, Lott MT et al. Familial mitochondrial encephalomyopathy (MERRF): Genetic, pathophysiological, and biochemical characterization of a mitochondrial DNA disease. Cell 1988; 55:601–610.

Zeviani M, Moraes CT, DiMauro S, Nakase H, Bonilla E, Schon EA, Rowland LP. Deletions of mitochondrial DNA in Kearns-Sayre syndrome. Neurology, 1988; 38:1339–1347.

Congenital Myopathies

Ambler MW, Neave C, Tutschka BG, Pueschel SM, Orson JM, Singer DB. X-linked recessive myotubular myopathy. Hum Pathol 1984; 15:566–574, 1107–1120.

Banker BQ. Congenital muscular dystrophy. In Engel AG, Banker BQ, eds. Myology. New York: McGraw-Hill, 1986, 367–1384.

Banker BQ. The congenital myopathies. In: Engel AG, Banker BQ, eds. Myology. New York, McGraw Hill, 1986:1527–1584.

Brooke MH, Carroll JE, Ringel SP. Congenital hypotonia revisited. Muscle Nerve 1979; 2:84–100.

Canal N, Comi GC, Comola M, Testa D, Mora M, Cornelio F. Centronuclear myopathy with unusual mitochondrial abnormalities. Clin Neuropathol 1985; 4:23–27.

Carpenter S, Karpati G, Holland P. New observations in reducing body myopathy. Neurology 1985; 35:818–827.

Clarren SK, Hall JC. Neuropathologic findings in the spinal cords of 10 infants with arthrogryposis. J Neurol Sci 1983; 58:89–102.

Dubowitz V, Brooke MH. Muscle Biopsy: A Modern Approach. Philadelphia: WB Saunders, 1973.

Dubowitz V. Muscle Disorders in Childhood, 2nd ed. Philadelphia: WB Saunders, 1979.

Gamble JG, Rinsky LA, Lee JH. Orthopedic aspects of central core disease. J Bone Joint Surg 1988; 70-A:1061–1066.

Glorieux J, Dussault JH, Letarte J, Guyda H, Morisette J. Preliminary results on the mental development of hypothyroid infants detected by the Quebec Screening Program. J Pediatr 1983; 102:19–22.

Goebel HH. Centronuclear myopathy with special consideration of the adult form. Eur Neurol 1984; 23:425–4343.

Goebel HH, von Loh S, Gehler J. Childhood neuromuscular disease with rimmed vacuoles. Eur J Pediatr 1986; 144:557–562.

Hall JG, Reed SD, Greene G. The distal arthrogryposes: delineation of new entities—review and nosologic discussion. Am J Med Genet 1982; 11:185–239.

Koch BM, Bertorini TE, Eng GD, Boehm R. Severe multicore disease associated with reaction to anesthesia. Arch Neurol 1985; 42:1204–1206.

Ledbetter DH, Riccardi VM, Airhart SD, Strobel RJ, Keenan BS, Crawford JD. Deletions of chromosome 15 as a cause of the Prader-Willi syndrome. N Engl J Med 1981; 304:325–358.

Leyten QH, Gabreels FJM, Joosten EMG, et al. An autosomal dominant type of congenital muscular dystrophy. Brain Dev 1986; 8:533–537.

Ortiz de Zarate JC, Maruffo A. The descending ocular myopathy of early childhood: myotubular or centronuclear myopathy. Eur Neurol 1970; 3:1–12.

Shuaib A, Paasuke BT, Brownell AKW. Central core disease: Clinical features in 13 patients. Medicine 1987; 66:389–396.

Shuper A, Weitz R, Varsano I, Mimouni M. Benign congenital hypotonia. A clinical study of 43 children. Eur J Pediatr 1987; 146:360–362.

Shy GM, Engel WK, Somars JE, Wanko T. Nemaline myopathy: a new congenital myopathy. Brain 1963; 86:793–810.

Shy GM, Engel WK, Wanko T. Central core disease: a myofibrillary and mitochondrial abnormality of muscle. Ann Intern Med 1962; 56:511–520.

Spiro AJ, Shy GM, Gonatas NK. Myotubular myopathy. Arch Neurol 1966; 14:1–14.

Stephansen JBP. Prader-Willi syndrome: neonatal presentation and later development. Dev Med Child Neurol 1980; 22:792–799.

Swinyard CA, Bleck EE. The etiology of arthrogryposis (multiple congenital contracture). Clin Orthop 1985; 194:15–29.

Wallgren-Pettersson C, Rapola J, Donner M. Pathology of congenital nemaline myopathy. A follow-up study. J Neurol Sci 1988; 83:243–257.

Zellweger H, Affifi A, McCormick WF, Mergner W. Benign congenital muscular dystrophy: a special form of congenital hypotonia. Clin Pediatr 1967; 6:655–660.

Zellweger H, Affifi A, McCormick WF, Mergner W. Severe congenital muscular dystrophy. Am J Dis Child 1967; 114:591–602.

133. CRAMPS AND STIFFNESS
Robert B. Layzer

The term *muscle stiffness* implies a state of continuous muscle contraction at rest; *cramps* or *spasms* are transient, involuntary contractions of a muscle or group of muscles. Table 133–1 lists some of the many disorders that cause stiffness or cramps.

Ordinary Muscle Cramps

The common muscle cramp is a sudden, forceful, often painful muscle contraction that lasts anywhere from a few seconds to several minutes. Cramps are provoked by a trivial movement or by contracting a shortened muscle. Cramps may occur during vigorous exercise, but are more likely to occur after exercise ceases. Unusually frequent cramps tend to accompany pregnancy, hypothyroidism, uremia, profuse sweating or diarrhea, hemodialysis, and lower motor neuron disorders, especially anterior horn cell diseases. Benign fasciculations or myokymia may be associated with frequent muscle cramps in apparently healthy persons.

Nocturnal cramps typically cause forceful flexion of the ankle and toes, but cramps can affect almost any voluntary muscle. A cramp often starts with fasciculations, after which the muscle becomes intermittently hard and knot-like as the involuntary contraction waxes and wanes, passing from one part of the muscle to another. EMG shows brief, periodic bursts of motor unit potentials discharging at a frequency of 200 to 300 Hz, appearing irregularly and intermingling with similar discharges from adjacent motor units. Several foci within the same muscle may discharge independently. This electrical activity clearly arises within the lower motor neuron, though whether it occurs in the soma, the peripheral nerve, or the intramuscular nerve terminals is still debated; the chemical mechanisms are not understood.

True cramps must be distinguished from crampy muscle pain unaccompanied by spasm. The cramps of McArdle disease occur only during intense or ischemic exercise and are silent on the EMG.

Stretching the affected muscle usually terminates a cramp. Information about prophylactic therapy is largely anecdotal, and no single agent appears to be uniformly effective. For nocturnal leg cramps, a bedtime dose of quinine, phenytoin, carbamazepine, or diazepam may be used. Frequent daytime cramps sometimes respond to maintenance therapy with carbamazepine or phenytoin.

Neuromyotonia (Isaacs Syndrome)

Neuromyotonia is a rare syndrome of continuous muscle stiffness, myokymia, and delayed muscle relaxation that is associated with a polyneuropathy that is usually mild or inapparent and identified only by electrodiagnostic study. Most cases are not hereditary, and no specific cause has been identified.

The symptoms begin insidiously, often in the second or third decade, and progress slowly for several years. Slow movement, clawing of the fingers, and toe-walking are later joined by stiffness of the proximal and axial muscles and occasionally of the oropharyngeal and respiratory muscles. Myokymia, a continuous rippling of the muscle surface, is usually evident in the distal extremities. The stiffness and myokymia are present at rest and continue during sleep. Voluntary contraction induces a prolonged muscle spasm that resembles myotonia, but myotonia usually cannot be elicited by percussion. Less constant features include excessive sweating, distal muscular wasting, hypoactive reflexes, and distal reduction of sensation.

Table 133–1. Motor Unit Disorders Causing Cramps and Stiffness

Location of Abnormality	Name of Disorder	Principal Manifestations	Treatment
Spinal cord and brain stem	Stiff-man syndrome	Rigidity and reflex spasms	Diazepam
	Tetanus	Rigidity and reflex spasms	Diazepam
	Progressive encephalomyelitis with rigidity and spasms	Rigidity and reflex spasms, focal neurological deficits	None
	Myelopathy with alpha rigidity	Extensor rigidity	None
	Spinal myoclonus	Segmental repetitive myoclonic jerks	Clonazepam
Peripheral nerves	Tetany	Carpopedal spasm	Correction of calcium, magnesium or acid base derangement
	Neuromyotonia	Stiffness, myokymia, delayed relaxation	Phenytoin, carbamazepine
Muscle	Myotonic disorders	Delayed relaxation, percussion myotonia	Phenytoin, carbamazepine, procainamide
	Schwartz-Jampel syndrome	Stiffness and myotonia	Phenytoin, carbamazepine
	Phosphorylase deficiency, phosphofructokinase deficiency	Cramps during intense or ischemic exercise	None
	Malignant hyperthermia	Rigidity during anesthesia	Dantrolene
Unknown	Ordinary muscle cramps	Cramps during sleep or ordinary activity	Quinine, phenytoin, carbamazepine

Nerve conduction tests and sural nerve biopsies usually furnish evidence of a diffuse neuropathy; in most cases, axonal degeneration is the principal finding, whereas occasionally there is chronic demyelination and remyelination with marked slowing of nerve conduction. The EMG recorded from stiff muscles reveals prolonged, irregular discharges of action potentials that vary in amplitude and configuration; some of them resemble fibrillations. Voluntary effort triggers more intense discharges that persist during relaxation, accounting for the myotonia-like after-contraction. The abnormal activity arises in the distal portions of motor nerves; it is reduced by peripheral nerve block and is abolished by blockade of neuromuscular transmission. Treatment with carbamazepine or phenytoin usually controls the symptoms and signs; there is little information about long-term prognosis.

Tetany

Tetany is a clinical syndrome characterized by convulsions, paresthesias, prolonged spasms of limb muscles, or laryngospasm; it is accompanied by signs of hyperexcitability of peripheral nerves. It occurs in patients with hypocalcemia, hypomagnesemia, or alkalosis; it occasionally represents a primary neural abnormality. Hyperventilation may unmask latent hypocalcemic tetany, but respiratory alkalosis itself only rarely causes outright tetany.

Intense circumoral and digital paresthesias generally precede the typical carpopedal spasms, which consist of adduction and extension of the fingers, flexion of the metacarpophalangeal joints, and equinovarus postures of the feet. In severe cases, the spasms spread to the proximal and axial muscles, eventually causing opisthotonus. In all forms of tetany, the nerves are hyperexcitable as manifested by the reactions to ischemia (Trousseau sign) and percussion (Chvostek sign). The spasms are due to spontaneous firing of peripheral nerves, starting in the proximal portions of the longest nerves. EMG shows individual motor units discharging independently at a rate of 5 to 25 Hz, each discharge consisting of a group of two or more identical potentials.

The treatment of tetany consists of correcting the underlying metabolic disorder. In hypomagnesemia, tetany does not respond to correction of the accompanying hypocalcemia unless the magnesium deficit is also corrected.

Stiff-Man Syndrome

The stiff-man syndrome is a rare disorder characterized by persistent muscular rigidity and painful spasms, resembling a chronic form of tetanus. The cause is unknown; no abnormality has been detected in the spinal cord or brain at autopsy. The symptoms develop over several months or years and may ether increase slowly or become stable. Aching discomfort and stiffness tend to predominate in the axial and proximal limb muscles, causing awkwardness of gait and slowness of movement. Trismus does not occur, but facial and oropharyngeal muscles may be affected. The stiffness diminishes during sleep and under general anesthesia. Later, painful reflex spasms occur in response to movement, sensory stimulation, or emotion. The spasms may lead to joint deformities and are powerful enough to rupture muscles or fracture bones. Passive muscle stretch provokes an exaggerated reflex contraction that lasts several seconds; Babinski signs have been described in a few cases, but muscle strength and sensation are usually normal.

EMG recordings from stiff muscles show a continuous discharge of motor unit potentials resembling normal voluntary contraction. As in tetanus, the activity is not inhibited by voluntary contraction of the antagonist muscles; however, a normal silent period is present during the stretch reflex, indicating that there is no impairment of recurrent spinal inhibition. The rigidity is abolished by spinal anesthesia, by peripheral nerve block, or by selective block of gamma motor nerve fibers. Some authors have postulated that both alpha and gamma motor neurons are rendered hyperactive by excitatory influences descending from the brain stem. EEG is normal. Routine CSF analysis is also normal, but IgG concentration may be increased, and oligoclonal IgG bands may be present. Serum and CSF antibodies to glutamic acid decarboxylase have been detected in several patients.

Administration of diazepam is the most effective symptomatic treatment; high doses may be required. Additional benefit can be obtained in some cases from administration of baclofen, phenytoin, clonidine, or tizanidine. The long-term prognosis is still uncertain.

A familial form of stiff-man syndrome, inherited in an autosomal dominant pattern, is manifested by muscular rigidity in the newborn period; the stiffness gradually lessens after early childhood. There have been a few reports of a chronic, progressive encephalomyelitis in which the stiff-man syndrome is associated with brain-stem and spinal cord signs and inflammatory changes in the spinal fluid. Some patients with destructive lesions of the cervical cord develop intense extensor rigidity of the arms, reflecting spontaneous activity of alpha motor neurons that are isolated from synaptic influences. Spinal myoclonus consists of segmental, repetitive jerking of limb or trunk muscles, often continuing for long periods. The activity may be unilateral or bilateral, and appears to result from segmental loss of inhibition of spinal reflexes due to tumor, infection, or other cord lesions.

References

Layzer RB. Motor unit hyperactivity states. In: Vinken PJ, Bruyn GW, eds. Handbook of Clinical Neurology, vol 41. New York: Elsevier-North Holland, 1979: 295–316.

Rowland LP. Cramps, spasms, and muscle stiffness. Rev Neurol (Paris) 1985; 141:261–273.

Solimena M, Folli F, Denis-Donini S, Comi GC, Pozza G, De Camilli P, Vicari AM. Autoantibodies to glutamic acid decarboxylase in a patient with stiff-man syndrome, epilepsy, and type I diabetes mellitus. N Engl J Med 1988; 318:1012–1020.

134. DERMATOMYOSITIS

Lewis P. Rowland

Dermatomyositis, a disease of unknown etiology, is characterized by inflammatory changes in skin and muscle.

Pathology and Pathogenesis. Dermatomyositis is thought to be an autoimmune disease, but there has been no consistent evidence of either antibodies or lymphocytes directed against muscle components. In the past few years, there has been growing agreement among muscle histologists that dermatomyositis is humorally mediated, characterized by more B cells than T cells in the muscle infiltrates and a vasculopathy with deposits of immunoglobulins in intramuscular blood vessels. This contrasts with the predominance of T cells in polymyositis, which is attributed to a disorder of lymphocyte regulation.

The acute changes of both skin and muscle are marked by signs of degeneration, regeneration, edema, and infiltration by lymphocytes. In muscle biopsies, however, lymphocytes may not be seen in 25% of cases. In muscle, the degenerative changes may be most marked at the periphery of muscle bundles *(perifascicular atrophy)*, but the distribution of lesions is not pathognomonic. Whether there is angiopathy is debatable. A similar myopathy, without skin lesions, can be induced in animals by immunization with muscle extracts. Virus-like particles have been seen in some cases, but no virus has been cultured from muscle.

Incidence. Dermatomyositis is rare. Together with polymyositis, the incidence has been estimated to be about seven cases each year for a population of one million. That figure may be too low; in our 1200-bed hospital, we see five new cases of dermatomyositis and 15 to 20 cases of polymyositis each year.

Dermatomyositis occurs in all decades of life, with peaks of incidence before puberty and at about age 40. In young adults, women are more likely to be affected. Although there are some views to the contrary, it is generally believed that about 10% of cases starting after age 40 are associated with malignant neoplasms, most often carcinoma of lung or breast. Typical findings, including the rash, have also been seen in patients with agammaglobulinemia, toxoplasmosis, hypothyroidism, sarcoidosis, ipepac abuse, hepatitis B infection, penicillamine reactions, or vaccination reactions. Cases have even been ascribed to azathioprine.

Symptoms and Signs. The first manifestations usually involve both skin and muscle at about the same time. The rash may precede weakness by several weeks, but weakness alone is almost never the first symptom.

The rash may be confined to the face in a butterfly distribution around the nose and cheeks but the edema and erythema are especially likely to affect the eyelids, periungual skin, and extensor surfaces of the knuckles, elbows, and knees. The upper chest is another common site. The initial redness may be later replaced by brownish pigmentation. Fibrosis of subcutaneous tissue and thickening of the skin may lead to the appearance of scleroderma. Later, calcinosis may involve subcutaneous tissues and fascial planes within muscle. The calcium deposits may extrude through the skin.

Affected muscles may ache and are often tender. Weakness of proximal limb muscles causes difficulty lifting, raising the arms overhead, rising from low seats, climbing stairs, or even walking on level ground. The interval from onset of weakness to most severe disability is measured in weeks. Cranial muscles are spared except that difficulty swallowing is noted by about a third of the patients. Some patients have difficulty holding the head up because neck muscles are weak. Sensation is preserved, tendon reflexes may or may not be lost, and there is no fasciculation.

Systemic symptoms are uncommon. Fever and malaise may characterize the acute stage in a minority of patients. Pulmonary fibrosis has been encountered and, rarely, there are cardiac symptoms. Arthralgia may be prominent but deforming arthritis and renal failure have never been documented.

In about 10% of cases, the cutaneous manifestations have features of both scleroderma and dermatomyositis, warranting the name *"sclerodermatomyositis."* These cases have sometimes been designated as *"mixed connective tissue disease,"* with a high incidence of antibody to extractable nuclear antigen, but it now seems unlikely that the "mixed" syndrome is unique in any way.

Diagnosis. The characteristic rash and myopathy usually make the diagnosis clear at a glance. Problems may arise if the rash is inconspicuous; in those cases the differential diagnosis is that of polymyositis (as described subsequently). Other collagen-vascular diseases may cause both rash and myopathy at the same time, but systemic lupus erythematosus is likely to affect kidneys, synovia, and central nervous system in patterns that are never seen in dermatomyositis. Similarly, there has never been a documented case of typical rheumatoid arthritis with typical dermatomyositis. The diagnosis of dermatomyositis is therefore clinical, based on the rash and myopathy. There is no pathognomonic laboratory test.

Except for the presence of lymphocytes in biopsied muscle and increased serum activity of creatine kinase (or other sarcoplasmic enzymes), there are no characteristic laboratory abnormalities. The EMG shows myopathic abnormalities and, often, evidence of increased irritability of muscle. Nonspecific serologic abnormalities include rheumatoid factor and several different kinds of antinuclear antibodies, none consistently present in patients with dermatomyositis.

Once the diagnosis is made, many clinicians set off on a "search for occult neoplasm." Callen, however, has shown that this activity is almost always fruitless. In patients with malignancy, the tumor is often recognized long before there are any manifesta-

tions of dermatomyositis. In other cases, the tumor is discovered by an abnormality of some simple routine test (blood count, erythrocyte sedimentation rate, test for heme pigment in stools, chest film) or findings on physical examination including pelvis and rectum. If the basic studies are done, there is no need for more extensive contrast studies or endoscopy, but CT of chest and abdomen might be advisable. Sometimes, no matter how exhaustive the search, the tumor is not discovered until an autopsy is performed.

Prognosis. The natural history of dermatomyositis is now unknown because the patients are automatically treated with steroids. Although the mortality rate 50 years ago was given as 33 to 50%, it is not appropriate to use those ancient figures for current comparison; antibiotics and respirators affect outcome as much as any presumably specific immunotherapy. Even so, in reviews published since 1982, mortality rates were 23%, 27%, and 35%. Because few fatalities have occurred in children, many of the deaths are probably due to associated malignancy. However, the myopathy itself may also be severe. In an analysis of survivors of childhood dermatomyositis, 83% were capable of self care, almost all were working, and half were married; 33% had persistent rash or weakness, and a similar number had calcinosis.

Treatment. The standard therapy for dermatomyositis is administration of prednisone. The recommended dosage for adults is at least 60 mg daily; higher doses are often given for severe cases. For children, the recommended dosage is higher: 2 mg/kg body weight. The basic dosage is continued for at least one month, perhaps longer. If the patient has improved by then, the dosage can be reduced slowly. If there has been no improvement, choices include prolonging the trial of prednisone in the same or higher dose, with or without addition of an immunosuppressive drug chosen according to local usage.

Within the past decade, improvement was reported in 80% of all steroid-treated patients in one series, but only 50% or fewer patients benefitted in other studies. Apparent response to treatment of individual cases or apparent relapses on attempted withdrawal of medication have been reported anecdotally many times. In one retrospective analysis, favorable outcome of childhood dermatomyositis seemed to be linked to early treatment (less than four months after onset) and use of high doses of prednisone. Dubowitz, however, reported just the reverse—better outcome and fewer steroid complications with low doses of prednisone (1 mg/kg body weight).

The value of steroid treatment is still unproved, however, because there has never been a prospectively controlled study. In one retrospective analysis, untreated patients were seen many years before treated patients. In another study there was no difference in outcome of patients treated with prednisone alone or with both prednisone and azathioprine. Moreover, it is not clear whether immunosuppressive drugs are more or less dangerous than steroids and there is no evidence that any single immunosuppressive drug is superior to others; azathioprine, methotrexate, cyclophosphamide, and cyclosporine have each been championed. Plasmapheresis has been of no value.

References

Arahata K, Engel AG. Mononuclear cells in myopathies. Hum Pathol 1986; 17:704–721.

Banker BQ, Victor M. Dermatomyositis (systemic angiopathy) in childhood. Medicine 1966; 45:261–289.

Bohan A, Peter JB, Bowman RL, Pearson CM. A computer-assisted analysis of 153 patients with polymyositis and dermatomyositis. Medicine 1977; 56:255–286.

Bowyer SL, Blane CE, Sullivan DB, Cassidy JT. Childhood dermatomyositis: factors predicting functional outcome and development of dystrophic calcification. J Pediatr 1983; 103:882–888.

Callen JP. The value of malignancy evaluation in patients with dermatomyositis. J Am Acad Dermatol 1982; 6:253–259.

Chalmers A, Sayson R, Walters K. Juvenile dermatomyositis: medical, social and economic status in adulthood. Can Med Assoc J 1982; 126:31–33.

Chou SM, Mike T. Ultrastructural abnormalities and perifascicular atrophy in childhood dermatomyositis. Arch Pathol Lab Med 1981; 105:76–85.

Dubowitz V. Prognostic factors in dermatomyositis. J Pediatr 1984; 104:336.

Henriksson K, Sandstedt P. Polymyositis. Treatment and prognosis. Acta Neurol Scand 1982; 65:280–300.

Hochberg MC. Mortalty from polymyositis and dermatomyositis in the United States, 1968–1978. Arthritis Rheum 1983; 26:1465–1472.

Hochberg MC, Feldman D, Stevens MB. Adult-onset polymyositis/dermatomyositis; an analysis of clinical and laboratory features and survival of 76 patients. Semin Arthritis Rheum 1986; 15:168–178.

Kelly JJ, Madoc-Jones H, Adelman LS, Andres PL, Munsat TL. Response to total body irradiation in dermatomyositis. Muscle Nerve 1988; 11:120–123.

Kissel JT, Mendell JR, Rammohan KW. Microvascular deposition of complement membrane attack complex in dermatomyositis. N Engl J Med 1986; 314:329–334.

Lakhanpal S, Bunch TW, Ilstrup DM, Melton LJ III. Polymyositis-dermatomyositis and malignant lesions: does an association exist? Mayo Clin Proc 1986; 61:645–653.

McKendry RJR. Influence of age at onset on the duration of therapy in idiopathic adult polymyositis and dermatomyositis. Arch Intern Med 1988; 147:1989–1991.

Manchal LA, Jin A, Pritchard KI, et al. Frequency of malignant neoplasms in patients with polymyositis-dermatomyositis. Ann Intern Med 1985; 145:1835–1839.

Mastaglia FL, Ojeda VJ. Inflammatory myopathies. Ann Neurol 1985; 17:215–227.

Mease PJ, Ochs HD, Wedgwood RJ. Successful treatment of ECHOvirus meningoencephalitis and myositis-fasciitis with intravenous immune globulin therapy in a patient with X-linked agammaglobulinemia. N Engl J Med 1981; 304:1278–1281.

Nimmelstein SH, Brody S, McShane D, Holman HR. Mixed connective tissue disease: a subsequent evaluation of the original 25 patients. Medicine 1980; 59:239–248.

Paljarvi L, Snall EV. Morphometric approaches to perifascicular atrophy in muscle biopsy; do they help to diagnose polymyositis? Neuropathol Appl Neurobiol 1984; 10:333–341.

Ringel SP, Carry MR, Aguilera AJ, Starcevich JM. Quantitative histopathology of the inflammatory myopathies. Arch Neurol 1986; 43:1004–1009.

Rowland LP, Clark C, Olarte MR. Therapy for dermatomyositis and polymyositis. Adv Neurol 1977; 17:63–97.

Rowland LP, Olarte MR, Penn AS, Lovelace RE, Jaretzki A III. Therapy of myasthenia gravis, dermatomyositis and polymyositis. In Serratrice G, et al (ed). Neuromuscular Diseases, Raven Press, New York, 1984, pp. 505–510.

Stehm ER. Intravenous immunoglobulins as therapeutic agents. Ann Int Med 1987; 107:367–382.

Whitaker JN. Inflammatory myopathy; a review of etiologic and pathogenetic factors. Muscle Nerve 1982; 5:573–792.

135. POLYMYOSITIS
Lewis P. Rowland

Definition. Polymyositis is a disorder of skeletal muscle, of diverse causes, characterized by acute or subacute onset, frequent improvement and, typically, infiltration of muscle by lymphocytes. Another name, no more precise, is "inflammatory myopathy."

Problems with this definition are indicated by two different views. According to one concept, polymyositis is a disease that is sometimes associated with a rash (dermatomyositis), sometimes with other manifestations of collagen-vascular diseases ("overlap syndromes"), and sometimes occurs alone (idiopathic polymyositis). This view does not recognize practical differences between dermatomyositis and polymyositis, nor does it recognize causes of polymyositis other than collagen-vascular disease or carcinoma.

In an alternative view, dermatomyositis is considered a reasonably well-defined disorder. Some cases of polymyositis may be manifestations of the same disease, differing only in that the rash is lacking. A few patients with chronic myopathy and no history of rash have developed subcutaneous calcinosis, implying that the skin had actually been involved. If there is no visible rash, however, an essential sign of dermatomyositis is missing and it then becomes impossible, in the acute stage, to define polymyositis as the same condition. Furthermore, other conditions (such as infection with influenza virus or toxoplasmosis, or disorders of uncertain cause such as sarcoidosis) can cause a similar clinical disorder with similar histologic changes. Some forms of polymyositis are also delineated primarily by unusual histologic structures; the best known in this class is *"inclusion body myopathy,"* which is difficult to recognize clinically but is identified by the presence in muscle of osmophilic whorls and intracytoplasmic or intranuclear filamentous inclusions. Whether the histologic change demarcates a specific disease is still uncertain because there are so many clinical variations, but Chou has championed the view that it may be due to persistent infection with mumps virus. Polymyositis is therefore viewed as a syndrome of diverse causes that can be identified by the following criteria.

Diagnosis. The symptoms are those of any disorder that causes weakness of proximal limb and trunk muscles. The weakness is deemed myopathic (rather than neurogenic) by conventional changes in electromyogram, muscle biopsy, and serum enzymes. The problem is then to identify qualities that are similar to those of the myopathy of dermatomyositis, attempting to distinguish this myopathy from others with which it might be confused: muscular dystrophies, metabolic myopathies, or disorders of the neuromuscular junction. The following criteria are suggested:

1. There is no family history of similar disease and the onset is usually after age 35; no familial limb-girdle dystrophy starts so late. Cases of younger onset are few, unless there is some associated collagen-vascular or other systemic disease.

2. Progression from onset to peak weakness is measured in weeks or months, not years as in the muscular dystrophies.

3. Symptoms may improve spontaneously or concomitantly with the administration of drugs, unlike any muscular dystrophy.

4. In addition to proximal limb weakness, there may be dysphagia or weakness of neck flexors but other cranial muscles are not affected. (If eyelids or ocular muscles were involved, it would be difficult or impossible to distinguish the disorder from myasthenia gravis.)

5. Arthralgia, myalgia, and Raynaud symptoms help to make the diagnosis, but lack of these symptoms does not exclude the diagnosis.

6. Muscle biopsy usually shows signs of degeneration, regeneration, and infiltration by lymphocytes, especially early in the course. As in patients with dermatomyositis, however, lymphocytic infiltration may be lacking in muscle biopsies in polymyositis. Typical histologic changes help to make the diagnosis; lack of these changes does not exclude the diagnosis. In histochemical stains, there must be no evidence of excess lipid or glycogen storage and there should be no signs of denervation.

7. In addition to conventional signs of myopathy in the electromyogram, increased irritability of muscle may be evident in the form of fibrillation waves or increased insertional activity.

The problem of diagnosis is exemplified by a patient with limb weakness at age 40 when EMG and muscle biopsy indicate that the disorder is a myopathy. Search must then be made for known causes of myopathy (Table 135–1). If none is found, the diagnosis of exclusion is idiopathic polymyositis.

It seems unlikely that this residual group is all due to one disease because there is clinical heterogeneity, such as differences in rapidity of progression, distribution of weakness, or severity of disorder. There is also histologic heterogeneity; some changes are deemed vacuolar, granulomatous, or marked by inclusion bodies. In addition, if there are so many known causes of similar syndromes, it is likely that others remain to be identified. A restricted concept of idiopathic polymyositis will emerge only when more is known about the disordered immunology of dermatomyositis itself.

Differences Between Dermatomyositis and Polymyositis. These conditions are usually

Table 135–1. Differential Diagnosis of Polymyositis

Etiology Unknown: Idiopathic polymyositis

Collagen-Vascular Diseases
SLE, rheumatoid arthritis, periarteritis nodosa, systemic sclerosis, giant cell arteritis, Sjögren syndrome

Infections
Toxoplasmosis, trichinosis, schistosomiasis, cysticercosis, Chagas disease, legionnaires' disease, candidiasis, acne fulminans, microspiradosis

Influenza virus, rubella, hepatitis B, Behcet, Kawasaki, mycoplasma, coxsackie, ECHOvirus, AIDS (human immunodeficiency virus)

Immunization

Drugs
Systemic: ethanol, penicillamine, clofibrate, steroids, emetine, chloroquin, kaluretics, aminocaproic acid, rifampicin, ipecac

Intramuscular: meperidine, pentazocine

Systemic Diseases
Carcinoma, thymoma, sarcoid, amyloid, psoriasis, hyperglobulinemia (plasma cell dyscrasia), celiac disease, papular mucinosis, graft vs. host disease after transplantation, alcoholism

Endocrine Diseases
Hyperthyroidism, hypothyroidism, hyperadrenocorticism, hyperparathyroidism, Hashimoto's, thyroiditis

Metabolic Diseases
Therapeutic starvation, total parenteral nutrition, anorexia nervosa
Hypocalcemia, osteomalacia, chronic renal disease
Chronic K^+ depletion
Carnitine deficiency in muscle
Lack of acid maltase, phosphorylase, phosphofructokinase
Iron overload on maintenance hemodialysis

---

considered together because of the similarities in course and muscle disease. There are, however, important differences, as follows:

1. Dermatomyositis is a homogeneous condition, only rarely associated with known cause other than carcinoma. Polymyositis is associated with some other systemic disease in about half the cases.
2. Polymyositis is often a manifestation of a specific collagen-vascular disease, such as systemic lupus erythematosus, systemic sclerosis, or different forms of vasculitis. Dermatomyositis, however, is rarely if ever associated with evidence of collagen-vascular disease other than scleroderma. When polymyositis occurs

in a patient with lupus erythematosus, for instance, it can be regarded as a manifestation of lupus, not a combination of two different disorders (or an "overlap syndrome").
3. Dermatomyositis occurs at all ages, including children. Polymyositis is rare before puberty.
4. As assessed by inability to walk, the myopathy of dermatomyositis is severe more often than the myopathy of polymyositis.
5. Dermatomyositis is far more likely to be associated with malignant neoplasm than myopathy without rash.

Therapy. For idiopathic polymyositis, standard therapy is the same as that described for dermatomyositis. When polymyositis is the manifestation of some other identifiable disease, therapy is altered appropriately. The possibility of steroid myopathy or some other drug-induced disorder must be considered, and endocrine disorders are treated by specific measures. Because of the differences between dermatomyositis and polymyositis, it seems advisable to consider them separately in experimental trials of therapy.

References

Arahata K, Engel AG. Monoclonal antibody analysis of mononuclear cells in myopathies. V. T8+ cytotoxic and suppressor cells. Ann Neurol 1988; 23:493–499.

Bautista J, Gil-Necija E, Castilla J, Chinchon I, Raffel E. Dialysis myopathy: 13 cases. Acta Neuropath (Berl) 1983; 61:71–75.

Benbassat J, Gefel D, Larholt K, et al. Prognostic factors in polymyositis. A computer-assisted analysis of 92 cases. Arthritis Rheum 1985; 28:249–255.

Carpenter S, Karpati G. The major inflammatory myopathies of unknown cause. Pathol Annu 1981; 16:205–237.

Chou SM. Inclusion body myositis: a chronic persistent mumps myositis? Hum Pathol 1986: 17:765–777.

Choucair AK, Ziter FA. Pentazocine abuse masquerading as familial myopathy. Neurology 1984; 34:524–527.

Crennan JM, Van Scoy RE, McKenna CH, Smith TF. Echovirus polymyositis in patients with hypogammaglobulinemia: failure of high-dose intravenous gamma globulin therapy. Am J Med 1986; 81:35–42.

Cumming WJK, Weiser R, Teoh R, Hudgson P, Walton JN. Localized nodular myositis: a clinical and pathological variant of polymyositis. Q J Med 1977; 184:531–546.

Doyle DR, McCurley TL, Sergent JS. Fatal polymyositis in D-penicillamine-induced nephropathy and polymyositis. N Engl J Med 1983; 308:142–145.

Eisen A, Berry K, Gibson G. Inclusion body myositis: myopathy or neuropathy? Neurology 1983; 33:1109–1114.

Giorno R, Barden MT, Kohler PF, Ringel SP. Immunohistochemical characterization of the mononuclear cells infiltrating muscle of patients with inflammatory and noninflammatory myopathies. Clin Immunol Immunopathol 1984; 30:405–412.

Haller RG, Knochel JP. Skeletal muscle disease in alcoholism. Med Clin North Am 1984; 68:91–103.

Hart FD. Polymyalgia rheumatica. Correct diagnosis and treatment. Drugs 1987; 33:280–287.

Isenberg DA. Immunoglobin deposition in skeletal muscle in primary muscle diseases. Q J Med 1983; 52:297–310.

Layzer RB, Shearn MA, Satya-Murti S. Eosinophilic polymyositis. Ann Neurol 1977; 1:65–71.

Martin F, Ward K, Slavin G, Levi J, Peters TJ. Alcoholic skeletal myopathy, a clinical and pathological study. Q J Med 1985; 55:233–251.

Mastaglia FL. Adverse effects of drugs on muscle. Drugs 1982; 24:304–321.

Munsat T, Cancilla P. Polymyositis without inflammation. Bull Los Angeles Neurol Soc 1974; 39:500–507.

Ojeda VJ. Necrotizing myopathy associated with steroid therapy. Report of two cases. Pathology 1982; 14:435–438.

Persellin ST. Polymyositis associated with jejunoileal bypass. J Rheumatol 1983; 10:637–639.

Pickens P. Myositis and collagen disease: a muscle biopsy study. Mt Sinai J Med 1978; 45:433–442.

Riddoch D, Morgan-Hughes JA. Prognosis in adult polymyositis. J Neurol Sci 1975; 26:71–80.

Ringel SP, Kenny CE, Neville HE, Giorno R, Carry MR. Spectrum of inclusion body myositis. Arch Neurol 1987; 44:1154–1160.

Ringel SP, Thorne EG, Phanuphak P, Lava NS, Kohler PS. Immune complex vasculitis, polymyositis, and hyperglobulinemic purpura. Neurology 1979; 29:682–689.

Rowland LP, Sagman D, Schotland DL. Polymyositis: a conceptual problem. Trans Am Neurol Assoc 1966; 91:332–334.

Schwartz HA, Slavin G, Ward P, Ansell BM. Muscle biopsy in polymyositis and dermatomyositis; a clinicopathological study. Ann Rheum Dis 1980; 39:113–120.

Sundaram MB, Ashenhurst EM. Polymyositis presenting with distal and asymmetrical weakness. Can J Neurol Sci 1981; 8:147–149.

Symmans WA, Beresford CH, Bruton D, et al. Cyclic eosinophilic myositis and hyperimmunoglobulin-E. Ann Intern Med 1986; 104:26–32.

Takahasi K, Ogita T, Okudaira H, et al. Penicillamine-induced polymyositis in patients with rheumatoid arthritis. Arthritis Rheum 1986; 29:560–564.

Tsokos GC, Moutsopoulos M, Steinberg AD. Muscle involvement in systemic lupus erythematosus. JAMA 1981; 246:766–768.

Uddenfeldt P, Bjelle A, Olsson T, Stjernberg N, Thunnell M. Musculoskeletal symptoms in early sarcoidosis. Acta Med Scand 1983; 214:279–284.

136. MYOSITIS OSSIFICANS

Lewis P. Rowland

The identifying characteristic of this rare disorder is the deposition of true bone in subcutaneous tissue and along fascial planes in muscle. McKusick believes that the primary disorder is in connective tissue and prefers to call the disorder "fibrodysplasia ossificans," rather than its traditional name, which implies a disease of muscle. Nevertheless, in some cases myopathic changes occur in muscle biopsy or electromyogram, and occasionally the serum enzymes are increased.

Symptoms start in the first year or two of life in most cases. Transient and localized swellings of the neck and trunk are the first abnormality. Later, minor bruises are followed by deposition of solid material beneath the skin and within muscles. Plates and bars of material may be seen and felt in the limbs (Fig. 136–1), paraspinal tissues, and abdominal wall. These concretions are readily visible on radiographic examination, and when they cross joints, a deforming ankylosis results. The cranial muscles are spared, but the remainder of the body may be encased in bone. The extent of disability depends upon the extent of ossification, which varies considerably.

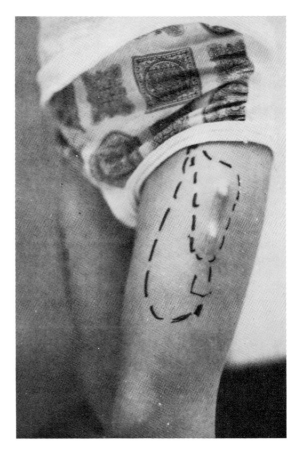

Fig. 136–1. Ossification of muscle biopsy scar in boy with myositis ossificans. The outer border of marks indicates extent of spontaneous ossification.

No abnormality of calcium metabolism has been detected.

Almost all cases are sporadic, but it is suspected that the disease is inherited because minor skeletal abnormalities occur in almost all patients, and these abnormalities seem to be transmitted in the family in an autosomal dominant pattern. The most common deformity is a short great toe (microdactyly), but curved fingers (clinodactyly) and other digital variations are also seen. Restricted ossification at the site of single severe injury may also occur in otherwise normal adults with no apparent genetic tendency.

In the past, there was no effective treatment, but the recent introduction of diphosphonates has given promise. These compounds seem to prevent the deposition of bone in the pathologic areas without interfering with normal growth. They do not correct established pathologic ossification, however, and the long-range hazards of the drugs are not known.

References

Amendola MA. Myositis ossificans circumscripta: computed tomography diagnosis. Radiology 1983; 149:775–779.

Connor JM, Smith R. The cervical spine in fibrodysplasia ossificans progressiva. Br J Radiol 1982; 55:492–496.

Connor JM, Evans DAP. Fibrodysplasia ossificans progressiva (myositis ossificans progressiva): clinical features and natural history of 34 UK patients. J Bone Joint Surg 1982; 64:76–83.

Lutwak L. Myositis ossificans progressiva. Mineral, metabolic and radioactive calcium studies of the effect of hormones. Am J Med 1964; 37:269–293.

McKusick VA. Hereditable Diseases of Connective Tissue, 4th ed. St Louis: C.V. Mosby Co., 1972:687–700.

Pitt P, Hamilton EBD. Myositis ossificans progressiva. J R Soc Med 1984; 77:68–70.

Smith R. Myositis ossificans progressiva: review of current problems. Semin Arthritis Rheum 1975; 4:369–380.

Chapter XVIII

Demyelinating Diseases

137. MULTIPLE SCLEROSIS

William A. Sibley
Charles M. Poser
Milton Alter

Multiple sclerosis (MS) is a disease of young adults that is characterized pathologically by numerous areas of demyelination and sclerosis in the CNS. Symptoms most often occur acutely and usually last for several weeks or longer, but may persist no longer than a few minutes or hours. Symptoms may seem bizarre and may not be substantiated by objective signs of neurologic abnormality.

The cause of the illness is unknown and the pathogenesis is poorly understood. There is no spontaneously occurring analogue in animals or a convincing experimental model; it seems likely that the disease is found only in humans.

An important characteristic of MS is that the number of lesions, or *plaques,* that are discovered scattered throughout the white matter (with occasional extension into gray matter) at autopsy is invariably larger than the number of lesions detected clinically or by means of laboratory tests. These silent lesions may be responsible for aspects of the disease that are poorly understood, especially mental and cognitive disturbances.

The course of MS is chronic, usually lasting for many years. Exacerbations and remissions occur in about 75% of patients. Complete recovery is almost universal after the first attack. Later, recovery is typically less complete after each attack, with a slow advance of disability. Exacerbations most commonly are recurrences of previous symptoms, although they often include new symptoms. Magnetic resonance imaging (MRI) shows that new symptoms lasting more than 24 to 48 hours, and associated with appropriate changes on neurologic examination (the definition of *ex-*

acerbation), are usually associated with one or more new MRI lesions, or enlargement of old lesions. Lesions of MS may be asymptomatic. Typical lesions of MS may be found at autopsy in people who die of other causes and never had any symptoms of MS. In addition, serial MRI scans in patients with stable MS show that new lesions often appear without symptoms, emphasizing the difficulty of judging "activity" without MRI monitoring. Slow progression is most likely due to gradual accumulation or enlargement of plaques, but progressive gliosis could also be a factor.

Pathogenesis. There are two major theories of pathogenesis. The first assumes direct infection of the CNS by a virus. Certainly, MS is not contagious; conjugal cases, for example, are rare. Support for the theory is derived from the occasional successful isolations of virus from the brains of MS patients. However, these isolations have usually not been repeatable, even in the same laboratory. The use of sensitive nucleic acid hybridization or immunofluorescent techniques for demonstration of a viral genome has also given inconsistent results. Many attempts to transmit MS to nonhuman primates have been unsuccessful after more than 15 years of observation.

The other theory, currently widely held, is that MS is due to altered immunity, probably genetically determined. Patients (and their siblings) tend to have higher antibody titers in serum and CSF for measles virus. Patients and siblings also have higher serum titers of antibodies to many other viruses, such as vaccinia, rubella, and varicella. This finding is generally assumed to imply greater immune responsiveness to infection. In one prospective study there were also 25 to 50% fewer common viral infections in MS patients than in controls, even in mildly affected MS patients with equal opportunity for infectious contacts.

Whereas direct viral infection seems unlikely, an abnormal immune response to common viruses may be an important trigger for exacerbations. Two prospective studies have now shown that about 30% of clinical exacerbations follow banal viral infections. The risk of worsening from any single infection is low—about 8%. MRI correlations with these common infections have not yet been made in large series, and the responsible viruses have not been cultured or otherwise identified.

Two theories have also been offered to explain the postinfectious triggering of some exacerbations. One proposes a cross-reaction between an antibody response to a virus and to the as-yet-unknown MS antigen, presumably a constituent of myelin. This is the *molecular mimicry* theory.

Another theory suggests that the infection activates T-lymphocytes, resulting in the production of gamma interferon, a substance that enhances antigenic recognition. Recombinant gamma interferon treatment, in one report, was associated with a dramatic increase in frequency of exacerbations. Gamma interferon promotes the expression of histocompatibility antigens on cell membranes, a condition necessary for destruction by a clone of sensitized lymphocytes, or by macrophages.

There is evidence of a genetic predisposition to MS, although most studies also emphasize the importance of one or more environmental factors. About 5% of patients have a sibling with MS and, overall, about 15% have some close relative with the illness. When one of a pair of monozygotic twins develops MS, the other member develops *clinical* MS in about 40% of cases. Recent MRI data suggest that the true figure may approach 70%; even this, however, would emphasize the importance of an environmental influence, in contrast to pure genetic control. The association of MS with specific histocompatibility types (HLA-A3, -B7, -DW2, -DR2), at least in northern European and North American populations, is relevant. About 55% of MS patients have the DR2 gene, in comparison to 18% of controls.

The HLA markers associated with MS are not the same in all populations, despite the similarity of MS in those populations. It is possible that different infectious agents of other environmental factors may cause or predispose to central demyelination in different populations.

Data on the ontogeny of human immunity indicate that adult levels of humoral and cellular immunity develop gradually during childhood and may not be mature until the second half of the first decade. In childhood, when there is a natural imbalance of immune components, individuals may be particularly susceptible to a demyelinating type of host response.

Experimental allergic encephalomyelitis (EAE) is often considered a model of multiple sclerosis. When young animals are inoculated with appropriate tissue or material and Freund's adjuvant, the course of EAE is likely to be exacerbating and remitting, with more central demyelination. Mature animals tend to show a monophasic illness with a greater inflammatory response. These patterns suggest that MS may be an age-dependent host response to childhood infection. This view fits with epidemiologic observations that when populations migrate to a region with a different frequency of MS, their risk of acquiring the disease is altered if they migrate before age 15, but not if they migrate as adults. In regions where MS is common, some childhood infections tend to occur later in childhood or in adolescence than in regions where MS is rare. Thus, early childhood infections may protect against MS, whereas later childhood infections may predispose to the disease.

Whereas the pathogenesis of the initial swelling and eventual destruction of the myelin sheath remains poorly understood, a better understanding exists regarding the possible mechanism for the very transient symptoms so characteristic of this disease. The naked axon is poorly suited for conduction of an action potential, and does it more slowly; if the demyelinated area is too long, conduction fails altogether. Marginal conduction through demyelinated areas may fail also in response to fatigue, increased calcium ion concentration, or elevated body temperature. This reduced margin of safety for conduction probably accounts for the rapid fluctuation in the intensity of symptoms from hour to hour noted by many patients.

The initial attack of MS or relapses in the course of the disease may follow acute viral infections, and prospective studies have shown that viral infection is an important environmental risk factor. Attacks may follow unusual fatigue, vaccination, or emotional upset, but the same studies have failed to demonstrate that these other influences are true risk factors. Often the relationship is fortuitous, because MS is a relatively common disease and bouts of worsening are even more common.

Numerous cases have been reported in which physical trauma was alleged to have precipitated or aggravated the disease. These anecdotal and uncontrolled observations cannot be considered as proof of a causal association between trauma and MS. The effect of pregnancy on MS is difficult to evaluate because the child-bearing age overlaps with the age when multiple sclerosis is likely to begin or exacerbate. However, if the pregnancy year is considered, exacerbations seem to cluster in the postpartum period rather then during the pregnancy. This tendency suggests that nonspecific factors such as fatigue may be important and that pregnancy itself may not have a deleterious effect. Therefore, it is necessary to consider the ability of the patient and family to care for the child as well as the desires of the patient and husband before interdicting or recommending termination of a pregnancy.

Pathology. The gross appearance of the external surface of the brain is usually normal. Occasionally there is atrophy of the cerebral convolutions with enlargement of the lateral and third ventricles. On sectioning the brain, numerous small irregular grayish areas are present in the cerebral hemispheres, particularly in the white matter and in the periventricular regions (Fig. 137–1). The white matter that forms the superior lateral angle of the body of the lateral ventricles is frequently and characteristically affected. Similar areas of discoloration are also found in the brain stem and cerebellum. These are the plaques of MS.

The external appearance of the spinal cord is usually normal. In a few cases, the cord may be slightly shrunken and the pia arachnoid may be thickened. The cord may occasionally be swollen over several segments if death follows soon after the onset of an acute transverse lesion of the cord. Plaques similar to those in the cerebellum can occasionally be seen on the external surface of the cord, but they are most easily recognized on cross sections. The optic nerves may be shrunken, but the external appearance of the other cranial nerves and the peripheral nerves is usually normal. In rare instances, necrotic areas may be present.

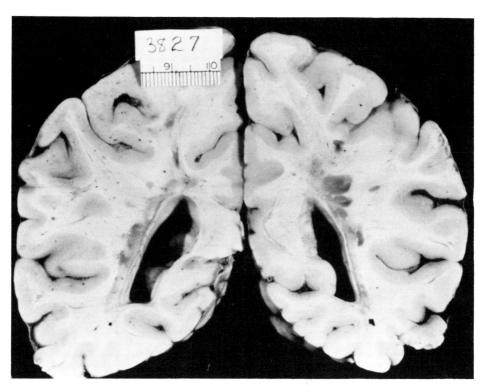

Fig. 137–1. Gross appearance, coronal section, occipital lobe. Note extensive periventricular lesions. Several small lesions are scattered elsewhere in the white matter. (Courtesy of Dr. Daniel Perl.)

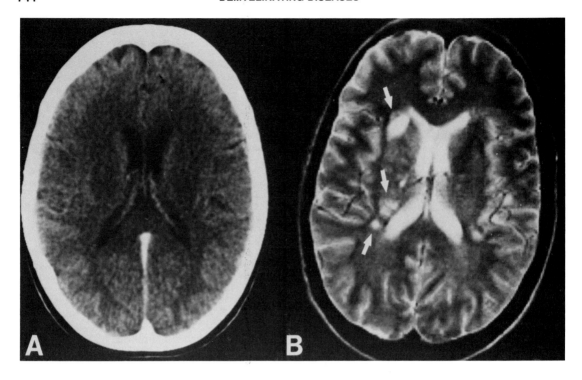

Fig. 137–2. The contrast-enhanced CT scan in *A* is normal. *B,* The axial T_2 MRI scan in the same patient during the same period shows multiple white matter lesions, the largest designated by arrows.

Myelin sheath stains of sections of the nervous system show areas of demyelination in the regions that were visibly discolored in the unstained specimen. In addition, many more plaques are apparent. These plaques are sharply circumscribed and are diffusely scattered throughout all parts of the brain and spinal cord. They are most numerous in the white matter of the cerebrum (Fig. 137–2), brain stem, cerebellum, and spinal cord. The lesions in the brain tend to be grouped around the lateral and third ventricles. The lesions in the cerebral hemisphere vary in size from that of a pinhead to large areas that encompass

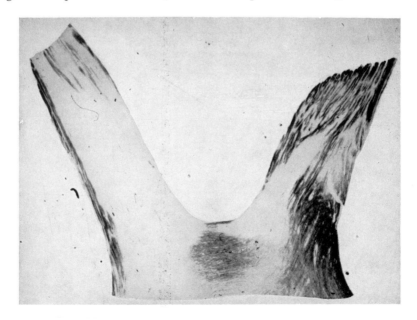

Fig. 137–3. Multiple sclerosis. Demyelinization of optic nerves and chiasm. (Courtesy of Dr. Abner Wolf.)

the major portion of one lobe of the hemisphere. Small lesions may be found in the gray matter and in the zone between the gray and white matter. Plaques of varying sizes may be found in the optic nerves, chiasm, or tracts (Fig. 137–3). Lesions in the corpus callosum are not uncommon (Fig. 137–4). The lesions in the brain stem are usually numerous (Fig. 137–5), and sections from this area when stained by the Weigert method have a characteristic "Holstein cow" appearance (Fig. 137–6).

In sections of the spinal cord, the areas of demyelination vary in size from small lesions involving a portion of the posterior or lateral funiculi to an almost complete loss of myelin in an entire cross section of the cord (Figs. 137–7 and 137–8).

Each individual lesion is characterized by its sharp delimitation from the surrounding normal tissue. Within the lesion is a complete or incomplete destruction of the myelin, a characteristically lesser degree of damage to the axis cylinders or neurons, proliferation of the glial cells, changes in the blood vessels, and relatively good preservation of the ground structure. Only rarely is the damage

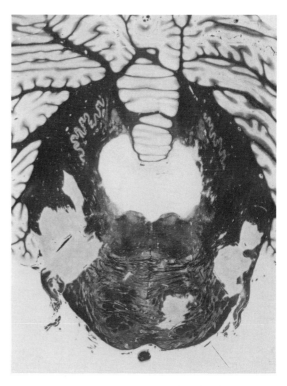

Fig. 137–5. Multiple sclerosis. Myelin sheath stain. Lesions in pons, middle cerebellum peduncle, and cerebellar white matter, typically near the dentate nuclei. (Courtesy of Dr. Charles Poser.)

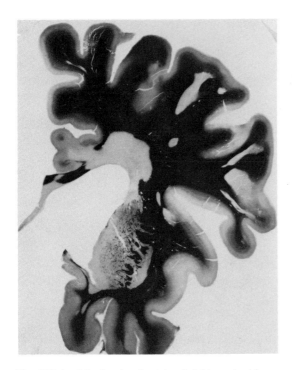

Fig. 137–4. Myelin sheath stain of right cerebral hemisphere in multiple sclerosis (celloidin). Note lesions in corpus callosum, superior lateral angle of the ventricle, and several plaques in the subcortical white matter. (Courtesy of Dr. Charles Poser.)

severe enough to affect the latter and produce a cyst (see Fig. 137–6).

Most myelin sheaths within a lesion are destroyed, and there is swelling and fragmentation of many of those that remain. The degree of damage to the axis cylinders is variable. In the more severe lesions, axons may be entirely destroyed, but more commonly only a few are severely injured and the remainder are normal or show only minor changes. Secondary degeneration of long tracts occurs when the axons have been destroyed.

When the lesion involves gray matter, nerve cells are less affected than myelin, but some cells may be completely destroyed and others may show degenerative changes.

Microglial cells proliferate and migrate into the lesion to phagocytize the debris. Compound granular cells laden with cholesterol esters (which have traditionally, although erroneously, been referred to as neutral fat) are present in great numbers in fresh lesions, in the perivascular spaces of the vessels and in the tissue adjacent to them. In older lesions, these cells are found chiefly in the perivascular spaces in and around the lesion. In or-

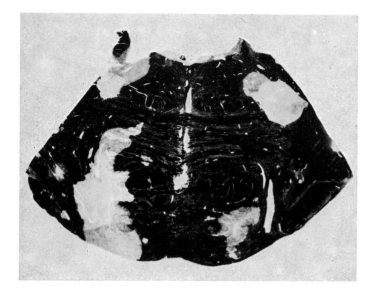

Fig. 137–6. Myelin sheath stain of brain stem in multiple sclerosis. Note sharp demarcation of lesions.

dinary cell stains (hematoxylin-eosin or Nissl), this perivascular accumulation of cells gives the appearance of a mild inflammatory reaction. The macroglia proliferate and produce fibrils that give the older lesions their characteristic sclerotic appearance and make them visible to the naked eye. Occasionally the extent of the gliosis exceeds the area of myelin loss.

Electron-microscopic examination of brain tissue obtained by cerebral biopsy in patients with MS reveals the following findings: there is evidence of both primary and segmental demyelination with short internodes and wide nodes of Ranvier; the myelin sheaths appear to be thin in relation to the axon diameter; and there is evidence of remyelination including unusual node of Ranvier configurations. The oligodendroglia reveal accumulation of dense bodies and myelin figures as well as vacuolization of cytomembrane systems. The astrocytes also show ac-

cumulation of dense bodies and myelin figures, increased numbers of glial filaments, and scattered cytoplasmic vacuoles. The endothelium of blood vessels contains dense bodies and lipid droplets. The same dense bodies are also seen in pericytes and, rarely, in the perivascular inflammatory cells as well as in the axons. There is a general increase in the extracellular spaces. There is no evidence of platelet or other thrombi in blood vessels nor are there any structural abnormalities of capillary or basement membrane. There is no evidence of peeling away of myelin lamellae by phagocytic cells; no unequivocal virus particles are seen. No myelin sheaths of the peripheral type are present.

Study of what appear to be old, inactive plaques has shown continued destruction of remaining myelin by macrophages. Axons that may have been thinly remyelinated are embedded in dense glial tissue and are distorted in shape and diameter. These findings

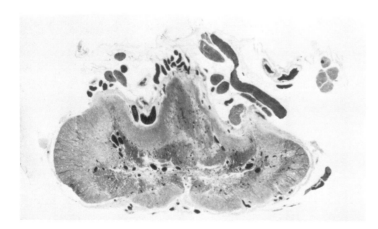

Fig. 137–7. Myelin sheath stain: tenth thoracic segment of spinal cord. Almost complete demyelination of the entire section. The gray matter is severely involved and there is cystic degeneration, causing obliteration of normal architecture.

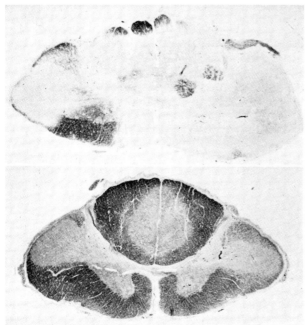

A

B

Fig. 137–8. Multiple sclerosis. *A*, Almost complete loss of myelin in transverse section of cord. *B*, Symmetric lesions in the posterior and lateral funiculi simulating distribution of lesions in combined system disease. (From Merritt HH, Mettler FA, Putnam TJ. Fundamentals of Clinical Neurology. Philadelphia: Blakiston, 1947.)

provide evidence that clinical progression of disability in MS may be due to secondary, nonspecific consequences of the disease rather than to the disease itself.

The peripheral nerves usually show no disease. However, some have reported subtle pathologic changes in sural nerve biopsies by electron microscopy. A few patients have had evidence of both MS and unequivocal demyelinating peripheral neuropathy. The significance of these unusual associations remains unclear.

Neurochemistry. The changes found most consistently in biochemical analysis of demyelinated areas are identical to those found in secondary demyelination or in experimental wallerian degeneration. There is a general decrease of all the characteristic myelin lipids (i.e., cerebrosides, sphingomyelin, cholesterol). In addition, cholesterol changes from the free form, which is the only one normally found in white matter, to esterified cholesterol.

Immunology. Although MS is thought to be an autoimmune disease, the evidence for this theory is indirect. The pathologic similarity to chronic EAE is often cited as a compelling analogy. Nonetheless, at present the MS antigen is unknown, and no antibody has been identified in serum or CSF shown to be specific for MS. Numerous attempts have been made to identify a specific antigen using a wide variety of humoral reactivity techniques and a number of methods for demonstrating cell-mediated hypersensitivity.

There are signs of lymphocyte abnormalities in MS. Several investigators have confirmed a decrease in numbers of suppressor T-lymphocytes just before an exacerbation in both blood and CSF. Lymphocytes in the CSF are mostly T-lymphocytes, and the total number and the relative number of T-helper cells rise with attacks. B-lymphocytes are found in the perivascular cuffs in the CNS, but are relatively uncommon in the CSF. They are the source of local immunoglobulin production.

Antibodies, including antiviral antibodies, can be found in the CSF but the patterns and titers differ in various patients. Antimyelin basic protein (MBP) antibody can be identified in the CSF in some MS patients; this finding is not restricted to MS but it could still play a part in pathogenesis. AntiMBP antibody cannot be demonstrated in MS serum, but has been found in immune complexes in serum. Free kappa light chains can be detected in the CSF of about 80% of MS patients—the same number that contain oligoclonal bands in CSF.

Incidence and Epidemiology. MS has an unequal geographic distribution. In general, the disease increases in frequency with latitude in both the northern and southern hemispheres. Near the equator, MS is virtually nonexistent. Farther from the equator, it reaches a prevalence of about 60/100,000 population. In some northerly areas, such as the Shetland and Orkney Isles off the coast of northern Scotland, reported prevalence rates exceed 150/100,000 population.

Because of variation in methods of case-finding and the need to rely on clinical and somewhat subjective criteria in diagnosing cases of MS in a population, the absolute numbers reported in any given area need to be accepted cautiously. It may therefore be best to consider the distribution of the disease in terms of zones of high, medium, and low frequency. Using this convention, most of northern Europe, northern United States, southern Canada, and southern Australia and New Zealand are high-incidence areas. Southern Europe, Asia Minor, North Africa, and northern Australia have moderate to low incidence rates. Central Africa appears to be a low-frequency zone for the disease; the disease is extremely rare or absent in black Africans. In a South African study, Afrikaaners had a higher incidence rate than blacks, but not as high as those South Africans of English descent; these, in turn, had a lower incidence rate than immigrants from Britain.

All of Japan has a low incidence rate of MS, as do Japanese living in Hawaii or on the west coast of the United States. Little is known about the distribution of MS in South America, but studies in Mexico and Guatemala showed a low prevalence. No formal population studies of MS have been carried out in China, but observations from neurologic clinics and hospitals indicate a low incidence. Taiwan, Indonesia, the Indian subcontinent, and the Pacific Isles also have a low incidence of the disease. A few observations among the sparse populations of the far north indicate that MS is uncommon and suggest that the direct relationship between frequency and geographic latitude may not hold at the northerly extremes. Occasional observations of foci of high frequency of MS are worthy of note, but chance or biased selection cannot be eliminated as explanations.

Whether Asian resistance to MS is genetic or environmental is unclear. In the United States, racial comparisons indicate a somewhat lower incidence among blacks, but northern blacks have a higher incidence of MS than southern blacks. Therefore, poorer ascertainment of MS in blacks and greater genetic resistance to demyelination are possible explanations for black-white differences in MS frequency. Blacks and whites with MS in

Philadelphia had the same increased frequency of HLA-A3, B7, and DW2.

There is a positive correlation between level of education and measures of good sanitation on the one hand and risk of MS on the other hand. The disease also correlates well with measures such as the percentage of literacy in the population and achievement on intelligence tests. In one study, intelligence tests were administered to military recruits before symptoms of MS became apparent, and therefore were unbiased. Although the ability to read and write cannot be of pathogenic significance, the life-style of more literate families may create conditions that increase the risk of MS. Infections in children of more affluent families tend to occur later than in less economically advantaged families. However, the more affluent also consume more animal fat and the association between risk of MS and increased socioeconomic status could support a dietary as well as an infectious cause of the disease. Perhaps both factors play a role. Eskimos have little if any MS, but they consume a high-fat diet. However, they also eat fish; their example may not challenge the significance of animal fat consumption as a factor in causing MS.

Studies of migrant populations allow an assessment of environmental changes on risk of MS while keeping genetic factors constant. Children born in Israel of immigrants from Asian and North African countries showed relatively higher incidence rates of MS, like European immigrants, rather than the low rates characteristic of their parents. This finding implies that an environmental factor is critically important in the etiology and pathogenesis of MS. This environmental factor may outweigh genetic resistance. Similar differences were noted among the native-born South African whites with a relatively low incidence, as opposed to the high incidence among immigrants from Great Britain. Refinement of these studies then revealed that age at immigration appeared to play an important role because an immigrant leaving the country of origin before the age of 15 would have nearly the same risk of acquiring MS as that of the native-born Israeli or South African. An individual immigrating after that age would have the risk factor of the country of origin. These findings have been confirmed by studies among various ethnic groups in Hawaii. These well-established data relating to the critical importance of the period at, or immediately after, puberty have been variously interpreted in terms of the acquisition at a critical period of an infectious agent with long latency, or conversely, the acquisition prior to that critical period of some temporarily effective protective, possibly immune mechanism.

The epidemic of MS reported from the Faroe Islands is further evidence of the importance of an environmental factor. Cases appeared in the Faroes shortly after the islands were occupied by British troops in World War II. The incidence of MS waned after the troops departed except for a short resurgence of the disease some years later, which may have been due to secondary cases. There was some evidence that close contact between the bivouac area of the troops and the residences of the patients may have been a causative factor. However, the paucity of cases of MS among conjugal pairs argues against direct transferability of a causative agent.

Although environmental factors may be important in etiology, the observation of increased risk of MS in families of an MS patient cannot be lightly dismissed; both environmental and genetic factors are probably important.

MS affects women more than men in a ratio of about 1.5 to 1 (Table 137–1). However, among patients with later onset, the sex ratio is closer to 1 to 1 or even reversed.

There are also clinical differences in different localities: acute syndromes of massive monophasic demyelination are uncommon in western countries with temperate climates and are more common in Asia. Painful tonic spasms and bilateral optic neuritis may also be more common in Asian populations.

MS is predominatly a disease of young adults. Although cases have been reported with onset of symptoms before the age of 10 and after the age of 60, these are rare; in the vast majority, symptoms begin in the period between 20 and 40 years of age. Although some series have reported as many as 3% of patients with onset of symptoms before the age of 10, pathologic verification has been obtained in only a few instances. Onset of symptoms in middle life is not rare. In one series, symptoms began after age 40 in 13% of 310 clinically studied cases and in 21% of 42 cases proved by necropsy. The oldest age at onset in that series was 63. In a series of 111 autopsy-proven cases, the oldest age at onset was 64.

Symptoms and Signs. The disease has been characterized by many authors as having dissemination of lesions in both time and space. Exacerbations and remissions occur frequently. In addition, the patient's signs and symptoms indicate the presence of more than one lesion. Symptoms and signs may be transient and some manifestations may seem bizarre. The patient may experience unusual subjective sensations that are difficult to describe and impossible to verify objectively by even an experienced examiner.

The symptoms and signs of MS (Tables 137–2 and 137–3) are so diverse that their enumeration would include all the symptoms that can result from injury to any part of the neur-

Table 137–1. Age and Sex Distribution of Autopsy-Proven Multiple Sclerosis

	Country of Origin			
	England	*Norway*	*U.S*	*Total*
Number of patients	55	31	71	157
Sex: male (%)	33	61	60	47
female (%)	67	39	40	53
Age of onset: range (years)	14–64	17–49	18–57	14–64
Mean (years)	34	31	28	32
males	37	32	28	33
females	33	29	27	31
Age groups				
<20 (%)	15	13	14	14
21–30 (%)	22	42	51	35
31–40 (%)	38	26	25	29
41–50 (%)	18	19	10	14
51–60 (%)	5	0	3	4
61–70 (%)	2	0	0	1
Duration of disease				
Mean (years)	12	17	14	14
Range	2 mo to 36 yrs	3 mo to 37 yrs	2 mo to 32 yrs	2 mo to 37 yrs

Table 137–2. Frequency of Various Symptoms in 157 Autopsy-Proven Cases of Multiple Sclerosis

	Country of Origin			
	England	Norway	U.S.	Total
Number of patients	55	31	71	157
		Percentage of Occurrence		
Muscle weakness	95	100	96	96
Ocular disturbance	84	81	92	85
Urinary disturbance	93	87	70	82
Gait ataxia	45	68	60	60
Paresthesias	69	55	52	60
Dysarthria or scanning speech	53	61	52	54
Mental disturbance	42	52	50	47
Pain	13	19	32	19
Vertigo	7	26	20	17
Dysphagia	14	13	9	12
Convulsions	5	6	7	6
Decreased hearing	3	6	10	6
Tinnitus	—	3	7	5

axis from the spinal cord to the cerebral cortex. The chief characteristics of the symptoms of MS are multiplicity and the tendency to vary in nature and severity with the passage of time. Complete remission of the first symptoms occurs frequently but, with subsequent attacks, remissions do not occur or are incomplete. The clinical course extends for one or many decades in most cases, but a few may terminate in death within a few months of onset.

There is no classic form of MS, and the clinical manifestations depend on the particular areas of the nervous system that are involved. For reasons that remain unknown, the disease frequently involves some areas and systems more than others; manifestations of lesions in the optic chiasm and nerves, brain stem, cerebellum, and spinal cord, in particular the corticospinal tracts and posterior column, are most frequent.

Because MS is primarily a disease of white matter and although the lesions may spill over into gray matter, signs and symptoms of nuclear involvement are uncommon, and signs and symptoms of basal ganglia involvement such as dystonia and athetosis are rare. Some clinicians like to classify MS into spinal, brain-stem, cerebellar, and cerebral forms, but there are many cases in which these forms are combined, making that classification of little clinical value. Similarly, the practice of designating as Devic disease a syndrome of coincidental involvement of optic nerve and spinal cord creates unnecessary confusion based on the erroneous belief that the epon-

Table 137–3. Frequency of Signs in 157 Autopsy-Proven Cases of Multiple Sclerosis

	Country of Origin			
	England	Norway	U.S.	Total
Number of patients	55	31	71	157
		Percentage of Occurrence		
Spasticity or hyperreflexia, or both	96	100	99	98
Babinski sign	95	100	86	92
Absent abdominal reflexes	73	94	84	82
Dysmetria or intention tremor	80	81	76	79
Nystagmus	73	68	73	71
Impairment of vibratory sensation	65	55	60	61
Impairment of position sensation	62	49	48	52
Impairment of pain sensation	51	39	43	44
Facial weakness	27	52	46	42
Impairment of touch sensation	22	29	36	29
Impairment of temperature sensation	16	19	20	17
Changes in state of consciousness	—	3	6	5

ymic condition differs in any way from MS. It is the combination of anatomically unrelated signs and symptoms that most commonly forms the basis for the clinical diagnosis of MS.

Visual disturbances include diplopia, blurring of vision, diminution or loss of visual acuity either unilaterally or bilaterally, visual field defects that may range from a unilateral central scotoma or field contraction (Fig. 137–9) to a homonymous hemianopia. These disturbances characteristically have an acute onset. Patients may also complain of a curious and quite distinctive problem in recognition of faces, a rather embarrassing matter that can be demonstrated to be due to the loss of contrast of shade and colors, causing blurring of vision. In early or very mild *optic* or *retrobulbar neuritis*, color vision may be decreased to some degree while black and white vision may remain normal. On rare occasions, when color vision is affected in both eyes, the patient may actually become aware of either transient or permanent color blindness, almost always of the red-green type. Examination of the visual fields with a red or green test object may reveal a relative central scotoma or field contraction that is not apparent with the usual white test object. *Optic neuritis* must be differentiated from papilledema because they may seem similar on funduscopic examination, but neuritis is characterized by more severe impairment of visual acuity. A central or cecocentral scotoma is most characteristic. *Retrobulbar neuritis*, which is a common manifestation of MS, may not be associated with any funduscopic abnormality, but is always manifested by loss or diminution of visual acuity.

Diplopia may be caused by lesions in the medial longitudinal fasciculus that cause *internuclear ophthalmoplegia.* Internuclear ophthalmoplegia is uncommon in any other condition and therefore constitutes an important sign in the diagnosis of MS. It is characterized by paresis of the medial rectus on one side, weakness of the lateral rectus on the other side, and nystagmus of the outwardly deviating eye (monocular nystagmus). This impairment of gaze may be present on attempt to deviate the eyes to one or both sides. In uncomplicated lesions of the medial longitudinal fasciculus, function of the medial rectus can be demonstrated by the preservation of its action in convergence. Mild diplopia may be reported as blurring of vision; only if the patient shuts either eye, with resulting improvement of visual acuity, is the true nature of the complaint discovered.

The sudden onset of optic or retrobulbar neuritis, without any other associated sign or symptom of CNS involvement, is often interpreted as being the first symptom of MS. However, it may also result from a postinfectious or postvaccinal reaction and other conditions. It is impossible to determine in any single individual whether isolated optic neuritis predicts later development of MS.

The most common pupillary abnormalities are irregularity in the outline of the pupil, partial constriction, and partial loss of the light reflex.

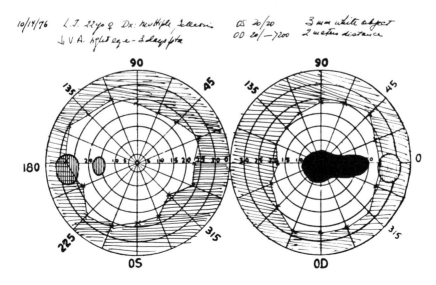

Fig. 137–9. Cecocentral scotoma in patient with acute right optic neuropathy: MS of three years duration.

Involvement of the descending root of the fifth cranial nerve occurs in few patients. There may be an impairment of pain sensation in the face, diminution or loss of the corneal reflex and, rarely, pain that is indistinguishable from that of trigeminal neuralgia.

Weakness of the facial muscles of the lower half of one side of the face is common, but complete peripheral facial palsy is rare. On the other hand, hemifacial spasm, consisting of spasmodic contractions of the facial muscles, may occur as one of the rare but characteristic paroxysmal disorders of MS. Fortunately, this condition may respond (as does trigeminal neuralgia) to treatments with carbamazepine. True vertigo, often lasting several days, may be severe in association with new lesions in the floor of the fourth ventricle; it is seldom a chronic symptom, however. The dysarthria and, rarely, the dysphagia seen in advanced cases of MS are most commonly due to cerebellar lesions or to lesions in the corticobulbar tracts that cause pseudobulbar palsy. In those instances, emotional lability or forced laughing or crying without the accompanying affect may also be present.

Limb weakness is the most common sign of the disease and may be manifested as monoplegia, hemiplegia, or tetraplegia (or pareses). Fatigability out of proportion to the demonstrable muscular weakness is a common complaint. The ataxia of gait proves to be one of the most disabling symptoms of MS. Most often, however, it is due to the combination of lesions in the cerebellum and loss of proprioception resulting from a lesion in the posterior columns of the spinal cord. Because it is so often combined with some spasticity of the legs, ambulation becomes extremely difficult.

In some patients, in particular those with a late onset, the disease may appear as a slowly progressive spastic paraplegia, with no abnormality except evidence of pyramidal tract involvement (i.e., spasticity, hyperreflexia, bilateral Babinski signs) and slight impairment of proprioceptive sensation.

The cerebellum or its connections with the brain stem are involved in most cases, with dysarthria, ataxia or gait, tremors, and incoordination of the muscles of the trunk and limbs. Tremor of the head and body is sometimes almost continuous when the patient is awake. The characteristic scanning speech of MS is a result of cerebellar incoordination of the palatal and labial muscles combined with dysarthria of corticobulbar origin.

Urinary disturbances are also extremely common, including incontinence and frequency or urgency of urination, which must be differentiated from those disturbances resulting from urinary tract infections or local conditions. Loss of libido and impotence are frequently found in men. Many sexual problems are psychologic rather than organic in origin. Sexual impairment may be due to fear of urinary incontinence during intercourse; control of this problem by propantheline may provide a partial solution.

Paresthesias include spontaneous feelings of numbness and tingling in the limbs, trunk, or face. The *Lhermitte symptom* is a sensation of "electricity" that is felt by the patient on passive or active flexion of the neck. It indicates a lesion of the posterior columns in the cervical portion of the spinal cord and may be seen in other diseases. In rare instances, Lhermitte symptom can be elicited by flexion of the trunk. Sharp shooting pains in the legs or in the abdomen, identical to those of tabes dorsalis, may also be encountered.

Mental symptoms occur frequently. Depression may be as common as the euphoria that is said to be characteristic of the disease. Disturbances of memory, subtle aphasic manifestations, or widespread cognitive defect may be elicited. It may not be possible to detect these changes by simple clinical examination. Special psychologic evaluations may be necessary and may explain some of the problems that patients report in their occupations, complaints that cannot be understood on the basis of clinically demonstrable neurologic abnormalities. Hysterical symptoms may be found in addition to those unquestionably due to anatomic lesions or physiologic alterations. The most common observation is the tendency of patients to exaggerate and extend symptoms that have a solid organic basis. For example, the patient with a right optic neuritis may complain of difficulty seeing with the other eye; numbness of the hand may be extended to involve the entire arm; or true diplopia may be transformed into triplopia, quadriplopia, or even monocular double vision. These instances of hysterical hyperbole seem to be more common in MS than in any other neurologic disease. A purely psychiatric presentation may occur and dementia may result.

The psychologic manifestations assume a particular importance in the genesis of exacerbations: whenever a previously experienced symptom recurs, it may result from physiologic alterations secondary to heat or some systemic or metabolic dysfunction or, alternately, it may be what can be called a "psychologically induced recall phenomenon." The very nature of MS, affecting young individuals who are often at the threshold of life-determining decisions or at the peak of professional productivity and who are then faced with the possibility of serious disability, increases the likelihood of psychologic alterations. The lack of specific treatment, uncertainty about long-term prognosis, and the frequent difficulty of establishing a definite diagnosis all complicate this serious problem.

In terms of frequency of signs and symptoms, the following occur in more than 75% of the patients at some time (see Tables 137–2 and 137–3): ocular disturbances, muscle weakness, spasticity and hyperreflexia, Babinski signs, absent abdominal reflexes, dysmetria or intention tremor, and urinary abnormality. Other combinations that occur in approximately 50 to 75% of the patients include nystagmus, gait ataxia, dysarthria or scanning speech, paresthesias, and objective alterations of vibratory and position senses. Mental disturbances of some kind, including both euphoria and depression, are seen in almost 50% of the patients (Table 137–4).

One of the characteristics of symptoms of MS is that they may be evanescent. Diplopia may last for minutes and paresthesias may last for seconds or hours; diminution of visual acuity may be equally short-lived. Transient loss of color vision may presage development of optic neuritis. Because of the transient and bizarre nature of some of these complaints, they are frequently called hysterical.

Remissions are also characteristic, but it is difficult for clinicians to agree on the nature or duration of these remissions. If one includes only the complete, or almost complete, disappearance of a major symptom such as loss of vision, marked weakness of a limb, or diplopia, significant clinical remissions occur in about 70% of the patients.

Mode of Onset. The onset is usually acute or subacute. There is no characteristic mode of onset, but several symptoms and signs frequently occur at the onset. Combinations of these are often helpful in establishing the presumptive diagnosis. Not infrequently, however, a thorough review of the past history reveals remote or recent episodes of other manifestations that had been ignored or not considered significant by the patient or physician. This is particularly true of transient paresthesias, mild urinary disturbances (often and erroneously diagnosed and treated as painless urinary tract infections), and mild ocular manifestations such as blurring of vision or transient diminution of monocular visual acuity. Muscle weakness, paresthesias, and ocular and cerebellar disorders are the most common symptoms at the onset of MS.

Laboratory Data. *Brain Imaging.* There is no pathognomonic test for MS, but the most valuable laboratory aid in the diagnosis is MRI, which shows multiple white matter lesions in 90% of patients with clinically definite MS as defined by traditional clinical criteria. Some lesions in brain and spinal cord are still missed by current MRI technology. Nevertheless, MRI has largely replaced CT in the diagnosis of MS because CT is much less sensitive, often seeming to be normal or showing only evidence of cerebral atrophy. Recent and old lesions can be differentiated by the injection of gadolinium, which appears in the MRI at the site of breakdown of the blood-brain barrier in acute lesions.

MRI, however, is not foolproof. Lesions similar to those of MS may be seen in encephalitis of any cause. As the age of the subject increases, MRI lesions of unknown significance appear more frequently. These *"unidentified bright objects"* or UBOs may be seen in asymptomatic individuals. Therefore, like the results of other laboratory tests, the findings of MRI must be considered together with the clinical manifestations.

CSF. Examination of the CSF is useful because any of five different measurements may indicate abnormality.

1. The number of white blood cells in CSF is often increased, up to 40 cells/mm^3 in about 30% of the patients. Although *CSF pleocytosis* is sometimes taken as a meas-

Table 137–4. Frequency of Mental Disturbances in Multiple Sclerosis in 46 Autopsy-Controlled Cases

Symptom	% of Cases
Disturbances of affect	54
Euphoria	31
Depression	7
Lability of mood	16
Psychotic episodes	4
Mental deterioration	26

(Modified from Carter S, Sciarra D, Merritt HH. Res Publ Assoc Res Nerv Ment Dis 1950; 28:471–511.)

ure of "activity" of the disease, the significance of these cells is uncertain, and it has not yet been determined whether the proportion of specific subsets of lymphocytes increases in CSF during exacerbations. In general, the number of T4- and T8-lymphocytes in CSF is similar to that in blood.

2. The *total protein content* is increased in about 40% of cases. However, levels over 100 mg/dl should raise doubts about the diagnosis of MS.

3. The *CSF gamma globulin content* is increased. In routine clinical laboratories, the determination of CSF IgG by electroimmunodiffusion or radioimmunodiffusion gives values over 13% of the total protein in 40 to 60% of the cases of MS. The lower figure is representative of ambulatory patients in the early years of illness and of most patients with minimal disability; the higher percentage is characteristic of patients with moderate or far-advanced MS.

Some clinicians find that the determination of the *gamma globulin index* is more useful than the simple determination of the total amount of gamma globulin. In this measurement, the amount of albumin in CSF is related to that in serum, to calculate the amount of gamma globulin actually arising in CSF.

4. *Oligoclonal bands* are found in CSF in MS. In electrophoretic patterns of normal CSF in agar gel, there is homogeneous staining in the IgG region. In the vast majority of patients with MS, however, there is heterogeneity in the IgG region with the appearance of several distinctly staining bands—so-called *oligoclonal* or *polyclonal bands*. Oligoclonal bands may be present even when the total CSF IgG content is normal; thus, oligoclonal bands may be expected in some patients with relatively little disability—exactly those cases with the most diagnostic uncertainty. Laterre and colleagues, for example, found banding in 87% of patients with advanced disability, but also in 73% of mildly disabled patients. Other laboratories have reported oligoclonal bands in virtually all patients with MS.

The changes in IgG are not specific for MS, however. Similar changes are seen in many patients with acute or chronic infections of the nervous system, and in

Table 137–5. CSF IgG Increase or Presence of Polyclonal Bands in Multiple Sclerosis and Other Diseases

Agar Gel Electrophoresis	%
Multiple sclerosis (323 cases)	78.6
Acute and chronic CNS infections (321 cases)	39.6
Peripheral neuropathies (273 cases)	5.1
CNS tumor, hydrocephalus (225 cases)	4.4
Cerebrovascular diseases (195 cases)	2.0
Miscellaneous (562 cases)	2.1

(From Laterre EC, Callewaert A, Heremans JF, and Sfaello Z. Neurology 1970; 20:982–990.)

2 to 5% of patients with degenerative diseases, neuropathies, tumors, or cerebrovascular disease (Table 137–5). Once the changes in immunoglobulins appear, they usually do not vary significantly, regardless of the subsequent course of the MS.

5. One other test of the CSF is measurement of the *content of myelin basic protein*, which has been used as a measure of activity of the disease by some investigators, but is of uncertain significance.

At this time no single absolutely reliable or completely pathognomonic laboratory examination exists for this disease. Too great reliance on the MRI, in the absence of characteristic symptoms and signs, can result in important errors. A typical MRI scan, however, coupled with the history, clinical examination, and characteristic changes in the CSF appears to be the most valuable diagnostic aid.

Evoked Responses. The recording of *cortical evoked responses* from visual, auditory, and somatosensory stimulation has proved to be of great value in demonstrating the existence of clinically unsuspected lesions. Visual evoked responses to both flash and pattern reversal stimuli have demonstrated abnormalities in many patients without history or signs of visual impairment. Similarly, auditory evoked responses have demonstrated unsuspected lesions in brain stem structures, and somatosensory evoked responses have suggested the presence of lesions in the spinal cord. Measurement of the delay of the blink reflex after electrical stimulation of the supraorbital nerve indicates the presence of a pontine lesion. The main advantage of these procedures is that they are simple, noninvasive, harmless, and relatively inexpensive with a remarkably high yield.

EEG. Abnormalities are found in about 35% of the patients in the acute stage of the disease, whereas slight changes may also be present in other stages. The abnormalities are chiefly in the form of slow waves and are considered to be a nonspecific reaction of the brain to an acute local pathologic process.

Psychologic Testing. These tests, especially in patients who have had no symptoms of mental or intellectual abnormality, may suggest impairment of cognitive function. Results, however, must be interpreted with caution.

Diagnosis. There is no specific test for MS; the diagnosis rests on the appearance of multiple signs and symptoms and the occurrence of the characteristic remissions and exacerbations (Table 137–6). The diagnosis can rarely be made with any degree of assurance at the time of the first attack. In day-to-day clinical practice, the diagnosis of MS is based on the ability to demonstrate, on the basis of the history, the neurologic examination, and laboratory tests, especially MRI, the existence of lesions involving different parts of the CNS. Thus, eliciting a history of mild, transient, and often overlooked or forgotten symptoms (e.g., transient diplopia, diminution of visual acuity, urinary urgency, weakness or numbness of a limb for a day or two) may provide such evidence.

Examination for monocular (and thus asymptomatic) disturbances of color vision with Ishihara or AO pseudoisochromatic color plates may demonstrate evidence of unsuspected subclinical optic neuropathy. The old aphorism that MS is a disease character-ized by dissemination in time and space is still the keystone of clinical diagnosis.

The advent of evoked potential tests has added a new dimension in the documentation of multiple lesions, and this has been even further amplified by MRI. Even in a patient who has had a single attack of optic neuritis or transverse myelitis, these tests may indicate more than one lesion, changing the diagnosis from "possible" to "probable" or even "definite." As more experience is gained with MRI, criteria may change again. At present, the following guidelines combine the clinical criteria of 1976 (see Table 137–6) and those of 1983 (Table 137–7), before there was much experience with MRI to document the presence of more than one lesion:

1. *Clinically definite MS* requires evidence from both history and neurologic examination of more than one lesion, or there may be history of two episodes, signs of one lesion on examination, and evidence from evoked responses or MRI or other lesions.

2. For *"laboratory-supported definite MS,"* there must be evidence of two lesions in either history or examination. If there is only one lesion in either of those categories, at least one more should be evident in evoked responses or MRI. In addition, CSF gamma globulin should be abnormal.

3. In the category of *clinically probable MS,* either history or examination, but not both, provides evidence of two lesions. If there is evidence of only one lesion by history and only one on neurologic ex-

Table 137–6. Criteria for Clinical Diagnosis of Multiple Sclerosis

Clinically Definite:	Consistent course
	Relapsing, remitting course; at least two bouts separated by at least one month
	Slow or stepwise progressive course for at least 6 months
	Documented neurologic signs of lesions in more than one site, of brain or spinal cord white matter
	Onset of symptoms between ages 10 and 50 years
	No better neurologic explanations
Probable:	History of relapsing, remitting symptoms but signs not documented and only one current sign commonly associated with MS
	Documented single bout of symptoms with signs of more than one white matter lesion; good recovery, then variable symptoms and signs
	No better neurologic explanation
Possible:	History of relapsing, remitting symptoms without documentation of signs
	Objective signs insufficient to establish more than one lesion of central white matter
	No better explanation

(From Rose AS, Ellison GW, Meyers LW, Tourtellotte WW. Neurology 1976; 26:20–22.)

Table 137–7.   Criteria for the Diagnosis of Multiple Sclerosis

	Number of Attacks	Evidence of More than One Lesion		CSF, OCB, or IgG
		Clinical	Laboratory	
A. Clinically Definite				
A1	2	2		
A2	2	1	and 1	
B. Laboratory-Supported Definite				
B1	2	1	or 1	+
B2	1	2		+
B3	1	1	and 1	+
C. Clinically Probable				
C1	2	1		
C2	1	2		
C3	1	1	and 1	
D. Laboratory-Supported Probable				
D1	2	0	0	+

(From Poser C, Paty DW, Scheinberg L, McDonald WI, Ebers GC. The Diagnosis of Multiple Sclerosis. New York: Thieme-Stratton, 1984.)

amination, the evoked potentials or MRI may provide evidence of the other one or more. (The diagnosis would change to "laboratory-supported definite" if there were also an abnormality of CSF IgG.)

Multiple lesions in the MRI may become accepted evidence of definite MS if the clinical manifestations are also compatible, so this elaborate scheme may not be necessary. However, the MRI is not absolutely reliable. Clinical judgment is still needed.

The 1983 classification eliminated the category of "possible" MS, but problem cases still arise, especially when MRI fails to document the presence of multiple lesions.

Although a suspicion of MS or a presumptive diagnosis can be made early in the course of the disease, reliable diagnosis depends on continued observation and numerous re-examinations over a period of months or years.

Differential Diagnosis. Because MS is almost exclusively a disease of the central white matter, signs and symptoms indicating involvement of the basal ganglia, cranial nerve nuclei, anterior horn cells, nerve roots, or peripheral nerves militate strongly against the diagnosis.

It is difficult, if not impossible, to differentiate between the first attack of MS and a postinfectious or postimmunization encephalomyelopathy. What has often been referred to as acute disseminated encephalomyelitis, commonly considered to be postinfectious or postimmunization in nature, turns out to be the first episode of MS in about 25% of patients. Familial incidence is unusual and should be considered as evidence against the diagnosis, as should age at onset after age 60.

Other conditions that may closely resemble the intermittent course of MS and the dissemination of lesions include: disseminated lupus erythematosus or polyarteritis nodosa; vascular malformation or hemangiomas of the brain stem or spinal cord; gliomas of the brain stem; cervical cord neoplasms; syringomyelia; cervical discs and spondylosis; and some lymphomas.

Progressive multifocal leukoencephalopathy, which is usually associated with a leukemia or lymphoma, may mimic an acute attack of MS.

Other conditions that need occasionally to be ruled out include neurosyphilis; spinocerebellar ataxias; malformations of the cervical spine and the base of the skull; tumors in the region of the foramen magnum; cerebellopontine angle tumors; tumors of the cerebral hemispheres; and combined system disease due to vitamin B$_{12}$ deficiency.

The rapid onset of paraplegia or quadriplegia with an appropriate sensory level, the syndrome of *acute transverse myelitis,* may be the first attack of MS or it may be an isolated episode, with no further neurologic disorder. This syndrome must be differentiated from compressive lesions such as tumor or acute epidural abscess. Spinal MRI is useful in the rapid exclusion of mass lesions. If MRI is normal, the syndrome may be the only manifestation of postinfectious encephalomyelitis. Anterior spinal artery thrombosis and meningovascular syphilis should also be considered. Viruses such as the herpes simplex B virus may cause acute myelitis in monkey handlers. Transverse myelitis may also occur as a rare manifestation of Epstein-Barr virus infection, and such cases often have negative monospot or heterophile antibody tests. Less rapidly progressive paraplegia may be due to tropical spastic paraplegia, an HTLV-1 virus infection, or it may be a manifestation of delayed radiation necrosis, or the syndrome of subacute necrotic myelopathy.

One of the most difficult differential diagnoses is that of conversion reaction. Because of the fleeting nature of symptoms, the absence or paucity of neurologic signs, especially at the onset of the disease, the not uncommon emotional disturbance, and the manifestation of the disease after physical or emotional trauma, this differential may tax the ingenuity of even the most astute physician. On the other hand, psychologic symptoms may mask the underlying disease for a long time and may delay the establishment of the correct diagnosis.

Course and Prognosis. MS follows an unpredictable course, but there are some reliable early prognostic guidelines. Exceptional cases are clinically silent for a lifetime; the typical pathologic findings are discovered as an incidental finding at autopsy. At the other extreme, some cases are so rapidly progressive that only weeks elapse between onset and death.

The usual patterns include the following forms: *benign*, with a few mild early exacerbations, complete or nearly complete remissions, and minimal or no disability (20%); *exacerbation-remitting*, with more frequent early exacerbations and less complete remissions, but with long periods of stability and some disability (25%); *chronic-relapsing*, with fewer remissions as the disease progresses and increasing (cumulative) disability (40%); and *chronic-progressive*, with insidious onset and steady progression of symptoms (15%).

The diagnostic use of evoked potentials, CT, and CSF oligoclonal IgG has changed some concepts of the course of MS. Some cases previously reported as "chronic progressive myelopathy" or "idiopathic optic neuritis" are now considered as probable or clinically definite MS (Table 137–8). These changes will also alter incidence data.

As a general rule, sensory symptoms at onset (e.g., blurred vision or paresthesias) tend to indicate a benign course, whereas early cerebellar and corticospinal signs imply a chronic-relapsing or chronic-progressive course.

In a report from MS clinic directors, the characteristics of a good prognosis in order of usefulness are the following: ambulatory ability, minimal corticospinal and cerebellar signs 5 years after onset; complete and rapid remission of initial symptoms; age 35 years or less at onset; only one symptom during the first year; acute onset of initial symptoms; brief duration of the most recent exacerbation; and absence of cerebellar signs on initial examination.

Pressure sores, intractable spasticity with contractures, and urinary tract infections are indicators of late stages with poor prognosis for significant recovery.

Death from the disease itself is rare. Intercurrent infection (urinary tract, respiratory tract, or decubitus ulcer) is the usual cause of death. Because about 75% of patients attain older age and are susceptible to the common fatal illnesses, there may be a lower incidence of myocardial infarction, perhaps because disabled patients are less exposed to occupational stress.

Average survival has increased from about 25 to 35 years after onset in the last few decades, probably a result of better management of infection and decubitus ulcers.

Disability and work capacity are extremely important in any chronic disease with onset from 15 to 55 years (see Table 137–8).

Treatment. The treatment and care of the patient with MS are two of the major clinical challenges for the physician. Too often "treatment" has been interpreted as "cure." This has resulted in the often heard statement "there is no treatment of MS," with resultant neglect of symptoms and complications that are amenable to management or prevention. It is literally true that there is no cure yet, and there is a long list of ineffective therapeutic regimens that have been tried. Anecdotal reports of "miracle responses" to therapy are often reported early in the disease, usually coincidental with spontaneous remissions. There is no way to arrest the natural course of MS, and restoration of long-standing physical impairment seems even more remote.

The therapeutic regimens that are now

Table 137–8. Working Capacity and Survival in 800 Patients with Multiple Sclerosis

Duration	1–5 yrs (%)	6–10 yrs (%)	11–15 yrs (%)	16–20 yrs (%)	21 yrs (%)
Working	71	50	31	30	28
Disabled	29	49	63	57	52
Dead	—	1	6	13	20

(From Bauer HJ. Neurology 1978; 28:8–20.)

widely employed are directed either toward shortening the intervals between remissions and halting progression (based on a viral-immunologic hypothesis of pathogenesis) or toward alleviating symptoms of disabling neurologic defects and assisting the patient and family in adaptation to the illness and rehabilitation.

Before making specific recommendations about treatment, we suggest some general guidelines: (1) the patient and family should be informed of the diagnosis by specific name when it is firmly established, so they can avail themselves of all available services, and to diminish the likelihood of fruitless search for unproven treatments; (2) the disease should be explained in clearly understandable terms, with a realistic but encouraging prognosis; (3) the patient should be re-evaluated at intervals for counseling, detection of early complications, and evaluation of progress; (4) the patient should be given realistic expectations for results from therapy and encouraged to ask questions and participate in decisions (e.g., adjustment of dosage of antispastic medicaton); and (5) the patient with MS has complex problems and may eventually require the assistance of several medical and nonmedical health-care specialists.

For the acute attack, many experienced clinicians give ACTH gel by daily intramuscular injection for 10 to 14 days, or they give oral steroids daily or on alternate days for up to one month. In a comparative study, methylprednisolone (1 gm by IV infusion daily for 7 days) gave more rapid improvement than ACTH gel.

Prophylactic therapy to reduce the frequency of exacerbations or to slow the rate of progression of disability has been attempted with a variety of immunosuppressive regimens. So far no treatment regimen has been devised that prevents clinical exacerbations or the MRI appearance of new plaques.

Daily or alternate-day steroid therapy, in doses that can be tolerated for long periods, does not alter the course of the illness. Azathioprine and cyclosporine have been used for long-term treatment but do not prevent

exacerbations; whether these immunosuppressive drugs are superior to placebo remains unclear. Cyclophosphamide therapy has been reported by some investigators to stabilize chronic progressive disease, but others have found no benefit. There is no consensus that long-term plasmapheresis, in combination with immunosuppressive regimens, is of benefit despite favorable reports.

In one controlled trial there were said to be fewer relapses in patients treated with injections of copolymer-I (a nonencephalitogenic peptide fragment of myelin basic protein) which was given in an attempt to desensitize patients to one of the putative MS antigens. However there were blinding problems in executing the trial, and the limited supply of copolymer did not permit wider testing; more time will be needed to evaluate this treatment.

Many experienced neurologists do not attempt to treat benign or slowly progressive cases. Steroids are often used for acute attacks. Patients with more rapidly progressive disease are sometimes treated with one of the immunosuppressive regimens or are referred to a clinical trial with a new agent.

Gait problems are the most common disability of MS. The problems respond to treatment if spasticity is the major cause. In these cases, careful use of baclofen is helpful, but if too much is administered, spasticity gives way to excessive flaccidity and makes the gait disorder worse. Ataxia and weakness are resistant to any therapy and rehabilitation is the only recourse. Spasticity of the legs, with resultant contractures and painful flexor and extensor spasms, often responds to baclofen and aids the application of physical therapy. Diazepam usually causes too much sedation and dantrolene has too many side effects. In severe problems of spasticity, intrathecal injection of phenol may be helpful, and even ethanol can be given by that route if urinary sphincter function is already sacrificed. Obturator nerve blocks or section may relieve adductor spasms.

Intention tremor occasionally responds to propranolol 320 mg per day in divided dosage. Cryothalamotomy has been used, but the complication of pseudobulbar palsy makes this procedure too hazardous.

Painful radiculopathies (e.g., trigeminal neuralgia) and painful paresthesias respond to the administration of carbamazepine.

Bladder management is extremely important to prevent debilitating and life-threatening infections and stone formation. The problem may be failure to retain urine, excessive urinary retention, or an alternating combination of the two. The symptoms are similar in all these cases. The most important measures are determination of postvoiding residuals, urine cultures and sensitivities and, occasionally, intravenous urograms. The atonic bladder with a large residual urine (over 100 ml) is easily managed by clean intermittent self-catheterization in conjunction with administration of urinary antiseptics, urinary acidifiers and, occasionally, anticholinergic agents (e.g., propantheline, imipramine). Bethanecol is not effective for long-term use. Small spastic bladder also responds to anticholinergic agents alone. Urinary symptoms are often reversible in early stages, but suprapubic cystostomy may be needed in late stages. The use of indwelling catheters often results in chronic infection and should be employed only for brief periods (e.g., while treating decubitus ulcers).

When there is a severe paraparesis, skin care to prevent decubitus ulcers is essential. Physical therapy and nursing care with adequate nutrition and hydration are valuable in preventing painful, disabling complications such as decubitus ulcers, renal and bladder calculi, contractures, and intercurrent infections. When these complications occur, aggressive attempts to relieve them often give gratifying results.

Diet therapy and vitamin supplements are frequently advocated, but no special supplementation or elimination diet has proven to be more beneficial than a well-balanced diet that maintains correct body weight and provides sufficient roughage for bowel management. Other therapies such as hyperbaric oxygen, plasmapheresis, neurostimulation, cobra venom, and acupuncture are absolutely unproven and any response to these treatments is usually a result of coincidental spontaneous remission so often seen early in the disease.

Counseling is highly important to provide emotional support, to encourage the patient to carry out usual activities, and to assist the patient in adapting to current or anticipated disabilities. Depression is common and often responds to tricyclic antidepressants. Lassitude and easy fatigability are little understood, but are frequent symptoms that may respond to short-term therapy with psychoactive drugs or corticosteroids. Bed rest should be discouraged to avoid chronic invalidism. There seems to be no basis for recommending relocation to warmer climates; in fact, warm humid weather makes most patients feel worse and air conditioning is almost essential in summer.

Physical therapy should be applied judiciously with the goals of maintaining mobility and avoiding contractures. Excessive active exercise may exhaust the patient and the increase in body temperature may cause transient symptoms. Swimming in cool water seems to be the best active physical therapy. Occupational therapy is important to assist patients in activities of daily living. In general, there are few diseases in which a comprehensive, continuing, judicious therapeutic regimen supervised by an experienced and sympathetic physician will give more rewarding results.

References

Allen I, McKeown S. A histological, histochemical and biochemical study of the macroscopically normal white matter in multiple sclerosis. J Neurol Sci 1979; 41:81–91.

Alter M, Zhen-xin Z, Davanipour Z, Sobel E, et al. Multiple sclerosis and childhood infections. Neurology 1986; 36:1386–1389.

Barnes MP, Bateman DE, Cleland PG, et al. Intravenous methylprednisolone for multiple sclerosis in relapse. J Neurol Neurosurg Psychiatry 1985; 48:157–159.

Bartlett PF, Wycherley K, Wong GH. Induction of histocompatibility antigens on neural cells by interferon-gamma. Neurosci Lett 1984; Suppl 15:S46.

Birk K, Rudick R. Pregnancy and multiple sclerosis. Arch Neurol 1986; 43:719–726.

Blaivas JG. Management of bladder dysfunction in multiple sclerosis. Neurology 1980; 30:12–18.

Bornstein MB, Miller A, Slagle S, Weitzman M, et al. A pilot trial of COP 1 in exacerbating-remitting multiple sclerosis. N Engl J Med 1987; 317:408–414.

Bye A, Kendall B, Wilson J. Multiple sclerosis in childhood: a new look. Dev Med Child Neurol 1985; 27:215–222.

Compston D, Vakarellis B, Paul E, McDonald W, et al. Viral infection in patients with multiple sclerosis and HLA-DR matched controls. Brain 1986; 109:325–344.

Compston A. HLA and neurologic disease. Neurology 1978; 28:413–414.

Cremer N, Johnson K, Fein G, Likosky W. Comprehensive viral immunology of multiple sclerosis. II. Analysis of serum and CSF antibodies by standard serologic methods. Arch Neurol 1980; 37:610–615.

Ebers G, Bulman D, Sadovnick A, Paty D, et al. A population-based study of multiple sclerosis in twins. N Engl J Med 1986; 315:1638–1642.

Eldridge R, McFarland H, Sever J, Sadowsky D, Krebs H. Familial multiple sclerosis: clinical, histocompatibility and viral serological studies. Ann Neurol 1978; 3:72–80.

Fazekas F, Offenbacher H, Fuchs S et al. Criteria for increased specificity of MRI interpretation in elderly subjects with suspected multiple sclerosis. Neurology 1988; 38:1822–1825.

Haile R, Hodge S, Iselius L. Genetic susceptibility to multiple sclerosis: a review. Int J Epidemiol 1983; 12:8–16.

Herndon R, Rudick R. Multiple sclerosis: the spectrum of severity. Arch Neurol 1983; 40:531–532.

Isayama Y, Takahashi T, Shimoyoma T, Yamadori A. Acute optic neuritis and multiple sclerosis. Neurology 1982; 32:73–76.

Johnson K, Likosky W, Nelson B, Fein G. Comprehensive viral immunology of multiple sclerosis. I. Clinical, epidemiological and CSF studies. Arch Neurol 1980; 37:537–541.

Johnson K. Cerebrospinal fluid and blood assays of diagnostic usefulness in multiple sclerosis. Neurology 1980; 30:106–109.

Kimura J. Abuse and misuse of evoked potentials as a diagnostic test. Arch Neurol 1985; 42:78–80.

Kurtzke JF. Epidemiologic contributions to multiple sclerosis: an overview. Neurology 1980; 30(2):61–79.

Kurtzke JF, Gudmundsson KR, Bergmann S. Multiple sclerosis in Iceland: I. Evidence of a postwar epidemic. Neurology 1982; 32:143–150.

McDonald W. The mystery of the origin of multiple sclerosis. J Neurol Neurosurg Psychiatry 1986; 49:113–123.

McDonald WI, Silberberg DH, eds. Multiple Sclerosis. London: Butterworths, 1986.

Mackay R, Hirano A. Forms of benign multiple sclerosis. Arch Neurol 1967; 17:588–600.

Matthews W, Acheson E, Batchelor J, Weller R, eds. McAlpine's Multiple Sclerosis. Edinburgh: Churchill-Livingstone, 1985.

Miller JR, Burke AM, Bever CT. Occurrence of oligoclonal bands in multiple sclerosis and other CNS diseases. Ann Neurol 1983; 13:53–58.

Murray T. Amantadine therapy of fatigue in multiple sclerosis. Can J Neurol Sci 1985; 12:251–254.

Myers LW, Ellison GW (eds). Rationale for immunomodulating therapies of multiple sclerosis. Neurology 1988; 38 (Suppl 2):4–89.

Myrianthopoulos N. Genetic aspects of multiple sclerosis. In: Koetsier C, ed. Handbook of Clinical Neurology. Amsterdam: Elsevier Science Publishing, 1985:289–317.

Ormerod IEC, Miller DH, McDonald WI, et al. The role of NMR imaging in the assessment of multiple sclerosis and isolated neurological lesions. A quantitative study. Brain 1987; 110:1579–1616.

Panitch HS, Hirsch RL, Schindler J, Johnson KP. Treatment of multiple sclerosis with gamma interferon: exacerbations associated with activation of the immune system. Neurology 1987; 37:1097–1102.

Paty D, Asbury A, Herndon R, McFarland H, et al. Use of magnetic resonance imaging in the diagnosis of multiple sclerosis: policy statement. Neurology 1986; 36:1575.

Paty DW, Jr, Oger JJF, Kastrukoff LF, et al. MRI in the diagnosis of MS: a prospective study with comparison of clinical evaluation, evoked potentials, oligoclonal banding, and CT. Neurology 1988; 38:180–185.

Peyser J, Poser C. Neuropsychological correlates of multiple sclerosis. In: Filskov S, Boll T, eds. Handbook of Clinical Neuropsychology. New York: John Wiley & Sons, 1986; 2:364–397.

Phadke J, Best P. Atypical and clinically silent multiple sclerosis: a report of 12 cases discovered unexpectedly at necropsy. J Neurol Neurosurg Psychiatry 1983; 46:414–420.

Poser C. Exacerbations, activity and progression in multiple sclerosis. Arch Neurol 1980; 37:471–474.

Poser C. The course of multiple sclerosis. Arch Neurol 1985; 42:1035.

Poser C. The pathogenesis of multiple sclerosis: a critical reappraisal. Acta Neuropathol 1986; 71:1–10.

Poser C. The peripheral nervous system in multiple sclerosis. J Neurol Sci 1987; 79:83–90.

Poser C, Paty DW, Scheinberg L, McDonald WI, Ebers GC. The Diagnosis of Multiple Sclerosis. New York: Thieme-Stratton, 1984.

Prineas J, Connell F. The fine structure of chronically active multiple sclerosis plaques. Neurology 1978; 28(2):68–75.

Rudick RA, Pallant A, Bidlack JM, Herndon RM. Free kappa light chains in multiple sclerosis spinal fluid. Ann Neurol 1986; 20:63–69.

Rudick RA, Schiffer R, Schwetz K, Herndon R. Multiple sclerosis: the problem of incorrect diagnosis. Arch Neurol 1986; 43:578–583.

Scheinberg L, Raine C, eds. Multiple sclerosis: experimental and clinical aspects. Ann NY Acad Sci 1984; 436:1–518.

Scheinberg L, Van den Noort S. Editorial on multiple sclerosis treatments. Neurology 1986; 36:703–704.

Scotti G, Sciaffa G, Biondi A, Landoni L, et al. Magnetic resonance in multiple sclerosis. Neuroradiol 1986; 28:319–323.

Sears ES, McCammon A, Bigelow R, Hayman LA. Maximizing the harvest of contrast enhancing lesions in multiple sclerosis. Neurology 1982; 32:815–820.

Sibley WA, ed. Nature and treatment of symptoms in multiple sclerosis. Neurology 1978; 29:6–139.

Sibley WA. Management of the patient with multiple sclerosis. Semin Neurol 1985; 5:134–145.

Sibley WA. Risk factors in multiple sclerosis—implications for pathogenesis. In: Serlupi Crescenzi G, ed. A Multidisciplinary Approach to Myelin Diseases. NATO Advanced Research Series. New York: Plenum Press, 1987.

Sibley WA, Bamford CR, Clark K. Clinical viral infections and multiple sclerosis. Lancet 1985; 1:1313–1315.

Warren KG, Catz I. A correlation between cerebrospinal fluid myelin basic protein and anti-myelin basic protein in multiple sclerosis patients. Ann Neurol 1987; 21:183–189.

Weiner HL, Hafler DA. Immunotherapy of multiple sclerosis. Ann Neurol 1988; 23:211–222.

138. DEVIC SYNDROME AND BALO DISEASE
William A. Sibley

Devic Syndrome

Devic syndrome (neuromyelitis optica) is a clinical syndrome characterized by acute bilateral optic neuritis and transverse myelitis. The two symptoms may occur simultaneously or may be separated by a few days or weeks. The syndrome may occur as a phase in otherwise typical disseminated MS, or it may be a manifestation of postinfectious encephalomyelitis; however, most cases are simply a variant of MS. The term *neuromyelitis optica* carries a connotation of severe disease because of the relatively frequent pathologic finding of necrosis of all structural elements of the nervous system in affected areas. Swelling of the spinal cord in such cases may lead to complete myelographic block. The prognosis for recovery in these patients is poor.

This syndrome is more common with MS in Asia or India than it is in the United States or western Europe.

Balo Disease

Balo disease (concentric sclerosis) is considered to be a variant of multiple (or, by some, of diffuse) sclerosis. It cannot be differentiated clinically from either multiple or diffuse sclerosis and the characteristic histologic picture of concentric areas of myelinoclasia may represent a peculiar local tissue reaction. Only a few cases have been reported in which a single, extensive area of demyelination exists with the characteristic concentric areas of alternating normal and demyelinized tissue (Fig. 138–1). Areas with such concentric appearance have been found in more classic cases of diffuse or disseminated sclerosis. In essence, it is strictly a histologic diagnosis without recognizable clinical concomitant.

References

Chien LT. Neuromyelitis optica (Devic's syndrome) in two sisters. Clin Electroencephalogr 1982; 13:36–39.

Cloys DE, Netsky MG. Neuromyelitis optica. In: Vinken PJ, Bruyn GW, eds. Handbook of Clinical Neurology, vol 9. New York: Elsevier-North Holland, 1970:426–436.

Courville CB. Concentric sclerosis. In: Vinken PJ, Bruyn GW, eds. Handbook of Clinical Neurology, vol 9. New York: Elsevier-North Holland, 1970:437–451.

Itoyama Y, Tateishi J, Kuroiwa Y. Atypical multiple sclerosis with concentric or lamellar demyelinated lesions: two Japanese cases studied post-mortem. Ann Neurol 1985; 17:481–487.

Kinney EL, Berdoff RL, Rao NS, Fox LM. Devic's syndrome and systemic lupus erythematosus: a case report with necropsy. Arch Neurol 1979; 36:643–644.

139. MARCHIAFAVA-BIGNAMI DISEASE
Charles M. Poser

Primary degeneration of the corpus callosum is a disease that occurs most frequently in middle-aged or elderly Italian men addicted to the use of wine. It is characterized by mental symptoms and signs of focal or diffuse disease of the brain. The disease was first described by Marchiafava and Bignami in 1903.

Etiology. The cause of the degenerative changes in the corpus callosum is not known. It is possible that the type of alcohol may be of importance because addiction to crude Italian wine is recorded in some of the isolated cases of nonItalian stock.

Experimental production of the characteristic lesion by administration of alcohol to dogs has been reported but not confirmed. The lesions are similar to those of chronic methyl alcohol intoxication, chronic arsenical encephalopathy, and chronic experimental cyanide poisoning, but these factors cannot account for the rare but well-documented occurrence of the disease in nonalcoholics.

The disease has been reported in teetotalers and in individuals who drank beverages other than Italian red wine. The importance of malnutrition as opposed to chronic intoxication, a theory favored by some, is not well documented, particularly because the disease was

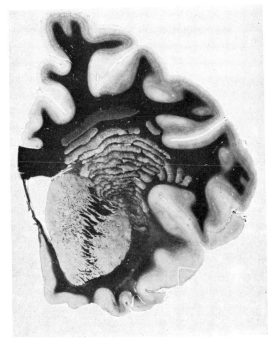

Fig. 138–1. Concentric areas of demyelination in centrum ovale. Myelin sheath stain of Balo disease. (Courtesy of Dr. H. Shiraki, Tokyo.)

not seen in survivors of German concentration camps or Japanese prisoner-of-war camps after World War II, despite their extreme undernourishment.

Pathology. The *sine qua non* of Marchiafava-Bignami disease is necrosis of the medial zone of the corpus callosum. The dorsal and ventral rims are spared. The necrosis varies from softening and discoloration (Fig. 139–1) to cavitation and cyst formation. Usually all stages of degeneration are found in any given case. In most cases, the rostral position of the corpus callosum is affected first. The lesions arise as small symmetric foci that extend and become confluent. Although medial necrosis of the corpus callosum is the principal pathologic finding, there may also be degeneration of the anterior commissure (Fig. 139–2), the posterior commissure, centrum semiovale, subcortical white matter, long association bundles, and middle cerebellar peduncles. All these lesions have a constant bilateral symmetry. Usually spared are the internal capsule, corona radiata, and subgyral arcuate fibers. The gray matter is not grossly affected.

Few diseases have such a well-defined pathologic picture. The corpus callosum may be infarcted as a result of occlusion of the anterior cerebral artery, but the symmetry of the lesions, the sparing of the gray matter, and the occurrence of similar lesions in the anterior commissure, long association bundles, and cerebellar peduncles are found only in Marchiafava disease.

The microscopic alterations are the result of a sharply defined necrotic process with loss of myelin but relative preservation of axis cylinders in the periphery of the lesions. There is usually no evidence of inflammation aside from a few perivascular lymphocytes. In most cases, fat-filled phagocytes are common. Gliosis is usually not well advanced. Capillary endothelial proliferation may be present in the affected area, but no thrombi are seen in the vessels.

The disease has been reported in association with central pontine myelinolysis and with Wernicke encephalopathy in alcoholics as well as in nonalcoholics, suggesting a possible common etiopathogenesis.

Incidence. More than 100 cases have been recorded in the literature since the original report in 1903. Most of the cases have been in men of Italian origin, but the disease has also been reported from China and Japan.

The disease was first observed in the United States in an Italian-born man in 1936, but it was not until 1943 that a second case was found in a native born, nonItalian-American who had developed a fondness for Italian red wine. An autopsy-proven case was seen by the author in a black man who drank bourbon and muscatel, and in a severely malnourished, nonalcoholic woman of German

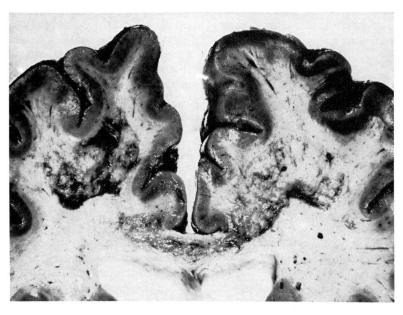

Fig. 139–1. Marchiafava-Bignami disease. Acute necrosis of corpus callosum and neighboring white matter of the frontal lobes. (From Merrit HH, Weisman AD. J Neuropathol Exp Neurol 1945; 4:155–163.)

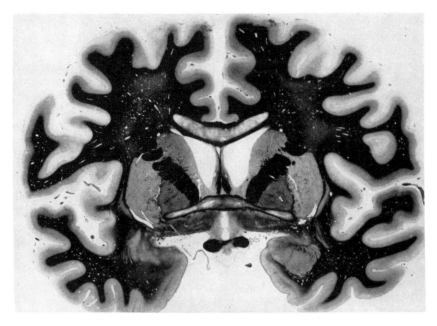

Fig. 139–2. Marchiafava-Bignami disease. Medial necrosis of the corpus callosum and anterior commissure with sparing of the margins. (Courtesy of Dr. P.I. Yakovlev.)

parentage. The onset of symptoms is in middle or late life.

Symptoms and Signs. The onset is usually insidious and the initial symptoms are so nonspecific that an accurate estimation of the exact time is difficult. The clinical picture is quite variable with a mixture of focal and diffuse signs of cerebral disease. The most common presentation is that of nonspecific dementia.

Mental symptoms are almost always present and are variously characterized by manic, paranoid, and delusional states, depression, extreme apathy, or dementia. Convulsions are common. Tremors, aphasia, apraxia, transitory hemiparesis, and other motor disabilities may be found.

Diagnosis. The diagnosis of Marchiafava-Bignami disease can rarely be made with certainty during life. CT and MRI may reveal typical callosal atrophy and the symmetric demyelinating lesions in the frontal white matter. It can be suspected, however, when an elderly man of Italian ancestry with a history of alcoholism develops an organic psychosis or dementia with convulsions, aphasia, or other focal cerebral symptoms.

Course. The disease is usually slowly progressive and results in death within three to six years. There is a rare acute fever lasting days or weeks. In an occasional patient there is a temporary remission.

Treatment. There is no adequate therapy.

References

Ghatak N, Hadfield N, Rosenblum W. Association of central pontine myelinolysis and Marchiafava-Bignami disease. Neurology 1978; 28:1295–1298.

Heepe P, Nemeth L, Brune F, et al. Marchiafava-Bignami disease. A correlative computed tomography and morphological study. Eur Arch Psychiat Neurol Sci 1988; 237:74–79.

Ironside R, Bosanquet FD, McMenemey WH. Central demyelination of the corpus callosum (Marchiafava-Bignami Disease). Brain 1961; 84:212–230.

Marchiafava E, Bignami A. Sopra un'alterazione del corpo calloso osservata in soggetti alcoolisti. Riv Patol Nerve 1903; 8:544–549.

Mayer J, de Liege P, Netter J, et al. Computerized tomography and nuclear magnetic resonance imaging in Marchiafava-Bignami disease. J Neuroradiol 1987; 14:152–158.

Poser CM. Demyelination in the central nervous system in chronic alcoholism, central pontine myelinolysis and Marchiafava-Bignami's disease. Ann NY Acad Sci 1973; 215:373–381.

140. CENTRAL PONTINE MYELINOLYSIS
Elliott L. Mancall

In 1959, Adams, Victor, and Mancall described a distinctive, previously unrecognized disease characterized primarily by the symmetrical destruction of myelin sheaths in the basis pontis. Numerous cases have since been reported. In most, there is a history of chronic alcoholism or other condition associated with malnutrition; in many, electrolyte disorders, especially hyponatremia, are observed. Histologically, the lesion, which appears to begin in the median raphe, may involve all or part of the base of the pons (Fig. 140–1). Direct spread of the lesion into the pontine tegmentum or superiorly into the mesencephalon has been recorded. Myelin sheaths are destroyed within the lesion, but the nerve cells and axis cylinders in the affected region remain relatively preserved. There is no inflammation. Microscopically, the lesion resembles the alterations of Marchiafava-Bignami disease. Similar myelinolytic lesions have been observed well beyond the confines of the brain stem, involving, for example, the cerebral cortex and subcortical white matter, basal ganglia, thalamus, subthalamus, amygdala, centrum ovale, corpus callosum, internal capsule, and cerebellum.

Most reported patients are young or middle-aged adults, although the disease can occur in children and in the elderly. Typically, there is a history of alcoholism and associated malnutrition, but other systemic disorders may be present. Central pontine myelinolysis is often associated with diseases of other organs, including the liver (cirrhosis, Wilson disease), kidney (vascular nephropathy, kidney transplant), and brain (Wernicke disease, tumors). Occasional cases have been associated with diabetes, amyloidosis, leukemia, and infections.

Although most cases have been diagnosed only at necropsy, the disorder has been increasingly recognized during life. The typical clinical presentation is one of a rapidly evolving corticospinal and corticobulbar syndrome, expressed as a flaccid tetraplegia with facial, glottal, and pharyngeal paralysis in a debilitated and nutritionally depleted alcoholic, often during an acute illness characterized by lethargy, seizures, and electrolyte imbalance. Overly rapid correction of hyponatremia seems to be the precipitating event in many patients, although perhaps not all. Supporting the notion of the importance of overly rapid correction of hyponatremia in pathogenesis is the observation that demyelination can be induced experimentally by rapid correction of hyponatremia. Changes in water content may also be significant. Although the patients are mute, they are usually not comatose; this is a form of the "locked-in" syndrome. Communication by blinking of the eyelids can sometimes be established. The clinical diagnosis is supported by documentation of abnormal brain-stem auditory evoked responses (BAER). Characteristic changes are found in the basis pontis with CT scanning or MRI.

The disease runs a rapid course; death generally ensues within days or weeks of the onset of symptoms. The principal pathologic change, demyelination, is potentially reversible, and some patients appear to have survived the acute illness.

The electrolyte changes in many cases in-

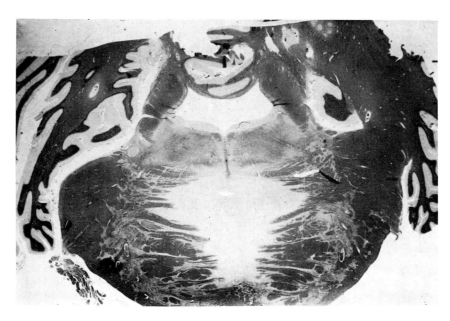

Fig. 140–1. Central pontine myelinolysis. Section through rostral pons showing characteristic lesion. (Courtesy of Dr. J. Kepes.)

clude hyponatremia, hypokalemia, and hypochloremia. Serum osmolality is low, but urine osmolality is normal. The changes are consistent with inappropriate secretion of antidiuretic hormone, perhaps a consequence of alcohol withdrawal, and are exaggerated by excessive fluid replacement. In some cases, hypoventilation and accumulation of CO_2 complicate the electrolyte disorder.

Therapy emphasizes the judicious use of normal saline and fluid restriction. Administration of dehydrating agents such as glycerol or urea has been advocated.

The cause of the disease remains unclear. Although a vascular cause has been suggested, most authors agree, as pointed out previously, that this is a metabolic disorder related either to malnutrition or, more likely in many cases, to severe electrolyte disturbance that is rapidly reversed (particularly hyponatremia).

References

Adams RD, Victor M, Mancall EL. Central pontine myelinolysis: a hitherto undescribed disease occurring in alcoholic and malnourished patients. Arch Neurol Psychiatry 1959; 81:154–172.

Ayus JC, Krothpalli RK, Arieff AI. Treatment of symptomatic hyponatremia and its relation to brain damage. N Engl J Med 1987; 317:1190–1195.

Kandt RS, Heldrich FJ, Moser HW. Recovery from probable central pontine myelinolysis associated with Addison's disease. Arch Neurol 1983; 40:118–119.

Kleinschmidt-Demasters BK, Norenberg MD. Rapid correction of hyponatrema causes demyelination: relation to central pontine myelinolysis. Science 1981; 211:1068–1071.

Laureno R. Central pontine myelinolysis following rapid correction of hyponatremia. Ann Neurol 1983; 13:232–242.

Messert B, Orrison WW, Hawkins MJ, Quaglieri CE. Central pontine myelinolysis. Neurology 1979; 29:147–160.

Norenberg MD, Leslie KO, Robertson AS. Association between rise in serum sodium and central pontine myelinolysis. Ann Neurol 1982; 11:128–135.

Schrier RW. Treatment of hyponatremia. N Engl J Med 1985; 312:1121–1122.

Stockard JJ, Rossiter VS, Wiederholt WC, Kobayashi RM. Brain stem auditory evoked responses in suspected central pontine myelinolysis. Arch Neurol 1976; 33:726–728.

Thompson DS, Hutton JT, Stears JC, Sung JH, Norenberg M. Computerized tomography in the diagnosis of central and extrapontine myelinolysis. Arch Neurol 1981; 38:243–246.

Wright DG, Laureno R, Victor M. Pontine and extrapontine myelinolysis. Brain 1979; 102:361–385.

Chapter XIX

Autonomic Nervous System

141. NEUROGENIC ORTHOSTATIC HYPOTENSION
Lucien J. Côté

The autonomic nervous system may fail in many medical disorders. Tests of autonomic function appear in Table 141–1. One classification separates primary and secondary disorders of the autonomic nervous system (Table 141–2).

Shy-Drager Syndrome

Shy and Drager described a distinct neurologic syndrome manifested by orthostatic hypotension and other autonomic disorders in combination with neurologic abnormalities due to degenerative changes in cerebellar, basal ganglia, or spinal motor neurons. Those with Shy-Drager syndrome show wide swings in blood pressure, which is often elevated above normal in the supine position and falls by more than 30/20 mm Hg within 2 minutes, without change in pulse rate, when the patient stands. They complain of light-headedness on standing and may note blurring of vision that starts peripherally and encroaches on central vision just before fainting. Unlike patients with vagotonic vasovagal

Table 141–1. Tests of Autonomic Function

Pupillary Response to Local Instillation	*Normal Response*	*Part of Reflex Arc Tested*
5% cocaine	Dilatation	Sympathetic innervation
5% tyramine	Dilatation	Sympathetic innervation
0.1–1.25% epinephrine	No mydriasis	Postganglionic sympathetic innervation
2.5% methacholine	No miosis	Parasympathetic innervation
Blood Pressure Response		
Ephedrine 25 mg IM	Blood pressure increases	Sympathetic innervation
Epinephrine 0.25 mg subcutaneous	No hypersensitivity of blood pressure	Adrenergic receptors
Cold pressor test	Blood pressure increases	Sympathetic efferent
Erect posture	Blood pressure maintained	Sympathetic afferent and efferent
Valsalva maneuver	Overshoot	Afferent and efferent limbs
Whole body heat	Perspiration	Sympathetic efferent limb
Pilocarpine iontophoresis (20 mg)	Local sweating	Intact sweat glands
Control of Heart Rate		
Atropine 1.0 mg IV	Heart rate increases	Parasympathetic efferent
Carotid sinus massage	Heart rate slows	Intact baroreceptors
Quantitative Measures		
Norepinephrine and epinephrine levels in plasma	Increase (175–200%) from supine to erect	Sympathetic efferent
Saliva flow test		
Schirmer test for lacrimal flow		

(Modified from Fujii N, Tabira T, Shibasaki H, Kuroiwa Y, Ohnish A, Nagaki J. J Neurol Neurosurg Psychiatry 1982; 45:656–657.)

Table 141–2.   Disorders of Autonomic Function

Primary
    Shy-Drager syndrome (multiple system atrophy or MSA)
    Primary autonomic failure (PAF) (idiopathic)
    Progressive autonomic failure with Parkinson disease
    Sympathotonic orthostatic hypotension
Secondary
    Spinal cord lesions
    Polyneuropathy—diabetes, amyloidosis, chronic renal failure
    Autoimmune disorders—Guillain-Barré syndrome, myasthenia gravis, dysautonomia (acute
        and subacute), rheumatoid arthritis, multiple sclerosis, systemic lupus erythematosus
    Metabolic disorders—porphyria, Tangier disease, Fabry disease, vitamin B_{12} deficiency
    Neoplasms—carcinomatous autonomic neuropathy; tumors involving the hypothalamus or
        midbrain
    Infections of the nervous system—tabetic neurosyphilis, Chagas disease
    Familial disorders—dysautonomia, hyperbradykinism
    Drugs—neuroleptics (tranquilizers, antidepressants), cardiovascular agents (prazosin, hydrala-
        zine, alpha-methyl-dopa, clonidine, guanethidine, phenoxybenzamine, hexamethonium
    Neurotoxins—alcohol, botulism, heavy metals, vincristine

syncope, patients with Shy-Drager syndrome do not experience pallor, nausea, increased sweating, or yawning before they black out.

The degenerative changes in central neurons usually cause parkinsonian features such as tremor at rest, cogwheel-like rigidity, bradykinesia, decreased associated movements, and impaired postural reflexes. Other changes include reduced sweating, iris atrophy, impaired eye movements, sexual impotence, and urinary and rectal incontinence due to failure of the innervation of the bladder and rectal sphincters. Often there is wasting and fasciculation of distal limb muscles with EMG evidence of anterior horn cell degeneration. Cerebellar signs such as intention tremor, ataxia, and dysarthria are seen frequently; there may be signs of corticobulbar and corticospinal tract involvement. Emotional lability is common late in the disease, but sensory impairment is rare. Patients with Shy-Drager syndrome are often depressed, but mental deterioration, if present, is usually mild and appears late.

Shy-Drager syndrome is uncommon, but Thomas and Schirger found 57 patients at the Mayo Clinic in 5 years; about 11% of all patients with orthostatic hypotension had the Shy-Drager syndrome. Age at onset of symptoms was between 37 and 75 years with a mean of 55 years. About 65% of patients were men and none was familial. The onset was insidious, often presenting wth postural light-headedness, extrapyramidal symptoms, urinary or bowel dysfunction, or impaired sexual function. The disease was usually progressive; patients became bedridden and de-

bilitated before they died about 8 years after onset. The common causes of death were cardiac arrhythmia, pulmonary embolism, and aspiration pneumonia.

Sung, Mastri, and Segal described the pathologic findings in 21 cases. Diffuse degenerative changes in the central (preganglionic) autonomic neurons were observed and there was degeneration of neurons in the extrapyramidal system, cerebellum, pyramidal tracts, and anterior horn cells. In more than 65% of the cases, the olivopontocerebellar and nigrostriatal systems were involved. In the others, the pathologic findings were mainly in the nigral system, as in Parkinson disease. The neurological disorder cannot be treated effectively, but orthostatic symptoms can be ameliorated.

Idiopathic Orthostatic Hypotension

Orthostatic hypotension of neurologic origin is seen in some patients without evidence of other neurologic disorder. Kontos and associates provided histologic and pharmacologic evidence that these patient have a defect in the postganglionic sympathetic neurons, whereas patients with Shy-Drager syndrome have degeneration of the preganglionic sympathetic neurons. These two neurogenic forms of orthostatic hypotension can be differentiated clinically and pharmacologically. Patients with idiopathic orthostatic hypotension, unlike those with Shy-Drager syndrome, show no clinical involvement of the CNS. In idiopathic orthostatic hypotension, the basal level of norepinephrine in the plasma is low; it is normal in Shy-Drager patients. In both disorders, supine plasma levels of norepinephrine fail to rise adequately when the patient stands. Patients with idiopathic orthostatic hypotension are supersensitive to intravenous administration of norepinephrine, which causes an abnormal rise in blood pressure; Shy-Drager patients show a normal response. On the other hand, an indirectly acting sympathomimetic agent that releases norepinephrine (i.e., tyramine) causes a blunted response in idiopathic orthostatic hypotension because the content of norepinephrine in the nerve endings is reduced. In Shy-Drager patients the response is normal.

Some patients with Parkinson disease experience a drop in blood pressure on standing without other obvious manifestations of autonomic nervous system failure. The cause of the drop in blood pressure is central in origin; it is often made worse by dopamine agonists such as L-DOPA (Sinemet) and bromocriptine.

Sympathotonic Orthostatic Hypotension

This rare form of orthostatic hypotension of neurogenic origin is associated with marked tachycardia when the patient stands. The sympathetic nervous system seems to react normally to postural changes, but there is an impaired response of the effector organ to norepinephrine, causing a drop of blood pressure despite the increased pulse rate.

Orthostatic Hypotension in Other Neurologic Diseases

Orthostatic hypotension may be seen in many diseases that affect the autonomic pathways and reflex arcs that normally adjust the blood pressure on change in posture. Polyneuropathy is a common cause of orthostatic hypotension in diabetes mellitus, amyloidosis, alcoholism, and porphyria. Orthostatic hypotension may be seen after spinal cord trauma, transverse myelitis, or syringomyelia.

Treatment. The treatment of orthostatic hypotension depends on the cause. In general, hypotension on standing, if asymptomatic, does not require treatment. Cerebral perfusion of the brain usually does not drop significantly until the systolic pressure is reduced below 80 mm Hg because of the effective autoregulation of the blood vessels in the brain.

Physical measures to reduce orthostatic drop in blood pressure are used first because they are simple and often control symptoms. These measures include maintaining the head and trunk at about 15 to 20° higher than the legs in bed, which promotes renin release and stimulates the autonomic nervous system. This can be achieved by using a hospital bed with head elevation, or by placing blocks under the head of an ordinary bed. Counterpressure support garments (such as Jobst half-body leotard) can reduce venous pooling when the patient is erect, but patients often find these garments too difficult to put on and wear, especially if they are disabled by the multiple neurologic abnormalities of the Shy-Drager syndrome. Daily tilt-table exercise is recommended by some physiatrists to stimulate the mechanisms that maintain blood pressure on change in posture. Although the drop in blood pressure often lessens with each successive tilt done a few minutes apart, no data suggest that the effect is lasting.

No single drug is specific for the treatment of orthostatic hypotension of neurogenic origin. Oral sympathomimetics such as ephedrine, phenylephrine, tyramine, or metaraminol are usually not helpful. Patients should be given supplemental sodium chloride to increase plasma volume and, if necessary, 9 α-fluorohydrocortisone to increase retention of salt and water. 9 α-fluorohydrocortisone should be started at a low dose (0.1 mg every few days) to 0.3 mg to 1.0 mg daily, depending on the blood pressure response and the plasma volume change. The patient must be watched carefully to avoid excessive water retention and blood pressure rise.

Recumbent hypertension in orthostatic hypotension of neurogenic origin is common even when the patient is taking no medication. Usually, no treatment is required because it can be controlled by elevating the patient's head and trunk 15 or 20°.

Other drugs often used in the treatment of orthostatic hypotension include indomethacin, β-adrenergic blockers such as propanolol, peripheral α-receptor agonists, ergot alkaloids, and levodopa. None of these drugs has proven consistently beneficial, but trials are justified because there is no specific treatment.

References

Bannister R, ed. Autonomic Failure. London: Oxford University Press, 1988.

Bradbury S, Eggleston C. Postural hypotension: a report of three cases. Am Heart J 1925; 1:73–86.

Gemmill JD, Venables GS, Ewing DJ. Noradrenaline response to edrophonium in primary autonomic failure: distinction between central and peripheral damage. Lancet 1988; 1:1018–1020.

Johnson RH, Lambie DG, Spalding JMK. Neurocardiology. Philadelphia: WB Saunders, 1984.

Kontos HA, Richardson DW, Norvell JE. Mechanisms of circulatory dysfunction in orthostatic hypotension. Trans Am Clin Climatol Assoc 1976; 87:26–33.

McLeod JD, Tuck RR. Disorders of the autonomic nervous system: Part I. Pathophysiology and clinical features. Ann Neurol 1987; 21:419–430.

McLeod JD, Tuck RR. Disorders of the autonomic nervous system: Part II. Investigation and treatment. Ann Neurol 1987; 21:419–529.

Polinsky RJ, Kopin IJ, Ebert MH, Weise V. Pharmacologic distinction of different orthostatic hypotension syndrome. Neurology 1981; 31:1–7.

Schatz IJ. Current management concepts in orthostatic hypotension. Arch Int Med 1980; 140:1152–1154.

Shy GM, Drager GA. A neurological syndrome associated with orthostatic hypotension: A clinical-pathologic study. Arch Neurol 1960; 2:511–527.

Sung JH, Mastri AR, Segal E. Pathology of Shy-Drager syndrome. J Neuropathol Exp Neurol 1979; 38:353–368.

Thomas JE, Schirger A. Idiopathic orthostatic hypotension: A study of its natural history in 57 neurologically affected patients. Arch Neurol 1970; 22:289–293.

142. ACUTE AUTONOMIC NEUROPATHY
Lewis P. Rowland

Acute autonomic neuropathy is rare and has been described in 12 cases since the first description by Young, Asbury, Corbett, and Adams in 1975. The autonomic manifestations include orthostatic hypotension, nausea and vomiting, constipation or diarrhea, bladder atony, impotence, anhidrosis, impaired lacrimation and salivation, and pupillary abnormalities. In pure dysautonomia, there are no motor or sensory abnormalities, although in a few cases with prominent autonomic manifestations, loss of cutaneous sensation is also severe and some patients have motor disorders.

In pure dysautonomia, the EMG, nerve conduction velocities, sural nerve biopsy, and CSF may be normal; in complicated cases, these studies may give abnormal results and may link the disorder to Guillain-Barré syndrome. Functional tests usually reveal widespread abnormality of autonomic function (see Table 141–1).

The cause is not known, but three of the 12 known cases were associated with high titers of antibody to Epstein-Barr virus. Symptoms may evolve for several weeks, plateau for many weeks, and then slowly improve. The differential diagnosis includes the follow-

ing neuropathies with prominent abnormalities of autonomic function:

Diabetes mellitus
Guillain-Barré syndrome
Alcoholic neuropathy
Amyloid neuropathy
Riley-Day syndrome (familial dysautonomia)
Acute intermittent porphyria
Botulism
Fabry disease
Paraneoplastic neuropathy

Treatment is symptomatic.

References

Appenzeller O. The Autonomic Nervous System, 3rd ed. New York: Elsevier, 1982.

Colan RV, Snead OC III, Oh SJ, Kashlan MB. Acute autonomic and sensory neuropathy. Ann Neurol 1980; 8:441–444.

Fagius J, Westerburg CE, Olsson Y. Acute pandysautonomia and severe sensory deficit with poor recovery. A clinical, neurophysiological and pathological case study. J Neurol Neurosurg Psychiatry 1983; 46:725–733.

Fujii N, Tabira T, Shibasaki H, Kuroiwa, Y, Ohnishi A, Nagaki J. Acute autonomic and sensory neuropathy associated with elevated Epstein-Barr virus antibody titer. J Neurol Neurosurg Psychiatry 1982; 45:656–657.

Hoyle C, Ewing DJ, Parker AC. Acute autonomic neuropathy with systemic lupus erythematosus. Ann Rheum Dis 1985; 44:420–424.

Laiwah ACY, MacPhee GJA, Boyle MR, Goldberg A. Autonomic neuropathy in acute intermittent porphyria. J Neurol Neurosurg Psychiatry 1985; 48:1025–1030.

Low PA, Dyck PJ, Lambert EH, Brimijoin WS, et al. Acute panautonomic neuropathy. Ann Neurol 1983; 13:412–417.

McLeod JG, Tuck RR. Disorders of the autonomic nervous system. Ann Neurol 1987; 21:419–430, 519–529.

Neville BG, Sladen OF. Acute autonomic neuropathy following primary herpes simplex infection. J Neurol Neurosurg Psychiatry 1984; 47:648–650.

van Lieshout JJ, Wieling W, von Montfrans GA, et al. Acute dysautonomia with Hodgkin disease. J Neurol Neurosurg Psychiatry 1986; 49(7):830–832.

Young RR, Asbury AK, Corbett JL, Adams RD. Pure pandysautonomia with recovery. Brain 1975; 98:613–636.

143. FAMILIAL DYSAUTONOMIA
Alan M. Aron

Familial dysautonomia was described by Riley and co-workers in 1949. The autonomic symptoms are prominent, but the condition also affects other parts of the nervous system and general somatic growth. It is transmitted as an autosomal recessive trait and virtually all patients are of Eastern European Jewish lineage. The frequency of the carrier state among relatives of affected patients in the United States is reported to be 1 in 50. The condition can be diagnosed at birth. Clinical manifestations tend to increase with age. Biochemical alterations point to decreased synthesis of noradrenaline. Hyperresponsitivity to sympathomimetic drugs suggests a denervation type of supersensitivity. The exact pathophysiology is yet to be elucidated.

The dysautonomic infant frequently has a low birth weight and breech presentation. Neurologic abnormality is detected in the neonatal period by decreased muscle tone, diminished or absent tendon reflexes, absent corneal reflexes, poor Moro response, poor cry, and inability to suck. The tip of the tongue is smooth because it lacks fungiform papillae. Feeding problems are common. Poor swallowing with resultant regurgitation may cause aspiration and pneumonia. Some infants require tube-feeding. Absence of overflow tears, normal during the first 2 or 3 months of life, persists thereafter; this is a consistent feature. Corneal ulceration may occur.

During the first 3 years of life, affected children have delayed physical and developmental milestones, episodic vomiting, excessive sweating, blotchy erythema, and breath-holding spells.

Dysautonomic crises occur after age 3, with irritability, self-mutilation, negativistic behavior, diaphoresis, tachycardia, hypertension, and thermal instability. The most outstanding symptom is episodic vomiting, which may be cyclic. Hospital admission may be required for parenteral hydration. Treatment is symptomatic using agents such as chlorpromazine or bethanecol.

The school age dysautonomic child tends to have short stature, awkward gait, and nasal speech. School performance may be poor. As a group, patents score in the average range on intelligence tests but they are frequently 20 or more points below unaffected siblings. Scoliosis may begin in childhood and progress most rapidly during preadolescence. Some underdeveloped patients show delayed puberty. Vomiting and vasomotor crises tend to decrease during adolescence. More frequent complaints center on decreased exercise tolerance, poor general coordination, emotional difficulties, and postural hypotension. Vasovagal responses may occur after micturition or during laryngeal intubation for anesthesia. About 40% of patents have sei-

zures early in life, usually associated with fever, breath-holding spells, or hypoxia. Less than 10% have subsequent seizure disorders.

Patients show abnormal responses to altered atmospheric air. Hypercapnia and hypoxia do not produce expected increases in ventilatory effort. Drowning has occurred, presumably because air hunger did not develop under water. Coma has occurred in patients at high altitudes.

Diagnosis. The most distinctive clinical sign is the absence or paucity of overflow tearing. Low doses of methacholine may restore transient tearing. Other clinical features include hyporeflexia, absent corneal responses, and absence of the fungiform papillae of the tongue. This is associated with impaired taste sensation. There is relative indifference to pain.

The diagnosis should be made on the constellation of clinical symptoms and genetic background. Intradermal histamine phosphate in a dose of 1:1000 (0.03 to 0.05 ml) normally produces pain and erythema. Within minutes, a central wheal forms and is surrounded by an axon flare, which is a zone of erythema measuring 2 to 6 cm in diameter. The flare lasts for several minutes. In dysautonomic patients, pain is greatly reduced and there is no axon flare. In infants, a saline dilution of 1:10,000 histamine should be used.

The methacholine test involves instillation of one drop of 2.5% methacholine into the eye. One drop of dilute pilocarpine (0.0625%) is the equivalent of 2.5% methacholine, which is currently unavailable. The other eye serves as control. The pupils are compared at 5-minute intervals for 20 minutes. The normal pupil remains unchanged, but the dysautonomic pupil develops miosis. This abnormality might not be due to parasympathetic denervation and hypersensitivity to methacholine. Instead, reduced tearing may be the source of a higher concentration of methacholine. There is reduced precorneal tear film and reduced drug washout by tears. The pupillary responses to light and accommodation in familial dysautonomia appear normal. The combination of absent flare response to intradermal histamine, miosis with methacholine or pilocarpine, and absent fungiform papillae on the tongue are diagnostic. Usually, there is an elevated urinary homovanillic acid–vanilylmandelic acid (HVA:VMA) ratio. This assay is not available in many laboratories and is not required for diagnosis.

Biochemical and Pathologic Data. The neuronal abnormality is probably present at birth, but slow degenerative changes seem to occur subsequently. The primary metabolic defect is unknown, but the biologic activity of nerve growth factor from cultured fibroblasts of patients seems much less than normal control. This could influence alterations of sensory and sympathetic nerves. DNA analysis has excluded the beta nerve growth factor gene region on chromosome 1p as the cause of familial dysautonomia. The nerve growth receptor gene on chromosome 17q has also been excluded. Serum levels of both norepinephrine and dopamine are markedly elevated during dysautonomic crises. Vomiting coincides with high dopamine levels; hypertension correlates with increased norepinephrine levels.

Pathologic data reveal hypoplastic cervical sympathetic ganglia with diminished volumes and neuronal counts. Sympathetic preganglionic spinal cord neurons seem to be reduced in number. The parasympathetic sphenopalatine ganglia have shown the most depleted neuronal populations with only minor reductions in the ciliary ganglia. The lingual submucosal neurons and sensory axons are reduced. Taste buds are scant; circumvallate papillae are hypoplastic.

Pathophysiology. Postural hypotension is explained by peripheral sympathetic denervation. Skin blotching and hypertension are attributed to denervation supersensitivity at the sympathetic effector sites. Lack of overflow tears correlates with the diminution of neurons in the sphenopalatine ganglia. Other symptoms can be explained as manifestation of a diffuse sensory deficit and autonomic insufficiency with hypersensitivity to acetylcholine and possibly to catecholamines.

Prognosis. Long-term survival has been reported. Surviving patients include several women who later became pregnant and had normal infants. Infant and childhood fatalities may be due to aspiration pneumonia, gastric hemorrhage, or dehydration. A second cluster of fatality is seen between the ages of 14 and 24 when pulmonary complications, sleep deaths, and cardiopulmonary arrests have occurred. The oldest patients are now in their late 30s or early 40s.

Treatment. Symptomatic treatment with agents such as chlorpromazine, bethanecol, and diazepam is indicated for crises. Parenteral fluids and sedation are other measures for symptomatic relief.

References

Axelrod FB, Nachtigall R, Dancis J. Familial dysautonomia: diagnosis, pathogenesis and management. Adv Pediatr 1974; 31:75–96.

Axelrod FB, Abularrage JJ. Familial Dysautonomia: A prospective study of survival. J Pediatr 1982; 101:234–236.

Axelrod FB, Pearson J. Congential sensory neuropathies: diagnostic distinction from familial dysautonomia. Am J Dis Child 1984; 138:947–954.

Axelrod FB, Porges RF, Seir ME. Neonatal recognition of familial dysautonomia. J Pediatrics 1987; 110:946–948.

Brant PW, McKusick VA. Familial dysautonomia, a report of genetic and clinical studies with a review of the literature. Medicine 1970; 49:343–374.

Breakefield XO, Orloff G, Castiglione C, Coussens L, Axelrod FB, Ullrich A. Structural gene for beta nerve growth factor not defective in familial dysautonomia. Proc Natl Acad Sci USA 1984; 81:4213–4216.

Breakefield XO, Ozeluis L, Bothwell MA, et al. DNA polymorphisms for the nerve growth factor receptor gene exclude its role in familial dysautonomia. Med Bull Med 1986; 3:483–494.

Gadoth N, Sokol J, Lavie P. Sleep structure and disordered breathing in familial dysautonomia. J Neurol Sci 1983; 60:117–125.

Gitlin SE, Bertani LM, Wilk E, Li BL, Dzaedzies S. Excretion of catecholamine metabolites by children with familial dysautonomia. Pediatrics 1970; 46:513–522.

Korczyn AD, Rubenstein AE, Yahr MD, Axelrod FB. The pupil in familial dysautonomia. Neurology 1981; 31:628–629.

Pearson J. Familial dysautonomia. J Auton Nerv Sys 1979; 1:119–126.

Pearson J, Axelrod F, Dancis J. Current concepts of dysautonomia: neuropathological defects. Ann NY Acad Sci 1974; 228:288–300.

Pearson J, Pytel B. Quantitative studies of sympathetic ganglia and spinal cord intermediolateral gray columns in familial dysautonomia. J Neurol Sci 1978; 39:47–59.

Pearson J, Pytel B. Quantitative studies of ciliary and sphenopalatine ganglia in familial dysautonomia. J Neurol Sci 1978; 39:123–130.

Riley CM, Day RL, Greely DM, Langford NS. Central autonomic dysfunction with defective lacrimation. I. Report of five cases. Pediatrics 1949; 3:468–478.

Smith AA, Dancis J. Responses to intradermal histamine in familial dysautonomia—a diagnostic test. J Pediatr 1963; 63:889–894.

Wilton W, Clayson D, Axelrod F, Levine DB. Intellectual development in familial dysautonomia. Pediatrics 1979; 68:708–712.

Ziegler MG, Lake RC, Kopin IJ. Deficient sympathetic neuron response in familial dysautonomia. N Engl J Med 1976; 294:630–633.

Chapter XX

Intermittent or Paroxysmal Disorders

144. MIGRAINE

Dewey K. Ziegler
Arnold P. Friedman

The most extensively studied common headache syndrome is vascular headache of the migraine type. Migraine, which is often familial, is characterized by recurrent attacks of headache that differ in intensity, frequency, and duration. Attacks are commonly unilateral and are usually associated with anorexia, nausea, and vomiting. They may be preceded by or associated with neurologic symptoms in *classic migraine*. Disorders of mood may also precede attacks. All these characteristics are not necessarily present in every patient. If there is no aura of preceding symptoms, the pattern is called *common migraine*.

Etiology. The primary cause of migraine still eludes us. Heredity is probably important, but the mode of transmission is uncertain; an autosomal dominant trait with incomplete penetrance cannot be excluded. There is, however, no biochemical or physiologic characteristic that can be consistently recognized in affected relatives.

Pathophysiology. The classic migraine attack itself is associated with changes in the intracranial or extracranial arteries. Direct measurements of cerebral blood flow, though relatively sparse, point to vasoconstriction during the preheadache phase. During the headache phase itself, there may be increased pulsations of extracranial arteries. In common migraine (without aura), changes in blood flow have not been demonstrated. Preheadache and headache phases are not sharply separated in classic migraine, where studies of cerebral blood flow may show vasodilation in some cortical areas and vasoconstriction in others. This could account for the cases of migraine in which symptoms of the aura continue into the headache phase, and for those cases in which the headache precedes the aura.

The migraine *aura* most often involves visual symptoms, probably because of ischemia in the occipital cortex. This may be associated with a secondary process of spreading cortical depression that accounts for the focal and other neurologic symptoms observed during an attack. Typically, the scotoma begins near the center of vision as a small gray area that expands into a horseshoe with bright zig-zag lines appearing at the outer edge of the gray area. The configuration of the zig-zag lines has been compared with a fortified wall, hence the term "fortification spectra." The rate of expansion of both the arch formed by the zig-zag lines and the associated band of blindness takes about 20 to 30 minutes to reach the outer limit of the visual field.

Although hypoxia is apparently not a cause of spreading depression, it may intensify the process and increase the sensitivity of cortical tissues to the depression of electrical activity.

An adequate theory of the pain of migraine must consider both the possible combined effect of large artery dilatation and the local or systemic biochemical changes. Implicated in local vasomotor control is neurokinin, a vasodilator that lowers the pain threshold.

During the attack-free interval, platelet aggregability increases and there is a low threshold of the platelets for release action. During the migraine headache, platelets undergo a release reaction that reduces serotonin content and increases the plasma content of thromboglobulin. The serotonin released from the platelets seems to be removed rapidly from the circulation and converted to 5-hydroxyindoleacetic acid (5-HIAA), which is excreted in the urine. The serotonin in plasma may exert a tonic influence on the cephalic vascular bed. Decrease in the plasma serotonin level would constrict the arterioles and dilate the larger arteries. Constriction of the arterioles would then cause tissue ischemia. A sterile inflammatory reaction has been reported, in which the dilatation and overdistention of the larger vessels become painful. Harold Wolff and his coworkers first suggested that a combination of vasodilatation and sterile inflammation may be responsible for the clinical syndrome of migraine. Several factors cannot be explained by these assumptions, including lack of evidence that plasma serotonin exerts a tonic influence on the cephalic vascular bed in humans, and the unilateral character of migraine.

An adequate theory of the pathogenesis of migraine must consider other biochemical changes, particularly the role of the endogenous or exogenous vasomotor agents that influence the tone of vascular smooth muscle and alter the caliber of vessels. Among the substances that could be involved are the amines, catecholamines, histamine, and tyramine; heparin; polypeptides; free fatty acids and prostaglandins; prolactin; and gamma aminobutyric acid (GABA). The exact role of the platelets in migraine and the significance of platelet aggregation are unknown.

An important factor appears to be the accumulation around the dilated arteries of substances that may sensitize them to pain. During a headache, the temporal artery on the painful side shows a greater catechol-uptake capacity than the same artery on the pain-free side.

Prostaglandin E_1 can trigger migraine in subjects who have never previously experienced migrainous headache and reserpine can precipitate an attack in patients who have had migraine headaches.

Tyramine, a pressor amine found in red wines and some cheeses, can evoke migraine in susceptible subjects. It is postulated that in dietary migraine the patient lacks the enzyme responsible for sulfate conjugation and that there is an inborn error of metabolism, but that has not been identified.

The physician must be cautious about interpreting changes in amines and other humoral agents found in venous blood as being primary factors in the initiation of a migraine attack. The mechanism underlying all trigger factors seems to be a sudden change in the external or internal milieu.

Biochemical approaches to migraine have been vigorously investigated; however, no clear picture has developed, particularly in regard to how the human organism responds biochemically to the stress that precedes and possibly provokes migraine.

Neurogenic Concept. According to the neurogenic concept of migraine, the primary event occurs in the CNS, and all the vascular phenomena are secondary. The evidence adduced includes the ties between the migraine attack and the sleep cycle, periods of relaxation after stress, and exposure to bright light. Depletion of endorphins has also been postulated. However, the relative importance of vascular and CNS events in the genesis of migraine pain is still debatable. Certainly, in many, but not all, attacks the pain has a pulsating quality and the external carotid arteries seem to be implicated. There is also controversy about the possible role of edema around the carotid arteries in lowering the pain threshold, and about the role of intracranial vessels, particularly the microcirculation.

It has been well-documented that cerebral blood flow decreases in classic migraine and that pattern persists into the headache phase. It is uncertain whether cerebral blood flow is also decreased in common migraine.

Diagnosis of Migraine. Migraine attacks, which freely occur in many complex patterns and settings, can be classified into the following types.

Classic Migraine. The headache of classic migraine is recurrent and periodic. Familial and personality factors are of major importance in pathogenesis. As a rule, the prodromes are sharply defined. Contralateral neurologic manifestations, usually visual, but occasionally motor or sensory, are common. The visual symptoms include scotomas, fortification spectra, visual-field defects, and transient amblyopia. The preheadache symptoms may appear transiently, inconstantly, or regularly, developing in 10 to 20 minutes. Visual prodromes may be accompanied by EEG slowing over the affected occipital lobe.

There is a high incidence of *ophthalmic migraine* in persons above age 50; unless the physician is acquainted with this partial syndrome and pursues the patient's description of the visual phenomena, erroneous diagnosis (e.g., TIA) is likely. Attacks of transient blindness in amaurosis fugax are brief (from a few seconds to 5 minutes), always monocular, and not accompanied by hemianopic fortification spectrum. The monocular visual loss may be total or partial, and occasionally includes photopsia or other types of scotoma. On the other hand, an older patient with migraine may have internal carotid artery disease, which makes it important to recognize transient monocular blindness. Intraoptic disorders and episodic blindness of giant-cell arteritis are other considerations in differential diagnosis. In some migraine patients, paresthesias may be noted simultaneously in the fingers and tongue. In about 20% of affected adults, the headache may be bilateral or occur on the same side as the visual or sensory deficit. The pain is usually throbbing and unilateral, and later may spread to other parts of the head. Anorexia, nausea, and vomiting are concomitant features. Classic migraine occurs in about 10% of all patients with migraine.

Common Migraine. This is the most frequent type of migraine, occurring in over 80% of migraine sufferers. The prodromes of common migraine are not sharply defined, and they may precede the attack by several hours or even days. These vary widely from patient to patient and include psychic disturbances, fatigue, nausea and vomiting, and changes in fluid balance. The actual headache is frequently longer than in the classic type of migraine; it may last hours or days. The pain is steady, unilateral or bilateral, and aching or throbbing in quality. Symptoms common to both classic and common migraines include irritability, chills, pallor, localized or general edema, sweating, and diuresis. Nasal signs and symptoms may lead the physician to ascribe the headache to involvement of nasal structures. Sensitivity to light and noise are prominent features. This type of migraine often occurs on weekends and holidays.

Cluster Headache. Cluster headache (e.g., ciliary or migrainous neuralgia, histamine cephalalgia, petrosal neuralgia) occurs in a series of closely spaced attacks that occur several or many times daily for several days or weeks. Cluster headaches may be followed by remission of months or years. Prodromes are uncommon. The pain may occur suddenly and wake the patient after an hour or two of sleep. Congestion of the conjunctivae, lacrimation, occasional ptosis of the eyelids, and sweating are associated manifestations. After 20 to 90 minutes, the pain stops as suddenly as it began. Cluster migraine is much more common in men than in women. Not all physicians agree that this type of headache should be considered a form of migraine.

In a few patients, attacks of paroxysmal and neuralgic pain in the distribution of the first division of the fifth cranial nerve are accompanied by *Raeder syndrome (paratrigeminal syndrome)* and may resemble cluster migraine. The mechanism is unknown, but it may be due to inflammation in the region of the eye, nose, or internal carotid artery, or there may be edema in and about the walls of the internal carotid artery.

A unique spotted pattern of hypothermia has been found by thermography in two thirds of patients with cluster headache. The pattern appears to be the result of a fixed vascular state because it does not change for years. The findings are not altered by the presence or absence of headache, nor by administration of vasoconstricting or vasodilating drugs. This thermographic picture is not found in other types of vascular headache.

Hemiplegic and Ophthalmoplegic Migraine. These rare types of migraine may occur in young adults. In ophthalmoplegic migraine, the pain is severe and occurs on the same side as the ophthalmoplegia (internal as well as external ophthalmoplegia), which may be partial or complete. Often the paralysis occurs as the headache subsides—3 to 5 days after the onset of persisting headache. Attacks may recur for months or years. Repeated ophthalmoplegic attacks may cause permanent injury to the third cranial nerve. The physician should be alert for the presence of a sphenoidal mucocele or an intracranial aneurysm on the main trunk of the internal carotid or at its junction with the posterior communicating artery.

The hemiplegic migraine complex is characterized by concomitant hemiparesis or even hemiplegia. The neurologic phenomena of both hemiplegic and ophthalmoplegic migraine may persist transiently after the headache has subsided.

Basilar Artery Migraine. Bickerstaff introduced the term "basilar artery migraine" to describe a recognized clinical disorder that can be a difficult diagnostic problem. It occurs in young women and girls, often in relation to menstrual periods. The first prodromal symptoms are usually visual and include visual loss or scintillations throughout both halves of the visual fields. This is quickly followed by vertigo, ataxia, dysarthria, and occasionally tinnitus or paresthesias in toes and fingers, not necessarily all or in this order. Consciousness may be lost in some patients. The symptoms last a few minutes or up to 45 minutes and are followed by a severe throbbing occipital headache and vomiting. Sometimes the symptom pattern is similar to that of classic or common migraine.

Complicated Migraine. The neurologic symptoms of classic migraine may persist beyond the headache phase. This variant has been called "complicated migraine." Permanent sequelae may occur after attacks of migraine and occasionally result in major or minor strokes. These include thrombosis of cerebral or retinal vessels during vasoconstriction and cerebral hemorrhage during the vasodilation phase. There is usually a family history of migraine in these patients and a history of migraine attacks in early life.

Disturbances of speech are more common in complicated migraine than is usually estimated. Dysarthria, repetitive expressions of single syllables or simple words, and complete aphasia have been noted. Receptive aphasia, dyslexia, dysgraphia, impaired word-finding, and amnesic aphasia have also been reported. This important condition may be misdiagnosed as some other cerebral disorder.

Migraine Equivalents. In some patients who have had migraine attacks, typical symptoms may be replaced by periodic occurrence of other bodily disturbances that have been called "migraine equivalents." These may consist of abdominal pain with nausea, vomiting, and diarrhea (abdominal migraine), pain localized in the thorax, pelvis, or limbs, bouts of fever, attacks of tachycardia, benign paroxysmal vertigo, and cyclic edema. Impairment of consciousness, altered mental states, confusion, lethargy, and disorders of mood, sleep, and behavior have also been reported as psychic equivalents of migraine. These "equivalents" are particularly frequent in children.

Complications. Arteriography excludes the presence of vascular malformations, but also indicates that permanent damage of neurologic structures may be associated with migraine. Lesions of the retina, cerebral hemispheres, and brain stem have been found in patients with migraine. The area most frequently affected is the occipital cortex, and hemianopsia may be permanent. CT indicates that there may be local changes, including edema and infarction of the cerebral hemisphere, in severe migraine attacks. Focal or nonfocal changes may occur in patients with migraine, depending in part on the severity of the episode.

Epidemiology. Migraine has been found in every society studied, with prevalence rates from 1 to 25% reported. Onset may be in childhood but most commonly occurs in adolescence or early adult life. Symptoms most commonly wane later in life. Sex incidence is equal in childhood, but in adult life a striking preponderance of females has been found in all epidemiological studies. Whether overall prevalence of headache or specific syndromes vary in prevalence from one society to another or from one socioeconomic group to another remains controversial; much of the uncertainty results from varied definitions of headache syndromes used in different studies. It is intriguing that there is a suggestion of high prevalence of classic migraine in the more highly educated.

Differential Diagnosis. Migraine must be differentiated from other conditions that cause chronic recurring headache. When headache continues steadily for weeks or months, it is probably caused by anxiety and depression.

In aneurysm or angioma, the recurrent headaches are always on the same side of the head and there may be focal neurologic signs or bleeding. Typical periodic headache that occurs for years is never caused by saccular aneurysm; that is, an aneurysm de novo does not cause or predispose to migraine headache and it is a coincidence if the two are associated. The occurrence of migraine in patients with unruptured angioma is not frequent and the migraine, with or without aura, is thought to be unrelated to the arteriovenous malformation.

Except for brain tumors in the pituitary, parapituitary, or occipital lobe, expanding lesions in the cranium, neoplasms, abscesses, and hematomas are rarely accompanied by a headache that simulates migraine. The finding of papilledema, focal neurologic signs, and abnormalities by the ancillary studies serves to direct attention to the possibility of a tumor.

Headache associated with temporal arteritis, carotid and basilar insufficiency, hypertension, and glaucoma must be considered in the differential diagnosis of migraine in older patients. Other disorders to be considered are pheochromocytoma, carcinoid, and mastocytosis.

The existence of a relationship between migraine and epilepsy is still controversial. There may be a higher incidence of epilepsy in unselected migraine sufferers than in the population as a whole. Headache is common after a major convulsion of any origin. Migraine differs from epilepsy in the timing of the attack; the onset of a migraine attack is rarely accompanied by loss of consciousness, although it may be followed by drowsiness or sleep. In epilepsy, the EEG frequently reveals specific abnormalities, whereas in migraine it is usually normal or shows nonspecific irregularities. Ergot preparations, which are specific in the treatment of acute migraine headache, are of no help in epilepsy. In a few patients, however, migraine and epilepsy are intimately associated.

Although allergy is common in migraine patients, it is also common in the general population. There is no good evidence that inhaled allergens play any but an occasional role in producing a migraine attack. There is more persuasive evidence that food allergens may be important precipitating causes in a few patients. True allergic headaches differ from migraine in history, physical characteristics, and response to allergic therapy.

Treatment. The array of therapeutic approaches proposed for migraine is more remarkable for diversity than for results. Management of the patient with migraine can, for practical purposes, be divided into three parts: general principles, symptomatic treatment of the acute attack, and prophylactic treatment.

General principles include eliminating the factors that precipitate or provoke an attack, including treatment of all underlying physiologic or structural abnormalities that may be discovered in the examination of the patient. Treatment includes correction of medical disorders, intercurrent infection, refractive errors, and dental problems, as well as removal or reduction of provoking factors. Examples of migraine-provoking factors include load of environmental stress at home, at work, or in social situations; ingestion of specific foods such as chocolate or caffeine, or foods that contain tyramine (cheese, red wine), monosodium glutamate, nitrites (hot dogs, bacon), phenylethyl amine; offending allergens; the missing of meals; exposure to glare or flickering lights; and drugs, such as oral contraceptives. Elimination of these provoking factors, however, does not completely eliminate attacks in most patients.

Physical activity should be regulated to provide routine daily exercise, well-balanced meals, and general avoidance of food or beverages that may trigger migraine attacks. A set time for retiring and rising, including weekends, may be beneficial. Adequate social activities and periods of relaxation should be encouraged.

Symptomatic Therapy for an Acute Attack. Symptomatic therapy for migraine includes analgesics, sedatives, and antianxiety agents. Of all the agents used, ergotamine tartrate is most effective in treating the acute attack. Analgesics combined with sedatives or tranquilizers may be helpful in the late stages of an attack or in mild attacks. If the pain is mild, dull, and aching, it may respond to aspirin (0.3 to 0.6 g) or phenacetin or acetaminophen and caffeine (50 mg). For patients who cannot take ergotamine tartrate or for whom the drug is not effective, meperidine hydrochloride may be necessary, especially in severe attacks in which the headache has been present for hours. The danger of addiction in the migraine patient who uses this agent must always be considered.

In an acute migraine attack, ergotamine tartrate is still the best pharmacologic agent to abort an attack. It constricts scalp arteries, causing a decrease in amplitude of cranial arteries that parallels the symptomatic relief. The vasoconstrictor effect of ergotamine tartrate is mediated by a direct effect on arterial serotonin receptors.

The medication must be administered early in an attack and the dosage has to be adjusted for each patient; however, caution should be used in giving ergotamine tartrate to patients who have experienced prolonged visual, sensory, or motor symptoms. Patients vary greatly in responses to ergotamine tartrate. Even in the same person, different physiologic states can cause different responses to the agent. Improper use of this drug has caused many treatment failures.

Caffeine acts synergistically with ergot alkaloids by potentiating the vasoconstrictor effect of the ergot, and by accelerating and enhancing intestinal absorption. This reduces the total dosage of ergotamine tartrate necessary to control an attack of migraine. Sedatives and antiemetics may help control the nausea and vomiting that occur during the migraine attack or that may be induced by ergotamine. Sedatives plus salicylates are of special value in treatment of a migraine attack in children.

Ergotamine tartrate can be given orally, sublingually, parenterally, or rectally. The recommended oral or rectal dose is 1 to 2 mg at the onset of headache followed by 2 mg within the hour; not more than 6 mg should be given for any single attack. The intramuscular dosage is 0.25 to 0.5 mg at onset. Rectal suppositories are more effective than oral preparations.

It is important to adjust the dosage for each patient to find the appropriate dose for later attacks. Most patients tolerate ergotamine tartrate well, but side effects include myalgia, paresthesias, nausea, vomiting, and, rarely, limb ischemia (even gangrene), angina pectoris, and thrombophlebitis. Moderately severe headache may require, in addition to less potent analgesics, codeine phosphate in doses of 60 mg every few hours.

The problem of drug dependence must be considered in the management of migraine, especially in patients who take ergotamine tartrate, narcotics, or other analgesics every day for years. Manifestations of withdrawal may be seen in patients who use opiates and other addicting analgesics in large doses for a long time. Even caffeine and ergotamine may lead to dependency states. Gradual withdrawal of the drug and management of the underlying depression are the basis of proper treatment. Analgesic nephropathy is a rare complication of prolonged and excessive use of analgesics.

Dihydroergotamine mesylate, an ergot derivative, moderately constricts the extracranial arteries; its side-effects (nausea and vomiting) are less severe than those of ergotamine tartrate, but the results are less predictable. It is administered only intravenously (0.5 mg).

Occasionally, an acute migraine attack is relieved by inhalation of 100% oxygen. The basis of this relief may be the reduction of cerebral blood flow after inhalation of the oxygen.

In an occasional patient, isometheptene mucate (65 mg) is a sympathomimetic agent that may be effective in combination with acetaminophen (325 mg) and dichloralphenazone (100 mg).

Prophylactic or Interval Treatment. There is no wholly effective treatment for prevention of migraine. The response to various treatments is highly individualized and the treatment must be tailored to individual needs. In prophylaxis or interval treatment, pharmacotherapy and psychotherapy are fundamental. Pharmacologic treatment is essentially the same for all types of migraine, including cluster headache.

The effect of drugs is difficult to assess; in some studies, placebo therapy reduced the frequency of migraine in over 40% of patients.

Drugs that block beta-adrenergic receptors have also been useful in preventing migraine attacks. Propranolol is used most often but other beta-blockers, such as metoprolol and nadolol, have also been effective. Dilatation of peripheral arteries in response to adrenalin is attributed to the uptake of adrenalin by beta-receptors in the vessel wall. Beta blockade could prevent dilatation in response to any humoral agent acting on these receptors. In addition, propranolol hydrochloride acts on platelet uptake of serotonin, on fatty acid metabolism, and on prostaglandins.

Propranolol, however, also has central nervous system effects. It relieves anxiety and patients often note a diminution in "drive," at times to an unpleasant degree.

Propranolol may precipitate or potentiate congestive heart failure, myocardial conduction defects, or asthma. Angina pectoris may follow sudden withdrawal of the drug, particularly in patients with pre-existing coronary disease. Adverse reactions may not be dose-dependent and rarely can occur at extremely low doses. It is preferable to begin therapy at low levels, 40 to 60 mg daily, in divided doses, increasing gradually to 200 mg daily. The half-life of propranolol hydrochloride is about 3 to 6 hours; effects may linger for 24 to 48 hours after the drug is stopped. The peak plasma levels of propranolol hydrochloride are reduced about 90 minutes after oral intake. The pulse rate should not be depressed below 60 beats per minute in a healthy individual with migraine with propranolol therapy.

Drugs that block entry of calcium ions into arterial walls are used extensively in cardiovascular disease and are thought to be effective by inducing dilatation of arteries. Calcium-blockers have also been found to be effective migraine prophylaxis. Efficacy and side effects seem to be similar in available compounds of this class, but verapamil may be superior to nifedipine and diltiazem. The oral dosage of verapamil for normal adults is 80 mg three times daily. Constipation is a common side effect, and there may also be pedal edema or other symptoms.

Amitriptyline has been reported to be effective in prophylactic treatment of migraine. Beneficial results do not appear to have any relationship to symptoms of depression. Amitriptyline may have a primary effect on migraine. It may act by inhibiting the uptake of norepinephrine and serotonin in peripheral and central neurons.

Platelet antagonists have been used in attempts to reduce the intensity and frequency of migraine. A platelet antagonist, naproxen, has proven effective against common migraine in doses of 300 to 400 mg given twice daily. Occasional side effects include irritation of the gastric mucosa and prolongation of bleeding time. There have been few studies of other drugs in this category, including aspirin given prophylactically in doses of 0.3 to 0.6 g daily and sulfinpyrazone in doses of 200 mg two to four times daily.

Methysergide maleate has proved to be an effective prophylactic agent in migraine. Methysergide maleate is chemically related to methylergonovine maleate and is a potent antagonist of serotonin. It may act by maintaining toxic vasoconstriction of scalp arteries if the plasma-serotonin level drops during a migraine attack.

Daily administration of 2 to 6 mg methysergide suppresses migraine completely or partially in about 60% of the patients. However, from 20 to 40% of these patients experience adverse side-effects such as abdominal discomfort, muscle cramps, paresthesias, edema, and depression. About 10% are unable to tolerate methysergide because of symptoms of peripheral vasoconstriction, intermittent claudication, or, rarely, angina pectoris that disappears when medication is discontinued. The patient should use the drug for 2 months, and then stop using it for 1 month, after which the medication can be resumed according to the pattern of 2 months of use and 1 month of nonuse. This cycle prevents the development of a syndrome of retroperitoneal fibrosis or pleuropulmonary and cardiac fibrosis, which is seen occasionally after long-term therapy with methysergide.

Cyproheptadine hydrochloride is antagonistic to both serotonin and histamine and may reduce the frequency and severity of headache in some patients. Side-effects include drowsiness (the most common), with stimulation of appetite and weight gain as secondary effects. The usual oral dosage is 4 mg 4 times daily, although this may be increased to a maximum of 24 mg daily. (This regimen has not been approved by the FDA.)

Pizotifen is structurally related to cyproheptadine and has similar antiserotonin and antihistamine effects. In clinical trials, the drug seems safe and effective in preventing migraine. It is now being used in Canada and Europe for prophylactic treatment.

Bellergal, a mixture of ergotamine tartrate, belladonna alkaloids, and phenobarbital, is also used for migraine prevention. The dosage is 1 tablet 3 or 4 times daily; a timed-release version, Bellergal-S, is given twice a day.

Diuretics have not proven useful in the treatment of migraine, although some patients with edema (especially before menses) feel more comfortable after fluid loss. There is no evidence that retention of water is related to the attack.

Other treatments for migraine include monoamine oxidase inhibitors which inhibit uptake of norepinephrine and serotonin in peripheral and central neurons. Use of these drugs is reserved for patients who are completely resistant to all other conventional forms of therapy. These antidepressants have potentially serious side-effects and elicit variable responses in migraine patients.

Miscellaneous agents include tranquilizers, sedatives, muscle relaxants, heparin compounds, lithium carbonate, levodopa, bromocriptine, indomethacin, prednisone, estrogens, serotonin precursors, papaverine, and anticonvulsants.

Clonidine, an antihypertensive drug, and indomethacin have not proven successful for the prophylaxis of migraine.

Use of the contraceptive pill may exaggerate migraine in some patients, increasing the frequency and severity of attacks. On the other hand, headache has been relieved in some young women who take oral contraceptives. Attacks of migraine occur as estrogen levels fall and may be delayed or abolished if levels are maintained artificially high by administration of estrogens; however, estrogen therapy has to be balanced with the risk of thrombotic and carcinogenic effects.

Daily use of ergotamine tartrate for migraine prophylaxis is not advisable; however, for patents with nocturnal attacks of cluster headache, an oral dose of 1 to 2 mg before retiring, taken over a period of 10 to 14 days, may help terminate the series of headaches.

Psychotherapy. The personality structure of the migraine patient, which needs careful evaluation, has been described as compulsive, with outstanding performance because of the emphasis on perfection, over-conscientiousness, and ambition. No doubt some migraine patients have anxiety, neurotic depressive reactions, conversion, and dissociative and phobic reactions. No single personality type describes all migraine patients.

It is not surprising that if the situations in which some headaches occur and recur are analyzed in relation to the psychological, social, and emotional significance to the patient, headache may be related to a psychological or emotional stress. For many patients, supportive doctor-patient relationships in the initial phase of therapy are important, and guidance, counseling, and situational insight are often needed continuously. Serious problems require the attention of a psychiatrist. Numerous relaxation treatments have reduced the number and severity of migraine attacks. These include demonstrating to patients how to increase control over some sensory function, e.g., muscle contraction (biofeedback).

References

Andermann F. Clinical features of migraine-epilepsy syndromes. In Andermann F, Lugarisi E (eds). Migraine and Epilepsy. Stoneham, MA: Butterworth, 1987:3–30.

Andermann F, Lugaresi E (eds). Migraine and epilepsy. Butterworth's, London, 1987.

Anonymous. Drugs for migraine. Medical Letter: 1987; 29:27–28.

Bille B. Migraine in school children. Acta Paediatr (Upps) 1962; 51(suppl 136):1–151.

Broderick JP, Swanson JW. Migraine-related strokes. Arch Neurol 1987; 44:868–871.

Bruyn GW. Biochemistry of migraine. Headache 1980; 20:235–246.

Chapman SL. A review and clinical perspective on the use of EMG and thermal biofeedback for chronic headaches. Pain 1986; 27:1–43.

Charcot JM. Sur un case de migraine ophtalmoplegique (paralysie oculomotrice periodique). Progr Med (Paris) 1890; 12:83–99.

Crisp AH, McGuinness B, Kalucy RS, Ralph PC, Harris G. Some clinical, social and psychological characteristics of migraine subjects in the general population. Postgrad Med J 1977; 53:691–697.

Dalessio D. Wolff's Headache and Other Head Pain, 4th ed. New York: Oxford University Press, 1980:123–126.

Doogan DP. Prophylaxis of migraine with beta-blockers. Practitioner 1983; 227:441–444.

Friedman AP. Medicine for migraine—What to use when. Mod Med 1980; 48:36–49.

Lance JW. Mechanism and Management of Headache, 4th ed. London: Butterworths, 1982.

Lanzi G, Grandi AM, Gamba G, et al. Migraine, mitral valve prolapse and platelet function in the pediatric age group. Headache 1986; 26:142–145.

Lauritzen M, Skyhoj OT, Lassen NA, Paulson OB. Changes in regional blood flow during the course of classic migraine attacks. Ann Neurol 1983; 13:633–641.

Lauritzen M, Skyhoj OT, Lassen NA, Paulson OB. Regulation of regional cerebral blood flow during and between migraine attacks. Ann Neurol 1983; 14:569–572.

Linet M, Stewart WF. Migraine headache: Epidemiologic perspectives. Epidemiol Rev 1984; 6:107–139.

Merskey H. Psychiatric aspects of migraine. In: Pearce J, ed. Modern Topics in Migraine. London: Wm Heinemann, 1975:52–61.

Olsen TS, Friberg L, Lassen NA. Ischemia may be the primary cause of the neurologic deficits in classic migraine. Arch Neurol 1987; 44:156–161.

Osuntokun BO, Bademosi O, Osuntokun O. Migraine in Nigeria. In: F.C. Rose (Ed.). Advances in Migraine Research and Therapy. New York, Raven Press (1982a): 25–38.

Pearce J. Complicated migraine. In: Pearce J, ed. Modern Concepts in Migraine. London: Wm Heinemann, 1975:30–44.

Price RW, Posner JB. Chronic paroxysmal hemicrania: disabling syndrome responding to indomethacin. Ann Neurol 1978; 3:183–184.

Raskin NH. Headache, 2nd Ed. New York, Churchill Livingstone, 1988.

Spierings ELH. The Pathophysiology of the Migraine Attack. Alphen aan den Rijn: Stafleu's Wetenschappelijke Vitgeversmaatschappij, 1980.

Ziegler DK, Ellis DJ. Naproxen in prophylaxis of migraine. Arch Neurol 1985; 42:582–584.

Ziegler DK, Hurwitz A, Hassanein RS, Kodanaz HA, Preskorn SH, Mason J. Migraine prophylaxis: A comparison of propranolol and amitriptyline. Arch Neurol 1987; 44:486–489.

---

145. EPILEPSY

Eli S. Goldensohn
Gilbert H. Glaser
Mark A. Goldberg

Epilepsy is characterized by sudden recurrent and transient disturbances of mental function or movements of the body that result from excessive discharging of groups of brain cells. The term *epilepsy* does not refer to a specific disease but rather to a group of symptom complexes that have many causes; some are static and others are progressive. All conditions that cause epilepsy have in common the quality of causing cerebral neurons to become excessively excited.

The signs and symptoms of epilepsy are manifold. Among the most common manifestations are episodes of partial or complete loss of consciousness, localized or generalized muscular spasms or jerks, or apparently purposeful behavior performed while awareness is depressed.

Epidemiology, Inheritance, and Survival

Epilepsy is common. Estimates based on epidemiologic studies indicate that up to 1% of the population (over 2 million people) in the United States have epilepsy and that new cases appear at an annual rate of about 40/ 100,000. This suggests that over 100,000 new patients are diagnosed annually. The rate is highest in children younger than 5, drops to a lower level between the ages of 20 and 50, and rises again in older people. The incidence and prevalence are higher for partial (focal) seizures than for generalized seizures (Table 145–1).

Epilepsy occurs with similar frequency in the United States and Europe. In most studies, the incidence is slightly higher in males than in females, which may be related to the greater frequency of head injuries in men. There is increasing evidence that socioeconomic factors play an important role in the development of epilepsy. For example, the incidence is higher in black children (1.96%) than in white children (0.95%) living in New Haven, Connecticut, but the cause of this difference is uncertain; the relative importance of perinatal factors, trauma, nutrition, and other environmental influences or genetics is unknown.

Chronic seizures often begin in early life; half start before age 20. Seizure-onset continues throughout life. As a rule, however, the later the onset of seizure is, the greater is the probability that the attacks are partial and associated with a structural lesion of the brain. The syndrome of benign febrile seizures, which occurs in about 4% of the population under the age of 5, is not considered epilepsy in most epidemiologic studies.

Seizures due to overt lesions of the brain may begin at any age. The distribution curve of incidence by age is broader in these cases than in the cases of unknown cause, but like the latter, there are two peaks: the first is in the early years in life and the second after the third decade. The first peak in incidence is related to the fact that the developing brain of an infant or young child may be more likely to react with seizures after cerebral injury by trauma, infections, or other illness. The second peak may be related to head injuries and neurologic diseases that appear in adults.

The long-term survival rate of patients with chronic seizures is somewhat lower than that of the general population. Patients with absence attacks accompanied by 3-Hz spike-and-wave discharges in the EEG have normal life expectancy. The increased risk of death within the first 10 years varies greatly depending on the etiology (Fig. 145–1). For individuals with seizures of unknown cause, there is a slight increase in risk of death within the first 10 years after diagnosis; later there is little evidence of increased risk of death. For those with epilepsy following insults such as stroke or head trauma, the risk of death is four-fold in the first 10 years. The greatest increase in mortality is among those with epilepsy who have abnormal neurologic signs at birth. It seems unlikely that the epilepsy per se accounts for the increased mortality in the latter two groups; rather it is associated with the underlying illnesses that also caused seizures.

The role of inheritance in cerebral seizures is controversial, because epilepsy is not a disease but a symptom of many different cerebral disorders. Also, it is difficult to distinguish social and economic factors from primary genetic predisposition. Poor nutrition and inadequate perinatal care frequently run in families; however, several studies indicate that, in patients with generalized epilepsy, near-relatives have a two- to four-fold increase in incidence of convulsive disorders (Table 145–2). A child of the average patient with epilepsy has about one chance in 30 of being affected. Familial incidence of epilepsy is greater in patients whose seizures begin early in life. Genetic predisposition may play a role in acquired epilepsy; the incidence of a family history of epilepsy is somewhat greater among relatives of patients with post-traumatic seizures, suggesting a possible minor secondary role of genetic predisposition. The higher occurrence of epileptiform dis-

Table 145–1. Incidence of Epilepsy by Type of Seizure (Rochester, Minnesota)

Seizure Type (by initial features)	No.	%	Rate/100,000 Person Years
Partial	384	52%	23
Generalized			
Tonic, tonic-clonic, or clonic	199	27%	13
Absence	58	8%	3
Myoclonic	61	8%	3
Total	318	43%	19
Other/Unclassified	30	4%	2
Total	732		43

(Modified from Hauser WE, Annegers JF, Andersen EV. Res Publ Assoc Res Nerv Ment Dis 1983; 61:267–294.)

Table 145–2.   Epilepsy in Offspring of Patients with 3-Hz Spike-and-Wave Discharge EEG

Study	Father with Epilepsy		Mother with Epilepsy	
	Sons	Daughters	Sons	Daughters
Janz & Beck-Mannagetta	189 6 (3.2%)	182 4 (2.2%)	211 10 (4.7%)	186 6 (3.2%)
Tsuboi & Endo	109 2 (1.8%)	124 2 (1.6%)	125 3 (2.4%)	148 5 (3.4%)
TOTAL	298 8 (2.7%)	306 6 (2.0%)	336 13 (3.9%)	334 11 (3.3%)

(From Hauser WA, Annegers JF, Anderson VE. Res Publ Assoc Res Nerv Ment Dis 1983; 61:267–294.)

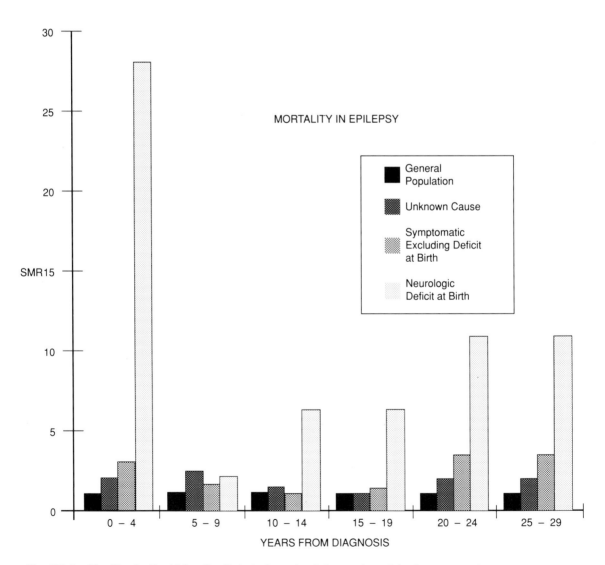

Fig. 145–1.   The Standardized Mortality Ratio is the ratio of the number of deaths in a population with epilepsy compared with the general population. (Derived from data in Hauser WA, Annegers JF, Elveback LR. Epilepsia 1980; 21:399–412.)

charges in the EEGs of relatives of patients with generalized epilepsy suggests a more prominent genetic background in patients with generalized seizures.

Pathophysiology, Anatomy, and Biochemical Considerations

Abnormal excitability of a localized group of neurons in the cerebral cortex is the crucial element in the genesis of partial seizures. Excessive excitability of neurons distributed throughout the entire cortical mantle is basic to generalized seizures. In generalized seizures, excessive excitability in deep gray-matter structures seems to play an important but secondary role. In cases of both partial and generalized seizures, the common dysfunction at the cellular level is manifested by abnormally excessive discharges of neurons. Normally, a balance of excitatory and inhibitory synaptic influences on normal neurons is maintained. In an epileptogenic area, however, transmembrane potentials recorded from single cells show that nearly all are receiving excessive excitatory synaptic influences. In some experimental foci, the excessive excitation appears to result from blockade of inhibition by gamma aminobutyric acid (GABA). The electrical phenomenon that occurs in single neurons that generates each interictal, epileptiform EEG spike is called a *paroxysmal depolarization shift* (PDS). The PDS is a prolonged large membrane depolarization of about 30 millivolts, having at its onset a superimposed high-frequency burst of action potentials. The PDS seems to be a universal epileptic phenomenon; it occurs in experimental lesions and has been demonstrated in the human epileptic cortex. It is initiated by strong excitatory synaptic inputs, but the characteristic form is probably intrinsic to the properties of the cell itself.

The cerebral cortex is the structure from which both focal and generalized seizures begin. Vertically oriented pyramidal cells have cell bodies in the deeper layers and their long apical dendrites are located in superficial layers where they receive mainly excitatory contacts, up to several thousand per dendritic tree. The cell body receives mostly inhibitory contacts, some 50 to 100 per cell body. Excitatory impulses on the pyramidal cells arrive near the cortical surface by the thousands, and inhibitory impulses are more deeply and strategically placed at the cell body to prevent firing. Impulses from any part of the cerebral cortex go predominantly to other regions of the cortex and only a small fraction are directed toward subcortical structures such as the specific and associational nuclei of the thalamus.

Vertical organization of the excitatory and inhibitory influences is in keeping with the idea that the structural design of the cortex rests upon complex interconnections among the large number of mosaic-like vertical columnar units. Functional vertical columns have been clearly demonstrated in the occipital lobe; the distribution of PDSs in discrete epileptogenic foci support this concept. This anatomic-physiologic analysis serves as the basis for the idea that the electrical activity of the cortex depends on small, vertically oriented columnar organizations in which excitation occurs at the apical dendrites, mainly near the surface and in which inhibition occurs predominantly in the deeper layers. In epileptogenic foci, the greatest EEG negativity is found about 1 mm below the surface, indicating that the negative spike is generated in superficial areas. Slow-wave areas of the experimental EEG spike-and-wave complexes are also surface-negative but seem to be generated at a deeper site. The intracellular correlates of the slow-wave portion appear to be deeply generated, inhibitory, postsynaptic potentials.

Biochemical Aspects. Seizures are accompanied by profound changes in cerebral metabolism; conversely, metabolic changes in the brain can cause seizures. In experimental animals, seizures stimulate cerebral metabolism. After a single seizure, cerebral oxygen and glucose consumption increase greatly as does rise of high energy phosphates. Cerebral blood flow increases in proportion to the rate of metabolism to provide adequate oxygenation of the brain. Nevertheless, an increase in tissue lactic acid indicates a shift to glycolytic metabolism. These alterations are readily reversed when the seizure ends. In human studies, during partial seizures, positron emission tomography (PET) demonstrates local increases in glucose metabolism, but, between seizures, there is hypometabolism of glucose in the same brain regions.

After prolonged or repetitive seizures (status epilepticus), correction of the biochemical abnormalities is delayed, and more profound and sometimes irreversible changes occur, including changes in nucleic acids and protein content. Systemic factors may also contribute to brain damage in prolonged seizures. These include lactic acidosis, hypotension, and hypoxia. The systemic factors were eliminated in experimental studies by artificially ventilating animals that were paralyzed with a neuromuscular blocking agent. Even then, abnormalities of cerebral metabolism were not completely corrected. These alterations in cerebral and systemic metabolism cause cellular damage that, in turn, may lead to further neurologic impairment and increased tendency for seizures.

Although the biochemical consequences of seizures are known, the biochemical causes of human seizures are poorly understood. In many patients, structural abnormalities are not detected and biochemical aberration is considered the epilepsy cause. This is particularly true of generalized seizures, where genetic factors are thought to produce a biochemical abnormality. Even when there is overt structural pathology, it is assumed that abnormal metabolism of damaged neurons gives rise to epileptic phenomena. In general, there are two major mechanisms: impaired membrane regulation of ion fluxes and abnormal synaptic transmission. Inhibition of Na^+-K^+ATPase, the enzyme believed to function as the Na^+-K^+ pump, results in seizures by allowing an increase in intracellular sodium and decrease of potassium content within the cell. Defective control of cation channels may cause unstable, readily depolarized neurons that are implicated in some forms of epilepsy. Drugs, such as phenytoin, are thought to stabilize the membranes. Possible abnormalities in Ca^{++} and Cl^- channels are being evaluated in epilepsy.

Impaired synaptic transmission may also cause depolarization of long chains of neurons leading to epileptic discharges. Several convulsant drugs (e.g., bicuculline) antagonize the inhibitory neurotransmitter, gamma aminobutyric acid (GABA), and may induce seizures by impeding normal inhibitory brain mechanisms. Other convulsants act by interfering with the synthesis of GABA; drugs are anticonvulsant if they are GABA agonists or increase cerebral GABA concentrations. Benzodiazepines and anticonvulsant barbiturates are agonists at the GABA-chloride receptor complex. Alterations in metabolism of other neurotransmitters affect seizure activity, but GABA is most important experimentally. However, no specific abnormalities of Na^+-K^+ATPase or in GABA metabolism have been found in human epilepsy.

Classification of Epileptic Seizures

The International Classification of seizures condenses the diverse manifestations of epileptic seizures into a concise scheme that has improved both professional communication and patient care. Better terms than *"grand mal," "petit mal," "psychomotor,"* and *"focal"* were needed as it became clear that most recurrent seizures begin in local areas of the cerebral cortex and present clinically as sequences of symptoms consequent to the spread of discharges to adjacent and distant regions (Table 145–3).

The International Classification emphasizes symptoms and signs that indicate the location of the initial brain dysfunction and its spread. The terminology is now used by all major neurologic journals. The fundamental criterion for classifying a given seizure is whether

Table 145–3.   International Classification of Epileptic Seizures

---

I   PARTIAL SEIZURES (seizures beginning locally)
   A. Simple partial seizures (consciousness not impaired)
      1. With motor symptoms
      2. With somatosensory or special sensory symptoms
      3. With autonomic symptoms
      4. With psychic symptoms
   B. Complex partial seizures (with impairment of consciousness)
      1. Beginning as simple partial seizures and progressing to impairment of consciousness
      2. With impairment of consciousness at onset
        a. With impairment of consciousness only
        b. With automatisms
   C. Partial seizures secondarily generalized
        a. Secondary to simple partial seizures
        b. Secondary to complex partial seizures
II   GENERALIZED SEIZURES (bilaterally symmetric and without local onset)
   A. Absence seizures
   B. Myoclonic seizures
   C. Clonic seizures
   D. Tonic seizures
   E. Tonic-clonic seizures
   F. Atonic seizures
III. UNCLASSIFIED EPILEPTIC SEIZURES (due to incomplete data)

(Modified from Proposal for Revised Clinical and Electroencephalographic Classification of Epileptic Seizures. Epilepsia 1981; 22:489–501.)

the abnormal discharges responsible for the onset of the seizure originate in a unilateral brain structure (a partial seizure) or in bilateral brain structures (a generalized seizure). A second important criterion is whether consciousness is retained. Accuracy in classification is improved greatly by using video tape recordings that simultaneously document clinical seizures and EEG changes.

Seizures are divided into two major categories, partial and generalized (see Table 145–3). Partial seizures begin in unilateral (focal or local) areas and may or may not spread bilaterally. Generalized seizures begin with immediate involvement of bilateral brain structures.

Partial seizures are divided into three types: simple partial attacks that arise from a local area and do not impair consciousness; complex partial attacks that begin in a local area but spread bilaterally and therefore impair consciousness; and simple or complex partial attacks that spread widely and secondarily evolve into generalized major motor seizures.

Generalized seizures begin with immediate involvement of both hemispheres and are associated with either bilateral body movements or changes in consciousness, or both. Generalized seizures are divided into six types: short absences with associated 3-Hz generalized spike-and-wave discharges in the EEG; atypical absences; myoclonic; clonic; tonic-clonic; and atonic. Seizures that cannot be classified because of incomplete data are listed as unclassified.

Symptoms

PARTIAL SEIZURES

Partial seizures are the most common type of epileptic seizures (Table 145–4). The first clinical and EEG features indicate they begin in unilateral structures. Partial seizures are divided into two types that are based primarily on whether consciousness is affected. If consciousness is unimpaired during the attack, it is a simple partial type. If there is a degree of altered awareness or unresponsiveness, or both, it is a complex partial seizure.

Simple Partial Seizures. Symptoms often indicate the area of the brain from which the attack begins, but this is not always the case. Simple partial seizures are divided into four types: partial motor attacks, autonomic attacks, somatosensory attacks, and special sensory attacks.

Partial motor attacks involve motor activity

Table 145–4. Prevalence of Epilepsy, Overall and by Initial Type

Type (by initial features)	No.	Rate*
Partial (focal origin)		
Sensory	9	0.2
Motor	24	0.6
Adversive	18	0.5
Temporal	64	1.7
Multiple types or unclassified	41	1.0
TOTAL	156	4.0
Generalized		
Tonic-clonic (grand mal) only	49	1.3
Incomplete†	14	0.4
Absence	17	0.4
TOTAL	80	2.1

*Per 1000 population—modified from census figures.
†With or without associated tonic-clonic convulsions.
(From Hauser WA, Kurland LT. Epilepsia 1975; 16:1–66.)

from any area of the body. They usually involve the limbs, face, or head and sometimes cause speech arrest. If a partial motor seizure progresses with sequential involvement of parts of the body that are represented by contiguous cortical areas, it is known as a *jacksonian seizure*. Localized paralysis or weakness that may last for minutes or days after a partial motor seizure is called *Todd paralysis* and indicates an underlying structural lesion. If partial motor seizures become continuous for hours or days, the condition is termed *epilepsia partialis continua*.

Autonomic symptoms (such as thirst or a desire to micturate) are rarely the sole manifestations of recurrent seizures.

Somatosensory attacks are usually described as feelings of numbness, deadness, or "pins and needles." Special sensory seizures include simple visual, auditory, olfactory, gustatory, and vertiginous feelings such as flashing lights, buzzing, or unpleasant odors. Nearly all special sensory seizures are, at one time or another, the aura or the earliest symptoms of a complex partial or generalized tonic-clonic seizure.

Symptoms of psychic seizures include dysmnesia of various types: déjà vu, jamais vu, flashback experiences of previous events, or forced thinking (i.e., a thought or series of recollections intrude upon the mind). Affective symptoms such as fear or depression may be experienced. Smiling and laughter sometimes occur. Intense fear is common and objective autonomic signs include pupillary dilatation, palpitations, pallor, and flushing. Illusions or distorted perceptions occur. Visual distortions affect the size, distance, symmetry, or shape of the object viewed. Distortions of sound include increased sensitivity to usual sounds and the imposition of a rhythmic crescendo-decrescendo quality to the sound. Feelings of floating or depersonalization, as if the person were "outside" the body, are common. Hallucinations may be complicated. The hallucinations may be realistic or distorted but the patient recognizes their basic unreality. Although psychic symptoms may occur alone, they are usually the aura of complex partial attacks and are sometimes the aura of secondarily generalized tonic-clonic attacks.

Complex Partial Seizures. Characteristically, complex partial seizures begin with emotional, psychic, illusory, hallucinatory, or special sensory symptoms. These are followed by clouding or consciousness with automatic behavior and amnesia. Sometimes, consciousness is clouded at the onset. Complex partial seizures occur in over 50% of adults with seizure disorders and used to be called *psychomotor seizures*. The auras or onsets of complex partial seizures include any of the signs and symptoms mentioned previously under Simple Partial Seizures, particularly illusory, psychic, hallucinatory, autonomic, and special sensory.

After the aura (which, if it occurs without further symptoms, is classified as a simple partial seizure), the patient becomes partially or completely unresponsive and may perform apparently purposeful activity. These automatisms are usually simple acts (e.g., picking at clothes, examining nearby objects, simply walking about) but more elaborate behavior may be seen during the period of impaired awareness. In the state of depressed awareness, patients may actively resist efforts to restrain them. A complete attack usually lasts from 1 to 3 minutes and, upon recovery, there is complete amnesia for the attack except for the aura or partial motor onset.

Complex partial seizures usually begin in the temporal lobe (Fig. 145–2), but may originate from the frontal, parietal, or occipital areas (Table 145–5). Those of frontal lobe origin usually begin with a blank stare and often occur in clusters. Attacks that begin with visual hallucinations frequently begin in the posterolateral part of the temporal lobe but may originate in the occipital lobe. Attacks

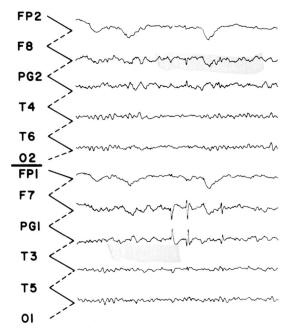

Fig. 145–2. Temporal lobe. Spikes in a patient with complex partial seizures. Focus in left anteromidtemporal area is higly localized to a nasopharyngeal electrode (PG1) that is common to channels 7 and 8.

beginning with unpleasant odors, however, uniformly begin in temporal structures and usually in the anteromedial portion. Automatic behavior or automatisms that are an integral part of a complex partial seizure may occur after abnormal discharges have spread bilaterally. Automatisms are also seen in seizures of nonfocal origin; automatic behavior and prolonged behavioral changes in generalized seizures are described below. Nevertheless, most complex automatisms seen clinically are associated with complex partial

Table 145–5. Location of Epileptiform Activity in 36 Patients with Complex Partial Seizures

	No. of Patients	Percentage
Anteromidtemporal	16	45
Mediotemporal	3	8
Posterotemporal	3	8
Occipital	3	8
Orbital-frontal	2	6
Multifocal	3	8
No epileptiform activity		
Normal EEG	2	6
Temporal slowing	4	11
Total	36	100

(Modified from White JC, Langston JW, Pedley TA. Neurology 1977; 27:1061–1068.)

seizures and most complex partial seizures have discharges that originate in the temporal lobe and spread to bilateral structures.

Automatisms. Behaviors that occur in association with a state of impaired consciousness and amnesia during or following a seizure are termed *automatisms.* The individual fails to recognize or distorts information and fails to imprint memories. Simple actions such as chewing, swallowing, and licking may be made. More complex automatisms include picking at and straightening one's clothes, walking from one room to another, or rearranging objects on a desk. More unusual behaviors include partial undressing or walking out of a building into the street. Nearly always there is complete amnesia for the automatism. The state of awareness is always impaired during automatic activity and the person is either unresponsive to verbal stimuli or can be recognized as in a confused state.

The amnesia, depressed responsiveness, and automatic activity all indicate dysfunction of bilateral structures. Ictal and postictal dysfunction of both hippocampi and related neuronal systems seem to be responsible for the amnesia. Prolonged behavioral changes and automatisms can occur with either complex partial or generalized absences with 3-Hz spike-and-wave discharges. Automatisms with absence attacks are usually shorter and simpler and are not associated with an aura, postictal confusion, or postictal sleepiness.

GENERALIZED SEIZURES

Absence Seizures. Absence seizures with 3-Hz spike-and-wave discharges are short interruptions of consciousness that last from 3 to 15 seconds each. They are not associated with auras or other evidence of focal onset. Absence seizures begin and end abruptly and recur from a few to several hundred times per day. Ongoing behavior stops. While otherwise immobile, the patient may show inconspicuous flickering of the eyelids or eyebrows at about 3 times/second; there may be simple automatic movements, such as rubbing the nose, putting a hand to the face, or chewing and swallowing. Falling or loss of muscle tone does not occur. Immediately after the short interruption of awareness, the individual is again mentally clear and fully capable of continuing previous activity.

In absence seizures of this type, bilaterally synchronous 3-Hz spike-and-wave discharges usually occur against otherwise normal background activity (Fig. 145–3). The age

at onset of these short absence seizures is almost always after the age of 2½ years; they almost never occur for the first time after age 20. Individuals with short absence seizures rarely have other neurologic problems, but 40 to 50% of patients have infrequent, easily controlled, generalized tonic-clonic seizures. Photic sensitivity is present in some cases (Fig. 145–4).

It is preferable to discard the term "petit mal"; if it is used, it should be reserved for these short absences. "Petit mal" has been widely used to describe many other types of seizures, a practice that often led to the improper choice of anticonvulsants. Absences clinically similar to the type described above may occur in brain-damaged patients, a combination called the *Lennox-Gastaut syndrome,* but the episodes occur less frequently and are of longer duration; the EEG includes slower (1.5–2 Hz) spike-and-wave discharges and continuous abnormalities in the background activity (Fig. 145–5). Short periods of unresponsiveness, which also occur in patients with complex partial seizures, are usually easily distinguished from the generalized absence seizures with 3-Hz spike-and-wave discharges because complex partial seizures are preceded by auras or special sensory symptoms, last longer, and are followed by confusion or sleepiness. In complex partial seizures, the EEG typically shows focal interictal spikes, most often from the temporal lobe.

Prolonged behavioral changes rarely continue for a day or more, though this is more likely to occur with absence seizures accompanied by continuous 3-Hz spike-and-wave discharges than with complex partial seizures. In either case, the patient performs activity in a confused manner with varying degree of depression of consciousness and amnesia.

Tonic-Clonic Seizures. Generalized tonic-clonic seizures occur at some time in the course of epilepsy in most patients with seizures regardless of the patient's usual clinical pattern. A tonic-clonic seizure is classified under generalized seizures if the attack itself, the neurologic examination, and the EEG all indicate that bilateral cerebral structures are simultaneously involved at the onset. A tonic-clonic seizure is classified as a partial seizure evolving to a secondarily generalized seizure if the criteria cited above indicate the attack began in one hemisphere and then spread to produce a major generalized attack.

Tonic-clonic convulsions usually last 3 to 5

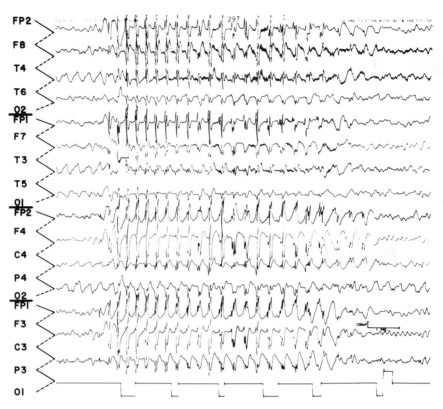

Fig. 145–3. EEG of patient undergoing absence seizure. 3-Hz spike-and-wave discharges begin and end abruptly. Patient involuntarily stopped hyperventilating at beginning of discharge and resumed hyperventilation when it was over. In the lowest line, auditory stimuli are signalled by downward deflection of the pen. When the patient recognizes the stimulus, he presses a button that deflects the pen upward. During the attack, the patient is unable to signal recognition of sound until 3-Hz spike-and-wave discharge has subsided.

minutes. Whether primarily or secondarily generalized following the spread of partial seizures, the convulsions are characterized by complete loss of consciousness and falling. The onset is sometimes accompanied by a high-pitched cry caused by forcible expiration against opposed vocal cords, which results from sudden involuntary contraction of the respiratory and laryngeal muscles. As the patient falls, the body stiffens because of generalized tonic contraction of the axial and limb muscles. The legs usually extend and the arms flex partially. The initial generalized contractions may be asymmetric, particularly if the attack had a partial beginning. During this tonic phase, which lasts less than a minute, respiration stops because of sustained contraction of the respiratory muscles; pallor or cyanosis may be seen. After the tonic stage, jerking or clonic (interrupted tonic) movements occur in all four limbs for less than a minute. The tongue is sometimes bitten because of involuntary contractions of the masticatory muscles. Urinary incontinence may

occur. Increased salivation and deep breathing may cause frothing at the mouth. A period of continued but more relaxed unconsciousness follows and lasts for about a minute. After this, the patient is confused, sleepy, and uncooperative for several minutes before full recovery. During the period of postictal confusion, the person sometimes performs actions automatically, such as undressing for bed or resisting restraint. There is amnesia for the seizure and for the behavior during the confused period.

Myoclonic Seizures. Myoclonic seizures are involuntary contractions of limb and truncal muscles that are sudden, brief, and recurrent. Like other seizure types, they occur with a variety of diseases including viral infections, anoxia, and progressive cerebral degenerations. Single myoclonic jerks that occur at or shortly after the onset of sleep are not seizures. Slight bilaterally symmetric myoclonic movements often occur in patients who have absence seizures with 3-Hz spike-and-wave complexes (petit mal), but rarely are severe

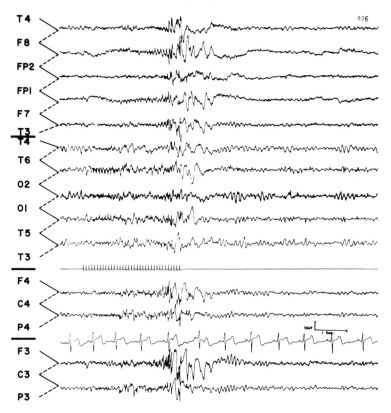

Fig. 145–4. EEG of patient with photic sensitive epilepsy. Stimuli at 10 flashes/second (line 11) precipitate generalized multiple spikes followed by spike-and-wave discharges that outlast photic stimulation.

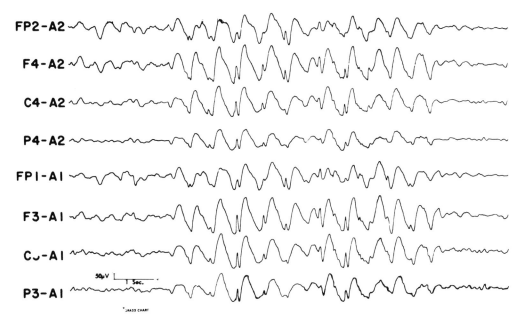

Fig. 145–5. Generalized major and atonic seizures with mental retardation. Slow spike-and-wave discharges (2 Hz) are superimposed on poorly organized background. This is typical of clinical condition sometimes called the Lennox-Gastaut syndrome.

bilaterally symmetric myoclonic jerks the predominant symptoms of individuals with 3-Hz spike-and-wave complexes. Generalized myoclonic movements are also seen in patients who have primarily generalized major attacks.

Randomly distributed asymmetric myoclonus usually indicates diffuse brain dysfunction, particularly including involvement of the upper brain stem. Myoclonus may occasionally occur from spinal lesions. Bilaterally symmetric myoclonic movements in infants with tonic spasms are discussed in the next section and other forms of myoclonus are discussed elsewhere in this volume.

Atonic Seizures. Atonic or astatic seizures usually begin in childhood and are characterized by sudden loss of postural tone. Sometimes this causes the child to drop abruptly to the ground. The episodes occur without warning, are extremely short, and frequently cause injury. Sometimes the decrease in muscle tone is less complete and causes only slumping or head-drop. If consciousness is lost, it is regained within a few moments of the loss of tone. The attacks are most often seen in retarded children with other evidence of brain abnormality; atonic seizures persist into adulthood. The interictal EEG usually shows slow-spike or multiple spike-and-wave complexes at 1 to 2.5 Hz between attacks (see Fig. 145–5). The seizures are particularly difficult to treat and do not respond to drugs that are effective in generalized short absence seizures. Atonic seizures are often associated with the Lennox-Gastaut syndrome.

Epileptic Syndromes

Febrile Convulsions. Single or recurrent primarily generalized seizures in infancy and early childhood may be associated only with fever in about 4% of the population and are usually benign. At first, it is difficult to separate these benign febrile convulsions (due to extracerebral infection) from seizures caused by brain damage due to unrecognized meningitis or by congenital brain defects. Signs of benign prognosis include onset between ages 6 months and 4 years, a normal EEG within a week after the seizure, absence of clinical signs of brain damage, and lack of atypical features or excessive duration of the attack. The chances of additional febrile seizures are about one in two if the first episode occurs before age 14 months. Recurrent attacks are much less likely (perhaps one in six) if the first attack occurs after age 33 months. The

movements are bilateral but may show unilateral elements. After recovery from febrile seizures, few children have attacks in later life, but it is not always possible to predict whether subsequent febrile or nonfebrile seizures will follow.

Neonatal Seizures. Seizures in the neonatal period differ in both the manifestations and cause from those seen later in infancy and childhood. They are characterized by variable, fragmentary, and migratory patterns and do not fit well into the International Classification. There are unilateral postural changes that vary from one side to another, mouth movements, deviation of the eyes, apnea, and shifting tonic or clonic movements. The most common causes of neonatal seizures are congenital malformations, hypoglycemia, hypocalcemia, anoxia, infections, and intracranial birth injuries. Focal seizures in neonates do not necessarily indicate focal damage; they also occur with metabolic causes. Neonatal seizures are often classified as minimal, multifocal clonic, tonic, and myoclonic. An EEG during the course of an attack may be normal, but shifting paroxysmal discharges associated with shifting patterns of clinical seizures are more usual. Taken together, the characteristic EEG abnormalities, the clinical attacks, and the cause are usually accurate indicators of the prognosis.

Infantile Spasms. Infantile spasms or West syndrome is a disorder of infancy and early childhood characterized by abrupt, short duration, flexions of the body, waist, and neck. It has a highly characteristic EEG pattern known as hypsarrhythmia (Fig. 145–6). The tonic spasms are bilaterally symmetric, last up to several seconds each, and occur many times a day, usually in clusters. The infants may also display more rapid generalized myoclonic jerks and abrupt head drops. In most cases, the onset is between ages 3 and 8 months, but rarely is as early as 1 week or as late as 2 years.

More than 75% of infants with infantile spasms and hypsarrhythmia are later found to be mentally defective. Causes of the syndrome include perinatal brain damage, metabolic disease (e.g., phenylketonuria, lipidosis, or pyridoxine deficiency), congenital malformations, anoxia, subdural hematoma, and infections or immunizations. In about half the patients, however, no cause is found.

Before age 5, the tonic spasms and the hypsarrhythmic EEG disappear. The consistency of the time of appearance and disap-

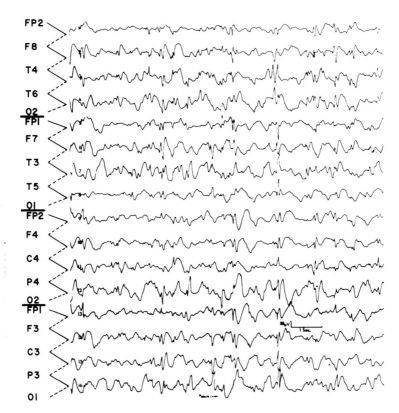

Fig. 145–6. EEG of infant with tonic spasms. High-voltage rhythmic and arrhythmic slow waves in delta range and spikes and irregular spike-and-wave discharges in generalized and random distribution appear in all areas. This constellation of abnormalities is called hypsarrhythmia. (Calibration: 50 μV and 1 second.)

pearance of the tonic spasms and of the hypsarrhythmic EEG with age indicates that maturation processes play a large part in the manifestations of this syndrome. Often, no further seizures occur and the EEG beomes normal. If seizures persist, they may be generalized tonic-clonic, atonic, or partial seizures with appropriate EEG abnormalities. A combination of such seizures with mental deficiency and associated with slow spike-and-wave discharges (see Fig. 145–5) is known as the *Lennox-Gastaut syndrome.*

Benign Rolandic Epilepsy. This relatively common disorder beomes manifest between the ages of 3 and 13 years and is associated with a typical EEG pattern (Fig. 145–7). Seizures occur infrequently and have a self-limited course, with no seizures after age 16 years. The seizures are characterized by unilateral paresthesias of the face and mouth or unilateral tonic or clonic movements of the facial muscles with speech arrest. Loss of consciousness and generalized convulsions may follow, particularly in attacks during sleep. The interictal EEG abnormalities are prominent in sleep but are not present in the awake

record in some 30% of cases. The background EEG activity is normal, but is interrupted by high voltage spikes that recur at short intervals in the central midtemporal areas (see Fig. 145–7). The spikes are usually unilateral but often shift in laterality during a single recording or become bilaterally synchronous. Generalized spike-and-wave discharges also sometimes occur during sleep. The diagnosis of benign rolandic epilepsy is made on the basis of the typical seizures and characteristic EEG in an otherwise intact child. The seizures disappear and the EEG becomes normal by age 16 years whether or not anticonvulsant medication is used. Carbamazepine in moderate dosage is used to prevent recurrent attacks but should be discontinued after 1 or 2 years if the EEG has returned to normal.

Juvenile Myoclonic Epilepsy. This entity usually begins between ages 12 and 19 years. Recurrent series of bilateral myoclonic jerks or spasms occur in the early morning after waking and sometimes are followed by generalized convulsions. The interictal EEG record is characteristic and shows bursts of generalized rapid (3 to 6 Hz) spike-and-wave and

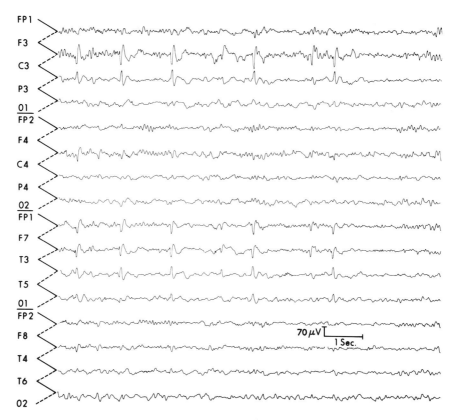

Fig. 145–7. A 9-year-old boy with benign rolandic epilepsy shows normal sleep patterns interrupted by high-voltage recurrent spikes in wide field over central temporal area. Field covered by spikes is sufficiently large to span left rolandic and sylvian fissures. Laterality of spikes may shift from side to side during recording.

multiple spike-and-wave complexes. During the actual myoclonic episodes, 10 to 16 Hz spikes occur. Valproic acid effectively controls both the myoclonus and the generalized convulsions in nearly all cases. However, even after several years of complete control, both types of attacks may recur after withdrawal of medication.

Reflex Epilepsy. Many stimuli (e.g., flickering light, touch, sound or music, the effort to read, speak, and write) may precipitate either focal or generalized seizures. Seizures can also be inhibited by sensory stimuli or conditioned reflexes. Although seizures may seem to occur only after a specific precipitating event, more often the specific stimulation is only one factor among others, recognized or unrecognized, that influence the convulsive disorder. In most patients with seizures that are precipitated by specific stimuli, few seizures are induced by the specific stimuli and more are spontaneous. Reflex epilepsy is extremely rare as an isolated entity.

Nonepileptic Syndromes with Convulsive Symptoms

Breathholding Spells. Pain, anger, and frustration cause some children to hold their breath until they become anoxic, lose consciousness, and fall. The anoxia and syncope result from one of two types of circulatory response, vasodepressor or cardiac asystole. The syncope is usually the only manifestation, but sometimes there are brief bilateral tonic or clonic movements, and sometimes generalized major convulsions ensue. The characteristic clinical feature of the breathholding spell that differentiates it from a true seizure disorder is that all attacks are precipitated by and are associated with apnea. Breathholding spells are not episodes of a true convulsive disorder, but rather of convulsive syncope with the convulsive features that result from anoxia. These spells rarely persist beyond age 3.

Tussive, Micturition, and Valsalva-Maneuver Syncope. Coughing, micturition, or forcibly exhaling against a closed glottis reduces cardiac output and results in cerebral anoxia with unconsciousness in susceptible individuals. Venous return to the right side of the heart is impeded by the raised intrathoracic pressure and vagal effects cause bradycardia and peripheral vasodilatation. The anoxic syncope is sometimes followed by brief tonic or clonic movements and rarely by generalized convulsions. This is not a convulsive disorder in the true sense and is called *"convulsive syncope."* Tussive syncope is most often seen in corpulent adults with cardiopulmonary disorders.

Other disorders may cause intermittent symptoms that may be confused with seizures; among them are paroxysmal choreoathetosis, migraine, benign paroxysmal vertigo, and TIAs.

Evaluating the Patient

An accurate history is critical when evaluating a patient with a seizure disorder of recent onset. Only rarely does the physician witness the seizures. Thus, it is necessary to rely on the patient's recollection and the observations of witnesses. Without both sources of information, it may be difficult or impossible to classify the seizure accurately. It is important to ask about premonitory symptoms; recollection of sensory, motor, or psychic experiences at onset; behavior during the seizure; evidence of lateralization; and postictal condition. A family history may indicate a genetic influence. Information about infancy and childhood is needed; adults often neglect to mention childhood seizures that may be of diagnostic importance. The review of systems should include questions about drug or alcohol abuse as well as systemic diseases. Physical examination, including neurologic, may point to a systemic disease or a focal neurologic disorder that causes seizures.

Laboratory Evaluation. It is not always possible to evaluate patients for every possible cause of seizures. Appropriate studies vary with the age and individual circumstances of the patient. Abnormalities noted in history or physical examination should be pursued; routine laboratory examinations evaluate possible metabolic abnormality and serve as baseline values for patients who are to be given medication. These include blood count, urinary analysis, fasting blood glucose, electrolyte determinations, and a measure of renal function.

Lumbar puncture should be performed for most infants with new-onset seizures and for older children or adults if intracranial infection is suspected or the etiology of seizures is unclear.

In patients with partial seizures or focal findings on neurologic or EEG examination, brain CT or MRI is mandatory because neoplasms, arteriovenous malformations, focal atrophy, or congenital abnormalities are found in about 30% of these patients. In contrast, patients with generalized seizures and no evidence of focal disease, CT and MRI abnormalities are found much less frequently. MRI may demonstrate structural brain disease even when CT is normal. Both are especially useful in evaluating patients if surgical therapy is considered. Radiographs of the skull may occasionally reveal intracranial calcifications or evidence of old trauma, but are normal in most patients and are not routinely obtained.

An EEG is essential for both diagnosis and treatment. The EEG is a record of potential changes that are generated by neurons in the cerebral cortex underlying each of 16 or more electrodes on the scalp. The potentials are amplified about a million times to activate a bank of writing arms that inscribe a permanent record on moving paper. The *International Placement* or *10–20 System* is standard for placement of scalp electrodes. Additional placements are used in evaluating convulsive disorders: *nasopharyngeal electrodes* are inserted through the nostrils and *sphenoidal needle electrodes* are inserted, using sterile technique, through the skin above the mandibular notch toward the foramen ovale. These placements often clarify abnormalities from the anterior and mediotemporal areas that are not clearly defined by scalp electrodes.

Although equipment with eight channels of simultaneous recording is sometimes adequate, 16 or more channels allow simultaneous comparison of activity from all or nearly all electrodes used. Most commercial equipment faithfully reproduces waves between 1 and 40 Hz and there are controls to diminish interference from noncerebral potentials. Although frequencies below 1 Hz occur in association with epileptiform discharges, higher-voltage slow artifacts from changes in skin resistance and electrode polarization prevent routine clinical recording of these slow potential changes.

In the normal relaxed adult, two frequency bands are usually seen: alpha activity at 8 to 13 Hz in the posterior regions of the head and beta activity at 14 to 35 Hz more anteriorly. Activity underlying the EEG from the cortex of an unanesthetized patient shows dominant alpha in the posterior temporal, parietal, and occipital areas. Continuous 25-Hz activity is seen in the perirolandic area and 17- to 20-Hz activity mixed with 6- to 8-Hz waves is found in the intermediate frontal areas. Some normal EEG activity can be confused with epileptiform discharges. For instance, runs of positive spikes at 6 and 14 Hz are common, particularly during sleep in normal children or young adults. They are most evident in the temporal and occipital areas, occurring bilaterally or independently on either side. Lambda waves are sharp waves generated in the occipital areas during visual scanning. The major phase is electropositive; these waves are also normal phenomena. Similar forms of the same distribution and polarity, called "lambdoid waves" or "positive occipital sharp waves of sleep," are found in early stage-II sleep and can be mistaken for epileptic activity. Spikes of unusual form and distribution, *small sharp spikes* (SSS) or *benign epileptiform transients* (BETs), are also normal and must be differentiated from true epileptogenic activity.

Interictal EEGs from Epileptogenic Foci. Interictal EEG epileptiform activity is helpful in confirming the presence of epilepsy but is not diagnostic. The interseizure EEG form that is most indicative of an epileptogenic focus is a focal spike. It is a localized triangular form that is distinct from the background and has a duration of 20 to 80 milliseconds. Triangular forms lasting 80 to 250 milliseconds, or *sharp waves*, are equally characteristic of an epileptogenic focus. Sharp waves and spikes may be monophasic, diphasic, or triphasic, with the largest phase usually electronegative. Spikes and sharp waves are often followed by slower waves and may take on the form of localized spike-and-wave complexes. Even though both the site of origin of a discharge and the underlying lesion may be discrete, the EEG may display abnormalities in remote areas. This is particularly true of discharges originating in the frontal and temporal lobes owing to the richness of commissural and deep connections.

Abnormal EEGs are usually found in epilepsy, but many patients with seizures have normal EEGs. The exact percentage varies depending on the seizure type and frequency, the circumstances under which the EEG is obtained, and the number of EEGs performed. Methods for increasing the likelihood of recording epileptiform discharges include obtaining records during sleep and after sleep deprivation, hyperventilation, and photic stimulation. If EEGs are still normal after these techniques have been used, the chances that the symptoms are epileptic are considerably reduced.

Only a small fraction of spikes and sharp waves that arise in a cortical focus are evident in the scalp EEG because of the distance between the electrode and the cortex and because only a small surface area is involved in generating the spike. Whether a spike at the cortex is seen at all in the EEG (and its amplitude if it is seen) is related more to the extent of projected synchronous discharging around the focus than to the size of the structural lesion itself. Thus, in a given patient, spikes may be seen in one EEG examination and not in another; spikes in the EEG from a single focus may shift to become maximal in different adjacent electrodes. In addition to spikes and sharp waves, focal rhythmic waves in the alpha-, beta-, or delta-frequency ranges may also suggest a local epileptogenic area. Areas of abnormal cortex may be extensive and an entire hemisphere may be epileptogenic with multiple independent foci.

Focal epileptiform discharges are easy to localize when they arise from the convexity of one hemisphere. Some focal discharges, however, are limited to the uncal region, insular cortex, and hippocampal gyrus, with little or no abnormal activity projected to the areas accessible to the scalp electrodes. Nasopharyngeal or sphenoidal electrodes are then useful. In some seizure patients, the EEG shows only focal nonparoxysmal abnormalities. Focal polymorphic delta or theta waves associated with local depression of usual alpha and beta waves indicate a structural lesion. When such focal patterns are evident, with or without spikes, in a patient with clinical seizures, the seizures almost always originate from that vicinity.

After surgical removal of an epileptogenic region, EEG abnormalities in the homologous area of the opposite hemisphere may persist for a time and then disappear. These discharges constitute a *"mirror focus."* The mirror focus before surgery often shows spikes that are independent in timing and form from the primary focus and at times may be more prominent than the primary focus. Although the differentiation of an independent contralateral focus from a mirror focus in surgical candidates has not been fully clarified by EEG techniques, useful EEG methods for this purpose include: asymmetry of barbiturate-induced fast activity (recorded from sphenoidal and nasopharyngeal electrodes), activation of the focus by intracarotid injections of rapidly acting barbiturates, and the use of depth electrodes and recording the EEG and seizures simultaneously on closed circuit television. Results of surgical treatment are usually better in patients with unilateral temporal lobe discharges than in bilateral foci, but this is not uniformly so. In one study, seven patients with apparently bilateral foci had small unilateral tumors and all benefited from operation. Spontaneous spiking in those cases did not lateralize sufficiently and lateralization was based on other factors including diminution of barbiturate-induced fast activity at the sphenoidal electrode on the side of the lesion.

EEGs During Partial Seizures. In a clinical seizure, electrical discharges begin locally and spread unilaterally or bilaterally. A common type of ictal EEG sequence is ushered in by a short period of local or generalized voltage depression, followed by localized low-voltage 10- to 13-Hz activity that progressively increases in amplitude to become spikes that spread throughout one or both hemispheres. As this electrical sequence continues, the intervals between spikes progressively increase and slow waves intervene, resulting in spike-and-wave complexes of increasing duration until the ictal discharge abruptly ceases. There are many variations on this basic sequence. One type begins with low-voltage rhythmic theta waves, followed locally by beta waves of increasing amplitude and decreasing frequency until spike-and-wave forms appear. Some focal seizures begin as low-voltage multiphasic spikes or spike-and-wave complexes that simply increase in amplitude and decrease in frequency of occurrence until the ictal discharge ends. Transition from interictal to ictal discharges can also be a burst of local monoformic theta waves followed by spike-and-wave complexes. In adults, a slow wave focus not previously present, which persists for hours after an attack, indicates there may be an underlying structural lesion.

The progression of electrical changes in focal seizures that originate in the temporal lobe, orbital gyrus, or insula correlates well with the clinical events. By the time automatisms become clinically apparent, bilateral subcortical structures are involved and normal background EEG activity is disrupted bilaterally. Paroxysmal activity is not always apparent in scalp recordings during clinical seizures. In one study, about 20% of patients who had seizures that were clinically typical of temporal-lobe origin and chemically activated showed no recognizable paroxysmal EEG changes at the scalp. In these cases, seizure discharges were often found in the medial-temporal structures by nasopharyngeal, sphenoidal, or depth electrodes.

Interictal and Ictal EEGs of Generalized Seizures. Interictal and ictal abnormalities in patients having 3-Hz spike-and-wave complexes with absence seizures differ only in the duration of the burst of spike-and-wave discharges. When discharges are longer than 3.5 seconds, a clinical absence is usually recognized and can be detected in 1 second using click stimuli (see Fig. 145–3). The bursts and clinical attacks usually last 3 to 15 seconds. The complexes initially occur at about 3 Hz and usually decrease to about 2.5 Hz in a few seconds. Interseizure patterns in generalized tonic-clonic seizures of unknown etiology often show bursts of more rapid spike-and-wave complexes that are bilaterally synchronous at 3.5 to 4.5 Hz. Interictal bilateral bursts at 4 to 7 Hz are also seen. In both cases, the EEG during a seizure usually begins with generalized suppression for a second or more, followed by spikes of low voltage that gradually increase in amplitude and decrease in frequency. Seconds later, the repetition rate of the spikes decreases and spike-and-wave complexes of increasing duration appear in a similar manner to that described after generalization of partial attacks.

Hyperventilation and photic stimulation frequently precipitate or increase the incidence of bilateral paroxysmal discharges in seizure disorders characterized by primary engagement of bilateral structures (see Fig. 145–4).

CONDITIONS ACCOMPANIED BY SEIZURES

In most cases of epilepsy, the cause or condition thought responsible for the seizures can be identified. Some diseases or injuries of the brain are associated with a high incidence of seizures; in others the incidence is only slightly higher than in the general population.

The list of conditions frequently accompanied by seizures is extensive and includes: cerebral dysgenesis, birth injuries, meningitis, encephalitis, cerebral trauma, tumors, abscesses, granulomas, parasitic cysts, degenerative diseases of the nervous system, metabolic disturbances or intoxications (e.g., uremia, water, and alcoholic), cerebral edema, cerebral vascular lesions, polycythemia, asphyxia, carbon-monoxide poisoning, protein shock, anaphylaxis, Raynaud disease, Stokes-Adams syndrome, carotid sinus sensitivity, tetany, insulin shock, hyperventilation, ingestion of convulsant drugs, and withdrawal from alcohol and drugs, particularly barbiturates. Seizures associated with alcohol withdrawal typically appear 9 to 48 hours after cessation of drinking; after barbiturate withdrawal, seizures occur in 24 to 72 hours. The frequency of the association of organic diseases with seizures that began before the age of 21 is given in Table 145–6.

Isolated seizures after drug withdrawal or other accidental causes do not justify a diagnosis of epilepsy, which requires recurrence of spontaneous seizures.

It is likely that the figure of 43.81% given in Table 145–6 for demonstrable causes of epileptic seizures is excessively low. Bergamini et al. found that only 30% of patients with complex partial seizures had evidence of a probable cause, but Falconer found obvious organic lesions (e.g., temporal sclerosis, small tumors, scars, and infarct) in 78% of patients with the same seizure type who were subjected to surgery for complex partial seizures of temporal-lobe origin.

The frequency of convulsive seizures in organic diseases of the brain is not directly related to the severity or degree of cerebral damage. The incidence of convulsive seizures, although significantly greater than in the general population, is low when brain damage spares the cerebral cortex, such as in parkinsonism and posterior fossa and diencephalic lesions.

Treatment

The treatment of patients with convulsive seizures can be considered in four parts: (1) identification and elimination of factors that might cause or precipitate attacks; (2) drug therapy to prevent attacks; (3) sustaining mental and physical health; and (4) surgical therapy in selected patients with seizures of focal origin.

Identification and Elimination of Factors. The elimination of factors that cause seizures requires the identification and treatment of structural or physiologic abnormalities discovered in the examination. Examples include removal of an operable brain tumor or vascular malformation, treatment of infections or metabolic abnormalities, and correction of drug dependence. Surgical removal of damaged tissue resulting from traumatic or vascular brain injuries will be discussed later.

PHARMACOLOGIC THERAPY

The basic approach to anticonvulsant therapy is to select an appropriate drug for the specific type of seizure disorder and to progressively increase the dose until seizures are controlled or toxic side effects limit further increments.

The size of the increment and the interval between dose adjustments should be guided by pharmacokinetic characteristics with sufficient time between dose adjustments to evaluate the prior change. Measurements of serum drug concentration during this period are helpful. If seizures are not controlled or toxicity is evident, a second drug can be carefully substituted or in some cases added to the first. Rarely, it may be necessary to use more than two drugs to achieve maximal control. Monotherapy, the use of a single agent, is always preferable to multidrug therapy, but can be unsuccessful. Prescribing more than one anticonvulsant at the onset of treatment

Table 145–6.   Etiology of Epilepsy in 782 Cases of Known Cause

Etiology	No. of Cases	Percentages*	
Brain injuries	318	40.7	(17.82)
Craniocerebral trauma	218	27.9	(12.21)
Infectious etiology (including postinfectious and postimmunization encephalitides)	213	27.2	(11.93)
CNS malformations and congenital metabolic diseases	33	4.2	(1.85)
TOTAL	782	100.00	(43.81)

*Percentages in parentheses refer to the entire sample of 1785 cases excluding cases with seizures secondary to tumors.
(From Bergamini L, Bergamasco B, Benna P, and Gilli M. Epilepsia 1977; 18:437–444.)

is not recommended because most patients can be controlled with a single drug; a second drug may be unnecessary and will increase toxicity and cost. Further, when two drugs are given simultaneously, adverse effects cannot accurately be ascribed to either one and both drugs may have to be withdrawn.

One of the major causes of drug therapy failure is noncompliance. Patients with persistently low anticonvulsant serum concentrations should be asked how they take the medication. Frequently, the patient has misunderstood directions, had unpleasant side-effects, or, for complex psychological reasons, failed to take prescribed doses. Education, simplification of the dosage schedule, or reducing the number of drugs often helps. It is important to recognize noncompliance because it serves no purpose to add a second or third medication if the patient is not taking the first one. Measurement of serum drug concentration helps in identifying noncompliance, but on occasion noncompliance must be distinguished from rapid metabolism.

Clinical Pharmacology. Anticonvulsant drug serum concentrations provide pharmacokinetic data on individual patients to guide dosage and to evaluate toxicity and drug interactions. The range of therapeutic concentrations has been established for most of the major anticonvulsants (Table 145–7). The upper levels usually are those of minimal toxicity rather than maximal therapeutic benefit and there is a wide variation of optimal dose in individual patients. Serum levels should be used as a guide in each case rather than as an absolute goal. If seizures have been completely controlled with no clinical toxicity, but a high serum concentration it is not appropriate to lower the dosage merely to achieve a "therapeutic level." It is also inappropriate to raise levels if complete control is obtained with lower than "therapeutic levels."

Drug Toxicity. All drugs used in the treatment of seizures have significant side effects. Table 145–8 lists the common manifestations of chronic use of anticonvulsants. The commonest toxic side effects associated with chronic anticonvulsant therapy are subtle impairments of cognition, alertness and motor function. A listing of all known side effects would be formidable. Fortunately, many are dose-related and can be eliminated by adjusting the dose. Serious side effects are rare, but physicians using antileptic drugs must be aware of the potential toxicity of each agent. Many chronic side effects can be treated by drug withdrawal, but occasionally, specific therapies are needed.

Acute allergic reactions can occur with any drug. An allergic manifestation is always an indication for immediate withdrawal of the offending drug. Diagnosis of dose-related symptoms is confirmed by measurement of drug serum concentration and may be due to excessive dose, peculiarities in individual rates of drug metabolism, or interactions with other drugs. Drug interactions may involve other anticonvulsant agents, drugs used to treat systemic diseases, or may be caused by interference with drug metabolism (e.g., isoniazid) or serum protein-binding (e.g., val-

Table 145–7. Antiepileptic Drugs

Generic Name	Common Trade Name	Serum Concentration* $\mu g/ml$	Elimination Half-Life† (hrs)	Time to Steady State (days)
Phenytoin	Dilantin‡	10–20	24 ± 6	7–8
Phenobarbital	————§	15–30	96 ± 24	>21
Primidone	Mysoline	8–12	6 ± 3	4–7
Ethosuximide	Zarontin	40–120	48 ± 12	7–10
Carbamazepine	Tegretol	6–12	20 ± 5	3–4
Clonazepam	Clonopin	13–72‖	30 ± 10	6
Valproate/ Divalproex	Depakene/ Depakote	50–100	6 ± 20	1–4

*Serum concentration usually associated with therapeutic effectiveness and minimal toxicity.

†Approximate half-life in adults. There may be considerable individual variation and values may be influenced by other drugs. Values tend to be age dependent, shortened in children and lengthened in neonates.

‡Because of substantial differences in bioavailability of generic preparations, phenytoin should be prescribed by brand name.

§Many manufacturers supply phenobarbital as the generic drug.

‖ng/ml

Table 145–8. Chronic Toxicity of Antiepileptic Drugs*

Drug	Side Effects
Phenytoin	Choreoathetosis
	Encephalopathy
	Hirsutism
	Gingival hyperplasia
	Peripheral neuropathy
	Pseudolymphoma
	Lupus erythematosus
	Hyperglycemia
	Megaloblastic anemia
	Hypocalcemia
Barbiturates	Depression
	Drowsiness
	Megaloblastic anemia
	Hyponatremia
Carbamazepine	Aplastic anemia
	Megaloblastic anemia
	Hyponatremia
Valproate	Platelet dysfunctions
	Hepatic necrosis
	Pancreatitis
	Menstrual irregularities
	Alopecia
	Weight gain
Clonazepam	Weight gain
Ethosuximide	Encephalopathy
	Lupus erythematosus

*Does not include acute, dose-related toxicity, allergic reactions, or drug interactions.

proic acid). Antiepileptic drugs may potentiate (e.g., warfarin) or diminish (e.g., oral contraceptives) the effectiveness of drugs used for other purposes. It is impossible to predict all interactions, but clinicians should be aware that drug interaction may be involved in producing increased serum drug concentrations and toxicity.

Pregnancy and Teratogenesis. Pregnancy does not significantly increase the frequency of seizures in most patients when serum levels are maintained. The rate of spontaneous abortions is higher in mothers with epilepsy and their children are 1.5 to 4 times more likely to have congenital malformations than are children of nonepileptic mothers. Most, if not all, anticonvulsants can contribute to teratogenic effects. For example, phenytoin and phenobarbital increase the incidence of cleft lip and cleft palate and can lead to a pattern of dysmorphic abnormalities. Valproic acid has been linked to neural tube and other defects and should be avoided when possible in women of childbearing age. Women who may

become pregnant should be advised about the increased incidence and types of congenital abnormalities due to either drugs or seizures. When feasible, anticonvulsant drugs should be discontinued before attempting to become pregnant and through at least the first trimester. Usually, however, seizure frequency and severity are too great to permit stopping drug therapy and an anticonvulsant should be continued. It is not known which anticonvulsant is safest in pregnancy, and prospective parents should be informed so they can participate in all decisions.

Treatment of Specific Seizure Types. Generalized tonic-clonic seizures usually respond to phenytoin, phenobarbital, primidone, carbamazepine, or valproic acid. In one controlled study comparing effectiveness of phenytoin, phenobarbital and carbamazepine, there was no clear advantage of one over the other so selection among the drugs depends on the physician's experience and the patient's response. Because phenytoin and carbamazepine are not sedative, they are usually preferred over phenobarbital. Usually carbamazepine is preferred in children and women because of gingival hyperplasia, hypertrichosis, and coarsening of features that can occur with phenytoin. Whether valproic acid is as effective as the other drugs in the treatment of generalized tonic-clonic seizures is not yet known. Unless other compounds have failed or are known to be ineffective, valproic acid should not be used in the first 2 years of life because of a relatively high incidence of fatal hepatic failure in infancy.

Generalized absence seizures can be treated with ethosuximide or valproic acid. Ethosuximide is the drug of choice in generalized absence seizures that meet typical clinical and EEG criteria as described earlier in this section. Atypical absence attacks do not usually respond to ethosuximide. Conversely, other than valproic acid, drugs effective in treating other seizure types have no effect in typical generalized absence attacks. Reduction or abolition of generalized 3-Hz spike-and-wave discharges in the EEG is the best laboratory index of effective treatment; monitoring serum drug concentrations helps in evaluating compliance and toxicity.

Partial seizures respond to the same drugs used for generalized tonic-clonic seizures. Carbamazepine and phenytoin are the most effective and have less bothersome side effects than the barbiturates. Valproic acid is less useful in treating partial seizures and should be reserved for resistant cases. Complex partial seizures tend to be difficult to treat and may require combinations of drugs. It is important to start with a single agent and gradually increase the dosage to the maximum tolerated before substituting or adding a new drug.

Tonic, myoclonic, atypical absence, and atonic seizures occur more frequently in children and may be due to several different causes, genetic or acquired. Typical tonic spasms (infantile spasms) respond to ACTH therapy (20 to 40 units/day) and resist most standard anticonvulsants. Tonic spasms and other myoclonic conditions may respond to valproic acid or clonazepam, but frequently resist all drug therapy, individually or in combination. The ketogenic diet may be helpful, but because 80% of total calories is derived from fats, it is unpalatable and difficult to maintain. However, it may provide a measure of control in otherwise uncontrolled children.

Between 2 and 5% of children aged 3 months to 5 years have a febrile convulsion that occurs without evidence of central nervous system infection or damage. In about one third, the seizures recur with fever but are gone before age 5 years. Typical cases are not considered subjects for anticonvulsant therapy as only 3% ever display nonfebrile attacks. Parents should be encouraged to treat developing fever vigorously with antipyretics and cooling. In atypical cases with abnormal neurologic examination, prolonged or focal seizures, or an immediate family history of afebrile seizures prophylactic treatment with appropriate doses of phenobarbital should be considered after careful weighing of risk and benefit.

Starting and Stopping Drugs. Instituting chronic anticonvulsant treatment is a major therapeutic intervention, undertaken only after careful evaluation of the patient. Seizures resulting from specific provocative events such as alcohol withdrawal or sleep deprivation do not require long-term therapy. Even after a single "unprovoked" seizure the patient may not have recurrent attacks and may not need treatment. The cause of the seizure, EEG findings, and personal views of the patient must be considered.

Stopping antiepileptic drugs may also be a difficult decision. A period of 2 to 4 seizure-free years on medication is usually a minimum requirement. Signs of brain damage, duration of epilepsy, type and number of seizures before control, EEG, and current circumstances are considered. Recent reports emphasize the value of the EEG in this determination. After several years of complete control in unselected cases the recurrence rate is about 30% in children. Criteria for discontinuing drug treatment seem more reliable for children than for adults. Withdrawal of anticonvulsants generates a risk that the patient must weigh against the potential benefits of successful termination of drug treatment.

The recurrence risk in adults is only slightly higher than in children, but the consequences of recurrence in terms of holding jobs and having a license to drive can be considerably more threatening to adults. Therefore, when considering withdrawal of medication, one must weigh not just the statistical risk of a recurrence but the significance to the patient. Recent studies indicate that adults with normal EEGs who have been completely free of seizures for 2 years and have no other risk factors have a 70% chance of no recurrence after discontinuing medication.

Use of Specific Drugs. An enormous literature on the pharmacology of each of the anticonvulsant agents has accumulated and detailed discussion of each agent can be found in the references.

Phenytoin. This drug was introduced for clinical practice in 1938 by Merritt and Putnam. They discovered the anticonvulsive activity in animals, established effectiveness in humans, and described the major toxic effects. Over the years, phenytoin has proven remarkably effective in the treatment of partial seizures and generalized tonic-clonic seizures. It prevents the spread of seizure activity from abnormally discharging neurons to normal surrounding cells. It is thought to act by reducing ion movements through cell membranes. Treatment of seizures in adults is usually started with 200 to 400 mg daily (5–7 mg/kg). The serum half-life is about 24 hours, so steady-state serum concentrations are not achieved for 5 to 7 days after oral therapy begins. Effective seizure control cannot be expected before that time. A serum concentration of 10 to 20 μg/ml correlates well with anticonvulsant effectiveness and minimum toxicity. Many patients can tolerate higher serum levels, but with an increasing incidence of side effects. Because of the long half-life, the total dose can be given once a day; some patients require two doses a day.

If more prompt control of frequent seizures is indicated, a loading dose of up to twice the usual initial dose may be given the first day and maintenance therapy then instituted. However, large doses are associated with gastrointestinal distress that may deter the patient from using the drug.

Phenytoin is metabolized to an inactive compound by hepatic microsomal oxidative enzymes that are saturated at serum levels not much higher than those needed for seizure control. As a consequence, a small increase in dose may result in enzymatic saturation, a disproportionate rise in serum drug concentration, and increased toxicity. Thus, only small increases in dosage should be made particularly when serum levels are in the upper therapeutic range but the saturation phenomenon can occur well within the therapeutic range. Other drugs that are metabolized by the same enzyme system may increase or decrease the metabolism and serum content of phenytoin. It is advisable to monitor phenytoin levels every time a new drug is added; drug interactions are often unpredictable.

Minor toxic symptoms occur frequently when phenytoin therapy starts. These manifestations are usually transient and disappear even with continued therapy. Gastric discomfort or nausea may be controlled by giving the drug after meals. Visual blurring or ataxia suggests dose-related toxicity and requires a decrease in dose. Allergic reactions may be severe and usually occur within several weeks after starting therapy. Pruritis, rash, or fever are indications for immediate drug withdrawal because continued therapy may lead to exfoliation, hepatic damage, or bone marrow suppression. These severe allergic reactions may be treated with corticosteroids.

A common chronic effect, especially in children, is gingival hyperplasia. Sometimes there is painful bleeding of the gums. This usually can be prevented by attention to oral hygiene, but surgery may be needed. Cognitive defects occur in children. Hirsutism occurs frequently, especially in young girls, and may be aesthetically distressing. More serious chronic effects include folic acid deficiency due to interference with intestinal absorption. Hypocalcemia may be due to drug-induced increased metabolism of vitamin D. A syndrome resembling systemic lupus erythematosus is usually reversed by discontinuing the drug. Peripheral neuropathy may occur after long term treatment with relatively high dosage.

Carbamazepine. This inostilbene is chemically related to the tricyclic antidepressants. It has the same clinical spectrum of activity as phenytoin and seems to have similar cellular actions.

Carbamazepine is effective in generalized tonic-clonic and partial seizures. It is comparable in efficiency to phenytoin but is more costly. Effective seizure control usually correlates with serum concentrations of 6 to 12 µg/ml. At higher concentrations, toxicity is common. There is considerable individual variation in the dosage required for effective serum concentrations; in practice, treatment begins with 200 mg the first day and increased over the first week to 600 mg daily in divided doses. Increases by 200 mg increments are made until seizures are controlled. In adults, the serum half-life is abut 20 hours under steady-state conditions; in children the half-life is less, so proportionately higher and more frequent doses are needed. It can be given once a day to many adults but, because of individual variation in half-life and the occurrence of blurred vision at peak levels, two or three times daily is usually preferred.

Carbamazepine is transformed into several metabolites. The 10,11-epoxide has anticonvulsant activity. Carbamazepine is metabolized by hepatic microsomal enzymes and there may be interaction with other drugs. For example, phenytoin frequently lowers carbamazepine levels while valproic acid frequently slows the rate of metabolism and raises carbamazepine levels. It is therefore necessary to determine serum concentration of carbamazepine whenever new drugs are added. In addition to the non-specific induction of liver enzymes common to all anticonvulsant drugs, carbamazepine specifically induces its own metabolism. Its half-life after a single dose is 30–36 hours whereas in the steady state after self-induction its half-life is reduced to 12–18 hours. It takes 2–3 weeks after the initiation of carbamazepine therapy to achieve a true steady state because during that period the half-life is constantly changing.

At serum concentrations exceeding 12 µg/ml, many patients experience blurred vision, a feeling of dysequilibrium or sedation. These symptoms are dose-related and can be eliminated by lowering the dose. Aplastic anemia is rare, occurs early in the course of treatment, and may be irreversible. Monitoring of blood count and platelets is recommended during the first 2 months of therapy and less frequently thereafter. Renal or hepatic toxicity and the syndrome of inappropriate antidiuretic hormone release are other rare toxic effects.

Barbiturates. Most barbiturates are too short-acting and too sedative for chronic therapeutic use. Phenobarbital and primidone, are the principal exceptions. They are long acting and depress abnormally discharging cortical neurons at dosages with tolerable sedative effect. They are effective against generalized tonic-clonic and partial seizures but not against generalized absence attacks. Phenobarbital is particularly useful in neonatal seizures, but may cause difficulty in concentration in older children. It exacerbates behavioral disturbances in hyperactive children, and causes hyperactivity in an appreciable number of normal children. Phenobarbital is effective in treatment of withdrawal from other sedative agents such as short-acting barbiturates and alcohol.

Phenobarbital has a half-life of about 4 days and requires 2 to 3 weeks of oral administration to reach steady-state concentrations. The usual starting dose is 1 mg/kg in adults and 3 mg/kg in children. Effectiveness is associated with serum concentrations of 15 to 30 μg/ml and many patients can tolerate surprisingly higher concentrations without sedation. Its long half-life allows phenobarbital to be taken as a single daily dose. The long half-life is advantageous in poorly compliant patients because adequate serum concentrations are maintained if a single dose is missed. In contrast to most other anticonvulsants, phenobarbital may be given intramuscularly and it is particularly useful when patients cannot take medication by mouth.

Primidone is metabolized almost quantitatively to phenobarbital and, under steady-state conditions, produces phenobarbital serum levels similar to that drug alone. The advantage, if any, of primidone is the anticonvulsant actions of the parent compound itself and its metabolites. Primidone has a half-life of 6 to 8 hours and should be given in divided doses three times daily. Serum concentrations of 8 to 12 μg/ml are associated with maximal therapeutic effect, and it is essential to monitor phenobarbital concentrations as most of the effect of primidone is from phenobarbital. Therapy can begin with 125 mg given at bedtime with a gradual increase to about 15 mg/ kg daily.

The limiting side effect of barbiturates is sedation, which is especially prominent with primidone early in therapy. Most patients tolerate the sedative effect after several weeks.

Ataxia and visual blurring are also dose related. Allergic reactions to phenobarbital include rash, leukopenia, and anemia. Chronic toxicity to barbiturates is rare, except for sedation, subtle impairment of cognitive function, and increased behavioral disturbances in hyperactive children.

Valproic Acid. Valproic acid differs both chemically and in mode of action from most other anticonvulsants. It is a branched chain fatty acid, which does not contain a nitrogen atom. It is usually given as divalproex sodium, a sodium-hydrogen dimer of valproic acid, in an enteric-coated tablet. It influences mitochondrial fatty acid metabolism and may affect the metabolism of amino acids. It is most useful in generalized seizures, but can be effective in partial seizures. It is particularly valuable in treating atypical absence seizures and myoclonus.

Valproic acid, taken orally, is rapidly absorbed and reaches peak levels in 1 to 2 hours. Serum half-life in adults is 6 to 8 hours; enteric-coated divalproex is more slowly absorbed, but has a longer plateau level. The usual starting dose is 10 mg/kg with gradual increases to as high as 60 mg/kg if needed. Because of its short half-life, correlation between successive serum level determinations and therapeutic effect depends on sampling times. Levels of 40 to 120 μg/ml are in the therapeutic range.

Valproic acid and divalproex are best given in divided doses, but are also effective in a single bedtime dose. Valproic acid is oxidized by both hepatic microsomal enzymes and mitochondria to form several metabolites that have little or no anticonvulsant activity. In general, valproic acid decreases the rate of metabolism of other drugs such as phenobarbital and carbamazepine, raising the serum concentration of those drugs. It displaces phenytoin from serum protein-binding sites, decreasing the total serum concentration of phenytoin although free phenytoin levels remain constant. Measurement of free levels is usually not available.

Nausea and gastrointestinal irritation are commonly dose related and can be minimized by increasing the dose slowly, by giving the drug with food, and by using enteric-coated tablets. Sedation and ataxia occur rarely. At high serum concentrations valproic acid may interfere with platelet function, so coagulation studies are indicated when surgery is planned for patients taking this drug. Fatal hepatic failure may occur in patients receiving valproic acid. This occurs most often in infants and young children and in individuals on polytherapy. Fatal hepatic failure occurs after a fulminant course in most cases. Thus, valproic acid should not be given to children under 2 years unless other medications are ineffective and the risk is clearly outweighed by the need for seizure control. In older children and adults who are taking other drugs, valproic acid should be used with caution. Frequent measurement of liver function is necessary during the early months of therapy. The reference list includes a study on the incidence of hepatic toxicity and fatalities. Valproic acid therapy should be avoided when feasible in women who may become pregnant.

Ethosuximide. This drug is highly effective and widely used to treat generalized absence seizures (petit mal). It is usually ineffective in other forms of epilepsy. Because its half-life is about 30 hours in children and much longer in adults, it can be taken only once daily but divided doses are usually preferable in order to avoid peak serum level side effects. Effectiveness is associated with serum concentrations of 40 to 120 µg/ml but monitoring of the EEG is frequently a more useful guide than serum levels in the treatment of generalized absence attacks. Treatment is usually started with 10 mg/kg and gradually increased to as high as 40 mg/kg, if needed.

Ethosuximide is relatively safe. Although transient leukopenia occurs, severe bone marrow depression is rare. Complete blood counts should be obtained regularly early in the course of therapy. Dose-related side effects include gastrointestinal upset, sedation, headache, and occasionally ataxia.

Benzodiazepines. Most of these compounds were introduced as antianxiety agents and hypnotics, but all have some anticonvulsant activity. Clonazepam is a widely-used effective oral anticonvulsant but shares with other drugs in this group the disadvantages of sedation and of tolerance to the anticonvulsant effect. Nevertheless, it is useful in treating otherwise refractory childhood seizures, including atypical absence and myoclonus attacks. Benzodiazepines are unique among anticonvulsants because there is a specific neuronal diazepine receptor that is part of the GABA-receptor complex. It is not known whether this receptor is abnormal in epilepsy.

Clonazepam is absorbed rapidly with a half-life of about 24 hours. It is transformed to several metabolites, some of which have anticonvulsive activity. There is little information about the correlation of serum concentration and therapeutic effectiveness. Clonazepam has little toxicity other than dose-related sedation and ataxia. Tolerance to the anticonvulsive effect is seen in many patients after prolonged use; it is often necessary to increase the dose to maintain the therapeutic efficacy of clonazepam.

Other Antiepileptic Drugs. Many other drugs have been used to treat epilepsy. Some are still available and are clinically useful. Generally, however, these drugs are either less effective or more toxic than those previously described, so they are reserved for refractory or otherwise unusual patients.

Treatment of Convulsive Status Epilepticus. Repetitive tonic-clonic convulsions, in which the patient does not recover normal alert state between attacks, is status epilepticus. It is a medical emergency that demands immediate and vigorous therapy. An organized, systematic approach to status epilepticus is necessary in order to avoid the severe brain damage which occurs with prolonged tonic-clonic status epilepticus. A monograph edited by Delgado-Escueta et al. that deals with all aspects of treatment of status is listed in the references.

Management starts with adequate ventilation, a secure intravenous line and, if possible, treatment of the precipitating causes. Blood should be taken for laboratory studies and serum drug concentration. Twenty-five to fifty grams of glucose, should be given intravenously (with 100 mg of thiamine for adults). After these preliminary steps, a large dose of an appropriate anticonvulsant is given intravenously. Only three drugs have gained widespread acceptance. (1) Diazepam, 10 mg administered over 2 minutes, is widely used as the initial agent. While this often stops the seizure, seizures may recur in a matter of minutes and it is therefore necessary to immediately begin further therapy. (2) Phenytoin may be given in doses of 15 to 18 mg/kg at a rate no greater than 50 mg/minute. This should be done with careful monitoring because if the rate of infusion is excessive, hypotension and cardiac arrhythmia may follow especially in patients with heart disease. Phenytoin has the advantage of producing less sedation than phenobarbital or diazepam. (3) If seizures persist phenobarbital or diazepam infusion may be given, but should not be given in conjunction with each other. A protocol for management of tonic-clonic status epilepticus is given in Table 145–9. Rarely, it may be necessary to induce prolonged general anesthesia with a barbiturate to control refractory status.

Status epilepticus in the neonate requires a more vigorous search for underlying precipitating factors (e.g. meningitis, hypoglycemia or hypocalcemia). Treatment begins with a loading dose of phenobarbital, 20 to 25 mg/kg followed by maintenance doses of 3 to 4 mg/kg. Successful treatment of neonatal status epilepticus depends on identification and treatment of the cause.

Mental and Physical Health. Usually it is not possible to eliminate the causative factors; in most patients, seizure control requires both the long-term adaptation of life style to a chronic disorder and the administration of an-

ticonvulsant drugs. Treatment is measured in years or a lifetime. Patients must be encouraged to overcome feelings of inferiority and self-consciousness and to live as normally as possible. Psychological support may be critical in adjusting to difficulties and may also affect the frequency of attacks. Relatives have to be educated about epilepsy. Over solicitousness should be avoided and the family should not make the subject a chronic invalid. The patient must learn that sleep deprivation may precipitate seizures.

Excessive restrictions should be avoided. Children with epilepsy should be encouraged to participate in sports. Swimming is permitted in most cases but only with continuous individual supervision. Any plan in adults must consider the type of seizure, details of

Table 145–9. Management of Tonic-Clonic Status Epilepticus

Time from initiation of observation and treatment (min)	Procedure
0	1. Assess cardiorespiratory function as the presence of tonic-clonic status is verified. If unsure of diagnosis, observe one tonic-clonic attack and verify the presence of unconsciousness after the end of the tonic-clonic attack. Insert oral airway and administer O_2 if necessary. Insert an indwelling intravenous catheter. Draw venous blood for anticonvulsant levels, glucose, BUN, electrolyte, and CBC stat determinations. Draw arterial blood for stat pH, Po_2, Pco_2, HCO_3. Monitor respiration, blood pressure, and electrocardiograph. If possible, monitor electroencephalograph.
5	2. Start intravenous infusion through indwelling venous catheter with normal saline, containing vitamin B complex. Give a bolus injection of 50 cc 50% glucose.
10	3. *Infuse diazepam intravenously* no faster than 2 mg/min until seizures stop or to total of 20 mg. *Also start infusion of phenytoin* no faster than 50 mg/min to a total of 18 mg/kg. If hypotension develops, slow down infusion rate. (Phenytoin 50 mg/ml in propylene glycol may be placed in a 100-ml volume control set and diluted with normal saline. The rate of infusion should then be watched carefully.) Alternately, phenytoin may be injected slowly by intravenous push.
30–40	4. If seizures persist, two options are available: iv phenobarbital *or* diazepam iv drip. The two drugs should *not* be given in the same patient, and an endotracheal tube should be inserted. *iv phenobarbital option:* Start infusion of phenobarbital no faster than 100 mg/min until seizures stop or to a loading dose of 20 mg/kg. *diazepam iv drip option:* 100 mg of diazepam is diluted in 500 cc D5/W and run in at 40 cc/hr. This ensures diazepam serum levels of 0.2 to 0.8 μg/ml.
50–60	5. If seizures continue, general anesthesia with halothane and neuromuscular junction blockade is instituted. If an anesthesiologist is not immediately available, start infusion of 4% solution of paraldehyde in normal saline; administer at a rate fast enough to stop seizures, *or* 50 to 100 mg of lidocaine may be given by intravenous push. If lidocaine is effective, 50 to 100 mg diluted in 250 cc of 5% D/W should be dripped intravenously at a rate of 1 to 2 mg/min.
80	6. If paraldehyde or lidocaine has not terminated seizures within 20 min from start of infusion, general anesthesia with halothane and neuromuscular junction blockade must be given.

(Modified from: Status epilepticus: summary. Delgado-Escueta et al. In Advances in Neurology Vol. 34. Status Epilepticus. Ed. AV Delgado-Escueta et al. Raven Press, NY, 1983.)

Table 145–10.   Results of Cortical Excision for Focal Epilepsy*

	No of Patients	%
Seizure-free since discharge	247	19
Seizure-free after some early postoperative attacks	178	14
Seizure-free Total	425	33
Seizure-free for 3 or more years, then occasional attacks	168	13
Marked reduction of seizure tendency	240	19
Seizure reduction Total	408	32
Moderate or slight reduction of seizure tendency	444	34
Inadequate follow-up data	87	
Death in first 2 years	25	
Postoperative deaths	18	
Total	1407	100

*Patients with nontumor lesions operated on between 1928 and 1974.
(Modified from Rasmussen T. Functional Neurosurgery. New York: Raven Press, 1979.)

occupation, and degree of seizure control. In most states, driving an automobile is restricted, but limitations can be modified when seizures are controlled. Consumption of alcohol should be limited but not prohibited. The physician should take a supportive role, not just present a list of dos and donts'. The risk of participating in most activities is usually justified to prevent chronic invalidism. Some patients with uncontrolled seizures or behavioral problems may benefit from sheltered workshops or even hospital long-term care. Local and state epilepsy societies and the Epilepsy Foundation of America provide educational materials and support services.

SURGICAL TREATMENT

Although surgical treatment for intractible partial (focal) epilepsy has proved successful in selected cases for many years (Table 145–9),

until recently it was not used extensively. In the past decade, however, increasing numbers of patients have been considered for the surgical removal of epileptogenic foci. Areas of the brain that are responsible for partial attacks can be reliably located in the more than 30% of individuals with partial seizures that have not been controlled with medical treatment. It is thought that many more patients could be relieved of seizures surgically if facilities were available.

The major criterion for surgical treatment is that medically treated uncontrolled seizures disrupt education, employment, and social or interpersonal affairs sufficiently to motivate the patient to seek help. Whether the patient is suitable for surgical treatment becomes a judgment based on locating a single epileptogenic area that is responsible for the seizures and whose removal will not seriously impair brain function. Evaluations are made in many centers in the U.S., using long-term EEG monitoring, closed circuit TV recording of seizures with simultaneous EEG, psychological evaluation, CT, MRI, and PET, chronic intracranial recording with depth electrodes or arrays of subdural electrodes, intracarotid amytal testing for speech lateralization and memory function, and electrocorticography. The results of surgical treatment obtained from the long-term Montreal Neurological Institute experience and from a worldwide survey of 40 centers are shown in Tables 145–10 and 145–11.

References

Browne TR: Clinical pharmacology of antiepileptic drugs. In: Epilepsy: Diagnosis, Management, Quality of Life. Penry JK (ed.), New York: Raven Press, 1986:22–27.
Consensus Development Conference on Febrile Seizures. Epilepsia 1981; 22:377–381.
Delgado-Escueta AV, Horan MP. Brain synaptosomes in epilepsy; organization of ionic channels and the Na^+K^+ pump. In: Glaser GH, Penry JK, Woodbury

Table 145–11.   Survey Results: Outcome with Respect to Epileptic Seizures

Classification	Hemispherectomy	Anterior Temporal Lobectomy	Extratemporal Resection	Corpus Callosum Section
Total patients	88	2,336	825	197
Total centers	17	40	32	16
No. seizure-free	68	1,296	356	10
Percent (range)	77.3 (0–100)	55.5 (26–80)	43.2 (0–73)	5.0 (0–13)
No. improved	16	648	229	140
Percent	18.2	27.7	27.8	71.0
No. not improved	4	392	240	47
Percent (range)	4.5 (0–33)	16.8 (6–29)	29.1 (17–89)	23.9 (10–38)

DM, eds. Antiepileptic Drugs: Mechanisms of Action. New York: Raven Press, 1980:85–126.

Delgado-Escueta AV, Enrile-Bacsal F. Juvenile Myoclonic Epilepsy of Janz. Neurology 1983; 34:285–294.

Delgado-Escueta AV, Wasterlain CG, Treiman DM, Porter RJ, eds. Advances in Neurology, vol 34, Status Epilepticus. New York: Raven Press, 1983.

Dreifuss FE, Santilli RN, Langer DH, Sweeney KP, Moline BA, Menander KB. Valproic acid fatalities: A retrospective review. Neurology 1987; 37:379–385.

Ebersole JS, Leroy RF. Evaluation of ambulatory cassette EEG monitoring; III Diagnostic accuracy compared to intensive inpatient EEG monitoring. Neurology 1983; 33:853–360.

Engel J Jr, ed. Surgical Treatment of Epilepsies. New York: Raven Press, 1987.

Goldberg MA. Costs of anticonvulsant therapy. Ann Neurol 1981; 9:95.

Goldensohn ES, ed. The non-convulsive epilepsies; clinical manifestations, diagnostic considerations, and treatment. Epilepsia 1983; 24:(suppl 1):s1–s82.

Goldensohn ES, Salazar AM. Temporal and spatial distribution of intracellular potentials during generation and spread of epileptogenic discharges. In Delgado-Escueta AV, et al. eds. Basic Mechanisms of the Epilepsies. Advances in Neurology 1986, vol 44. New York: Raven Press, 1986.

Hauser WA, Annegers JF, Andersen EV. Epidemiology and genetics of epilepsy. Res Publ Assoc Res Nerv Ment Dis 1983; 61:267–294.

Janz D. On major malformations and minor anomalies in the offspring of parents with epilepsy: Review of the literature. In: Janz D, Dam M, Richens A, Bossi L, Helge H, Schmidt D, eds. Epilepsy, Pregnancy, and the Child. New York: Raven Press, 1982:211–222.

Loiseau P, Duche B, Cordova S, Dartigues JF, Cohadon S. Prognosis of Benign Childhood Epilepsy with Centotemporal Spikes: A follow-up Study of 168 Patients. Epilepsia, 1988; 29(3):229–235.

Mattson RH, Cramer JA, Collins JF, et al. Comparison of carbamazepine, phenobarbital, phenytoin and primidone in partial and secondarily generalized tonic-clonic seizures. N Engl J Med 1985; 313:145–151.

Reynolds EH, Shorvon SD, Galbraith AW, et al. Phenytoin monotherapy for epilepsy: A long term prospective study, assisted by serum level monitoring in previously untreated patients. Epilepsia 1981; 22:475–488.

Schmidt D. Adverse effects In: Frey HH, Janz D, eds. Handbook of Experimental Pharmacology, vol 74. New York: Springer Verlag 1985:791–829.

Schmidt D, Einice I, Haenel F. The influence of seizure type on the efficacy of plasma concentrations of phenytoin, phenobarbital and carbamazepine. Arch Neurol 1985; 42.

Shinnar S, Vining EPG, Mellits ED, et al. Discontinuing antiepileptic medication in children with epilepsy after two years without seizures. N Engl J Med 1985; 313:976–980.

146. TRANSIENT GLOBAL AMNESIA

John C.M. Brust

Transient global amnesia (TGA) is characterized by sudden inability to form new memory traces (anterograde amnesia) plus retrograde memory loss for events of the preceding days, weeks, or even years. During attacks, which affect both verbal and nonverbal memory, there is often bewilderment or anxiety and a tendency to repeat one or several questions (e.g., "Where am I?"). Physical and neurologic examination, including mental status, is otherwise normal. Immediate registration of events (e.g., serial digits) is intact, and self-identification is preserved. Attacks last minutes or hours, rarely longer than a day, with gradual recovery. Retrograde amnesia clears in a forward fashion, often with permanent loss for events occurring within minutes or a few hours of the attack; there is also permanent amnesia for events during the attack itself. TGA sometimes seems to be precipitated by physical or emotional stress, such as sexual intercourse, driving an automobile, or swimming in cold water. Because amnesia can accompany a variety of neurologic disturbances, such as head trauma, intoxication, partial complex seizures, or dissociative states, criteria for diagnosing TGA should include observation of the attack by others.

Patients are usually middle-aged or elderly and otherwise healthy. Recurrent attacks occur in less than 25% of cases and fewer than 3% have more than three. Intervals between attacks range from 1 month to 19 years. Permanent memory loss is rare, although subtle defects have been reported after only one attack. The frequency of both seizures and subsequent stroke, including transient ischemic attacks, is probably no different than in a comparable age-matched population.

The cause of TGA is controversial. The benign prognosis, variety of precipitating circumstances, and reports of EEG abnormalities have suggested epileptic origin. Evidence against that theory includes the following: Attacks last hours rather than minutes. Also, the most frequently observed EEG changes have been small sharp spikes of questionable significance. Moreoever, other seizure phenomena are rarely encountered, recurrent attacks are infrequent, and isolated memory impairment is not a feature of other types of seizure.

In support of a vascular origin, i.e., transient ischemic attacks involving the inferomedial temporal lobes, is a high prevalence of risk factors (hypertension, prior cerebral ischemia, arteriosclerotic heart disease) among TGA patients, who are usually over 50 years old. Attacks have been associated with cerebral angiography (especially vertebral), polycythemia, and cardiac valvular disease. However, it is unclear why recurrent spells, signs of cerebral infarction, and subsequent TIA are so infrequent. Moreover, patients with amnestic stroke due to documented posterior cerebral artery occlusion have not reported previous TGA; their neurologic signs have included more than simple amnesia (e.g., visual impairment), and they have not exhibited repetitive queries.

There have been reports of TGA in patients with migraine. Sometimes both amnestic and migrainous attacks (including visual symptoms and vomiting) have occurred simultaneously or followed one another. Spreading depression of Leao, possibly the pathophysiologic basis of cerebral symptoms in migraine, could, by affecting the hippocampus, explain some cases of TGA as well.

These mechanisms are not mutually exclusive, and it is possible that even when strict diagnostic criteria for TGA are applied, it will have diverse origins. Theoretical considerations support treatment with antiplatelet agents, but the benign natural history makes it difficult to evaluate any "preventive" treatment.

References

Bender MB. Syndrome of isolated episodes of confusion with amnesia. J Hillside Hosp 1956; 5:212–215.

Caplan LB. Transient global amnesia. In: Vinken P, Bruyn G, Klawans H, eds. *Handbook of Clinical Neurology, vol 45, part 1.* Amsterdam: Elsevier Science, 1985:205–218.

Fisher CM, Adams RD. Transient global amnesia syndrome. Acta Neurol Scand 1964; 40(suppl 9):7–82.

Hinge HH, Jensen TS, Kjaer M, et al. The prognosis of transient global amnesia. Results of multicenter study. Arch Neurol 1986; 43:673–676.

Kushner MJ, Hauser WA. Transient global amnesia: A case-control study. Ann Neurol 1985; 18:684–691.

Miller JW, Petersen RC, Metter EJ, Millikan CH, Yangihara T. Transient global amnesia. Neurology 1987; 37:733–737.

Olesen J, Jorgensen MB. Leao's spreading depression in the hippocampus explains transient global amnesia. A hypothesis. Acta Neurol Scand 1986; 73:219–220.

147. MENIERE SYNDROME

Elliot D. Weitzman
June M. Fry

Meniere syndrome, or paroxysmal labyrinthine vertigo, was first described by Prosper Meniere in 1861. It is characterized by recurrent sudden attacks of severe vertigo accompanied by tinnitus and sensorineural hearing loss. Early in the course of the disease, vertigo may occur without tinnitus or hearing loss, but the final diagnosis should not be made until all three symptoms are present.

Symptoms. Isolated and recurrent attacks of sudden, severe vertigo are the cardinal features of the syndrome. There is no vertigo or instability between attacks. An attack of vertigo may last for 10 minutes or several hours; attacks have occasionally lasted as long as 24 hours. Continuous vertigo that lasts for days or weeks is almost never due to Meniere syndrome. Loss of consciousness for a few seconds occurs in a small percentage of cases. Perception of whirling or spinning objects in the environment is characteristic, but occasionally there is only a sensation of giddiness or nonrotational motion. Most episodes are associated with nausea, vomiting, and profuse perspiration, but nausea may occur without vomiting in mild attacks.

Tinnitus and hearing loss occur in most cases during the acute attack of vertigo and usually persist between attacks. Tinnitus is usually a low buzzing sound that becomes louder before or during the attack of vertigo. Hearing loss in the involved ear is sensorineural in type, usually with a decrease in the perception of low tones. The hearing loss typically fluctuates, often abruptly, but if the condition is not treated, it progresses slowly to severe cochlear damage and total deafness.

Signs. Except for signs of involvement of the eighth cranial nerve, general physical and neurologic examinations are normal between attacks. Nystagmus is always present during an attack and is horizontal and rotary toward the bad ear. Nystagmus may persist for several days after the attack subsides. The audiogram reveals a low-tone loss, and loudness recruitment is almost always present to some degree. About 65% of cases are unilateral; the others are bilateral. Permanent reduction of the caloric response with directional preponderance and other vestibular dysfunction usually appears during the first few years. These abnormal vestibular findings often parallel the hearing loss.

Incidence and Age of Onset. Meniere syndrome is common, with an estimated prevalence of 1 to 2 cases/10,000 population. The syndrome develops during the fifth and sixth decades in 65% of patients and occurs only rarely before the third or after the seventh decade. Men are affected two or three times more often than women.

Course and Prognosis. Meniere syndrome

is a chronic disease; symptoms recur unpredictably for many years. The attacks may occur weeks or months apart and, if not treated, typically become more frequent and severe until they occur once every 2 to 4 days. Attacks occasionally occur daily, with complete relief between attacks. The condition may disappear spontaneously after many years. Complete loss of hearing is sometimes followed by cessation of the attacks of vertigo. The disease becomes bilateral in 10 to 15% of patients.

Laboratory Data. Routine examinations of blood, urine, and CSF are normal both during and between attacks. Audiometric and vestibular tests are abnormal as described above.

Etiology, Pathogenesis, and Pathology. The cause of Meniere syndrome is not known. However, dilation or hydrops of the endolymphatic labyrinth was found in two patients with Meniere disease by Hallpike and Cairns in 1938; this observation has been confirmed by many investigators. It is not known what causes this distention of the endolymph space, nor is it entirely clear that it is the cause of the clinical symptoms. Additional pathologic changes in some patients include dilation and rupture of the saccule, dilation of the utricle, atrophy of the stria vascularis, loss of spiral ganglion cells, and degeneration of sensory and neural elements in the cochlea. Tomographic radiographs of the vestibular aqueduct and periaqueductal pneumatization have been correlated with autopsy examination of the temporal bone to show decreased or absent pneumatization that is associated with a short and narrow vestibular aqueduct.

Mechanical, physiologic, and biochemical theories have been advanced to explain the development and symptoms of hydrops. Possibilities include mechanical blockage of inner ear cochlear and endolymphatic ducts; autonomic dysfunction with vasospasm of vessels of the stria vascularis; rupture of the Reissner membrane that separates the endolymph and perilymph; vitamin deficiency; allergy; altered hypothalamic neurovascular mechanisms; and psychosomatic factors.

Diagnosis. The diagnosis of Meniere syndrome is not difficult in most cases with a characteristic history of acute attacks of vertigo associated with tinnitus and hearing loss but with no other neurologic abnormality. There should be no vertigo between attacks; tinnitus and sensorineural hearing loss are required for a definitive diagnosis. Meniere syndrome must be differentiated from acute labyrinthitis, which is more prolonged and usually not recurrent. Tumors of the posterior fossa, especially neuromas of the acoustic nerve, often cause tinnitus, hearing loss, and vertigo; however, the vertigo rarely occurs in explosive attacks and is usually present constantly. Several other conditions may cause episodic dizziness, but the diagnosis of Meniere syndrome should be made only when tinnitus and hearing loss are present. Multiple sclerosis may cause paroxysmal vertigo, but not with nausea and vomiting; hearing loss and tinnitus are rare in multiple sclerosis, and there are other neurologic signs that are not associated with Meniere syndrome.

Treatment. Because Meniere syndrome is both intermittent and unpredictable, it is difficult to assess therapies. The acute episode is self-limited and may not require treatment other than reassurance; however, a severe vertiginous attack can often be stopped by subcutaneous injection of atropine, slow intravenous infusion of epinephrine, histamine diphosphate, or diphenhydramine. Cervical sympathetic block on the affected side has been reported to curtail an acute attack. Prophylactic treatment of frequent attacks includes a diet with severe restriction of salt intake and the addition of ammonium chloride capsules, which are reported to control attacks in more than 75% of patients. Vasodilators (e.g., nicotinic acid, tolazoline hydrochloride, diphenhydramine hydrochloride, dimenhydrinate) have been used to control vertigo and methantheline has been used for tinnitus and hearing loss; the value of these treatments is uncertain.

Surgery for Meniere syndrome has included general destructive procedures, selective nerve section, and endolymphatic sac operations. Disabling vertigo has been treated by deafferentation of the vestibular apparatus by selective section of the vestibular nerve, surgical labyrinthectomy, cryosurgery, and ultrasonic treatment of the semicircular canal. Endolymphatic sac operations have been used to treat both vertigo and hearing loss. Modifications include opening the sac, removing the bone around the sac without entering the lumen, insertion of a plastic tube into the sac to drain endolymph into a mastoidectomy cavity, and placing a temporalis flap into the sac to enhance endolymph resorption.

Operative intervention can prevent recurrent attacks of vertigo but, because of a significant number of complications and the irreversibility of these procedures, it should be reserved for patients with severe and intractable symptoms for whom medical therapy is ineffective.

References

Arenberg IK. Endolymphatic hypertension and hydrops in Meniere's disease: Current perspectives. Am J Otol 1982; 4:52–65.

Baloh RW. Dizziness, Hearing Loss, and Tinnitus. Essentials of Neurology. Philadelphia: FA Davis, 1984.

Brookes GB, Hodge RA, Booth JB, Morrison AW. The immediate effects of acetazolamide in Meniere's disease. J Laryngol Otol 1982; 96:57–72.

Drachman DA, Hart CW. An approach to the dizzy patient. Neurology 1972; 22:323–334.

Goin DW, Staller SJ, Asher DL, Mischke RE. Summating potential in Meniere's disease. Laryngoscope 1982; 92:1383–1389.

Hallpike CS, Cairns H. Observations on the pathology of Meniere's syndrome. J Laryngol 1938; 53:625–654.

Kanzaki J, Ouchi T, Yokobori H, Ino T. Electrocochleographic study of summating potentials in Meniere's disease. Audiology 1982; 21:409–424.

Meniere P. Sur une forme particulière de surdité grave dependant d'une lesion de l'oreille interne. Gaz Med Paris 1861; 16:29.

Pulec JL. Meniere's disease: Etiology, natural history, and results of treatment. Otolaryngol Clin North Am 1973; 6:25–39.

Snow JB Jr, Kimmelman CP. Assessment of surgical procedures for Meniere's disease. Laryngoscope 1979; 89:737–747.

Stahle, J, Wilbrand HF, Rask-Andersen H. Temporal bone characteristics in Meniere's disease. Ann NY Acad Sci 1981; 374:794–807.

Wilmot TJ. Meniere's disorder. Clin Otolaryngol 1979; 4:131–143.

---

148. SLEEP DISORDERS

Elliot D. Weitzman
June M. Fry

Although disorders of sleep and the daily sleep-wake cycle have been recognized by physicians since the earliest medical writings, only in 1979 has a medical and scientific discipline emerged with an explicit nosology that attempts to include all clinical syndromes (Table 148–1). Sleep disorders occur throughout the human life span, with specific clinical conditions associated with specific ages, from the prematurely born infant to the elderly individual. Each age group has its specific clinical entities that relate to maturational aspects (e.g., nocturnal enuresis, night terrors, head banging and body rocking, and somnambulism), age, and sex-related conditions (e.g., hypersomnia, Kleine-Levin syndrome, sleep apnea syndrome). Certain clinical conditions of special importance to neurologists may be lifelong, such as the narcolepsy syndrome and nocturnal seizures that begin in childhood or adolescence, but these are usually adequately controlled by appropriate medication. In the past 15 years, the scope of the sleep disorders problem has been recognized and, although data are fragmentary, certain recent statistics are striking. It appears that 8 to 15% of the adult population have frequent and chronic complaints about the quality and amount of sleep. Also, estimates of sleeping-pill use range from 3 to 11% of the adult population with 39% of all hypnotic prescriptions being written for people over age 60. There is evidence of increased mortality risk in the population who complain of a chronic sleep disorder and who often use a hypnotic.

The classification of sleep disorders, with few exceptions, is based on the natural clustering of clinical signs, symptoms, age incidence, and natural history, but not on tissue pathology (Tables 148–1 and 148–2). An important advance has been the development of clinical polysomnography for the objective polygraphic measurement of physiologic and autonomic changes in patients and normal subjects during prolonged or recurrent sleep periods. Continuous polygraphic recordings of the EEG, EMG of facial and limb muscles, electro-oculogram (EOG), respiration, oxygen saturation (ear oximetry), heart rate, and other special measurements (blood pressure, esophageal pH, blood hormone concentrations) are now routinely used in all "sleep disorders centers," and increasingly in "clinical neurophysiologic laboratories."

Normal Physiology of Sleep

The normal sleep pattern of the night consists of three to five short-term sleep cycles consisting of alternating periods of rapid eye movement (REM) and nonREM sleep, each lasts 85 to 100 minutes. The normal, healthy adult typically falls asleep within 10 minutes of lying down to sleep and then goes through a sequence of Stages 1, 2, 3, and 4 sleep, followed by the reverse (Stages 4, 3, 2), after which REM sleep occurs, lasting 10 to 20 minutes. This first cycle takes about 90 to 100 minutes, the next three cycles are about the same length, with a small reduction to 85 or 90 minutes for the last two sleep cycles. The duration and percentage of REM sleep increases during the latter half of the night's sleep, accounting for some 40% of sleep time during the 2 hours before final awakening. Stages 3 and 4 occur predominantly during

Table 148–1. Outline of Diagnostic Classification of Sleep and Arousal Disorders

DIMS: Disorders of Initiating and Maintaining
    Sleep (Insomnias)
  Psychophysiologic
    Transient and situational
    Persistent
  Associated with psychiatric disorders
    Symptoms and personality disorders
    Affective disorders
    Other functional psychoses
  Associated with use of drugs and alcohol
    Tolerance to or withdrawal from CNS
        depressants
    Sustained use of CNS stimulants
    Sustained use of or withdrawal from other
        drugs
    Chronic alcoholism
  Associated with sleep-induced respiratory
        impairment
    Sleep apnea syndrome
    Alveolar hypoventilation syndrome
  Associated with sleep-related (nocturnal)
        myoclonus and "restless legs"
    Sleep-related (nocturnal) myoclonus
        syndrome
    "Restless legs" syndrome
  Associated with other medical, toxic, and
        environmental conditions
  Childhood-onset DIMS
  Associated with other DIMS conditions
    Repeated REM-sleep interruptions
    Atypical polysomnographic features
    Not otherwise specified
DOES: Disorders of Excessive Somnolence
  Psychophysiologic
    Transient and situational
    Persistent
  Associated with psychiatric disorders
    Affective disorders
    Other functional disorders
  Associated with use of drugs and alcohol
    Tolerance to or withdrawal from CNS
        stimulants
    Sustained use of CNS depressants
  Associated with sleep-induced respiratory
        impairment
    Sleep apnea syndrome
    Alveolar hypoventilation syndrome
  Associated with sleep-related (nocturnal)
        myoclonus and "restless legs"
    Sleep-related (nocturnal) myoclonus
        syndrome
    "Restless legs" syndrome
  Narcolepsy

  Idiopathic CNS hypersomnolence
  Associated with other medical, toxic, and
        environmental conditions
  Associated with other DOES conditions
    Intermittent (periodic) syndromes
      Kleine-Levin syndrome
      Menstrual-associated syndrome
    Insufficient sleep
    Sleep drunkenness
    Not otherwise specified
  No DOES abnormality
    Longer sleeper
    Subjective DOES complaint without
        objective findings
    Not otherwise specified
Disorders of the sleep-wake schedule
  Transient
    Rapid time-zone change syndrome ("jet
        lag")
    Work-shift change in conventional sleep-
        wake schedule
  Persistent
    Frequently changing sleep-wake schedule
    Delayed sleep phase syndrome
    Advanced sleep phase syndrome
    Non-24-hour sleep-wake syndrome
    Irregular sleep-wake pattern
    Not otherwise specified
Dysfunctions associated with sleep, sleep stages,
        or partial arousals (parasomnias)
  Sleepwalking (somnambulism)
  Sleep terror (pavor nocturnus, incubus)
  Sleep-related enuresis
  Other dysfunctions
    Dream anxiety attacks (nightmares)
    Sleep-related epileptic seizures
    Sleep-related bruxism
    Sleep-related head banging
    Familial sleep paralysis
    Impaired sleep-related penile tumescence
    Sleep-related painful erections
    Sleep-related cluster headaches and chronic
        paroxysmal hemicrania
    Sleep-related abnormal swallowing
        syndrome
    Sleep-related asthma
    Sleep-related cardiovascular symptoms
    Sleep-related gastroesophageal reflux
    Sleep-related hemolysis (paroxysmal
        nocturnal hemoglobinuria)
    Asymptomatic polysomnographic finding
    Not otherwise specified

Table 148–2.   **Distribution of Major Diagnostic Entities in 3900 Patients***

Type of Disorder	Percent of Total
Disorders of initiating and maintaining sleep	31
Psychiatric disorders (affecting personality and psychoses)	11
Psychophysiological	5
Drug and alcohol dependency	4
Sleep-related myoclonus and restless-legs syndrome	4
Other DIMS	7
Disorders of excessive daytime somnolence	51
Sleep apnea syndrome	22
Narcolepsy	13
Idiopathic hypersomnolence	5
Other disorders of daytime somnolence	11
Disorders (dyssomnias) of the sleep-wake cycle	3
Disorders (parasomnias) associated with sleep	15

*Patients were evaluated in 11 sleep-disorder centers during a 2-year period.
(From Coleman R, et al. JAMA 1982; 247: 997–1003.)

the first one third of the sleep period. The approximate percentage of each sleep stage is: Stage 1, 5 to 10; Stage 2, 50; Stage 3, 15; Stage 4, 10; and REM, 20.

Stage 1 sleep is characterized by low-voltage mixed-frequency EEG activity, associated with slow, rolling eye movements. The mentalis muscle (chin) EMG is of moderately high amplitude but less than that seen in quiet waking. Stage 2 sleep is represented by a moderately low-voltage background EEG, intermixed with brief (0.2 to 1.0 sec.) high-voltage discharges (K-complexes) and 12 to 15 Hz low to moderate amplitude coherent discharges (spindles). Stage 3 sleep consists of high-amplitude background activity of theta (5–7 Hz) and delta (1 to 3 Hz) waves as well as K-complexes and spindle activity. Stage 4 sleep is high-voltage delta waves at a frequency of 0.5 to 3.0 Hz. Tonic mentalis muscle (but not extremity or axial muscle) activity is present during the nonREM sleep of Stages 1 through 4. REM sleep is represented by low-voltage mixed-frequency EEG activity, similar to that found in Stage 1. However, "sawtooth waves" consisting of 3 to 5 Hz triangular waveforms are seen in REM sleep. The EOG shows groups ("bursts") of conjugate REM in all directions of gaze. Tonic EMG activity from

the chin is either totally absent or markedly suppressed and phasic muscle potential discharges are prominent and also occur in irregular bursts.

Recent advances in the field of human chronobiology have also been important for the understanding of clinical disorders of the daily sleep-wake cycle. When humans are not entrained by 24-hour time cues, they develop daily sleep-wake cycles with periods slightly greater than 24 hours. Studies carried out in an environment free of time cues for weeks to months in both laboratories and caves have consistently demonstrated a preferred "free-running" period of about 25 hours. The conclusion derived from these studies is that the normal daily sleep-wake cycle (one third sleep, two thirds waking) requires an active process of entrainment to maintain a 24-hour rhythm. Each day, therefore, the normal person advances the phase of sleep by 1 hour to hold the cycle to a 24-hour period. On weekends or days off, most people show a phase delay of several hours but then re-entrain for a short time at a new phase (clock time). Measurements of physiologic indices (e.g., body temperature, urinary electrolytes, hypothalamic-pituitary hormones, psychological performance measures, sleep stages, blood pressure, heart rate) have shown that different variables can develop independent cycle lengths in time-isolated conditions. These results have led to the concept that there are multiple oscillators, normally synchronized with each other, that can become desynchronized under free-running conditions. Studies of imposed phase shifts of the sleep-wakefulness cycle in the laboratory and after rapid transmeridian flights demonstrate that sleep is disturbed, thereby suggesting that the sleep-wake cycle itself has component rhythms.

Specific Disorders of Sleep

In this section, only selected disorders are described, primarily those relevant to neurology, plus those for which new understanding or treatment regimens have been recently described. (For a more complete review of the sleep disorders the reader is referred to *Sleep*, volume 2, 1979, and to Weitzman ED. Ann Rev Neurosci; 1981.)

DISORDERS OF INITIATING AND MAINTAINING SLEEP (INSOMNIAS)

Emotional disorders represent one of the largest clinical categories associated with insomnia complaints. There is increasing evidence that *major depressive and bipolar disorders* are organic diseases of the brain, although their diagnosis and treatment are primarily managed within the discipline of psychiatry. The neurologist should be familiar with certain key features reflected in a clinical sleep disorder. The major sleep abnormalities consist of a chronic and recurrent inability to maintain sleep through the expected sleep period, usually with premature early morning arousal and, less often, difficulty initiating sleep. Wakefulness is characteristically intrusive; complaints of severe and persistent restlessness are common during the nocturnal sleep episode. Most depressed patients also complain of daytime insomnia and are unable to take "refreshing naps." They report a tired, "washed-out," dysphoric feeling during the day. In both monopolar and bipolar major depression, the latency from sleep onset to the first REM period may be shortened and there is a major reduction of Stages 3 and 4 sleep. Insomniacs with secondary depression or personality disorders (e.g., generalized anxiety, neurotic phobias, obsessive-compulsive disorders) usually do not have a shortened REM latency, but do show fragmented sleep with a reduction in Stages 3 and 4. Polysomnographic recordings often show the presence of coherent alpha activity (e.g., 9–11 Hz) superimposed on sleep EEG patterns (e.g., 1–3 Hz), and a mixture of REM and sleep spindles. These polygraphic patterns are less common during normal sleep and may indicate internal dissociative sleep features of chronic insomnia syndromes.

The widespread *use and abuse of CNS depressant drugs* (hypnotic and sedative drugs, tranquilizers, bedtime use of alcohol) without a rational pharmacologic basis has been emphasized. The effectiveness of long-term hypnotic drug use has not been scientifically established beyond 30 days of study. In addition, although one third of all sedative drugs are used by people older than 60, there have been few objective studies of their effectiveness in elderly patients. Nightly use of alcohol is sometimes recommended by physicians, but its effectiveness has not been established. With heavy and sustained alcohol use, sleep is disrupted with shortened REM periods and intrusive awakenings. Acute alcohol withdrawal produces a major sleep disturbance with a decrease in nonREM and an increase in REM sleep and, if severe, merges with the acute toxic withdrawal syndrome (delirium tremens).

A major advance has been the recognition that tolerance to or withdrawal from CNS depressants may produce significant insomnia (i.e., drug dependency insomnia). The short-term sleep inducing and maintenance effects are lost and both the patient and physician often either increase the dose or add other drugs. After chronic use, sleep is interrupted by frequent awakenings lasting more than 5 minutes; a consequent partial withdrawal syndrome with arousals in the second half of the night (early morning awakenings) is then erroneously viewed as persistent insomnia. If the hypnotic is withdrawn too rapidly, a severe sleep disturbance occurs, which may again be misinterpreted as the return of an underlying insomnia. Polysomnographic recording during chronic, heavy drug use shows that Stages 3 and 4 and REM sleep are decreased, stage demarcations are less clear with frequent stage changes, and K-complexes, delta waves, and REM are all decreased. A rapid withdrawal from chronic high-dose use of hypnotics (especially barbiturates) produces a disrupted sleep pattern, often with a high percentage of REM sleep and intense phasic activity. Periodic movements during sleep ("nocturnal myoclonus," see below) may also temporarily occur during the withdrawal period. Withdrawal from the chronic use of high-dose hypnotics should be done gradually and under clinical supervision. However, many patients have remarkable improvement in their sleep after withdrawal from the chronic use of hypnotics.

Another cause of a chronic nightly sleep disturbance is *sleep apnea*, or hypoventilation, during sleep. Although most patients with sleep apnea complain of excessive daytime somnolence, some complain primarily of frequent awakenings and restless, unrefreshing sleep. Such patients are more likely to have nonobstructive (central), rather than obstructive, apnea. In some cases, a mixed upper-airway obstructive and central apnea pattern may be present. (See "Disorders of Excessive Somnolence," later in this section for a discussion of upper-airway obstructive sleep apnea syndromes.)

The *central alveolar hypoventilation* syndrome is associated with major changes in respiratory function during sleep, including central sleep apnea and hypopnea associated with recurrent hypoxemia, hypercapnia, and a decreased tidal and minute volume. REM sleep is the time of greatest abnormality with the longest apneic episodes and the greatest fall in oxygen saturation. This syndrome occurs in association with chronic residual poliomyelitis, muscle diseases (e.g., myotonic dystrophy, anterior horn cell disease), involvement of thoracic cage bellows action or diaphragmatic muscle weakness, cervical spinal cordotomy, brain-stem lesions of structures that control ventilation, dysautonomia syndromes, and massive obesity.

PERIODIC MOVEMENTS DURING SLEEP (NOCTURNAL MYOCLONUS)

Many patients who complain of chronically disturbed sleep have stereotyped periodic movements of one or both legs and feet during sleep. The movement, which occurs primarily in nonREM sleep, consists of a dorsiflexion of the foot, extension of the big toe, and often flexion of the leg at the knee and hip. This triple flexion movement lasts 1.5 to 2.5 seconds (Fig. 148–1).

Although originally described as "myoclonic" by Sir Charles Symonds in 1953, these movements are not as brief as true myoclonic contractions and do not occur in isolated muscles. They are remarkably periodic

(20- to 30-second intervals) and may continue for 30 minutes to even several hours. In contrast to most movement disorders, which are inhibited by sleep (e.g., cerebellar and extrapyramidal tremors, chorea, dystonia, hemiballism), *periodic movements during sleep* (PMS) are initiated by sleep. PMS are different from *hypnic jerks* (sleep starts), which are nonperiodic, isolated myoclonic movements, that occur at sleep onset and simultaneously involve the muscles of the trunk and extremities. Hypnic jerks are considered normal because most children and adults experience them occasionally.

PMS are found in most cases of *restless-legs syndrome* that are studied with polysomnographic recordings. In the restless-legs syndrome, the patient feels an irresistible urge to move the legs, especially when sitting or lying down. There is a nonpainful discomfort deep inside the leg, most commonly between the knee and ankle, that makes the patient move the legs or walk about vigorously. The symptoms interfere with and delay sleep onset and may recur during the night. Thus, the condition may lead to an insomnia complaint in its own right, independent of PMS. Restless legs symptoms usually disappear by early

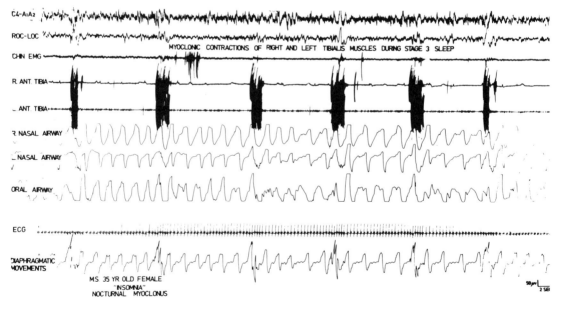

Fig. 148–1. Nocturnal myoclonus in a 52-year-old woman with a 20-year complaint of insomnia, which had increased over the past 3 years. She reported great difficulty in falling asleep upon retiring at 10:00 p.m. Often she would lie awake for 3 or 4 hours, sleep eventually 1 to 2 hours before awakening, and then have trouble returning to sleep for the rest of the night. She denied any history of restless-legs syndrome, was not aware of abnormal movements during sleep, and was unable to nap during the day. She had not taken medication for this problem for many years. Polysomnography during two consecutive nights demonstrated severe nocturnal myoclonus occurring in prolonged episodes, each lasting several hours. The myoclonus was synchronous in both legs. (From McGregor PA, Weitzman ED, Pollak CP. Am J EEG Technol 1978; 18:107.)

morning and the patient can obtain more refreshing sleep.

PMS occur in association with many sleep disorders, including sleep apnea, narcolepsy-cataplexy, drug dependency, and other chronic insomnia syndromes. PMS may develop in patients being treated with antidepressants, during withdrawal from drugs (e.g., barbiturates, benzodiazepines), and occasionally in patients with chronic uremia, anemia, and iron deficiency.

These findings suggest that PMS do not cause insomnia but rather develop from chronic daily sleep-wake disturbances of any origin. The neurophysiologic mechanisms responsible for PMS are unknown, but the suggestion has been made that a chronic disturbance of the temporal organization of the sleep-wake schedule and sleep stages may disinhibit an underlying CNS pacemaker.

Many drugs have been tried, but none have been clearly effective in eliminating PMS. In most cases, treatment is not indicated, but when the movements themselves disturb sleep, clonazepam has met with some success.

DISORDERS OF EXCESSIVE SOMNOLENCE

The clinical neurologist is asked to evaluate symptoms of excessive daytime sleepiness more than any other major category of sleep complaint. It is therefore important that the patient's complaint and symptoms be well defined to provide the physician with a rational basis for a diagnostic and treatment decision. The major symptoms include sleepiness and napping during a time of day when the patient wishes to be awake. The complaint has often been present for weeks or years, and presumes a regular (i.e., entrained) 24-hour sleep-wake cycle. The patient complains of an increased amount of unavoidable napping, apparent increase in total sleep during the 24-hour day, or difficulty in achieving full alertness after awakening in the morning. These symptoms should not be confused with complaints of tiredness, lack of energy, motivation or drive, or decreased alertness. The latter may reflect alterations of mood and affect and, although they may accompany true sleepiness, are more appropriately considered to be dysphoric symptoms such as might accompany depression. Also, the clinician should attempt to separate complaints of remaining in bed from true sleep. A shift of sleep time with extended morning sleep in a

"night person" may also be mistaken for a sleep disorder.

The list of disorders of excessive somnolence is large but, from a clinical point of view, two major syndromes are involved in some 80% of patients in this category who are seen in sleep-disorders centers: the hypersomnia-sleep-apnea (HSA) syndrome and narcolepsy.

The Hypersomnia-Sleep-Apnea Syndrome (HSA). The patient with the HSA syndrome complains of excessive daytime somnolence, which may vary in severity from day to day. Major complaints are the inability to sustain wakefulness occurring at inappropriate or dangerous times (e.g., driving a car, waiting for a red light, while eating), a pervasive sleepiness throughout the day, serious interference with work needs, and a major reduction of leisure or family time. Almost all patients have loud, intermittent snoring. Many cannot sleep at any time without snoring. The snoring pattern is recurrent with pauses between snores of 20 to 50 seconds. Each cycle comprises a series of three to six loud snores and gasps followed by a relatively silent period. During the nonsnoring period, the patient may either have quiet apnea (diaphragmatic arrest) or make ineffective respiratory efforts because of an obstructed upper airway.

In addition to loud cyclic snoring, there are other nighttime symptoms. Sleep is restless, with frequent brief arousals and unusual sleeping postures. The patient may sleep in a chair or in other nonsleeping areas of his or her home, talk during sleep, have nocturnal enuresis, fall out of bed, and wake in the morning with a generalized severe headache and a feeling of having had an unrefreshing night.

In the adult, the syndrome occurs predominantly between the fourth and sixth decades; the ratio of incidence of men versus women is 20 to 1. The syndrome in women usually occurs after the menopause. About 65% of patients are obese and symptoms often increase dramatically with a rapid weight gain. Numerous congenital and acquired abnormalities of the upper airway are associated with the HSA syndrome. These include micrognathia, deviated nasal septum, narrow nasal passages from a previous fracture, chronic rhinitis, enlarged adenoids or tonsils, palatopharyngeal abnormalities (e.g., Pierre-Robin syndrome, post cleft-palate repair, Treacher-Collins syndrome), enlarged tongue in acromegaly, hypothyroidism with myxedema of the upper-airway soft tissues, temporomandibular joint abnormalities, and others.

Sleep apnea also occurs in infants and children. In infants, it has been associated with the "near miss for sudden infant death syndrome," as well as familial, congenital, and acquired dysautonomia syndromes, adenotonsillar hypertrophy, and craniofacial disorders. In adults, sleep apnea is present in some patients with chronic obstructive pulmonary disease. The HSA syndrome occurs more often among elderly patients.

In addition to the daytime hypersomnia and nighttime sleep disturbances, many sleep apnea patients have systemic hypertension, primarily diastolic, and a wide variety of cardiac arrhythmias during sleep. Recognized systemic complications of HSA syndrome are pulmonary hypertension, cardiac enlargement, elevated hematocrit, and an increased risk of sudden death during sleep.

An all night polygraphic recording is used to diagnose the condition and to quantify the frequency, severity, and type of sleep apnea (Fig. 148–2). *Nonobstructive sleep apnea* (central) is the cessation of all respiratory movements (diaphragmatic arrest); *obstructive apnea* is the absence of upper airway air flow (from nose and mouth) in the presence of respiratory effort; *mixed apnea* consists of an initial nonobstruction followed by obstructive apnea; *hypopnea* is a partial decrease of respiratory effort and air flow by greater than 50%; *subobstructive apnea* is a partial decrease of air flow in the presence of respiratory effort (usually indicating a partial pharyngeal obstruction). The subobstructive apnea is the abnormality present in common snoring and can be associated with a mild degree of oxygen desaturation. During the recurrent apnea episodes in severe cases, oxygen desaturation often falls below 50% and a bradycardia (<60 beats/minute) alternates with a tachycardia (>110 beats/minute) for each snoring cycle. Stages 3 and 4 sleep are diminished or absent, Stages 2 and REM are present; there are many stage changes and brief arousals. The duration of apneic episodes and the degree of oxygen desaturation increase in REM sleep.

When severe the most effective treatment for the hypersomnia-sleep-apnea syndrome is to provide the patient with an open tracheal airway (tracheostomy), thereby bypassing the upper airway obstruction during sleep. This treatment immediately reverses the daytime sleepiness, improves mood, restores noctur-

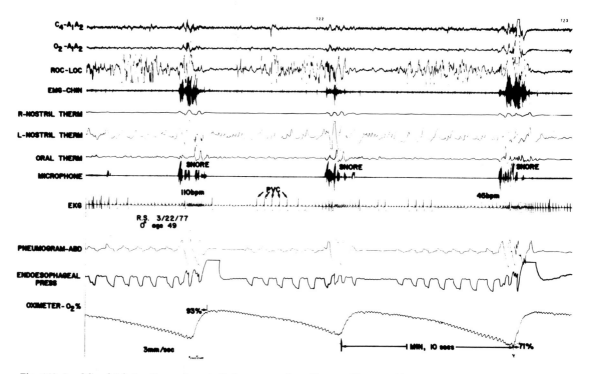

Fig. 148–2. Mixed (obstructive and central) sleep apnea in a 49-year-old man with progressive sleepiness of 4 years' duration. Note bradytachycardia pattern associated with multiple premature ventricular contractions. There were frequent falls in oxygen saturation below 75% ($P_{O_2} \approx 40$ mm Hg). (From Weitzman ED, Pollak C, McGregor P. In: Aminoff M, ed. Electrodiagnosis in Clinical Neurology. Edinburgh: Churchill-Livingstone, 1980.)

nal sleep toward a normal pattern, either fully or partially improves the sleep-treated cardiac arrhythmia, restores high oxygen saturation values, decreases the blood hematocrit, and in some cases, decreases the systemic hypertension.

Nasal continuous positive airway pressure (CPAP), a recently available nonsurgical treatment, now replaces tracheostomy for about 80% of patients with severe obstructive sleep apnea. Air pressure is generated by a small blower, delivered via tubing to a nasal mask, and controlled by a pressure valve. Each patient must have a treatment trial during polysomnography to determine the pressure required to alleviate airway obstruction during sleep. If successful and well tolerated, a commercially available nasal CPAP unit is prescribed for home use.

In some cases, especially in children and young adults, the removal of enlarged tonsils and adenoids relieves the obstruction. The surgical procedure, uvulopalatopharyngoplasty, has been an inconsistently beneficial treatment and selection criteria are not well established. Hyoidplasty and mandibular advancement have successfully treated patients with structural abnormalities causing hypopharyngeal obstruction.

Other treatments for less severe cases have been sustained weight loss in the obese patient, tricyclic drugs, and progesterone, but these have met with only limited success.

Narcolepsy-Cataplexy Syndrome. Narcolepsy is a distinct clinical syndrome of unknown cause that has well-defined symptoms, age of onset, and natural history. The two major symptoms are recurrent episodes of excessive and uncontrollable *daytime somnolence* and sleep during the normal waking part of the day, and *cataplexy*, which is characterized by brief, sudden episodes of muscle weakness without loss of consciousness. Cataplexy develops at some point in the history of the illness in some 79 to 90% of cases. The episodes of weakness vary; they may be total, with flaccid paralysis of all somatic musculature (except diaphragmatic and extraocular muscles) with a sudden fall to the ground, or partial, with weakness of isolated muscle groups. A careful history often reveals frequent episodes of dropping of the head or jaw, dysarthric speech, weakness of facial muscles, leg muscle weakness, and sudden dropping of objects from the hands, all lasting only seconds or minutes. These episodes are characteristically triggered by a sudden emotional surge (e.g., amusement, anger, excitement, startle, surprise, sadness). Many patients attempt to avoid emotional situations and to control emotions to avoid embarrassment and the discomfort of cataplexy. The other characteristic symptoms are hypnagogic hallucinations, sleep paralysis, brief lapses of memory, and automatic behavior episodes.

Hypnagogic (predormital) hallucinations characteristically occur at the onset of the daytime sleep episode or on falling asleep at night. Less commonly, they occur at the end of the sleep episode (hypnopompic postdormital hallucinations). The narcoleptic's hallucination is almost always visual and may involve a scene or story sequence or only simple forms. The imageries have all the characteristics of a vivid dream sequence in which the patient is frequently personally involved. At times, the patients may be aware of the ongoing real world around them while simultaneously experiencing the hallucination-dream sequence.

Sleep paralysis is a brief episode during which the patient is unable to perform any voluntary movement and occurs on falling asleep and on awakening. The individual is unable to move, speak, or open the eyes, but is fully aware of his condition and can recall it at a later time. When it first occurs, especially when it is accompanied by frightening hallucinations, the patient may be extremely anxious; however, as the episodes occur more frequently, the patient learns to accept them as brief and benign. If the patient attempts to cry out or move, he may produce faint moans or gasps and appear to an observer to be deeply asleep or dreaming. An episode usually lasts 1 to 2 minutes, and typically ends spontaneously and completely; rarely do they last more than 10 minutes. If the patient is lightly touched, shaken, or even spoken to, an episode may be abruptly terminated. Sleep paralysis occurs occasionally in normal persons, especially during adolescence and young adulthood. There is a rare syndrome of independent familial sleep paralysis in which other symptoms of narcolepsy never develop. It is presumed that sleep paralysis is due to similar brain stem-spinal neuron inhibitory mechanisms, as has been shown during normal REM sleep. Thus, it may be viewed as a fragment of the complex neurophysiologic changes of REM sleep, although associated temporally and extending into the wakeful, conscious state.

Automatic behavior in narcoleptic patients consists of a wide variety of episodes lasting from only a few seconds of altered consciousness to prolonged periods (several minutes to 1 hour) to bizarre, complex behavioral sequences. At times, hallucinatory experiences may accompany the episodes. These behaviors tend to occur in association with performance of motor activities such as driving a car, writing, typing, conversing, and performing monotonous tasks. When writing or typing, the patient may misspell a few words or write an entire page without sense or syntax. Patients may drive long distances and then be aware that they are in a strange place and be amnestic for the sequence of behavior that brought them there. Continuous polygraphic recordings of narcoleptic patients have demonstrated frequent "microsleep" episodes with reduced responsiveness in performance tests. The presumption is that automatic behavior represents a "twilight" sleep state when consciousness, awareness, and memory consolidation is deficient, but sufficient awareness is present that complex and protective motor behavior continue to be performed.

These behaviors are to be differentiated from automatisms of complex partial seizures and epileptic experiential hallucinations, fugue states, and transient global amnesia.

Although sleep attacks, cataplexy, hypnagogic hallucinations, and sleep paralysis usually happen at different times, they may occur in combination or in rapid succession in such a way that REM sleep is immediately preceded by cataplexy, is associated with hypnagogic hallucinations (vivid dream), and then ended with muscle paralysis. Too often, these symptoms are neither understood nor appreciated by physicians, and the disorder remains undiagnosed for many years.

The symptoms produce major social, familial, educational, and economic consequences to both patient and family. Patients do not achieve their intellectual potential and suffer frequent failures of occupation, education, and marriages. Family members, friends, and even the patient often interpret the symptoms as indicating laziness, lack of ambition, delayed maturation, or psychological defects. Because these symptoms begin during the crucial period of maturation from puberty to adulthood, misinterpretation and lack of a diagnosis can greatly impact the patient's personality and feelings of self-esteem.

Narcolepsy begins toward the end of puberty and early adulthood (ages 15 to 25); 80% of patients develop their first symptoms before age 35. It can be recognized before puberty (ages 7 to 12) and occasionally begins after age 40. Neither gender is more prone to the disorder than the other. Once present, it is a life-long illness. It is estimated that narcolepsy occurs at a rate of 4/10,000.

There is now evidence that narcolepsy is a genetic disorder. The major histocompatibility complex located on the short arm of chromosome 6 contains one or more genetic markers for narcolepsy. The strongest association found thus far is between human leukocyte antigen (HLA) DR2 and narcolepsy. In addition, the narcolepsy-cataplexy syndrome occurs in dogs and other animals in whom it is transmitted as an autosomal recessive trait.

A major advance in our understanding of narcolepsy has been the recognition that the daytime sleep attacks, cataplexy, hypnagogic hallucinations, and sleep paralysis are all manifestations and fragments of the REM sleep process (Fig. 148–3). Most of the sleep episodes during the day are REM periods; at night there is a sleep-onset REM period about 70% of the time in patients with narcolepsy-cataplexy. It almost never occurs in normal subjects. A recent diagnostic procedure has been developed in sleep disorders centers based upon the probability of having a REM period immediately after sleep onset. The *multiple sleep latency test* calls for the patient to lie in a quiet darkened room 4 or 5 times during the day at 2-hour intervals; sleep patterns are then recorded by polysomnographic techniques. The latency from "lights out" to sleep onset and the sleep stage that develops is determined. Patients with narcolepsy consistently have a very short sleep latency (1–5 minutes) and most include REM sleep. Patients who do not have narcolepsy but who have daytime hypersomnia due to sleep apnea also have abnormally short sleep latency, but only rarely develop sleep-onset REM periods.

The cause and localization of narcolepsy has not been determined. There are several clinical reports of structural disease in the upper brain stem-hypothalamus area with narcoleptic symptoms and cataplectic-like behavior. This has been produced in cats after microinjection of cholinergic drugs in the pontine recticular formation; however, no pathology has been reported thus far in animals with genetic narcolepsy-cataplexy.

The present treatment for the narcolepsy

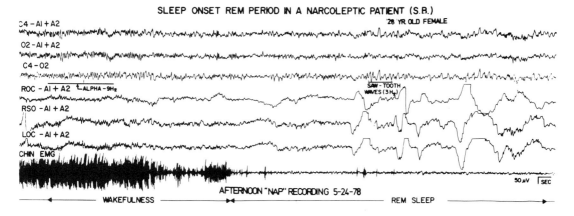

Fig. 148–3. Sleep onset REM period during an afternoon nap in a 28-year-old woman with a clear history of narcolepsy. Polysomnographic recordings also demonstrated REM onset of the nocturnal sleep period. (From McGregor PA, Weitzman ED, Pollak CP. Am J EEG Technol 1978; 18:107.)

syndrome is the use of adrenergic stimulant drugs (pemoline, methylphenidate, amphetamines) for the sleepiness and sleep attacks, and tricyclic compounds (imipramine, chlorimipramine) for cataplexy. The use of stimulant drugs should be carefully monitored; the patient and physician should cooperate in adjusting the amount and timing of doses to meet the functional daytime needs and scheduling of the patient's activities. Cataplexy, when present to a significant degree, is usually well controlled with tricyclics (e.g., imipramine, 25 mg, 3 times daily); however, impotence can be an undesirable side-effect in men. Other drugs, such as gamma-hydroxy butyrate, given nightly, and propranolol, given during the day, have been reported to be effective, but their usefulness has not been determined. Monoamine oxidase inhibitors such as phenelzine sulfate (Nardil) totally suppress REM sleep in patients with narcolepsy but, because of the risk of serious side-effects, are not often used. An important adjunctive treatment is the rational scheduling of daytime naps and the maintenance of proper sleep hygiene in accord with the patient's 24-hour functional activities. The physician's role in providing the patient with a clear understanding of the nature of the symptoms and with emotional support in coping with the many adaptive difficulties cannot be overemphasized.

Kleine-Levin Syndrome. A syndrome of periodic hypersomnia in young males (ages 10 to 21) was first described by Kleine in 1925 and extended to include bulimia by Levin in 1936. Gallinek in 1954, and Critchley in 1962, emphasized the marked behavioral and psy-

chological changes that accompany the periodic excessive sleep and bizarre food ingestion *(megaphagia)*. These consist of serious disturbances in social interaction, sexual hyperactivity and exhibitionism, compulsive eating, depression, hallucinations, disorientation, memory deficits, and sometimes frank delusions. The hypersomnolence-bulimia episode usually lasts 1 to 2 weeks with an interval of 3 to 6 months between episodes. During the intervening period, the patient is usually normal, although some patients have a persistent personality disorder. Although most cases occur in adolescent and young adult males, rare cases have been described in girls. The condition decreases in frequency and severity as a function of age and rarely is present beyond the fourth or fifth decade.

Polysomnographic recording has been reported during a typical hypersomniac episode in several cases. The reports have described a variety of changes. These include extended sleep periods, multiple sleep-onset REM periods, disturbed sleep with decreased stages 3 and 4, frequent intrusive arousals, and sleep apneic episodes.

A definitive treatment for Kleine-Levin syndrome is not known, but there are reports of limited success with amphetamines and methylphenidate. Because of similarities between Kleine-Levin syndrome and bipolar depression, lithium has been used.

Other Conditions Associated with Excessive Daytime Somnolence. Various neurologic and medical conditions are associated with excessive daytime sleepiness including endocrine and metabolic disorders, liver failure, uremia, chronic pulmonary disease (with hypercapnia), hypothyroidism (severe with myxedema), incipient coma with diabetes mellitus, and severe hypoglycemia. Neurologic disorders such as tumors in the area of the third ventricle (e.g., glioma, craniopharyngioma, dysgerminoma, pinealoma, pituitary adenomas), obstructive hydrocephalus, increased intracranial pressure, viral encephalitis, and other infections of the brain and surrounding membranes can cause increased daytime somnolence. The postconcussion syndrome has been associated with increased sleepiness; however, complaints of tiredness, fatigue, depression, lethargy, malaise, and lack of interest must be carefully distinguished from sleepiness.

Disorders of the Sleep-Wake Schedule

A major advance in our understanding of the physiology of the daily sleep period and its disorders derives from the investigation of biologic rhythms and, specifically, from studies of human circadian timekeeping systems. Many functions, including body temperature, plasma and urine hormones, renal functions, psychological performance measures, and internal sleep-stage organization all participate in this circadian rhythm. Studies of these cyclic physiologic systems using time isolated and nonscheduled human laboratories have shown that different variables develop nonsynchronized but mutually coupled cycle lengths. These findings have gven rise to the concept that there are multiple biologic oscillators that are normally synchronized but that can become desynchronized under free-running conditions. Evidence for the importance of biologic-rhythm function in sleep disturbances comes from studies of acute phase shifts such as occur after transmeridian air flights or in shiftwork. The daily sleep period is disturbed after acute shifts in such a way that intrusive awakenings take place, sleep length is shortened, and REM-phase advances relative to sleep onset. Adaptation is slower after an eastward flight or a phase advance in the laboratory than after a phase delay (westward flight).

Disorders of the circadian sleep-wake cycle are divided into two major categories, transient and persistent. The transient disorders include the temporary sleep disturbance following an acute workshift change and a rapid time zone change ("jet lag"). Both sleep deprivation and the circadian phase shift produce a complex of symptoms including an inability to have sustained sleep; frequent arousals, especially at the end of sleep episodes; excessive sleepiness; and falling asleep at inappropriate times in relation to social or economic requirements. Affected individuals are fatigued, sleepy, and intermittently inattentive when they should be awake, and have partial insomnia during the daily time for sleep. A wide range of important occupations are involved in these acute phase-shift syndromes (e.g., doctors, nurses, police, firemen, airline pilots, air-traffic controllers, diplomats, international business executives, radar operators, postal workers, long distance truck drivers).

Persistent sleep-wake cycle disorders are divided into several major clinical categories. The person who frequently changes his sleep-wake schedule (e.g., shiftworker) has a mixed pattern of excessive sleepiness alternating with arousal at inappropriate times of the day. Sleep is typically shortened and disrupted. Waking is associated with a decrease in performance and vigilance. The physician caring for such patients should be aware that the syndrome often disrupts social and family life and becomes intolerable.

The *delayed-sleep-phase syndrome* has been recognized as a specific chronobiologic sleep disorder. Patients suffering this syndrome describe a chronic inability to sleep at a desired time to meet their required work or study schedules. They are typically unable to fall asleep until some time between 2 and 6 a.m. On weekends and vacation days, they sleep until late morning or early afternoon and feel refreshed, but have great difficulty awakening at the required 7 or 8 a.m. on workdays. They score high as "night persons" on a standard questionnaire of this tendency. These patients have a normal sleep length and internal organization of sleep when the clock time of sleep onset and sleep end coincides with the circadian timing of the endogenous oscillator that controls daily sleep (e.g., 5 a.m. to 1 p.m.).

If sleep onset is attempted at earlier times (e.g., midnight) there is usually a long latency to sleep onset. Patients describe a long history of many unsuccessful attempts to sleep at an earlier hour, and the "sleep-onset insomnia" has inappropriately been treated by many prescribed and self-administered hypnotic drugs. Other common forms of treatment that fail include behavior modification, psychotherapy, alcohol, and home remedies.

Successful treatment has been a phase shift of the time of the daily sleep episode by progressive phase delay of the sleep time. By delaying the time of going to sleep and awakening by 2 or 3 hours each day (i.e., a 26- or 27-hour sleep-wake cycle), the patient's sleep timing can be successfully reset to the clock time preferred by the patient. Because this form of therapy can be more easily achieved by a phase delay than by a phase advance, it has been postulated that differences in the shape of the "phase-response curve" may underlie these patients' chronobiologic problems. The phase-advance part of the curve may be weak, whereas the phase-delay portion may be normal in these patients compared with normal individuals. Normal persons phase advance the sleep time each day by about 1 hour to hold to a 24-hour day and prevent a free-running rhythm of 25 hours. This daily, active entrainment process also requires a well-functioning advance capability and a range of entrainment sufficiently broad on both sides of 24 hours to enable a normal person to adjust to variations in sleep onset and waking times, which is necessary to maintain an appropriately synchronized phase of sleep to the 24-hour schedule.

An *advanced sleep-phase syndrome* has not yet been clearly identified, but a person with this syndrome would complain of undesirably early sleep onset and wake times. Aging leads to such a characteristic change in the timing of sleep; older people awaken spontaneously earlier in the morning and go to sleep earlier in the evening. Maturational alterations in the shape of the phase response curve might underlie these changes and in fact produce an advanced sleep-phase syndrome in the elderly. However, other sleep-wake changes occur as a function of aging, including intrusive nocturnal awakenings, fragmentation of the sleep pattern, reduction of stages 3 and 4 sleep, and repeated daytime brief sleep periods. Some of these changes can be attributed to aging but other factors also affect sleep, including occult sleep disorders, changes in other physiologic systems, chronic diseases, and socioeconomic changes.

The *hypernyctohemeral syndrome* is a disorder of the sleep-wake cycle in which the patient is completely out of touch with the 24-hour cycle of the rest of society. These rare individuals maintain a 25- to 27-hour biologic day despite all attempts to entrain themselves to a 24-hour cycle. A personality disorder or blindness may predispose to this condition. Repeated attempts to entrain to a 24-hour pattern in patients with the hypernyctohemeral syndrome produce cyclic periods of nonsynchronization to society's rhythm and cyclic (3–4-week) disrupted and delayed sleep with an associated daytime sleepiness. Delayed sleep-phase and hypernyctohemeral syndromes may differ only in degree because the former also demonstrates a tendency to a progressive phase delay. The hypernyctohemeral person may have an even further altered phase response curve with essentially no phase advance capablity.

An "irregular sleep-wake pattern" syndrome is also included within the general category of *disorders of the sleep-wake schedule*. The pattern consists of considerable irregularity without an identifiable persistent sleep-wake rhythm. There are frequent daytime naps at irregular times and a disturbed nocturnal sleep pattern. When severe, it may be impossible to identify a circadian sleep-wake cycle. Descriptions of the severe sleep disorders of patients with encephalitis lethargica during the historic influenza epidemic of 1918–1920 conform in many respects to such a severe dysfunction. Encephalitic lesions in these patients were localized to the periventricular group, particularly in the hypothalamus, and formed the neuropathologic basis of considering the junction of the diencephalon and the mesencephalon as a "sleep-regulating center." Many lesions in and around the third ventricle, hypothalamus, and mesencephalon produce an altered daily sleep-wake cycle in addition to excessive daytime somnolence. Of considerable interest, therefore, are recent studies that have shown that bilateral destruction of the suprachiasmatic nuclei (SCN) in animals (i.e., rats, hamsters, monkeys) produces an abnormal daily sleep-wake cycle. These animals no longer demonstrated a circadian rhythm under free-running conditions. The retinohypothalamic tract is the presumed pathway mediating light-dark entrainment of the SCN.

The Parasomnias

The parasomnias comprise a group of neurologic and medical conditions in which an undesirable behavioral and physiologic event occurs during or in association with sleep, however, the sleeping-and-waking process is not abnormal. The disturbing symptom specifically affects either motor behavior, autonomic dysfunction, psychological state, or a combination. The range of symptoms is broad and encompasses all age groups. The disorders are described individually, and an attempt has been made to organize several around the concept of "disorders of the state of partial arousal" (e.g., sleep terror, sleep-related enuresis, somnambulism). This list of parasomnias will certainly be augmented as cases of disturbing sleep dysfunction are increasingly referred to specalized sleep disorders centers.

Somnambulism (Sleepwalking). An episode of sleepwalking is a sudden behavioral sequence that interrupts sleep. It consists of either sitting up in bed or leaving the bed and walking, without full awareness. It selectively emerges from Stages 3 or 4 sleep and not from REM sleep. The behavior may be quite complex, including automatic and semipurposeful motor acts (e.g., walking, opening and closing doors, opening a window, climbing stairs, dressing, and even preparing food). A subgroup of patients, usually young adult men, perform acts that are destructive or harmful to themselves (e.g., breaking furniture, throwing objects about the room, climbing out or walking through a window). The patient is not easily aroused to full consciousness during the episode and often strongly resists arousal attempts. Voice communication is either not possible or is fragmentary. The individual episode generally lasts no more than 15 minutes and is terminated by returning to bed, going to sleep in another place, or spontaneous arousal with confusion regarding his location. The patient awakens in the morning either unaware of the somnambulist episode or surprised to find himself in another place with only a dim fragmented recollection of the episode. Dreaming is not present and, when aroused during the episode, the patient does not report strong emotions or hallucinatory imagery, but, usually, only brief nonsustained thoughts. Some patients who perform destructive acts describe a recurrent dream of feeling overwhelmed and unable to escape a powerful destructive force.

Somnambulism episodes occur normally in children; 15% of all children have had one or more episodes. In a small percentage of children (1–6%) episodes occur frequently (at times nightly). If the episodes persist, recur, or begin in adolescence or adulthood, there is a high association with serious psychopathology.

Polysomnographic studies have demonstrated that a somnambulist episode emerges from typical Stages 3 and 4 sleep, usually preceded by high-amplitude delta waves; however, there is no change in heart rate or respiration just before onset of the motor behavior. There is no evidence of seizure activity in the EEG, either preceding or during the episode of somnambulism. It is important to distinguish somnambulism from recurrent nocturnal seizure disorders such as partial complex seizures (psychomotor epilepsy). A standard EEG during waking and daytime sleep, using nasopharyngeal leads, may be indicated. In addition, a videotape of the complex behavior during a nocturnal episode in a sleep-recording laboratory can be extremely useful to help differentiate a somnambulist episode from a seizure arising from sleep. Somnambulism may occur in the same patient and in families with other episodic parasomnias, including nocturnal enuresis and sleep-terror attacks. Diazepam in nightly doses of 5 to 20 mg or shorter acting benzodiazepines are useful for control of attacks, especially when violent behavior is present.

Sleep Terror (Pavor Nocturnus, Incubus). A sleep-terror episode is a sudden arousal during Stages 3 and 4 sleep during the first third of the night. Typically, it is initiated by a sudden, loud, high-pitched scream, and sitting up in bed. The patient behaves in an agitated, frightened manner. Polygraphic recordings have not shown autonomic changes before the attack; however, after the onset, there are major autonomic changes including rapid pulse, rapid respiration, sweating, and pupillary dilation (the pupils are normally meiotic during sleep). Sleep-terror attacks occur mainly in children, but may persist into adulthood and rarely begin in adulthood. During the attack (5–15 minutes) the patient is usually inconsolable and may repeat cries for help or call for a close family member. It is usually not possible to elicit complex dream imagery at the end of the event. The patient returns to sleep quickly and has amnesia for the event the next morning. Sleep terrors differ from recurrent nightmares because of the lack of complex hallucinatory imagery and remembered strong emotions and their association with nonREM Stages 3 and 4 sleep. By contrast, nightmares occur during REM sleep during the middle and latter thirds of the night and can usually be recounted in a vivid, emotionally charged, and detailed story full of personal fears and threats. As with somnambulism, recurrent sleep-terror attacks should be differentiated from nocturnal sleep-related seizures. There is no evidence that sleep terrors are harmful in and of themselves. If they are persistent, a thorough psychological evaluation of the child and family may be indicated.

Sleep-Related Enuresis. Sleep-related enuresis occurs during Stages 3 and 4 nonREM sleep in the first third of the night. It is often associated with a brief arousal; the individual is confused and disoriented, but does not describe a complex dream sequence or a feeling of terror or anxiety. "Primary" enuresis is the persistence of sleep-related bedwetting from infancy to childhood. "Secondary" enuresis is the reappearance of bedwetting after successful bladder training. These idiopathic forms are to be distinguished from symptomatic enuresis, which is caused by a known organic condition. Most children with idiopathic enuresis stop bed-wetting by age 10 or 12, although emotional stress can reactivate the problem. There is no evidence that there is an epileptic discharge associated with idiopathic enuresis; of course, sleep-related seizures, particularly of the major motor type, may also be accompanied by urinary incontinence and additional symptoms and signs such as tongue or cheek biting, blood on the pillow, or tonic-clonic movements. Polysomnographic and EEG recording is useful in identifying this condition.

Treatment of nocturnal enuresis is generally done with behavioral modification and bladder-training techniques. In selected cases in which bed-wetting may have psychosocial consequences (e.g., attending a summer camp, visiting friends, living in a college dormitory arrangement), short-term use of imipramine hydrochloride, 25 mg nightly, may be helpful.

Sleep-Related Headaches. Patients with cluster headaches, migraine, and chronic paroxysmal hemicrania characteristically have attacks during sleep. These attacks awaken the patient with severe pain, either directly out of REM sleep or in the immediate postREM period. Phase shifts of the daily sleep period demonstrate that the timing of the headache follows the timing of REM sleep itself. A patient with cluster headaches usually awakens with severe, unilateral eye and upper facial pain, tearing, rhinorrhea, conjunctival vasodilation, and often, Horner syndrome. Nausea and vomiting may occur. The attack may last from 30 minutes to several hours and may recur periodically, several times per night, in association with REM sleep. Chronic paroxysmal hemicrania attacks occur more frequently, up to 24 episodes/24 hours, are brief (5–15 minutes), and occur equally during waking and sleeping periods; however, during sleep, the attacks are synchronized with REM sleep episodes.

Sleep-Related Gastroesophageal Reflux Syndrome. Patients with gastroesophageal reflux may be awakened from sleep with burning substernal pain (heartburn), a sour taste, coughing, choking, and even respiratory stridor. During the day, they may also have postprandial regurgitation, esophagitis, and laryngopharyngitis; when severe, it may lead to esophageal ulceration or stricture. The mechanism of gastroesophageal reflux is related to lower esophageal sphincter incompetence. The course of this sphincter incompetence has not been determined, but several regulatory factors are under active investigation. These include serum gastrin-cholecystokinin secretion, prostaglandins, substance P, and other gut and pancreatic polypeptides, plus cholinergic, adrenergic, and histamine-controlled neural functions. It has been shown that in association with the incompetence of the lower esophageal sphincter, there is decreased acid clearance in the lower esophagus during sleep, with recurrent reflux of low-pH gastric juice into the esophagus. A specific sleep-stage relationship has not been established. Treatment should include simple, general therapeutic measures such as dietary restriction of alcohol, high-fat foods, and chocolate, sleeping with the head of the bed raised, and calcium-free antacids taken 1 hour after meals and at bedtime. The use of cimetidine or ranitidine (histamine-receptor antagonists) at bedtime may be especially useful.

Other Parasomnias. There is a growing list of other pathologic events that occur during sleep. The bibliography contains several recent reviews and specialized classification schemes. A partial list includes dream-anxiety attacks, sleep-related epileptic seizures, bruxism (teeth grinding), head banging, body rocking, familial sleep paralysis, abnormal swallowing syndrome, sleep-related asthmatic attacks, sleep-related angina and other cardiovascular symptoms, and sleep-related hemolysis (paroxysmal nocturnal hemoglobinuria).

References

Anders TF, Carskadon MA, Dement WC. Sleep and sleepiness in children and adolescents. Pediatr Clin N Am 1980; 27:29–43.

Association of Sleep Centers. Diagnostic classification of sleep and arousal disorders. Sleep 1979; 2:1–154.

Chiles JA, Wilkus RJ. Behavioral manifestations of the

Kleine-Levin syndrome. Dis Nerv Syst 1976; 11:646–648.

Coleman R, Pollak CP, Weitzman ED. Periodic movements in sleep (nocturnal myoclonus): relation to sleep disorders. Ann Neurol 1980; 8:416–421.

Coleman R, Roffwarg H, Kennedy S, et al. A national cooperative study of sleep-wake disorders based upon a polysomnographic diagnosis. JAMA 1982; 247:997–1003.

Critchley M. Periodic hypersomnia and megaphagia in adolescent males. Brain 1962; 85:627–656.

Dement W, Rechtschaffen A, Gulevich G. The nature of the narcoleptic sleep attack. Neurology 1966; 16:18–33.

Dexter JD, Weitzman ED. The relationship of nocturnal headaches to sleep stage patterns. Neurology 1970; 20:513–518.

Ekbom RA. Restless legs syndrome. Neurology 1960; 10:868–873.

Ferber R. Sleep disorders in infants and children. In: Riley I, ed. Clinical Aspects of Sleep and Sleep Disturbances. Stoneham, MA: Butterworth, 1985:113–157.

Fry JM. Sleep disorders. In: Bardo DM, ed. Symposium on the Post Menopausal Woman. Med Clin N Am 1987; 71:95–110.

Guilleminault C, ed. Narcolepsy. Sleep 1986; 9:99–291.

Guilleminault C, ed. Sleeping and Waking Disorders. Indications and Techniques. Menlo Park, CA: Addison Wesley, 1981.

Guilleminault C, Lugaresi E, eds. Sleep Wake Disorders. Natural History, Epidemiology, and Long-term Evolution. New York: Raven Press, 1983.

Jeffries JJ, Lefebuvre A. Depression and mania associated with Kleine-Levin-Crutchley syndrome. Can J Psychiatry 1973; 18:439.

Kales A, Allen C, Scharf MB, Kales JD. Hypnotic drugs and their effectiveness: allnight EEG studies of insomniac subjects. Arch Gen Psychiatry 1970; 23:226.

Kokkoris CP, Weitzman ED, Pollak CP, Spielman AJ, Czeisler CA, Bradlow H. Long-term ambulatory temperature monitoring in a subject with a hypernyctohemeral sleep-wake cycle disturbance. Sleep 1978; 1:177–190.

Lavie P, Gadoth N, Gordon CR, Goldhammer G, Bechar M. Sleep patterns in Kleine-Levin syndrome. Electroencephalogr Clin Neurophysiol 1979; 47:369–371.

Levin M. Narcolepsy (Gelineau's syndrome) and other varieties of morbid somnolence. Arch Neurol Psychiatry 1929; 22:1172–1200.

Mendelson WB. Human sleep: research and clinical care. New York: Plenum Medical Book Co. 1987.

Moore RY. The retinohypothalamic tract, suprachiasmatic hypothalamic nucleus and central neural mechanisms of circadian rhythm circulation. In: Suda M, Hayaishi O, Nakagawa H, eds. Biological Rhythms and their Central Mechanism. New York: Elsevier-North Holland, 1979:343–354.

National Institute of Mental Health Consensus Development Conference. Drugs and insomnia. The use of medication to promote sleep. JAMA 1984; 251:2410–2414.

Orlosky MJ. The Kleine-Levine syndrome: A review. Psychosomatics 1982; 23:609–621.

Phillipson EA. Respiratory adaptations in sleep. Annu Rev Physiol 1978; 40:133–156.

Pressman MR, Fry JM. What is normal sleep in the elderly? Clin Geriatric Med 1988; 4:71–81.

Prinzmetal M, Bloomberg W. The use of benzedrine for the treatment of narcolepsy. JAMA 1935; 105:2051.

Reynolds CF, Black RS, Coble P, Holzer B, Kupfer DJ. Similarities in EEG sleep findings for the Kleine-Levin syndrome and unipolar depression. Am J Psychiatry 1980; 137:116–118.

Sanders MH, Moore SE, Eveslage J. CPAP via nasal mask. A treatment for occlusive sleep apnea. Chest 1983; 83:144–145.

Sullivan CE, Berthon-Jones M, Issa FG, et al. Reversal of obstructive sleep apnea by continuous positive airway pressure applied through the nares. Lancet 1981; 1:862–865.

Weitzman ED, Pollak CP, McGregor P. The polysomnographic evaluation of sleep disorders in man. In: Aminoff M, ed. Electrophysiological Approaches to Neurological Diagnosis. Edinburgh: Churchill-Livingstone, 1979:496–524.

Weitzman ED. Sleep and aging. In: Katzman R, Terry R, eds. Neurology of Aging. Philadelphia, FA Davis, 1983:167–188.

Weitzman ED, Czeisler CA, Zimmerman JC, Moore-Ede M. Biological rhythms in man: relationship of a sleep-wake, cortisol, growth hormone and temperature during temporal isolation. In: Martin JB, Reichlin S, Bick K, eds. Neurosecretion and Brain Peptides. New York: Raven Press, 1981:475–499.

Weitzman ED. Sleep and its disorders. Annu Rev Neurosci 1981; 4:381–417.

Weitzman ED, Czeisler CA, Coleman RM, et al. Delayed sleep phase syndrome. Arch Gen Psychiatry 1981; 38:737–746.

Wever R. The Circadian System of Man. New York: Springer-Verlag, 1979.

Williams RL, Karacan I, eds. Sleep Disorders: Diagnosis and Treatment. New York: John Wiley, 1978.

Chapter XXI

Systemic Diseases

149. ENDOCRINE DISEASES
Earl A. Zimmerman

The secretions of the endocrine glands have a profound influence on the metabolism of the nervous system. Disturbances of consciousness and mental activity plus various neurologic symptoms may occur with dysfunction of the glands. This article considers the clinical manifestations that occur with hyper- and hypofunction of these glands. (The mass effects of tumors on the endocrine glands are considered in Chapter V, Tumors.)

Pituitary

HYPOPITUITARISM

Hypofunction of the pituitary may occur because of undersecretion of unknown cause or damage to the gland by tumors, inflammatory processes, vascular lesions, or trauma. The location of the lesion can be the pituitary itself, the stalk that connects it with the hypothalamus, or the hypothalamus. Destruction of the hypophyseal portal system in the stalk, or the median eminence above by a tumor (such as a craniopharyngioma), or sarcoidosis will deprive the anterior pituitary of hypothalamic regulating hormones. As in pituitary disease itself, all the anterior pituitary hormones may be reduced in peripheral blood except prolactin (PRL) which is increased because regulation of PRL secretion is mainly under inhibitory control by hypothalamic dopamine. Another indication that the problem may be above the pituitary is the presence of diabetes insipidus, which rarely occurs with an intrasellar tumor unless the mass extends upward to involve the hypothalamus.

Diseases of the pituitary that cause endocrine deficiencies include pituitary tumor, Simmonds disease, pituitary dwarfism, and diabetes insipidus.

Pituitary Tumor. A variable degree of hypopituitarism is present in most patients with pituitary adenomas, particularly when the tumors are a considerable size. It is important to emphasize, however, that some patients with microadenomas will have preserved function; this is why early recognition and treatment of these lesions are imperative. Secretion of gonadotropins is affected first; in women, this leads to irregularities of the menstrual periods and amenorrhea, and in men to loss of libido and decreased potency. In late cases, oligospermia or azoospermia and testicular atrophy may be present. The skin is often thin, smooth, and dry; the peculiar pallor (alabaster skin) and inability to tan have been related to loss of the melanocyte-stimulating hormone. There is a decrease in axillary and pubic hair, and in the frequency of shaving. Due to decrease in adrenocorticotropic hormone (ACTH) and thyroid-stimulating hormone (TSH) production, patients frequently complain of lethargy, weakness, fatigability, intolerance of cold, and constipation. Acute adrenal crisis with nausea, vomiting, hypoglycemia, hypotension, and circulatory collapse occasionally occurs, particularly in response to stress, but less often than in primary adrenal failure (Addison disease).

Evaluation of patients with pituitary insufficiency due to an intrasellar disease or a suprasellar lesion involving the hypothalamic-pituitary system depends on the assessment of function of the target organs, and the direct assay in the blood of the anterior pituitary hormones. The basic endocrine evaluation usually includes initially a thyroid screen (T_3, T_4), a PRL assay, and a 24-hour urine collection for adrenal steroids. The PRL assay is obtained because there is hypersecretion of the hormone in most pituitary adenomas. Like the gonadotropins (luteinizing hormone

[LH] and follicle-stimulating hormone [FSH]) and TSH, low PRL values are found in the blood of normal individuals by radioimmunoassay and are of little help in detecting hypopituitarism in postmenopausal patients, however, LH and FSH should be normally elevated, and low values are diagnostically helpful in these individuals. In men, sperm counts and testosterone determinations are useful indicators of gonadotropin deficiency. Elevated LH and FSH or TSH suggest primary gonadal or thyroid failure, respectively, rather than hypothalamic-pituitary disease, except in the rare cases of pituitary tumors that oversecrete these hormones. Dynamic testing of pituitary reserve is occasionally necessary to detect more subtle forms of hypopituitarism. The most commonly used tests are the insulin hypoglycemia test to stimulate growth hormone (GH) and the intravenous ACTH infusion test for cortisol response. Along with the thyroid screen, the ACTH infusion test is also useful if rapid evaluation of the most critical functions is needed in a sick patient who might require immediate replacement therapy or surgery. Stimulation tests with the releasing factors, thyrotropin-releasing hormone (TRH) and gonadotropin-releasing hormone (LHRH), are occasionally useful in differentiating between hypothalamic and pituitary disease.

Simmonds Disease. Simmonds disease, or pituitary cachexia, is the result of total destruction of the anterior lobe. Destruction of the gland may result from infarction, hemorrhage, trauma, tuberculosis, and other infections.

Pituitary cachexia occurs most commonly in middle life and in women of childbearing age, especially after parturition. The syndrome is pluriglandular, and is probably due to hypofunction of the thyroid, adrenals, and gonads as a consequence of loss of the trophic hormones of the pituitary.

Symptoms include severe asthenia and progressive wasting of fat and subcutaneous tissue. The skin becomes thin, dry, and wrinkled, nails become brittle, hair is shed, and teeth fall out. Body temperature is subnormal. Blood pressure may be low, the basal metabolic rate reduced, and the blood sugar content decreased. Psychotic symptoms may develop.

The syndrome of pituitary cachexia is closely imitated by anorexia nervosa, which occurs in young women who abstain from eating.

The course of Simmonds disease varies. Death may result when the failure of function of the anterior pituitary is severe. Treatment of pituitary cachexia consists of a high-protein, high-salt diet and replacement therapy with cortisone, thyroid, and testosterone or estrogen.

Pituitary Dwarfism. Growth retardation may occur because of a reduction in the secretion of growth hormone. The degree of growth retardation varies from frank dwarfing to slightly less than normal development. Stunting of development may occur in children when the gland is injured by suprasellar tumors.

Pituitary dwarfs may be normal in size at birth or they may be abnormally small when born. They are usually the children of normal-size parents. Mental development is normal. In infancy and childhood, except for the smallness, the body configuration is normal. With increasing age they develop the wizened appearance of a dwarfish old man (*progeria*). Genitals are underdeveloped and there is a lack of development of secondary sexual characteristics. Occasionally, however, sexual development is normal and the dwarf is able to produce offspring; an example is Barnum's famous dwarf, Tom Thumb.

Other forms of dwarfism not related to hypofunction of the pituitary gland include achondroplasia and those forms associated with Potts disease and nutritional disorders of infancy (pancreatic insufficiency or celiac disease). The dwarfing of cretinism is attributed to primary hypofunction of the thyroid, but it is likely that associated pituitary dysfunction is partly responsible for the underdevelopment in these cases.

Diabetes Insipidus. Diabetes insipidus is a clinical syndrome characterized by the excessive excretion of urine and an abnormally large fluid intake.

Diabetes insipidus is caused by impaired production of the antidiuretic hormone (arginine vasopressin) of the posterior lobe of the pituitary. There are two general groups of cases. In the so-called "primary type," there is no known lesion in the pituitary or hypothalamus. The "secondary type" is associated with lesions in the hypothalamus, either in the supraoptic and paraventricular nuclei or in their tracts in the medial eminence or upper pituitary stalk. Among the conditions that affect this region are tumors (e.g., pituitary adenomas, craniopharyngiomas, meningiomas, aneurysms), xanthomatosis (Schüller-Christian disease), sarcoidosis, trauma, infections, and vascular disease.

Primary diabetes insipidus is rare. It affects chiefly young people and is seen in boys more frequently than in girls. Heredity is a factor in some cases. Secondary or symptomatic diabetes insipidus is more frequent, but uncommon. It is present in many patients with xanthomatosis and in some patients with tumors or other lesions in the hypothalamic region. Its appearance is an important symptom of hypothalamic disease.

Unless complicated by symptoms associated with the lesion, which is also the cause of the diabetes insipidus, the symptoms are limited to polyuria and polydipsia. Eight to 20 L or even more urine is passed in 24 hours and there is a comparably high level of water intake. The necessity of frequent voiding and the excessive water intake may interfere with normal activities and disturb sleep. Usually, however, general health is maintained if this is an isolated deficiency of the hypothalamus. The symptoms and signs in patients with tumors or other lesions in the hypothalamic region are those usually associated with these conditions and are considered elsewhere.

The laboratory findings are normal with the exception of the low specific gravity of the urine (1.001 to 1.005) and an increase in the osmolality of the serum in many of the cases.

The diagnosis of diabetes insipidus is made on the basis of the excretion of large quantities of urine and insatiable thirst. It is distinguished from the polyuria of diabetes mellitus by the glucosuria and high specific gravity of the urine in diabetes mellitus. A large amount of urine may be passed by patients with chronic nephritis, but not the large volumes (more than 8 L/day) often found in patients with diabetes insipidus. The presence of albumin, casts in the urine, and other associated findings should prevent any confusion in the diagnosis. Psychogenic polydipsia may simulate diabetes insipidus, and must be differentiated.

A rare cause of diabetes insipidus is failure of the kidney to respond to vasopressin. This has been reported as a hereditary defect in infant boys. The defect in some familial cases of diabetes insipidus may be in the osmoreceptor mechanism.

Because absence of vasopressin is difficult to determine in blood by radioimmunoassay, the diagnosis is made by clinical tests, which include antidiuretic responses to exogenous vasopressin and dehydration. Administration of 5 pressor units of aqueous vasopressin rapidly results in a marked decrease in urinary output and an increase in osmolality (specific gravity greater than 1.011) in a patient with diabetes insipidus, and no response in nephrogenic disease. However, patients with psychogenic polydipsia may also have a limited response. Unlike in diabetes insipidus, however, there is a normal response to dehydration in psychogenic polydipsia, although the time required for an increase in urinary concentration may be 12 to 18 hours. Normal subjects dehydrated for 6 to 8 hours will reduce urinary volumes and concentrated urinary osmolality to roughly twice that of plasma (specific gravity greater than 1.015). Patients with severe diabetes insipidus will not respond and should be observed closely and not be allowed to lose more than 3% of their body weight during the test. Otherwise they may become severely ill due to dehydration. A useful clinical test that combines dehydration with the response to exogenous vasopressin has been devised by Moses and Miller; it can distinguish between these disorders and detect patients with partial diabetes insipidus as well.

The diagnosis of diabetes insipidus carries with it the necessity of determining the cause. This means a thorough examination of the nervous system with particular attention to the visual acuity and the fields of vision. Radiographs of the skull and CT or MRI should be a routine part of the examination.

Diabetes insipidus of the primary type may persist for years. Diabetes insipidus due to known lesions in the hypothalamus may also be permanent, but remissions with complete cessation of symptoms are not infrequent.

The treatment of diabetes insipidus associated with tumors or other remediable lesions in the hypothalamus is that appropriate to the lesion (i.e., surgical removal or radiation therapy). Symptomatic therapy of the diabetes insipidus, if it persists in these cases and in patients with diabetes insipidus of unknown cause, is directed toward suppression of the diuresis. No effort should be made to limit the fluid intake. Aqueous pitressin can be administered hypodermically in 5 pressor-unit doses 1 to 4 times daily; it may be sprayed intranasally in the form of lysine vasopressin or placed high in the nasopharynx on cotton pledgets. Pitressin tannate in oil injected intramuscularly is slowly absorbed and may be effective for several days. Dried posterior pituitary extract may be inhaled as snuff.

The drug of choice is the new analog of vasopressin, dDAVP (1-desamino-8-D arginine vasopressin). Because it has no smooth muscle effects, it produces no pressor or cardiac complications. The nasal irritation associated with administration of lysine vasopressin nasal spray and other preparations is also avoided. It is given by nasal instillation and provides good control for about 8 hours. Partial diabetes insipidus may require no therapy or may be ameliorated by oral administration of clofibrate or chlorpropamide. Chlorpropamide occasionally causes hypoglycemia and, in rare cases, water intoxication.

EXCESSIVE SECRETION OF ANTIDIURETIC HORMONE

Inappropriate secretion of the antidiuretic hormone (cerebral salt wasting) may occur with injury to the hypothalamohypophyseal system by head injury, infections, tumors, and other causes. It has been reported in association with carcinomas of the lung and occasionally with other tumors that elaborate vasopressin.

The salient features of the syndrome are hyponatremia and hypotonicity of body fluids, urinary excretion of significant quantities of sodium despite hyponatremia, normal renal and adrenal function, absence of edema, hypotension, azotemia or dehydration, and improvement of the electrolyte disturbance and clinical symptoms on restriction of fluids.

Evidence of cerebral dysfunction related to the electrolyte disturbance may occur. Headache, confusion, somnolence, coma, convulsive seizures, weakness or transient focal neurologic signs, and an abnormal EEG have been reported in rare cases. Mild forms clear with simple fluid restriction. In severe cases with seizures or coma, furosemide diuresis with electrolyte replacement (3% NaCl) should be carried out.

HYPERPITUITARISM

It is now recognized that most pituitary tumors are associated with oversecretion of one or more anterior pituitary hormones. The most commonly affected hormone is PRL, which is elevated in the peripheral blood in about 75% of tumor cases. Growth hormone (GH) overproduction, which causes acromegaly, occurs in about 15% of pituitary tumors; half of these also produce PRL. Tumors that secrete ACTH, which cause Cushing disease, are less common. Tumors that produce TSH or gonadotropins are rare.

Prolactin-Secreting Adenomas. The association of the syndrome of amenorrhea and galactorrhea with pituitary adenoma was recognized almost 3 decades ago by Forbes and Albright, but the oversecretion of PRL was not fully established until this decade by the development of a radioimmunoassay for PRL. It is now recognized that nearly all the men and many of the women with PRL oversecretion by a pituitary adenoma *(prolactinoma)* do not exhibit galactorrhea. A significant number of women with galactorrhea have normal PRL values and no evidence of a pituitary tumor.

Normal PRL values range from 1 to 20 ng/ml in men, and 1 to 25 ng/ml in women. Causes of elevated plasma values are given in Table 149–1. In PRL-secreting adenomas, values are usually less than 200 ng/ml. Higher plasma concentrations are nearly always associated with prolactinomas, although they may also be slightly elevated. There is a rough positive correlation between the PRL level and the size of the tumor.

Large tumors (macroadenomas) that secrete prolactin may involve the visual pathways and may cause some degree of hypopituitarism. In the past these patients were managed by surgical decompression, often by the transsphenoidal route, radiotherapy, or both. It has become common to treat these patients with the dopamine agonist, bromocriptine, as the primary therapy. Such tumors frequently respond to daily maintenance doses of 7.5 mg, although larger doses may be necessary. Long-term therapy is needed, since the tumor may recur when bromocriptine is withdrawn. More experience with this type of therapy is needed to determine the total duration of drug maintenance. In the last decade, another group of patients has been recognized; these are usually women in the childbearing age with infertility and breast discharge who often have a small isolated adenoma within the pituitary gland (microadenoma). In many of these patients, the only abnormality found on complete endocrine evaluation is hyperprolactinemia. These small tumors also occur in men. Until recently, the therapy of choice was total removal of the microadenoma by transsphenoidal surgery, which is relatively safe and has a high apparent-cure rate. Plasma PRL fell in many of these cases and menses returned in 30%. On the other hand, the natural history of these common tumors is not fully known. The patient's endocrine history often suggests that a very small tumor has been

Table 149–1. Causes of Elevated Prolactin Levels

Normal	Drugs	Diseases
Sleep	Phenothiazines	Pituitary adenoma
Stress	Butyrophenones	Chiari-Frommel syndrome
Exercise	Benzamides	Pituitary stalk section
Coitus	Reserpine	Hypothalamic diseases
Nipple stimulation	α-methyl	Sarcoidosis
Pregnancy	dopa	Tumors (e.g., craniopharyngioma)
Nursing	Morphine	Histiocytosis X
	Prostaglandin F2α	Primary hypothyroidism
	Thyrotropin-releasing hormone	Renal failure
	Estrogens	Partial seizures

present for decades. Patient observation for a number of years has revealed progressive enlargement in 4–11%, but no change in the remaining patients. There is also a recurrence rate of 10 to 20% after transsphenoidal surgery. Bromocriptine is now generally considered the therapy of choice for prolactin microadenoma. Return of fertility usually occurs soon after institution of low doses of the drug. After pregnancy occurs, the medication is usually withdrawn. Nearly all the resulting pregnancies have been uneventful, although a few women have had tumor swelling and visual difficulties in the last trimester. In such situations readministration of the drug often rapidly reduces the size of the tumor obviating the need for emergency surgery.

Growth Hormone-Secreting Adenomas. Excessive secretion of GH causes gigantism if it begins before closure of the epiphysis occurs, or *acromegaly* (Figs. 149–1 through 149–3) if it starts later. When fully developed, acromegaly is easily recognized by excessive skeletal and soft tissue growth. Facial features are coarse, with a large bulbous nose, prominent supraorbital ridges, a protruding mandible, separated teeth, and thick lips. Hands and feet are enlarged, and the patient frequently has a slightly kyphotic posture. The voice is harsh, and increased sweating is frequently noticed. Visceromegaly is also part of the clinical picture. These changes are usually slowly progressive. Patients complain of headaches, fatigue, muscular pain, paresthesias that are sometimes manifested as a carpal tunnel syndrome, visual disturbances, and impairment of gonadal function. Generalized arthritis and diabetes mellitus are frequent components; thyroid enlargement and hirsutism may also be present. Increased mortality associated with acromegaly is well documented.

Hypersecretion of GH is associated with active disease. Although GH blood values may be only slightly elevated in patients with the disease, they may also be elevated in normal patients by physical stress or sleep. A glucose tolerance test with GH determinations may be necessary to prove hypersecretion of GH. In normal individuals, GH should be suppressed to less than 5 ng/ml in a glucose tolerance test; in patients with acromegaly it is not, however, it may rise paradoxically during the test. There may also be a paradoxic increase in GH in acromegaly in response to the administration of TRH, or a decrease in the response to dopaminergic drugs.

In some patients, the GH-secreting adenoma is small and can be totally removed by transsphenoidal surgery with immediate return of GH to normal levels. In other patients, the tumor is large, requiring decompression and radiotherapy. GH may require years to return to normal levels after radiotherapy. Some tumors respond to bromocriptine. Somatostatin analogs are being introduced as a means of controlling GH secretion in patients unresponsive to other forms of therapy.

Cushing Syndrome. Seventy percent of patients with Cushing syndrome have bilateral adrenal hyperplasia, 25% have an adrenal adenoma or carcinoma, and 5% have ectopic ACTH production by a lung tumor or other neoplasm. High plasma ACTH values measured by radioimmunoassay are associated with ectopic syndromes and adrenal hyperplasia caused by a hypersecreting pituitary tumor. Only half the patients with proven pituitary tumors have elevated morning ACTH values, although elevated corticoid levels and loss of the diurnal rhythm are usually found. Although it is now generally accepted that adrenal hyperplasia is due to ACTH overproduction by the pituitary, it remains difficult to demonstrate a tumor in half the cases. Suspicion remains high and a tumor ultimately appears in at least 15% of patients after bilat-

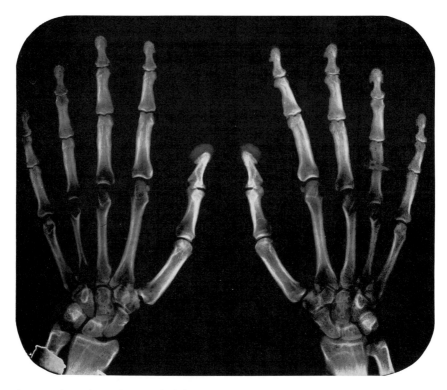

Fig. 149–1.   Acromegaly. Tufting of terminal phalanges. (Courtesy of Dr. Juan Taveras.)

eral adrenalectomy when there is hyperpigmentation *(Nelson syndrome)* and excessive
ACTH secretion despite adrenocorticoid steroid replacement therapy. Inability to detect
a tumor could also be explained if the disease
originates in the hypothalamus with oversecretion of corticotropin-releasing factor. Administration of cyproheptadine has been followed by reduction of ACTH and resolution
of the clinical disease in some patients with
Cushing disease and Nelson syndrome. This
drug inhibits serotonergic pathways in the
brain that stimulate secretion of the releasing
factors.

Although helpful, the development of the
radioimmunoassy for ACTH has not solved
all problems associated with the differential
diagnosis of Cushing syndrome. Primary obesity may also mimic the clinical disease due
to secondary hypercortisolism. In these patients, the urinary free cortisol is normal, and
the overnight dexamethasone test (0.5–1 mg)
suppresses the morning blood cortisol value
to normal (less than 5 mg/dl). The use of the
overnight and 2-day dexamethasone (8 mg/24
hrs) tests in the differential diagnosis are
given in Table 149–2. The treatment of choice
for these usually small adenomas is total removal by transsphenoidal surgery. These tu-

mors have a greater tendency to recur in
Cushing disease than in the other hyperse-
cretory states. Thus, radiotherapy is more often used in these patients. Cyproheptadine is
used as an initial trial of therapy in some patient, and for control of the disease after surgery and radiotherapy. As in acromegaly, the
response to radiotherapy may be slow in
Cushing disease. Ketoconazole, an inhibitor
of adrenal steroidogenesis, may be useful in
inhibiting the hypercortisolism, but it has no
effect on the tumor.

SOTOS SYNDROME

In 1964, Sotos and his associates described
five children with a syndrome characterized
by gigantism that began in utero or in the first
few years of life and was thought to be of
cerebral origin. Other features of the syndrome, in addition to high stature, include
macrocrania, hypertelorism, dolichocephaly,
high arched palate, macroglossia, large hands
and feet, syndactyly of toes, and scoliosis.

The neurologic abnormalities are nonprogressive and include clumsiness, convulsive
seizures, and mental retardation. The ventricles are enlarged without evidence of cortical
atrophy.

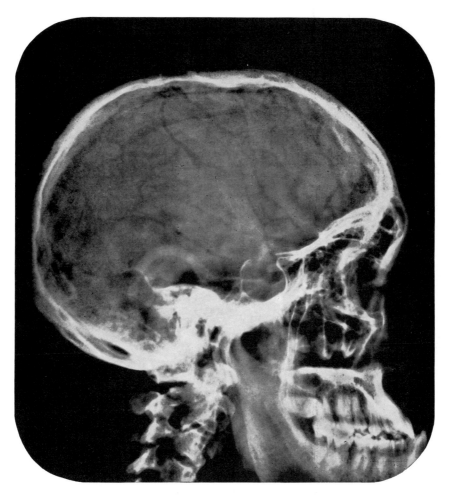

Fig. 149–2. Pituitary tumor. Chromophile adenoma with ballooning of sella turcica, prognathism, and enlargement of skull bones. (Courtesy of Dr. Juan Taveras.)

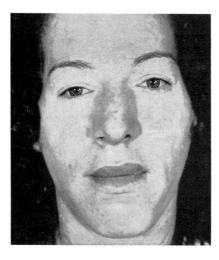

Fig. 149–3. Chromophile adenoma of pituitary. Prognathism and enlargement of nose in acromegaly. (Courtesy of Dr. E. Herz.)

The cause of the overgrowth is not known. GH values are normal.

Thyroid

HYPOTHYROIDISM

Hypothyroidism is the functional state that results from deficiency or complete lack of the thyroid hormone. It may develop before birth or in infancy, childhood, or adult life. Thyroid hormone is important in early growth and development and the syndromes that occur as a result of deficiency depend upon the age of the patient at the time of onset of the deficiency. These can be divided into three categories: cretinism, juvenile myxedema, and adult myxedema.

When severe thyroid deficiency develops in utero or in early life, there is retardation of physical and mental development. Soon after birth, subcutaneous tissue thickens, the cry

Table 149–2. Evaluation of Hypercortisolism (Cushing Syndrome)

Clinical Presentation	Morning Cortisol after Overnight Dexamethasone	Urinary Corticosteroids after High-dose Dexamethasone (8 mg/24h)	Plasma ACTH
Obesity	Suppress to normal	Suppress	—
Adrenal hyperplasia (Cushing disease)	Does not suppress	Suppress	Often elevated
Adrenal tumor (adenoma or carcinoma)	Does not suppress	Does not suppress	Low
Ectopic ACTH secretion	Does not suppress	Does not suppress	High

becomes hoarse, the tongue enlarges, and the infant has widely spaced eyes, pot-belly, and an umbilical hernia. If treatment is not given promptly, dwarfism and a severe degree of mental deficiency result.

The clinical picture in juvenile myxedema is similar to that of cretinism with variations that depend on the patient's age at onset of thyroid deficiency. The degree of physical and mental retardation is usually less severe than in infantile myxedema. Enlargement of the sella turcica has been reported in juvenile myxedema.

Adult myxedema is characterized by lethargy, weakness, slowness of speech, nonpitting edema of the subcutaneous tissues, coarse and pale skin, dry brittle hair, thick lips, enlargement of the tongue, decreased sweating, and excessive sensitivity to cold.

The neurologic complications of myxedema include: headache, cranial nerve palsies, peripheral neuritis, myopathy, reflex changes, psychotic episodes, and coma with convulsions.

The incidence of cranial nerve palsies is low. Some hearing loss occurs in about 15% of patients. Vertigo and tinnitus may also be present. Unilateral or bilateral facial palsy is recorded in a higher percentage of patients than would be expected by the coincidence of the two conditions. Dysarthria or hoarseness is common but is probably related to myxedematous infiltration of the tongue and palate and not to involvement of the twelfth or tenth cranial nerves.

A mild polyneuritis has been reported in rare patients. This is characterized mainly by paresthesias in the arms and legs. Paresthesias accompanied by thenar atrophy are usually due to involvement of the median nerve in the carpal tunnel. Unexplained slow relaxation of muscles and *myoedema* (mounding

phenomenon) on percussion of the muscles are not infrequent.

Characteristic of the hypothyroid state is slow relaxation of the Achilles tendon reflexes. Generalized enlargement, or hypertrophy, of muscles has been reported in a few children (*Kocher-Débre-Sémélaigne syndrome*). The enlarged muscles give the affected individual an athletic appearance (infant Hercules—Fig. 149–4); the size of the muscles decreases with replacement therapy.

Episodes of delirium, uncontrolled excitability, depression, and other psychotic states are infrequent complications. Coma of sudden onset is rare. If untreated, this complication has a high mortality rate. Cerebellar ataxia and choreoathetosis sometimes occur.

The coincidence of myxedema and myasthenia gravis occasionally has been noted.

The characteristic laboratory findings in myxedema are elevated serum cholesterol (300–700 g), low circulating thyroid hormones (T_3, T_4), elevated TSH, a low radioiodine uptake, and an increased CSF protein content; plasma PRL may also be elevated. An absence of alpha waves and a decrease in the amplitude of the waves in the EEG have been reported. The protein content of the CSF is increased; values in excess of 100 mg/dl are not uncommon. All laboratory findings revert to normal after adequate therapy.

The diagnosis of myxedema is usually made from the patient's characteristic appearance and laboratory tests. Any physical or mental retardation in infants should lead to a consideration of hypothyroidism.

The treatment of myxedema is 12.5 to 25 μg levothyroxine. The hormone should be given cautiously because rapid administration may precipitate angina and heart failure. There may be a relative adrenal cortical insufficiency requiring replacement therapy. The dose is gradually increased every 1 to

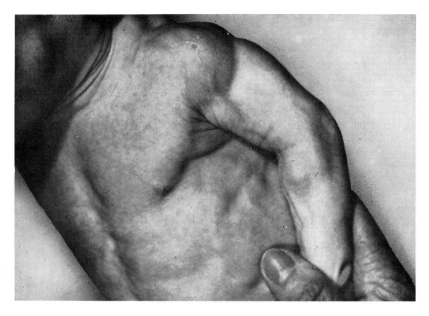

Fig. 149–4. Enlargement of muscles in myxedema, Kocher-Débre-Sémélaigne syndrome. (Courtesy of Dr. Arnold Gold.)

2 weeks if there are no toxic symptoms and the desired effects are not obtained with the previous dose. Prophylactic treatment of cretinism is important in goiter districts, where iodine should be given to all pregnant women.

HYPERTHYROIDISM (GRAVES DISEASE)

Hyperthyroidism results from excessive secretion of the thyroid gland. Clinically, it is associated with an increased metabolic rate, abnormal autonomic functions, tremor, exophthalmos and other ocular abnormalities, and myopathy.

The neurologic symptoms are usually limited to tremor of the hands, exophthalmos, lid lag, infrequency of winking, weakness of convergence, and weakness of limb muscles. Mental disturbances may occur, ranging from mild emotional instability to psychotic syndromes.

In addition to the common signs of Graves disease, other neurologic syndromes may occur in association with thyrotoxicosis, namely, myasthenia gravis, chronic thyrotoxic myopathy, familial periodic paralysis, and exophthalmic ophthalmoplegia.

It is clear that there is no causative relationship between hyperthyroidism and myasthenia gravis, but the coincidence of the two diseases is inordinately frequent; about 5% of patients with myasthenia gravis have hyperthyroidism. In most patients, the two diseases occur simultaneously; in others, myasthenia gravis precedes or follows the thyrotoxicosis by months or years. The differential diagnosis between the muscular weakness of hyperthyroidism and myasthenia gravis is made on the basis of the characteristic serologic, pharmacologic, and physiologic abnormalities of myasthenia. The distinction is usually made clinically because oropharyngeal weakness or ophthalmoparesis almost always signifies the presence of myasthenia. Treatment of patients with hyperthyroidism and myasthenia gravis consists of a combination of the modern therapies for each of the two diseases.

Thyrotoxic Myopathy. This muscle disease was first described about four decades ago. Weakness and wasting are greatest in the muscles of the pelvic girdle, particularly the iliopsoas, and to a lesser extent in the muscles of the shoulder girdle. The reflexes are normal or hyperactive and sensation is normal. Gross muscular twitching may be seen, but fibrillation potentials are not seen in the EMG. Diagnosis is made by the characteristic distribution of the muscular weakness and wasting in a patient with thyrotoxicosis. Myasthenia gravis is excluded by the lack of cranial symptoms, AChR antibodies, and response to edrophonium. Improvement of the affected muscles follows effective treatment of the hyperthyroidism.

The occurrence of hyperthyroidism and periodic paralysis in the same patient is rare but is much more frequent than would be anticipated on chance occurrence (see Article 131, Periodic Paralysis).

Exophthalmic Ophthalmoplegia. This is a syndrome in which there is both exophthalmos and weakness of the extraocular muscles. There may be chemosis of the lids, edema of the conjunctiva, and papilledema.

The relationship of exophthalmic ophthalmoplegia to diseases of the thyroid is not clear. The condition may appear in patients with hyperthyroidism, in patients who have had a thyroidectomy but who are euthyroid, and in euthyroid patients with no previous history of hyperthyroidism.

The pathologic changes are confined to the orbit. There is an increase in the orbital contents with edema, hypertrophy, infiltration, and fibrosis of the extraocular muscles.

The onset of symptoms is gradual; exophthalmos is often accompanied by diplopia due to paresis of one or more ocular muscles. Both eyes may be involved at the same time or the exophthalmos in one eye may precede that in the other by several months. With advance of exophthalmos, paresis of the extrinsic muscles of the eye increases until finally the eyeball is almost totally fixed. Papilledema sometimes occurs, and ulcerations of the cornea may develop due to failure of the lid to protect the eye. The paralysis may involve all eye muscles or those muscles concerned with the movement of the eyes in a particular plane, particularly upward. The symptoms progress rapidly for a few months and may lead to complete ophthalmoplegia. Occasionally there is spontaneous improvement; as a rule the symptoms persist unchanged throughout the life of the patient unless they are relieved by therapy.

Syndromes similar to Graves ophthalmopathy may occur in patients who have no evidence of thyroid disease; *orbital myositis* and *orbital pseudotumor* are terms used to describe these syndromes, to which the *Tolosa-Hunt syndrome* is related. It has not been possible to develop tests that would distinguish these conditions from euthyroid Graves disease; immunologic, endocrine, ultrasound, and CT criteria have all been recommended.

Treatment of Graves ophthalmopathy is controversial. Radiation therapy of the pituitary or thyroid has no effect on the syndrome; neither does the surgical removal of the thyroid. The roof of the orbit and canal of the optic nerve can be removed from above,

through an anterior craniotomy. The exophthalmos may be relieved by this operation, but if the condition has been of extended duration, little improvement in the ophthalmoplegia results because irreversible changes have already developed in the extraocular muscles. Some authors state that the operation is rarely needed, because the exophthalmos usually does not progress to a serious degree before it comes to a spontaneous arrest. Partial suturing of the lids is recommended to protect the eyeball. The use of prednisone is favored by many clinicians.

Parathyroid

HYPOPARATHYROIDISM

The disturbance in the calcium and phosphorus metabolism that results from a deficiency in the activity of the parathyroid gland produces a train of neurologic symptoms described by the term *parathyroid tetany.*

Hypoparathyroidism may be due to the removal of the glands in the course of a thyroid operation. Rarely, hypoparathyroidism may occur without any obvious cause or it may be associated with either Addison disease or moniliasis. Idiopathic hypoparathyroidism may develop at any age, but is uncommon in children. A form of hypoparathyroidism (pseudohypoparathyroidism), described in 1942 by Albright and his associates, is characterized by hyperphosphatemia and hypocalcemia, similar to that of true hypoparathyroidism, but the parathyroids are histologically normal or hyperplastic, and the administration of parathyroid hormone does not cause significant phosphaturia or an increase in the serum calcium content. In addition to the usual signs of hypocalcemia, there is a characteristic habitus in these patients. There is shortening of the stature, the physique is stocky, the face is round, and there is shortening of the metacarpal and metatarsal bones. Occasionally, subcutaneous ossification also occurs. Convulsive seizures occur in more than 65% of these patients (Table 149–3). A form of pseudohypoparathyroidism has been described in which the serum calcium and phosphorus are normal and tetany is absent. This has been described by the unwieldy term *pseudopseudohypoparathyroidism* and proably represents a forme fruste of pseudohypoparathyroidism.

The symptoms of hypoparathyroidism include muscle cramps, carpopedal spasm, laryngeal stridor, and convulsive seizures. All

Table 149–3. Incidence of Signs and Symptoms in Pseudohypoparathyroidism

Characteristics	% of Patients
Biochemical	
Hypocalcemia	96
Increased alkaline phosphatase	20
Body habitus	
Short stature	80
Round face	92
Stocky or obese	50
Ocular	
Lenticular opacities	49
Dental	
Hypoplasia, enamel defects	51
Calcification	
Subcutaneous	55
Basal ganglia	50
Skeletal	
Short metacarpals	68
Thickened calvarium	62
Neurologic	
Mental retardation	75
Seizures	59
Muscle cramps, twitches	38

(From Drezner MK, Neelon FA. In: Stanbury JB, Wyngaarden JB, Fredrickson DS, Goldstein JL, Brown MS, eds. The Metabolic Basis of Inherited Disease, 5th ed. New York: McGraw-Hill, 1982.)

these symptoms or any one or two may be present. The convulsive seizures of hypoparathyroidism are usually of the grand mal type. Sometimes, however, they are bizarre and are apt to be called "hysterical attacks." They tend to occur frequently and respond poorly to anticonvulsant drugs. Although hypoparathyroidism is a rare cause of seizures, this diagnosis should be considered in patients who have frequent or bizarre seizures that do not respond to anticonvulsant medication, even when no signs of tetany can be elicited. Psychotic manifestations may occur in connection with or independent of the convulsive seizures.

Tetany is present in nearly all patients with hypoparathyroidism. It may be manifested by carpopedal spasm or only in latent form. Latent tetany can be demonstrated by contraction of the facial muscles on tapping the facial nerve in front of the ear (Chvostek sign), the production of carpal spasm by reducing the circulation in the arm by means of a blood pressure cuff (Trousseau sign), and lowered threshold of electrical excitability of the nerve (Erb sign).

Other findings with hypoparathyroidism include cataracts, symmetric bilateral punctate calcifications in the basal ganglia (Fig. 149–5), multiple ectodermal lesions (i.e., dry scaly skin, alopecia, atrophic changes in the nails), and aplasia or hypoplasia of the teeth. Papilledema and increased intracranial pressure sometimes occur, but the mechanism is unexplained. Chorea, torticollis, athetosis, dystonia, paralysis agitans, oculogyric crises, and other basal ganglia symptoms have been reported in isolated cases. These symptoms do not appear to have any relationship to the presence or absence of calcifications in the basal ganglia.

The level of blood calcium depends on the degree of hypofunction of the glands. It will fall as low as 4.5 mg/dl with complete absence of activity of the parathyroids, but values in the range of 6 to 8 mg/dl are most commonly enountered. These figures are below the threshold for calcium excretion and there is an absence of calcium in the urine. The serum phosphorus is elevated. Values in adults are considerably lower than those in children, in whom the serum phosphorus content may be as high as 12 mg/dl. Alkaline phosphatase is usually low. The CSF findings are normal except in rare cases with papilledema, in which the pressure may be moderately increased. The EEG shows various abnormalities, particularly 2 to 5 Hz waves occurring in short bursts. Minute symmetric areas of calcification in the cerebral substance may be seen in skull radiographs.

The diagnosis of hypoparathyroidism is made on basis of the clinical symptoms, the hypocalcemia and the absence of calcium in the urine and low or undetectable plasma parathormone. In pseudohypoparathyroidism, parathormone values are elevated.

Hypoparathyroidism must be differentiated from other causes of tetany and hypocalcemia. In patients with convulsive seizures or papilledema, the differential must include other causes of these signs. The relationship of these signs to the hypocalcemia is determined by the effects of therapy with dihydrotachysterol.

Tetany may occur in association with alkalosis resulting from excessive loss of gastric content or the ingestion of large amounts of alkali. The tetany of these conditions is distinguished from that of hypoparathyroidism by the presence of calcium in the urine, the normal serum calcium content and changes in the CO_2 content of the blood or the CO_2-combining power of the serum.

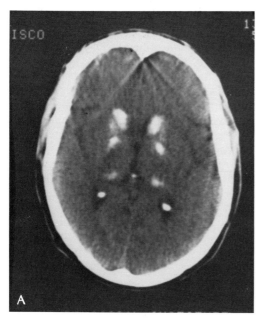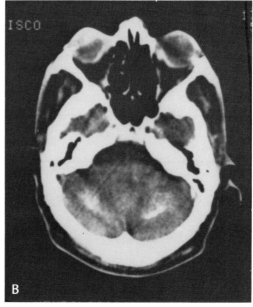

Fig. 149–5. Pseudohypoparathyroidism. *A.* Dense areas of calcification are in head of caudate nucleus (anterior), putamen and globus pallidus (middle pair), and pulvinar (posterior). The fine densities in occipital horns are calcifications in choroid plexus. *B.* Calcification is also seen in subcortical areas of cerebellar hemispheres. (Courtesy of Drs. S.K. Hilal and M. Mawad.)

Other causes of hypocalcemia are hypomagnesemia, rickets, osteomalacia, and renal insufficiency with urea and phosphate retention. Hypomagnesemia may result from malabsorption, alcoholism, and prolonged parenteral therapy. Magnesium replacement therapy corrects the hypocalcemia. In rickets and osteomalacia, the decrease in the serum calcium is not accompanied by an increase in the phosphorus content. Rickets can also be diagnosed by the characteristic findings of this condition. The decrease in serum calcium and the concomitant increase in serum phosphorus are less severe in renal failure than in hypoparathyroidism.

The hypoparathyroidism that follows damage to the gland by thyroidectomy is frequently transient; the symptoms disappear with regeneration of the damaged glands. The symptoms and signs of idiopathic hypoparathyroidism may be mild and occur only in connection with active exercise gastrointestinal disturbances, or acute infections. In other cases, the symptoms are constant. Fatalities are rare but mental deterioration may occur, particularly in patients with convulsive seizures.

Parathormone is effective in relieving the symptoms and in restoring the serum levels of calcium and phosphorus to normal, but its effect diminishes with prolonged administration. In addition, it is entirely ineffective in the rare form of hypoparathyroidism labeled by Albright as pseudohypoparathyroidism.

Dihydrotachysterol aids in the absorption of calcium from the intestines and increases the excretion of phosphorus. It is effective in relieving the symptoms of tetany and in restoring the serum calcium and phosphorus levels to normal. The dose should be regulated according to the needs of the patient. Overdosage will cause abnormally high levels of calcium in the serum. Dihydrotachysterol is taken orally in a dosage of 1.25 mg 3 times daily until the blood calcium is normal. The drug is then administered in a suitable dosage to maintain the serum calcium at a normal level as determined by direct estimation of the serum content or the excretion of calcium in the urine.

HYPERPARATHYROIDISM

An excess of the parathyroid hormone causes thinning of the bones, muscular weakness, and the formation of renal stones.

It was not until 1925 that the role of the parathyroid as the cause of the bone disease in von Recklinghausen osteitis fibrosa cystica was known. It soon became obvious that all the symptoms were related to the presence of a tumor or hyperplasia of the gland. Albright postulated that hyperplasia or adenoma formation may be caused by some situation that tends to lower the serum calcium levels with stimulation of germinal centers; these centers then may lose their property of being controlled by normal stimuli. Adenomas or hyperplasia of the gland has been reported in association with eosinophilic or basophilic adenomas of the pituitary, adenomas of the islets of Langerhans, pancreatitis, and gastric ulcers.

Overactivity of the parathyroids is due to the presence of an adenoma or to a diffuse enlargement of the glands. The tumors are usually simple adenomas, but carcinomatous involvement of the gland has been reported. The adenomas usually occur singly, but two or more tumors were found in 6% of the 89 cases collected by Albright. In simple hyperplasia, all parathyroids are enlarged as the result of proliferation of the wasserhelle cells.

The changes in the bones are described by the term *osteitis fibrosa cystica*. The bones are decalcified and there is a great increase in the number of osteoclasts. As a result, there may be bone tumors (osteoclastomas) or multiple cysts with fibrous walls. Nephrolithiasis is present in more than 75% of the cases and nephrocalcinosis is less common.

The disease was formerly considered to be quite rare, but Cope and his associates have collected 343 cases at the Massachusetts General Hospital. The condition may occur in patients at any age, but seldom appears before age of 20. Women are affected about twice as frequently as men.

Table 149–4. Clues to the Diagnosis of Hyperparathyroidism in the First 343 Cases at the Massachusetts General Hospital

Clue	No. of Cases
Bone disease	80
Renal stones	195
Peptic ulcer	27
Pancreatitis	9
Fatigue	10
Hypertension	6
Mental disturbance	3
CNS signs	7
Multiple endocrine abnormalities	3
Lumps in neck	1
No symptoms	2

(From Cope O. N Engl J Med 1966; 274: 1174–1182.)

The initial symptoms (Table 149–4) may be pains in the back and limbs and weakness of skeletal muscle. Loss of appetite, nausea, or constipation may occur as a result of hypotonia of the smooth muscles of the intestines. Spontaneous fractures and shortening of stature may result from changes in the bones. Renal stones are common and symptoms of chronic nephritis develop when calcium is deposited in the renal tubules. Polyuria and polydipsia are common.

Weakness of the trunk and limb muscles may be severe. There may be mild or moderate atrophy due to Type II fiber atrophy. Tendon reflexes are decreased or absent. Psychotic episodes or periods of coma may occur.

All kinds of bone deformities may occur. The long bones may be bent, the pelvis may be deformed, or various deformities of the vertebral column may develop. In advanced cases, the stature is shortened, the neck disappears into the thorax and the chest takes on a pigeon-breast appearance. Cyst formation in the vertebrae is a rare cause of spinal cord or root compression.

The blood calcium content is high, usually greater than 12 mg/dl; the phosphorus content is low or normal except when the renal function is impaired. A determination of the renal tubular reabsorption of phosphate may be of additional value in borderline cases. The serum phosphatase is elevated. Anemia and leukopenia may occur when there is extensive fibrosis in the bone marrow. The volume of the urine is increased. Albumin and casts may be present.

Radiographic changes in the bones are characteristic. There is general decalcification except for the teeth. Thickness of the skull is not affected, but the calvarium has a ground-glass appearance. Tumor and cysts of the bone may be seen.

Hyperparathyroidism may be manifested by the combination of bone and kidney disease or by either alone. The development of typical skeletal deformities or recurrent attacks of nephrolithiasis should lead to the consideration of hyperparathyroidism. The diagnosis is confirmed by the findings of a high calcium and low phosphorus content in the serum, elevated plasma parathormone by radioimmunoassay, and increased urinary excretion of cyclic 3′,5′-AMP.

The differential diagnosis includes diseases of the bone with changes that may be mistaken for those of hyperparathyroidism and other causes of hypercalcemia. These can usually be distinguished without difficulty from the clinical picture, the character and distribution of the radiographic changes, and the blood chemistry.

When the disease is discovered early and treated, there is a prompt improvement of symptoms. The giant cell tumors disappear and the bone cysts fill in slowly.

If untreated, the disease progresses slowly. The bones become thin and there are spontaneous fractures and collapse of the vertebrae. Patients become bedridden and die of renal failure.

Treatment is surgical removal of the adenomas. All glands should be visualized because of the possibility that more than one adenoma is present or that the condition is due to hyperplasia of the glands. In the latter case, subtotal resection should be performed. Postoperative tetany may develop in patients with severe bone decalcification. This complication is treated by a high-calcium, low-phosphorus regimen.

Pancreas

HYPOGLYCEMIA

The nervous system depends entirely on glucose for its metabolism; dysfunction develops rapidly whenever the amount of glucose in the blood falls below critical levels. Low blood sugar levels may be associated with overdosage of insulin in the treatment of diabetes mellitus. Spontaneous hypoglycemia is usually the result of an excessive secretion of insulin by the pancreas (hyperinsulinism).

According to Conn, 80 to 90% of all cases of spontaneous hypoglycemia are due to one of three causes: functional hypoglycemia, hyperinsulinism with demonstrable pancreatic lesion, or organic disease of the liver. Hypoglycemia may occur with tumors of the islet cells, or it may be associated with functional overactivity of the cells. In the 27 cases reported by Hoefer, Guttman, and Sands, an adenoma was present in 21, carcinoma in four, and hyperplasia in two cases. Islet cell tumors occur most frequently in the body or tail of the pancreas. Multiple tumors, which are present in more than 10% of cases, are rarely associated with adenomas of the parathyroid. The tumors are 1 to 2 cm in diameter, although occasionally they are much larger. Functioning β-cell islet tumors of the pancreas may also coexist with other forms of multiple endocrine adenomatosis (MEA) such as the following: Type I—pancreas, parathyroid, pituitary; Type II A—medullary thyroid carcinoma, pheochromocytoma, parathyroid; Type II B—mucosal and ganglial neuromatosis.

Hypoglycemia may occur when the function of the liver is severely impaired or when the pituitary or adrenal is seriously damaged. Little is known about the cause of the functional hypoglycemia that occurs in patients with no demonstrable lesion of the liver, pancreas, or other endocrine glands.

Spontaneous hypoglycemia occasionally occurs in infants. The cause is still unknown. In some 50% of the cases, the fall in the blood glucose level can be related to the administration of casein hydrolysate or L-leucine (leucine sensitive hypoglycemia). It is probable that the appearance of spontaneous hypoglycemia in some of these infants may be an early manifestation of an inherited metabolic abnormality associated with diabetes mellitus. The symptoms associated with the hypoglycemia include muscular twitchings, myoclonic jerks, and convulsive seizures. Failure of mental development results if the condition is not recognized and adequately treated at onset.

The pathologic changes associated with hypoglycemia include those related to the underlying cause and include tumors of the pancreas, tumors and atrophy of the pituitary, cirrhosis and other diseases of the liver, and atrophy of the adrenals. In addition, there may be degenerative changes in the brain after one or more severe and prolonged attacks of hypoglycemia. In these cases there is a loss of neurons of the third and fourth layers of the cortex of the cerebral hemispheres. There is glial proliferation in the affected areas.

Hyperinsulinism is rare. Whipple collected 32 cases at the Presbyterian Hospital in New York. Islet cell tumors were present in 27 of the cases. The age at time of operation in Whipple's patients ranged from 20 to 65 years. The duration of symptoms before operation varied from a few months to 20 years. Women were affected twice as frequently as men.

The symptoms in infantile hypoglycemia usually begin in the first 6 to 12 months of life. There is a tendency for the condition to be familial.

The symptoms of hyperinsulinism are paroxysmal, tending to occur when the blood sugar could be expected to be low (i.e., in the morning before breakfast, after a fast of several or many hours, and after heavy exercise). Occasionally, however, the symptoms occur only a few hours after an apparently adequate meal. The duration of symptoms varies from a few minutes to hours. Their severity is also variable. There may be only nervousness, anxiety, or tremulousness that is readily relieved by the ingestion of food. Severe attacks last for several hours, during which the patient may perform automatic activity with complete amnesia for the entire period, or there may be convulsive seizures followed by a prolonged coma. Rarely, the latter will not respond to therapy. The frequency of attacks varies from several per day to one in many months.

Hypoglycemic symptoms may be divided into two groups, autonomic and cerebral.

Sympathetic disturbances are present in most patients at the onset of hypoglycemia and usually precede the development of the more serious cerebral symptoms. These include lightheadedness, sweating, nausea, vomiting, pallor, palpitation, precordial oppression, headache, abdominal pain, and ravenous hunger.

Cerebral symptoms usually occur in association with the sympathetic phenomena, but may be the only manifestations of hypoglycemia. The most common symptoms are paresthesias, diplopia, and blurred vision. These may be followed by generalized weakness, tremors, transient hemiplegia, aphasia, periods of abnormal behavior, confusion, incoherence, irritability, minor or major convulsive seizures, or periods of coma without a preceding convulsive seizure. The periods of confusion and abnormal behavior may simulate psychomotor epilepsy. Convulsive seizures, when they occur, may be jacksonian or grand mal. Although convulsions are a common manifestation of severe hypoglycemia, hyperinsulinism is a rare cause of recurrent convulsive seizures (epilepsy), probably representing less than 0.1% of cases.

The neurologic examination is usually normal except during attacks of hypoglycemia when there may be oculomotor weakness, nystagmus, hemiparesis, or hemianesthesia. The reflexes may be hyperactive or depressed. Plantar responses are extensor whenever convulsive seizures or coma occur. Amyotrophy, resulting from damage to ventral horn cells, has been reported. Retardation of mental development is common in untreated cases of infantile hypoglycemia.

The fasting blood sugar is usually low, but it may be normal and remain normal for many days or months in patients who suffer infrequent attacks. In the 27 cases with proven lesions of the pancreas reported by Hoefer, Guttman, and Sands, the fasting blood sugar level ranged from 30 to 71 mg/dl. It was below 40 mg/dl in 28% and below 50 mg/dl in 68%. The blood sugar is always low at the onset of an attack. It may return to normal if the specimen is not withdrawn until after a convulsive seizure or if the patient has been in coma for several hours. The level at which symptoms appear varies; some patients do not develop symptoms until the level is below 40 mg/dl; others present classic symptoms with blood sugar levels between 50 and 60 mg/dl. The glucose tolerance test gives variable results. It may be flat or of the diabetic type, but low values are more commonly found, especially if specimens are taken 5 to 8 hours after the stimulating dose of glucose. The EEG shows focal or widespread dysrhythmia during an attack of hypoglycemia and in some cases even in the interval between attacks.

The diagnosis of hyperinsulinism is made by the paroxysmal appearance of signs of autonomic and cerebral dysfunction in association with a low blood sugar and an inappropriately high insulin level by radioimmunoassay. The paroxysms usually appear when the blood sugar would be expected to be low; practically all patients know their symptoms can be relieved by eating.

If it is not possible to obtain a specimen of blood during an attack, the blood should be tested during fasting. After 12 to 14 hours, 80% of patients with islet tumors have low glucose and high insulin levels. The fast, however, may need to be continued up to 72 hours to enable diagnosis. An intravenous tolbutamide test, determination of proinsulin levels, and insulin suppression tests may also be helpful. Tumor visualization procedures should be used to search for other neoplasms that occasionally produce hyperinsulinism.

The differential diagnosis includes other causes of symptoms of sympathetic overactivity and convulsive seizures. These are usually excluded by the lack of relationship of the attacks to fasting and by normal blood sugar levels.

Hypoglycemia associated with diseases of the liver, pituitary, or adrenal usually can be distinguished by other signs and symptoms of disease in these organs.

Because pancreatic tumors may be small, surgical exploration may be indicated. A negative exploration does not absolutely exclude the presence of a tumor because small adenomas can be present in the depth of the gland and not be palpated by the surgeon.

Mild attacks of spontaneous hypoglycemia may occur at infrequent intervals for many years, but they tend to become progressively more frequent and severe. Occasionally, there may be remission of the attacks for months or years. Death may result from coma during an attack. Rarely, a patient may remain in coma for days or weeks even though blood sugar returns to normal, because of severe irreversible damage to the cerebral cortex. This unusual sequence of events may also occur in psychotic patients treated with large doses of insulin.

Treatment of spontaneous hypoglycemia is separated into treatment of the acute attack and the treatment of the underlying cause.

Early and intensive treatment of an acute attack is important to prevent anoxic damage to the brain. If the patient is conscious, sugar can be administered in the form of candy, orange juice, or milk. Comatose patients should be given glucose intravenously.

When the episodes of hypoglycemia cannot be explained on any other basis, the presumptive diagnosis is adenoma of the islets of Langerhans and an exploratory operation is indicated. This should not be delayed because the frequent feedings that are needed to ward off the attacks often lead to obesity. The attacks of hypoglycemia usually disappear after operative removal of the tumor. A second operation may be necessary if two or more tumors are present and are not all removed at the first operation.

Functional hyperinsulinism is treated by a diet that is high in proteins and low in carbohydrates in order to avoid the stimulatory effect of the latter on the pancreas. Diazoxide may help control hypoglycemia. In persistent cases, streptozocin may be given intravenously to destroy β cells, but it is also nephrotoxic.

HYPOINSULINISM

Hypoinsulinism, or diabetes mellitus, may be accompanied by a variety of lesions in the nervous system. These are mainly in the form of a mono- or polyneuritis. Other neurologic complications include diabetic coma associated with an extreme degree of hyperglycemia and acidosis. Vascular lesions may occur in the brain as a result of the vascular disease associated with diabetes mellitus.

Adrenal

The adrenal is composed of two parts, the cortex and the medulla. The cortex secretes numerous steroid hormones, which can be classified into three groups: *mineralocorticoids*, the most potent of which is aldosterone, the major action of which is to cause sodium conservation and potassium loss from the kidney; *glucocorticoids*, including cortisol, which is most active in humans in elevating the blood sugar; and *sex steroids*, androgens and estrogens, which make a very small contribution to these hormones in the body compared to the gonads under normal circumstances. The glucocorticoids have additional important actions including anti-inflammatory activity, effects on protein and fat metabolism, and suppression of ACTH and melanocyte-stimulating hormone secretion from the pituitary gland. Excess secretion of the melanocyte-stimulating hormone accounts for the hyperpigmentation seen in primary adrenal failure, which is not seen in hypoadrenalcorticism due to hypopituitarism.

The hormone elaborated by the adrenal medulla is composed of two fractions, epinephrine and norepinephrine. Epinephrine has a stimulatory effect on the CNS and acts as a vasodilator of peripheral blood vessels. Norepinephrine constricts peripheral blood vessels and elevates the systemic blood pressure.

ADRENAL HYPOFUNCTION

There is no known disease that results from hypofunction of the adrenal medulla. Adrenal cortical hypofunction may develop acutely in the presence of severe overwhelming infections, particularly meningococcemia or staphylococcemia. Acute or chronic adrenal cortical insufficiency may also be a feature of hypofunction of the pituitary.

Hypofunction of the adrenal cortex is usually due to an atrophy of the gland of unknown cause. The gland may be destroyed by tuberculosis, neoplasms, amyloidosis, hemachromatosis, and fungal infections. Chronic insufficiency of the adrenal cortex, or *Addison disease*, is characterized by weakness, easy fatigability, weight loss, increased pigmentation of the skin, hypotension, anorexia, nausea, vomiting, diarrhea, irritability, anxiety, and episodes of hypoglycemia. Psychotic symptoms develop in rare cases. The syndrome of pseudotumor cerebri has been reported as a complication of Addison disease. Addison disease is quite rare and the symptoms usually have their onset in middle or late life. The diagnosis is suggested by the appearance of characteristic symptoms and it can be confirmed by low plasma cortisol, decreased 24-hour urinary output of 17-hydroxy corticosteroids, and failure of an injection of corticotropin to produce a significant rise in plasma cortisol.

The prognosis of Addison disease is poor without substitution therapy. The average life expectancy is 1 to 2 years. The course is punctuated by a series of crises, which may be precipitated by overexertion, acute infections, surgical procedures, or administration of laxatives. Death is often due to severe hypoglycemia. With adequate hormone therapy, the symptoms can be relieved and life expectancy greatly increased.

The treatment of Addison disease consists of regulation of sodium metabolism by the administration of fludrocortisone and a high-salt diet. Glucocorticoid is replaced in divided doses with cortisol or an equivalent steroid, often cortisone.

ADRENAL HYPERFUNCTION

Adrenal Virilism and Adrenogenital Syndrome. Hyperfunction of the adrenal cortex produces the syndrome described by Cushing and attributed by him to the presence of a basophilic adenoma of the pituitary.

The clinical symptoms of Cushing disease can be reproduced by the administration of corticosteroids. Myopathy or increased intracranial pressure may also result. The syndrome of pseudotumor with headache, nausea, vomiting, and papilledema tends to occur on withdrawal of therapy, particularly in children who were given steroid therapy for asthma, eczema, arthritis, and nephrosis. Treatment is reinstated with later gradual withdrawal of the steroid therapy.

Overproduction of the steroid hormones with androgenic activity by hyperplasia or tumors of the adrenal cortex may produce the syndrome of masculinization in women. Its biologic counterpart, a tumor with excessive production of estrogenic substances causing feminization in men, has been recognized, but is extremely rare. Adrenal virilism is relatively rare but may occur at any time from the prenatal period to old age. The syndromes that develop depend on the patient's gender and age at onset. Many inherited errors of steroid metabolism cause congenital adrenal hyperplasia. The most common is 21-hydroxylase deficiency, which results in relative deficiencies in aldosterone and corticoid secretion and excessive adrenal androgen production, resulting in virilization. Deficiency of 11-β-hydroxylase also produces oversecretion of adrenal androgens and virilization, some cortisol deficiency, and hypertension. Both disorders can be treated with glucocorticoid therapy, which corrects the excessive androgen production.

Androgenic hyperplasia of the adrenal cortex before birth leads to pseudohermaphroditism in the female and pubertas praecox with macrogenitosomia in the male. Precocious puberty may result from injury to the hypothalamus by hamartomas or other tumors in that region. Tumor or hyperplasia of the gland occurring before the age of puberty causes macrogenitosomia in boys and virilization in girls. Virilization in girls is characterized by enlargement of the clitoris, hirsutism, retarded breast development, rapid growth, amenorrhea, and an increase in the excretion of the 17-ketosteroids. Virilism after the age of puberty is not uncommon. Symptoms may vary from that of the classic adrenogenital syndrome to a moderate degree of hirsutism.

Adrenal virilism is usually suspected from the history and physical examination. There is invariably an increased excretion of urinary 17-ketosteroids. In tumors associated with feminization, there is an increase in the estrogenic substances in the blood and urine. In some cases, a tumor in the adrenal region can be palpated. Changes in the pyelogram are often of value in establishing the diagnosis. Arrhenoblastoma of the ovary, tumors of the testes, pineal tumors, and Cushing syndrome are to be considered in the differential diagnosis.

Treatment is surgical removal of the tumor or steroid therapy for inborn errors in steroid metabolism.

Primary Aldosteronism. In 1955, Conn reported a new syndrome due to production of aldosterone by a tumor of the adrenal cortex. Since the original report, a small number of cases have been recorded in the literature. The clinical syndrome is characterized by recurrent attacks of severe muscular weakness simulating familial periodic paralysis, tetany, polyuria, hypertension, inability of the kidneys to concentrate urine, and a striking imbalance of serum electrolytes with hypokalemia, hypernatremia, and alkalosis. Changes consistent with those of hypokalemia are found in the EKG. Conn reported that hypertension can result from adrenocortical tumors that produce hyperaldosteronism without concomitant hypokalemia. Aldosterone secretion and excretion are elevated and plasma renin activity is reduced. This combination is pathognomonic of primary aldosteronism.

Treatment is removal of the adrenal tumor or subtotal adrenalectomy in cases where the hyperaldosteronism is due to functional overactivity of the gland. If the disease persists after surgery, it may be controlled by administration of spironolactone.

Pheochromocytoma. Hyperfunction of the adrenal medulla as a result of a tumor of the chromaffin cells is characterized by an increased secretion of epinephrine and norepinephrine with signs and symptoms of hyperadrenalism. Tumors of the chromaffin cells of the adrenal medulla are rare, but they are important because they are one cause of hypertension that can be cured. They may occur in association with von Recklinghausen disease, Lindau disease, hereditary ataxia with telangiectasia of the conjunctiva, Sturge-Weber disease, tuberous sclerosis, and tumors of other endocrine glands. Glucose intolerance is often present.

Hypertension of a moderate or severe degree is the characteristic feature. This may be sustained or intercurrent. The persistent hypertension is indistinguishable on routine examinations from other types of benign or malignant hypertension. The intercurrent type is characterized by paroxysmal attacks of palpitation, precordial pain, severe headache, dizziness, sweating, weakness, anxiety, nausea, vomiting, diarrhea, dilated pupils, paresthesias, rapid pulse, and a rise in blood pressure, which may attain levels between 200 and 300 mm Hg. Death may result from cerebral hemorrhage, pulmonary edema, or cardiac failure in one of the acute attacks or as a result of one of these complications in the sustained type.

Initial screening tests should include determinations of 24-hour urinary excretion of catecholamine metabolites: vanillylmandelic acid, normetanephrine, and metanephrine, which will confirm the diagnosis in up to 90% of patients with pheochromocytoma. Determination of the relative amounts of epinephrine and norepinephrine excreted in the urine may aid in localizing the tumor. If more than 20% of the total catecholamine is epinephrine, the tumor is either located in the adrenal medulla or in an organ of Zuckerkandl. Prefer-

ential secretion of norepinephrine is associated with tumors in other intra-abdominal and extra-abdominal sites, as well as with tumors in the adrenal. Pharmacologic tests are occasionally used to confirm the diagnosis, particularly in those in which there is a high index of suspicion on clinical grounds and in which the catecholamine determinations are equivocal. There are risks involved in all these provocative tests. Hypertensive patients harboring these tumors are abnormally sensitive to the hypotensive effects of phentolamine. Histamine or tyramine is administered to normotensive patients to precipitate an attack of hypertension so that catecholamines can be evaluated.

Ovary

Estrogen-containing compounds have been widely used as contraceptives for more than 10 years and there are many reports in the literature describing untoward side-effects. These include hypertension, migraine, cerebrovascular lesions, optic neuritis, and papilledema with increased intracranial pressure (pseudotumor cerebri).

In view of the large number of patients taking these hormones and the occasional occurrence of these conditions in women of the age groups concerned, it is difficult to assess the role of the hormone in the development of the morbid condition under consideration.

There is no doubt, however, that the taking of estrogenic hormones for contraceptive purposes is accompanied by the risk of certain complications. This risk must be measured against the importance of preventing pregnancy.

References

Pituitary

Hypopituitarism

Abrams GM, Schipper HM. Neuroendocrine syndromes of the hypothalamus. In: Zimmerman EA, Abrams GM, eds. Neuroendocrinology and Brain Peptides. Neurologic Clinics, vol. 4. Philadelphia: WB Saunders, 1986:769–782.

Bauer HG. Endocrine and other clinical manifestations of hypothalamic disease: a survey of 60 cases with autopsies. J Clin Endocrinol Metab 1954; 14:13–31.

Coggins CH, Leaf A. Diabetes insipidus. Am J Med 1967; 42:807–813.

Daughaday WH. The adenohypophysis. In: Wilson JD, Foster DW, eds. Textbook of Endocrinology. 7th ed. Philadelphia: WB Saunders, 1985:568–613.

Farquharson F. Simmond's disease; extreme insufficiency of the adenohypophysis. Springfield, IL: Charles C Thomas, 1950.

Klingmuller D, Dewes W, Krane J, Brecht G, Schweikert

W-V. Magnetic resonance imaging of the brain in patients with anosmia and hypothalamic hypogonadism (Kallmann's syndrome). J Clin Endocrinol Metab 1987; 65:581–584.

Locke S, Tyler HR. Pituitary apoplexy: Report of two cases with pathological verification. Am J Med 1961; 30:643–648.

Martin FIR. Familial diabetes insipidus. Q J Med 1959; 28:573–582.

Martin JB, Reichlin S, Brown GM. Clinical Neuroendocrinology. Philadelphia: FA Davis, 1977.

Moses AM. Clinical and laboratory features of central and nephrogenic diabetes insipidus and primary polydipsia. In: Reichlin S, ed. The Neurohypophysis, Physiological and Clinical Aspects. New York: Plenum Medical, 1984:115–138.

Plum F, Van Uitert R. Nonendocrine diseases and disorders of the hypothalamus. In: Reichlin S, Baldessarini RJ, Martin JB, eds. The Hypothalamus. New York: Raven Press, 1978:415–473.

Robinson AG, Verbalis JG. Treatment of central diabetes insipidus. Front Horm Res 1985; 13:292–303.

Todd J. A case of Simmond's disease with mental symptoms. Br Med J 1951; 2:569–571.

Weisberg LA, Zimmerman EA, Frantz AG. Diagnosis and evaluation of patients with an enlarged sella turcica. Am J Med 1976; 61:590–596.

Antidiuretic Hormone

Burrows FA, Shutack JG, Crone RK. Inappropriate secretion of antidiuretic hormone in a postsurgical pediatric population. Crit Care Med 1983; 11:527–531.

Decaux G, Unger J, Brimioulle S, Mockel J. Hyponatremia in the syndrome of inappropriate secretion of antidiuretic hormone: rapid correlation with urea, sodium chloride, and water restriction therapy. JAMA 1982; 247:471–474.

Lester MC, Nelson PB. Neurological aspects of vasopressin release and the syndrome of inappropriate secretion of antidiuretic hormone. Neurosurgery 1981; 8:735–740.

Moses AM, Notman DD. Diabetes insipidus and syndrome of inappropriate antidiuretic hormone secretion (SIADH). Adv Intern Med 1982; 27:73–100.

Hyperpituitarism

Bertrand G, Tolis G, Montes J. Immediate and long-term results of transsphenoidal microsurgical resection of prolactinomas in 92 patients. In: Tolis G, Stefanis C, Mountokalakis T, Labrie F, eds. Prolactin and Prolactinomas. New York: Raven Press, 1983:441–452.

Comi RJ, Gorden P. The response of serum growth hormone levels to the long-acting somatostatin analog SMS 201-995 in acromegaly. J Clin Endocrinol Metab 1987; 64:37–42.

Forbes AP, Henneman PH, Griswold GC, Albright F. Syndrome characterized by Galactorrhea, amenorrhea, and low urinary FSH: comparison with acromegaly and normal lactation. J Clin Endocrinol Metab 1954; 14:265–271.

Hemmingytt S, Kalkhoff RK, Daniels DL, et al. CT study of hormone-secreting microadenomas. Radiology 1983; 146:65–69.

Kleinberg DL, Noel GL, Frantz AG. Galactorrhea: A study of 235 cases including 48 with pituitary tumors. N Engl J Med 1977; 296:589–600.

Koppelman MCS, Jaffe MJ, Reith KG, Caruso RC, Loriaux DL. Hyperprolactinemia, amenorrhea, and galactorrhea. Ann Intern Med 1984; 100:115–121.

Krieger DT. Pituitary ACTH hyperfunction: Physiopathology and clinical aspects. In: Camanni F, Muller EE, eds. Pituitary Hyperfunction: Physiopathology and Clinical Aspects. New York: Raven Press, 1984:221–234.

Lee BCP, Deck MDF. Sellar and juxtasellar lesion detection with MR. Radiology 1985; 157:143–147.

Loli P, Berselli ME, Tagliaferri M. Use of ketoconazole in the treatment of Cushings syndrome. J Clin Endocrinol Metab 1986; 63:1365–1371.

McGregor AM, Scanlon MK, Hall K, Cook DB, Hall R. Reduction in size of a pituitary tumor by bromocriptine therapy. N Engl J Med 1979; 300:291–293.

Montini M, Pagani G, Gianola D, et al. Long-lasting suppression of prolactin secretion and rapid shrinkage of prolactinomas after a long-acting injectable form of bromocriptine. J Clin Endocrinol Metab 1986; 63:266–268.

Nicolis G, Shimshi M, Allen C, Halmi N, Kourides IA. Gonadotropin-producing pituitary adenoma in a man with long-standing primary hypogonadism. J Clin Endocrinol Metab 1988; 66:237–241.

Sperling MR, Pritchard PB, Engel J Jr, Daniel C, Sagel J. Prolactin in partial epilepsy: An indicator of limbic seizures. Ann Neurol 1986; 20:716–722.

Thomas JP. Treatment of acromegaly. Br Med J 1983; 286:330–332.

Tyrrell JB, Brooks RM, Fitzgerald PA, Cofoid PB, Forsham PH, Wilson CB. Cushing's disease: selective transsphenoidal resection of pituitary adenomas. N Engl J Med 1978; 298:753–758.

Sotos Syndrome

Abraham JM, Snodgrass GJ. Sotos' syndrome of cerebral gigantism. Arch Dis Child 1969; 44:203–210.

Dodge PR, Holmes SJ, Sotos JF. Cerebral gigantism. Dev Med Child Neurol 1983; 25:248–252.

Hook EB, Reynolds JW. Cerebral gigantism. Endocrinological and clinical observations of six patients. J Pediatr 1967; 70:900–914.

Ott JE, Robinson A. Cerebral gigantism. Am J Dis Child 1969; 177:357–368.

Smith A, Farrar JR, Silink M, Judzewitch R. Investigations in dominant Sotos' syndrome. Ann Genet 1981; 24:226–228.

Sotos JF, Dodge PR, Muirhead D, et al. Cerebral gigantism in childhood. N Engl J Med 1964; 271:109–116.

Tindall GT, Barrow DL, Martin JB. Disorders of the Pituitary. St. Louis: CV Mosby, 1986.

Weiss MH, Teal J, Gott P, et al. Natural history of microprolactinomas: Six-year follow-up. Neurosurgery 1983; 12:180–183.

Thyroid

Barnard RD, Campbell MJ, McDonald MI. Pathologic findings in a case of hypothyroidism with ataxia. Neurol Neurosurg Psychiatry 1971; 34:755–760.

Brain WR, Turnbull HM. Exophthalmic ophthalmoplegia. Q J Med 1938; 7:293–323.

Brody IE, Dudley AW Jr. Thyrotoxic hypokalemic periodic paralysis. Arch Neurol 1969; 21:1–6.

Brown J, Coburn JW, Wigod RA, Hiss JM Jr, Dowling J. Adrenal steroid therapy of severe infiltrated ophthalmopathy of Graves' disease. Am J Med 1963; 34:786–795.

Bulens C. Neurologic complications of hyperthyroidism. Arch Neurol 1981; 38:669–670.

Bursten B. Psychoses associated with thyrotoxicosis. Arch Gen Psychiatry 1961; 4:267–273.

Catz B, Russel S. Myxedema, shock and coma. Arch Intern Med 1961; 108:407–417.

Cronstedt J, Carling L, Ostbert H. Hypothyroidism with subacute pseudomyotonia. An early form of Hoftmann's syndrome? Acta Med Scand 1975; 198: 137–139.

Day RM, Carroll FG. Corticosteroids in treatment of optic nerve involvement associated with thyroid dysfunction. Trans Am Ophthalmol Soc 1967; 65:41–51.

Dyck PJ, Lambert EH. Polyneuropathy associated hypothyroidism. J Neuropathol Exp Neurol 1970; 29:631–658.

Fidler SM, O'Rourke RA, Buchsbaum W. Choreoathetosis as a manifestation of thyrotoxiosis. Neurology 1971; 21:55–57.

Fort P, Lipshitz, Pugliese M, Klein I. Neonatal thyroid disease: differential expression in three successive offspring. J Clin Endocrinol Metab 1988; 66:645–647.

Gamblin GT, Harper DG, Galentine P, Buck DR, Chernow B, Eil C. Prevalence of increased intraocular pressure in Graves' disease—evidence of frequent subclinical ophthalmopathy. N Engl J Med 1983; 308:420–424.

Garcia CA, Flening H. Reversible corticospinal tract disease due to hyperthyroidism. Arch Neurol 977; 34:647–648.

Glorieux J, Dussault JH, Letarte J, Guyda H, Morissette J. Preliminary results on the mental development of hypothyroid infants detected by the Quebec Screening Program. J Pediatr 1983; 102:19–22.

Gorman CA. Extrathyroid manifestations of Graves' disease. In: Ingbar SH, Braverman LE, eds. The Thyroid. A Fundamental and Clinical Text. Philadelphia: JB Lippincott, 1986:1015–138.

Gorman CA, DeSanto LW, MacCarty CS, Riley FC. Optic neuropathy of Graves' disease. N Engl J Med 1974; 290:70–75.

Hagberg B, Westphal O. Ataxic syndrome in congenital hypothyroidism. Acta Paediatr Scand 1970; 59:323–327.

Kennerdell JS, Rosenbaum AE, El-Hoshy MH. Apical optic nerve compression of dysthyroid optic neuropathy on computed tomography. Arch Ophthalmol 1982; 100:324–328.

Klein I, Parker M, Shebert R, Ayyar DR, Levey GS. Hypothyroidism presenting as muscle stiffness and pseudo hypertrophy: Hoffmann's syndrome. Am J Med 1981; 70:891–894.

Kodama K, Bandy-Dafoe P, Sikorska H, Bayly R, Wall JR. Circulating autoantibody against a soluble eye-muscle antigen in Graves' ophthalmopathy. Lancet 1982; 2:1353–1356.

Lindberger K. Myxoedema coma. Acta Med Scand 1975; 198:87–90.

Nordgren L, von Scheele C. Myxedematous madness without myxedema. Acta Med Scand 1976; 199:233–236.

Ramsay I. Thyroid Disease and Muscle Dysfunction. Chicago: Year Book Medical Publishers, 1974.

Rao SN, Katiyar BC, Nair KRP, Misra S. Neuromuscular status in hypothyroidism. Acta Neurol Scand 1980; 61:167–177.

Rosman NP. Neurological and muscular aspects of thyroid dysfunction in childhood. Pediatr Clin North Am 1976; 23:575–594.

Sanders V. Neurologic manifestations of myxedema. N Engl J Med 1962; 266:547–552, 599.

Satoyoshi E, Murakami K, Kowa H, Kinoshito M, Nishyama Y. Periodic paralysis in hyperthyroidism. Neurology 1963; 13:746–752.

Savoic JC, Fardeau M, Leger F, Quichaud J. Hyperthyroidism without hypermetabolism in two cases of diffuse muscular atrophy. Ann Endocrinol 1975; 36:175–176.

Slavin ML, Glaser JS. Idiopathic orbital myositis, report of 6 cases. Arch Ophthalmol 1982; 100:1261–1265.

Solomon DJ, Chopra IJ, Smith FJ. Identification of subgroups of euthyroid Graves' ophthalmopathy. N Engl J Med 1977; 296:340–349.

Spiro AJ, Hirano A, Beilin RL, Finkelstein JW. Cretinism with muscular hypertrophy (Kocher-Débre-Sémélaigne syndrome). Arch Neurol 1970; 23:340–349.

Strakosch CR, Wenzel BE, Row VV, Volpe R. Immunology of autoimmune thyroid diseases. N Engl J Med 1982; 307:1499–1507.

Swanson JW, Kelly JJ Jr, McConahey WM. Neurologic aspects of thyroid dysfunction. Mayo Clin Proc 1981; 56:504–512.

Teng CS, Yeo PPB. Ophthalmic Graves' disease: natural history and detailed thyroid function studies. Br Med J 1977; 1:273–275.

Trobe JD, Glaser JS, Laflamme P. Dysthyroid optic neuropathy. Arch Ophthalmol 1978; 96:1199–1209.

Trokel SL, Hilal SK. Recognition and differential diagnosis of enlarged extraocular muscles in computed tomography. Am J Ophthalmol 1979; 87:503–512.

Wall JR, Henderson J, Strakosch CR, Joyner DM. Graves' ophthalmopathy: a review. Can Med Assoc J 1981; 124:855–866.

Werner SC. Prednisone in emergency treatment of malignant exophthalmos. Lancet 1966; 1:1004–1007.

Parathyroid

Albright F, Reifenstein EC Jr. The Parathyroid Gland and Metabolic Bone Disease. Baltimore: Williams & Wilkins, 1948.

Anonymous. Anticonvulsant osteomalacia [Editorial]. Br Med J 1976; 2:1340–1341.

Burch WM, Posillico JT. Hypoparathyroidism after I-131 therapy with subsequent return of parathyroid function. J Clin Endocrinol Metab 1983; 57:398–401.

Cogan MG, Covey CM, Arieff AI, Wisniewski A, Clark OH. Central nervous system manifestations of hyperparathyroidism. Am J Med 1978; 65:563–630.

Cope O. The story of hyperparathyroidism at the Massachusetts General Hospital. N Engl J Med 1966; 274:1174–1182.

Drezner MK, Neelon FA. Pseudohypoparathyroidism. In: Stanbury JB, Wyngaarden JB, Fredrickson DS, Goldstein JL, Brown MS, eds. The Metabolic Basis of Inherited Disease, 5th ed. New York: McGraw-Hill: 1982; 1508–1527.

Frame B, Heinze EG Jr, Block MA, Manson GA. Myopathy in primary hyperparathyroidism. Ann Intern Med 1968; 68:1022–1027.

Houssain M. Neurological and psychiatric manifestations in idiopathic hypoparathyroidism: Response to treatment. J Neurol Neurosurg Psychiatry 1970; 33:153–156.

Mallette LE, Bilezikian JP, Heath DA, Aurbach GD. Primary hyperparathyroidism. Clinical and biochemical features. Medicine 1974; 53:127–146.

Mallette LE, Patten BM, Engel WK. Neuromuscular disease in secondary hyperparathyroidism. Ann Intern Med 1975; 82:474–483.

McKinney AS. Idiopathic hypoparathyroidism presenting as chorea. Neurology 1962; 12:485–491.

Newman JH, Neff TA, Ziporin P. Acute respiratory failure associated with hypophosphatemia. N Engl J Med 1977; 296:1101–1103.

Nusynowitz ML, Frame B, Kolb PO. The spectrum of hypoparathyroid states. Medicine 1976; 55:105–119.

Parfitt AM, Kleerkoper M. Clinical disorders of calcium, phosphorus and magnesium metabolism. In: Maxwell MH, Kleeman CT, eds. Clinical Disorders of Fluid and Electrolyte Metabolism. New York: McGraw-Hill, 1980; 947–1000.

Patten BM, Bilezikian JP, Mallette LE, Prince A, Engel WK, Aurbach GD. Neuromuscular disease in primary hyperparathyroidism. Ann Intern Med 1974; 80:182–194.

Pierides AM, Edwards WG Jr, Cullum UX Jr, McCall JT, Ellis HA. Hemodialysis encephalopathy with osteomalacic fractures and muscle weakness. Kidney Int 1980; 18:115–124.

Roisin AJ. Ectopic calcification around joints of paralyzed limbs in hemiplegia, diffuse brain damage and other neurological diseases. Ann Rheum Dis 1975; 34:499–505.

Rubenstein A, Brust JCM. Parkinsonian syndrome as complication of post-thyroidectomy hypoparathyroidism. NY State J Med 1974; 74:2029–2030.

Scott GD, Wills MR. Muscle weakness in osteomalacia. Lancet 1976; 1:626–629.

Tabaee-Zadeh MJ, Frame B, Kappahn K. Kinesiogenic choreoathetosis and idiopathic hypoparathyroidism. N Engl J Med 1972; 286:762–763.

Pancreas

Anderson JM, Milner RDG, Strich SJ. Effects of neonatal hypoglycaemia on the nervous system: A pathological study. J Neurol Neurosurg Psychiatry 1967; 30:295–310.

Bell WE, Samaan NA, Longnecker DS. Hypoglycemia due to organic hyperinsulinism in infancy. Arch Neurol 1971; 23:330–339.

Courville CB. Late cerebral changes incident to severe hypoglycemia (insulin shock): Their relation to cerebral anoxia. Arch Neurol Psychiatry 1957; 78:1–14.

Cryer PE. Glucose homeostasis and hypoglycemia. In: Williams Textbook of Endocrinology, Wilson JD, Foster DW, eds. 7th Ed. Philadelphia: WB Saunders, 1985:989–1017.

Gale E. Hypoglycaemia. Clin Endocrinol Metab 1980; 9:461–475.

Harrison MJG. Muscle wasting after prolonged hypoglycemic coma: Case report with electrophysiological data. J Neurol Psychiatry 1976; 39:465–470.

Kalimo H, Olsson Y. Effects of severe hypoglycemia on the human brain: Neuropathologic case reports. Acta Neurol Scand 1980; 62:345–356.

Mabry CC, DiGeorge AM, Auerbach VH. Leucine-induced hypoglycemia. J Pediatr 1960; 57:526–538.

Merimec TJ. Spontaneous hypoglycemia in man. Adv Intern Med 1977; 22:301–307.

Pagliara AS, Karl IE, Haymond M, Kipnis DM. Hypoglycemia in childhood. J Pediatr 1973; 82:365–379, 558–577.

Richardson JC, Chambers RA, Heywood PM. Encephalopathies of anoxia and hypoglycemia. Arch Neurol 1959; 1:178–190.

Richardson ML, Kinard RE, Gray MB. CT of generalized gray matter infarction due to hypoglycemia. AJNR 1981; 2:366–367.

Seltzer HS. Severe drug-induced hypoglycemia. A review. Compr Therap 1979; 5:21–29.

Silas JH, Grant DS, Maddocks JL. Transient hemiparetic attacks due to unrecognized nocturnal hypoglycemia. Br Med J 1981; 282:132–133.

Turkington RW. Encephalopathy induced by oral hypoglycemia drugs. Arch Intern Med 1959; 137:1082–1083.

Wassner SJ, Li JB, Sperouto A, Norman ME. Vitamin D deficiency, hypocalcemia and increased skeletal muscle degradation in rats. J Clin Invest 1983; 72:102–112.

Whipple AO. Hyperinsulinism in relation to pancreatic tumors. Surgery 1944; 16:289–305.

Wilkinson DS, Prockop LD. Hypoglycemia: Effects on the nervous system. In: Vinken PJ, Bruyn GW, eds. Handbook of Clinical Neurology (vol 27). New York: Elsevier-North Holland, 1976:53–78.

Adrenal

Adrenal Hypofunction

Abbas DH, Schlagenhauff RE, Strong HE. Polyradiculoneuropathy in Addison's disease: Case report and review of literature. Neurology 1977; 27:494–495.

Addison T. On the Constitutional and Local Effects of Diseases of the Suprarenal Capsules. London: D Highley, 1855.

Doppman JL. CT findings in Addison's disease. J Comput Assist Tomogr 1982; 6:757–761.

Drake FR. Neuropsychiatric-like symptomatology of Addison's disease: A review of the literature. Am J Med Sci 1957; 234:106–113.

Kandt RS, Heldrich FJ, Moser HW. Recovery from probable central pontine myelinolysis associated with Addison's disease. Arch Neurol 1983; 40:118–119.

Krautli B, Muller J, Landolt AM, von Schulthess F. ACTH-producing pituitary adenomas in Addison's disease: Two cases treated by transsphenoidal microsurgery. Acta Endocrinol 1982; 99:357–363.

Neufeld M, Maclaren NK, Blizzard RM. Two types of autoimmune Addison's disease associated with different polyglandular autoimmune (PGA) syndromes Medicine 1981; 60:355–362.

Van Dellen RG, Purnell DC. Hyperkalemic paralysis in Addison's disease. Mayo Clin Proc 1969; 44:904–914.

Walker DA, Davies M. Addison's disease presenting as a hypercalcemic crisis in a patient with idiopathic hypoparathyroidism. Clin Endocrinol 1981; 14:419–423.

Adrenal Hyperfunction

Aron DC, Findling JW, Fitzgerald PA, Forsham PH, Wilson CB, Tyrrell JB. Cushing's syndrome: Problems in management. Endocr Rev 1982; 3:229–244.

Askari A, Vignos PJ Jr, Moskowitz RW. Steroid myopathy in connective tissue disease. Am J Med 1976; 61:485–492.

Azarnoff DL, ed. Steroid Therapy. Philadelphia: WB Saunders, 1975.

Crapo L. Cushing's syndrome: A review of diagnostic tests. Metabolism 1979; 28:955–977.

Gabliloue JL, Seman AT, Sabet R, Mitty HA, Nicolis GL. Virilizing adrenal adenoma with studies on the steroid content of the adrenal venous effluent and a review of the literature. Endocr Rev 1981; 2:462–470.

Gold EM. The Cushing syndromes: changing views of diagnosis and treatment. Ann Intern Med 1979; 90:829–844.

Greenwald RA. Complications of steroid therapy. Del Med J 1981; 53:451–460.

Krieger DT. Pathophysiology and treatment of Cushing disease. Prog Clin Biol Res 1982; 87:19–32.

Krieger DT. The central nervous system and Cushing's syndrome. Mt Sinai J Med 1972; 39:416–428.

List CF, Dowman CE, Bagchi BK, Bebin J. Posterior hypothalamic hamartomas and gangliomas causing precocious puberty. Neurology 1959; 8:164–174.

Lüdecke DK, Schabet M, Saeger W. In vitro secretion of adenoma and anterior lobe cells in two typical cases of Cushing's disease. Neurosurgery 1983; 12:549–554.

New MI, Dupont B, Pang S, Pollack M, Levine LS. An update of congenital adrenal hyperplasia. Recent Prog Horm Res 1981; 37:105–181.

Rimsza ME. Complications of corticosteroid therapy. Am J Dis Child 1978; 132:806–810.

Sheehan JP. Hormone replacement treatment and benign intracranial hypertension. Br Med J (Clin Res) 1982; 284:1675–1676.

Vyas CK, Tallwar KK, Bhatnagar V, Sharma BK. Steroid-induced benign intracranial hypertension. Postgrad Med J 1981; 57:181–182.

Walker AE, Adamkiewicz JJ. Pseudotumor cerebri associated with prolonged corticosteroid therapy. JAMA 1964; 188:779–784.

Primary Aldosteronism

Atsumi T, Ishikawa S, Miyatake T, Yoshida M. Myopathy and primary aldosteronism: Electron microsopic study. Neurology 1979; 29:1348–1358.

Conn JW. Presidential address: II primary aldosteronism, new clinical syndrome. J Lab Clin Med 1955; 45:6–17.

Ferriss JB, Brown JJ, Fraser R, Lever AF, Robertson JI. Primary hyperaldosteronism. Clin Endocrinol Metab 1981; 10:419–452.

Ganguly A, Grim CE, Weinberger MH. Primary aldosteronism. The etiologic spectrum of disorders and their clinical differentiation. Arch Intern Med 1982; 142:813–815.

Ganguly A, Pratt JH, Weinberger MG, Grim CE, Fineberg NS. Differing effects of metoclopramide and adrenocorticotropin on plasma aldosterone levels in glucocorticoid-suppressible hyperaldosteronism and other forms of hyperaldosteronism. J Clin Endocrinol Metab 1983; 57:388–392.

Scoggins BA, Coghlan JP. Primary hyperaldosteronism. Pharmacol Ther (B) 1980; 9:367–394.

Vaughan NJA, Slater JD, Lightman SL, et al. The diagnosis of primary aldosteronism. Lancet 1981; 1:120–125.

Weinberger MH, Grim CE, Hollifield JW, et al. Primary aldosteronism: Diagnosis, localization and treatment. Ann Intern Med 1979; 90:386–395.

Pheochromocytoma

Bowerman RA, Silver TM, Jaffe MH, Stuck KJ, Hinerman DL. Sonography of adrenal pheochromocytomas. AJR 1981; 137:1227–1231.

Bridgwater GR, Starling JR. Pheochromocytoma: Paroxysmal hypertensive headaches. Headache 1982; 22:84–85.

Goldfien A. Phaeochromocytoma. Clin Metab 1981; 10:607–630.

Hoffman RW, Gardner DW, Mitchell FL. Intrathoracic and multiple abdominal pheochromocytomas in von Hippel-Landau disease. Arch Intern Med 1982; 142:1962–1964.

Howard JE, Barker WH. Paroxysmal hypertension and other clinical manifestations associated with benign chromaffin cell tumors. Bull Johns Hopkins Hosp 1937; 61:371–410.

Lance JW, Hinterberger H. Symptoms of pheochromocytoma, with particular reference to headache, correlated with catecholamine production. Arch Neurol 1976; 33:281–288.

Manger WM. Psychiatric manifestations in patients with pheochromocytoma. Arch Intern Med 1985; 145: 229–230.

Ram CV, Engelman K. Pheochromocytoma. Recognition and management. Curr Probl Cardiol 1979; 4:1–37.

Reeves RA, Kiss JE, Meess M, Levey GS, Shapiro AP. Pseudopseudohypoparathyroidism and pheochromocytoma. Association or coincidence? Arch Intern Med 1983; 143:1619.

Thomas JE, Rooke ED, Kvale WF. The neurologist's experience with pheochromocytoma: A review of 100 cases. JAMA 1966; 197:754–758.

Ovary

Andrews WC. Oral contraception. Clin Obstet Gynecol 1979; 6:3–26.

Collaborative Group for the Study of Stroke in Young Women. Oral contraception and increased risk of cerebral ischemia or thrombosis. N Engl J Med 1973; 288:871–878.

Collaborative Group for the Study of Stroke in Young Women. Oral contraceptives and stroke in young women: Associated risk factors. JAMA 1975; 231:718–722.

Estanol B, Rodriquez A, Conte G, Aleman JM, Loyo M, Pizzuto J. Intracranial venous thrombosis in young women. Stroke 1979; 10:680–684

Mattson RH, Cramer JA, Darney PD, Naftolin F. Use of oral contraceptives by women with epilepsy. JAMA 1986; 256:238–240.

Suginami H, Hamada K, Yano H, Kuroda G, Matsuura S. Ovulation induction with bromocriptine in normoprolactinemic anovulatory women. J Clin Endocrinol Metab 1986; 62:899–903.

Roberts JM. Oestrogens and hypertension. Clin Endocrinol Metab 1981; 10:489–512.

Schoenberg BS, Whisnant JP, Taylor WF, Kempers RD. Strokes in women of childbearing age. A population study. Neurology 1970; 20:181–189.

Stadel BV. Oral contraceptives and cardiovascular disease. N Engl J Med 1981; 305:612–618, 672–677.

Tooke JE, McNichol GP. Thrombotic disorders associated with pregnancy and the pill. Clin Haematol 1981; 10:613–630.

150. HEMATOLOGIC AND RELATED SYSTEMIC DISEASES

Leonard Berg
Octavio de Marchena

Sickle Cell Anemia

Sickle cell anemia is an inherited disease of the blood related to the presence of abnormal hemoglobin (Hb S) patterns in which the red cells assume a "sickle" or oat-shaped form. It occurs predominantly in blacks. Affected subjects are frequently asthenic, have a chronic hemolytic anemia, and are prone to develop bacterial infections and chronc ulcers on the legs. The clinical course usually begins in infancy or in childhood and is punctuated by crises that are characterized by fever and pain in the abdomen or limbs. Multiple thromboses and painful infarctions in the bones and viscera give rise to a variety of clinical manifestations.

Neurologic complications include bacterial meningitis, thrombosis of the dural sinuses, subdural or subarachnoid hemorrhage, and hemorrhage from or thromboses of the large vessels within the cranium or the smaller vessels in the substance of the brain. Small and large infarctions are found principally in the boundary zones between the distributions of major cerebral and cerebellar arteries. Infarction of the spinal cord and cranial neuropathies may also result. Changes in blood vessels include fusiform narrowing, intimal hyperplasia, occlusions, and neovascularization of the moyamoya variety. Corresponding radiologic abnormalities have been visualized by angiography, which carries special risk in this disease and which should only be performed after special precautions (e.g., transfusion, hydration).

The sickling phenomenon is important in the pathogenesis of the circulatory disorder. These red cells assume the sickled form (at first reversibly but later irreversibly) in response to hypoxia. Sickling results in stiffening of the red cells, loss of their deformability in transit through capillaries, increased viscosity, and sludging. These phenomena lead to stagnation and further hypoxia, which increases the number of sickled cells.

The neurologic manifestations, which are usually those of a stroke, may coincide with or be independent of the crises. Psychotic manifestations and convulsions may occur. When subarachnoid hemorrhage appears, a ruptured berry aneurysm is frequently found.

How sickling produces the changes in the large vessels, which in turn, cause strokes is not clear. However, involvement of the small nutrient vessels of arteries, the vasa vasorum, by sickled cells has been suggested as a precipitating event for the large vessel changes.

The diagnosis of sickle cell anemia should be suspected when signs and symptoms of an acute cerebrovascular accident occur in a young black. The usual stained blood smear may not reveal the typical anomaly of the red cells, which will be evident if a drop of blood is mixed with a drop of 2% sodium metabisulfate on a glass slide under a cover slip and allowed to deoxygenate for 10 to 15 minutes. Proper identification of the disorder requires demonstration of Hb S by electrophoresis or biochemical means. Radiographic findings of infarcts in the bones provide clues to the diagnosis. Marrow expansion in vertebral bodies results in a biconcave or "fishmouth" radiologic appearance. In the skull, extension of the marrow through the outer table of bone gives the characteristic "hair-on-end" appearance. These radiologic changes in the skull are usually more striking in thalassemia (Fig. 150–1), another chronic hemolytic anemia of children and young adults.

Palliative measures consist of proper hygiene to avoid hypoxia and ischemia, prevention of dehydration, and correction of electrolyte disturbances. The role of exchange transfusions or repeated simple transfusions is still being explored, with attention to the hazards attendant upon repeated transfusions in a chronic disease. Prenatal detection of the disease is now possible in the first trimester of pregnancy by restriction-enzyme analysis of trophoblast DNA.

Pernicious Anemia

See Article 125, Subacute Combined Degeneration of the Spinal Cord, for a discussion of pernicious anemia.

Polycythemia Vera

Polycythemia vera is a chronic progressive disease characterized by excessive activity of the bone marrow with a persistent elevation of the number of red blood cells in the circulation and splenomegaly.

Etiology. The disorder is now accepted as a neoplastic proliferation of the erythropoietic tissues analogous to leukemia. The overproduction of red cells is autonomous, as indicated by decreased production and excretion of erythropoietin, the hormone that stimulates red cell production.

Incidence. Polycythemia vera is a rare disease of all races. The onset of symptoms is usually in the fifth to sixth decades of life. Men are affected more frequently than women.

Symptoms and Signs. In addition to the plethoric facies, and reddish or purple color of the mucous membranes and skin of the neck and limbs, there are diverse symptoms: lassitude, increased sweating, loss of weight, headache, vertigo, tinnitus, visual disturbances, paresthesias in the limbs, dyspnea, and gastrointestnal symptoms. Dilated retinal veins and enlargement of the spleen are regularly present.

Hemiplegia, aphasia, or other focal neu-

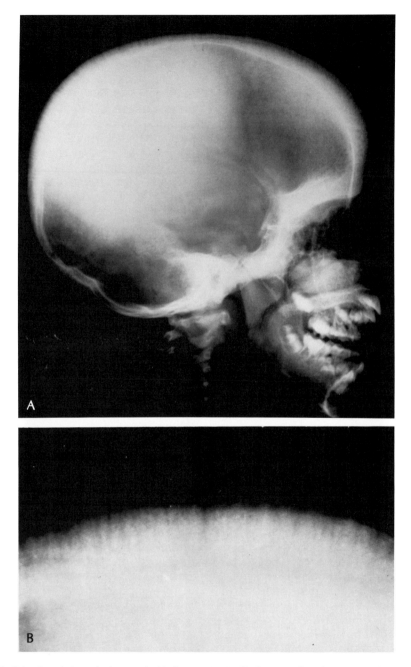

Fig. 150–1. Skull in chronic hemolytic anemia (thalassemia). *A.* Thickening of vault. *B.* Magnified view of "hair-on-end" appearance due to extramedullary hematopoiesis in the widened diploic space. (Courtesy of Dr. William H. McAlister.)

rologic signs may occur when there is thrombosis or rupture of intracranial vessels. Papilledema may occur as a result of changes in the circulation of the retina or because of increased intracranial pressure, possibly due to thrombosis of one of the dural sinuses. TIAs in the cerebral or retinal circulation are not uncommon. As in other diseases marked by extramedullary hematopoiesis, spinal cord compression by intraspinal hematopoietic tissue is a possible complication. Despite the frequency of paresthesias, objective signs of polyneuropathy are rare.

Laboratory Data. The total volume of the blood is increased. The red cell mass per kg of body weight is constantly high in contrast to symptomatic polycythemia in which it is normal. The blood is abnormally dark and thick with delay in the clotting time. The red count is usually in the range of 7 to 11 million/mm³. The hemoglobin content is proportionately increased but occasionally it is less markedly elevated than the red count because of hypochromia of the red cells. The white cell count is commonly about 15,000/mm³ and the number of platelets is increased. Immature red cells and leukocytes may be present in the blood. Bone marrow is hyperplastic.

The CSF is normal unless there has been an intracranial hemorrhage; then it may be bloody. The pressure is increased when there is papilledema associated with venous sinus thrombosis.

Pathophysiology. Thromboembolic complications result from the thrombocytosis and hyperviscosity due to the elevated red blood cell mass. Bleeding tendencies arise from hypervolemia and platelet dysfunction that may be present.

Diagnosis. The diagnosis of polycythemia vera as the cause of neurologic symptoms can usually be made without difficulty on the basis of the plethoric appearance of the patient, the splenomegaly, and the examination of the blood. Occasionally tumors of the brain, particularly cerebellar hemangioblastomas, may be accompanied by a high red cell count in the blood. Distinction between these and cases of polycythemia vera with papilledema may be difficult without CT. Symptomatic polycythemia must be excluded by studies of red cell mass and arterial oxygen saturation.

Course. Polycythemia vera is a slowly progressive disease that, when untreated, usually leads to death in a few years. Only rarely is there a spontaneous remission. With treatment, the median survival has improved to more than 12 years. Causes of death include vascular complications in the brain and other organs, acute leukemia, and myelofibrosis.

Treatment. Venesection (phlebotomy), "spray x-ray therapy," radioactive phosphorus, and other marrow suppressants (e.g., melphalan, busulfan, chlorambucil) have all been used in therapy. There is still disagreement regarding the choice of therapies. One concern is the possibility of increased incidence of acute leukemia associated with some of these agents. Anticoagulant therapy is indicated when the red cell count is high and there are signs or symptoms suggesting insufficiency of the circulation of one or more of the cerebral vessels.

Essential Thrombocythemia

This disorder is analogous to polycythemia vera and leukemia in that it represents a neoplastic proliferation of the megakaryocyte/platelet cell line. The clinical picture includes splenomegaly, excessive bleeding due to platelet dysfunction, and thromboembolic events, especially painful occlusive syndromes in the fingers and toes. Characteristic laboratory findings include persistent thrombocytosis (usually over 1 million/mm³), circulating platelet aggregates, platelet dysfunction, elevated white blood cell count, and some degree of anemia. The neurologic complications are often present without other clinical manifestations and are mainly the result of retinal, cerebral, or brainstem ischemic events. Amaurosis fugax, confusion, and focal neurologic disorders result. Thrombosis of the superior sagittal sinus has been reported.

The thrombotic tendency in essential thrombocythemia appears to be greater than expected from the platelet count alone. Patients with secondary thrombocytosis, such as following splenectomy, do not appear to be at increased risk of thrombosis. The factor responsible for the thrombotic tendency in these patients may be abnormal platelet function rather than the increased numbers of platelets.

Initial therapy includes administration of aspirin and dipyridamole and platelet removal by plasmapheresis. Marrow suppressant drugs are then used as described for polycythemia vera.

Hypereosinophilic Syndrome

The idiopathic hypereosinophilic syndrome is characterized by persistent eosinophilia without obvious cause. Multiple organ damage has been reported in this syndrome, most commonly endomyocardial fibrosis. Neurologic dysfunction occurs in over half the patients. A sensory polyneuropathy is the most common neurologic syndrome, occurring in about 50% of those with the disorder, and brain embolism occurs in about 10%. There is also a distinctive encephalopathy with behavioral disturbances and upper motor neuron signs.

Lymphomas

Malignancies of the lymphoreticular system include the disorders called Hodgkin disease and the nonHodgkin lymphomas. The Hodgkin lymphomas, derived from the Reed-Sternberg cell, are classified as lymphocytic predominant, mixed cellularity, lymphocytic depleted, and nodular sclerosis. There is less agreement about classification of the non-Hodgkin lymphomas, which are sometimes characterized according to histologic growth pattern (nodular or diffuse) and cytology (lymphocytic, lymphoblastic, large cell or histiocytic, undifferentiated, or mixed). There are efforts to identify the lymphocytic lymphomas according to surface markers (T-cell, B-cell, or null-cell), monoclonal antibodies, and morphology (convoluted or noncleaved follicular center cells). The subclassifications bear clinical correlates with regard to age of predilection, rapidity of course, response to treatment, and frequency of various types of neurologic syndromes. Despite the differing incidences of neurologic syndromes according to age of patient and histologic type of neoplasm, one can view the neurologic complications of the lymphomas as follows:

Primary
Metastatic
  Intracranial (rarely intraparenchymal, usually epidural or subdural)
  Intraspinal (usually epidural)
  Leptomeningeal (including cranial and spinal nerves)
  Peripheral nerves and plexuses
Nonmetastatic
  Infectious
  Vascular
  Metabolic
  Remote effects
  Iatrogenic

The *primary* lymphomas of brain, formerly called *reticulum cell sarcoma* or *microglioma*, may be of the lymphocytic or histiocytic (non-Hodgkin) cell type. They occur more often than metastatic lymphomas in brain and may be single or multifocal. These tumors are being encountered more frequently because immunosuppressed hosts (e.g., organ transplant recipients) are particularly susceptible to their development.

Metastatic involvement of the nervous system in the lymphomas usually takes the form of invasion of the extradural space by granulomatous masses that compress the spinal cord or occlude its blood supply. Invasion of the parenchyma of the brain or spinal cord is rare.

A rare, predominantly intravascular, malignant B-cell lymphoma appears as one form of malignant angioendotheliomatosis. Most patients with this illness have neurologic involvement, which presents with progressive confusion, obtundation, and multifocal involvement of the brain.

Pathology. Metastatic cerebral involvement in the lymphomas is so rare that for many years its existence was doubted. Isolated patients with convulsions or other cerebral symptoms have been recorded in the literature, but in most the symptoms were due to the presence of nodules in the dura. A few patients with lymphomas within the brain have been reported. Mycosis fungoides, a primary cutaneous lymphoma of T-cell origin, occasionally metastasizes to the brain, where the infiltrative lesions may be accompanied by demyelination.

Metastatic tumors may damage the spinal cord by direct compression of its substance, by compression of its vascular supply, or by collapse of affected vertebrae.

Leptomeningeal invasion may be focal but it is more often diffuse. Cranial and spinal nerves are frequently infiltrated as they traverse the subarachnoid spaces. Involvement of the peripheral nerves and plexuses is due to compression by tumor masses or infiltration by the malignant cells.

Incidence. The overall incidence of epidural spinal cord compression in the lymphomas is about 5%. Metastatic cerebral and peripheral nerve syndromes are less common. Diffuse leptomeningeal invasion, previously a rare complication, is being encountered more often. It is seen most frequently in the diffuse histiocytic and undifferentiated non-Hodgkin lymphomas because of increased longevity from systemic therapy.

Signs and Symptoms. When lymphomas occur in brain parenchyma the focal and general symptoms are those of any brain tumor. Compression of the spinal cord by epidural lymphomatous masses leads to a subacute transverse cord syndrome, usually at a thoracic level. Local back or radicular pain is frequently an early manifestation, but because paraspinal lymphomas often gain access to the epidural space through the spinal foramina sparing the vertebrae, bone pain is sometimes absent. By contrast, with other metastatic malignancies of the spinal epidural space, back pain is almost uniform because the pain arises from metastatic lesions of the vertebral column. If the spinal cord compression is not appropriately diagnosed and treated, spastic paraplegia, sensory loss below the level of the lesion, and urinary bladder dysfunction result.

In rare cases, the lesion in the thoracic spinal cord is due to compression of its vascular supply by the lymphoma, resulting in flaccid paraplegia, sensory loss below the level, and paralysis of the urinary bladder and sphincters.

When lymphomas invade the leptomeninges diffusely, a variety of syndromes may result: headache, meningeal irritation, papilledema, cranial neuropathies, confusion, seizures, and symmetric or asymmetric polyradiculopathies, which clinically mimic the Guillain-Barré syndrome. Invasion or compression of peripheral nerves and plexuses leads to appropriate painful and nonpainful focal signs and symptoms.

Diagnosis. Intracerebral masses are recognized on CT, but the opportunistic abscesses to which these patients with lymphomas are susceptible may mimic cerebral lymphomas both clinically and by CT. Diagnostic biopsy is often necessary. Leptomeningeal invasion can at times be detected by contrast enhancement of the intracranial subarachnoid spaces on CT (Fig. 150–2).

The CSF dynamics and content are normal when the damage to the spinal cord is caused by vascular occlusion. Dynamic block and increased protein content in the CSF are the characteristic findings when the symptoms are due to compression of the cord. When spinal cord compression is suspected, myelography should be performed at the time of lumbar puncture. When spinal puncture is suspected lumbar puncture should not be performed alone. MRI, myelography, or both would be appropriate.

Diffuse leptomeningeal seeding of lymphomas is characterized by increased protein and decreased sugar content of the CSF with malignant cells present. Demonstration of lymphoma cells in the CSF by millipore or cytocentrifuge techniques is essential for the identification of leptomeningeal disease, which may often occur as a relapse when systemic lymphoma remains in remission.

Treatment. Many patients with the more localized stages of systemic lymphomas respond to combined irradiation and chemotherapy with long-lasting remissions and apparent cure. Drug regimens include nitrogen mustard, cyclophosphamide, vincristine, and prednisone in various combinations. Therapies now being tested for the more aggressive malignant lymphomas include bleomycin, doxorubicin, and total body irradiation followed by bone marrow transplantation.

The metastatic neurologic complications of lymphomas can also be effectively reversed by proper treatment. Long-term "cures" of the primary brain lymphomas may follow radiation therapy. Intraspinal lymphomas must be treated as an emergency with large doses of dexamethasone and appropriate dosage of radiation therapy to prevent a spinal cord catastrophe. Laminectomy is only rarely needed unless the diagnosis of lymphoma has not previously been established.

Leptomeningeal metastases of lymphoma carry a worse prognosis because they usually accompany late and more widespread systemic disease (especially bone marrow invasion). Neurologic remissions may still be induced by craniospinal irradiation and intrathecal or intraventricular administration of methotrexate, thiotepa, or cytosine arabinoside.

Nonmetastatic neurologic complications of the lymphomas include syndromes discussed in other chapters (infections, and vascular, neuromuscular, oncologic diseases). They are mentioned briefly here because the clinician dealing with the lymphoma patient must always be alert to the need for accurate differentiation of metastatic from nonmetastatic causes of neurologic manifestations. Among the infections, herpes zoster occurs in about 20% of patients with Hodgkin lymphoma, less often in non-Hodgkin lymphomas. The zoster may be localized or generalized. Cryptococcal and listerial meningitis, fungal and toxoplasmic abscesses, and viral encephalitis (especially progressive multifocal leukoencephalopathy) occur with increased frequency in patients with systemic lymphoma.

The vascular syndromes include cerebral infarcts from intravascular coagulation, embolism from nonbacterial thrombotic endocarditis, and granulomatous angiitis. Hemorrhagic complications occur from thrombocytopenia, hepatic failure, or intravascular coagulation. A particular risk is that of spinal subdural hematoma that complicates lumbar puncture in lymphoma patients with a bleeding tendency. Paralysis of the cauda equina may result.

Metabolic causes of neurologic syndromes in lymphoma patients include hypoxic, hypoglycemic, hepatic and uremic encephalopathies, and Wernicke encephalopathy in the setting of malnutrition. The remote neurologic effects of lymphoma are rare, but may present widely diverse manifestations: polymyositis, Eaton-Lambert syndrome, Guillain-

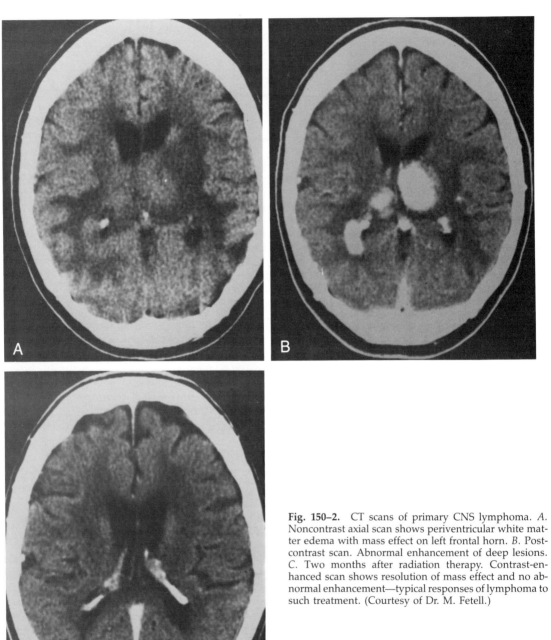

Fig. 150–2. CT scans of primary CNS lymphoma. *A.* Noncontrast axial scan shows periventricular white matter edema with mass effect on left frontal horn. *B.* Postcontrast scan. Abnormal enhancement of deep lesions. *C.* Two months after radiation therapy. Contrast-enhanced scan shows resolution of mass effect and no abnormal enhancement—typical responses of lymphoma to such treatment. (Courtesy of Dr. M. Fetell.)

Barré syndrome, peripheral neuropathies, radiculopathies, subacute necrotic myelopathy, subacute motor neuronopathy, subacute cerebellar degeneration, and dementia.

Neurologic complications of therapy for lymphoma include radiation injury to the nervous system (especially radiation myelopathy), radiation injury to carotid arteries in the neck, radiation-methotrexate damage to the brain, corticosteroid psychosis or myopathy, toxic neuropathies of chemotherapy, especially vincristine, and thrombocytopenic bleeding tendencies in bone marrow suppressed from chemotherapy and irradiation.

Leukemia

Malignancies of the white blood cells include acute lymphocytic, acute nonlymphocytic (e.g., granulocytic, myelogenous or myelocyctic, and monocytic), chronic lymphocytic, and chronic granulocytic leukemias. There are efforts to subclassify the disorders according to chromosomal or surface markers. Neurologic manifestations in the acute leukemias are common and are of the metastatic or nonmetastatic varieties. In the chronic leukemias, the nervous system is involved less commonly, mainly by nonmetastatic complications, especially infection.

Metastatic involvement is typified by meningeal leukemia, the principal cause of relapse after remissions were induced by systemic therapy alone in acute lymphocytic leukemia of childhood and acute nonlymphocytic leukemia of children and young adults. Other metastatic syndromes include cranial and spinal neuropathies (often a part of meningeal disease), epidural compression of the spinal cord, and hypothalamic invasion. Only rarely are other regions of the brain or spinal cord invaded, usually by microscopic infiltrates that are not large enough to produce focal neurologic signs.

Small or large hemorrhages in the brain may occur in blastic crises, especially when the peripheral white blood cell count is over 300,000/mm³. In this setting, white blood cells lodge in small vessels ("leukostasis"), damage the walls, and lead to hemorrhage, which is frequently fatal. Hemorrhages may also result from meningeal leukemia as it compresses and damages blood vessels deep in the sulci of the brain.

Incidence. Pathologic reports indicate that the meninges or parenchyma of the nervous system are invaded by leukemic infiltrations in more than 65% of patients with acute leukemia. Although there are no clinical signs of nervous system disease in many of these patients, symptomatic involvement of the nervous system increased during the years when systemic acute leukemia began to respond to chemotherapy. Reasons cited include increased longevity and sequestration of leukemic cells in the nervous system where they are protected by the blood-brain barrier from systemic antileukemic drugs. Symptomatic meningeal leukemia developed in 50 to 70% of patients with systemically treated acute lymphocytic leukemia in the years before prophylactic or "presymptomatic" therapy of the CNS became standard.

Symptoms and Signs. Meningeal leukemia may be asymptomatic, detectable only by a diagnostic spinal puncture. More often it presents with headache, vomiting, seizures, visual disturbances, papilledema, cranial or spinal nerve deficits, and signs of meningeal irritation. Focal signs of cerebral damage are infrequent except for hypothalamic syndromes, such as diabetes insipidus. Separation of the sutures is common in infants and young children. Isolated cranial or spinal nerve palsies without diffuse meningeal syndromes and paraplegia from spinal epidural leukemic masses may also be seen.

Laboratory Signs. The findings in the blood are those associated with leukemia. With infiltration of the meninges the CSF pressure rises. The protein content of the fluid increases and there is a pleocytosis in the fluid. The cells are sometimes normal lymphocytes or polymorphonuclear leukocytes, but leukemic cells are usually present by millipore or cytocentrifuge techniques. The CSF sugar content may be moderately or greatly reduced. CT may show hydrocephalus or subarachnoid enhancement in meningeal leukemia. Intracerebral hemorrhages are readily visualized.

Treatment and Prognosis. Before the advent of modern therapy, acute leukemia was uniformly fatal within a few months. Remission can now be induced in more than 90% of patients with acute lymphocytic leukemia. This induction therapy usually consists of prednisone and vincristine, but asparaginase is sometimes added. Because meningeal leukemia intervened so frequently while there was systemic (bone marrow) remission, it has become standard practice to follow induction therapy with prophylactic treatment of the CNS. Various protocols are being compared, including craniospinal irradiation plus intrathecal or intraventricular chemotherapy, irradiation plus intravenous chemotherapy, and intrathecal or intraventicular chemotherapy without irradiation. Methotrexate is the drug chosen most often for injection into the CSF, but drugs employed intravenously include methotrexate, mercaptopurine, cytosine arabinosde, thioguanine, vincristine, and asparaginase. Intermittent maintenance therapy is required to prevent bone marrow or nervous system relapse.

Symptomatic meningeal leukemia can often be cleared by craniospinal irradiation plus intrathecal or intraventricular administration of methotrexate. With these forms of vigorous treatment and meticulous supportive care, many patients have been apparently cured of acute lymphocytic leukemia. They have remained free of disease for a few years off treatment after 3 or 4 years of maintenance therapy.

The outlook for acute nonlymphocytic leukemia is less favorable. Remissions can be induced with cytosine arabinoside plus daunorubicin or doxorubicin, often with another drug such as mercaptopurine or thioguanine, and sometimes with adjuvants such as immunotherapy. The incidence of meningeal leukemia is lower in these patients than in those with acute lymphocytic leukemia, but some centers are exploring the use of prophylactic treatment of the nervous system for nonlymphocytic disease. Meningeal nonlymphocytic leukemia is treated with intrathecal methotrexate or cytosine arabinoside, with or without craniospinal irradiation.

Nonmetastatic neurologic complications of leukemia were well-known before the modern era of therapy. Large or small hemorrhages may be found in the brain due to the bleeding tendency associated with thrombocytopenia. Many of the nonmetastatic neurologic complications described in the section on the lymphomas are also encountered in leukemic patients. Progressive multifocal leukoencephalopathy occurs in a few patients with either acute or chronic leukemia. Leukemia patients are particularly susceptible to infections with cryptococci and other fungi.

Soon after the introduction of prophylactic cranial radiation for acute lymphocytic leukemia, patients were encountered who developed lethargy, confusion, behavioral changes, seizures, dysarthria, ataxia, spasticity, and sometimes coma. When their brains were examined, there were usually no signs of leukemia. Instead, the pathologic findings sometimes were those of a leukoencephalopathy (i.e., demyelination and astrogliosis) in the frontal and parietal lobes. In other instances, a microangiopathy with calcification and micronecrosis was found in the lenticular nuclei and cerebral cortex. The calcification can be detected in these locations by CT. There is general agreement that both the leukoencephalopathy and the microangiopathy are associated with therapy for the leukemia. Most authors consider that irradiation alone, especially in larger doses, is a major cause, but the offending roles of large-dose intravenous methotrexate, chemotherapy delivered directly to the nervous system, duration of therapy, and the presence of episodic CNS leukemia are still being evaluated. These nonmetastatic complications are a major reason why many protocols have been employed and compared for use in acute leukemia, including attempts to avoid prophylactic cranial irradiation.

Multiple Myeloma

This disorder of older adults is a disseminated malignancy of plasma cells or their anaplastic precursors in the B-cell line. Proliferation of the malignant cells leads to widespread bone destruction, bone marrow failure, production of large amounts of an abnormal monoclonal immunoglobulin (paraprotein, M component), and decreased production of normal immunoglobulins. Signs and symptoms include bone pain, weakness, cachexia, and bleeding tendency. Secondary manifestations are susceptibility to infections and clinical results of hypercalcemia and renal failure. Amyloidosis (in 15% of patients), macroglobulinemia, hyperviscosity, and cryoglobulinemia may accompany multiple myeloma. Anemia and marked elevation of the erythrocyte sedimentation rate are characteristic.

Neurologic disorders are seen in 30 to 40% of patients with multiple myeloma. As is true with the lymphomas and leukemias, the neurologic complications may be metastatic or nonmetastatic. Characteristic syndromes include compression of spinal cord, spinal roots, cauda equina, cranial nerves, or (rarely) brain by myelomatous masses arising from adjacent bone. The cord may also be compromised by a pathologic vertebral fracture (Fig. 150–3). The overall incidence of cord compression in multiple myeloma is 5 to 15%. Clinical syndromes occasionally result from infiltration of the meninges or brain by my-

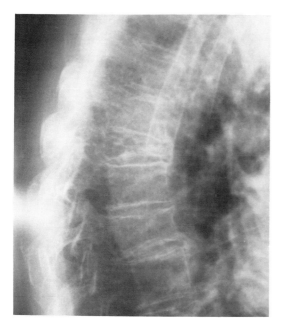

Fig. 150–3. Multiple myeloma. Diffuse osteopenia, complete collapse of a midthoracic vertebra, and anterior wedging of another, two levels below. (Courtesy of Dr. Lowell G. Lubic.)

eloma cells. The peripheral nerves may be invaded focally or diffusely.

The nonmetastatic neurologic complications of multiple myeloma are similar to the neurologic complications of lymphomas, but a few bear special attention here. Hypercalcemia encephalopathy and uremic neurologic disorders are common. The hyperviscosity syndrome is described under macroglobulinemia. Amyloidosis in multiple myeloma may lead to spinal cord compression by extradural amyloid masses or infiltrative neuropathies (Gasserian ganglion syndrome, carpal tunnel syndrome, diffuse polyneuropathies). A solitary myeloma (plasmacytoma) of bone is often accompanied by paraproteinemia and may lead to a polyneuropathy as a remote effect. Patients with the rare osteosclerotic variant of multiple myeloma are particularly prone to develop nonmetastatic polyneuropathy.

Diagnosis. Characteristic multiple osteolytic lesions are seen on radiographs of the skull and other bones (Fig. 150–4). Bone marrow aspiration or biopsy of a skeletal lesion reveals the sheets of plasma cells; paraprotein may be detected by electrophoretic analysis of blood. The abnormal proteins may also be detected in urine (Bence Jones protein) and CSF.

When the leptomeninges are invaded, myeloma cells may be found in the CSF.

Treatment. Compressive lesions are excised and irradiated. For systemic diseases, chemotherapy (usually melphalan or cyclophosphamide, often with prednisone) has been effective. Plasmapheresis is effective for the hyperviscosity syndrome. Supportive care and treatment for infection, hypercalcemia, and renal failure must be included. Before the availability of chemotherapy, survival in multiple myeloma varied from 6 to 18 months after onset. Current therapy has prolonged the median survival several-fold.

Macroglobulinemia and Monoclonal Gammopathy

In 1944, Waldenström described a disease of unknown cause characterized by the presence in the serum of globulins of enormous molecular size. Since the original report, several hundred cases have been reported, usually in older adults. It is now recognized as a plasma cell (B-cell) dyscrasia leading to accumulation in the serum of a high-molecular-weight IgM paraprotein. In addition to the large globulins, there are relative lymphocytosis, thrombocytopenia, splenomegaly, and lymphoid hyperplasia. The symptoms include weakness and weight loss, and those associated with hemorrhage into skin or viscera. The neurologic complications include hemorrhagic and ischemic lesions, collections of lymphocytes and plasma cells in the CNS, and polyneuropathy. A useful screening procedure for macroglobulinemia is the Sia test, in which a white flocculus results when one drop of macroglobulinemic serum is added to a test tube of distilled water.

Serum hyperviscosity is a common result of the macroglobulinemia and presents mainly with neurologic manifestations. Sludging of the microcirculation leads to headache, vertigo, tinnitus, poor hearing, nystagmus, blurred vision, retinopathy, seizures, confusion, delirium, and minor focal signs. Sausage-shaped veins, resulting from a series of local beadings and intervening marked dilatations, accompanied by numerous flame hemorrhages and exudates, constitute a characteristic funduscopic appearance. Plasmapheresis is essential to reduce the viscosity of the circulating blood and may remove antibodies against myelin-associated glycoprotein. Some patients with macroglobulinemia run a quite benign course. Neurologic manifestations usually indicate a more serious disorder and call for treatment, which

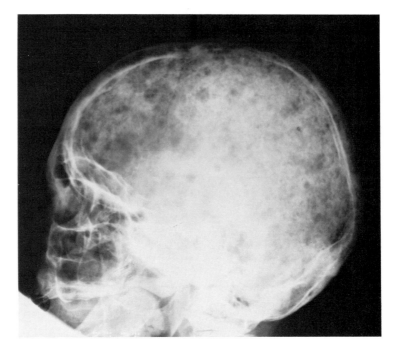

Fig. 150–4. Multiple myeloma. Myriads of osteolytic lesions. (Courtesy of Dr. Lowell G. Lubic.)

is usually accomplished with chlorambucil and prednisone.

Monoclonal Gammopathies

Persons who have an M component (a monoclonal immunoglobulin) in the serum but lack evidence of multiple myeloma or macroglobulinemia are said to have monoclonal gammopathy of unknown significance (formerly known as benign monoclonal gammopathy). Some of these patients go on to develop multiple myeloma or macroglobulinemia, but most do not. Even with low serum levels of immunoglobulins these patients may develop nonmetastatic complications including neuropathies, some mimicking motor neuron disease, and other paraneoplastic syndromes. The role of the M component in pathogenesis is still not clear. Although immunoglobulin binding to nerve and myelin components can be demonstrated, a cause and effect relationship between the immunoglobulin and the neuropathy has not been proven.

Chediak-Higashi Disease

Chediak-Higashi disease is a rare autosomal recessive disease with onset usually in early childhood. Giant peroxidase-positive cytoplasmic granules occur in leukocytes. Disseminated focal infiltrations by lymphocytes and large mononuclears with similar inclusions may be present in many organs including the peripheral nerves. Cytoplasmic inclusions resembling lysosomes and lipofuscin have been found in neurons of the central and peripheral nervous systems. Manifestations include albinism, photophobia, generalized lymphadenopahy, hepatosplenomegaly, fever, and susceptibility to infection. Decreased activity of the "natural killer" subset of T-cells has been documented. Cranial and peripheral polyneuropathy, nystagmus, and ataxia may develop. Anemia, leukopenia, and thrombocytopenia are frequently noted. The diagnosis is readily made by recognition of the giant cytoplasmic granules in leukocytes on Wright's or peroxidase stain. The administration of prednisone and vincristine has been reported to be of value in the acute phases. Death usually occurs in childhood as a result of recurrent pyogenic infections or the development of an accelerated phase resembling lymphoma.

Thrombotic Thrombocytopenic Purpura

Thrombotic thrombocytopenic purpura is a rare disorder of unknown etiology in which three pathogenetic mechanisms have been identified: (1) occlusion of small arteries, arterioles, and capillaries by amorphous hyaline material (Fig. 150–5) of fibrin-platelet origin, especially in the heart, kidney, and brain; (2) microangiopathic hemolytic anemia due to an extracorpuscular mechanism and associated with increased mechanical and osmotic fragility of the red blood cells; and (3) thrombocytopenia. In a few cases, pathologic features have suggested a relationship to lupus erythematosus or polyarteritis nodosa.

The disease is usually acute, lasting from a few days to several months. The hematologic abnormalities give rise to pallor, hematuria, purpura, and jaundice. In nearly all patients, there are cerebral symptoms, fever, abdominal pain, nausea, vomiting, arthralgias, and signs of renal involvement.

The cerebral symptoms in order of frequency are: mental confusion progressing to coma; seizures, usually generalized but occasionally focal; aphasia; hemiplegia; and papilledema. The focal neurologic signs are likely to be transient, lasting only for hours or a few days. Within days or weeks, similar or other symptoms may occur.

Diagnosis is based upon the triad of microangiopathic hemolytic anemia, thrombocytopenia, and cerebral symptoms and signs. The platelet count is almost always decreased, but may be normal in the interval between attacks. Typical lesions are found on gingival biopsy in about 50% of patients. This disorder must be differentiated from the symptomatic

hemolytic anemias of malignancy, leukemias, lymphomas, bacteremia, lupus erythematosus, and disseminated intravascular coagulation. Clinical features and appropriate laboratory studies usually identify these conditions.

In the past, most patients ran a brief course terminating in death. Although there is no general agreement as to optimum therapy, complete remissions have been induced with standard and high-dose corticosteroid therapy, vincristine, splenectomy, antiplatelet agents (e.g., aspirin, dipyridamole, average-molecular-weight dextran), exchange transfusions, plasma transfusions, and plasmapheresis. Relapses often respond to additional therapy. Prompt improvement without neurologic residual has occurred even in comatose patients.

Multifocal Eosinophilic Granuloma

Histiocytosis X is the term proposed by Lichtenstein to include eosinophilic granuloma of bone, Hand-Schüller-Christian disease, and Letterer-Siwe disease. There has been an increasing tendency since then to separate the disorders. Solitary and multifocal eosinophilic granulomas are recognized as a nonneoplastic reaction of well-differentiated his-

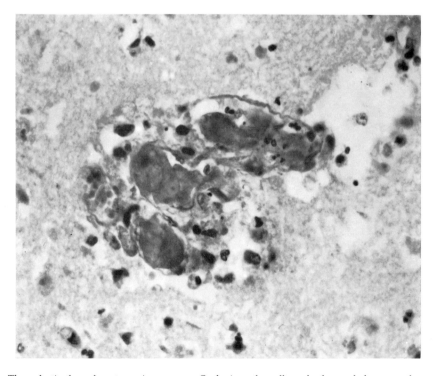

Fig. 150–5. Thrombotic thrombocytopenic purpura. Occlusion of small cerebral vessels by amorphous hyaline material. (Courtesy of Dr. Abner Wolf.)

tiocytes, whereas Letterer-Siwe disease is a malignant disorder of infancy characterized by lymphomatous proliferation of poorly differentiated histiocytes. This discussion focuses on multifocal eosinophilic granulomas.

Pathology and Pathogenesis. The cause of the disease is unknown. An infectious agent has been suggested as the most likely cause, with some evidence for an immune disorder. The essential feature of the pathologic changes is the presence of focal or widespread chronic inflammatory granulomas in the involved organs. The microscopic pathology consists of proliferation of histiocytic cells of the Langerhans type with an associated proliferation of fibroblasts and an infiltration of lymphocytes, eosinophlic leukocytes, and mature plasma cells. The presence in Langerhans histiocytes of an antigen that cross-reacts with S-100, the glial protein, has been useful in histopathologic differential diagnosis. In the chronic stages of the disease large collections of foamy macrophages containing cholesterol are conspicuous within the granulation tissue. These lipid-laden macrophages represent a secondary effect of the destructive process and not a primary storage of lipid.

Incidence. The disease is rare. There is no evidence that it is inherited, but familial occurrence has been reported. Generally, it first appears in childhood or adolescence; solitary eosinophlic granuloma of bone usually becomes symptomatic in young adult life.

Symptoms and Signs. The signs and symptoms of the disease depend on the location of the granulomas (Table 150–1). A solitary focus in one of the long bones produces a painful bony swelling (eosinophilic granulomas of bone). When the histiocytic lesions are localized in the membranous bones, defects in the skull (Fig. 150–6), exophthalmos, and diabetes insipidus are the principal features of the disease. Periodic malaise, fever, adenopathy, respiratory infections, hepatosplenomegaly, and skin lesions are seen. Involvement of the alveolar process may cause loss of teeth. Spontaneous pneumothorax has been reported with the development of granulomas in the lungs.

Neurologic signs may be produced by nodular infiltration of the dura with extension to the underlying brain or by the development of histiocytic granulomas within the substance of the nervous system. Granulomas within the hypothalamus and third ventricle may result in retardation of growth, diabetes insipidus, and organic dementia. Pyramidal tract signs, cranial nerve palsies, and cerebellar ataxia may be present and may be related to corresponding lesions in the base of the skull, cerebellum, and brain stem. Increased intracranial pressure and hydrocephalus may result from granulomas and chronic inflammatory changes in the dural sinuses, ventricular cavities, and subarachnoid cisterns. Lesions of the spinal cord and cauda equina are rare. Several patients have had only involvement of the nervous system with no evidence of visceral or skeletal lesions.

Laboratory Data. A mild or moderate degree of anemia may occur. The CSF may be normal or show an elevated protein content and increased cells, usually lymphocytes.

Diagnosis. Little difficulty is encountered when visceral and skeletal lesions are present. Radiographs of the skull and other bones, radionuclide scans of the skeleton, and biopsy of the liver, spleen, or lymph nodes are usually sufficient to establish the diagnosis. CT has demonstrated lesions in the hypothalamus and cerebellum. Surgical biopsy may be necessary in cases showing only involvement of the nervous system.

Course. The course of the disease, when untreated, is variable but progressive. Remissions may occur.

Treatment. Lesions of the bone respond to radiation therapy or surgical curettage. Corticosteroids, nitrogen mustard, methotrexate and the vinca alkaloids have been used with caution for systemic disease. Focal lesions of the nervous system have been treated with

Table 150–1. The Frequency of Clinical Manifestations in 180 Cases of Multifocal Eosinophilic Granuloma

	No. of Cases	%
Skeletal lesions	147	81
Diabetes insipidus	102	56
Exophthalmos	89	49
Growth retardation	54	30
Skin	45	25
Gingivitis	42	23
Adenopathy	32	18
Otitis media	28	15
Splenomegaly	27	15
Pulmonary infiltration	26	15
Hepatomegaly	26	15
Anemia	22	12

(Modified from Avioli LV, Lasersohn JT, Lopresti JM. Medicine 1963; 42:119–147.)

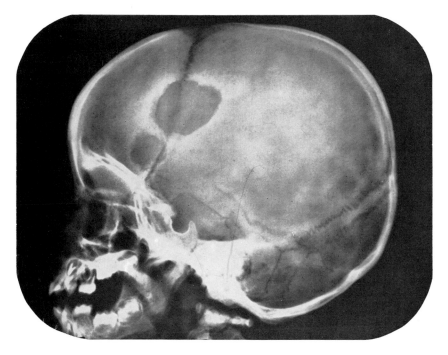

Fig. 150–6. Eosinophilic granuloma. Multiple lytic lesions in skull. (Courtesy of Dr. Juan Taveras.)

low dosage irradiation. Diabetes insipidus and septicemia are treated by standard techniques.

Coagulation Disorders

This section groups several rare disorders that mainly have non-neurologic manifestations.

PAROXYSMAL NOCTURNAL HEMOGLOBINURIA

This disorder of the bone-marrow stem cell is characterized by episodes of hemolytic anemia and thrombosis, mainly in the venous system. Sagittal sinus and other intracranial venous thromboses occur.

HEPARIN-INDUCED THROMBOCYTOPENIA WITH THROMBOSIS

Thrombocytopenia during heparin therapy is thought to result from heparin-dependent antibodies that cause platelet aggregation, platelet thrombus formation, and clearance of platelets from the circulation. Both arterial and venous thromboses occur, usually after several days of heparin therapy. Because the amount of heparin given is not important, the disorder has been seen with both subcutaneous heparin and flushing of intravenous lines with heparin solutions. Ceasing heparin adminstration leads to rapid correction of the thrombocytopenia.

ANTITHROMBIN III DEFICIENCY

Antithrombin III is the primary physiologic antagonist of thrombin and other activated clotting factors. Homozygous deficiency has not been described and may be lethal in the prenatal period. Heterozygotes have reduced levels of antithrombin III. The most common clinical feature is recurrent venous thrombosis, although thrombotic events may occur at other sites. Patients may show "heparin resistance" because heparin cannot function normally without antithrombin III. Occasionally, low levels of antithrombin III are seen in the nephrotic syndrome or liver disease and may contribute to the hypercoagulable states seen in those conditions.

PROTEIN C DEFICIENCY

Protein C is a vitamin K-dependent factor that dampens hemostatic reactions. A homozygous deficiency leads to extensive thromboses and death during the neonatal period. Heterozygotes have recurrent venous thromboses. A rare complication of warfarin therapy, coumarin skin necrosis, has been associated with protein C deficiency. Presumably the cause is rapid decrease in the level of protein C before other vitamin K-dependent coagulation factors are affected.

References

Sickle Cell Anemia

Dean J, Schechter AN. Sickle-cell anemia: Molecular and cellular bases of therapeutic approaches. N Engl J Med 1978; 299:752–763, 804–811, 863–870.

Goossens M, Dumez Y, Kaplan L, et al. Prenatal diagnosis of sickle-cell anemia in the first trimester of pregnancy. N Engl J Med 1983; 309:831–833.

Greer M, Schotland D. Abnormal hemoglobin as a cause of neurologic disease. Neurology 1962; 12:114–123.

Haruda F, Friedman JH, Ganti SR, Hoffman N, Chutorian AM. Rapid resolution of organic mental syndrome in sickle cell anemia in response to exchange transfusion. Neurology 1981; 31:1015–1016.

Konotey-Ahulu FID. The sickle cell diseases: Clinical manifestations including the sickle crisis. Arch Intern Med 1974; 133:611–619.

Nagel RL, Chang H. The status of the development of antisickling agents. In: Fried W, ed. Comparative Clinical Aspects of Sickle Cell Disease. New York: Elsevier-North Holland, 1982:163–170.

Pavlakis SG, Bello J, Prohovnik I et al. Brain infarction in sickle cell anemia: magnetic resonance imaging correlates. Ann Neurol 1988; 23:125–131.

Powars D, Wilson B, Imbus C, Pegelow C, Allen J. The natural history of stroke in sickle cell disease. Am J Med 1978; 65:461–471.

Rothman SM, Fulling KH, Nelson J. Sickle cell anemia and central nervous system infarction: A neuropathological study. Ann Neurol 1986; 20:684–690.

Rowland LP. Neurological manifestations in sickle cell disease. J Nerv Ment Dis 1952; 115:456–457.

Stockman JA, Nigro MA, Mishkin MM, Oski FA. Occlusion of large cerebral vessels in sickle-cell anemia. N Engl J Med 1972; 287:846–849.

Wilimas J, Goff JR, Anderson HR Jr, Langston JW, Thompson E. Efficacy of transfusion therapy for one to two years in patients with sickle cell disease and cerebrovascular accidents. J Pediatr 1980; 96:205–208.

Polycythemia Vera

Berk PD, Goldberg JD, Silverstein MN, et al. Increased incidence of acute leukemia in polycythemia vera associated with chlorambucil therapy. N Engl J Med 1981; 304:441–447.

Christian HA. The nervous symptoms of polycythemia vera. Am J Med Sci 1917; 154:547–554.

Golde DW. Polycythemia: Mechanisms and management. Ann Intern Med 1981: 95:71–87.

Loman J, Dameshek W. Plethora of intracranial venous circulation in case of polycythemia. N Engl J Med 1945; 232:394–397.

Millikan CH, Siekert RF, Whisnant JP. Intermittent carotid and vertebral-basilar insufficiency associated with polycythemia. Neurology 1960; 10:188–196.

Pearson TC, Wetherly-Mein G. Vascular occlusive episodes and venous hematocrit in primary proliferative polycythemia. Lancet 1978; 2:1219–1222.

Reed RE. Polycythemia vera and agnogenic myeloid metaplasia. Med Clin North Am 1980; 64:667–681.

Rice GP, Assis LJ, Barr RM, Ebers GC. Extramedullary hematopoiesis and spinal cord compression complicating polycythemia rubra vera. Ann Neurol 1980; 7:81–84.

Silverstein A, Gilbert H, Wasserman LR. Neurologic complications of polycythemia. Ann Intern Med 1962; 57:909–916.

Stahl SM, Ellinger G, Baringer JR. Progressive myelopathy due to extramedullary hematopoiesis: Case report and review of the literature. Ann Neurol 1979; 5:485–489.

Yiannikas C, McLeod JG, Walsh JC. Peripheral neuropathy associated with polycythemia vera. Neurology 1983; 33:139–143.

Essential Thrombocythemia

Hehlmann R, Jahn M, Baumann B, Kopcke W. Essential thrombocythemia; 61 cases. Cancer 1988; 61: 2487–2496.

Iob I, Scanarini M, Andrioli GC, Pardatscher K. Thrombosis of the superior sagittal sinus associated with idiopathic thrombocytosis. Surg Neurol 1979; 11:439–441.

Jabaily J, Iland HJ, Laszlo J, et al. Neurologic manifestations of essential thrombocythemia. Ann Intern Med 1983; 99:513–518.

Jamshidi K, Ansari A, Windschitl HE, Swaim WR. Primary thrombocythemia. Geriatrics 1973; 28:121–133.

Levine J, Swanson PD. Idiopathic thrombocytosis: A treatable cause of transient ischemic attacks. Neurology 1968; 18:711–713.

Mundall J, Quintero P, von Kaulla KN, Harmon R, Austin J. Transient monocular blindness and increased platelet aggregability treated with aspirin. Neurology 1972; 22:280–285.

Ozer FL, Truax WE, Miesch DC, Levin WC. Primary hemorrhagic thrombocythemia. Am J Med 1960; 28:807–823.

Preston FE, Martin JF, Stewart RM, Davies-Jones GAB. Thrombocytosis, circulating platelet aggregates and neurological dysfunction. Br Med J 1979; 2: 1561–1563.

Hypereosinophilic Syndrome

Monaco S, Lucci B, Laperchia N, et al. Polyneuropathy in hypereosinophilic syndrome. Neurology 1988; 38:494–496.

Moore PM, Haley JD. Fauci AS. Neurologic dysfunction in the idiopathic hypereosinophilic syndrome. Ann Intern Med 1985; 102:109–114.

Lymphomas

Aisenberg AC. Cell lineage in lympho-proliferative disease. Am J Med 1983; 74:679–685.

Ascherl GF Jr, Hilal SK, Brisman R. Computed tomography of disseminated meningeal and ependymal malignant neoplasms. Neurology 1981; 31:567–574.

Brazis PW, Biller J, Fine M, Palacios E, Pagano RJ. Cerebellar degeneration with Hodgkin's disease: Computed tomographic correlation and literature review. Arch Neurol 1981; 38:253–256.

Cabanillas F, Burgess MA, Bodey GP, Freireich EJ. Sequential chemotherapy and late intensification for malignant lymphomas of aggressive histologic type. Am J Med 1983; 74:382–388.

Cairncross JG, Posner JB. Neurological complications of malignant lymphoma. In: Vinken PJ, Bruyn GW, Klawans HL, eds. Handbook of Clinical Neurology (vol 39). New York: Elsevier-North Holland, 1980:27–62.

Collins RC, Al-Mondhiry H, Chernik NL, Posner JB. Neurologic manifestations of intravascular coagulation in patients with cancer. Neurology 1975; 25:795–806.

DeReuck JL, Sieben GJ, Sieben-Praet MR, Ngendahayo P, DeCoster WJ, Vander Eecken HM. Wernicke's encephalopathy in patients with tumors of the lymphoid-hemopoietic systems. Arch Neurol 1980; 37:338–341.

Dujovny M, McBride D, Segal R. Intracranial manifestations of Hodgkin's disease. Surg Neurol 1980; 13:258–265.

Ernerudh J, Olsson T, Berlin G, Gustafsson B, Karlsson H. Cell surface markers for diagnosis of central nervous system involvement in lymphoproliferative diseases. Ann Neurol 1986; 20:610–615.

Greenberg HS, Kim J-H, Posner JB. Epidural spinal cord compression from metastatic tumor: Results with a new treatment protocol. Ann Neurol 1980; 8:361–366.

Hauch TW, Shelbourne JD, Cohen HJ, Mason D, Kremer WB. Meningeal mycosis fungoides: Clinical and cellular characteristics. Ann Intern Med 1975; 82:499–505.

Hautzer NW, Aiyesimojou A, Robertaille Y. Primary spinal intramedullary lymphomas. Ann Neurol 1983; 14:62–66.

Herman TS, Hammond N, Jones SE, Butler JJ, Byrne GE Jr, McKelvey EM. Involvement of the central nervous system by non-Hodgkin's lymphoma. Cancer 1979; 43:390–397.

Levitt JL, Dawson DM, Rosenthal DS, Moloney WC. CNS involvement in the non-Hodgkin's lymphomas. Cancer 1980; 45:545–552.

Litam JP, Cabanillas F, Smith TL, Bodey GP, Freirich EJ. Central nervous system relapse in malignant lymphomas: Risk factors and implications for prophylaxis. Blood 1979; 54:1249–1257.

Oken MM, Costello WG, Johnson GJ, et al. The influence of histologic subtype on toxicity and response to chemotherapy in non-Hodgkin's lymphoma. Cancer 1983; 51:1581–1586.

Patchell R, Perry MC. Eosinophilic meningitis in Hodgkin disease. Neurology 1981; 31:887–888.

Quinn JJ, Taylor CR, Swanson V, et al. Childhood leukemia and lymphoma: Correlation of clinical features with immunological and morphological studies. Med Pediatr Oncol 1979; 7:35–47.

Rajjoub RK, Wood JH, Ommaya AK. Granulomatous angiitis of the brain: A successfully treated case. Neurology 1977; 27:588–591.

Rodichok LD, Harper GR, Ruckdeschel JC, et al. Early diagnosis of spinal epidural metastases. Am J Med 1981; 70:1181–1188.

Rosenblum WI, Hadfield MG. Granulomatous angiitis of the nervous system in cases of herpes zoster and lymphosarcoma. Neurology 1972; 22:348–354.

Schaumburg HH, Plank CR, Adams RD. The reticulum cell sarcoma-microglioma group of brain tumours. Brain 1972; 95:199–212.

Schold SC, Cho E-C, Somasundaram M, Posner JB. Subacute motor neuronopathy: A remote effect of lymphoma. Ann Neurol 1979; 5:271–287.

Sheibani K, Battifora H, Winberg CD. Further evidence that "malignant angioendotheliomatosis" is an angiotropic large cell lymphoma. N Engl J Med 1986; 314:943–948.

Somasundaram M, Posner JB. Neurologic problems in patients with Hodgkin's disease. In: Lacher MJ, ed. Hodgkin's Disease. New York: John Wiley & Sons, 1976:325–370.

Weber MB, McGavran MH. Mycosis fungoides involving the brain. Arch Neurol 1967; 16:645–650.

Whitehouse JMA, Kay HE, eds. CNS Complications of Malignant Disease. Baltimore: University Park Press, 1979:113–156.

Young RC, Howser DM, Anderson T, Fisher RI, Jaffe E, DeVita VT Jr. Central nervous system complications of non-Hodgkin's lymphoma: The potential role for prophylactic therapy. Am J Med 1979; 66:435–443.

Leukemia

Baker RD. Leukopenia and therapy in leukemia as factors predisposing to fatal mycoses. Am J Clin Pathol 1962; 37:358–373.

Bleyer WA. Central nervous system leukemia. Pediat Clin No Am 1988; 35:789–814.

Bleyer WA, Poplack DG. Intraventricular versus intralumbar methotrexate for central-nervous-system leukemia: Prolonged remission with the Ommaya reservoir. Med Pediatr Oncol 1979; 6:207–213.

DeVivo DC, Malas D, Nelson JS, Land VJ. Leukoencephalopathy in childhood leukemia. Neurology 1977; 27:609–613.

Freireich EJ, Thomas LB, Frei E III, Fritz RD, Forkner CE Jr. A distinctive type of intracerebral hemorrhage associated with "blastic crisis" in patients with leukemia. Cancer 1960; 13:146–154.

Geiser CF, Bishop Y, Jaffe N, Furman L, Traggis D, Frei E. Adverse effects of intrathecal methotrexate in children with acute leukemia in remission. Blood 1975; 45; 189–195.

Inati A, Sallan SE, Cassady JR, et al. Efficacy and morbidity of CNS "prophylaxis" in childhood acute lymphoblastic leukemia: Eight years' experience with cranial irradiation and intrathecal methotrexate. Blood 1983; 61:297–303.

Kretzchmar K, Gutjahr P, Kutzner J. CT studies before and after CNS treatment for acute lymphoblastic leukemia and malignant non-Hodgkin's lymphoma in childhood. Neuroradiology 1980; 20:173–180.

Miller DR, Leikin S, Albo V, Sather H, Karon M, Hammond D. Prognostic factors and therapy in acute lymphoblastic leukemia of childhood: CCG-141. Cancer 1983; 51:1041–1049.

Ochs JJ, Berger P, Brecher ML, Sinks LF, Kinkel W, Freeman AI. Computed tomography brain scans in children with acute lymphocytic leukemia receiving methotrexate alone as central nervous system prophylaxis. Cancer 1980; 45:2274–2278.

Pochedly C. Neurologic manifestations in acute leukemia. NY State J Med 1975; 75:575–580, 715–721, 878–882.

Price RA, Birdwell DA. The central nervous system in childhood leukemia. III. Mineralizing microangiopathy and dystrophic calcification. Cancer 1978; 42:717–728.

Price RA, Johnson WW. The central nervous system in childhood leukemia. I. The arachnoid. Cancer 1973; 31:520–533; II. Subacute leukoencephalopathy. Cancer 1973; 35:306–318.

Shapiro WR, Young DF, Mehta BM. Methotrexate: Distribution in cerebrospinal fluid after intravenous, ventricular and lumbar injections. N Engl J Med 1975; 293:161–166.

Sibley WA, Weisberger AS. Demyelinating disease of the brain in chronic lymphatic leukemia. Arch Neurol 1961; 5:300–307.

Whitehouse JMA, Kay HE, eds. CNS Complications of Malignant Disease. Baltimore: University Park Press, 1979:3–109.

Williams HM, Diamond HD, Craver LF. The pathogenesis and management of neurological complications in patients with malignant lymphomas and leukemia. Cancer 1958; 11:76–82.

Multiple Myeloma

Abramsky O. Neurologic manifestation of cryoglobulinemia. In: Vinken PJ, Bruyn GW, Klawans HL. Handbook of Clinical Neurology (vol 38). New York: Elsevier-North Holland, 1980; 181–188.

Bardick PA, Zvaifler NJ, Gill GN, Newman D, Greenway GD, Resnick DL. Plasma cell dyscrasia with polyneuropathy, organomegaly, endocrinopathy, M protein, and skin changes: The POEMS syndrome. Medicine 1980; 59:311–322.

Benson WJ, Scarffe JH, Todd IDH, Crowther D. Spinal cord compression in myeloma. In: Whitehouse JMA, Kay HEM, eds. CNS Complications of Malignant Disease. Baltimore: University Park Press, 1979; 159–172.

Dalakas MC, Engel WK. Polyneuropathy with monoclonal gammopathy: Studies of 11 patients. Ann Neurol 1981; 10:45–52.

Kelly JJ Jr, Kyle RA, Latov N, Eds. Polyneuropathies and Plasma Cell Dyscrasias. Martinus Nijhol, Boston, 1987.

Kelly JJ Jr, Kyle RA, Miles JM, Dyck PJ. Osteosclerotic myeloma and peripheral neuropathy. Neurology 1983; 33:202–210.

Kyle RA. Multiple myeloma: Review of 869 cases. Mayo Clin Proc 1975; 50:29–40.

Nemni R, Galassi G, Latov N, Sherman WH, Olarte MR, Hays AP. Polyneuropathy in nonmalignant IgM plasma cell dyscrasia: A morphological study. Ann Neurol 1983; 14:43–54.

Paredes JM, Mitchell BS. Multiple myeloma: Current concepts in diagnosis and management. Med Clin North Am 1980; 64:729–742.

Pruzanski W, Russell ML. Serum viscosity and hyperviscosity syndrome in IgG multiple myeloma: The relationship to Sia test and to concentration of M component. Am J Med Sci 1976; 271:145–150.

Reitan JB, Pape E, Fosså SD, Julsrud O-J, Slettnes ON, Solheim ØP. Osteosclerotic myeloma with polyneuropathy. Acta Med Scand 1980: 208:137–144.

Spaar FW. Paraproteinaemias and multiple myeloma. In: Vinken PJ, Bruyn GW, Klawans HL, eds. Handbook of Clinical Neurology (vol 39). New York: Elsevier-North Holland, 1980:131–179.

Spiers ASD, Halpern R, Ross SC, Neiman RS, Harawi S, Zipoli TE. Meningeal myelomatosis. Arch Intern Med 1980; 140:256–259.

Trotter JL, Engel WK, Ignaczak TF. Amyloidosis with plasma cell dyscrasia: An overlooked cause of adult onset sensorimotor neuropathy. Arch Neurol 1977; 34:209–214.

Victor M, Banker BQ, Adams RD. The neuropathy of multiple myeloma. J Neurol Neurosurg Psychiatry 1958; 21:73–88.

Macroglobulinemia and Monoclonal Gammopathy

Abramsky O. Neurologic manifestations of macroglobulinemia. In: Vinken PJ, Bruyn GW, Klawans HL, eds. Handbook of Clinical Neurology (vol 39). New York: Elsevier-North Holland, 1980:188–199.

Bajada S, Mastaglia FL, Fisher A. Amyloid neuropathy and tremor in Waldenström's macroglobulinemia. Arch Neurol 1980; 37:240–242.

Dalakas MC, Flaum MA, Rick M, Engel WK, Gralnick HR. Treatment of polyneuropathy in Waldenström's macroglobulinemia: Role of paraproteinemia and immunologic studies. Neurology 1983; 33:1406–1410.

Edgar R, Dutcher TF. Histopathology of the Bing-Neel syndrome. Neurology 1961; 11:239–245.

Fahey JL, Barth WF, Solomon A. Serum hyperviscosity syndrome. JAMA 1965; 192:464–467.

Kelly JJ, Adelman LS, Berkman E, Bahn I. Polyneuropathies and IgM monoclonal gammopathies. Arch Neurol 1988; 45:1355–1360.

Latov N, Hays AP, Sherman. Peripheral neuropathy and anti-MAG antibodies. CRC Crit Rev Neurobiol 1988; 3:301–332.

Latov N, Hays AP, Donofrio PD, et al. Monoclonal IgM with unique specificity to gangliosides GM1 and GD1b and to lacto-N-tetraose associated with human motor neuron disease. Neurology 1988; 38:763–768.

Mackenzie MR, Lee TK. Blood viscosity in Waldenström macroglobulinemia. Blood 1977; 49:507–510.

Pestronk A, Cornblath DR, Ilyas AA et al. A treatable chronic multifocal motor polyneuropathy with antibodies to a defined neural antigen. Ann Neurol 1988; 24:73–78.

Shy ME, Rowland LP, Smith TS, et al. Motor neuron disease and plasma cell dyscrasia. Neurology 1986; 36:1429–1436.

Smith BR, Robert NJ, Ault KA. In Waldenström's macroglobulinemia the quantity of detectable circulating monoclonal B lymphocytes correlates with clinical course. Blood 1983; 61:911–914.

Chediak-Higashi Syndrome

Blume RS, Wolff SM. The Chediak-Higashi syndrome: Studies in four patients and a review of the literature. Medicine 1972; 51:247–280.

Creel D, Boxer LA, Fauci AS. Visual and auditory anomalies in Chediak-Higashi syndrome. Electroencephalogr Clin Neurophysiol 1983; 55:252–257.

Gallin JI, Elin RJ, Hubert RT, Fauci AS, Kaliner MA, Wolff SM. Efficacy of ascorbic acid in Chediak-Higashi syndrome (CHS): Studies in humans and mice. Blood 1979; 53:226–234.

Higashi O. Congenital gigantism of peroxidase granules: First case ever reported of qualitative abnormality of peroxidase. Tohoku J Exp Med 1954; 59:315–332.

Lockman LA, Kennedy WR, White JG. The Chediak-Higashi syndrome: Electrophysiological and electron microscopic observation on the peripheral neuropathy. J Pediatr 1967; 70:942–951.

Pezeshkpour G, Kurent JS, Krarup C, et al. Peripheral neuropathy in the Chediak-Higashi syndrome (abstract). J Neuropathol Exp Neurol 1986; 45:353.

Roder JC, Todd RF, Rubin P, et al. The Chediak-Higashi gene in humans. III. Studies on the mechanisms of NK impairment. Clin Exp Immunol 1983; 51:359–368.

Sheramata W, Kott HS, Cyr DP. The Chediak-Higashi-Steinbrinck syndrome: Presentations of three cases with features resembling spinocerebellar degeneration. Arch Neurol 1971; 25:289–294.

Sung JH, Meyers JP, Stadlan EM, Gowen D, Wolf A. Neuropathological changes in Chediak-Higashi disease. J Neuropathol Exp Neurol 1969; 28:86–118.

Thrombotic Thrombocytopenic Purpura

Amorosi EL, Ultmann JE. Thrombotic thrombocytopenic purpura: Report of 16 cases and review of the literature. Medicine 1966; 45:139–159.

Aster RH. Plasma therapy for thrombotic thrombocytopenic purpura: Sometimes it works, but, why? N Engl J Med 1985; 312:985–987.

Cuttner J. Thrombotic thrombocytopenic purpura: A ten-year experience. Blood 1980; 56:302–306.

Gutterman LA, Stevenson TD. Treatment of thrombotic thrombocytopenic purpura with vincristine. JAMA 1982; 247:1433–1436.

Moshcowitz E. An acute febrile pleiochromic anemia

with hyaline thrombosis of the terminal arterioles and capillaries. Arch Intern Med 1925; 36:89–93.

Myers TJ, Wakem CJ, Ball ED, Tremont SJ. Thrombotic thrombocytopenic purpura: combined treatment with plasmapheresis and antiplatelet agents. Ann Intern Med 1980; 92:149–155.

O'Brien JL, Sibley WA. Neurologic manifestations of thrombotic thrombocytopenic purpura. Neurology 1958; 8:55–64.

Silverstein A. Thrombotic thrombocytopenic purpura: The initial neurologic manifestations. Arch Neurol 1968; 18:358–362.

Washington University School of Medicine in St. Louis. Clinicopathologic conference: Thrombocytopenia, hemolytic anemia and transient neurologic deficits. Am J Med 1980; 68:267–274.

Multifocal Eosinophilic Granuloma (Histiocytosis X)

Adornato BT, Eil C, Head GL, Loriaux DL. Cerebellar involvement in multifocal eosinophilic granuloma: Demonstration by computerized tomographic scanning. Ann Neurol 1980; 7:125–129.

Christian HA. Defects in membranous bones, exophthalmos and diabetes insipidus: an unusual syndrome of dyspituitarism. Med Clin North Am 1919–1920; 3:849–871.

Hand A Jr. Polyuria and tuberculosis. Arch Pediatr 1893; 10:673–675.

Hewlett RH, Ganz JC. Histiocytosis X of the cauda equina. Neurology 1976; 26:472–476.

Jinkins JR. Histiocytosis X of the hypothalamus. Comput Radiol 1987; 11:181–184.

Kepes JJ. Histiocytosis X. In: Vinken PJ, Bruyn GW, Klawans HL, eds. Handbook of Clinical Neurology (vol 38). New York: Elsevier-North Holland, 1979; 93–117.

Lahey ME, Histiocytosis X: An analysis of prognostic factors. J Pediatr 1975; 87:184–189.

Lichtenstein L. Histiocytosis X: Integration of eosinophilic granuloma of bone, "Letterer-Siwe disease" and "Schüller-Christian disease" as related manifestations of a single nosologic entity. Arch Pathol 1953; 56:84–101.

Lieberman PH, Jones CR, Dargeon HWK, Begg CF. A reappraisal of eosinophilic granuloma of bone, Hand-Shüller-Christian syndrome and Letterer-Siwe syndrome. Medicine 1969; 48:375–400.

Osband ME. Histiocytosis X (review). Hematol Oncol Clin No Am 1987; 1:737–751.

Osband ME, Lipton JM, Lavin P, et al. Histiocytosis X: Demonstration of abnormal immunity, T-cell histamine H2-receptor deficiency, and successful treatment with thymic extract. N Engl J Med 1981; 304:146–153.

Risdall RJ, Dehner LP, Duray P, Kobrinsky N, Robison L, Nesbit ME Jr. Histiocytosis X (Langerhans' cell histiocytosis). Prognostic role of histopathology. Arch Pathol Lab Med 1983; 107:59–63.

Rowden G, Connelly EM, Winkelmann RK. Cutaneous histiocytosis X. The presence of S-100 protein and its use in diagnosis. Arch Dermatol 1983; 119:553–559.

Sawhny BS, Dohn DF. Neuroendocrinological aspects of histiocytosis X of the central nervous system. Surg Neurol 1980; 14:237–239.

Schüller A. Ueber eigenartige Schädeldefekte im Jugendalter. Forschr Geb Röntgenstrahlen 1915–1916; 23:12–18.

Sims DG. Histiocytosis X: Follow-up of 43 cases. Arch Dis Child 1977; 52:433–440.

Coagulation Disorders

King DJ, Kelton JG. Heparin associated thrombocytopenia. Ann Intern Med 1984; 100:535–540.

McGehee WG, Klotz TA, Epstein DJ, Rapaport SI. Coumarin necrosis associated with hereditary protein C deficiency. Ann Intern Med 1984; 100:59–60.

Schafer AI. The hypercoagulable states. Ann Intern Med 1985; 12:814–828.

---

151. HEPATIC DISEASE
Neil H. Raskin

Persistence of the terms *hepatic coma* and *encephalopathy* has led to imprecision of both clinical and pathophysiologic concepts. The often fatal comatose state associated with acute hepatic necrosis is often attended by striking elevations of serum ammonia; coma here is usually a single event of rapid onset and fulminant course that is characterized by delirium, convulsions, and occasionally, decerebrate rigidity. The mechanism of encephalopathy in this circumstance is not clear.

Usually, hepatic encephalopathy develops in patients with chronic liver disease when portal hypertension induces an extensive portal collateral circulation; portal venous blood bypasses the detoxification site, which is the liver, and drains directly into the systemic circulation to produce the cerebral intoxication that is properly termed *portal-systemic encephalopathy.* Several examples of portal-systemic encephalopathy have been reported in which the hepatic parenchyma was normal, underlining the anatomic importance of bypassing the liver as the mechanism. The offending nitrogenous substance arising in the intestine has not been identified with precision, but ammonia is the prime suspect.

The clinical syndrome resulting from shunting is an episodic encephalopathy comprising admixtures of ataxia, action tremor, dysarthria, sensorial clouding, and asterixis. The episodes are usually reversible, although they may recur. Cerebral morphologic changes are few except for an increase in large Alzheimer Type-II astrocytes. In a few patients with this disorder, a relentlessly progressing neurologic disorder occurs in addition to the fluctuating intoxication syndrome, including dementia, ataxia, dysarthria, intention tremor, and a choreoathetotic movement. The brains of these patients show zones of pseudolaminar necrosis in cerebral and cerebellar cortex, cavitations and neuronal loss in the basal ganglia and cerebellum, and glycogen-staining inclusions in enlarged astrocytes. This irreversible disorder has been termed "acquired chronic hepatocerebral degeneration," but it is probably the ultimate morphologic destruction that may result from the chronic metabolic defect that attends portal-systemic shunting.

Clinical Features. Thought processes usually are compromised insidiously, although an acute agitated delirium occasionally may usher in the syndrome. Mental dullness and drowsiness are usually the first symptoms; patients yawn frequently and drift off to sleep easily, yet remain arousable. Cognitive defects eventually appear. Asterixis almost always accompanies these modest changes of consciousness. As encephalopathy progresses, bilateral paratonia appears and the stretch reflexes become brisk; bilateral Babinski signs are usually obtained when obtundation becomes more profound. Convulsions are decidedly uncommon in this disorder unlike uremic encephalopathy. Spastic paraparesis may eventually be seen. Decerebrate and decorticate postures and diffuse spasticity of the limbs frequently accompany deeper stages of coma.

In the patient with overt hepatocellular failure with jaundice or ascites, the diagnosis of this disorder is not difficult. However, when parenchymal liver disease is mild or nonexistent, an elevated serum ammonia level or an elevation of CSF glutamine has high diagnostic sensitivity. The CSF is otherwise bland. The ultimate diagnostic test is clinical responsiveness to ammonium loading; the risks of this procedure in patients with intact hepatocellular function are minimal. Ten grams of ammonium chloride is given in daily divided doses for 3 days; the appearance or worsening of asterixis, dysarthria, or ataxia, or a further slowing of EEG frequency, is diagnostic.

Pathophysiology. Several substances have been considered the putative neurotoxin in portal-systemic encephalopathy. These include methionine, other amino acids, short-chain fatty acids, biogenic amines, indoles and skatoles, and ammonia. None of these has succeeded in explaining the condition better than ammonia.

Ammonia, a highly neurotoxic substance, is ordinarily converted to urea by the liver; when this detoxification mechanism is bypassed, levels of ammonia in the brain and blood increase. Occasionally, blood ammonia levels are normal or only slightly elevated in the face of full-blown coma. This has been used as a powerful argument against the implication of ammonia in this disorder; however, at physiological pH almost all serum ammonia in the $NH_4^+ \rightleftarrows NH_3 + H^+$ system is in the form of NH_4^+, with only traces of NH_3 present. It is NH_3 that crosses membranes with facility and is far more toxic than NH_4^+; thus it is possible that when methods become available to measure circulating free ammonia levels in portal-systemic encephalopathy, they will be strikingly and consistently elevated. Ammonia is detoxified in brain astrocytes by conversion to the nontoxic glutamine.

Following up on the observation that levodopa benefited patients in hepatic coma, Fischer and Baldessarini proposed their false neurotransmitter hypothesis to explain the mechanism of this effect and other features of the disorder. They suggested that amines such as octopamine (or their aromatic amino acid precursors tyrosine and phenylalanine), which are derived from protein by gut bacterial action, might escape oxidation by the liver and flood the systemic and cerebral circulations. Octopamine could then replace norepinephrine and dopamine in nerve endings and act as a false neurotransmitter; the accumulation of false neurotransmitters might then account for the encephalopathy, and the amelioration could be achieved by restoring "true" neurotransmitters through an elevation of tissue dopamine levels. However, L-dopa administration has a powerful peripheral effect, inducing the renal excretion of ammonia and urea; this probably accounts for the beneficial effects of L-dopa in some encephalopathic patients. Further, octopamine concentration in rat brain has been elevated more than 20,000-fold, along with depletion of both norepinephrine and dopamine, without any detectable alteration of consciousness. Whereas false neurotransmitters do accumulate in portal-systemic encephalopathy, there is little reason to hold them responsible for the encephalopathy. It has also been suggested that increased sensitivity to inhibitory neurotransmitters such as GABA and glycine may underlie the encephalopathy.

Treatment. Administration of antibiotics (especially neomycin or metronidazole) decreases the population of intestinal organisms to decrease production of ammonia and other cerebrotoxins. Lactulose is also beneficial for reasons that are not clear, but it lowers colonic pH, increases incorporation of ammonia into bacterial protein, and is a cathartic. The effects of neomycin and lactulose, given together, seem better than the effects either gives alone.

References

Asconapé JJ. Use of antiepileptic drugs in the presence of liver and kidney diseases: a review. Epilepsia 1982; 23(suppl 1): S65–S79.

Bower RH, Fischer JE. Nutritional management of hepatic encephalopathy. Adv Nutr Res 1983; 5:1–11.

De Groen PC, Aksamit AJ, Rakela J, et al. Central nervous system toxicity after liver transplantation: Role of cyclosporin and cholesterol. N Engl J Med 1987; 317:861–866.

Ferenci P, Pappas SC, Munson PJ, et al. Changes in the status of neurotransmitter receptors in a rabbit model of hepatic encephalopathy. Hepatology 1984; 4:186–191.

Fischer JE, Baldessarini RJ. False neurotransmitters and hepatic failure. Lancet 1971; 2:75–80.

Hoyumpa AM Jr, Schenker S. Perspectives in hepatic encephalopathy. J Lab Clin Med 1982; 100:477–487.

Lockwood AH, Ginsberg MD, Rhoades HM, Gutierrez MT. Cerebral glucose metabolism after portacaval shunting in the rat. J Clin Invest 1986; 78:86–95.

Lunzer M, James IM, Weinman J, Sherlock S. Treatment of chronic hepatic encephalopathy with levodopa. Gut 1974; 15:555–561.

Raskin NH, Bredesen D, Ehrenfeld WK, Kerland RK. Periodic confusion caused by congenital extrahepatic portacaval shunt. Neurology 1984; 34:666–669.

Ritt DJ, Whelan G, Werner DJ, Eigenbrodt EH, Schenker S. Combes B. Acute hepatic necrosis with stupor or coma. Medicine 1969; 48:151–172.

Shady H, Lieber CS. Blood ammonia levels in relationship to hepatic encephalopathy after propanolol. Am J Gastroenterol 1988; 83:249–255.

Sherlock S. Chronic portal systemic encephalopathy: Update 1987. Gut 1987; 28:1043–1048.

Summerskill WHJ, Davidson EA, Sherlock S, Steiner RE. The neuropsychiatric syndrome associated with hepatic cirrhosis and an extensive portal collateral circulation. Q J Med 1956; 25:245–266.

Victor M, Adams RD, Cole M. The acquired (non-Wilsonian) type of chronic hepatocerebral degeneration. Medicine 1965; 44:345–396.

Zieve L, Doizai M, Derr RF. Reversal of ammonia coma in rats by L-dopa: a peripheral effect. Gut 1979; 20:28–32.

152. BONE DISEASE
Roger N. Rosenberg

Osteitis Deformans

Osteitis deformans (Paget disease) is a chronic disease of the adult skeleton, characterized by bowing and irregular flattening of the bones. Any or all of the skeletal bones may be affected, but the tibia, skull, and pelvis are the most frequent sites. Except for the production of skeletal deformities and pain,

the disease causes disability only when the skull or spine is involved.

Pathology. In affected bones, there is an imbalance between formation and resorption of bone. In most cases, there is a mixture of excessive bone formation and bone destruction. The areas of bone destruction are filled with hyperplastic vascular connective tissue. New bone formation may occur in the destroyed areas in an irregular, disorganized manner. The metabolic disturbance that causes the bone abnormality is unknown.

Incidence. Osteitis deformans is a common bone disorder in adult life. A postmortem incidence of 3% in patients over 40 years of age was reported by Schmorl. Men and women are equally affected. The common age of onset is in the fourth to sixth decades; it is rare before age 30.

Symptoms and Signs. There are two types of neurologic symptoms that appear in patients with Paget disease: (1) those due to the abnormalities in bone, and (2) those due to arteriosclerosis, which is a common accompaniment. The cerebral signs and symptoms that occur with arteriosclerosis are no different from those that occur in patients with arteriosclerosis in the absence of Paget disease.

The neurologic defects of osteitis deformans are usually related to pressure on the CNS or the nerve roots by the overgrowth of bone. Convulsive seizures, generalized or neuralgic head pain, cranial nerve palsies, and paraplegia occur in a few cases. Deafness caused by pressure on the auditory nerves is the most common symptom; unilateral facial palsy is the next most common symptom. Loss of vision in one eye, visual-field defects, or exophthalmos may occur when the sphenoid bone is affected. Compression of the spinal cord is more common than compression of the cerebral substance by the bony overgrowth, which is extremely rare except when there is sarcomatous degeneration of the lesions. Platybasia may occur in advanced cases.

Laboratory Data. The serum calcium content is normal and the serum phosphorus is normal or only slightly increased. The serum alkaline phosphatase is increased; the level varies with the extent and activity of the process. It may be only slightly elevated when the disease is localized to one or two bones.

Diagnosis. The diagnosis of Paget disease is made from the patient's appearance and the characteristic radiographic changes. Involvement of the skull in advanced cases is manifested by a generalized enlargement of the calvarium, anteroflexion of the head, and depression of the chin on the chest. When the spine is involved, the patient's stature is shortened; the spine is flexed forward and its mobility is greatly reduced.

Radiographically, osteitis deformans in the skull appears as areas of increased bone density with loss of normal architecture, mingled with areas in which the density of the bone is decreased (Fig. 152–1). The margins of the bones are fuzzy and indistinct. The general appearance is that of an enormous skull with the bones of the vault covered with "cotton wool." In advanced cases, there may be a flattening of the base of the skull on the cervical vertebrae (*platybasia*) with signs of damage to the lower cranial nerves, medulla, or cerebellum. Both CT and magnetic resonance imaging aid diagnosis (Fig. 152–2).

Diagnosis may be difficult if the clinical symptoms are mainly neurologic. In these instances, radiographs of the pelvis and legs, or a general survey of the entire skeleton, may establish the diagnosis. Rarely, it may be impossible to distinguish monophasic Paget disease of the skull from osteoblastic metastases. A careful search for a primary neoplasm, particularly in the prostate, or biopsy of one of the lesions in the skull, may be necessary in those cases.

Course. The course of Paget disease is variable, but usually extends over several decades. The neurologic lesions seldom lead to any serious degree of disability other than deafness, convulsive seizures, or compression of the spinal cord.

Treatment. There is no specific therapy. Radiation therapy for the affected bones may temporarily relieve pain. Bauer recommended the administration of a high-calcium, high-vitamin diet with the addition of large doses of vitamin D and cevitamic acid to aid in the formation of new bone. The latter is especially important when there is involvement of weight-bearing bones. Thyrocalcito-

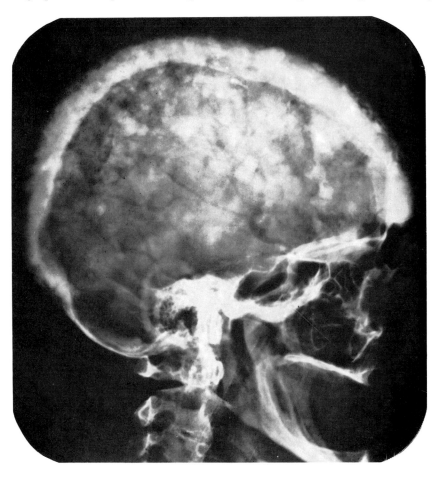

Fig. 152–1.   Osteitis deformans (Paget disease) of the skull. (Courtesy of Dr. Juan Taveras.)

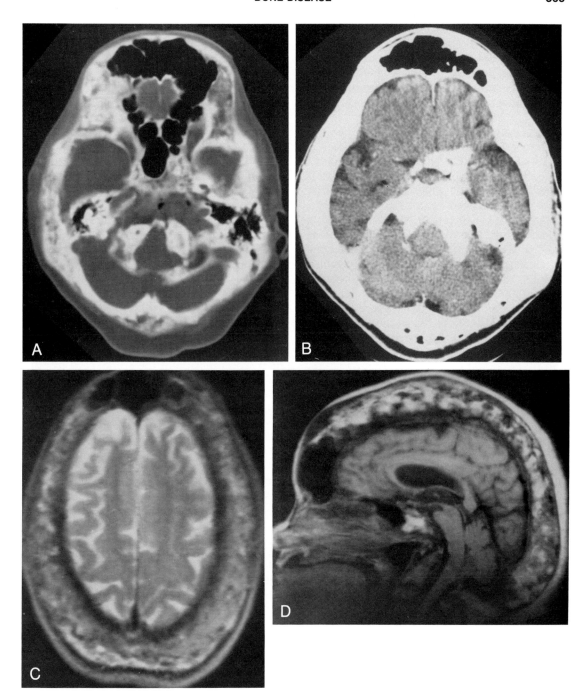

Fig. 152–2. Paget disease. Basilar invagination. *A.*Using bone windows, axial CT scan shows the foramen magnum projected within the posterior fossa. Intradiploic calcific density with "cotton wool" appearance is typical of Paget disease. *B.* Higher section, using soft-tissue windows, demonstrates obliteration of basal cisterns and brainstem compression due to basilar invagination. *C.* Axial T2-weighted MR scan shows prominent mottled signal in the diploic space. *D.* Sagittal T1-weighted MR scan confirms impingement of brainstem by dens. (Courtesy of Drs. J.A. Bello and S.K. Hilal.)

nin is now being given to inhibit the osteolytic process. Decompression of the cord may be necessary when it is compressed by involved vertebrae. Decompression of the posterior fossa gives temporary relief of symptoms in cases with platybasia.

Fibrous Dysplasia

The skull and the bones in other parts of the body are occasionally involved by a process characterized by small areas of bone destruction or massive sclerotic overgrowth.

The clinical picture of fibrous dysplasia is related to the site and extent of the bony overgrowth. Sassin and Rosenberg reported the incidence of involvement of the various bones of the skull in 50 cases: frontal, 28; sphenoid, 24; frontal and sphenoid, 18; temporal, 8; facial, 15; parietal, 6; and occipital, 8. Diffuse involvement of the entire skull produces a condition termed *leontiasis ossea*. In this condition, there is exophthalmos, optic atrophy, and other cranial nerve palsies (Fig. 152–3).

In addition to the disfiguration of the skull in the polyostotic form, symptoms of the monostotic form of the disease include headache, convulsions, exophthalmos, optic atrophy, and deafness. Symptoms may begin at any age, but onset usually occurs in early adult life. The family history is negative and there is no racial or sexual predominance.

A polyostotic form of the disease characterized by café-au-lait spots, endocrine dysfunction with precocious puberty in girls, and involvement of the femur (shepherd's crook deformity) was described by Albright and associates.

Achondroplasia

Achondroplasia (chondrodystrophy) is a form of dwarfism characterized by short arms and legs, lumbar lordosis, and enlargement of the head due to an inherited defect in the ossification of cartilage.

The disease is rare and is estimated to occur in 15 of 1 million births in the United States. It is usually inherited as an autosomal dominant trait.

Symptoms of involvement of the nervous system sometimes develop as a result of hydrocephalus, compression of the medulla and cervical cord at the level of the foramen magnum, compression of the spinal cord by ruptured intervertebral disk, and bony compression of the lower thoracic or lumbar cord. Convulsive seizures, ataxia, and paraplegia are the most common symptoms. Mental development is usually normal.

The diagnosis is made from the character-

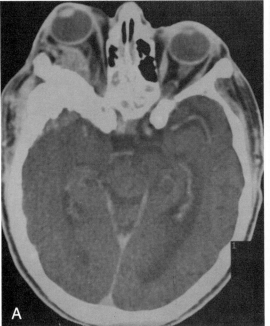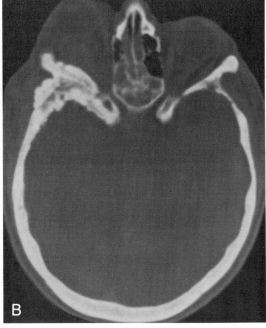

Fig. 152–3. Fibrous dysplasia. CT scans. *A.* Axial, contrast-enhanced scan shows proptosis on right with abnormal soft tissue enhancement within orbit and middle cranial fossa. *B.* Bone window depicts pronounced thickening of sphenoid bone. (Courtesy of Dr. T.L. Chi.)

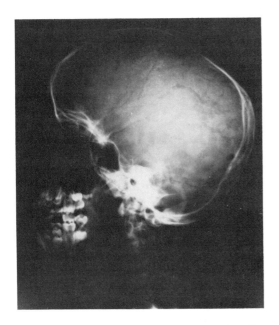

Fig. 152–4. Skull radiograph showing typical malformation of achondroplasia. The clivus is shortened.

istic body configuration of short arms and legs, normal-size trunk, enlargement of the head, and changes in the radiographs of the skeleton (Fig. 152–4).

Many affected infants die in the perinatal period, although a normal life span is possible for patients with less severe involvement of the bones.

Shunting procedures may be necessary in patients with hydrocephalus caused by involvement of the bones at the base of the skull. Laminectomy is indicated when signs of cord compression appear.

References

Osteitis Deformans

Chen J-R, Rhee RSC, Wallach S, Auramides A, Flores A. Neurologic disturbances in Paget disease of bone: Response to calcitonin. Neurology 1979; 29:448–457.

Douglas DL, Duckworth T, Kanis JA, Jefferson AA, Martin TJ, Russell RG. Spinal cord dysfunction in Paget's disease of bone. Has medical treatment a vascular basis? J Bone Joint Surg (Br) 1981; 63B:495–503.

Douglas DL, Kanis JA, Duckworth T, Beard DJ, Paterson AD, Russell RG. Paget's disease: Improvement of spinal cord dysfunction with diphosphate and calcitonin. Metab Bone Dis Relat Res 1981; 3:327–335.

Gandolfi A, Brizzi R, Tedesghi F, Cusmano F, Gabrielli M. Fibrosarcoma arising in Paget's disease of the vertebra: Review of the literature. Surg Neurol 1983; 13:72–76.

Goldhammer Y, Braham J, Kosary IZ. Hydrocephalic dementia in Paget's disease of the skull: Treatment by ventriculoatrial shunt. Neurology 1979; 29:513–516.

Wallach S. Treatment of Paget's disease. Adv Neurol 1982; 27:1–43.

Weisz GM. Lumbar spinal canal stenosis in Paget's disease. Spine 1983; 8:192–198.

Fibrous Dysplasia

Albright F. Polyostotic fibrous dysplasia: A defense of the entity. J Clin Endocrinol Metab 1947; 7:307–324.

Cole DE, Fraser FC, Glorieux FH, et al. Panostotic fibrous dysplasia: A congenital disorder of bone with unusual facial appearance, bone fragility, hyperphosphatasemia, and hypophosphatemia. Am J Med Genet 1983; 14:725–735.

Daffner RH, Kirks DR, Gehweiler JA Jr, Heaston DK. Computed tomography of fibrous dysplasia. AJR 1982; 139:943–948.

Finney HL, Roberts JS. Fibrous dysplasia of the skull with progressive cranial nerve involvement. Surg Neurol 1976; 6:341–343.

Reid CS, Pyeritz RE, Kopits SE et al. Cervicomedullary compression in young patients with achondroplasia. J Pediatr 1987; 110:522–530.

Saper JR. Disorders of bone and the nervous system: The dysplasias and premature closure syndromes. In: Vinken PJ, Bruyn GW, eds. Handbook of Clinical Neurology (vol 38). New York: Elsevier-North Holland, 1979: 381–429.

Sassin JF, Rosenberg RN. Neurologic complications of fibrous dysplasia of the skull. Arch Neurol 1968; 18:363–376.

Achondroplasia

Dandy WF. Hydrocephalus in chondrodystrophy. Bull Johns Hopkins Hosp 1921; 32:5–10.

Denis JP, Rosenberg HS, Ellsworth CA Jr. Megalocephaly, hydrocephalus and other neurological aspects of achondroplasia. Brain 1961; 84:427–445.

Duvoisin RC, Yahr MD. Compressive spinal cord and root systems in achondroplastic dwarfs. Neurology 1962; 12:202–207.

Kahandovitz N, Rimoin DL, Sillence DO. The clinical spectrum of lumbar spine disease in achondroplasia. Spine 1982; 7:137–140.

Wynne-Davies R, Walsh WK, Gormley J. Achondroplasia and hypochondroplasia. Clinical variation and spinal stenosis. J Bone Joint Surg (Br) 1981; 63B:508–515.

153. RENAL DISEASE
Neil H. Raskin

Uremia is a term used to describe a constellation of signs and symptoms in patients with severe azotemia due to acute or chronic renal failure; symptomatic renal failure is an acceptable definition. The clinical features of the neurologic consequences of renal failure do not correlate well with any single biochemical abnormality, but seem to be related to the rate of development of renal failure. This section summarizes the features of uremic encephalopathy and neuropathy and the distinctive neurologic complications of dialysis and renal transplantation.

Uremic Encephalopathy

In uremia, as in other metabolic encephalopathies, there is a continuum of signs of neurologic dysfunction including dysarthria, instability of gait, asterixis, action tremor, multifocal myoclonus, and sensorial clouding. One or more of these signs may predominate, but fluctuation of clinical signs from day to day is characteristic. The earliest and most reliable indication of uremic encephalopathy is sensorial clouding. Patients appear fatigued, preoccupied, and apathetic, and have difficulty concentrating. Obtundation then becomes more apparent as perceptual errors, defective memory, and mild confusion become evident. Illusions and perceptions sometimes progress to frank visual hallucinations.

Asterixis is almost always present once sensorial clouding appears: it is most effectively elicited by having the patient hold the arms outstretched in fixed hyperextension at the elbow and wrist, with the fingers spread apart. After a latency of up to 30 seconds, flexion-extension ("flapping") of the fingers at the metacarpophalangeal joints and at the wrist appears arrhythmically and at irregular intervals.

Multifocal myoclonus refers to visible twitching of muscles that is sudden, arrhythmic, and asymmetric, involving muscles first in one locus, then in another, and affecting chiefly the face and proximal limbs. It is a strong indication of a severe metabolic disturbance and usually does not appear until stupor or coma has supervened. In uremia, asterixis and myoclonus may be so intense that muscles appear to fasciculate, giving rise to the term *"uremic twitching."* This form of myoclonus probably signifies cortical irritability; it is, at times, difficult to distinguish from a multifocal seizure. Tetany is commonly associated with myoclonus and other signs of encephalopathy. It may be overt, with spontaneous carpopedal spasms, or latent, manifested by a positive Trousseau sign. The spasms originate in abnormal peripheral nerve discharges. In uremic patients, tetany does not usually respond to injections of calcium and occurs despite metabolic acidosis (which usually inhibits hypocalcemic tetany).

Alterations in limb tone appear as encephalopathy progresses and brain-stem function becomes compromised. Muscle tone is usually heightened and is sometimes asymmetric. Eventually, decorticate posturing may appear in preference to decerebrate attitudes. Focal motor signs are present in about 20% of patients; these signs often clear after hemodialysis.

Convulsions are usually a late manifestation of uremic encephalopathy. In the older literature, convulsions were thought to occur far more often than is now reported; this may have been the result of failing to distinguish hypertensive encephalopathy from uremia, which are disorders that may coexist. Hypertensive retinopathy and papilledema are major signs that distinguish the two conditions; further, focal signs such as aphasia or cortical blindness are much more common in hypertensive brain disease than in uremia. The treatment of recurring uremic convulsions is not straightforward because the pharmacokinetics of phenytoin are altered in uremic patients. In uremia, plasma protein binding of phenytoin is decreased so much that the unbound fraction of the drug is two to three times greater than that found in normal plasma. However, in uremic patients, the volume of distribution of the drug is larger and there is an increased rate of conversion of phenytoin to hydroxylated derivatives, resulting in lower total serum concentrations of the drug for any given dose. This combination of factors allows the physician to administer the usual dosage of phenytoin (300–400 mg daily) to a uremic patient and attain therapeutic unbound levels of the drug despite lower total serum levels (i.e., 5–10 mg/L rather than 10–20 mg/L).

Meningeal signs occur in about 35% of uremic patients; half of those affected have CSF pleocytosis. CSF protein elevations greater than 60 mg/dl occur in 60% of uremic patients; in 20%, the CSF protein exceeds 100 mg/dl. CSF protein content may return to normal in the immediate posthemodialysis period. The increase in CSF protein is caused by an alteration in the permeability properties of the brain's capillary endothelial cells adjacent to the CSF, which have tight intercellular junctions.

There are no specific pathologic alterations of brain in uremic encephalopathy; cerebral use of oxygen is depressed, as it is in other metabolic encephalopathies, due to a primary interference with synaptic transmission. Depressed cerebral metabolic rate and clinical state usually change together, but are probably independent reflections of generally impaired neuronal functions. The profundity of uremic encephalopathy correlates only in a general way, and sometimes poorly, with biochemical abnormalities in the blood. Cerebral acidosis has been suggested as a possible mechanism, but CSF pH is usually normal.

Brain calcium is increased by 50% and seems to be due to excess circulating parathyroid hormone, which is nondialyzable. It is not clear whether calcium changes are related to the cerebral dysfunction.

The rapid clearing of uremic encephalopathy after dialysis suggests that small-to-moderate sized water-soluble molecules are responsible for the encephalopathy. Excessive accumulation of toxic organic acids overwhelms the normal mechanisms for excluding such compounds from the brain and may be important. These organic acids may block transport systems of the choroid plexus and of glia that normally remove metabolites of some neurotransmitters in brain. Furthermore, there is a nonspecific increase in cerebral membrane permeability in uremia and this may permit greater entry into brain of uremic toxins such as the organic acids, which further derange cerebral function.

Uremic Neuropathy

Peripheral neuropathy is the most common neurologic consequence of chronic renal failure. It is a distal, symmetric, mixed sensorimotor neuropathy affecting the legs more than the arms. It is clinically indistinguishable from the neuropathies of chronic alcohol abuse or diabetes mellitus. The rate of progression, severity, prominence of motor or sensory signs, and prevalence of dysesthesia vary. It is several times more common in men than in women. The symptom of burning feet was considered a common feature of uremic neuropathy but probably resulted from removal of water-soluble thiamine by hemodialysis and, with near-universal B-vitamin replacement, this syndrome is now rare. The restless-legs syndrome occurs in 40% of uremic patients and probably heralds peripheral nerve involvement by the uremic disorder. This syndrome comprises creeping, crawling, prickling, and pruritic sensations deep within the legs. These sensations are almost always worse in the evening; they are relieved by movement of the limbs. Clonazepam is effective in terminating this syndrome.

The rate of progression of uremic neuropathy varies widely; in general, it evolves over several months, but may be fulminant. Among most patients who enter chronic hemodialysis programs the neuropathy stabilizes or improves slowly. Patients with mild neuropathy often recover completely, but those who begin dialysis with severe neuropathy rarely recover even after several years.

Successful renal transplantation has a clear, predictable, and beneficial effect on uremic neuropathy. Motor-nerve conduction velocities increase within days of transplantation. There is progressive improvement for 6 to 12 months, often with complete recovery, even in patients with severe neuropathy before transplantation.

Pathologically, this neuropathy is usually a primary axonal degeneration with secondary segmental demyelination, probably due to a metabolic failure of the perikaryon; there is also a predominantly demyelinative type. Because uremic neuropathy improves with hemodialysis, it seems evident that the neuropathy results from the accumulation of dialyzable metabolite. These substances may be in the "middle molecule" (300–2000 dalton) range; compounds of this size cross dialysis membranes more slowly than smaller molecules such as creatinine and urea, which are the usual measures of chemical control of uremia. Supporting this contention are observations that control of neuropathy in some cases depends on increased hours of dialysis each week (beyond that necessary for chemical control of uremia) and that peritoneal dialysis seems to be associated with a lower incidence of neuropathy. The peritoneal membrane seems to permit passage of some molecules more readily and selectively than the cellophane membrane used in hemodialysis. The transplanted kidney deals effectively with substances of different molecular size; the resulting elimination of middle molecules could explain the invariable improvement of the neuropathy after transplantation.

There is a parathormone-induced increase in calcium in peripheral nerves in experimental uremia, which causes slowed nerve conduction velocity; these changes can be prevented by prior parathyroidectomy. In human uremic patients, circulating parathormone levels correlate inversely with nerve conduction velocities. However, it seems unlikely that parathoromone is involved in uremic neuropathy because the hormone is nondialyzable and hyperparathyroidism itself is not usually associated with neuropathy.

Dialysis Dysequilibrium Syndrome

Headache, nausea, and muscle cramps attend hemodialysis in over 50% of patients; in somewhat over 5% obtundation, convulsions, or delirium may occur. The cerebral sequelae are usually seen with rapid dialysis at the outset of a dialysis program; symptoms usually appear toward the third or fourth hour of a dialysis run, but occasionally appear 8 to 24 hours later. The syndrome is usually self-limited, subsiding in hours, but delirium may persist for several days. Some patients become exophthalmic because of increased intraocular pressure at the height of the syndrome. Other clinical correlates include increased intracranial pressure, papilledema, and generalized EEG slowing.

Shift of water into brain is probably the proximate cause of dysequilibrium. Rapid reduction of blood solute content cannot be paralleled by brain solutes because of the blood-brain barrier. An osmotic gradient is produced between blood and brain causing movement of water into brain, which results in encephalopathy, cerebral edema, and increased intracranial pressure. The osmotically active substances retained in brain have not yet been identified.

Dialysis Dementia

A distinctive, progressive, usually fatal encephalopathy may occur in patients who are chronically dialyzed for periods that exceed 3 years. The first symptom is usually a stammering, hesitancy of speech, and at times, speech arrest. The speech disorder is intensified during and immediately after dialysis and, at first, may be seen only during these periods. A thought disturbance is usually evident and there is a consistent EEG abnormality, with bursts of high voltage slowing in the frontal leads. As the disorder progresses, speech becomes more dysarthric and aphasic; dementia and myoclonic jerks usually become apparent (Table 153–1) at this time. The other

Table 153–1.   Clinical Features of Dialysis Dementia

Feature	Totals in 42 Patients
Age at onset (yr)	21–68 (average, 45)
Months on hemodialysis at onset	9–84 (average, 37)
Duration of illness until death (mo)	1–15 (average, 6)
Sex	21 M, 21 F
Dementia	98%
Speech impairment	95%
Myoclonus	81%
Seizures	57%
Behavioral abnormalities	52%
Gait disorder	17%
Tremor	7%

(Modified from Lederman RJ, Henry CF. Ann Neurol 1978, 4:199–204.)

elements of the encephalopathy include delusional thinking, convulsions, asterixis, and occasionally focal neurologic abnormalities. Early in the course, diazepam is effective in lessening myoclonus and seizures, and in improving speech; it becomes less effective later. The CSF is unremarkable. Increased dialysis time and renal transplantation do not seem to alter the course of the disease. No distinctive abnormalities have been found in brain at autopsy.

The geographical variation in the incidence of dialysis dementia suggests that there could be a neurotoxin. Aluminum content is consistently elevated in the cerebral gray matter of patients who die from this condition. Municipal water supplies heavily contaminated with aluminum have been linked to the appearance of the syndrome in epidemiologic studies. Another possible source is absorption of aluminum from orally administered phosphate-binding agents that are given to uremic patients. Plasma protein binding of aluminum retards the removal of aluminum during dialysis even when an aluminum-free dialysate is used. Nevertheless, there have been several reports of remission of dialysis dementia when aluminum was removed from the diet, from the dialysate or from patients with deferoxamine. Cerebral aluminum intoxication, still an unconfirmed hypothesis, seems to be the most likely possibility at this time. Brain GABA levels are reduced in numerous regions, but the meaning of this finding is not clear.

Neurologic Complications of Renal Transplantation

A curious vulnerability to certain brain tumors and unusual infections of the nervous system occurs in patients who have undergone transplantation; however, cerebral infarction is the most common neurologic complication.

The risk that a lymphoma will develop after a transplant is about 35 times greater than normal; this increased risk depends almost entirely on the increased incidence of primary lymphoma (formerly called reticulum-cell sarcoma) in brain. Brain tumors appear between 5 and 46 months after transplantation. The resulting clinical syndromes include increased intracranial pressure, rapidly evolving focal neurologic signs, or combinations of these. Convulsions are a rare feature of these tumors. A remarkable characteristic of primary lymphomas is the response to radiotherapy; survivals of 3 to 5 years are not unusual.

Systemic fungal infections are found at autopsy in about 45% of patients who have been treated with renal transplantation and immunosuppression; brain abscess formation occurs in about 35% of these patients. In almost all cases, the primary source of infection is in the lung. Chest radiographs and the presence of fever aid in differentiating fungal brain abscess from brain tumor in recipients of transplants. Aspergillus has a unique predilection for dissemination to brain and accounts for most fungal brain abscesses; candida, nocardia, and histoplasma are found in the others. The clinical syndrome resulting from these infections is usually delirium accompanied by seizures. Headache, stiff neck, and focal signs also occur, but not commonly. The CSF is often remarkably bland, and brain biopsy may be the only reliable way to establish a diagnosis. The distinction of fungal brain abscess from possibly radiosensitive brain tumor makes it important to consider this procedure.

References

Adams HP, Dawson G, Coffman TJ, Corry RI. Stroke in renal transplant recipients. Arch Neurol 1986; 43:113–115.

Alfrey AC. Aluminum. Adv Clin Chem 1983; 23:69–91.

Altmann P, Al-Salihi F, Butter K, et al. Serum aluminum levels and erythrocyte dihydropteridine reductase activity in patients on hemodialysis. N Engl J Med 1987; 317:80–84.

Babb AL, Ahmad S, Bergström J, Scribner BH. The middle molecule hypothesis in perspective. Am J Kidney Dis 1981; 1:46–50.

Healton EB, Brust JCM, Feinfeld DA, Thomson GE. Hypertensive encephalopathy and the neurologic manifestations of malignant hypertension. Neurology 1982; 32:127–132.

Lederman RJ, Henry CF. Progressive dialysis encephalopathy. Ann Neurol 1978; 4:199–204.

Raskin NH, Fishman RA. Neurologic disorders in renal failure. N Engl J Med 1976; 294:143–148, 204–210.

Said G, Boudier L, Selva J, et al. Patterns of uremic polyneuropathy. Neurology 1983; 33:567–574.

Sweeney VP, Perry TL, Price JDE, et al. Brain γ-aminobutyric acid deficiency in dialysis encephalopathy. Neurology 1985; 35:180–184.

---

154. RESPIRATORY CARE: DIAGNOSIS AND MANAGEMENT

Matthew E. Fink

Many different neurologic problems are encountered in a neurologic intensive care unit (ICU) (Table 154–1); all patients share a common need for intensive nursing care and car-

diorespiratory monitoring to prevent a life-threatening complication. The overall mortality of ICU patients is 10%. Some 80% of the survivors eventually return to their homes able to function independently.

Diagnosis is rarely a problem; the major concern in the ICU is treatment of neurologic disease and the medical complications that determine survival and recovery. The usual disorders that require ICU treatment are intracranial hypertension, acute cerebral ischemia, and respiratory failure (see Sections 36 and 41, Treatment and Prevention of Stroke; and Brain Edema and Disorders of Intracranial Pressure). Respiratory failure is the most common reason for admission of neurologic patients to the ICU.

Respiratory Physiology

Respiratory failure occurs when gas exchange is impaired. The diagnosis of respiratory failure depends on arterial blood gas analysis. $PaO_2 < 60$ torr or $PaCO_2 > 50$ torr unequivocally defines respiratory failure. However, there are warning signs of deteriorating ventilatory function before respiratory failure is overt. Patients with neurologic disease rarely complain of dyspnea. The premonitory signs of mild respiratory failure are restlessness, insomnia, confusion, tachycar-

Table 154–1. Analysis of 272 Admissions to Neurologic Intensive Care Unit in 3-Month Period

Type of Admission	%	No.
Medical:		
Intracerebral or subarachnoid hemorrhage	8	21
Head trauma	5	13
Brain infarction	5	13
Neuromuscular disease	2	6
CNS infections	2	5
Status epilepticus	1	4
Medical complication	1	4
Spinal cord injury	<1	2
Other	<1	1
Surgical:		
Craniotomy for tumor	25	69
Craniotomy for aneurysm or vascular malformation	16	44
Carotid endarterectomy	14	38
Spinal surgery for tumor or vascular malformation	6	17
Ventricular shunt	6	16
Craniotomy for hematoma	4	10
Medical complication	3	9

Note. Admissions to The Neurological Institute of New York, October–December, 1983.

dia, tachypnea, diaphoresis, and headache. When ventilation is severely affected, there may be central cyanosis, hypotension, asterixis, poor chest expansion, miosis, papilledema, and coma. It is impossible to accurately predict arterial oxygen tension (PaO_2) and arterial carbon dioxide tension ($PaCO_2$) from clinical signs; measurement of arterial blood gases is essential. Normal PaO_2 is a function of age. A healthy 20-year-old has a PaO_2 of 90 to 95 torr. With each decade, PaO_2 decreases by three torr. Normal $PaCO_2$ is 37 to 43 torr and is not affected by age.

Hypoxemia is caused by five conditions: (1) a low inspired oxygen concentration (PiO_2), (2) hypoventilation, (3) ventilation-perfusion mismatching, (4) right-to-left shunting, and (5) impaired diffusion. Clinically, only conditions two, three, and four, are important. The accurate interpretation of PaO_2 depends on the alveolar-arterial (A-a) oxygen tension difference. The alveolar PO_2 (PaO_2) can be calculated from the equation $PaO_2 = PiO_2 - PaCO_2/0.8$. An A-a gradient of greater than 20 torr always indicates intrapulmonary pathology. Hypoxemia with an A-a gradient less than 10 torr strongly suggests extrapulmonary causes of hypoxemia (hypoventilation). Ventilation-perfusion mismatching can often be distinguished from right-to-left shunting by observing the effects of breathing 100% oxygen. Patients with ventilation-perfusion mismatching (i.e., bronchospasm) show a dramatic rise in PaO_2, often greater than 500 torr, but patients with intrapulmonary shunting (i.e., severe pulmonary edema) show little or no improvement in PaO_2.

Hypercapnia is caused by three conditions: (1) breathing a CO_2-containing gas, (2) hypoventilation, and (3) severe ventilation-perfusion mismatch. Hypoventilation is identified by high $PaCO_2$ with a normal A-a gradient. In ventilation-perfusion mismatching, there is arterial hypoxemia before arterial hypercapnia because of differences in O_2 and CO_2 dissociation curves. It is impossible to increase O_2 saturation beyond 100% in well-ventilated areas of the lung to make up for poorly ventilated areas. In neuromuscular disease with primary hypoventilation, mild hypoxemia is a marker of impending ventilatory failure, before arterial pCO_2 increases.

Acid-base disturbances may be respiratory or metabolic and acute or chronic. An acute change in pCO_2 of 10 torr results in a pH change of 0.08 units. A chronic change in pCO_2 of 10 torr causes a pH change of only 0.03 units. An acute base change of 10 mEq/L leads to a pH change of 0.15 units. Respiratory alkalosis may be divided into disorders with a normal A-a gradient (CNS disorders, drugs, hormones, pregnancy, high altitude, severe anemia, psychogenic hyperventilation, endotoxemia, mechanical ventilation) or an elevated A-a gradient (gram-negative sepsis, endotoxemia, hepatic failure, interstitial lung disease, pulmonary edema, pulmonary emboli, pneumonia, asthma). Respiratory acidosis may be part of any disorder causing respiratory failure.

The cause of respiratory failure can be determined by identifying the component of the system that is malfunctioning. Usually, hypercapnic respiratory failure is due to abnormalities in the extrapulmonary compartment (brainstem respiratory center, efferent nerves, neuromuscular junction, respiratory muscles, chest wall, pleura, upper airway). Nonhypercapnic, hypoxemic respiratory failure is always caused by abnormalities in the pulmonary compartment (lower airway, pulmonary circulation, interstitium, alveolocapillary area).

Pulmonary function tests are essential in the treatment of patients with neurologic diseases. Bedside spirometry is usually sufficient to provide the basic information to formulate a diagnosis and treatment plan. Measurements of minute ventilation, maximum breathing capacity, inspiratory and expiratory muscle pressures, vital capacity and forced expiratory volumes can quickly and painlessly differentiate obstructive airway disease from neuromuscular disease. Pulmonary function testing is a reliable and objective way to follow the course of many neuromuscular diseases and assess response to therapy.

Neurologic Diseases with Primary Respiratory Dysfunction

BRAINSTEM DISEASE

Reticular formation neurons, sensitive to hypoxemia and hypercarbia, are located in the brainstem and may be affected by ischemia, hemorrhage, inflammation, or neoplasms. The medullary center is responsible for initiation and maintenance of spontaneous respirations while the pontine pneumotaxic center helps to coordinate cyclic respirations. Forebrain damage causes Cheyne-Stokes respirations (regular, cyclic respiratory pattern with crescendo-decrescendo apnea) and transient posthyperventilation apnea, as respiratory drive becomes dependent on changes in pCO_2. There may be loss of voluntary deep breathing or breath holding. Hypothalamic or midbrain damage may cause central neurogenic hyperventilation (low pCO_2 with normal A-a gradient). Damage to the base of the pons may cause paralysis of voluntary breathing with bursts of rapid deep respirations when pCO_2 rises. Lower pontine tegmental damage may lead to apneustic (inspiratory breath holding) or cluster breathing (irregular bursts of rapid breathing alternating with apneic periods). Medullary damage may cause ataxic breathing (irregular pattern with hypoxemia and hypercarbia), gasping or apnea (brain death). Apnea is determined by ventilating the patient with 100% oxygen for 20 minutes, turning off the ventilator and allowing the pCO_2 to rise above 50 torr. Arterial blood gases are checked at both the beginning and end of the test to confirm hyperoxemia and hypercarbia. The physician must stand at the bedside during the apnea test to observe chest wall and diaphragm movements and to confirm the absence of respiratory muscle movement.

In addition to abnormalities in respiratory rate and pattern and synchronization of diaphragm and intercostal muscles, brainstem damage often alters consciousness and causes paralysis of pharyngeal and laryngeal musculature, predisposing to aspiration pneumonitis. Patients with severe brainstem dysfunction should have nasotracheal or orotracheal intubation, electively, to prevent respiratory complications.

Brainstem respiratory centers may be depressed (lose responsiveness to CO_2 and/or O_2) by narcotics or barbiturates, metabolic abnormalities such as hypothyroidism, and by starvation or metabolic alkalosis. Idiopathic primary alveolar hypoventilation and "central sleep apnea syndrome" are due to brainstem malfunction. These disorders are easily distinguished from structural brainstem pathology by the lack of associated neurologic signs.

SPINAL CORD DISEASE

The respiratory system is affected depending on the segmental level and severity of the spinal injury. In spinal cord trauma, the most common cause of death is acute respiratory failure due to apnea, aspiration pneumonia, tension pneumothorax, or pulmonary embolism. The chronic care of a quadraplegic patient is heavily dependent on the degree of respiratory impairment.

A lesion at C_3 abolishes both diaphragmatic and intercostal muscle activity, leaving only accessory muscle function. The result is severe hypercapnic respiratory failure. Acute spinal cord lesions at the C_5 to C_6 level produce an immediate fall in vital capacity to 30% of normal. Several months after injury, however, the vital capacity will increase to 50 to 60% of normal. High thoracic lesions will compromise intercostal and abdominal muscles, causing a limitation of inspiratory capacity and active expiration. Midthoracic lesions have little impact on respiratory muscle function because only the abdominal muscles are affected.

Most spinal cord diseases cause respiratory impairment by interrupting the suprasegmental impulses that drive the diaphragm and intercostal muscles. However, there are two notable exceptions: strychnine poisoning and tetanus. Both of these toxins block the inhibitory interneurons within the spinal cord, causing simultaneous increases in the activity of muscles that are normally antagonists. Episodes of apnea may lead to hypoxemic death because of the intense muscle spasms of the upper airway muscles, diaphragm, and intercostal muscles.

MOTOR NEURON DISEASES

Amyotrophic lateral sclerosis (ALS) is the most common form of motor neuron diseases that cause respiratory failure. Respiratory failure is the leading cause of death, usually developing late in the disease because of ventilatory limitation and impaired cough due to respiratory muscle weakness. If symptoms begin with limb weakness the disorder may progress to respiratory failure in 2 to 5 years. If oropharyngeal symptoms appear first, respiratory complications may be caused by recurrent aspiration pneumonitis. Rarely, respiratory failure is the first clinical manifestation of ALS.

Frequent pulmonary function testing can identify patients at risk of respiratory complications. The earliest changes are decreases in maximum inspiratory and expiratory muscle pressures, followed by reduced vital capacity and maximum breathing capacity. When vital capacity falls to 25 ml/kg of body weight, the ability to cough is impaired, increasing the risk of aspiration pneumonia. Blood gases remain normal until the patient is near respiratory arrest.

New cases of poliomyelitis are now rare in industrialized countries, but an occasional patient with the postpoliomyelitis syndrome of late progressive weakness may develop ventilatory failure. This is attributed to a combination of factors, including the "normal" loss of lung volume and compliance with aging and loss of ventilatory drive, superimposed on respiratory muscle weakness.

PERIPHERAL NEUROPATHIES

The Guillain-Barré syndrome is the prototype of neuropathies with respiratory complications (see Section 108). Of patients with this syndrome, 20% require some ventilatory support; 50% of severe cases (unable to walk) require tracheal intubation and mechanical ventilation. There is a 3% mortality with the best possible treatment. Most deaths are due to pulmonary embolism and severe pneumonia. Some degree of respiratory insufficiency must be expected in all patients with severe disease; therefore, during the 2 to 4 week period of progression, there should be frequent measurements of inspiratory and expiratory pressures and vital capacity. Normal vital capacity is 65 ml/kg; a fall to 30 ml/kg is associated with a poor cough and accumulation of oropharyngeal secretions. At a level of 25 ml/kg, the sigh mechanism is impaired, atelectasis develops, and mild hypoxemia may result. If the vital capacity falls below 15 ml/kg, endotracheal intubation is necessary to provide positive pressure ventilation. Do not wait for signs of hypercarbia before proceeding with tracheal intubation. When pCO_2 rises, the patient is near respiratory arrest and delay will cause major morbidity and mortality.

Disorders of Neuromuscular Transmission

Myasthenia gravis (MG), botulism and neuromuscular blocking drugs may affect respiratory muscles (see also Sections 23 and 127). Myasthenia almost always affects cranial muscles, causing ptosis, weakness in the ocular and oropharyngeal muscles, plus symmetric facial weakness. Respiratory muscle weakness usually accompanies oropharyngeal weakness, further increasing the tendency for aspiration pneumonia. As in Guillain-Barré syndrome and other neuromuscular diseases, blood gas abnormalities are a late manifestation of respiratory failure. Frequent measurement of inspiratory and expiratory pressures and vital capacity is essential; tracheal intubation is carried out if the vital capacity is less than 15 ml/kg. MG is a treacherous disease because fluctuations may be sudden and unpredictable. Patients with severe dysarthria and dysphagia are at greatest risk.

Myasthenic crisis is defined as deterioration of respiratory failure that requires mechanical ventilation. It occurs in 12 to 16% of new patients seen with MG and accounts for most mortality. However, the overall mortality has significantly declined in the past four decades. In my hospital, during the 1940s and 1950s, the mortality was more than 30%; this declined to about 12% during the 1960s, and to 3% in the 1970s. Some 90% of patients with crisis had dysarthria and dysphagia, predisposing them to aspiration pneumonia; 25% had clear evidence of pneumonia or upper respiratory tract infections. However, 40% of patients with crisis had no evident exacerbating factors other than spontaneous worsening of myasthenia; it is likely that some of these also had aspiration-induced worsening. There was no evidence that cholinesterase inhibitors played any role in the acute deterioration (cholinergic crisis). The median duration of mechanical ventilatory support during a single crisis episode was 2 weeks. There was no specific proven therapy to shorten the duration of crisis. A multicenter controlled trial is needed to determine whether plasmapheresis, corticosteroids, or other measures might shorten the duration of mechanical ventilation.

MUSCLE DISEASE

Muscular dystrophies, myotonic disorders, inflammatory myopathies, periodic paralyses, metabolic myopathies, endocrine disorders, infectious myopathies, toxic myopathies, myoglobinuria, and electrolyte disorders may cause widespread skeletal muscle weakness (see also Chapter XVII). Respiratory failure may appear in acute fulminant attacks or after a period of progression. Rarely, respiratory failure may be the first manifestation of a generalized myopathy. As in other neuromuscular disorders, hypercapnic respiratory failure is always preceded by a severely impaired cough mechanism; the patient has difficulty clearing respiratory tract secretions. Atelectasis with ventilation-perfusion mismatching and mild hypoxemia usually precedes hypercarbia. Pulmonary function tests show respiratory muscle weakness (decreased inspiratory and expiratory pressures) and decreased vital capacity as the disease progresses. Pulmonary function tests are often abnormal, even though there are no clinical symptoms of respiratory muscle involvement.

The myopathic diseases that are complicated by respiratory failure are Duchenne dystrophy, acute hypokalemic paralysis, polymyositis or dermatomyositis, adult-onset acid maltase deficiency, and cytoplasmic inclusion body myopathy.

Treatment of Respiratory Failure in Neurologic Diseases

MECHANICAL VENTILATION

Mechanical ventilation may be positive pressure or negative pressure. Until the mid-1950s, all mechanical ventilation was negative pressure. The most common device was the Drinker tank respirator ("iron lung"), which created a cyclical subatmospheric pressure around the patient's chest, causing chest expansion. Today, there are several types of negative-pressure devices, cuirass ventilators, that can be used on a chronic basis to assist the patient's own respiratory efforts without tracheal intubation. Patients with motor neuron disease and chronic myopathies are sometimes able to live at home with these devices.

Positive-pressure ventilation can be delivered for short periods with the use of a tight fitting face mask. However, tracheal intubation with a cuffed tube is necessary to prevent leakage of air around the tube. Small suitcase-sized portable and battery-powered volume-cycled ventilators are available for ambulatory use. Ventilator-dependent patients may go home and remain mobile.

Mechanical ventilation is the primary treatment for respiratory failure. Indications for intubation and positive pressure ventilation are respiratory rate > 35/minute, vital capacity < 15 ml/kg, inspiratory force < 25 cm of water, PaO_2 < 70 torr with maximum oxygen by face mask or $PaCO_2$ > 50. Endotracheal intubation is always performed initially; tracheostomy is considered later. Indications for tracheostomy are listed in Table 154–2.

Positive pressure ventilators are pressure cycled or volume cycled; the latter are preferable because they deliver a precise tidal volume over a wide range of pressures. The initial tidal volume is 10 ml/kg with a respiratory rate of 12 to 15 breaths/minute. A recommended starting level is 90% inspired oxygen; the inspired concentration is gradually adjusted downward until the PaO_2 is 70 to 90 torr.

Weaning from the ventilator can be considered when pulmonary function tests show improvement and there are no significant medical complications (Table 154–3). Weaning can be accomplished in two ways: (1) a gradual reduction of the mandatory ventilator rate enabling the patient to take over the spontaneous respirations (weaning with IMV [intermittent mandatory ventilation]); (2) complete removal of the patient from the respirator, allowing free breathing for short periods with oxygen supplementation alone (weaning with a T-tube). Weaning on a ventilator (IMV) requires more work for the patient due to the internal resistance of the machine. Thus, some patients with respiratory muscle weakness wean more easily on a T-tube. At best, the process of weaning from a respirator is trial and error and requires constant adjustment. When weaning is successful, the endotracheal tube is removed when the patient demonstrates the ability to cough and swallow oropharyngeal secretions. If there is persistent oropharyngeal muscle weakness, a patient may need a tracheostomy tube to prevent aspiration, even though there is excellent respiratory muscle function (see Table 154–2).

Table 154–2. Indications for Tracheostomy

1. Need for definitive airway for more than 3 weeks
2. Chronic upper airway obstruction
3. Inadequate suctioning through endotracheal tube
4. Poor patient tolerance of endotracheal tube
5. Unsuccessful tracheal intubation
6. Chronic neurologic disorder with continued risk for aspiration

Table 154–3. Criteria for Weaning from Ventilator

1. Vital capacity > 15 ml/kg
2. Inspiratory pressure > 25 torr
3. Expiratory pressure > 40 torr
4. PaO_2 > 80 torr with 40% oxygen
5. PCO_2 < 42 torr
6. Spontaneous respiratory rate < 20
7. No adverse medical conditions—fluid overload, anemia, diminished consciousness, fever, acidosis, alkalosis, gastric distension, sedative drugs, cardiac arrhythmias, renal failure, hypovolemia

References

American Thoracic Society Symposium Summary. Respiratory muscles: Structure and function. Am Rev Respir Dis 1986; 134:1078–1093.

Bach JR, O'Brien J, Krotenberg R, Alba A. Management of end stage respiratory failure in Duchenne muscular dystrophy. Muscle Nerve 1987; 10:177–182.

Cohen MS, Younger D. Aspects of the natural history of myasthenia gravis: Crisis and death. In: Grob D, ed. Myasthenia Gravis: Pathophysiology and Management. Ann NY Acad Sci 1981; 377:670–677.

Gracey DR, Divertie MB, Howard FM. Mechanical ventilation for respiratory failure in myasthenia gravis. Mayo Clin Proc 1983; 58:597–602.

Guillain-Barré Study Group. Plasmapheresis and acute Guillain-Barré syndrome. Neurology 1985; 35: 1096–1104.

Guilleminault C, Tilkian A, Dement WC. The sleep apnea syndromes. Ann Rev Med 1976; 27:465–484.

Hall JB, Wood LDH. Liberation of the patient from mechanical ventilation. JAMA 1987; 257:1621–1628.

Hill NS. Clinical applications of body ventilators. Chest 1986; 90:897–905.

Karpel JP, Aldrich TK. Respiratory failure and mechanical ventilation: Pathophysiology and methods of promoting weaning. Lung 1986; 164:309–324.

Kreitzer SM, Saunders NA, Tyler HR, et al. Respiratory muscle function in amyotrophic lateral sclerosis. Am Rev Respir Dis 1978; 117:437–447.

Ledsome JR, Sharp JM. Pulmonary function in acute cervical cord injury. Am Rev Respir Dis 1981; 124:41–44.

Make BJ, Gilmartin ME. Rehabilitation and home care for ventilator-assisted individuals. Clin Chest Med 1986; 7:679–691.

Narins RG, Emmett M. Simple and mixed acid-base disorders. A practical approach. Medicine 1980; 59:161–187.

Petty TL. Intensive and Rehabilitative Respiratory Care, 3rd ed. Philadelphia: Lea & Febiger, 1982.

Plum F, Posner JB. The Diagnosis of Stupor and Coma, 3rd ed. Philadelphia: FA Davis, 1980.

Ropper AH, Kehne SM. Guillain-Barré syndrome: Management of respiratory failure. Neurology 1985; 35:1662–1665.

Rosenow RC, Engel AG. Acid maltase deficiency in adults presenting as respiratory failure. Am J Med 1975; 64:485–491.

Rowland LP. Controversies about the treatment of myasthenia gravis. J Neurol Neurosurg Psychiatry 1980; 43:644–659.

West JB. Pulmonary Pathophysiology—The Essentials. 3rd ed, Baltimore: Williams & Wilkins, 1987.

155. PARANEOPLASTIC SYNDROMES
Michael R. Fetell

Neurologic paraneoplastic syndromes (NPS) have been described in patients with systemic neoplasms. Some, such as the Eaton-Lambert syndrome (ELS) or opsoclonus, are so characteristic that the clinician first considers an occult malignancy. Other syndromes, such as sensorimotor neuropathy, are nonspecific and association with a primary neoplasm may be difficult to prove or simply coincidental. The diagnosis is then made by excluding other causes.

NPS may be evident years before symptoms of the primary tumor or may evolve during treatment of the tumor. The oft quoted figure that 7% of patients with systemic tumor have NPS is likely an overestimate of these rare syndromes. The importance of these disorders, however, exceeds their frequency; the neurologic signs may signal the presence of a tumor, even the type of tumor. For example, small-cell or ovarian carcinoma are the two most likely tumors in patients with ELS. Hodgkin and non-Hodgkin lymphomas are most often associated with subacute motor neuronopathy. Several NPS may be found in the same patient, e.g., ELS and subacute cerebellar degeneration, ELS and subacute sensory neuropathy, or limbic encephalitis and subacute sensory neuropathy.

These disorders provide fertile ground for speculation about pathophysiology. Attention has been drawn to antibodies against neural tissues in cerebellar degeneration, Eaton-Lambert syndrome, subacute sensory neuronopathy, and retinal ganglion cell degeneration. However, the precise mechanism is obscure. Recently an antineuronal autoantibody has been identified in patients with small cell lung carcinoma and a variety of neurologic paraneoplastic syndromes, suggesting that subacute sensory neuropathy, encephalomyelitis, and autonomic dysfunction may represent different expressions of a single autoimmune paraneoplastic process. Treatment of the primary neoplasm or immunosuppressive therapy may ameliorate these disorders, but too often is ineffective.

NPS are classified according to organ or tissue of primary manifestations (Table 155–1). Small-cell lung cancer (also called oat cell carcinoma) probably arises from neural crest cells, and is by far the most common tumor associated with NPS. It also causes many other paraneoplastic syndromes such as Cushing syndrome, inappropriate ADH secretion, and presumably due to ectopic peptide secretion. Workup of a suspected case of NPS should include careful scrutiny of the chest radiograph. If physical examination (including pelvic examination), screening chemistries, blood count, and stool for occult blood are negative, the next step should probably be a CT scan of the chest, followed by a mammogram and a pelvic CT scan in women.

Diagnosis requires exclusion of other neu-

Table 155–1. Neurological Paraneoplastic Syndromes

Organ or Site	Syndrome Signs	Clinical Signs	Pathology	Primary Tumors	Evidence for Improvement of NPS with Control of Primary Tumor*	Other Treatment
Cerebrum	"Limbic encephalitis"	Seizures, myoclonus, memory loss out of proportion to dementia	Inflammation	Small cell lung Ca, Hodgkin	+	Plasmapheresis
Cerebellum	Subacute cerebellar degeneration	Ataxia, nystagmus, dysarthria	Loss of Purkinje cells; inflammation (variable)	Small cell lung Ca, ovarian Ca, Hodgkin	++	None
	Opsoclonus	Opsoclonic eye movements, myoclonus, ataxia	? Inflammation cerebellum	Neuroblastoma, ganglioneuroblastoma, small cell lung Ca	+++	ACTH
Brainstem	Brainstem encephalitis	Cranial nerve palsies	Inflammation	Small cell lung Ca	?	None
Spinal cord	Subacute necrotic myelitis	Paraplegia, quadriplegia	Myelomalacia	Lung, breast Ca, lymphoma	–	None
Anterior horn cells	Subacute motor neuronopathy	Asymmetric limb pareses, fasciculations	Degeneration of anterior horn cells	Hodgkin, other lymphomas	–	Often stabilizes
Dorsal root ganglion	Subacute sensory neuronopathy	Profound sensory (especially proprioceptive) loss	Inflammation and degeneration dorsal root ganglion cells, secondary degeneration of posterior columns	Small cell lung Ca	–	None
Peripheral nerve	Sensorimotor peripheral neuropathy	Distal weakness and sensory loss	Variable: axonal vs. demyelinating	Hodgkin, non-Hodgkin lymphoma, myeloma	–	None
Neuromuscular junction	Lambert-Eaton myasthenic syndrome	Proximal limb weakness, legs > arms, areflexia, dry mouth, impotence, muscle aches	Degeneration and atrophy presynaptic motor nerve terminals	Small cell lung Ca, ovarian Ca	+	Plasmapheresis, immunosuppression, guanidine
Muscle	Dermatomyositis	Quadriparesis, skin rash	Inflammation of muscle, perifascicular atrophy	Small cell lung Ca	+	Corticosteroids
Autonomic nervous system	Autonomic failure	Orthostatic hypotension	?	Small cell lung Ca	?	?
Eye	Photoreceptor degeneration	Visual loss, ring-like scotomata	Degeneration of photoreceptors	Small cell lung Ca, Small cell cervical Ca	+/–	+/– Corticosteroids

*+ = slight; ++ = moderate; +++ = strong; +/– = conflicting; – = none; ? = no data.

rologic disease that may be related to the tumor directly, or by metastasis, chemotherapy, radiotherapy, immunotherapy, or opportunistic infection. CT and MRI are necessary to exclude parenchymal metastasis, myelography and MRI exclude spinal metastasis, and CSF examination excludes meningeal carcinomatosis.

Limbic Encephalitis and Brainstem Encephalitis

Patients with limbic encephalitis present with dementia; characteristically, with marked impairment in memory function. Gliosis, perivascular cuffing, and microglial infiltrates with profound neuronal loss are present to various degrees at multiple levels of the neuraxis. In this sense, brainstem encephalitis (which may be manifest by central hypoventilation) is not a discrete pathologic entity, but may be a focal emphasis of a more widespread disorder. Many of the original cases of subacute cerebellar degeneration, for example, also showed evidence of brainstem or dorsal root ganglion inflammation. These pathologic findings prompt speculation of viral etiology, but no organism has been found.

The diagnosis is made clinically. It is suspected when parenchymal and meningeal metastases and metabolic encephalopathy have been excluded. CT is usually normal or reveals cortical atrophy.

Reversibility of limbic encephalitis with treatment of the primary tumor with chemotherapy implies that early diagnosis is of benefit. The syndrome has also been reported to improve with plasmapheresis.

Paraneoplastic Cerebellar Degeneration

This striking clinical syndrome develops subacutely, over days or weeks, in patients with oat cell lung carcinoma, ovarian carcinoma, or Hodgkin disease. Ataxia of trunk and limbs, dysarthria, nystagmus, and occasionally vertigo are present in varying degrees. In Brain and Wilkinson's original report, the CNS disorder preceded the discovery of the primary malignancy by up to 3 years in almost 60% of cases. Rarely, the onset of symptoms is so abrupt that it simulates encephalitis or even vascular disease, making diagnosis difficult in a patient without known malignancy. CT is normal at first, but may show cerebellar atrophy later. CSF may reveal a mild lymphocytic pleocytosis.

Pathologic examination reveals striking loss of Purkinje cells, with variable degrees of in-

flammation; anti-Purkinje cell antibodies have been identified in numerous patients but antibodies are not always present in this disorder and there are nagging questions about the specificity of the antibody reaction. One study suggested that patients with antibodies were more likely to have neurologic symptoms synchronous with, or before diagnosis of the tumor. These patients also tended to have a more severe and progressive cerebellar syndrome. These data, combined with the frequently observed improvement in the cerebellar syndrome with control of the primary tumor, make a strong case for autoimmunity in the pathogenesis. However, immunosuppression and plasmapheresis have yet to prove beneficial.

Opsoclonus

The word opsoclonus is derived from a Polish word that means "eyes dancing." It is a recognizable clinical syndrome, with chaotic conjugate saccadic eye movements often in association with myoclonus. Although it is seen with metabolic disorders, intoxications, and encephalitis, the association with occult neoplasms has drawn greatest attention. In infants and children, more than 50% of cases of opsoclonus are associated with a peripheral neuroblastoma, usually in the thorax. These children usually have less advanced neoplastic disease, but even those with higher stages of neoplasm have much better prognosis for survival than patients with equivalent-stage neuroblastoma without opsoclonus. This observation led to the hypothesis that autoimmunity both controls the tumor and leads to the paraneoplastic syndrome. However, ACTH suppresses both tumor and nontumor opsoclonus/myoclonus equally well, and even after removal or control of the neuroblastoma, ACTH may be needed to suppress opsoclonus.

In adults, opsoclonus/myoclonus occurs most often with small-cell carcinoma of lung, and usually relents when the primary tumor is controlled. Other tumors such as breast and nonsmall-cell lung carcinoma, and medullary thyroid carcinoma may produce the syndrome. Some cases show cerebellar lesions at autopsy, with degeneration of Purkinje cells, but the neurologic locus for opsoclonus is unknown. Antibodies to Purkinje cells and peripheral nerve were identified in one patient with nonneoplastic opsoclonus, and antineuronal nuclear antibodies were found in some patients with paraneoplastic opsoclonus associated with breast carcinoma.

Subacute Necrotic Myelopathy (Paraneoplastic Myelopathy)

This subacute progressive necrotic myelopathy usually affects the thoracic spinal cord. Pathologic examination frequently reveals severe myelomalacia extending over several spinal segments. It may be seen with various tumors, including carcinoma of breast and lung and lymphomas. Initially, there was some skepticism about the validity of this entity because some patients were included who had received spinal radiotherapy. The principal differential diagnoses are epidural spinal cord compression and radiation myelopathy. For diagnosis the following must be normal: myelography, spinal MRI, and CSF examination. Clinical evidence should indicate the spinal level of the lesion, which must lie outside sites of earlier radiotherapy. Although IgG antibodies reacting against tumor and normal spinal cord were found in one case, there is no evidence that the syndrome can be reversed by immunosuppression or treatment of the primary neoplasm.

Subacute Motor Neuronopathy or Paraneoplastic Anterior Horn Cell Disease

Unlike most NPS, this disorder may spontaneously arrest. It is seen in patients with lymphoma, principally Hodgkin disease, but it may also occur with non-Hodgkin lymphomas. It is the only neurologic paraneoplastic syndrome that is not to be associated with oat-cell lung cancer.

The clinical features are those of a lower motor neuron syndrome with weakness, wasting, and fasciculation in one or more limbs. Bowel and bladder functions remain unaffected. Myelography and CSF examination are normal; electromyography shows acute and chronic denervation, muscle fasciculations, and normal nerve conduction velocities. The latter two features help differentiate this disorder from motor peripheral neuropathy. On neuropathologic examination there is striking degeneration of anterior horn cells, often in a patchy fashion involving segmental areas of the spinal cord. Mild neuronal degeneration of posterior columns and intermediolateral columns is seen in some cases. There is no known treatment, but fortunately the weakness often stabilizes before disability is severe; reinervation probably explains why some patients seem to recover.

Patients with subacute motor neuronopathy lack signs of upper motor neuron disease. Reports of an ALS-like NPS and carcinoma have not been confirmed in epidemiologic studies, and the association in reported cases is probably coincidental. However, there is a growing number of patients with both upper and lower motor neuron disease in association with plasma cell dyscrasias.

Subacute Sensory Neuronopathy

Denny-Brown first described subacute sensory neuronopathy (SSN) in 1948, calling it a "unique example of deafferentation." He also appreciated the salient pathologic features of degeneration of dorsal root ganglion cells, posterior roots, and secondary degeneration of the posterior columns. Also, there may be inflammation in the dorsal root ganglions.

Patients note severe dysesthesias, loss of sensation in limbs and sometimes in the face and tongue. Sensory ataxia may be disabling. Strength is preserved if patients are asked to concentrate or look at the limb before attempting to contract the muscles. Other NPS may coexist with SSN, especially polymyositis, limbic encephalitis, or cerebellar degeneration. An antibody has been identified in patients with small-cell carcinoma of lung, which reacts with nuclei of dorsal root ganglion and other CNS nerve cells.

Peripheral Neuropathy

Symptoms of sensorimotor peripheral nerve dysfunction in patients with cancer are common, and are most often due to neurotoxicity of chemotherapeutic drugs. Distal weakness, sensory loss, and areflexia are described most often in association with Hodgkin and non-Hodgkin lymphoma. However, there is nothing clinically unique about peripheral neuropathy. Diagnosis is made by excluding other causes. There is no known treatment.

Photoreceptor Degeneration or Carcinoma-Associated Retinopathy (CAR Syndrome)

Most patients with this disorder are elderly and have subacutely progressive bilateral blindness, with ringlike scotomas. The visual loss may be episodic at first, and patients sometimes complain of bizarre visual sensations. Visual loss may precede symptoms of the malignancy by several months and may progress to blindness. Examination reveals marked narrowing of retinal arterioles. The electroretinogram (ERG) is flat.

Pathologic examination in all cases shows loss or degeneration of photoreceptors, with variable loss of cells in the outer nuclear layer. Most cases are associated with small-cell carcinoma of the lung, although it has been reported with other carcinomas of lung, histiocytic lymphoma, and carcinoma of the cervix. Antibodies against retinal ganglion and photoreceptor cells have been found in the serum; in two patients antibody reactivity was shared by similar antigens isolated from the tumor and retina. Antibody against tumor antigens may cross-react with retinal tissue to cause this disorder. Only one case has been reported with transient improvement.

Miscellaneous NPS

Many neurologic syndromes are attributed to neoplasms when no other cause is found, but their paraneoplastic basis is unproved. "Paraneoplastic" myotonia, neuromyotonia, optic neuritis, progressive supranuclear palsy, or internuclear ophthalmoplegia, either are rare forms of NPS or merely coincidental. Autonomic dysfunction in the form of orthostatic hypotension, on the other hand, has been seen with oat-cell lung cancer and pancreatic carcinoma, and may be a sympathetic nervous system analog of the cholinergic dysautonomia seen in Lambert-Eaton syndrome.

LAMBERT-EATON MYASTHENIC SYNDROME

This disorder is described in Section 128, Other Disorders of Neuromuscular Transmissions.

DERMATOMYOSITIS

This entity is discussed in detail in Section 134.

Nonmetastatic Cerebrovascular Diseases

Cancer may affect the nervous system secondarily, by predisposing to cerebral thrombosis, embolism, or hemorrahge. Some causes are considered briefly here and are discussed more fully in Chapter V, Tumor, or the effects of chemotherapy, may cause thrombocytopenia that may lead to intracerebral, subarachnoid, subdural, or spinal hemorrhage. Hepatic disease can depress production of clotting factors and lead to a hemorrhagic diathesis.

Thrombosis of small intracerebral vessels due to sludging occurs in leukemias when the leukocyte count is over 150,000. Mucin-producing adenocarcinomas are particularly prone to cause marantic endocarditis or nonbacterial thrombotic vegetations on heart valves. *Disseminated intravascular coagulopathy* (DIC) is often present, diagnosed by an elevation of serum fibrin degradation products. The brain is a site for embolism in nonbacterial endocarditis in 33 to 50% of cases. Even when diagnosed during life, there is no known treatment that can inhibit further embolization, although heparin may be of benefit if DIC is present.

A hypercoagulable state is suspected to be the cause of the nonmetastatic cerebral venous sinus thrombosis. The disorder occurs mostly in patients with hematologic malignancies. Patients develop acute signs and symptoms of increased intracranial pressure, with headache, papilledema, lethargy, and seizures and hemipareses due to superior sagittal sinus thrombosis. The CSF may be mildly hemorrhagic, with a moderate number of red blood cells. Angiography was long considered the only definitive diagnostic study, but sometimes CT can show a "delta sign" in the region of the torcula, and sagittal MRI may clearly delineate the site of sinus occlusion.

References

General

Anderson NE, Rosenblum MK, Graus F, Wiley RG, Posner JB. Antibodies in paraneoplastic syndromes associated with small-cell lung cancer. Neurology 1988; 38:1391–1399.

Brain L, Norris FH, eds. The Remote Effects of Cancer on the Nervous System. New York: Grune & Stratton, 1965.

Chad DA, Recht L. Neurological paraneoplastic syndromes. Cancer Investigation 1988; 61:67–82.

Henson RA, Urich H. Cancer and the nervous system: The neurological manifestations of systemic malignant disease. Boston: Blackwell, 1982.

Markman M. Response of paraneoplastic syndromes to antineoplastic therapy. West J Med 1986; 144: 580–585.

Spence AM, Sumi SM, Ruff R. Remote effects of cancer in the CNS. Curr Cancer 1983; 8(3):4–43.

Limbic Encephalitis

Jaeckle K, Rogers L, Wong M. Autoimmune paraneoplastic limbic encephalitis. Neurology 1988; 38(Suppl 1):390.

Brennan LV, Craddock PR. Limbic encephalopathy as a nonmetastatic complication of oat cell lung cancer. Its reversal after treatment of the primary lung lesion. Am J Med 1983; 75:518–520.

Case Records of the Massachusetts General Hospital. Case #30-1985. N Engl J Med 1985; 313:249–257.

Corsellis JAN, Goldberg GJ, Norton AP. Limbic encephalitis and its association with carcinoma. Brain 1968; 91:481–496.

Dorfman LJ, Forno LS. Paraneoplastic encephalomyelitis. Acta Neurol Scand 1972; 48:556–574.

Glaser GH, Pincus JH. Limbic encephalitis. J Nerv Ment Dis 1969; 149:59–67.

Shapiro WR. Remote effects of neoplasm on the central nervous system: Encephalopathy. Adv Neurol 1976; 15:101–117.

Brainstem Encephalitis

Dietl HW, Pulst SM, Engelhardt P, et al. Paraneoplastic brainstem encephalitis with acute dystonia and central hypoventilation. J Neurol 1982; 227:229–238.

Kaplan AM, Itabashi HH. Encephalitis associated with carcinoma: Central hypoventilation syndrome and cytoplasmic inclusion bodies. J Neurol Neurosurg Psychiatry 1974; 37:1166–1176.

Paraneoplastic Cerebellar Degeneration

Anderson NE, Rosenblum MK, Posner JB. Paraneoplastic cerebellar degeneration; clinical-immunologic correlations. Ann Neurol 1988; 24:559–567.

Brain L, Wilkinson M. Subacute cerebellar degeneration associated with neoplasms. Brain 1965; 88:465–478.

Cocconi G, Ceci G, Juvarra G, et al. Successful treatment of subacute cerebellar degeneration in ovarian carcinoma with plasmapheresis. A case report. Cancer 1985; 56:2318–2320.

Cunningham J, Graus F, Anderson N, et al. Partial characterization of the Purkinje cell antigens in paraneoplastic cerebellar degeneration. Neurology 1986; 36:1163–1168.

Greenberg HS. Paraneoplastic cerebellar degeneration. J Neurooncol 1984; 2:377–382.

Greenlee JE, Brashear HB. Antibodies to cerebellar Purkinje cells in patients with paraneoplastic cerebellar degeneration and ovarian carcinoma. Ann Neurol 1983; 14:609–613.

Jaeckle KA, Graus F, Houghton A, et al. Autoimmune response of patients with paraneoplastic cerebellar degeneration to a Purkinje cell cytoplasmic protein antigen. Ann Neurol 1985; 18:592–600.

Kearsley JH, Johnson P, Halmagyi GM. Paraneoplastic cerebellar disease: Remission with excision of the primary tumor. Arch Neurol 1985; 42:1208–1210.

Paone JF, Jeyasingham K. Remission of cerebellar dysfunction after pneumonectomy for bronchogenic carcinoma. N Engl J Med 1980; 302:156.

Ridley A, Kennard C, Scholtz CL, et al. Omnipause neurons in two cases of opsoclonus associated with oat cell carcinoma of the lung. Brain 1987; 110:1699–1710.

Tanaka K, Yamazaki M, Sato S, et al. Antibodies to brain proteins in paraneoplastic cerebellar degeneration. Neurology 1986; 36:1169–1172.

Trotter JL, Hendin BA, Osterland CK. Cerebellar degeneration with Hodgkin Disease. Arch Neurol 1976; 33:660–661.

Opsoclonus

Altman AJ, Baehner RL. Favorable prognosis for survival in children with coincident opso-myoclonus and neuroblastoma. Cancer 1976; 37:846–852.

Bray PF, Ziter FA, Lahey ME, et al. The coincidence of neuroblastoma and acute cerebellar encephalopathy. J Pediatr 1969; 75:983–990.

Budde-Steffen C, Anderson NE, Rosenblum MK, et al. An antineuronal antibody in paraneoplastic opsoclonus. Ann Neurol 1988; 23:528–531.

Cawley LP, James VL, Minart BJ, et al. Antibodies to Purkinje cells and peripheral nerve in opsoclonia. Lancet 1984; 1:509–510.

Digre KB. Opsoclonus in adults: Report of three cases and review of the literature. Arch Neurol 1986; 43:1165–1175.

Dropcho E, Payne R. Paraneoplastic opsoclonus-myoclonus: Association with medullary thyroid carcinoma and review of the literature. Arch Neurol 1986; 43:410–415.

Ellenberger C, Campa JF, Netsky MG. Opsoclonus and parenchymatous degeneration of the cerebellum. Neurology 1968; 18:1041–1046.

Graus F, Cordon-Cardo C, Cho ES, et al. Opsoclonus and oat cell carcinoma of lung: Lack of evidence for anti-CNS antibodies. Lancet 1984; 1:1479.

Paraneoplastic Myelopathy

Babikian VL, Stefansson K, Dieperink ME, et al. Paraneoplastic myelopathy: Antibodies against protein in normal spinal cord and underlying neoplasm. Lancet 1985; 2:49–50.

Lester EP, Feld E, Kinzie JJ, et al. Necrotizing myelopathy complicating Hodgkin's Disease. Arch Neurol 1979; 36:583–585.

Mancall EL, Rosales RK. Necrotizing myelopathy associated with visceral carcinoma. Brain 1964; 87:639–656.

Ojeda VJ. Necrotizing myelopathy associated with malignancy. Cancer 1984; 53:1115–1123.

Renkawek K, Kida E. Combined acute necrotic myelopathy (ANM) and cerebellar degeneration associated with malignant disease. Clin Neuropathol 1983; 2:90–94.

Richter RB, Moore RV. Non-invasive central nervous system disease associated with lymphoid tumors. Johns Hopkins Med J 1968; 122:271–283.

Subacute Motor Neuronopathy and Motor Neuron Disease

Rowland LP, Schneck SA. Neuromuscular disorders associated with malignant neoplastic disease. J Chronic Dis 1963; 16:777–795.

Schold SC, Cho E-S. Somasundaram M, et al. Subacute motor neuronopathy; A remote effect of lymphoma. Ann Neurol 1979; 5:271–287.

Shy ME, Rowland LP, Smith T, et al. Motor neuron disease and plasma cell dyscrasia. Neurology 1986; 36:1429–1436.

Walton JN, Tomlinson BE, Pearce GW. Subacute "poliomyelitis" and Hodgkin's disease. J Neurol Sci 1968; 6:435–445.

Subacute Sensory Neuropathy

Denny-Brown D. Primary sensory neuropathy with muscular changes associated with carcinoma. J Neurol Neurosurg Psychiatry 1948; 11:73–87.

Graus F, Elkon KB, Cordon-Cardo C, et al. Sensory neuronopathy and small cell lung cancer. Antineuronal antibody that also reacts with the tumor. Am J Med 1986; 80:45–52.

Horwich MS, Cho L, Porro RS, et al. Subacute sensory neuropathy: A remote effect of carcinoma. Ann Neurol 1977; 2:7–19.

Ohnishi A, Ogawa M. Preferential loss of large lumbar primary sensory neurons in carcinomatous sensory neuropathy. Ann Neurol 1986; 20:102–104.

Vick N, Schulman S, Dau P. Carcinomatous cerebellar degeneration, encephalomyelitis, and sensory neuropathy (radiculitis). Neurology 1969; 19:425–441.

Wilkinson PC. Serological findings in carcinomatous neuromyopathy. Lancet 1964; 1:1301–1303.

Carcinomatous Photoreceptor Degeneration

Grunwald GB, Kornguth SE, Towfighi, et al. Autoimmune basis for visual paraneoplastic syndrome in patients with small cell lung carcinoma. Cancer 1987; 60:780–787.

Grunwald GB, Klein R, Simmonds MA, et al. Autoimmune basis for visual paraneoplastic syndrome in patients with small-cell carcinoma. Lancet 1985; 1:658–661.

Keltner JL, Roth AM, Chang RS. Photoreceptor degeneration: Possible autoimmune disorder. Arch Ophthalmol 1983; 101:564–569.

Kinglele TG, Burde RM, Rapazzo JA, et al. Paraneoplastic retinopathy. J Clin Neuro Ophthalmol 1984; 4:239–245.

Kornguth SE, Klein R, Appen R, et al. Occurrence of anti-retinal ganglion cell antibodies in patients with small cell carcinoma of the lung. Cancer 1982; 50:1289–1293.

Sawyer RA, Selhorst JB, Zimmerman LE, et al. Blindness caused by photoreceptor degeneration as a remote effect of cancer. Am J Ophthalmol 1976; 81:606–613.

Thirkill CE, Roth AM, Keltner JL. Cancer-associated retinopathy. Arch Ophthalmol 1987; 105:372–375.

Autonomic Dysfunction

Chiappa KH, Young RR. A case of paracarcinomatous pandysautonomia. Neurology 1973; 23:423.

Green GJ, Breckenridge AM, Wright FK. Severe orthostatic hypotension associated with carcinoma of the bronchus. Postgrad Med J 1979; 55:426–429.

Khurana RK, Koski CL, Mayer RF. Dysautonomia in Eaton-Lambert syndrome. Ann Neurol 1983; 14:123.

Park DM, Johnson RH, Crean GP, et al. Orthostatic hypotension in bronchial carcinoma. Br Med J 1972; 3:510–511.

Thomas JP, Sheilds R. Associated autonomic dysfunction and carcinoma of the pancreas. Br Med J 1970; 4:32–.

Lambert-Eaton Myasthenic Syndrome

Dau PC, Denys EH. Plasmapheresis and immunosuppressive drug therapy in the Eaton-Lambert syndrome. Ann Neurol 1982; 11:570–575.

Kim Y. Passively transferred Lambert-Eaton Syndrome in mice receiving purified IgG. Muscle Nerve 1986; 9:52?–5?0.

Lauritzen M, Smith T, Fischer-Hansen B. Eaton-Lambert syndrome and malignant thymoma. Neurology 1980; 30:634–638.

Lennon WA, Lambert EH, Whittingham S, et al. Autoimmunity in the Lambert-Eaton myasthenic syndrome. Muscle Nerve 1982; 5:S21–S25.

Newson-Davis J, Murray NMF. Plasma exchange and immunosuppressive drug treatment in the Lambert-Eaton myasthenic syndrome. Neurology 1984; 34:480–485.

O'Neill JH, Murray NMF, Newsom-Davis J. The Lambert-Eaton myasthenic syndrome. A review of 50 cases. Brain 1988; 111:577–596.

Dermatomyositis

Barnes BE. Dermatomyositis and malignancy. A review of the literature. Ann Intern Med 1976; 84:68–76.

Bohan A, Peter JB, Bowman RL, et al. A computer-assisted analysis of 153 patients with polymyositis and dermatomyositis. Medicine 1977; 56:255–286.

Lakhanpal S, Bunch TW, Ilstrup DM, et al. Polymyositis-dermatomyositis and malignant lesions: Does an association exist? Mayo Clin Proc 1986; 61:645–653.

Nonmetastatic Cerebrovascular Diseases

Bedikian A, Valdivieso M, Luna M, et al. Nonbacterial thrombotic endocarditis in cancer patients: Comparison of characteristics of patients with and without concomitant disseminated intravascular coagulation. Med Ped Oncol 1978; 4:149–157.

Biller J, Challa VR, Toole JF, et al. Nonbacterial thrombotic endocarditis. A neurological perspective of clinicopathological correlations of 99 patients. Arch Neurol 1982; 39:95–98.

Case Records of the Massachusetts General Hospital: Case #27-1980. N Engl J Med 1980; 303:92–100.

CPC: The consequences of the inconsequential: marantic (nonbacterial thrombotic) endocarditis. Am Heart J 1979; 98:513–522.

Graus F, Rogers LR, Posner JB. Cerebrovascular complications in patients with cancer. Medicine 1985; 64:16–35.

Hickey WF, Garnick MB, Henderson IC, et al. Primary cerebral venous thrombosis in patients with cancer— a rarely diagnosed paraneoplastic syndrome. Am J Med 1982; 73:740–750.

Johnson PC, Rolak LA, Hamilton RH, et al. Paraneoplastic vasculitis of nerve: A remote effect of cancer. Ann Neurol 1979; 5:437–444.

Kooker JG, MacLean JM, Sumi SM. Cerebral embolism, marantic endocarditis, and cancer. Arch Neurol 1976; 33:260–264.

McKee LC Jr, Collins RD. Intravascular leukocyte thrombi and aggregates as a cause of morbidity and mortality in leukemia. Medicine 1974; 53:463–478.

Ondrias F, Slugen I, Valach A. Malignant tumors and embolizing paraneoplastic endocarditis. Neoplasma 1985; 35:135–140.

Reagan TJ, Okazaki H. The thrombotic syndrome associated with carcinoma. A clinical and pathological study. Arch Neurol 1974; 31:390–395.

Sigsbee B, Deck MDF, Posner JB. Non-metastatic superior saggital sinus thrombosis complicating systemic cancer. Neurology 1979; 29:139–146.

---

156. NUTRITIONAL DEFICIENCY AND GASTROINTESTINAL DISEASE
Lewis P. Rowland

Malnutrition is still a serious problem throughout the world. In poor countries, dietary deficiency is common. In industrial countries, nutritional syndromes are more likely to be seen in alcoholics, in patients with chronic bowel disease, or after some medical treatment that interferes with essential elements of diet (Table 156–1). Even if the acute disorders are corrected, there may be long-term effects: maternal malnutrition may affect the fetus to cause mental retardation; on another level, chronic neurologic syndromes persisted in World War II prisoners long after they had resumed a normal diet.

Dietary therapy may be important to the management of some inborn errors of metabolism to prevent accumulation of some toxic substances (as in phenylketonuria) or to am-

Table 156–1.   Neurologic Syndromes Attributed to Nutritional Deficiency

Site of Major Syndrome	Name
Encephalon	Hypocalcemia (lack of vitamin D), tetany, seizures
	Mental retardation (protein-calorie deprivation)
	Cretinism (lack of iodine)
	Wernicke-Korsakoff syndrome (thiamine)
Corpus callosum	Marchiafava-Bignami disease
Optic nerve	Tobacco-alcohol amblyopia
Brain stem	Central pontine myelinolysis
Cerebellum	Alcoholic cerebellar degeneration
	Vitamin E deficiency in bowel disease
Spinal cord	Combined system disease (B_{12} deficiency)
	Tropical spastic paraparesis (some forms ?)
Peripheral nerves	Beriberi (thiamine), pellagra (nicotinic acid)
	Hypophosphatemia (?)
	Tetany (vitamin D deficiency)
Muscle	Myopathy of osteomalacia

plify the activity of a mutant enzyme (as in vitamin B_6-responsive homocystinuria).

Diseases due to malnutrition may arise if essential nutrients are not provided because the diet is inadequate. The result may be the same if nutrients are lost by vomiting or diarrhea, if there is malabsorption, if use of a nutrient is impaired, or if the target organ is unresponsive to a mediating hormone.

Examples of different syndromes are found in other chapters of this book; a simple listing or table is a gross oversimplification for two reasons. First, vitamin deficiency is likely to be multiple and often accompanied by protein-calorie malnutrition; thus, the resulting syndromes are complex. Second, it is possible to tabulate the major target system of a particular syndrome, although most involve more than one system; spinal cord syndromes and encephalopathy, for example, may be more prominent than the peripheral neuropathy of pellagra. In contrast, peripheral neuropathy, optic neuropathy, or dementia may be seen in patients with combined system disease of the spinal cord due to vitamin B_{12} deficiency. Some neurologic syndromes are attributable to dietary excess (Table 156–2). For this reason, too, the syndromes are likely to be complex.

Only a brief overview will be offered of disorders of the stomach and intestine. The major neurologic syndrome of stomach disease results from lack of intrinsic factor and B_{12} deficiency. There are no major neurologic consequences of peptic ulcer (other than those that might result from shock after massive hemorrhage), but treatment of the ulcer may

lead to a neurologic disorder. Antacids may cause a partial malabsorption syndrome. Cimetidine therapy avoids these problems but may cause an acute confusional state. Surgical therapy may cure the ulcer, but may also create a neurologic disorder due to malabsorption.

Malabsorption syndromes may arise for any of several reasons (Table 156–3). In patients with these disorders, neurologic abnormalities seem to be disproportionately frequent. Alone, or in combinations, there may be evidence of myopathy, sensorimotor peripheral neuropathy, degeneration of corticospinal tracts and posterior columns, and cerebellar abnormality. Optic neuritis, atypical pigmentary degeneration of the retina, and dementia are less common signs of malabsorption syndromes.

There seem to have been three waves of explanation. First, the syndromes were attributed to vitamin B_{12} deficiency, which probably accounted for some but not all cases; many patients had normal serum B_{12} levels and did not respond to vitamin B_{12} therapy. Then there was considerable interest in the relation of the neurologic abnormality to osteomalacia, which often appeared in the same patients. Osteomalacia also accompanied similar neurologic syndromes in patients who had dietary problems other than malabsorption (e.g., lack of sunlight or dietary vitamin D, resistance to vitamin D, renal disease, ingestion of anticonvulsant drugs). However, osteomalacia or vitamin D deficiency was hard to prove in some cases and there was often no response to vitamin D therapy. Now

Table 156–2. Neurologic Syndromes Attributed to Dietary Excess

Syndrome	Condition	Agent
Increased intracranial pressure	Self-medication	Vitamin A
Encephalopathy	Phenylketonuria	Phenylalanine
	Water intoxication	Water
	Hepatic encephalopathy	Protein (and NH_3)
	Ketotic or nonketotic coma in diabetes	Glucose
Strokes	Hyperlipidemia	Lipid
Peripheral neuropathy	Hypochondriasis	Pyridoxine

there is growing evidence that some of these syndromes are due to lack of vitamin E, and although the pathogenesis is not known, the neurologic disorders can sometimes be corrected by administering large doses of vitamin E (up to 4 g daily of alpha tocopherol). The diagnosis can be suspected if autofluorescent inclusions of lipochrome pigment are seen in muscle biopsy.

Another unusual syndrome of malabsorption is episodic abnormality of sleep, thirst,

Table 156–3. Some Causes of Neurologic Disorder Due to Malabsorption

Defective intraluminal hydrolysis	Gastric resection
	Pancreatic insufficiency
	Exclusion or deficiency of bile salts
Primary mucosal cell abnormality	Celiac disease
	A-beta-lipoproteinemia
Inadequate absorption surface	Massive small gut resection
	Ileal resection or by-pass
	Jejunal bypass
	Jejunocolic fistula
	Gastroileostomy
Abnormalities of intestinal wall	Ileojejunitis
	Amyloidosis
	Radiation injury
Lymphatic obstruction and stasis	Lymphoma
	Tuberculosis
Bacterial overgrowth and parasitic infections	Blind loops
	Jejunal diverticula
	Scleroderma
	Whipple disease
	Tropical sprue
	D-lactic acidosis
Miscellaneous	Diabetic neuropathy
	Hypoparathyroidism
	Hypothyroidism

(From Glickman R. In: Wyngaarden JB, Smith LH Jr, eds. Cecil's Textbook of Medicine, 16th ed. Philadelphia: WB Saunders, 1982:678–690.)

hunger, and mood, a combination that suggests a hypothalamic disorder. This has been attributed to bacterial overgrowth with production of D-lactic acid. Whether D-lactic acid or something else is the actual neurotoxin is uncertain, but treatment with oral antibiotics has abolished the syndrome in several patients.

Chronic diarrhea from any cause, including malabsorption or abuse of laxatives, may cause hypokalemia with resulting chronic myopathy, acute paralysis, or acute myoglobinuria. Acute hypophosphatemia may arise in alcoholics who are being treated for loss of fluids and electrolytes, and it may follow hyperalimentation. In these circumstances, limb weakness may simulate Guillain-Barré syndrome, or the acute electrolyte disorder may actually precipitate the neuropathy; seizures and coma may be part of the picture.

There are some conditions in which diarrhea accompanies (but is not thought to cause) the neurologic disorder. The combination of diarrhea, orthostatic hypotension, and peripheral neuropathy suggests the possibility of amyloid disease or diabetes mellitus. The combination of chronic diarrhea, arthritis, and dementia or other cerebral disorder suggests *Whipple disease*.

References

Carr DB, Shih VE, Richter JM, Martin JB. D-lactic acidosis simulating a hypothalamic syndrome after bowel bypass. Ann Neurol 1982; 11:195–197.

Dahlquist NR, Perrault J, Callaway CW, Jones JD. D-lactic acidosis and encephalopathy after jejunoileostomy: Response to overfeeding and to fasting in humans. Mayo Clin Proc 1984; 59:141–145.

Dodge PR, Prensky SL, Feigin R. Nutrition and the developing nervous system. St. Louis: CV Mosby, 1977.

Feurle GE, Volk B, Waldherr R. Cerebral Whipple's disease with negative jejunal histology. N Engl J Med 1979; 300:907–909.

Gill GV, Bell DR. Persisting nutritional neuropathy amongst former war prisoners. J Neurol Neurosurg Psychiatry 1982; 45:861–865.

Glickman R. Malabsorption syndromes. In: Wyngaarden JB, Smith LH Jr (eds). Cecil's Textbook of Medicine, 16th ed. Philadelphia: WB Saunders, 1982: 678–690.

Guggenheim MA, Ringel SP, Silverman A, Grabert BE. Progressive neuromuscular disease in children with chronic cholestasis and vitamin E deficiency; diagnosis and treatment with alpha tocopherol. J Pediatr 1982; 100:51–58.

Harding AE, Muller DPR, Thomas PK, Willison HJ. Spinocerebellar degeneration secondary to chronic intestinal malabsorption: a vitamin E deficiency syndrome. Ann Neurol 1982; 12:419–424.

Insogna KL, Bordley DR, Caro JF, Lockwood DH. Osteomalacia and weakness from excessve antacid ingestion. JAMA 1980; 244:2544–2546.

Kaplan JG, Pack D, Hourupian D, DeSousa T, Brin M, Schaumberg H. Distal axonopathy associated with chronic gluten enteropathy: A treatable disorder. Neurology 1988; 38:642–645.

Krendel DA, Gilchrist JM, Johnson AO, Bossen EH. Isolated deficiency of vitamin E with progressive neurologic deterioration. Neurology. 1987; 37:538–540.

Kinney HC, Burger PC, Hurwitz BJ, Hijmans JC, Grant JP. Degeneration of the central nervous system associated with celiac disease. J Neurol Sci 1982; 53:9–22.

Malouf R, Brust JCM. Hypoglycemia: Causes, neurological manifestations, and outcome. Ann Neurol 1985; 17:321–430.

Mitchell JE, Seim HC, Colon E, Pomeroy C. Medical complications and medical management of bulimia. Ann Int Med 1987; 107:71–77.

Muller DPR, Lloyd JK, Wolff OH. Vitamin E and neurological function. Lancet 1983; 1:225–228.

Pallis CA, Lewis PD. The Neurology of Gastrointestinal Disease. Philadelphia: WB Saunders, 1974.

Parry GJ, Bredsen DE. Sensory neuropathy with low-dose pyridoxine. Neurology 1985; 35:1466–1468.

Rippe DJ, Edwards MK, D'Amour PG, Holden RW, Roos KL. MR imaging of central pontine myelinolysis. JCAT 1987; 11:724–726.

Roos D. Neurological complications in patients with impaired vitamin B_{12} absorption following partial gastrectomy. Acta Neurol Scand 1978; 59 (suppl 69):1–77.

Rosenberg M, McCarten JR, Snyder BD, Tulloch JW. Hypophosphatemia with reversible ataxia and quadriparesis. Am J Med Sci 1987; 293:261–264.

Schott GD, Wills MR. Muscle weakness in osteomalacia. Lancet 1976; 1:626–629.

Sitrin MD, Lieberman F, Jensen WE, Noronha A, Milburn C, Addington W. Vitamin E deficiency and neurologic disease in adults with cystic fibrosis. Ann Intern Med 1987; 107:51–54.

Smiddy WE, Green WR. Nutritional amblyopia. A histopathologic study with retrospective clinical correlation. Graefe's Arch Clin Exp Ophthalmol 1987; 225:321–324.

Sokol RJ, Kayden NJ, Bettis DB et al. Isolated vitamin E deficiency in the absence of fat malabsorption: familial and sporadic cases. J Lab Clin Med 1988; 111:548–559.

Traber MG, Sokol RJ, Ringel SP, Neville HE, Thellman CA, Kayden HJ. Lack of tocopherol in peripheral nerves of vitamin E-deficient patients with peripheral neuropathy. N Engl J Med 1987; 317:262–265.

Weintraub MI. Hypophosphatemia mimicking acute Guillain-Barré-Strohl syndrome. A complication of parenteral alimentation. JAMA 1980; 235:1040–1041.

Winick M. Malnutrition and the Brain. New York: Oxford University Press, 1976.

Yokota T, Wada Y, Furukawa T, Tsukagoshi H, Uchihara T, Watabiki S. Adult-onset spinocerebellar syndrome with idiopathic vitamin E deficiency. Ann Neurol 1987; 22:84–87.

157. COLLAGEN-VASCULAR DISEASE
Lewis P. Rowland

Several different syndromes are commonly linked because they are characterized by the combination of arthritis, rash, and visceral disorders. Because arthritis is common to all, and because fibrinoid degeneration of blood vessels is common, they are frequently called *collagen-vascular diseases*. However, inflammatory lesions of the blood vessels also characterize syndromes in which the vascular lesions are the dominant pathologic change. Periarteritis nodosa was the model vasculitis, but classification of related syndromes depended on autopsy evaluation of histologic changes in the arteries, whether large or small vessels were involved, and which organs were most affected. Similar classifications were applied to clinical diagnosis, but overlap between syndromes and lack of knowledge of pathogenesis obscure the area. Some of these diseases seem due to the deposition of circulating immune complexes within vessel walls, and some may be due to persistent viral infection. Nevertheless, the classification of Christian and Sergent is useful (Table 157–1), and some syndromes have such characteristic clinical and neurologic manifestations that they warrant individual discussion (Table 157–2). Clinical disorders of brain, spinal cord, peripheral nerve, and muscle are prominent in these diseases.

Polyarteritis Nodosa

Polyarteritis nodosa is a form of inflammatory arteritis affecting any of the small, medium, and occasionally even large arteries. It is characterized by nonspecific symptoms commonly associated with an infection or signs and symptoms involving abdominal organs, joints, peripheral nerves, muscles, or CNS.

Etiology. The cause of polyarteritis nodosa is unknown. Streptococcus infections, Australia antigen or other viral causes such as hepatitis B virus or bacterial hyperergy have been suggested as possible causes. The disease is occasionally associated with a rheumatic fever diathesis. The coincidence of this

**Table 157–1. Clinical Classification of
Vasculitis Syndromes**

Characterized by Necrotizing Vasculitis:

Temporal arteritis	Henoch-Schonlein
Wegener	purpura
granulomatosis	Periarteritis nodosa
Aortic arch arteritis	Cogan syndrome

Occasionally Complicated by Necrotizing Vasculitis:

Rheumatic diseases: rheumatoid arthritis; systemic lupus erythematosus; rheumatic fever.

Infections: hepatitis B; acute respiratory infections; streptococcal infection; poststreptococcal glomerulonephritis; bacterial endocarditis.

Respiratory diseases: Loeffler syndrome; asthma; serous otitis media.

Hypersensitivity: serum sickness; drug allergy; amphetamine abuse.

Plasma cell dyscrasias: essential cryoglobulinemia; myeloma; macroglobulinemia.

Others: dermatomyositis; dermal vasculitis; ulcerative colitis; colon carcinoma.

(From Christian CL, Sergent JS. Am J Med 1976; 60:549–550.)

condition with asthma, serum sickness, and reactions to drugs speaks strongly for hypersensitivity as an etiologic factor. This hypothesis was supported by the work of Rich, who years ago reproduced the lesions in rabbits by repeated injection of horse serum. Antigen-antibody complexes (immune complex disease) may be an important contributing cause of polyarteritis nodosa. In experimental studies of immune complex disease, the vascular lesions in animals that follow injections of heterologous serum (serum sickness model) are pathologically similar to those of human polyarteritis nodosa. The role of hepatitis B virus in causing immune complex disorders or polyarteritis nodosa is uncertain; immune complexes have been demonstrated in vessels in the absence of vasculitis, but with evidence of chronic aggressive hepatitis.

Pathology. There is widespread panarteritis. The pathology in the nervous system includes infiltrates in the adventitia and vasa vasorum; polymorphonuclear leukocytes, and eosinophils. Necrosis of the media and elastic membrane occurs and may lead to formation of multiple small aneurysms. As these become fibrotic, they may rupture; proliferation of intima may lead to thrombosis of vessels. Repair and fibrosis of the aneurysms lead to a characteristic beading appearance caused by the nodules.

Incidence. Polyarteritis nodosa is rare, but when it occurs, the CNS is involved in about 25% of cases. Both genders are affected. The disease may occur at any age, but more than 50% of the reported cases are in the third or fourth decades of life.

Signs and Symptoms. Onset may be acute or insidious. Fever, malaise, tachycardia, sweating, fleeting edema, weakness, and pains in the joints, muscles, or abdomen are common early symptoms (Tables 157–3 and 157–4). Blood pressure may be elevated and there may be a moderate or severe anemia with leukocytosis.

Visceral lesions occur in most cases. Kidney involvement produces symptoms and signs similar to acute glomerular nephritis. Cutaneous hemorrhages, erythematous eruptions, and tender reddened subcutaneous nodules may appear in the skin of the trunk or limbs. Gastrointestinal, hepatic, renal, or cardiac symptoms may develop.

Involvement of peripheral nerves is most common. This may take the form of mononeuritis multiplex or a diffuse symmetric sensorimotor neuropathy. Sympathetic nerves may be affected with changes in the size and shape of the pupils and impairment of the reaction to light. Damage to the nerves is presumably due to ischemia secondary to involvement of the nutrient arteries.

Damage to cerebral arteries may lead to thrombosis or hemorrhage. Large vessels are rarely affected but rupture of the basilar artery has been reported. Symptoms of involvement of the spinal vessels are rare.

The most common manifestations of cerebral involvement are headache, convulsions, blurred vision, vertigo, sudden loss of vision in one eye, and confusional states or organic psychosis.

A disorder characterized by keratitis and deafness in nonsyphilitic individuals is called the *Cogan syndrome.* It occurs predominantly in young adults with negative blood and CSF tests for syphilis and no stigmata of congenital syphilis. The cause of the keratitis and deafness is not known, but cases have been reported in which the syndrome was one feature of polyarteritis nodosa. Symptoms begin suddenly, involving the cornea and both divisions of the eighth nerve. The eye and the eighth nerve are usually involved simultaneously, but there may be several weeks or months between the onset of symptoms in the eye and the ear. Affection of the eighth nerve is usually signaled by nausea, vomiting, tinnitus, and loss of hearing. With progression of the hearing loss to complete deafness, the vestibular symptoms subside.

Table 157–2.   Syndromes Associated With Systemic Vasculitis

Syndrome	Systemic Manifestations	Laboratory Abnormalities	Neurologic Syndromes
Systemic vasculitis (periarteritis nodosa)	Skin, kidneys, joints, lungs, hypertension; abdominal pain; heart	Serum complement decreased; immune complexes; hepatitis B antigen and antibody; rheumatoid factor	Peripheral neuropathy; mononeuritis multiplex; stroke; polymyositis
Wegener granulomatosis	Nose, paranasal sinuses, lungs, other viscera	As above; also increased serum IgE	Peripheral or cranial neuropathy; encephalopathy
Churg-Strauss vasculitis	Lungs, other viscera	As above; also eosinophilia	
Temporal arteritis (giant cell arteritis)	Fever, malaise, myalgia, weight loss, claudication of chewing	Increased ESR	Visual loss due to lesions of optic nerve or retina; papilledema; stroke rare
Polymyalgia rheumatica	Fever, malaise; myalgia, weight loss	Increased ESR	None
Cogan syndrome	Interstitial keratitis, aortic insufficiency; occasionally other viscera	Increased ESR; CSF pleocytosis	Vestibular or auditory loss; peripheral neuropathy; stroke; encephalomyelopathy
Takayasu syndrome (aortic arch disease; pulseless disease)	Cataracts, retinal atrophy; cranial muscular wasting; claudication loss of peripheral pulses; heart	Increased ESR	Stroke; amaurosis fugax; visual loss
Granulomatous angiitis of the brain	None	CSF pleocytosis, increased protein content, normal sugar	Somnolence, confusion; encephalomyelopathy; myeloradiculoneuropathy
Systemic lupus erythematosus	Skin, lungs, kidneys, joints, liver, heart, Raynaud, fever	Leukopenia, multiple autoantibodies, increased ESR; evidence of renal or hepatic disease	Organic psychosis; seizures; chorea; myelopathy; peripheral neuropathy; polymyositis; aseptic meningitis
Systemic sclerosis	Skin, lungs, GI tract, kidneys, heart, joints, Raynaud	None characteristic except disordered mobility of esophagus and bowel	Polymyositis
Rheumatoid arthritis	Joints; viscera occasionally	Rheumatoid factor	Polymyositis; mononeuritis multiplex, peripheral neuropathy
Dermatomyositis	Skin, by definition; lungs; GI tract, rare	Inflammatory cells in muscle	Polymyositis
Mixed connective tissue disease (sclerodermatomyositis?)	Skin lesions of dermatomyositis or scleroderma; joints; Raynaud; lungs; esophagus	Antibody to extractable nuclear ribonucleoprotein	Polymyositis

(From Cupps TR, Fauci AS. Adv Intern Med 1982; 27:315–324.)

Laboratory Data. There is a leukocytosis with an inconstant eosinophilia. Nontreponemal serologic tests for syphilis may be positive and there may be positive skin and serologic tests for trichinosis. CSF is normal unless there has been a meningeal hemorrhage.

Diagnosis. Diagnosis of polyarteritis nodosa should be considered in all patients with an obscure febrile illness with symptoms of involvement of the nervous system (particularly chronic peripheral neuropathy) and other organs. The diagnosis can often be established by biopsy of sural nerve, muscle, or testicle.

Course and Prognosis. Prognosis is poor. Death usually occurs because of lesions of the kidneys, other abdominal viscera, or the heart; occasionally, lesions in the brain or peripheral nerves may cause death. Duration of life after onset of symptoms varies from a few months to several years. Spontaneous healing of the arteritis may occur and is followed by remission of all symptoms and signs, including those due to involvement of the peripheral nerves.

Table 157–3. Clinical Features in Patients* with Polyarteritis Nodosa

Clinical Manifestation	%	Number of Patients
Fever	71	460
Weight loss	54	405
Organ System Involvement		
Kidney	70	375
Musculoskeletal system	64	301
Arthritis/arthralgia	53	301
Myalgias	31	238
Hypertension	54	356
Peripheral neuropathy	51	495
Gastrointestinal tract	44	507
Abdominal pain	43	122
Nausea/vomiting	40	30
Cholecystitis	17	64
Bleeding	6	205
Bowel perforation	5	64
Bowel infarction	1.4	140
Skin	43	476
Rash/purpura	30	259
Nodules	15	369
Livedo reticularis	4	194
Heart	36	413
Congestive heart failure	12	204
Myocardial infarct	6	64
Pericarditis	4	204
Brain	23	184
Stroke	11	90
Altered mental status	10	90
Seizure	4	90

*Mean age of patients was 45; the male–female ratio was 2.5:1.
(From Cupps TR, Fauci AS. Adv Intern Med 1982; 27:315–324.)

Table 157–4. Symptoms at Onset in Patients with Polyarteritis Nodosa

Symptoms	Percent of Patients
Malaise/weakness	13
Abdominal pain	12
Leg pain	12
Neurologic signs/symptoms	10
Fever	8
Cough	8
Myalgias	5
Peripheral neuropathy	5
Headache	5
Arthritis/arthralgia	4
Skin involvement	4
Painful arms	4
Painful feet	4

(From Cupps TR, Fauci AS. Adv Intern Med 1982; 27:315–324.)

Treatment. There is no specific therapy. Treatment is chiefly supportive, including blood transfusions and symptomatic therapy for associated conditions. Corticosteroids may be of temporary or permanent benefit in some cases.

Temporal Arteritis and Polymyalgia Rheumatica

A special form of periarteritis limited to the temporal artery was described by Horton, Magath, and Brown in 1934. Since then, many cases have been recorded. The pathologic condition is similar to that of periarteritis nodosa except that the inflammatory reaction around the vessels is more severe and many multinucleated giant cells are found in the media (giant-cell arteritis). It is usually restricted to the temporal arteries, but occasionally other arteries of the head and, rarely, those elsewhere in the body may be involved. The syndrome occurs in both sexes and is most common in the sixth to eighth decades of life.

Symptoms include headache, centered about the involved temporal artery, together with the general systemic reactions of a low-grade infection, i.e., fever, anorexia, weight loss, and a leukocytosis in the blood. The erythrocyte sedimentation rate almost always exceeds 50 mm/hour. The affected temporal artery is prominent, nodular, tortuous, tender to pressure, and noncompressible. Blindness occurs in about 35% of cases, presumably due to thrombosis of the central artery of the retina. The affected disc may be swollen with retinal hemorrhages, pale and ischemic, or normal. There may be multifocal signs including other cranial nerve palsies and evidence of arteritis involving noncranial arteries such as coronary arteries and arteries in the limbs. Confusion, hemiplegia or other focal neurologic signs my occur when the inflammatory reaction involves the internal carotid artery or its branches. The brain may be affected by giant cell arteritis, with or without involvement of extracranial arteries. This process may occur in the absence of pathologic changes in biopsies of the temporal artery.

The course is self-limited with remission of symptoms after a prolonged course of several months. Partial or complete loss of vision is usually the only residual. Prednisone seems of value in shortening the course and preventing blindness in the unaffected eye if started while symptoms are unilateral. Restoration of vision is variable and not clearly benefited by steroid therapy.

Diffuse myalgia may be a prominent symptom in elderly patients with malaise, weight loss, and increased erythrocyte sedimentation rate, a syndrome called *polymyalgia rheumatica*. In many of these patients, the temporal artery may show the same pathologic alterations as in temporal arteritis, even when there are no cranial symptoms. Thus, these two poorly defined syndromes overlap. (In polymyalgia, there is no weakness, serum enzymes are normal, and there are no pathologic changes in muscle biopsy or electromyogram; if there were, the syndrome would be indistinguishable from polymyositis.)

The long-term survival of patients with either temporal arteritis or polymyalgia is good. In one study in Sweden, life expectancy of these patients was about the same as others of the same age in the general population; there was no increase in death rates due to vascular disease or malignancy.

Granulomatous Giant Cell Arteritis

Several types of granulomatous, giant cell, necrotizing, or allergic angiitis have been described in the literature. Various names have been given to the slightly different types of arteritis, including Wegener granulomatosis, Zeek necrotizing angiitis, and allergic granulomatosis of Strauss, Churg, and Zak. Most publications have described lesions in the upper respiratory tract, lungs, and kidneys. It is now evident that any organ system may be affected and that neurologic symptoms and signs are not rare. It is postulated that granulomatous arteritis is allergic in nature and possibly related to bacterial sensitivity, drug or chemical toxicity, or autoimmune mechanisms.

Vascular changes may occur at any age, but most patients are 30 to 60 years old. There is a slight predominance of women.

Neurologic symptoms may result from involvement of the vessels of the peripheral nerves or brain. There may then be clinical evidence of mononeuritis multiplex, polyneuropathy, or focal cerebral symptoms.

GRANULOMATOUS ANGIITIS OF THE BRAIN

In one form of granulomatous angiitis, clinical manifestations are restricted to the brain. Thus, this is appropriately called *granulomatous angiitis of the brain*. In a few cases, the spinal cord is similarly affected, alone or with cerebral lesions. Therefore, the more compre-

hensive term is *granulomatous angiitis of the nervous system (GANS)*.

This disorder is essentially defined by the characteristic histologic lesion, a granulomatous change that includes multinucleated giant cells. The lesion affects small or larger named cerebral blood vessels.

Lesions of this nature are found in some patients who have clinical evidence of a cerebral infarct ipsilateral to herpes zoster ophthalmicus. Otherwise, there is no clinical clue to the nature of the disease. A few patients have had evidence of immunosuppression by sarcoidosis, Hodgkin disease, or AIDS.

After herpes zoster, the clinical manifestations may be those of an uncomplicated stroke, with severe or mild manifestations in different cases. When there is no evidence of zosterian infection, the symptoms include two invariable but nonspecific sets, focal cerebral signs and mental obtundation, which may be preceded by dementia. The course is subacute, so this can be regarded as a progressive encephalopathy.

Characteristically, there is a CSF pleocytosis, up to 500 mononuclear cells/high power field. CSF protein content is usually increased, exceeding 100 mg/dl in 75% of cases, but CSF sugar content is normal.

Some researchers suggest that the syndrome is sufficiently characteristic to warrant clinical diagnosis, especially if there is angiographic evidence of "beading" of arteries, presumably evidence of vasculitis. Cases so diagnosed have been treated with cyclophosphamide and, if the outcome was favorable, the authors concluded that catastrophic outcome had been averted. However, in autopsy-proven cases, the arteriogram is usually normal or shows evidence of the infarct or local tissue swelling, but not "beading." Moreover, the clinical and CSF manifestations can be caused by infiltration of meninges by tumor cells and also by viral infection—and "beading" of cerebral arteries is a nonspecific finding.

The consensus is that diagnosis in living patients can be verified only by a brain biopsy that includes meningeal vessels. In histologically proven cases (without zoster), the outcome has been fatal in most or all cases within a few years. About half the patients die within 6 weeks, but a third live longer than 1 year after onset. Treatment with corticosteroids and immunosuppressive drugs has not been effective.

Systemic Lupus Erythematosus

Systemic lupus erythematosus (SLE) is a disease in which there is widespread inflammatory change in the connective tissue (collagen) of the skin and systemic organs. The primary damage is to the subendothelial connective tissue of capillaries, small arteries, and veins, the endocardium, and the synovial and serous membranes.

Etiology and Incidence. The cause of the disease is not known, but increasing evidence suggests that immune complexes are deposited in small vessels. The initiating event could be a persistent viral infection, but sometimes serologic and clinical manifestations follow administration of drugs, such as procainamide. Although rare, the incidence may be increasing. Most cases begin between ages 20 and 40, but the disease may be seen in children. Some 95% of adult patients are women.

Symptoms and Signs. The chief clinical manifestations are: prolonged, irregular fever, with remissions of variable duration (weeks, months, or even years); erythematous rash; recurrent attacks with evidence of involvement of synovial and serous membranes (polyarthritis, pleuritis, pericarditis); depression of bone marrow function (leukopenia, hypochromic anemia, moderate thrombocytopenia); and, in advanced stages, clinical evidence of vascular alteration in the skin, kidneys, and other viscera.

The neurologic syndromes are diverse and include convulsions, functional psychosis or organic dementia, cerebral blindness, chorea, cranial nerve palsies, polyneuritis, hemiplegia, transverse myelopathy, or polymyositis (Table 157–5). These symptoms are often attributed to thrombosis of small vessels or petechial hemorrhages, but the evidence of "vasculitis" is actually meager and there is growing belief that the neurologic manifestations are due to the direct effects of some type of neuronal antibodies. However, that theory may also be presumptuous. In fact, the pathogenesis of SLE itself is not well understood, and the pathogenesis of the cerebral or peripheral lesions is another enigma. In some cases cerebral emboli arise from endocarditis or thrombotic thrombocytopenia.

Laboratory Data. Changes in the blood have been mentioned above. Hematuria, albuminuria, and other signs of damage to the kidneys may be present. Serum γ-globulin is often increased and biologic false-positive serologic tests for syphilis may be encountered.

Table 157–5. Neurologic Manifestations in 140 Patients with SLE

Manifestation	Number of Patients
Psychiatric disorders	24
Dementia	22
Seizures	17
Long tract signs	16
Cranial nerve abnormalities	16
Peripheral neuropathy	15
Cerebellar signs	5
Scotomata	4
Papilledema (pseudotumor)	2
Chorea	2
Myelitis	1

(From Feinglass EJ, Arnett FC, Dorsch CA. Medicine 1976; 55:323–339.)

Phagocytic polymorphonuclear leukocytes (LE cells) are found in the bone marrow or in the buffy coat of centrifuged heparinized blood of most, but not all, cases. These cells reflect antibody to whole nucleoprotein, one of numerous different antibodies found in the serum of these patients and reacting with autologous tissue constituents. LE cells are present in about 80% of all cases and are considered by some to be pathognomonic of SLE, although they are occasionally found in other diseases. The fluorescent antinuclear-antibody test is positive in virtually all cases of SLE, but this greater sensitivity is gained at the expense of specificity because antinuclear antibodies may be encountered in many other diseases. Serum complement may be decreased especially in patients with renal disease; deposits of globulin and complement may be found in renal biopsies. CSF is usually normal, but there may be an increase in the protein content and an abnormal colloidal gold reaction when peripheral nerves or CSF are involved. For reasons that are not clear, the CSF sugar content may be depressed in patients with myelitis.

Diagnosis. Diagnosis may be difficult. Fever, weight loss, arthritis, anemia, leukopenia, pleuritis, and cardiac, renal, or neurologic symptoms in a young woman should lead to a consideration of this diagnosis. An erythematous rash on the bridge of the nose and the malar eminences in a butterfly-like distribution facilitates the diagnosis. Finding LE cells or antinuclear antibodies in the blood is of value in establishing the diagnosis.

Course and Prognosis. Death usually is the outcome of renal failure or intercurrent infection. The course may be prolonged for many months or years. In some cases there are remissions of months' or years' duration.

Treatment. There is no satisfactory treatment. Administration of corticosteroids or immunosuppressive drugs may reduce the severity of symptoms and may be followed by a remission of symptoms, but more commonly long-term therapy is needed. Treatment of cerebral manifestations is especially disappointing and has led to the use of large doses, which may themselves be deleterious.

Other Collagen-Vascular Diseases

Neurologic syndromes may complicate other collagen-vascular diseases, usually when the systemic disorder is evident. Sometimes there are characteristic syndromes. For instance, an aggressive polyneuropathy may be seen in patients with rheumatoid arthritis. Some clinicians believe the neuropathy may be precipitated by steroid therapy. Another neurologic syndrome of rheumatoid arthritis is atlantoaxial dislocation with resulting cord compression; the syndrome is attributed to resorption of the odontoid process.

In Sjogren syndrome, peripheral neuropathy and polymyositis may be prominent. Peripheral neuropathy is also seen in more than half the patients with the idiopathic hypereosinophilic syndrome, and there may be evidence of vasculitis in the nerve biopsy. Subacute encephalopathy also occurs in patients with that rare disorder.

References

Polyarteritis Nodosa

Bicknell JM, Holland JV. Neurologic manifestations of Cogan syndrome. Neurology 1978; 28:278–281.

Cheson BD, Blunming AZ, Alroy JA. Cogan's syndrome. A systemic vasculitis. Am J Med 1976; 60:549–555.

Christian CL, Sergent JS. Vasculitis syndromes: clinical and experimental models. Am J Med 1976; 61:511–553.

Cogan DG. Syndrome of nonsyphilitic interstitial keratitis and vestibuloauditory symptoms. Arch Ophthalmol 1945; 33:144–149—1949; 42:42–49.

Cupps TR, Fauci AS. The vasculitic syndromes. Adv Intern Med 1982; 27:315–344.

Ford RG, Siekert RG. Central nervous system manifestations of periarteritis nodosa. Neurology 1965; 15:114–122.

Lande A, Rossi P. The value of total aortography in diagnosis of Takayasu arteritis. Radiology 1975; 114:287–297.

Lovelace RE. Mononeuritis multiplex in polyarteritis nodosa. Neurology 1964; 14:434–442.

Moore PM, Cupps TR. Neurological complications of vasculitis. Ann Neurol 1983; 14:155–167.

Moore PM, Fauci AS. Neurologic manifestations of systemic vasculitis. Am J Med 1981; 71:517–523.

Reik L. Disseminated vasculomyelinopathy: an immune complex disease. Ann Neurol 1980; 7:291–296.

Rose AG, Sinclair-Smith CC. Takayasu's arteritis? A study of 16 autopsy cases. Arch Pathol Lab Med 1980; 104:231–234.

Schwartzman RJ, Parker JC Jr. The aortic arch syndrome. In: Vinken PJ, Bruyn CW, eds. Handbook of Clinical Neurology (vol 39). New York: Elsevier-North Holland, 1980:213–238.

Sergent JS, Lockshin MD, Christian CL, Gocke DJ. Vasculitis with hepatitis B antigenemia. Medicine 1975; 55:1–18.

Temporal Arteritis and Polymyalgia Rheumatica

Andersson R, Malmvall BE, Bengtsson BA. Long-term survival in giant cell arteritis including temporal arteritis and polymyalgia rheumatica. Acta Med Scand 1986; 220:361–364.

Ayoub WT, Franklin CM, Torretti D. Polymyalgic rheumatica: Duration of therapy and long-term outcome. Am J Med 1985; 79:309–315.

Barricks ME, Traviesa DB, Glaser JS, Levy IS. Ophthalmoplegia in cranial arteritis. Brain 1977; 100:209–221.

Bengtsson BA, Malmvall BE. Alternate-day corticosteroid regimen in maintenance therapy of giant cell arteritis. Surv Ophthalmol 1976; 20:247–260.

Biller J, Asconape J, Weinblatt ME, Toole JR. Temporal arteritis associated with normal sedimentation rate. JAMA 1982; 247:486–487.

Calamia KT, Hunder GG. Giant cell arteritis (temporal arteritis) presenting as fever of undetermined origin. Arthritis Rheum 1981; 24:1414–1418.

Caselli RJ, Hunder GG, Whisnant JP. Neurologic disease in biopsy-proven giant cell (temporal) arteritis. Neurology 1988; 38:352–357.

Chumbley LC, Harrison EG, DeRemee RA. Allergic granulomatosis and angiitis (Churge-Strauss Syndrome): 30 cases. Mayo Clin Proc 1977; 52:477–484.

Cullen JF, Coleiro JA. Ophthalmic complications of giant cell arteritis. Surv Ophthalmol 1976; 20:247–260.

Goodman BW. Temporal arteritis. Am J Med 1979; 67:839–852.

Hall S, Hunder CC. Is temporal artery biopsy prudent? Mayo Clin Proc 1984; 59:309–314. 1985; 79:793–796.

Hamilton CR Jr, Shelley WM, Tumulty PA. Giant cell arteritis: including temporal arteritis and polymyalgia rheumatica. Medicine 1971; 50:1–27.

Hauser WA, Ferguson RH, Holley KE, Kurland LT. Temporal arteritis in Rochester, Minnesota. Mayo Clin Proc 1981; 46:597–602.

Hollenhorst RW, Brown JR, Wagener HP, Shick RM. Neurologic aspects of temporal arteritis. Neurology 1960; 10:490–498.

Horton BT, Magath TB, Brown GE. Arteritis of the temporal vessels. Arch Intern Med 1934; 53:400–409.

Hunder GG, Sheps SG, Allen GL, Joyce JW. Daily and alternate-day corticosteroid regimens in treatment of giant cell arteritis. Comparison in a prospective study. Ann Intern Med 1975; 82:613–618.

Klein RG, Hunder GG, Stanson AW, Sheps SG. Large artery involvement in giant cell (temporal) arteritis. Ann Intern Med 1975; 83:806:812.

Love DC, Rapkin J, Lesser GR, et al. Temporal arteritis in blacks. Ann Int Med 1986; 103:387–388.

Malmvall BE, Benstsson BA. Giant cell arteritis: clinical features and involvement of different organs. Scand J Rheumatol 1978; 7:154–158.

Ostberg G. On arteritis with special reference to polymyalgia arteritica. Acta Pathol Microbiol Scand [A] 1973; 237(suppl):1–59.

Park JR, Hazleman BL. Immunological and histological

study of temporal arteritis. Ann Rheum Dis 1978; 37:238–243.

Rewcastle NB, Tom MI. Non-infectious granulomatous angiitis of the nervous system associated with Hodgkin's disease. J Neurol Neurosurg Psychiatry 1962; 25:51–58.

Samantray SK. Takayasu arteritis: 45 cases. Aust NZ J Med 1978; 8:68–73.

Tribe CR, Scott SGI, Bacon PA. Rectal biopsy in the diagnosis of systemic vasculitis. J Clin Pathol 1981; 34:843–850.

Vilaseca J, Gonzalez A, Cid MC, Lopez-Vivancos J, Orrtega A. Clinical usefulness of temporal artery biopsy. Ann Rheum Dis 1987; 46:282–285.

Granulomatous Giant Cell Arteritis

Cupps TR, Moore PM, Fauci AS. Isolated angiitis of the central nervous system. Prospective diagnostic and therapeutic experience. Am J Med 1983; 74:97–105.

Fauci AS, Haynes BF, Katz P, Wolff SM. Wegener's granulomatosis: prospective clinical and therapeutic experience with 85 patients for 21 years. Ann Intern Med 1983; 98:76–85.

Harrison PE Jr. Granulomatous angiitis of the central nervous system. J Neurol Sci 1976; 29:335–341.

Kroneman OC, Pevzner M. Failure of cyclophosphamide to prevent cerebritis in Wegener's granulomatosis. Am J Med 1986; 80:526–527.

Russell RWR. Giant-cell arteritis: a review of 35 cases. Q J Med 1959; 28:471–489.

Sigal LH. The neurologic presentation of vasculitic and rheumatologic syndromes. A review. Medicine 1987; 66:157–180.

Warrell DA, Godfrey S, Olsen EGJ. Giant-cell arteritis with peripheral neuropathy. Lancet 1968; 1:1010–1013.

Younger DS, Hays AP, Brust JCM, Rowland LP. Granulomatous angiitis of the brain: An inflammatory reaction of diverse etiology. Arch Neurol 1988; 45:514–518.

Systemic Lupus Erythematosus

Andrianakos AA, Duffy J, Suzuki M, Sharp JT. Transverse myelopathy in systemic lupus erythematosus. Ann Intern Med 1973; 83:616–624.

Asherson RA, Lubbe WF. Cerebral and valve lesion in SLE: association with antiphospholipid antibodies. J Rheumatol 1988; 15:539–543.

Bluestein HG, Pischel KD, Woods VL Jr. Immunopathogenesis of the neuropsychiatric manifestations of systemic lupus erythematosus. Springer Semin Immunopathol 1986; 9:237–249.

Brandt KD, Lessell S, Cohen AS. Cerebral disorders of vision in systemic lupus erythematosus. Ann Intern Med 1975; 83:163–169.

Canoso JJ, Cohen AS. Aseptic meningitis in systemic lupus erythematosus. Report of 3 cases. Arthritis Rheum 1975; 18:369–374.

Clark EC, Bailey AA. Neurological and psychiatric signs associated with systemic lupus erythematosus. JAMA 1956; 160:455–459.

Devinsky O, Petito CK, Alonso DR. Clinical and neuropathlogical findings in systemic lupus erythematosus: The role of vasculitis, heart emboli, and thrombotic thrombocytopenic purpura. Ann Neurol 1988; 23:380–384.

Feinglass EJ, Arnett FC, Dorsch CA. Neuropsychiatric manifestations of systemic lupus erythematosus; diagnosis, clinical spectrum, and relationship to other features of the disease. Medicine 1976; 55:323–339.

Foote RA, Kimbrough SM, Stevens JC. Lupus myositis. Muscle Nerve 1982; 5:65–68.

Johnson RT, Richardson EP. The neurological manifestations of systemic lupus erythematosus. Medicine 1968; 47:337–369.

Penn AS, Rowan AJ. Myelopathy in systemic lupus erythematosus. Arch Neurol 1968; 18:337–349.

Prockop LD. Myotonia, procaine amide, and lupus-like syndrome. Arch Neurol 1966; 14:326–330.

Sergent JS, Lockshin MD, Klempner MS. Central nervous system disease in systemic lupus erythematosus. Am J Med 1975; 58:644–654.

Zvaifler NJ, Bluestein HG. Pathogenesis of CNS manifestations of systemic lupus erythematosus. Arthritis Rheum 1982; 25:862–866.

Other Collagen-Vascular Syndromes

Alexander EL, Alexander GE. Aseptic meningoencephalitis in primary Sjogren's syndrome. Neurology 1983; 33:593–598.

Fox RI, Robinson CA, Curd JG, Kozin F, Howell FV. Sjogren's syndrome. Proposed criteria for classification. Arth Rheum 1986; 29:577–585.

Krieg T, Meurer M. Systemic scleroderma; clinical and pathophysiologic aspects. J Am Acad Dermatol 1988; 18:457–484.

Mikulowski P, Wolheim FA, Rotmil P, Olsen I. Sudden death in rheumatoid arthritis with atlanto-axial dislocation. Acta Med Scand 1975; 198:445–451.

Moore PM, Harley JB, Fauci AS. Neurologic dysfunction in the idiopathic hypereosinophilic syndrome. Ann Int Med 1985; 102:109–114.

Smith CH, Sauino PJ, Beck RM, Schatz NJ, Sergott RC. Acute posterior multifocal placoid pigment epitheliopathy with cerebral vasculitis. Arch Neurol 1983; 40:48–50.

Stiehm ER, Ashida E, Kim KS, et al. Intravenous immunoglobulins as therapeutic agents. Ann Int Med 1987; 107:367–382.

Sundaran MBM, Rajput AH. Nervous system complications of relapsing polychondritis. Neurology 1983; 33:513–515.

Vollersten RS, Conn DL, Ballard DJ, et al. Rheumatoid vasculitis: Survival and associated risk factors. Medicine 1986; 65:365–374.

158. NEUROLOGIC ASPECTS OF PREGNANCY

Charles W. Olanow

Virtually any neurologic disorder, except those confined to children or the elderly, can be encountered during pregnancy. The development of even a minor neurologic problem during pregnancy may affect its significance and management. The impact of pregnancy on the disease, the effect of the disease on pregnancy, labor, delivery and the fetus must all be considered. One must also consider the consequences of diagnostic and therapeutic procedures on both the fetus, and the patient. In prescribing treatment to a pregnant patient, the physician must consider the effects of the pregnancy, the placenta, and the fetus on drug metabolism plus the teratogenic potential of the drug. Unnecessary drugs should be avoided or eliminated. One must keep in mind that complications of pregnancy are more likely to be associated with neurodevelopmental disabilities in the offspring and that the patient must deal with the prospect of caring for a newborn child.

Neuromuscular Disorders

No neuropathies are restricted to pregnant women, but several occur with increased frequency, especially in the last trimester: Bell palsy, carpal tunnel syndrome, neuralgia paresthetica, brachial neuritis, peroneal neuropathy, femoral neuropathy, and obturator neuropathies. Possible mechanisms include allergic reactions and compression during pregnancy, or during vaginal delivery or cesarean section. EMG and nerve conduction studies are helpful in differentiating these conditions; in general, the prognosis for recovery is good with conservative treatment.

Acute inflammatory polyneuropathy or the Guillain-Barré syndrome probably does not appear with increased frequency during pregnancy; however, women who have previously had the syndrome tend to have relapses, particularly in the first trimester. The development of a severe polyneuropathy in a pregnant woman is alarming, but can usually be managed satisfactorily with careful monitoring of autonomic function, respiratory status, and fetal growth. Ventilatory, nutritional, and psychological support are provided as needed. High dose steroids and plasma exchange can be used without adverse effects on the infant, but are generally not necessary. Labor, delivery, and the fetus are not affected by the disease. Uterine contractions remain normal.

Polyneuropathy due to thiamine deficiency may result from hyperemesis gravidarum or extreme nutritional deprivation. Sensory fibers are primarily involved, and treatment consists of thiamine and nutritional replacement. Administration of intravenous glucose solutions without supplemental thiamine aggravates the deficiency and may lead to Wernicke syndrome or even death.

Lumbar disk disease and sciatica are common during pregnancy, usually in those with a history of previous attacks. Conservative treatment is usually sufficient. Surgery should be avoided or deferred, although successful laminectomies have been performed during pregnancy.

Myasthenia gravis frequently affects women of childbearing age. Symptoms may begin, remit, or worsen during pregnancy. Individual patients may respond differently in successive pregnancies. Patients with malignant thymoma may have an increased risk of extrathoracic metastasis during pregnancy; therapeutic abortion may be considered in these rare cases. Myasthenia does not influence the routine management of pregnancy, but drugs that interfere with neuromuscular transmission are specifically contraindicated. Uterine contractions, labor, and delivery are usually normal and cesarean section is required only for obstetrical reasons. General anesthesia is to be avoided, as are sedatives and narcotics that may interfere with maternal and fetal respiration. Transient neonatal myasthenia may appear in infants of myasthenic mothers due to transplacental transfer of maternal antibody to acetylcholine receptor. Symptoms improve within a few weeks as the antibody disappears. Supportive treatment, anticholinesterase agents and, occasionally, plasma exchange may be required.

Women with myopathies may become pregnant, especially those with myotonic dystrophy. Pregnancy usually occurs in less severely afflicted women and myotonic dystrophy may not be diagnosed until after delivery. Exacerbations of myotonia and muscle weakness, increase in fetal and neonatal loss, and obstetrical complications have all been observed. The high incidence of spontaneous abortions in the first trimester has been attributed to abnormalities in the sperm or ovum. Second and third trimester abortions are due to functional abnormalities of the uterus, which cannot retain the fetus. Polyhydramnios may develop due to the inability of the affected fetus to swallow; prenatal detection of polyhydramnios suggests that the fetus is affected. All stages of labor may be prolonged due to uterine inertia and voluntary muscle weakness. Postpartum hemorrhage can occur because of the inability of the uterus to contract.

Multiple Sclerosis

Multiple sclerosis (MS) may begin, worsen, relapse, or remit during pregnancy. Some 20 to 40% of women have a relapse or worsen during pregnancy or shortly thereafter, usually within 3 months of delivery. A state of natural immunosuppression may occur during pregnancy as manifested by decreased numbers of helper T-cells, decreased lymphocyte response to mitogens, and suppression of lymphocyte and antibody responses to plasma and amniotic fluid. Animal studies suggest that experimental allergic encephalitis is less severe in pregnant animals, and the appearance of symptoms may be delayed until after delivery or spontaneous abortion. Uncomplicated MS has no effect on pregnancy, labor or delivery. There is no change in fertility and no reported increase in congenital malformations. Occasionally specific problems such as frequent urinary tract infections and coexisting paraparesis warrant attention. Some authorities suggest that MS patients should avoid pregnancy. Most now recommend that the decision for pregnancy should be based on the functional capacity of the mother to care for a child. She should be prepared for possible worsening of symptoms, particularly in the puerperium.

Tumors

Virtually every type of brain and spinal cord tumor has been reported during pregnancy. The incidence of most is no more frequent than in nonpregnant women of the same age. However, tumors are frequently diagnosed during pregnancy because they tend to enlarge, particularly during the second or third trimester. This increase in size has been attributed to enlargement of individual tumor cells and to an increase in blood volume. Small benign tumors, such as acoustic neuromas or meningiomas, may only become symptomatic in the third trimester, disappear in the postpartum period, and recur in a later pregnancy.

Choriocarcinoma is a highly invasive tumor of trophoblastic origin. It may cause irregular uterine bleeding and an enlarged uterus in the months after a molar pregnancy or abortion, but may also occur during or after a normal pregnancy. Cerebral metastases are common, usually accompanied by pulmonary metastases. They may present as single or mutiple lesions, stroke, or hemorrhage. The trophoblastic tissue tends to penetrate the vascular wall and to proliferate, occluding the artery and causing infarction or rupture of the artery with subsequent hemorrhage. Rarely, there is local invasion of the sacral plexus and cauda equina. Persistent elevation of serum and CSF levels of chorionic gonadotrophin aid the diagnosis.

The management of tumors in a pregnant woman varies with the individual patient. If necessary, surgery can be performed; however, it is best to delay intervention until after pregnancy or at least until the fetus has a chance for survival if the pregnancy must be terminated. Interruption of pregnancy is seldom necessary unless the tumor is malignant. Hyperventilation, hypothermia, and steroids have all been used safely. However, mannitol increases the osmolarity of maternal plasma, causing amniotic fluid and free water to flow from fetus to mother. Experimental studies suggest this may result in severe fetal dehydration. Thus, mannitol should be avoided in pregnancy if possible.

The pituitary gland normally enlarges during pregnancy, probably due to increased vascularity and proliferation of prolactin-secreting cells. Occasionally, this may compromise vision and necessitate surgical decompression. Pituitary size declines after delivery and conservative treatment is desirable.

Spinal cord tumors occur only rarely during pregnancy and most "tumors" are due to arteriovenous malformations (AVMs). Spinal AVMs usually present with sudden onset of a myelopathy or subarachnoid hemorrhage but, in pregnancy, they may have a relapsing and remitting course and can be confused with MS. MRI may aid the diagnosis. An increased incidence of AVM during pregnancy may be related to hormonal effects on abnormal blood vessels, with dilatation of arteriovenous shunts, or compression of epidural veins and enlargement of venous angiomas.

Benign intracranial hypertension occurs with increased frequency during pregnancy, particularly in the third, fourth, and fifth months of gestation. Symptoms disappear spontaneously in most cases but may persist until delivery; they may recur in subsequent pregnancies. Conservative treatment, with weight reduction and repeated lumbar puncture is usually adequate.

Cerebrovascular Disease

INTRACRANIAL HEMORRHAGE

Intracranial and, particularly, subarachnoid hemorrhage are prone to occur during pregnancy, endangering the lives of both mother and fetus. Cerebral hemorrhage occurs with an incidence of 1 to 5/10,000 pregnancies and causes 10% of maternal deaths. AVMs and berry aneurysms produce most intracranial hemorrhages of pregnancy. AVMs are particularly common in women under age 25, and tend to bleed during the second trimester or at delivery. The risk of bleeding from a berry aneurysm increases with each trimester and remains high in the weeks after delivery but, in contrast to AVMs, not at parturition.

The treatment of vascular malformations and aneurysms is basically the same as in nonpregnant patients, unless the patient is in labor. A quiet room, sedatives, stool-softeners, and efforts to avoid Valsalva maneuvers are important. There is an increased risk of rebleeding for both AVMs and aneurysms, which argues for surgical intervention when feasible. If there are multiple aneurysms, only the one responsible for the hemorrhage should be clipped. If the aneurysm is inoperable, vaginal delivery may be elected if the bleeding occurs in the first trimester, but cesarean section is preferred if the bleed occurs in the third trimester. Patients with inoperable AVMs often have an elective cesarean section because of the high incidence of rebleeding during delivery.

Other causes of intracranial hemorrhage in pregnancy include placental abruptio with disseminated intravascular coagulation, leukemia, thrombocytopenia, vasculitis (systemic lupus erythematosus may be exacerbated during pregnancy), metastatic choriocarcinoma, eclampsia (see below), and cerebral venous thrombosis.

ISCHEMIC CEREBROVASCULAR DISEASE

The risk of focal ischemic cerebrovascular disease is 13 times greater in pregnant than in nonpregnant women of the same age. In the Glasgow study, 35% of women between 15 and 45 years with ischemic stroke were pregnant or puerperal. Cerebral vein thrombosis was once considered the most common cause, but more recent data suggest that arterial occlusion accounts for 60 to 80% of strokes. This disorder occurs more frequently in the second and third trimesters or in the first week after delivery. Venous occlusion, by contrast, occurs 3 days to 4 weeks after childbirth. Arterial infarction is generally in the internal carotid artery territory; middle cerebral artery lesions are twice as frequent as in nonpregnant women. There is an increased risk of infarction of the anterior pituitary gland (Sheehan syndrome), at or near delivery, due to the vulnerability of the enlarged pituitary gland to ischemia.

The differential diagnosis of stroke in pregnant women differs considerably from the general population. Embolism is the most common cause. Atherosclerosis is a much less frequent cause of stroke in women of childbearing age, particularly among pregnant women. Rheumatic fever tends to flare during pregnancy with increased risk of cerebral embolization, so antibiotic prophylaxis is recommended. There is an increased incidence of subacute bacterial endocarditis. Streptococcus viridans is the most frequent infecting agent, but there is a high incidence of infection with enterococcus after delivery or abortion.

A cardiomyopathy of unknown origin occurs in the late stages of pregnancy or during the puerperium. Like other cardiomyopathies, there is a risk of mural thrombi with cerebral embolization. Multiparous black women older than 30 years are at greatest risk. In most, the heart returns to normal after delivery.

Paradoxical embolus through a patent foramen ovale is a risk because of the increased incidence of thrombophlebitis in pelvic and leg veins. Amniotic fluid emboli should be considered in multiparous women older than age 30 who have uterine or vaginal tears that might allow amniotic fluid to enter the systemic circulation. Most patients present with acute pulmonary symptoms, but paradoxical cerebral emboli may be seen. Diagnosis can be established by demonstrating fetal epithelial-squamous cells above the buffy coat of blood withdrawn from the right atrium. Air embolization is rare but may follow cesarean section or complex vaginal delivery, vaginal douching or air insufflation, and knee-chest exercises during the puerperium. Fat emboli and metastatic choriocarcinoma may also cause focal infarction.

Treatment is based on a precise definition of the underlying mechanism and follows the principles of management employed in the general population. Angiography and carotid endarterectomy can be performed safely. Prospective studies suggest that aspirin does not increase the risk of congenital malformations. No data are available on the use of dipyridamole. Warfarin should be avoided, particularly in the first trimester, because of increased risk of teratogenic complications and fetal wastage. Heparin is not known to cause these problems and is recommended when anticoagulants are required in the first trimester or in the weeks preceding delivery.

Epilepsy

Some 0.3 to 0.5% of pregnancies are complicated by epilepsy. Patients with pre-existing epilepsy experience increased seizure frequency in about 40% of cases. This has been attributed to fluid and electrolyte imbalance, weight gain, hormonal alterations, and increased clearance or decreased absorption of anticonvulsant drugs but, in most instances, poor compliance is responsible. Drug monitoring and patient counseling are important. Epilepsy is associated with an increased risk of obstetrical complications, fetal wastage, and congenital malformations. Genetic predisposition, seizure frequency, and anticonvulsant drugs may all play a role. A two-fold increase in congenital malformations is seen in untreated epileptics without seizures and the incidence is doubled when anticonvulsants are used. A *fetal hydantion syndrome* includes craniofacial anomalies (particularly cleft palate), growth and mental retardation, and limb abnormalities. This syndrome is probably not specific for phenytoin but many physicians consider carbamazepine the drug of choice to treat grand mal seizures because of a possible reduction in teratogenicity. Trimethadione is associated with a high incidence of congenital malformations and valproic acid has been implicated in neurotube defects. The free fraction of an anticonvulsant drug crosses the placenta and is present in the mother's milk. This creates a potential problem for patients treated with phenobarbital because a large proportion of the drug is in the free state, which may depress neonatal respiration and consciousness, and may cause a withdrawal syndrome in the neonate. Neonatal bleeding in the first few days of life may follow use of phenobarbital or phenytoin because of interference with vitamin K metabolism. Phenobarbital and phenytoin also cause a macrocytic anemia, which responds to folic acid. Ethosuximide (Zarontin) is the preferred drug in women with petit mal seizures.

The goals of treatment are to maintain the patient in a seizure-free state while minimizing adverse effects on the pregnancy and fetus. Only one anticonvulsant should be used, if possible, and serum concentrations should be maintained within the therapeutic range. If a woman anticipates pregnancy and has been free of seizures for 5 years, attempts should be made to discontinue anticonvulsant drug therapy. Generally, women with seizure disorders are not discouraged from having children, but they should understand that there is an increased risk of congenital malformations.

The differential diagnosis of seizures that begin during pregnancy includes eclampsia (see below) and thrombotic thrombocytopenic purpura, which occurs with increased frequency in pregnancy and may present with seizures. A seizure at delivery may indicate water intoxication due to abuse of oxytocin or a reaction to local anesthetics. Seizures in the immediate postpartum period suggest the possibility of cerebral venous thrombosis.

Eclampsia

Eclampsia is a disorder of unknown origin that occurs in the second half of pregnancy. The syndrome is characterized by hypertension, seizures, and coma. It is more common in poorly nourished young primiparous women and in those with advanced extrauterine pregnancies. In most, it is preceded by a pre-eclampsia syndrome: hypertension, proteinuria, edema, overactive tendon reflexes, and headache. Aggressive treatment of the pre-eclampsia syndrome usually prevents development of true eclampsia. In a few cases, postpartum eclampsia has been associated with retained placental fragments, suggesting that a toxin liberated by the placenta causes the disorder.

The cerebral manifestations of eclampsia result from hypertension and include cerebral hemorrhage and hypertensive encephalopathy. Some 30 to 50% of patients have visual problems, which may be primarily ocular (arteriolar spasm, central retinal artery occlusion, retinal edema and hemorrhages, and retinal detachment) or cerebral (papilledema and cortical blindness). Pathologically, the brain shows gross hemorrhage in a hypertensive distribution or microinfarcts with punctate hemorrhages in the cortical gray matter, particularly in the occipital regions.

Prompt termination of the pregnancy is essential once the diagnosis has been established, although it is preferable to control blood pressure and convulsions beforehand, if possible. Hydralazine is an effective antihypertensive drug that can be given intravenously and does not compromise uterine blood flow. The treatment of seizures is controversial. Obstetricians have employed magnesium for more than 50 years, even though it has no anticonvulsant properties, is not known to cross the blood-brain barrier, and may depress respiration in both mother and infant. It acts by blocking neuromuscular transmission, which presumably prevents tonic and clonic movements. Obstetricians use it because "it works," although most neurologists believe that conventional anticonvulsants would be preferable.

Miscellaneous

Chorea gravidarum is defined as any form of chorea that occurs during pregnancy. Commonly, it begins in the first half of pregnancy and disappears during pregnancy or in the puerperium. Of affected women, 60% have a history of previous chorea; 20% have chorea in subsequent pregnancies. There is a strong correlation with rheumatic fever and consequently it is less frequently encountered now than in the past. It is important to exclude Wilson disease, drugs, lupus erythematosus, Huntington disease, polycythemia, hyperthyroidism, hypoparathyroidism, and acanthocytosis. Treatment consists of sedation, rest, nutrition and, if necessary, phenothiazines or haloperidol. Pregnancy is generally not affected by chorea, and it is not an indication for abortion.

Rarely, patients with *Parkinson disease* may become pregnant. They have been maintained uneventfully on levodopa and dopamine-agonist therapy without adverse effects to the pregnancy or to the fetus. However, congenital malformations have occurred in experimental animals treated with levodopa.

Headaches are a common neurologic symptom and have the same differential diagnosis as in nonpregnant women. Supportive therapy is usually adequate. Ergot agents are generally avoided because they may increase uterine contractions. Propanolol can be used, but it may cause fetal bradycardia and may mask fetal distress.

Infection in pregnant women raises the possibility of transplacental transmission to the fetus. Poliomyelitis was once a common problem in pregnancy and was associated with an increased risk of first trimester abortion. Infection with listeria monocytogenes is now an increasing problem in pregnant women, associated with increased risk of abortion and neonatal meningitis. It tends to occur in women who are immunocompromised and may reflect the state of altered immunity in pregnant women. Congenital syphilis is becoming a problem once again and cases of neonatal AIDS are now well recognized.

There is increasing interest in prenatal DNA testing of women who carry a fetus at risk for the development of an inherited neurologic disorder. Chorionic villus biopsy provides an opportunity to examine genetic material of the fetus as early as 8 or 9 weeks into pregnancy. Linkage studies between the gene for the disease and a known marker can be assessed to determine the likelihood that the fetus is affected. With current probes and informative mating, Duchenne muscular dystrophy and myotonic dystrophy can be predicted in more than 95% of cases. Developments in these disorders have fueled enthusiasm for similar approaches to other heritable neurologic diseases.

References

Barnes JE, Abbott KH. Cerebral complications incurred during pregnancy and puerperium. Am J Obstet Gynecol 1961; 82:192–207.

Birk K, Rudick R. Pregnancy in multiple sclerosis. Arch Neurol 1986; 43:719–726.

Dalessio DJ. Seizure disorders and pregnancy. N Engl J Med 1985; 312:559–563.

Donaldson JO. Neurology of pregnancy. In: Major Problems in Neurology Series. Philadelphia: WB Saunders, 1978.

Fennell DF, Ringel SP. Myasthenia gravis and pregnancy. Obst Gynecol Survey 1987; 41:414–421.

Hachinski V, Dinsdale HB, Kaplan PW et al. Controversies in neurology: magnesium sulfate in the treatment of eclampsia. Arch Neurol 1988; 45:1360–1366.

Roelvink NCA, Kamphorst W, Alphen HAMV, Rao BR. Pregnancy-related primary brain and spinal tumors. Arch Neurol 1987; 44:227–231.

Wiebers DO. Ischemic cerebrovascular complications of pregnancy. Arch Neurol 1985; 42:1106–1113.

Chapter XXII

Environmental Neurology

159. ALCOHOLISM
John C.M. Brust

In the US, 7% of all adults and 19% of adolescents are "problem drinkers"—addicted to ethanol or, even if abstinent most of the time, likely to get into trouble when they drink. Ethanol-related deaths exceed 100,000 each year, accounting for 5% of all deaths in the United States. The devastation is direct (from intoxication, addiction, and withdrawal) or indirect (from nutritional deficiency or other ethanol-related diseases).

Ethanol Intoxication

To obtain a mildly intoxicating blood ethanol concentration (BEC) of 100 mg/dL, a 70 kg person must drink about 50 g (2 oz) of 100% ethanol. Following zero-order kinetics, ethanol is metabolized at about 70 to 150 mg/kg of body weight/hour with a fall in BEC of 10 to 25 mg/dL/hour. Thus, most adults require 6 hours to metabolize a 50 g dose, and the ingestion of only 8 g of additional ethanol/hour would maintain the BEC at 100 mg/dL.

Symptoms and signs of acute ethanol intoxication are due to cerebral depression, possibly at first of the reticular formation with cerebral disinhibition, and later of the cerebral cortex itself. Manifestations depend not only on the BEC but on the rate of climb and the person's tolerance, which is related less to increased metabolism than to poorly understood adaptive changes in the brain. At any BEC, intoxication is more severe when the level is rising than when it is falling, when the level is reached rapidly, and when the level has only recently been achieved. A single BEC determination, therefore, is not a reliable indicator of drunkenness, and the correlations of Table 159–1 are broad generalizations. Death from respiratory paralysis may occur with a BEC of 400 mg/dL, and survival

Table 159–1. Correlation of Symptoms with Blood Ethanol Concentration (BEC)

BEC	Symptoms
50–150 mg/dL	Euphoria or dysphoria, shyness or expansiveness, friendliness or argumentativeness. Impaired concentration, judgment, and sexual inhibitions
150–250 mg/dL	Slurred speech and ataxic gait, diplopia, nausea, tachycardia, drowsiness, or labile mood with sudden bursts of anger or antisocial acts
300 mg/dL	Stupor alternating with combativeness or incoherent speech, heavy breathing, vomiting
400 mg/dL	Coma
500 mg/dL	Respiratory paralysis

at 700 mg/dL; a level of 500 mg/dL would be fatal in 50% of subjects.

Low-to-moderate BECs cause slow saccadic eye movements and interrupted, jerky pursuit movements that may impair visual acuity. Esophoria and exophoria cause diplopia. With a BEC of 150 to 250 mg/dL, there is increased EEG beta activity ("beta buzz"); higher concentrations cause EEG slowing. During sleep, suppression of the rapid eye movement (REM) stage is followed, after a few hours, by REM "rebound."

The term *pathologic intoxication* refers to sudden extreme excitement, with irrational or violent behavior, after even small doses of ethanol. Episodes are said to last for minutes or hours, followed by sleep and, upon awakening, amnesia for the events that took place. Delusions, hallucinations, and homicide may occur during bouts of pathologic intoxication. Some cases are probably psychological dissociative reactions; others may be due to the kind of paradoxic excitation that sometimes follows barbiturate administration.

The term *alcoholic blackout* refers to amnesia for periods of intoxication, sometimes lasting several hours, even though consciousness at the time did not seem to be disturbed. Although sometimes considered a sign of physiologic dependence, blackouts also occur in occasional drinkers. Their nature is uncertain.

Acute ethanol poisoning causes more than 1000 deaths each year in the United States. In stuporous alcoholic patients, subdural hematoma, meningitis, and hypoglycemia are important diagnostic considerations, but it is equally important to remember that ethanol intoxication alone can be fatal.

Blood ethanol causes a rise of blood osmolality, about 22 mOsm/L for every 100 mg/dL of ethanol; however, there are no transmembrane shifts of water and the hyperosmolarity does not cause symptoms. Ethanol overdose should be considered in any comatose patient when serum osmolarity is higher than predicted by calculating the sum of serum sodium, glucose, and urea.

Patients stuporous or comatose from ethanol intoxication are generally managed like those poisoned by other depressant drugs (Table 159–2). Death comes from respiratory depression, and artificial ventilation in an intensive care unit is the mainstay of treatment. Hypovolemia, acid-base or electrolyte imbalance, and abnormal temperature require attention, and, if there is any uncertainty about the blood sugar, 50% glucose is given intravenously, along with parenteral thiamine. Because ethanol is rapidly absorbed, gastric lavage does not help unless other drugs have been ingested. In obstreperous or violent patients, sedatives (including phenothiazines and haloperidol) should be avoided because they may push the patient into stupor and respiratory depression. When the patient is being addressed he may be alert, but then lapse into stupor or coma when stimuli are decreased.

In a nonhabitual drinker, a BEC of 400 mg/dL takes 20 hours to return to zero. The only practical agent that might accelerate ethanol metabolism and elimination is fructose, but this causes gastrointestinal upset, lactic acidosis, and osmotic diuresis. (An imidazobenzodiazepine drug has been developed that reverses symptoms of mild-to-moderate ethanol intoxication; it is available for experimental use only.) Hemodialysis or peritoneal dialysis can be used for BECs over 600 mg/dL; for severe acidosis; for concurrent ingestion of methanol, ethylene glycol, or other dialyzable drugs; and for severely intoxicated children. Analeptic agents such as ethamivan, caffeine, or amphetamine have no useful role and can cause seizures and cardiac arrhythmia. Although patients are often depleted of magnesium, administration of magnesium sulfate may further depress the sensorium in an intoxicated patient. Reports suggesting that naloxone benefits patients with ethanol intoxication require confirmation.

Ethanol-Drug Interactions

The combination of ethanol with other drugs, often in suicide attempts, causes 2500 deaths annually, or 13% of all drug-related fatalities. Ethanol is often taken with marijuana, barbiturates, opiates, cocaine, hallucinogens, and inhalants—with varying interactions. Alcoholics often abuse barbiturates, and, although they are cross-tolerant, ethanol and barbiturates taken acutely in combination lower the lethal dose of either alone. Ethanol with chloral hydrate ("Mickey Finn") may be especially dangerous.

Impaired judgment and respiratory depression are also hazards when ethanol is combined with hypnotics such as methaqualone, sedating antihistamines, antipsychotic agents, and tranquilizers such as meprobamate and benzodiazepines. Because of its long half-life (up to 100 hours), flurazepam, the most widely used prescription sleeping pill in the United States, may accumulate with repeated use, causing potentially dangerous in-

---

Table 159–2.   Treatment of Acute Ethanol Intoxication

For obstreperous or violent patients
  Isolation, calming environment, reassurance—avoid sedatives
  Close observation

For stuporous or comatose patients
  If hypoventilation, artificial respiration in an intensive care unit
  If serum glucose in doubt, intravenous 50% glucose with parenteral thiamine
  Careful monitoring of blood pressure; correction of hypovolemia or acid-base imbalance
  Consider hemodialysis if patient apneic or deeply comatose
  Avoid emetics or gastric lavage
  Avoid analeptics
  Do not forget other possible causes of coma in an alcoholic

coordination when ethanol is consumed the following day.

The cross-tolerance of ethanol with general anesthetics such as ether, chloroform, or fluorinated agents raises the threshold to sleep induction, but synergistic interaction then increases the depth and length of the anesthetic stage reached. Tricyclic antidepressants do not have a consistent effect; desipramine antagonizes the effects of alcohol and amitriptyline potentiates them. Ethanol and morphine, repeatedly used, can increase each other's potency, and methadone addicts not only frequently become alcoholics, but can then develop a characteristic encephalopathy. Death has followed ethanol taken with propoxyphene. A mild reaction resembling that caused by disulfiram occurs when patients combine ethanol with sulfonylureas such as tolbutamide or with some antibiotics, including chloramphenicol, griseofulvin, isoniazid, metronidazole, and quinacrine.

Ethanol Dependence and Withdrawal

The term *hangover* refers to the headache, nausea, vomiting, malaise, nervousness, tremulousness, and sweating that can occur in anyone after brief but excessive drinking. Hangover does not imply ethanol addiction, but "ethanol withdrawal" does, and encompasses several disorders (Table 159–3), which may occur alone or in combination after reduction or cessation of drinking. Severity depends on the length and degree of a particular binge.

Tremulousness, the most common ethanol withdrawal symptom, usually appears in the morning after several days of drinking. It is promptly relieved by ethanol, but if drinking cannot continue, tremor becomes more intense, with insomnia, easy startling, agitation, facial and conjunctival flushing, sweating, anorexia, nausea, retching, weakness, tachypnea, tachycardia, and systolic hypertension. Except for inattentiveness and inability to fully recall the events that occurred during the binge, mentation is usually intact.

Table 159–3.   Ethanol Withdrawal Syndromes

Early
Tremulousness
Hallucinosis
Seizures
Late
Delirium tremens

Symptoms subside in a few days, but it may be 2 weeks before they completely disappear.

Perceptual disturbances, with variable insight, occur in about 25% of these patients and include nightmares, illusions, and hallucinations, which are most often visual, but may be auditory, tactile, olfactory, or a combination. Imagery includes insects, animals, or people. Hallucinations are usually fragmentary, lasting minutes at a time for several days. Sometimes, however, auditory hallucinations of threatening content last much longer, and occasional patients develop a persistent state of auditory hallucinosis with paranoid delusions that resembles schizophrenia and may require care in a mental hospital. Repeated bouts of acute auditory hallucinosis may predispose to the chronic form.

Ethanol can precipitate *seizures* in any epileptic; seizures usually occur the morning after weekend or even single-day drinking rather than during inebriation. The term *"rum fits"* refers to seizures occurring during withdrawal in alcoholic patients who are not otherwise epileptic; they usually occur within 48 hours after drinking ceases. There may be a single seizure, a brief cluster, or infrequently, status epilepticus. Although focal features characterize nearly 25% of patients, few have evidence of earlier head injury or other structural cerebral pathology. Rum fits may occur in otherwise asymptomatic patients or may accompany tremulousness or hallucinosis. Seizures or hallucinations sometimes occur during intoxication, perhaps because reduction of intake and increasing tolerance produce relative withdrawal.

The diagnosis of rum fits depends on an accurate history and exclusion of other cerebral lesions. Because reliable follow-up is unlikely, a seizure workup should be done, including CT and examination of CSF. Early in withdrawal, the EEG may demonstrate fleeting spikes or sharp waves, but after 2 weeks, less than 10% of patients with rum fits have spontaneous EEG abnormalities, compared with 50% of those with idiopathic epilepsy.

In contrast to tremor, hallucinosis, or seizures, which usually occur within 1 or 2 days of abstinence, *delirium tremens* usually begins from 48 to 72 hours after the last drink. Patients with delirium tremens often are hospitalized for other reasons. Delirium tremens may follow withdrawal seizures, either before the postictal period has cleared or after 1 or 2 asymptomatic days, but when seizures occur during a bout of delirium tremens, some other diagnosis (such as meningitis) should be considered.

Symptoms typically begin and end abruptly, lasting from hours to a few days. There may be alternating periods of confusion and lucidity. Infrequently, relapses may prolong the disorder for a few weeks. A typical patient is agitated, inattentive, and grossly tremulous, with fever, tachycardia, and profuse sweating. The patient picks at the bed clothes or stares wildly about and intermittently shouts at or tries to fend off hallucinated people or objects. "Quiet delirium" is infrequent. Mortality is as high as 15%; death is usually due to other diseases (such as pneumonia or cirrhosis), but it may be attributed to unexplained shock, lack of response to therapy, or no apparent cause.

Treatment of ethanol withdrawal includes prevention or reduction of early symptoms, prevention of delirium tremens, and management of delirium tremens after it starts (Table 159–4). Sedatives have been recommended for recently abstinent alcoholics or those with mild early withdrawal symptoms, with theoretical consideration given to cross-tolerance with ethanol. Popular agents include paraldehyde, barbiturates, and benzodiazepines. With any, the aim is to give a loading dose likely to cause symptoms of mild intoxication (calming, dysarthria, ataxia, fine nystagmus) and then to adjust subsequent doses to avoid intoxication and tremulousness. After 1 or 2 days, dosage is gradually tapered, with reinstitution of intoxicating doses should withdrawal symptoms reappear. Beta-adrenergic blocking agents dampen alcohol withdrawal tremor and have been reported to decrease agitation and autonomic signs as well, reducing the need for benzodiazepines or other sedatives.

Ethanol, when used parenterally, has the disadvantage of a low therapeutic index. Because ethanol is directly toxic to many organs, it should be avoided during hospitalization even though most patients resume drinking on discharge. Neither phenothiazines nor haloperidol have a specific effect on hallucinations; theoretically, they are less likely to prevent hallucinosis or delirium tremens than drugs cross-tolerant with ethanol, and they can exacerbate seizures.

Status epilepticus during ethanol withdrawal is treated as in other situations; intravenous phenobarbital or diazepam has an advantage, compared to phenytoin, of reducing other withdrawal symptoms when the patient awakens. Long-term anticonvulsants in patients with ethanol withdrawal seizures are superfluous; abstainers do not need them, and drinkers do not take them. An epileptic whose seizures are often precipitated by ethanol abuse unfortunately does need treatment, even though compliance is unlikely.

Hypomagnesemia is common during early ethanol withdrawal, and although it may not be the primary cause of symptoms, magnesium sulfate should be given to hypomagnesemic patients. Hypokalemia and hypocalcemia may also be present, and the latter may respond to treatment only when hypomagnesemia is corrected. Parenteral thiamine and multivitamins are given even if there are no clinical signs of depletion.

Delirium tremens, once appearing, cannot be reversed abruptly by any agent, and specific cross-tolerance of a sedative with ethanol is less important in full-blown delirium tremens than in early abstinence. Parenteral diazepam is more effective than paraldehyde in

Table 159–4. Treatment of Ethanol Withdrawal

Prevention or Reduction of Early Symptoms
  Diazepam 10–40 mg or chlordiazepoxide 25–100 mg, PO or IV, repeated hourly until sedation or mild intoxication. Successive daily doses tapered by about one fourth of preceding day's with resumption of higher dose if withdrawal symptoms recur.
  Alternatively, pentobarbital 200 mg, PO, IM, or IV, and then 100 mg hourly prn. Maintenance dose and duration determined by symptoms. Subsequent tapering at about 100 mg/day.
  Alternatively, paraldehyde 5–15 mg, PO or PR, repeated hourly prn. Maintenance and tapering titrated with symptoms. Thiamine 100 mg and multivitamins, IM or IV.
  Magnesium, potassium, and calcium replacement as needed.

Delirium Tremens
  Diazepam 10 mg IV, then 5 mg or more (up to 40 mg) every 5 minutes until calming. Maintenance diazepam IV (or IM) 5 mg or more every 1 to 4 hours, prn.
  Careful attention to fluid and electrolyte balance; several liters of saline/day, or even pressors, may be needed.
  Cooling blanket or alcohol sponges for high fever.
  Prevent or correct hypoglycemia.
  Thiamine and multivitamin replacement.
  Consider coexisting illness (e.g., liver failure, pancreatitis, meningitis, subdural hematoma).

rapid calming and has fewer adverse reactions (including apnea) and lower mortality. The required doses might be fatal in a normal person (see Table 159–4), but one cannot predict in an individual patient how high the tolerable dose is. Liver disease decreases the metabolism of diazepam, and patients with cirrhosis may be more vulnerable to the depressant effects of sedatives; as delirium tremens clears, hepatic encephalopathy takes its place.

General medical management in delirium tremens is intensive. Although dehydration may be severe enough to cause shock, patients with liver damage may retain sodium and water. Hypokalemia can cause cardiac arrhythmias. Hypoglycemia may be masked, as may other serious coexisting illnesses such as alcoholic hepatitis, pancreatitis, meningitis, or subdural hematoma.

Wernicke-Korsakoff Syndrome

Although pathologically indistinguishable, Wernicke and Korsakoff syndromes are clinically distinct. Wernicke syndrome, when full-blown, consists of mental, eye movement, and gait abnormalities. Korsakoff syndrome is only a mental disorder that differs qualitatively from that of the Wernicke syndrome (Table 159–5). Both are the result of thiamine deficiency.

In acute Wernicke syndrome mental symptoms most often consist of a "global confusional state," appearing over days or weeks; there is inattentiveness, indifference, decreased spontaneous speech, disorientation, impaired memory, and lethargy. Stupor and coma are unusual, as is selective amnesia. Disordered perception is common; a patient might identify the hospital room as his apartment or a bar. In less than 10% is mentation normal.

Abnormal eye movements include nystag-mus (horizontal with or without vertical or rotatory components), lateral rectus palsy (bilateral but usually asymmetric), and conjugate gaze palsy (horizontal, with or without vertical), progressing to complete external ophthalmoplegia. While sluggishness of pupillary reaction is common, total loss of reactivity to light does not seem to occur and ptosis is rare. Whether mental symptoms in acute Wernicke syndrome ever occur without abnormal eye movements is uncertain.

Truncal ataxia, present in over 80% of patients, may prevent standing or walking. Dysarthria and limb ataxia, especially in the arms, are infrequent. Peripheral neuropathy, which occurs to some degree in most patients, may cause weakness sufficient to mask the ataxia. Abnormalities of caloric testing are common, with gradual improvement, often incomplete, in several months.

Patients with Wernicke syndrome frequently have signs of nutritional deficiency (e.g., skin changes, tongue redness, cheilosis) or liver disease. Autonomic signs are common. Although beri-beri heart disease is rare, acute tachycardia, dyspnea on exertion, and postural hypotension unexplained by hypovolemia are common, and sudden circulatory collapse may follow mild exertion. Hypothermia is less frequent; fever usually indicates infection.

In acute Wernicke syndrome, the EEG may show diffuse slowing or it may be normal. CSF is normal except for occasional mild protein elevation. Elevated blood pyruvate, falling with treatment, is not specific. Decreased blood transketolase (which requires thiamine pyrophosphate as cofactor) more reliably indicates thiamine deficiency.

In most cases, the more purely amnestic syndrome of Korsakoff emerges as the other mental symptoms of Wernicke syndrome respond to treatment. Korsakoff syndrome

Table 159–5. Major Nutritional Disturbances in Alcoholics

Disorder	Clinical Features	Deficiency
Wernicke syndrome	Dementia, with lethargy, inattentiveness, apathy, and amnesia Ophthalmoparesis Gait ataxia	Thiamine
Korsakoff syndrome	Dementia, mainly amnesia, with or without confabulation	Thiamine
Cerebellar degeneration	Gait ataxia; limb coordination relatively preserved	?
Polyneuropathy	Distal limb sensory loss and weakness; less often autonomic dysfunction	?
Amblyopia	Optic atrophy, decreased visual acuity, central scotomata; total blindness rare	?

rarely occurs without a background of Wernicke syndrome. The amnesia is both anterograde, with inability to retain new information, and retrograde, with rather randomly lost recall for events months or years old. Alertness, attentiveness, and behavior are relatively preserved, but there tends to be a lack of spontaneous speech or activity. Confabulation is not invariable and, if initially present, tends gradually to disappear. Insight is usually impaired, and there may be flagrant anosognosia for the mental disturbance.

The histopathologic lesions of Wernicke-Korsakoff syndrome consist of variable degrees of neuronal, axonal, and myelin loss, prominent blood vessels, reactive microglia, macrophages, and astrocytes, and, infrequently, small hemorrhages. Nerve cells may be relatively preserved in the presence of extensive myelin destruction and gliosis, and astrocytosis may predominate chronically. Lesions affect the thalamus (especially the dorso-medial nucleus and the medial pulvinar), the hypothalamus (especially the mammillary bodies), the midbrain (especially the oculomotor and periaqueductal areas), and the pons and medulla (especially the abducens and medial vestibular nuclei). In the anterior-superior vermis of the cerebellum, severe Purkinje cell loss and astrocytosis accompany lesser degrees of neuronal loss and gliosis in the molecular and granular layers.

The traditional view that the memory impairment of Korsakoff syndrome is the result of lesions in the mammillary body has been challenged by others who attribute amnesia to lesions in the dorsomedial nucleus of the thalamus. The global confusion of Wernicke syndrome, on the other hand, may occur without visible thalamic lesions, and may be a biochemical disorder. Periaqueductal, oculomotor, or abducens nucleus lesions may explain ophthalmoparesis, which also is seen in patients whose eye movement disorders resolved before death. The cerebellar and vestibular lesions probably contribute to ataxia.

Experimental and clinical evidence ascribes a specific role to thiamine in the Wernicke-Korsakoff syndrome. A genetic influence is implied because only a few alcoholic or otherwise malnourished people are affected and Caucasians seem more susceptible.

Untreated Wernicke-Korsakoff syndrome is fatal, and the mortality rate is 10% among treated patients. Concomitant liver failure, infection, or delirium tremens may make the cause of death unclear. Postural hypotension and tachycardia call for strict bed rest; associated medical problems may require intensive care. The cornerstone of treatment is thiamine, 50 to 100 mg daily until a normal diet can be taken; intramuscular or intravenous administration is preferred because thiamine absorption is impaired in chronic alcoholics. Hypomagnesemia may retard improvement after thiamine treatment; magnesium is therefore replaced, along with other vitamins. Protein intake may have to be titrated against the patient's liver status.

With thiamine treatment, the ocular abnormalities (especially abducens and gaze palsies) improve within a few hours and usually resolve within a week; in about 35% of the patients, horizontal nystagmus persists indefinitely. Global confusion may improve in hours or days and usually resolves within a month, leaving Korsakoff amnesia in over 80%. In less than 25% of these patients, there is eventual clearing of the memory deficit. Ataxia may improve in a few days but recovery is complete in less than 50% of patients, and nearly 35% do not improve at all.

Alcoholic Cerebellar Degeneration

Cerebellar cortical degeneration may occur in nutritionally deficient alcoholics without Wernicke-Korsakoff syndrome (see Table 159–5). Instability of the trunk is the major symptom, often with incoordination of leg movements. Arm ataxia is less prominent; nystagmus and dysarthria are rare. Symptoms evolve in weeks or months and eventually stabilize, sometimes even with continued drinking and poor nutrition. Ataxia without Wernicke disease is less likely to appear abruptly or to improve.

Pathologically, the superior vermis is invariably involved, with nerve cell loss and gliosis in the molecular, granular, and especially the Purkinje cell layers. There may be secondary degeneration of the olives and of the fastigial, emboliform, globose, and vestibular nuclei. Involvement of the cerebellar hemispheric cortex is exceptional and limited to the anterior lobes. Pathologic evidence of Wernicke disease may coexist even though it is unsuspected clinically. CT and autopsies, moreover, have revealed cerebellar atrophy in alcoholics who were not clinically ataxic.

Alcoholic cerebellar degeneration is probably nutritional in origin. Identical lesions occur in malnourished nonalcoholics, and ataxia may begin in malnourished alcoholics after weeks of abstinence. The clinical and pathologic similarity to the cerebellar component of Wernicke syndrome suggests shared mechanisms, but most patients with alcoholic cerebellar degeneration do not have pathologic evidence of Wernicke disease.

Alcoholic Polyneuropathy

Alcoholic polyneuropathy is a sensorimotor disorder, probably of nutritional origin, that stabilizes or improves with abstinence and an adequate diet (see Table 159–5). Neuropathy is found in most patients with Wernicke-Korsakoff syndrome, but more often occurs alone. Paresthesias are usually the first symptom; there may be burning or lancinating pain and exquisite tenderness of the calves or soles. Impaired vibratory sense is usually the earliest sign; proprioception tends to be preserved until other sensory loss is substantial. Loss of ankle jerks is another early sign; eventually there is diffuse areflexia. Weakness appears at any time, and may be severe. Distal leg muscles are affected first, although proximal weakness may be marked. Radiologically demonstrable neuropathic arthropathy of the feet is common, as are skin changes (e.g., thinning, glossiness, reddening, cyanosis, hyperhidrosis). Peripheral autonomic abnormalities are usually less prominent than in diabetic neuropathy, but may cause urinary and fecal incontinence, hypotension, hypothermia, cardiac arrhythmia, dysphagia, dysphonia, impaired esophageal peristalsis, altered sweat patterns, or abnormal Valsalva ratio. Pupillary parasympathetic denervation is rare. The CSF is usually normal except for occasional mild elevation of protein.

Pathologically, there is degeneration of both myelin and axons; it is not certain which occurs first. Clinical and experimental evidence suggest that alcoholic polyneuropathy is nutritional in origin, and that more than thiamine may be lacking.

Peripheral nerve pressure palsies, especially radial and peroneal, are common in alcoholics. Nutritional polyneuropathy may increase the vulnerability of peripheral nerves to compression injury in intoxicated subjects, who tend to sleep deeply in unusual locations and positions. Recovery usually takes days or weeks; splints during this period can prevent contractures.

Alcoholic Amblyopia

Alcoholic amblyopia is a visual impairment that progresses over days or weeks, with development of central or centrocecal scotomas and temporal disc pallor (see Table 159–5). Demyelination affects the optic nerves, chiasm, and tracts, with predilection for the maculopapular bundle. Retinal ganglion cell loss is secondary. Ethanol (or tobacco) toxicity plays little or no role; amblyopia clears in patients who receive dietary supplements but continue to smoke and drink ethanol. Alcoholic amblyopia does not progress to total blindness; it may remain stable without change in drinking or eating habits. Improvement, which is often incomplete, nearly always follows nutritional replacement.

Alcoholic Liver Disease

Cirrhosis is the sixth leading cause of death in the United States, and nearly all cirrhosis deaths in people older than 45 are caused by ethanol. Altered mentation in an alcoholic therefore always raises the possibility of hepatic encephalopathy, which may accompany intoxication, withdrawal, Wernicke syndrome, meningitis, subdural hematoma, hypoglycemia, or other alcohol states. Hepatic encephalopathy is discussed in detail in Section 151, "Hepatic Disease." Other neurologic disorders encountered in alcoholic cirrhotics include a poorly understood syndrome of altered mentation, myoclonus, and progressive myelopathy following portacaval shunting, and "acquired (non-Wilsonian) chronic hepatocerebral degeneration," a characteristic syndrome of dementia, dysarthria, ataxia, intention tremor, choreoathetosis, muscular rigidity, and asterixis, which usually occurs in patients who have had repeated bouts of hepatic coma.

Hypoglycemia

Metabolism of ethanol by alcohol dehydrogenase and of acetaldehyde by mitochondrial aldehyde dehydrogenase utilize NAD. The resulting elevated NADH/NAD ratio impairs gluconeogenesis and, if food is not being eaten and liver glycogen is depleted, there may be severe hypoglycemia with altered behavior, seizures, coma, or focal neurologic deficit. Residual symptoms are common, including dementia. Even after appropriate treatment with intravenous 50% dextrose, these patients require close observation; blood glucose may fall again, with the return of symptoms and possibly permanent brain damage.

Ethanol stimulates intestinal release of secretin, which, by enhancing glucose-stimulated insulin release, aggravates reactive hypoglycemia, especially in children.

Alcoholic Ketoacidosis

In alcoholic ketoacidosis, beta-hydroxybutyric acid and lactic acid accumulate in association with heavy drinking. The mechanism is unclear. Typical patients are chronic alcoholic young women who increase their ethanol consumption for days or weeks and then stop drinking when they are overcome by anorexia. Vomiting, dehydration, confusion, obtundation, and Kussmaul respiration ensue. Blood glucose may be normal, low, or moderately elevated, with little or no glycosuria. A large anion gap is accounted for by beta-hydroxybutyrate, lactate, and lesser amounts of pyruvate and aceto-acetate. Serum insulin levels are low, and serum levels of growth hormone, epinephrine, glucagon, and cortisol are high, but glucose intolerance usually clears without insulin and is not demonstrable upon recovery. It is not unusual for patients to have repeated attacks of alcoholic ketoacidosis.

Alcoholics may have other reasons for metabolic acidosis with a large anion gap (e.g., methanol or ethylene glycol poisoning). When beta-hydroxybutyrate is the major ketone present, the nitro-prusside test ("Acetest") may be negative. Treatment includes infusion of glucose (and thiamine), correction of dehydration or hypotension, and replacement of electrolytes such as potassium, magnesium, and phosphate. Small amounts of bicarbonate may be given. Insulin is usually not needed.

Infection in Alcoholics

Alteration of white blood cell function contributes to the alcoholic's predisposition to infection (e.g., bacterial and tuberculous meningitis). Infectious meningitis must always be considered in alcoholics with seizures or altered mental status, even when the clinical picture seems to be that of intoxication, withdrawal, thiamine deficiency, hepatic encephalopathy, hypoglycemia, or other alcoholic disturbances.

Trauma in Alcoholics

Thrombocytopenia, a direct effect of ethanol and a consequence of cirrhosis, increases the likelihood of intracranial hematomas after head injury. Abnormalities of clotting factors also increase the possibility of intracranial hematomas. Experimentally, moreover, acute ethanol enhances blood-brain barrier leakage around areas of cerebral trauma. Close observation is essential after even mild head injury in intoxicated patients; an abnormal sensorium must not be dismissed as drunkenness.

Alcohol and Stroke

Although some data suggest that moderate ethanol ingestion protects against coronary artery disease, case-control and cohort studies have shown an increased risk of both occlusive and hemorrhagic stroke (especially rupture of saccular aneurysm) among drinkers. There are several possible mechanisms. Heavy drinkers have an increased prevalence of hypertension. Ethanol may cause cerebral vasodilatation or cerebral arteriolar and venular spasm; studies have described both inhibition and facilitation of platelet aggregation. There are also effects, independent of liver damage, on coagulation factors. Alcoholic cardiomyopathy predisposes to embolic stroke.

Alcoholic Myopathy

In every large series of patients with myoglobinuria, a disproportionate number of patients are alcoholic. The biochemical abnormality that predisposes alcoholics to myoglobinuria is not understood. Chronic myopathy with progressive proximal limb weakness and elevated serum creatine kinase (CK) has also been reported, although the specific relationship to alcohol has been questioned.

Central Pontine Myelinolysis and Marchiafava-Bignami Disease

Central pontine myelinolysis occurs in both alcoholics and nondrinkers, appears related to abnormalities of sodium and water, and causes symptoms consistent with the pathologic findings. Marchiafava-Bignami disease, on the other hand, is nearly always associated with alcoholism (including wine, beer, and whiskey). It is of unknown origin and causes symptoms, including death, that are scarcely explained by the characteristic callosal lesions. Central pontine myelinolysis and Marchiafava-Bignami disease are discussed in detail in Sections 137 and 138.

Alcoholic Dementia

Alcoholic dementia refers to progressive mental decline in alcoholics, without apparent cause, nutritional or otherwise. Although probably common, the pathologic basis is unclear, but ventricles and cerebral sulci are often enlarged. Whether mental function and atrophy improve with abstinence is controversial.

Fetal Alcohol Syndrome

The association of maternal alcoholism with congenital malformations and delayed psychomotor development has been known for only 20 years. Major clinical features of the "fetal alcohol syndrome" include cerebral dysfunction, growth deficiency, and distinctive facies (Table 159–6); less often there are abnormalities of the heart, skeleton, urogenital organs, skin, and muscles. Neuropathologic abnormalities include absence of corpus callosum, hydrocephalus, and abnormal neu-

Table 159–6. Clinical Features of the Fetal Alcohol Syndrome

Feature	Majority	Minority
CNS	Mental retardation Microcephaly Hypotonia Poor coordination Hyperactivity	
Impaired growth	Prenatal for length and weight Postnatal for length and weight Diminished adipose tissue	
Abnormal face		
Eyes	Short palpebral fissures	Ptosis Strabismus Epicanthal folds Myopia Microphthalmia Blepharophimosis Cataracts Retinal pigmentary abnormalities
Nose	Short, upturned Hypoplastic philtrum	
Mouth	Thin vermilion lip borders Retrognathia in infancy Micrognathia or prognathia in adolescence	Prominent lateral palatine ridges Cleft lip or palate Small teeth with faulty enamel
Maxilla	Hypoplastic	
Ears		Posteriorly rotated Poorly formed concha
Skeletal		Pectus excavatum or carinatum Syndactyly, clinodactyly, or campodactyly Limited joint movements Nail hypoplasia Radiolunar synostosis Bifid xiphoid Scoliosis Klippel-Feil anomaly
Cardiac		Septal defects Great vessel anomalies
Cutaneous		Abnormal palmar creases Hemangiomas Infantile hirsutism
Muscular		Diaphragmatic, inguinal, or umbilical hernias Diastasis recti
Urogenital		Labial hypoplasia Hypospadias Small rotated kidneys Hydronephrosis

ronal migration, with cerebellar dysplasia, heterotopic cell clusters, and microcephaly. These changes occur independently of other potentially incriminating factors such as maternal malnutrition, smoking, caffeine, or age. Binge-drinking, which may produce high ethanol levels at a critical fetal period, may be more important than chronic ethanol exposure, and early gestation appears to be the most vulnerable period.

Children of alcoholic mothers are often intellectually borderline or retarded without other features of the fetal alcohol syndrome; fetal effects of ethanol may thus cover a broad spectrum. Stillbirths and minimal brain damage (attention deficit disorder) seem especially frequent among offspring of heavy drinkers, and each anomaly of the fetal alcohol syndrome may occur alone or in combination with others. The face of a typical patient with the fetal alcohol syndrome is distinctive and as easily recognized at birth as that of the infant with Down syndrome. Irritability and tremulousness, with poor suck reflex and hyperacusis, are usually present at birth and last weeks or months. Of these children, 85% perform more than two standard deviations below the mean on tests of mental performance; those who are not grossly retarded rarely have even average mental ability. Older children are often hyperactive and clumsy, and there may be hypotonia or hypertonia. Except for neonatal seizures, epilepsy is not a component of the syndrome.

Ethanol is directly teratogenic to many animals, but the mechanism is not known. In humans, this risk of alcohol-induced birth defects is established above 3 oz of absolute alcohol daily. Below that, the risk is uncertain; a threshold of safety has not been defined. The incidence of fetal alcohol syndrome may be as high as 1 to 2/1000 live births, with partial expressions of 3 to 5/1000. It may affect 1% of infants born to women who drink 1 oz of ethanol daily early in pregnancy. About 35% of the offspring of heavy drinkers are affected by fetal alcohol syndrome. Fetal alcohol syndrome may be the leading teratogenic cause of mental retardation in the Western world.

Treatment of Chronic Alcoholism

The literature on the treatment of alcoholism is voluminous, and strong opinions outweigh scientific data. Not all problem drinkers consume physically addicting quantities of ethanol; no personality type defines an alcoholic; and the relative roles of genetics and social deprivation vary from patient to patient. Such variability of alcoholic populations means, of course, that no treatment modality (e.g., psychotherapy, group psychotherapy, family or social network therapy, drug therapy, behavioral [aversion] therapy) and no single therapeutic setting (e.g., general hospital, a halfway house, a vocational rehabilitation clinic, Alcoholics Anonymous) is appropriate for all. For example, the success rate of Alcoholics Anonymous has been estimated to be 34%.

The use of tranquilizing and sedating drugs is especially controversial, because they may lead to switching of dependency or to drug-ethanol interactions. Some clinicians espouse short-term use of these drugs in doses high enough to reduce the psychological tensions that lead to ethanol use, but low enough not to block symptoms of ethanol withdrawal.

Disulfiram inhibits aldehyde dehydrogenase and reduces the rate of oxidation of acetaldehyde, accumulation of which may account for most symptoms that appear soon after someone taking disulfiram drinks ethanol. Within 5 to 10 minutes of ethanol ingestion, there is warmth and flushing of the face and chest, throbbing headache, dyspnea, nausea, vomiting, sweating, thirst, chest pain, palpitations, hypotension, anxiety, confusion, weakness, vertigo, and blurred vision. The severity and duration of these symptoms depend on the amount of ethanol drunk; a few milliliters can cause mild symptoms followed by drowsiness, sleep, and recovery; severe reactions can last hours or be fatal, and require hospital admission, with careful management of hypotension and cardiac arrhythmia.

Taken in the morning, when the urge to drink is least, disulfiram 0.25 to 0.5 g daily does not alter the taste for ethanol and helps only patients who strongly desire to abstain. In the United States 150,000 to 200,000 patients are maintained on disulfiram, although controlled studies demonstrating substantial long-term benefit are lacking. Side-effects of disulfiram that are unrelated to ethanol ingestion include drowsiness, psychiatric symptoms, and cardiovascular problems. Paranoia, impaired memory, ataxia, dysarthria, and even major motor seizures may be difficult to distinguish from ethanol effects, as may peripheral neuropathy. Hypersensitivity hepatitis may also occur.

Clinical studies on the use of lithium in

chronic alcoholism have been promising, but it is not yet accredited therapy for this condition. The same can be said for most other recommended psychotherapeutic and drug treatments.

References

Blass JP, Gibson GE. Abnormality of a thiamine-requiring enzyme in patients with Wernicke-Korsakoff syndrome. N Engl J Med 1977; 297:1367–1370.

Brust JCM. Stroke and drugs. In: Toole JF (ed), Vascular Diseases, part 2. Handbook of Clinical Neurology (vol II). Amsterdam: Elsevier Science, 1988.

Donahue RP, Abbott RD, Reed DM, Yano K. Alcohol and hemorrhagic stroke. The Honolulu Heart Program. JAMA 1986; 255:2311–2314.

Fuller RK, Branhey L, Brightwell DR, et al. Disulfiram treatment of alcoholism. A Veterans Administration cooperative study. JAMA 1986; 256:1449–1455.

Goldstein DB. Effects of alcohol on cellular membranes. Ann Emerg Med 1986; 15:1013–1018.

Isbell H, Fraser HF, Wikler A. An experimental study of the etiology of "rum fits" and delirium tremens. Q J Stud Alcohol 1955; 16:1–33.

Kraus ML, Gottlieb LD, Horwitz RI, Anseher M. Randomized clinical trial of atenolol in patients with alcohol withdrawal. N Engl J Med 1985; 313:905–909.

Lishman WA. Alcoholic dementia: A hypothesis. Lancet 1986; 1:1184–1186.

Mendelson JH, Mello NK, eds. The diagnosis and treatment of alcoholism. New York: McGraw-Hill, 1979.

Ng SKC, Hauser WA, Brust JCM, Susser M. Alcohol consumption and withdrawal in new-onset seizures. N Engl J Med 1988; 319:666–673.

Ravenholt RT. Addiction mortality in the United States 1980: Tobacco, alcohol, and other substances. Popul Dev Rev 1984; 10:697–724.

Rubin E. Alcoholic myopathy in heart and skeletal muscle. N Engl J Med 1979; 301:28–33.

Sellers EM, Kalant H. Alcohol intoxication and withdrawal. N Engl J Med 1976; 294:757–762.

Streissguth AP, Clarren SK, Jones KL. Natural history of the fetal alcohol syndrome: A 10-year follow-up of eleven patients. Lancet 1985; 2:85–91.

Suzdak PD, Glowa JR, Crawley JN, et al. A selective imidazobeno-diazepine antagonist of ethanol in the rat. Science 1986; 234:1243–1247.

Thompson WL, Johnson AD, Maddrey WL, et al. Diazepam and paraldehyde for treatment of severe delirium tremens. A controlled trial. Ann Intern Med 1975; 82:175–180.

Victor M, Adams RD. The effect of alcohol on the nervous system. Res Publ Assoc Res Nerv Ment Dis 1953; 32:526–573.

Victor M, Adams RD, Mancall EL. A restricted form of cerebellar cortical degeneration occurring in alcoholic patients. Arch Neurol 1959; 1:579–688.

Victor M, Dreyfus PM. Tobacco-alcohol amblyopia. Further comments on its pathology. Arch Ophthalmol 1965; 74:649–657.

Victor M, Adams RD, Collins GH. The Wernicke-Korsakoff Syndrome. Philadelphia: FA Davis, 1971.

160. DRUG ABUSE
Ralph W. Richter

Cannabis

The hemp plant cannabis sativa has been used for its euphoric properties for several thousand years. Delta 9 tetrahydrocannabinol (Δ9 THC) is the most prevalent psychoactive substance in the plant. *Marihuana,* or "grass," is a mixture of flowering tops, leaves, small stems, and grains containing 1% to 2% THC. *Hashish* contains the resin of the flowering tops and contains 5% to 10% THC. There are other forms as well.

Marihuana use has increased in all age groups and is linked to the use of other drugs; marihuana has emerged as a boundary drug between licit drugs (tobacco and alcohol) and illicit drugs.

The psychic effects of cannabis include a general feeling of pleasure, increased excitement, and distortion of time and space. As the dose is increased, ideas may verge to paranoia, irresistible impulses, illusions, and hallucinations. Autonomic effects include dry mouth, tachycardia, hypertension, and enhanced tendon reflexes. There are no marked or consistent pupillary changes but tremors, miosis, drowsiness, and stupor can occur.

The primary physiologic changes produced by marihuana occur in the limbic-diencephalic structures but vary from stimulation of limbic activity to depression, or from disinhibition to inhibition, depending on the dose, time, previous experience, and current mood. The cellular mechanisms are uncertain. A major acute interaction of THC with other psychoactive drugs is mutual potentiation of depressant properties and antagonism of any stimulant properties; when THC is added to any of these drugs, the resultant effect either becomes more depressant or shifts to the depressant side.

Frequent (daily) users of cannabis develop tolerance to both physical and psychological effects of the drug so that dosage increases or the user seeks more potent psychotropic drugs. Cannabis users do not present physical dependence as manifest by specific withdrawal symptoms. After discontinuation of cannabis, anorexia, insomnia, and irritability are well tolerated, but psychological dependence is an obstacle to discontinued usage. Animal experiments point to permanent damage of the mammalian brain but it has not been possible to document damage to the human limbic system or to appraise changes in personality.

Lysergic Acid Diethylamide

Since medieval times, psychotic experiences have resulted from eating ergot-contaminated bread. Lysergic acid diethylamide (LSD-25) is a partially synthetic amide of lysergic acid, the basic structure of many important ergot alkaloids. Amides of lysergic acid are also found in morning glory seeds. These compounds readily pass the blood-brain barrier and the blood-placental barrier.

Psychic alterations affect mood and perception, causing visual hallucinations, distortions of body image, acute panic reactions or schizophrenia-like reactions, and acute paranoid states. Recurrent drug state effects (flashbacks) may occur in the absence of the drug and may be precipitated in former LSD-25 users who take other psychotomimetic substances including marihuana. Chronic LSD-25 users may be severely depressed or suicidal. LSD-25 rarely causes convulsions. Most bad acid trips can be treated on an outpatient basis. If a toxic psychosis occurs and there is immediate danger, hospitalization is indicated and haloperidol by oral or intramuscular route is used.

Mescaline

Peyote or mescal-buttons are still used in religious ceremonies by Indians of the southwestern United States and Mexico. Mescaline is said to be the active ingredient in the peyote obtained from cactus and chemically related to amphetamine; other hallucinogenic phenethylamines have close structural relationships to LSD-25.

Belladonna

Drugs from belladonna plants include atropine and scopolamine. Synthetic atropine derivatives are glycolate esters. These substances are readily absorbed after ingestion and the duration of action may last from 8 to more than 24 hours. They depress the cholinergic brain stem activating system, producing slow waves in the EEG.

These agents cause marked auditory hallucinations, memory loss (in contrast to LSD-25), clouding of consciousness, incoherence, and hyperthermia.

Phencyclidine

Phencyclidine (PCP) is an arylcycloalkylamine used in veterinary medicine. The street drug ("angel dust") is synthesized inexpensively in illegal laboratories. It is one of the most frequently abused drugs. It is taken by smoking, swallowing, or "snorting." The drug acts rapidly after ingestion. The duration of the drug's influence is dose-dependent, usually minutes or hours, although some patients have been affected for several days. The drug seems to act especially on thalamo-neocortical and limbic systems; autonomic effects are sympathomimetic. The psychic actions of PCP resemble sensory isolation. Sensory impulses reach the neocortex, but the neural signals are grossly distorted. Psychotic states may resemble schizophrenia. For treatment of this toxic psychosis, haloperidol is recommended; phenothiazines may potentiate the anticholinergic actions of PCP.

Seizures and agitation after PCP intoxication can be treated with diazepam. Hypertension, if marked, should be treated with diazoxide or hydralazine. Severe intoxication may necessitate use of assisted respiration or antiarrhythmic drugs. To enhance excretion, continuous gastric suctioning, urinary acidification, and augmenting urine output with fluids and diuretics have been recommended; oral administration of activated charcoal may bind with PCP secreted into stomach.

Amphetamines and Anorectics

Amphetamines and related synthetic stimulants include dextroamphetamine, methamphetamine, phenmetrazine, and methylphenidate. Stimulants do not induce severe physiologic dependence or withdrawal, but "reinforcing effects" may contribute to the use of these drugs in combination with others.

Acute high-dose amphetamine use may induce a toxic hallucinatory state; chronic amphetamine psychosis includes paranoid symptoms; visual, auditory, and olfactory hallucinations; delusions of persecution; and body-image changes.

Intravenous administration of methamphetamine ("speed") is used for a "rush." The acute overdose hypertensive crisis may precipitate a stroke. Microvascular insults may follow chronic intoxication; "angiitis" can be demonstrated on angiograms by arterial "beading." Hemorrhagic or thrombotic strokes may occur in chronic intravenous abusers.

Sudden death has been ascribed to cardiac arrhythmias. Other direct effects include grand mal convulsions and choreoathetoid dyskinesia. Symptoms of sympathomimetic stimulation such as anxiety, tremulousness, hypertension, and tachycardia are controlled with diazepam or chlorpromazine. Barbiturates should be avoided becaused they may produce an excited-delirious state. Alpha-adrenergic blockers may be required to treat acute hypertension. Seizures and hyperthermia require vigorous control because the latter may precipitate disseminated intravascular coagulation.

Cocaine

Cocaine is a local anesthetic of high efficiency and a powerful CNS stimulant of short duration with a low margin of safety. It is legally classified as a Schedule II drug with high abuse potential and small recognized medical use.

Cocaine is the most widely used illegal drug in the U.S. The cocaine alkaloid *("freebase")* is called *"crack"* because of the sound made by crystals popping when it is heated or *"rock"* because of its appearance. Cocaine can be snorted or injected intravenously. Smoking of freebase delivers large quantities of cocaine to the lung vascular bed producing effects comparable to intravenous injection.

Euphoria, restlessness, excitability, and increased heart rate and blood pressure are seen. Hyperpyrexia, tonic-clonic convulsions, angina pectoris, ventricular arrhythmias, and myocardial infarction have occurred. Cerebrovascular accidents related to cocaine abuse have been described, including subarachnoid hemorrhage. Treatment of overdose is symptomatic with respiratory and cardiovascular monitoring and support systems.

The intensity of the euphoric psychological experience may lead to delirium, paranoid ideation, and assaultive behavior that is followed by a dysphoric "crash." Repeated doses may then be tried and often are used with alcohol, marihuana, or opiates to decrease irritability.

Cocaine dependency has reached all social classes. Adequate treatment methods are lacking. Residential therapeutic communities or treatment in an inpatient hospital unit may be needed.

Inhalants

Commercially available volatile solvents include model airplane glue, fingernail polish remover, gasoline, paint thinner, plastic cements, cleaning fluids, and aerosol propellants. Intentional inhalation of volatile agents is often peer-originated and peer-perpetuated. The "high" includes euphoria, drowsiness, and ataxia; it may lead to delirium and toxic psychosis. Psychic dependence may develop.

In glue-sniffers, chronic toxicity may include peripheral neuropathy; "huffer's" neuropathy is predominantly motor and is attributed to n-hexane. N-hexane neuropathy is also seen in industrial workers and has been produced experimentally in rats. Amyl nitrite and isobutylnitrite have become popular among adults as producers of brief altered-states-of-consciousness and as orgasm "expanders."

Sedative Hypnotics

Barbiturates and other sedative hypnotics are the most widely prescribed psychoactive drugs in the United States. Some individuals are prone to overuse any drug that lessens anxieties; most of these persons have no identification with drug subcultures. Episodes of acute intoxication with slurred speech and ataxic gait should draw the physician's attention to drug abuse. Development of physical dependence to barbiturates occurs after continuous intoxication for periods of 92 to 144 days. After abrupt withdrawal, an abstinence syndrome is characterized by disappearance of signs of intoxication, weakness, tremor, anxiety, anorexia, nausea and vomiting, rapid weight loss, increased pulse and respiration rates, fever, increased blood pressure, difficulty in making cardiovascular adjustments in standing, grand mal seizures, and delirium. Death may follow acute withdrawal, delirium, or hyperpyrexia.

After prolonged use, nonbarbiturate sedative hypnotics can also provide physical dependence and a barbiturate-like withdrawal syndrome with possible convulsions. These agents include meprobamate (Miltown, Equanil), glutethimide (Doriden), ethchlorvynol (Placidyl), methyprylon (Noludar), ethinamate (Valmid), chlordiazepoxide (Librium), diazepam (Valium), oxazepam (Serax), and methaqualone (Quaalude). Methaqualone may also cause peripheral neuropathy.

Detoxification from barbiturates and other sedative hypnotic dependence should be carried out in the hospital because of possible life-threatening complications and because cross-dependence barbiturates may be substituted by other drugs, followed by gradual dose reduction. The equivalent daily dose of phenobarbital substitutes for the total estimated daily tolerance dose of short-acting sedatives by administering one "sedative dose" (30 mg) of phenobarbital for each "hypnotic dose" of the short-acting barbiturate or sedative the patient has been using.

Overdose with sedative hypnotics may be life-threatening. Gastric lavage is indicated for patients who have ingested overdoses of soporific or hypnotic drugs, regardless of the time elapsed since ingestion. Endotracheal intubation should precede gastric lavage in unresponsive patients. The rate of onset of coma is usually an indication of the quantity of drug absorbed. Forced diuresis may promote the excretion of drugs that have significant renal excretory rates. Patients in prolonged severe coma and patients who have ingested potentially lethal doses may benefit from hemodialysis if the ingested drug is dialyzable. Larger molecular structures may be removed by plasmapheresis.

Designer Drugs and MPTP

A number of narcotics and stimulants have been structurally redesigned in clandestine laboratories to escape current laws. Examples include analogs of fentanyl and an anesthetic dubbed "China white," which are several thousand times more potent than heroin.

A product of meperidine analog synthesis (MPTP) produced chronic parkinsonism in a group of addicts after intravenous use. Symptoms occurred, on a delayed basis, after drug use had stopped and progressed. The most severely affected patients had rigidity, masked facies, flexed posture, and abnormal gait. MPTP in animal studies has been found to be selectively toxic to cells of the zona compacta of the substantia nigra. Thus, an animal model for Parkinson disease has inadvertently become available.

Opiates

Opiates are derived from the seed pods of poppies. They were used as sedatives and analgesics by the ancient Egyptians and have long been used for pleasure in Eastern cultures. Morphine is the major alkaloid base of opium and was named in honor of Morpheus, the Greek god of dreams. Morphine combines analgesia with the capacity to relieve anxiety, but repeated use produces tolerance and physical dependence. Sudden withdrawal of morphine or other opiates or the administration of antagonists leads to an imbalanced enkephalinergic system resulting in the exaggerated sympathetic autonomic phenomena

that form the clinical withdrawal or abstinence syndrome.

Heroin is the synthetic 3,6-diacetate ester of morphine. It was introduced in 1898 as a "nonaddicting" cough medicine. Not only is heroin highly addictive, but it crosses the blood-brain barrier much more readily than morphine. In the United States, heroin (diacetylmorphine) has been the opioid drug most frequently associated with nonmedical opioid dependency; heroin can be taken through sniffing or by intradermal, intramuscular, or intravenous injection. Methadone, another synthetic compound, was originally used as a heroin substitute in addicts under medical supervision, but methadone has also been distributed illicitly and is now a major toxic hazard in nontolerant persons.

In New York City, narcotic abuse has become the leading cause of death in the 15 to 35 age group: more than 50% of the deaths followed acute reactions, 40% were a result of violence related to drug use, and about 5% were caused by infection. In one ghetto hospital, 6.7% of all patients had narcotic addiction recorded as one of the diagnoses. Neurologic abnormalities were encountered in 2.6% of the addicts. Newborns of addicted mothers made up 4.3% of total addict discharges.

The addict usually injects an unsterile mixture of heroin adulterated by quinine, lactose, or other diluents. Illicitly obtained methadone may be taken with the adulterated heroin. Opiate overdose causes coma, depressed respiration, tachycardia, and contracted pupils. In deeper levels of coma or with severe hypoxia, the patient's pupils may be dilated. The overdose may be complicated by increased intracranial pressure and convulsive seizures. An oral airway is inserted and the patient is ventilated. Naloxone, an opiate antagonist, is administered intravenously, 0.4 mg every 5 minutes. Careful observation is needed in methadone overdose because the drug action lasts more than 24 hours. With the increasing incidence of multidrug ingestion (including alcohol, tranquilizers, and sedatives) in addiction to narcotics, respiratory depression may alternate with episodes of hyperactivity and delirium.

OPIATE WITHDRAWAL

Signs and Symptoms. Physiologic or pharmacologic dependence is manifested by signs and symptoms produced either by termination of the drug (withdrawal abstinence or abrupt withdrawal) or by administration of narcotic antagonists such as naloxone (precipitated or acute abstinence). The frequency with which certain signs and symptoms of narcotic withdrawal were observed in a group of 320 heroin-using soldiers in Vietnam is presented in (Table 160–1). The subgroup of intravenous users had the highest frequency of withdrawal signs and symptoms.

Non-narcotic Medical Regimen. A non-narcotic medical regimen frequently can provide symptomatic relief for the four primary problems associated with narcotic withdrawal: pain, gastrointestinal symptoms, insomnia, and nervousness.

Pain. Muscle, bone, and joint pain and aches may be controlled adequately with analgesics such as propoxyphene (Darvon), 65 or 130 mg every 3 to 4 hours. Milder symptoms may be treated with aspirin or phenacetin. Muscle spasms usually can be managed with diazepam (Valium), 10 mg; chlorzoxazone (Paraflex), 500 to 750 mg; or 250 mg chlorzoxazone plus 300 mg acetaminophen (Parafon Forte) every 4 to 6 hours.

Gastrointestinal Symptoms. Nausea may be controlled by prochlorperazine (Compazine), 10 mg, or trimethobenzamide (Tigan), 250 mg every 4 hours. If vomiting persists, the patient should be hospitalized or started on methadone detoxification. Diarrhea and gastrointestinal cramps usually can be managed by diphenoxylate with atropine (Lomotil), 2.5 to 5 mg every 4 hours. Propantheline (Pro-Banthine), 15 to 30 mg or dicyclomine (Bentyl), 10 mg every 4 to 6 hours also is helpful in controlling gastrointestinal cramps and diarrhea, and the pharyngeal congestion, sialorrhea, rhinorrhea, and lacrimation associated with opiate withdrawal.

Isomnia. This is frequently one of the most difficult symptoms to control without narcotic substitution therapy. Chloral hydrate in relatively large doses (2 to 2.5 g) with or without diphenhydramine (Benadryl), 100 mg at bedtime, frequently is helpful. Barbiturates should be avoided, especially in an outpatient withdrawal program, because of the potential for abuse.

Methadone for Detoxification. Methadone should be used only in the treatment of patients who have objective evidence of physical dependence; it should be initiated only after objective signs of opiate withdrawal. Whether detoxification is carried out on an inpatient or outpatient basis depends on the individual situation. During the past several years, a number of treatment programs have successfully used outpatient methadone detoxification.

Different methadone reduction schedules have been employed. In most patients, an initial dose of 15 to 20 mg of oral methadone is adequate to control symptoms. If the patient is hospitalized, the next dose can be given when symptoms return. If treatment is car-

Table 160–1. Observed and Reported Signs and Symptoms During Heroin Withdrawal

Sign/Symptom	Smoking N = 200 (%)	Sniffing N = 60 (%)	Injection (IV) N = 60 (%)
Rhinorrhea	56.5	65.0	73.3
Lacrimation	53.0	60.0	68.3
Diaphoresis	41.5	40.0	61.7
Piloerection	42.0	40.0	63.3
Chilliness	52.0	58.3	70.0
Hot/cold flashes	45.0	48.3	56.7
Muscle cramps	25.0	35.0	46.7
Back/leg/joint pains	63.5	73.3	90.0
Muscle twitching/tremor	26.5	30.0	40.0
Restlessness	84.0	85.0	96.7
Double-blurred vision	19.0	10.0	18.3
Headaches	32.0	28.3	31.7
Insomnia	74.5	71.7	81.7
Abdominal cramps	60.5	58.3	93.3
Nausea	32.5	41.7	55.0
Vomiting	16.5	25.0	45.0
Diarrhea	37.0	46.7	48.3
No signs or symptoms	6.0	0.0	0.0

(From Richter RW. Medical Aspects of Drug Abuse. Hagerstown, Maryland. Harper and Row. 1975. With permission.)

ried out on an outpatient basis, only enough methadone should be given to last 24 hours. The patient should be seen and re-evaluated daily. Generally, 30 to 40 mg of methadone during the first 24 hours is adequate. Because the effects of methadone last more than 12 hours, no more than two doses in a 24-hour period are required.

If symptoms are controlled adequately by 30 to 40 mg during the first 24 hours of withdrawal, a daily reduction of 5 to 10 mg/day can be initiated. The rate of reduction must be individualized. Most patients can be completely withdrawn from the drug in 3 to 10 days.

Clonidine for Detoxification. Clonidine hydrochloride, the alpha$_2$ adrenergic agonist, has substantial antiwithdrawal effects; it replaces opiate-medicated inhibition of brain noradrenergic activity, and has been found particularly effective in methadone withdrawal. Usually 5 μg/kg/day (0.35 mg/day for a 70 kg man) in two equal doses is sufficient. Six to 10 days of inpatient therapy, with tapering to avoid rebound hypertension, usually is required. Clonidine should never be given concomitantly with opiates of any type. The combination causes dizziness, oversedation, and severe hypotension.

COMPLICATIONS OF ADDICTION TO OPIATES

Cerebral Complications. Cerebral sequelae of a drug overdose may include acute delirium with agitation, tremors, and hallucinations that last for hours or days. Chronic dementia may result from prolonged anoxia or cardiorespiratory arrest. Rare postoverdose complications in opiate addicts include stroke, parkinsonian tremors, hemiballism, and dystonia (Table 160–2).

In acute reactions, cerebral edema is frequent when comatose patients survive for a prolonged period. There may be evidence of diffuse myelin breakdown in cerebral deep white matter, marked depletion of astrocytes of deep white matter, or neuronal depletion of the globus pallidus.

Transverse Myelitis. Acute transverse myelitis may occur after heroin is taken intravenously after a period of abstinence (e.g., in prison or hospital). The acute myelitis may be due to systemic reaction (to the heroin, quinine, or other adulterants), transient ischemia (in the vulnerable thoracic cord circulation), hypersensitivity reaction, or direct toxicity of the drug.

Nerve and Muscle Disorders. Peripheral

Table 160–2. Neurologic Complications of Addiction to Opiates

Cerebral complications of narcotic overdose

  Coma without complications
  Coma with neurologic sequelae
    Seizures (focal, generalized, status epilepticus)
    Increased intracranial pressure
    Acute delirium
    Chronic organic brain damage
    Delayed postanoxic encephalopathy
    Stroke
    Involuntary movement disorder

Transverse myelitis

Toxic (quinine) amblyopia

Deafness

Peripheral nerve lesions
  Brachial and lumbosacral plexitis
  Atraumatic and traumatic mononeuropathy
  Acute or subacute polyneuropathy

Muscle disorders
  Acute myoglobinuria
  Chronic myopathy
  Crush syndrome after coma

Addiction-related infections with neurologic complications
  Endocarditis and other septic states
  Osteomyelitis
  Tuberculosis
  Local abscesses, pyomyositis or fasciitis
  Malaria
  Tetanus

Acquired immune deficiency syndrome (AIDS)*

*AIDS is transmitted by shared use of intravenous needles.

nerve lesions in opiate addicts may result from drug injections into nerves or from the pressure of the tourniquet used to make a target vein swell. Atraumatic mononeuritis, brachial and lumbosacral plexitis, and fulminating symmetric polyneuropathy resembling Guillain-Barré syndrome have also been observed. Hypersensitivity reactions are a possible cause of these disorders.

Fibrosing myopathy is common among "skin-poppers" due to repeated superficial intramuscular injections of opiates and adulterants. The clinical features of "crush syndrome" (i.e., myoglobinuria and local injury of skin and muscle of the dependent side of comatose patients) may appear after narcotic overdose. Myoglobinuria may also follow venous injection of heroin-adulterant mixtures with no evidence of trauma, compression, or ischemia.

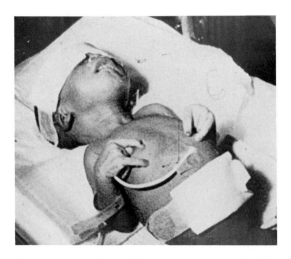

Fig. 160–1. Newborn infant undergoing narcotic withdrawal with muscle rigidity, tremors, and seizures.

Fetal Addiction. Opiates freely cross the placenta. Signs of withdrawal may be detected in the fetus in utero following abrupt discontinuation of drug use in the mother. The newborn infant, deprived of the maternal source of narcotics, may show withdrawal symptoms, especially a unique type of coarse flapping tremor and irritability. Muscular rigidity is common (Fig. 160–1). Diarrhea and vomiting are common. A shrill, high-pitched cry, sneezing, and yawning are often present. Convulsions and myoclonic jerks may occur. Neonatal withdrawal symptoms may be partly controlled with phenobarbital and chlorpromazine. Respiratory center changes related to intrauterine exposure to narcotics are considered contributing factors in sudden infant death, also reported in these infants.

Maternal heroin addiction is associated with a high incidence of intrauterine growth retardation and prematurity. These children stand a high risk of developing some degree of psychomotor retardation.

Endocarditis and Other Septic States. Abuse of narcotics often involves parenteral injection of unsterile substances through makeshift apparatus. Addicts with unrecognized subacute bacterial endocarditis may present with embolic stroke, meningitis, brain abscess, or subarachnoid hemorrhage from mycotic aneurysms (Fig. 160–2). Cutaneous infections and multiple vascular injection sites provide excellent routes for systemic inoculation by Staphylococcus aureus, gram-negative saprophytes, or candida. Resistant bacterial organisms require rigorous treatment. Surgical intervention and intensive

chemotherapy are necessary for candida endocarditis and some gram-negative infections. Septic states without endocarditis may also lead to bacterial meningitis, brain abscess, and subdural or epidural abscesses. Cerebral mucormycosis has been documented in heroin addicts.

Bone, Muscle, and Fascial Injections. Hematologic osteomyelitis in narcotic addicts usually involves lumbar or cervical vertebrae or the sacrum. The intervertebral disks are affected, narrowing joint spaces and causing bone destruction and sclerosis. Back pain is accompanied by low-grade fever. Predominant organisms are Pseudomonas aeruginosa, Staphylococcus aureus, and candida. Potts (tuberculous) abscess may present in similar manner. Needle aspiration under fluoroscopic control may suffice for obtaining a culture, but open surgery to obtain a good diagnostic bone sample may be necessary. Long-term antibiotic treatment is necessary and recovery is slow. Radiographic changes may persist, making criteria for progress mainly clinical. Decreased pain or progressive ambulation are the most useful criteria.

Fulminating onset of fever and swollen, tender deep muscles may be due to infections similar to tropical pyomyositis. Rapid spread of the infection along fascial planes may create medical and surgical emergencies.

Malaria. Falciparum malaria, frequently with acute brain lesions, was common among heroin addicts in New York in the 1930s. Quinine was then added to the opiates and artificially transmitted malaria disappeared; it surfaced again in California in 1973 when drug mixtures omitted quinines.

Hepatitis. Acute viral hepatitis due to use of contaminated needles may progress to coma, seizure phenomena, decerebrate rigidity, and death.

Tetanus. Tetanus in addicts may be atypical in onset. Multiple skin abscesses are commonly seen. Myalgias may be attributed to drug withdrawal rather than to onset of tetanus. By the time help is obtained, tetanus may be established. The most common presenting symptoms are trismus and paraspinal rigidity; generalized muscle spasms last for seconds or minutes. Adequate respiratory management of tetanus in these patients invariably requires tracheostomy and controlled ventilation. For control of convulsions, intravenous administration of phenobarbital with intramuscular chlorpromazine is useful, but curare may have to be given intrave-

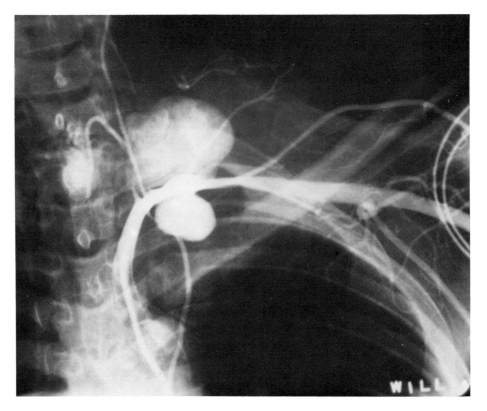

Fig. 160–2. Left subclavian arteriogram of addict who had left brachial plexus compression by a large myoctic aneurysm arising from subclavian artery. There are at least two contrast-filled compartments to the aneurysm.

nously. Use of curare requires continuous sedation of the patient and rigorous ventilatory therapy. Cardiovascular complications, including sympathetic overactivity, are common. The frequency of tetanus among addicts dropped after extensive immunization programs among clients of addiction treatment programs.

Intravenous drug abusers in this country and Europe are particularly vulnerable to infection by retroviruses, the agents of the acquired immunodeficiency syndrome (AIDS). The human immunodeficiency virus (HIV) has neurotropic properties and acute meningitis is seen as well as progressive dementia. Many other neurologic complications including myelopathies, peripheral neuropathies, opportunistic CNS infections, and CNS neoplasms may also be seen in HIV-infected addicts.

TREATMENT IN A THERAPEUTIC COMMUNITY

Narcotic dependence is a complex psychosocial illness with cultural, historical, and socioeconomic dimensions. Success in treatment is highly dependent on the motivation of each addicted person. Self-interest, desire,

and will are major characteristics of human nature that can be directed creatively toward restorative therapy.

The therapeutic community approach depends on the concept that an individual's environment can be used as an instrument of therapy. A number of community-based, drug-free, long-term residential treatment and rehabilitation centers are available. Some programs also employ outpatient treatment successfully.

The emphasis in therapy is on present behavior, interpersonal relationships, and attitudes. The individual learns to accept the unchangeable reality of the past and is required to think in terms of "what can be done now." The addict then examines the internal resources that release effective coping skills. Group situations subject the addict to scrutiny and confrontation by peers. No single client can play one staff member against another or against the community. This forces openness in therapy and honesty in interpersonal relationships and behavior. There is a constant refusal to "do for" the addict. The emphasis is on helping him to explore himself and to obtain group identity. Exaddicts develop pride; whatever is accomplished has more meaning under these circumstances and affords the stimulus needed for growth. Many of the basic pathologic features of the addict—loneliness, isolation, dependency, low self-esteem—thus may be gradually overcome.

References

Cregler LL, Mark H. Medical complications of cocaine abuse. N Engl J Med 1987; 315:1495–1500.

DeGans J, Stam J, Van Wijngaarden GK. Rhabdomyolysis and concomitant neurological lesions after intravenous heroin abuse. J Neurol Neurosurg Psychiatry 1985; 48:1057–1059.

Heurich AE, Brust JCM, Richter RW. Management of urban tetanus. Med Clin North Am 1973; 57:1373–1381.

Khantzian EJ, McKenna GJ. Acute toxic and withdrawal reactions associated with drug use and abuse. Ann Intern Med 1979; 90:361–372.

Koppel BS, Tuchman AJ, Mangiardi JR, et al. Epidural spinal infection in intravenous drug abusers. Arch Neurol 1988; 45:1331–1340.

Langston JW, Langston EB, Irwin I. MPTP-induced parkinsonism in human and non-human primates. Acta Neurol Scand 1984; 70(Suppl 100):49–54.

Misken DBW, Lorenz MA, Pearson RL, Dankovich AM. Pseudomonas aeruginosa bone and joint infection in drug abusers. J Bone Joint Surg [Am] 1983; 65-A:829–832.

Pearson J, Richter RW. Addiction to opiates: Neurologic aspects. In: Vinken PJ, Bruyn GW, eds. Handbook of Clinical Neurology (vol 37). New York: Elsevier-North Holland, 1979:365–400.

Prockop L, Couri D. Nervous system damage from mixed organic solvents. Review of inhalants: Euphoria to dysfunction. In: Sharp CW, Brehm MC, eds. Rockville, MD: USDHEW National Institute for Drug Abuse, 1977:185–196.

Richter RW, ed. Medical Aspects of Drug Abuse, Hagerstown: Harper & Row, 1975.

161. IATROGENIC DISEASE
Lewis P. Rowland

The growing number of drugs used to treat human disease and the growing number of invasive procedures used for diagnosis and therapy have generated a new class of illness. 15 years ago, 3% of admissions to Boston hospitals were due to adverse drug reactions and 30% of all patients in those hospitals had at least one adverse drug reaction. The figures may be higher now. Neurologic reactions were not prominent in that list, although they accounted for 20% of all adverse reactions in another study.

A partial list of the neurologic syndromes (Table 161–1) seems formidable at first glance, and it is important to put that list in perspective. The drugs listed do not cause an adverse reaction every time they are used. For example, penicillin is high on the list of drugs that cause convulsive encephalopathies, but only a few cases have been recorded. Most of the other disorders are rare.

Some reactions, however, are common. Tardive dyskinesia is a price paid by many individuals for control of mental disorders, and levodopa-induced dyskinesia is the exchange many make for control of parkinsonism. Cerebral hemorrhage or femoral neuropathy due to retroperitoneal hemorrhage is the price a few patients pay for the prevention of stroke in many other patients. Drug-induced confusion and ataxia are common effects of anticonvulsants, and mental dulling or poor school performance are matters of concern for those who treat epilepsy. The adverse effects of radiotherapy limit our treatment of brain tumors. Control or elimination of these effects by alternative agents or procedures therefore has high priority in the therapeutic needs of neurology. The same must be said for the adverse effects of drugs that are used to treat neurologic disease but which may damage other organs (e.g., corticosteroids, immunosuppressive drugs, antineoplastic drugs).

It is sometimes difficult to list the rare side-effects of a drug without inappropriately frightening the patient or physician. When considering the list of adverse reactions one must consider the relative risks and the benefits expected from the use of specific drugs or specific procedures; patients must understand the trade-offs involved if they are to be able to give *informed consent*.

There is another aspect of these drug reactions; some have what might be considered beneficial effects. For instance, the neuroparalytic accidents that followed the use of rabies vaccine led to the discovery of experimental autoimmune encephalomyelitis, and this, in turn, has had a lasting impact on our concepts of multiple sclerosis. In the meantime, vaccines have been improved and now rarely lead to neurologic disease. Similarly, penicillamine-induced myasthenia is a rare syndrome, but it has led to valuable observations about the nature of myasthenia. Penicillin has also become important in the study of experimental epileptic neurons. Other drugs have been used to analyze the nature of peripheral neuropathies; some act on Schwann cells or myelin, others on the perikaryon, others distally on the axon. Understanding the pathogenesis of some adverse reactions may lead to improved medical care in areas beyond the direct impact of the drugs involved.

Table 161–1. Adverse Neurologic Reactions Due to Drugs or to Procedures for Diagnosis or Therapy

Adverse Reaction	Drug or Procedure	Adverse Reaction	Drug or Procedure
Basal ganglia syndromes (parkinsonism, tardive dyskinesia, dyskinesias)	Reserpine Phenothiazines Butyrophenones Levodopa	Muscle fibrosis	Pentazocine Meperidine
Leukoencephalopathy	Vaccines Radiation Methotrexate	Myotonia	Diazacholesterol
		Malignant hyperthermia	Succinylcholine Halothane, other anesthetics
Encephalopathy	Penicillin Lithium Monoamine oxidase inhibitors Insulin (hypoglycemia) Propoxyphene Pentazocine Phenytoin Carbamazepine Hemodialysis Metrizamide Methotrexate Vincristine Corticosteroids Insulin-induced hypoglycemia Overhydration (water intoxication) Cimetidine Radiotherapy	Neuroleptic malignant syndrome	Neuroleptic drugs
		Myelopathy	Intrathecal injections (methotrexate, iophendylate) Spinal anesthesia Spinal angiography Arachnoiditis after myelography Radiotherapy Iodochlorhydroxyquin Vaccination
		Stroke	Massage of carotid sinus Chiropractic manipulation of neck Overcorrection of high blood pressure Induced hypotension for surgery Procedures that cause cardiac arrest Cerebral angiography Open heart surgery Oral contraceptives Insulin-induced hypoglycemia Amphetamines Anticoagulants Radiotherapy of neck or head
Central pontine myelinolysis	Rapid correction of hypernatremia		
Brain tumor	Immunosuppression (sarcoma) Radiotherapy (meningioma)		
Meningoencephalitis (viral, yeast, toxoplasmosis)	Immunosuppression		
Pseudotumor cerebri	Corticosteroids Tetracycline Naldixic acid Vitamin A	Peripheral neuropathy	Isoniazid Nitrofurantoin Ethambutol Phenytoin Vincristine Procarbazine Disulfiram Nitrous oxide
Myopathies and myoglobinuria	Corticosteroids Penicillamine Anticonvulsants (with osteomalacia) Emetine Ipepac Thiazides, furosemide, and other kaliuretics Chloroquin Epsilon caproic acid Bacterial toxins due to tampon use (toxic shock syndrome)	Hypophosphatemia	Vaccination Anticoagulants (compression of nerve by hematoma) Barbiturates (in acute porphyria) Perihexilene Disopyramide Metronidazole
Myasthenia	Penicillamine Anticonvulsants	Optic neuropathy	Penicillamine Chloroquine Isoniazid Ethambutol Vincristine
Other neuromuscular block	Aminoglycoside antibiotics Succinylcholine		

References

Allain T. Dialysis myelopathy; Quadriparesis due to extradural amyloid of beta-microglobulin origin. Brit Med J 1988; 296:752–753.

Anonymous. Drugs that cause psychiatric symptoms. Med Lett Drugs Ther 1986; 28:81–86.

Atkinson JLD, Sundt TM, Jr, Kazmier FJ, Bowie EJW, Whisnant JP. Heparin induced thrombocytopenia and thrombosis in ischemic stroke. Mayo Clin Proc 1988; 63:353–361.

Baker GL, Kahl LE, Zee BC, Stolzer BL, Agarawal AK, Medsger TA Jr. Malignancy following treatment of rheumatoid arthritis with cyclophosphamide. Long-term case-control follow-up study. Am J Med 1987; 83:1–10.

Bowyer SL, LaMothe MP, Hollister JR. Steroid myopathy: Incidence and detection in a population with asthma. J Allergy Clin Immunol 1985; 76:234–242.

Caranasos GJ, Stewart RB, Cluff LE. Drug-induced illness leading to hospitalization. JAMA 1974; 228:713–717.

Critchley EMR. Drug-induced neurological disease. Br Med J 1979; 1:862–865.

Cybulski GR, D'Angelo CM. Neurological deterioration after laminectomy for spondylotic cervical myeloradiculopathy: The putative role of spinal cord ischaemia. J Neurol Neurosurg Psychiatry 1988; 51:717–718.

Dahlquist NR, Perrault J, Callaway CW, Jones JD. D-lactic acidosis and encephalopathy after jejunoileostomy: Response to overfeeding and to fasting in humans. Mayo Clin Proc 1984; 59:141–145.

Denicoff KD, Rubinow DR, Papa MZ, et al. The neuropsychiatric effects of treatment with interleukin-2 and lymphokine-activated killer cells. Ann Intern Med 1987; 107:293–300.

Dyck PJ, Classen SM, Stevens JC, Obrien PC. Assessment of nerve damage in the feet of long-distance runners. Mayo Clin Proc 1987; 62:56–57.

Evans CDH, Lacey JH. Toxicity of vitamins: Complications of a health movement. Br Med J 1986; 292:509–510.

Fadul CE, Lemann W, Thaler HT, Posner JB. Perforations of the gastrointestinal tract in patients receiving steroids for neurologic disease. Neurology 1988; 38:348–352.

Hohlfeld R, Michels M, Heininger H, Besinger U, Toyka KV. Azathioprine toxicity during long-term immunosuppression of generalized myasthenia gravis. Neurology 1988; 38:258–262.

Hunter JM. Adverse effects of neuromuscular blocking drugs. Br J Anaesth 1987; 59:46–60.

Junck L, Marshall WH. Neurotoxicity of radiological contrast agents. Ann Neurol 1983; 13:469–484.

Kramer J, Klawans HL. Iatrogenic neurology: Neurologic complications of nonneuropsychiatric agents. Clin Neuropharmacol 1979; 4:175–198.

Lane RJM, Mastaglia F. Drug-induced myopathies in man. Lancet 1978; 2:562–566.

Laschinger JC, Izumoto H, Kouchoukos NT. Evolving concepts in prevention of spinal cord injury during operations on the descending thoracic and thoraco—abdominal aorta. Ann Thorac Surg 1987; 44:667–674.

Levenson JL. Neuroleptic malignant syndrome. Am J Psychiatry 1985; 142:1132–1145.

McWey RE, Curry NS, Schabel SI, Reines HD. Complications of nasoenteric feeding tubes. Am J Surg 1988; 155:253–257.

Malouf R, Brust JCM. Hypoglycemia: Causes, neurological manifestations and outcome. Ann Neurol 1985; 17:421–430.

Marton KI, Gean AD. The spinal tap: A new look at an old test. Ann Int Med 1986; 104:840–848.

Miller RR. Hospital admissions due to adverse drug reactions. A report from the Boston Collaborative Drug Surveillance Program. Arch Intern Med 1974; 134:219–223.

Rosenberg M, McCarten JR, Snyder BD, Tulloch JW. Case report; hypophosphatemia with reversible ataxia and quadriparesis. Am J Med Sci 1987; 293:261–261.

Schaumberg H, Kaplan J, Windebank A, et al. Sensory neuropathy from pyridoxine abuse: A new megavitamin syndrome. N Engl J Med 1983; 309:445–448.

Seale JP, Compton MR. Side-effects of corticosteroid agents. Med J Aust 1986; 144:139–142.

Silverstein A, ed. Neurological Complications of Therapy. Mt. Kisco, NY: Futura, 1982.

Smith BH, ed. Symposium on iatrogenic disorders of the nervous system. NY State J Med 1977; 77:1090–1117.

Sterns RH, Riggs JE, Schochet SS Jr. Osmotic demyelination syndrome following correction of hyponatremia. N Engl J Med 1986; 314:1535–1542.

Sury MRJ, Russell GN. Hydrocortisone myopathy. Lancet 1988; 2:515.

Swash M, Schwartz MS. Iatrogenic neuromuscular disorders: A review. J Roy Soc Med 1983; 76:149–151.

Toshniwal PK, Glick RP. Spinal epidural lipomatosis; report of a case secondary to hypothyroidism and review of the literature. J Neurol 1987; 234:172–176.

Watanabe T, Trusler GA, Williams WG, Edmonds JF, Coles JG, Hosokawa Y. Phrenic nerve paralysis after pediatric cardiac surgery. J Thorac Cardiovasc Surg 1987; 94:383–388.

Zampella EJ, Duvall ER, Sekar RC, et al. Symptomatic spinal epidural lipomatosis as a complication of steroid immunosuppression in cardiac transplantation patients. J Neurosurg 1987; 67:760–774.

---

162. POLLUTANTS AND INDUSTRIAL HAZARDS
David Goldblatt

Accidental acute exposure to a large amount of a toxic material usually causes a well-defined syndrome that often involves other organs and the nervous system. On the other hand, if chronic exposure to potentially toxic materials is followed by illness, it may be difficult to establish toxicity as the cause. For example, amyotrophic lateral sclerosis (ALS) has developed in persons exposed to lead, mercury, and selenium, but a cause-effect relationship has not been established. These problems become even greater for people who are exposed to hazardous materials that are released as pollutants into the environment away from the place of manufacture or primary use. For example, it is uncertain what harm, if any, has come to North American Indians who consume large amounts of fish contaminated with methyl mercury. Even more equivocal are situations such as the Love Canal incident of chemical dumping near Niagara Falls, defoliant spraying in Vietnam, and the aerial distribution of organophosphorus pesticides in the western states. In the latter, the mass media have created "a cause in search of a disease." This statement is meant to emphasize the need for objectivity and a scientific approach, including dose-response data. Methods such as behavioral testing and electrophysiologic measurements are being added to the more traditional toxicologic and biochemical techniques to discover possible consequences of chronic low-dose exposure to diverse materials such as lead, aluminum, and food additives. The possible food additive-induced hyperactivity in children and similar putative toxic effects of low-dose environmental exposure are not sufficiently established to be discussed in this text. The possibility that Guam ALS-parkinsonism-dementia is caused by an amino acid excitotoxin in sago flour, however, keeps the interest in toxic food substances as slow neurotoxins high.

Table 162–1 summarizes the principal manifestations of some common occupational and environmental hazards to health. The table should be read from left to right, because each agent listed in the right-hand column is not found in every environment mentioned, and does not account for every manifestation listed.

Aluminum

Encephalopathy has been reported to result from inhalation of aluminum dust. Patients undergoing chronic renal dialysis may develop a progressive, fatal encephalopathy that has been more common in treatment centers where aluminum-containing water is not deionized. Clinically, the condition is characterized by dysarthric-dyspractic speech, myoclonus, dementia, and focal seizures. The EEG is abnormal. There are no specific histologic changes in the brain, and neurofibrillary degeneration is not present.

In cats and rabbits, aluminum induces a progressive encephalopathy with neurofibrillary degeneration resembling that seen in Alzheimer disease. The aluminum content of brains from patients with Alzheimer disease is elevated in patchy distribution. In both the experimental and human disorders, the metal accumulates within cell nuclei, and likely influences the genetic apparatus. In contrast, although the overall alumimum content of cerebral gray matter is abnormally high in dialysis encephalopathy, it is actually lower than control values within cell nuclei. These complexities indicate that, at present, a causative role for aluminum in human disease has not been established. A possible relationship exists between long-term exposure to particulate alumina in a smelting plant and the development of incoordination, intention tremor, cognitive changes, and spastic paraparesis in exposed workers.

Arsenic

Arsenic poisoning may result from occupational or environmental exposure. Arsenic is used in insecticides, weed killers, and wood preservatives. It has accounted for deaths from contaminated beer. It is not widely used in rat poisons today, and has little current medicinal use, although it is employed in treatment of trypanosomiasis.

The symptoms of arsenic poisoning are related mainly to the gastrointestinal tract and to the nervous system, usually as painful polyneuropathy. Skin changes also occur; white striae in the fingernails (Mees bands) may be present. Injected and inhaled arsenicals have caused acute encephalopathy. Arsenic ingested in large doses causes vomiting, diarrhea, and convulsions; it may be lethal. Polyneuropathy may develop after an interval of several weeks in patients who recover.

The treatment of acute poisoning includes emesis or gastric lavage and osmotic cathartics. Fluid and electrolyte balance and plasma volume must be maintained; 2,3-dimercaptopropanol (BAL) is given intramuscularly in doses of 4 to 5 mg/kg of body weight every 4 hours for 24 hours, then at 6-hour intervals for 2 or 3 days, and finally in tapering doses for a total of 10 days. The clinical benefit of treatment of encephalopathy remains unproved. For chronic poisoning, 2.5 mg/kg of body weight is given 4 times daily for 2 days, twice on the third day, and then continued by daily injection to complete a 10-day course.

Barium

Barium is used in depilatories and some pesticides. Its soluble salts (unlike the barium sulfate used in radiologic examinations) are absorbed systemically and can lower serum potassium, producing a clinical picture resembling periodic paralysis.

Bismuth

Bismuth in soluble form is no longer used to treat systemic disorders such as syphilis, but prolonged use of insoluble bismuth salts for gastrointestinal disorders can result in absorption. It has been held responsible for a reversible encephalopathy with mental derangement.

Lead

Lead has no biologic or medicinal use and is considered potentially harmful when taken into the body in any amount, although many apparently asymptomatic persons have a measurable level of lead in their bodies. Lead poisoning (plumbism) may result from occupational exposure or from the accidental ingestion of lead compounds or lead-containing paint.

Lead encephalopathy occurs chiefly in children who ingest lead-containing paint chips and putty, which are still found in old houses. Beverages that have been stored in lead-glazed earthenware pottery are a potential hazard; fatal encephalopathy developed in a child who habitually drank apple juice from an earthenware pitcher. Encephalopathy has also been reported in adults who drank whiskey that had been distilled in automobile radiators.

Pathologic Changes. The classic alteration in lead encephalopathy is swelling of the brain with flattened gyri and small ventricles. This is associated with a vasculopathy in which protein-containing edema fluid surrounds the abnormally permeable capillaries. The capillaries have swollen and proliferated endothelial cells and may show thrombi and focal necrosis. Cortical neuronal necrosis may be focal or laminar, and appears to be ischemic in origin, although lead may have a direct toxic effect on neurons and an indirect toxic effect through a vascular mechanism. None of these changes is constant, however, and there may be no discernible alterations in fatal cases. Even when the brain is swollen, herniation is rare and the mechanism of death is usually unclear.

Symptoms and Signs. The onset of cerebral symptoms is usually abrupt and may be coincidental with the onset of acidosis. Convulsive seizures of a generalized or focal nature are common. Paralysis may follow the seizures. Any type of neurologic sign may develop, including cerebellar ataxia, hemiplegia, or decerebrate rigidity. Lethargy, delirium, and coma are not uncommon. The optic disks may be swollen or there may be optic atrophy. Cranial nerve palsies are uncommon, although facial or oculomotor paralysis may develop. The sutures of the skull are sep-

arated and the fontanelles, if still open, are bulging. Polyneuropathy may accompany the encephalopathy in older children, but in infants there is usually no evidence of this. The body temperature is usually normal, but may be elevated in association with convulsions or in the terminal stages of the disease.

Laboratory Data. Lead in blood and urine indicates recent exposure. Even if they have no definite symptoms, children with blood levels of lead higher than 30 μg/dL should be considered intoxicated. Zinc protoporphyrin accumulates in red blood cells, and erythrocyte porphyrin above 60 μg/dL supports the diagnosis of lead intoxication. In adults, an undue body burden is associated with a plasma lead level of 60 μg/dL or more. Damage to the proximal tubule may lead to excretory loss of glucose, phosphate, and amino acids. Urinary excretion of delta-aminolevulinic acid is an indirect measure of toxicity. Hypochromic anemia and basophilic stippling of red cells develop. Radiography may disclose lead in the intestines and in the epiphyseal plates of long bones. The CSF may be under greatly increased pressure, with elevated protein. The CSF white blood cell count may be normal, but is more commonly in the range of 20 to 40 cells/mm^3, and cell counts of several hundred may occur.

Diagnosis. The diagnosis of lead encephalopathy in infants is made from the history of pica, the anemia, and the laboratory data described. Brain tumor, subdural hematoma, tetany, metachromatic leukodystrophy, and other causes of convulsions and paralysis should be considered in the differential diagnosis. CT reveals cerebral edema.

Treatment and Prognosis. Although mortality in acute lead encephalopathy is now low, common residual effects include dementia, seizures, ataxia, and spasticity. Treatment involves the use of 2,3-dimercaptopropanol (BAL) and edetate ethylenediaminetetraacetic acid (EDTA) for chelation of lead. General supportive measures include maintenance of ventilation, control of seizures, cleansing the bowel of residual lead, and cautious administration of fluids because inappropriate secretion of ADH often occurs. Use of steroids in conjunction with edetate ethylenediaminetetraacetic acid (EDTA) has been questioned. Mannitol may be needed to reduce intracranial pressure. Oral penicillamine (with supplemental pyridoxine) may suffice in milder cases of lead poisoning and is also

Table 162–1.   Environmental and Occupational Health Hazards and Manifestations

Organ System Primarily Affected	Manifestations Acute and Chronic	Environments and Practices Conveying Increased Risk of Developing Disease	Chemical and Physical Agents
Skin	Dermatitis Chloracne Skin cancer	Electroplating, photoengraving, metal cleaning, wood preserving, food preserving, contact with foods and cosmetics, use of household chemicals and soaps.	Hydrocarbon solvents; beryllium; arsenic, zinc oxide, PCB, nickel, dioxane, soap, pentachlorophenol, bismuth, alcohol, drugs.
Respiratory system	Acute pulmonary edema and pneumonitis Asthma Chronic lung disease Lung cancer	Construction and insulation; textile manufacturing; painting; arc-welding; meat wrapping; animal handling; in-flight airline services; radiological work; exposure to traffic exhausts, dust, and industrial air pollution; improper ventilation and heating.	Arsenic, asbestos, chromium, iron oxide, ionizing radiation, beryllium, ozone, nitrogen oxides, textile dusts, nickel, carbonyl, aerosolized plastics (e.g., vinyl chloride, teflon), dusts, fumes, vapors.
Cardiovascular system	Arrhythmias Angina Intermittent claudication Arteriosclerosis	Exposure to traffic exhaust, diesel engine operation, sewage treatment, cellophane and plastic manufacturing, motor vehicle repairing, extreme hot/cold, contact with synthetic film and hazardous agents in art and hobby supplies, pest extermination.	Carbon monoxide, hydrogen sulfide, barium, organophosphates, freon, glues and solvents, heat and cold.
Gastrointestinal system	Abdominal pain, nausea Vomiting, diarrhea, bloody stools Hepatic necrosis Hepatic cancer Hepatic fibrosis	Jewelry making, dry cleaning, refrigerant manufacturing, food processing, chemical handling, printing, contact with lead-based paints and components of batteries and electrical equipment, consumption of improperly handled food.	Heavy metals (e.g., lead, cadmium); carbon tetrachloride, chlorinated hydrocarbons, phosphorus, beryllium, arsenic, nitrosamines, vinyl chloride, aflatoxin, bacterial toxin.

System	Health effects	Occupations/sources	Pollutants/hazards
Genitourinary system	Aminoaciduria Chronic renal disease Bladder cancer	Plumbing, soldering, exterminating, textile manufacturing, contact with components of batteries.	Cadmium, lead, mercury, organic dyes, halogenated hydrocarbons.
Nervous system	Headache/convulsions/coma Extrapyramidal disorders Peripheral neuropathy	Wood working, painting, exposure to traffic exhaust, fireproofing, plumbing, soldering, manufacturing of textiles and petrochemicals, contact with pesticides and battery components, consumption of improperly prepared food.	Mercury, manganese, lead, carbon monoxide, boron, fluoride, organophosphates, hexane, organic solvents, wood preservatives (pentachlorophenol).
Auditory system	Hearing loss (and stress reactions)	Subway operations, metal working, construction, activities involving loud music.	Loud noise, high frequency noise.
Ophthalmic system	Eye irritation Cataracts	Petroleum refining, chemical handling, paper production, laundering, contact with photographic films, glass blowing.	Nitrogen oxides, acetic acid, formaldehyde, radiation.
Reproductive system	Spontaneous abortions Birth defects Infertility	Operating room procedures, contact with pesticides, contact with battery components.	Anesthetic gases, ionizing and non-ionizing radiation, lead, chemicals (dioxane), pesticides (DBCP).
Hematologic system	Pancytopenia and aplasia Acute myelogenous leukemia Lymphadenopathy, anemia, buboes	Dye manufacturing; dry cleaning; chemical handling; contact with hazardous agents in art and hobby supplies; contact with rodent excreta, rodent bites.	Benzene, arsenic, organic dyes, arsine, nitrates, drugs, lead.
Nasal cavity and sinuses	Inflammation Cancer	Welding; photoengraving; manufacturing of glass, pottery, linoleum, textile, wood and leather products; contact with battery components.	Arsenic, selenium, chromium, nickelcarbonyl, wood.

(Modified from Health Systems Agency of New York City, Inc., 111 Broadway, New York, NY 10006.)

useful for chronic treatment once a course of chelating agents has been completed.

Lithium

Lithium is used to treat mania, to prevent pathologic mood swings in manic-depressive illness, and for prophylaxis of chronic cluster headache. Systemic toxicity involves the gastrointestinal tract and heart. Neurotoxicity is prominent but reversible; its severity is related to drug levels in serum. Twitching, tremor, ataxia, dysarthria, and brisk reflexes are features.

Manganese

Manganese has poisoned miners in many countries. Prolonged exposure to this metal, which is used in alloys and in unleaded gasoline, leads to behavioral changes and, later, to parkinsonism caused by widespread damage to basal ganglia. Rigidity and hypokinesia can be improved by the use of L-dopa.

Mercury

Mercury is potentially injurious in three forms: inorganic salts, metallic mercury (mercury vapor), and organomercurials. Mercuric chloride, formerly employed as a disinfectant, was sometimes ingested with suicidal intent. The brunt of damage was sustained by the kidneys, resulting in uremia with delirium, coma, and convulsions. There was no damage to the nervous system if the patient recovered.

Ingested mercury metal (from broken thermometers or ruptured intestinal tubes) is not ordinarily harmful. Brief exposure to mercury vapor is dangerous only under special circumstances, as when it volatilizes at a high temperature, causing pulmonary edema. Chronic poisoning by mercury vapor sometimes occurs among miners and among workers employed in the chlor-alkali industry, as well as among persons who make switches, thermometers, and barometers, or who calibrate scientific glassware. Chronic poisoning by inorganic mercuric salts is clinically similar to poisoning by mercury vapor, although, experimentally, mercury levels in the brain are lower in mercuric salt poisoning, which suggests that the CNS is less prominently involved.

Gastrointestinal complaints such as gingivitis, stomatitis, excessive salivation, anorexia, abdominal pains, constipation, and diarrhea develop as a result of mercurial poisoning. Neurologic complications usually take the form of tremors and personality changes. There is circumoral tremor resembling that seen in syphilitic general paresis, tremor of the tongue, and tremor of the limbs on posture-holding, which increases with voluntary movement. The psychological changes, which include timidity, seclusiveness, and irritability, have been referred to as "erethism" and the "Mad Hatter syndrome." The syndrome is reversible if the patient is removed from the contaminated environment.

Organomercurials (alkyl compounds) become more toxic as their organic moiety becomes smaller and simpler. Regulations now ban the use of methyl and ethyl mercury fungicides in many countries, after devastating incidents in the Middle East in which widespread poisoning occurred when treated grain was distributed for planting but was instead consumed by farmers who did not understand the hazard.

Biomethylation of mercury metal by microorganisms in the ocean or in polluted streams and lakes introduces deadly methyl mercury into the food chain that leads eventually to humans, but biomethylation alone has not produced definite toxicity in North Americans who eat a large amount of fish (e.g., dieters, Indians). Biosynthesis, however, may have added more methyl mercury to the preformed methyl mercury discharged by manufacturing plants in Japan, where outbreaks of poisoning in Minamata and Niigata were traced to the ingestion of fish from contaminated waters (Minamata disease).

Symptoms of methyl mercury poisoning, which may develop several weeks or months after ingestion, include paresthesias of the mouth, tongue, and limbs, constriction of the visual field, blindness, loss of hearing, weakness, inability to concentrate, dysarthria, tremors, and incoordination. When large amounts of methyl mercury have been ingested, spastic weakness may be followed by coma or death. The fetus is especially vulnerable.

Because of its propensity for combining with sulfhydryl groups in or on cellular membranes, mercury blocks sodium currents and inhibits the transport of sugars. It interferes, as well, with intracellular enzymes. Focal cerebral atrophy, perhaps on a vascular (anoxic) basis, most severely affects the precentral and striate cortex. Granule cell degeneration in the cerebellum occurs in chronic mercurialism.

Treatment of acute mercury poisoning is

carried out with 2,3-dimercaptopropanol (BAL), but this is not effective in chronic poisoning. Poisoning with mercury vapor is a syndrome that is reversible even without treatment, but mercury appears to fall more rapidly, and urinary excretion increases with the administration of penicillamine or N-acetyl penicillamine.

Thallium

Thallium therapy is now obsolete. Thallium poisoning in many cases can be traced to accidental ingestion. Swallowing a large amount of a thallium-containing rat poison usually causes death.

Gastrointestinal symptoms, epigastric pain, colic, nausea, vomiting, and diarrhea develop within 24 hours. The gastrointestinal symptoms are followed within 2 to 5 days by numbness and weakness of the limbs, delirium, convulsions, cranial nerve palsies, and blindness. The hair falls out, ecchymoses appear in the skin, and bleeding may develop from the skin. The urine contains albumin and casts. Death usually occurs within a few days.

In the chronic form of intoxication, formerly caused by small amounts of thallium absorbed from salves for ringworm or from depilatory creams, the most common symptoms are alopecia, optic neuritis, or generalized polyneuropathy. Blurring or dimness of vision develops after several weeks or months of exposure. There is loss of central vision with some constriction of the peripheral fields. The optic disks become atrophic. A generalized polyneuritis may develop coincidentally with optic neuritis; either may occur independently. Paresthesias, limb weakness, and loss of reflexes with little or no impairment of cutaneous sensibility are characteristic of involvement of the peripheral nerves by thallium.

The prognosis is poor and death usually occurs in acute poisoning when large amounts of the toxin are ingested. In the chronic form of poisoning, the prognosis for life is good. The polyneuritis is usually of only a mild or moderate degree and complete recovery is the rule. There may be improvement in vision in the patients with optic neuritis, but there is always some reduction in visual acuity. Treatment depends on making the diagnosis, which may be obscure. The hair can be tested within a few days after exposure. Chelating agents are not useful in treatment. Diethyldithiocarbamate, which increases uri-

nary excretion of thallium in the rat, may actually increase the level of thallium in the brain and has had adverse effects in human use. Prussian blue administered orally, intravenous potassium chloride, and hemodialysis have been helpful.

Methyl Alcohol

Methanol (methyl alcohol), which is metabolized to formaldehyde and formic acid, produces acute poisoning in persons who drink methanol-containing fuel in place of ethanol. The ingestion of 2 to 8 oz is lethal. Atmospheric exposure can also produce symptoms (e.g., while cleaning machinery with a methanol-containing solvent). Eyes, liver, kidney, and heart are damaged, and petechiae and edema occur in the brain, lungs, and gastrointestinal tract. Severe acidosis develops.

The symptoms of poisoning, which usually develop within a few hours of ingestion, are drunkenness, drowsiness, headache, blurring of vision, nausea, vomiting, abdominal pain, dyspnea, and cyanosis. Delirium and coma may ensue if a large amount has been ingested. Blindness is the most common symptom and persists after recovery from the acute intoxication. The occurrence of visual loss is probably related in part to individual idiosyncrasy to the drug, because it does not occur in all cases of intoxication.

When large amounts of methanol are ingested, death usually occurs within 3 days. Recovery has occurred after a coma of 3 or 4 days. Visual loss is the only neurologic sequel in patients who recover from acute poisoning. The visual acuity is greatly reduced. There is a central scotoma with constriction of the peripheral fields. The pupils may be large and may react poorly to light. The optic disk may be congested or normal in appearance. There is usually complete or nearly complete restoration of vision in the course of a few months.

The diagnosis of methanol poisoning in a comatose, hospitalized patient is difficult unless there is a history of ingestion of the poison or unless its odor can be detected on the breath. Blood methanol can be tested. The diagnosis is not difficult in patients with visual loss after acute intoxication.

Treatment involves gastric lavage, general supportive measures, and administration of alkali (sodium bicarbonate). Concomitant administration of ethanol, intravenously or orally, antagonizes the oxidation of methanol in the liver and aids in its unchanged excretion, in that way reducing exposure to its toxic metabolites. Hemodialysis is effective.

Organic Solvents

Organic compounds used as solvents and in numerous other industrial applications can cause acute encephalopathy and chronic polyneuropathy. Toxic encephalopathy is produced by methyl chloride and bromide, carbon disulfide, toluene, and ethylene glycol. Toluene also causes cerebellar atrophy with ataxia, but its neurologic effects have been associated with abuse rather than occupational exposure. Toxic neuropathy is caused by n-hexane (glue-sniffer's neuropathy), methyl n-butyl ketone, carbon disulfide, styrene, trichloroethylene, acrylamide, polychlorinated biphenyls (PCB), and triorthocresyl phosphate (TCP). Highly toxic dioxin is present as a contaminant in the herbicide TCP, and also in 2,4,5-T, an herbicide used in Vietnam in the defoliant, "Agent Orange."

Pesticides

The pesticide chlordecone (Kepone), which controls weevils, ants, and roaches, was responsible for tremor ("Kepone shakes") and other symptoms in heavily exposed industrial workers in Virginia. Considerable environmental contamination occurred but, as yet, no direct evidence of disease has been adduced among those secondarily exposed.

Organophosphate insecticides can cause polyneuropathy of delayed onset. Parathion has been considered an exception, but produced delayed polyneuropathy in one instance when a large amount was ingested with suicidal intent. Because it inhibits cholinesterase, parathion produces a cholinergic crisis after acute exposure, with symptoms including giddiness, coma, and convulsions. There are no fully accepted data concerning chronic low-dose exposure in humans, although there have been reports of psychiatric, visual, and electrophysiologic disturbances.

References

General

Arena JM. Poisoning—Toxicology, Symptoms, Treatments, 4th ed. Springfield: Charles C Thomas, 1979.

Baker EL Jr. Neurologic and behavioral disorders. In: Levy BS, Wegman DH, eds. Occupational Health. Boston: Little, Brown, 1983:317–330.

Friberg L, Nordberg GF, Vouk VB, eds. Handbook on the Toxicology of Metals. New York: Elsevier-North Holland, 1979.

He F. Occupational toxic neuropathies—an update. Scand J Work Environ Health 1985; 11:321–330.

Hunter D. The Diseases of Occupations, 6th ed. Boston: Little, Brown, 1978.

Juntunen J, ed. Occupational neurology. Acta Neurol Scand 1982; 66(suppl 92):1–218.

Last JM. Maxcy-Rosenau Public Health and Preventive Medicine, 12th ed. Norwalk, CT: Appleton-Century-Crofts, 1986.

Le Quesne PM. Toxic substances and the nervous system: The role of clinical observation. J Neurol Neurosurg Psychiatry 1981; 44:1–8.

Spencer PS, Nunn PB, Hugon J, Ludolph AC, Ross SM, Roy DN, Robertson RC. Guam amyotrophic lateral sclerosis-parkinsonism-dementia linked to a plant excitant neurotoxin. Science 1987; 237:517–522.

Spencer PS, Schaumburg HH. Experimental and Clinical Neurotoxicology. Baltimore: Williams & Wilkins, 1980.

Vinken PJ, Bruyn GW, eds. Handbook of Clinical Neurology (vol 36). New York: Elsevier-North Holland, 1979.

Aluminum

Cannata JB, Briggs JD, Junor BJR, Fell GS. Aluminium hydroxide intake: Real risk of aluminium toxicity. Br Med J 1983; 286:1937–1938.

Longstreth WT Jr, Rosenstock L, Heyer NJ. Potroom palsy? Neurologic disorders in three aluminum smelter workers. Arch Int Med 1985; 145:1972–1975.

Marlowe M, Stellern J, Errera J, Moon C. Main and interaction effects of metal pollutants on visual-motor performances. Arch Environ Health 1985; 40:221–225.

Arsenic

Alpers BJ. So-called "brain purpura" or "hemorrhagic encephalitis." Arch Neurol Psychiatry 1928; 20:497–523.

Aposhian HV. DMSA and DMPS—Water soluble antidotes for heavy metal poisoning. Annu Rev Pharmacol Toxicol 1983; 23:193–215.

Beckett WS, Moore JL, Keogh JP, Bleecker ML. Acute encephalopathy due to occupational exposure to arsenic. Br J Ind Med 1986; 43:66–67.

Blackwell M, Robbins A. Arsine (arsenic hydride) poisoning in the workplace. Am Ind Hyg Assoc J 1979; 40A:56–61.

Gerhardt RE, Crecelius EA, Hudson JB. Moonshine-related arsenic poisoning. Arch Intern Med 1980; 140:211–213.

Barium

Morton W. Poisoning by barium carbonate. Lancet 1945; 2:738–739.

Ott DJ, Gelfand DW. Gastrointestinal contrast agents. Indications, uses and risks. JAMA 1983; 249:2380–2384.

Bismuth

Buge A, Supino-Viterbo V, Raucurel G, Metzger J, Deghy H, Gardeur D. Evolutive correlations with clinical, electrical, CT scan and toxicological data in five cases of oral bismuthic encephalopathies (author's translation). Sem Hop Paris 1979; 55:1466–1472.

Stahl JP, Gaillat J, Leverve X, Carpentier F, Guignier M, Micoud M. Encephalites au sel insoluble de bismuth. Nouv Presse Méd 1983; 11:3856.

Lead

American Academy of Pediatrics Subcommittee on Accidental Poisoning: Prevention, diagnosis and treatment of lead poisoning in childhood. Pediatrics 1969; 44:291–298.

Aub, JC, Fairhall LT, Minot A, Retnikoff P. Lead poisoning. Medicine 1925; 4:1–250.

Boothby JA, deJesus PV, Rowland LP. Reversible forms of motor neuron disease—lead "neuritis." Arch Neurol 1974; 31:18–23.

Byers RK. Lead poisoning, review of the literature and report of 45 cases. Pediatrics 1959; 23:585–603.

Chisholm JJ Jr. The use of chelating agents in the treatment of acute and chronic lead intoxication in childhood. J Pediatr 1968; 73:1–38.

Chisholm JJ Jr, Kaplan E. Lead poisoning in childhood—comprehensive management and prevention. J Pediatr 1968; 73:942–950.

Klein M, Namer R, Harpur E. Earthenware containers as a source of fatal lead poisoning. N Engl J Med 1970; 283:669–672.

Needleman HL. Lead at low dose and the behavior of children. Acta Psychiatr Scand 1983; 303(suppl): 38–48.

Neggers YH, Stitt KR. Effects of high lead intake in children. J Am Diet Assoc 1986; 86:938–940.

Rutter M. Raised lead levels and impaired cognitive/behavioural functioning: A review of the evidence. Dev Med Child Neurol 1980; 42 (suppl):1–36.

Weissberg JB, Lipschutz F, Oski FA. Delta aminolevulinic acid dehydralase activity in circulatory blood cells. A sensitive laboratory test for the detection of childhood lead poisoning. N Engl J Med 1971; 284:565–569.

Lithium

El-Mallakh RS, Kantesaria AN, Chaikovsky LI. Lithium toxicity presenting as mania. Drug Intell Clin Pharm 1987; 21:979–981.

Gaby NS, Lefowitz DS, Israel JR. Treatment of lithium tremor with metoprolol. Am J Psychiatry 1983; 140:593–595.

Schou M, Amdisen A, Trap-Jensen J. Lithium poisoning. Am J Psychiatry 1968; 125:520–527.

Manganese

Abd El Naby S, Hassanein M. Neuropsychiatric manifestations of chronic manganese poisoning. J Neurol Neurosurg Psychiatry 1965; 28:282–288.

Canavan MM, Cobb S, Drinker CK. Chronic manganese poisoning. Arch Neurol Psychiatry 1934; 32:501–512.

Chandra SV. Psychiatric illness due to manganese poisoning. Acta Psychiatr Scand 1983; 303(suppl):49–54.

Florence TM, Stauber JL. Neurotoxicity of manganese. Lancet 1988; 1:363.

Rosenstock HA, Simons DG, Meyer JS. Chronic manganism. Neurologic and laboratory studies during treatment with levodopa. JAMA 1971; 217:1354–1358.

Schuler P, Oyanguren H, Maturana V, et al. Manganese poisoning. Environmental and medical study at a Chilean mine. Ind Med Surg 1957; 26:167–173.

Szobor A. Contribution à la question du manganisme. Psychiatr Neurol 1957; 133:221–232.

Mercury

Adams CR, Ziegler DK, Lin JT. Mercury intoxication simulating amyotrophic lateral sclerosis. JAMA 1983; 250:642–643.

Albers JW, Kallenbach LR, Fine LJ et al. Neurologic abnormalities and remote occupational elemental mercury exposure. Ann Neurol 1988; 24:651–659.

Eyl TB. Organic-mercury food poisoning. N Engl J Med 1971; 284:706–709.

Goldblatt D, Greenwood MR, Clarkson TW. Chronic metallic mercury poisoning treated with N-acetylpenicillamine (abstract). Neurology 1971; 21:439.

Hay WJ, Rickards AG, McMenemey WH, Cumings JN. Organic mercurial encephalopathy. J Neurol Neurosurg Psychiatry 1963; 26:199–202.

Kurland LT, Faro SN, Siedler H. Minamata disease. World Neurol 1960; 1:370–390.

Marsh DO. Organic mercury: Methylmercury compounds. In: Vinken PJ, Bruyn GW, eds. Handbook of Clinical Neurology (vol 36). New York: Elsevier-North Holland, 1979; 73–81.

Marsh DO, Myers GJ, Clarkson TW, Amin-Zaki L, Tikriti S, Majeed MA. Fetal methylmercury poisoning: Clinical and toxicological data on 29 cases. Ann Neurol 1980; 7:348–353.

Pierce PE, Thompson JF, Likosky WH, et al. Alkyl mercury poisoning in humans. Report of an outbreak. JAMA 1972; 220:1439–1442.

Snyder RD. Congenital mercury poisoning. N Engl J Med 1971; 284:1014–1016.

Thallium

Bank WJ, Pleasure DE, Suzuiki K, Nigro M, Katz R. Thallium poisoning. Arch Neurol 1972; 26:456–464.

Mahoney W. Retrobulbar neuritis due to thallium poisoning from depilatory cream. JAMA 1932; 98:618–620.

Passarge C, Wieck HH. Thallium polyneuritis. Fortschr Neurol Psychiatr 1965; 33:477–557.

Rambar AC. Acute thallium poisoning. JAMA 1932, 98:1372–1373.

Rauws AG, van Heyst AN. Check of Prussian blue for antidotal efficacy in thallium intoxication [letter]. Arch Toxicol 1979; 43:153–154.

Saddique A. Thallium poisoning: A review. Vet Hum Toxicol 1983; 25:16–22.

Shabalina LP, Spiridonova VS. Thallium as an industrial poison (review of literature). J Hyg Epidemiol Microbiol Immunol 1979; 23:247–255.

Smith DH, Doherty RA. Thallotoxicosis: Report of three cases in Massachusetts. Pediatrics 1964; 34:480–490.

Stein MD, Perlstein MA. Thallium poisoning. Am J Dis Child 1959; 98:80–85.

Methyl Alcohol

Bennet IL Jr, Cary FM, Mitchell GL, Cooper MN. Acute methyl alcohol poisoning: A review based on experience in an outbreak of 323 cases. Medicine 1953; 32:431–463.

Cytryn E, Futeral B. Lactate accumulation in methanol poisoning. Lancet 1983; 2:56.

Harrop GA Jr, Benedict EM. Acute methyl alcohol poisoning associated with acidosis. JAMA 1920; 74:25–27.

Organic Solvents

Allen N, Mendell JR, Billmaier DJ, Fontaine RE, O'Neill J. Toxic polyneuropathy due to methyl n-butyl ketone. Arch Neurol 1975; 32:209–218.

Baker EL, Fine LJ. Solvent neurotoxicity: The current evidence. J Med 1986; 28:126–129.

Bennett RH, Forman HR. Hypokalemic periodic paralysis in chronic toluene exposure. Arch Neurol 1980; 37:673.

Juntunen J, Matikainen E, Antti-Poika M, Suoranta H, Valle M. Nervous system effects of long-term occupational exposure to toluene. Acta Neurol Scand 1985; 72:512–517.

Scelsi R, Poggi P, Fera L, Gonella G. Toxic polyneuropathy due to n-hexane. J Neurol Sci 1980; 47:7–19.

Schaumburg HH, Spencer PS. Toxic neuropathies. Neurology 1979; 29:429–431.

Schaumburg HH, Spencer PS. Clinical and experimental studies of distal axonopathy—a frequent form of brain and nerve damage produced by environmental chemical hazards. Ann NY Acad Sci 1979; 329:14–29.

Struwe G. Psychiatric and neurological symptoms in workers occupationally exposed to organic solvents—results of a differential epidemiological study. Acta Psychiatr Scand 1983; 303(suppl): 100–104.

Waldron HA. Solvents and the brain. Br J Ind Med 1986; 43:73–74.

Pesticides

de Jager AEJ, van Weerden TW, Houthoff HJ, de Monchy JGR. Polyneuropathy after massive exposure to parathion. Neurology 1981; 31:603–605.

Goulding R. Poisoning on the farm. J Soc Occup Med 1983; 33:60–65.

Matsumura F. Toxicology of Insecticides, 2nd ed. New York: Plenum Press, 1985.

Taylor JR, Selhorst JB, Houff S, Martinez J. Chlordecone intoxication in man. Neurology 1978; 28:626–630.

Index

Page numbers in *italics* indicate figures; numbers followed by *t* indicate tables.